Brief Contents

Prepare for the real world of nursing practice

Safe Maternity & Pediatric Nursing Care

An OB/Peds textbook that focuses on what you must know.
You'll find just the right depth and breadth of content to master the knowledge and skills that you need to practice safely and effectively.

Real-World Case Studies with questions are a great way to assess your knowledge before and/ or after reading each chapter. You can find suggested answers online at Davis*Plus*.com.

---

14 Assessment and Care of the Family After Birth

KEY TERMS

anhedonia
endometritis
hematoma
hematuria
mastitis
orthostatic hypotension
psychosis
sitz bath
subinvolution
thromboembolism
thrombus

Davis*Plus* For audio pronunciation guide, visit www.DavisPlus.com

CHAPTER CONCEPTS

Assessment
Infection
Mood
Nursing role
Perfusion

LEARNING OUTCOMES

1. Define the key terms.
2. Demonstrate the correct method of uterine massage for postpartum assessment.
3. Discuss possible causes of uterine atony.
4. Outline postpartum care in the first hour after delivery.
5. Demonstrate a focal postpartum assessment using the BUBBLE LE mnemonic.
6. Plan patient-centered care that addresses the special needs of the adolescent postpartum patient.
7. Describe a therapeutic approach for managing the psychosocial needs of a patient who is relinquishing her infant for adoption.
8. Plan discharge teaching for the postpartum patient.
9. Identify the signs and symptoms of postpartum hemorrhage (PPH) and review appropriate management of PPH.
10. Discuss the causes, signs and symptoms, and management of a patient with a hematoma.
11. Recognize signs and symptoms of a postpartum infection and discuss appropriate management of the infection.
12. Identify women at risk for thrombophlebitis, as well as nursing interventions to prevent thromboembolism in the postpartum patient.
13. Differentiate between postpartum depression and postpartum psychosis and identify appropriate nursing interventions for each disorder.

REAL-WORLD CASE STUDY

Alice

■ Alice delivered her fourth child, a baby boy weighing 10 pounds and 2 ounces, 1 hour ago and has been transferred to the postpartum unit. The nurse reports that Alice was 42 weeks gestation and had her labor induced with oxytocin. She had a long second stage, pushed

---

REAL-WORLD CASE STUDY

Alice

■ Alice delivered her fourth child, a baby boy weighing 10 pounds and 2 ounces, 1 hour ago and has been transferred to the postpartum unit. The nurse reports that Alice was 42 weeks gestation and had her labor induced with oxytocin. She had a long second stage, pushed for 2 hours, and then required an assisted delivery with forceps. Her uterus became soft and boggy between assessments and has required massage and an increase in the rate of the IV oxytocin to maintain a firm fundus. The postpartum nurse begins the physical assessment and notes that the uterus is boggy and her peripad is saturated with blood.

1. What risk factors does Alice have for PPH?
2. What additional information should the postpartum nurse collect about Alice?
3. What actions should the nurse take at this time?

to provide physical care and to monitor for complications. Nurses also teach the woman about self-care before discharge.

Uterine Assessment

After delivery and expulsion of the placenta, the uterus is about the size of a grapefruit and is located midline in the abdomen, halfway between the umbilicus and symphysis pubis. Slowly, over the next several hours, the fundus (ie, the top portion of the uterus) will rise on the midline of the abdomen to the level of or slightly above the umbilicus. Thereafter, the height of the fundus decreases by at least 1 cm or 1 finger-breadth daily as the uterus goes through the process of involution. By the 10th day, the fundus is usually not palpable.

To palpate the fundus, the nurse should position one hand at the base of the uterus just above the symphysis pubis and the other hand at the umbilicus. The nurse should press downward with the hand at the umbilicus until the fundus is palpated as a firm, hard, globular mass in the abdomen (Fig. 14.1). The nurse will note the position of the fundus and document the location.

CONCEPTUAL CORNERSTONE

Infection

An infection occurs when a host is invaded by microorganisms that enter the body, multiply, and cause illness or even death. When an infection occurs, it can be acute or chronic. It can be a localized infection in one area of the body, such as in a wound, or it can become systemic, which means the infection affects the entire body. In postpartum, infections are usually localized and can occur in uterine tissue, wound tissue, the urinary tract, and the breast. However, a localized infection that is not identified and treated early can progress into a systemic infection, which could have debilitating effects for the patient.

The nurse needs to be alert for patients with risk factors that predispose them to infection in the postpartum period. Regardless of the location of the infection, there are similarities in the signs and symptoms of an infection, such as fever, redness, ecchymosis, and drainage. Prompt recognition of signs of infection and initiation of antimicrobials, fluids, and nutrition can change the course of the infection and the length of stay for the patient.

Conceptual Cornerstone expands on principles, generalizations, classifications, or ideas discussed in each chapter, tying the concept to what you're about to read.

SAFETY *STAT!*

Never palpate a uterus without supporting the lower segment because the uterus could invert if not stabilized.

Next, the nurse will assess the consistency of the mass. If it is soft or "boggy," the nurse will support the lower uterine segment and gently massage in a circular pattern with the other hand until the uterus becomes firm. If massage is not effective, there may be a large blood clot in the uterus or extreme uterine atony. *Atony* refers to a lack of muscle tone, which could lead to PPH. Many women receive oxytocin after delivery to promote uterine contractions. If the uterus does not remain firm with the administration of oxytocin and massage, the health-care provider should be notified.

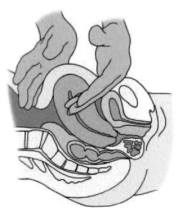

FIGURE 14.1 Fundal massage. To palpate the uterus, the upper hand is cupped over the fundus; the lower hand stabilizes the uterus at the symphysis pubis.

Safety *STAT!* in each chapter alerts you to the most important safety precautions.

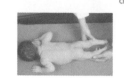

FIGURE 35.12 Inspecting an infant's gluteal folds for congenital hip dysplasia.

For older children with DDH, immobilization using traction or surgical interventions to produce a reduction may be needed. The surgical procedure of an osteotomy has an aim of reconstructing an acetabulum with a shallow angle so that the femoral head stays in place. A period of time in postsurgical casting may also be needed.

Legg-Calve-Perthes Disease

A child who presents with an aseptic necrosis of the femoral head is diagnosed with Legg-Calve-Perthes. Confirmed via radiography, the child is typically between the ages of 2 and 12 upon diagnosis. The pathophysiology of the disorder remains unknown but the mechanism stems from a disrupted circulation pattern affecting the femoral head. Occurring over a period of 1 to 3 years, there is a slow disruption to the surrounding tissues, including to the femoral head and the region of the growth plate (ie, epiphysis).

Assessments of Legg-Calve-Perthes Disease

The disorder is one of the older child, often the school-aged children may present with pain, joint discomfort, or hip joint stiffness, especially upon ambulation. The child may or may not have experienced pain in the area. The most effective method of diagnosis is radiography or a CAT scan.

Interventions for Legg-Calve-Perthes Disease

The child is put on rest because activity may worsen the disorder by causing microfractures to the weakened epiphysis. Traction, bracing, and surgical options may be warranted to restore hip ROM and allow revascularization of the affected area. Treatment options vary for children younger than age 10; older children have a significant degenerative arthritis with the disease.

Nursing Considerations for Legg-Calve-Perthes Disease

Pediatric nurses should be aware of the immobilization programs that require parents to adhere to. Families need support when the treatment plan includes a period of reduced activity for healing. Working with child-life personnel to adapt a physical education program can assist with the adherence needed for appropriate care.

Slipped Capital Femoral Epiphysis

Also known as a *coxa vara*, a slipped femoral epiphysis occurs as a spontaneous displacement of the capital epiphysis of the femoral head in an inferior direction. Occurring most commonly during an accelerated growth episode, the child presents with a sudden or a progressive slip of the functional abilities, a disability, a limp, and complaints of hip pain.

Assessments of Slipped Capital Femoral Epiphysis

If idiopathic, the diagnosis is accompanied...

Interventions for Congenital Hip Dysplasia or Dislocation

After DDH is confirmed via radiographic examination, the severity of the shallowness of the acetabulum is determined. Immediate treatment is started to stop the progression of the deformity. In young infants, the femoral head is placed into the acetabulum and the child is splinted in a flexed and abducted position, using one of a variety of abduction devices, such as the popular Pavlik harness. Use of an abduction device must continue for up to 6 months. Parent education is vital and frequent assessments with strap length adjustments are warranted as the infant is experiencing rapid growth.

Nursing Considerations for Congenital Hip Dysplasia or Dislocation

Early newborn screening is an essential aspect of early identification of DDH. With screening of all newborns, early identification and rapid placement of an abduction device will allow up to a 95% cure rate without the need for surgical interventions.

HEALTH PROMOTION

Parental education is essential because the family must understand the importance of 24-hour-a-day use of the harness and the assessment of the child's skin and circulation around the sites of the straps.

PATIENT TEACHING GUIDELINES

The family needs to understand how to assess for the integrity of the abduction device and what complications are associated with a poor fit, slipping of the straps, or a loss of skin integrity under the strap contact sites. Assessments that need attention include straps that are not snug enough to keep the infant in an abducted position (ie, knees up and out), straps that easily fall away from their required position, and skin that is red, raw, or open. It is important to keep a layer of cotton under the straps to prevent skin chaffing and skin sores from developing. If these complications are found, the family should report them to their care provider for assistance and...

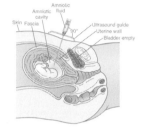

FIGURE 5.6 Amniocentesis testing for genetic disorders.

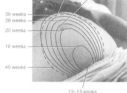

FIGURE 5.7 Fundal height measurements as the pregnancy progresses. Fundal measurement should approximately equal the number of weeks of gestation.

appropriate care. During each visit, the health-care provider and nurse will:

- Evaluate any physical or psychological patient concerns and answer questions.
- Weigh the patient to monitor for appropriate weight gain.
- Monitor vital signs for increasing blood pressure.
- Perform urinalysis to monitor for:
  - Glucose: may indicate gestational diabetes.
  - Ketones: produced when the body is breaking down fat for energy.
  - Protein: may be a sign of pre-eclampsia, kidney damage, or urinary infection.
  - Nitrates: indicates urinary tract infection.
- Measure fundal height:
  - The distance between the top of the pubic bone to the top of the uterus.
  - The fundus reaches the level of the umbilicus at ~20 weeks and measures ~20 cm (Fig. 5.7).
  - Each subsequent visit to the health-care provider should indicate growth of the uterus.

heard as early as 8 weeks, but more commonly at 10 to 12 weeks.
- Perform a psychological assessment.
  - Warning Signs:
    - Increasing anxiety about the pregnancy
    - Inappropriate responses or preoccupations about the pregnancy
    - Failure to acknowledge quickening
    - Signs of substance abuse
    - Inability to cope with stress
    - Failure to prepare for the baby, such as preparing clothing and selecting feeding method.

LEARN TO C.U.S.

During a prenatal visit with a Lauren, she acknowledges that she has not prepared any clothes or a crib for her newborn. Lauren "can't decide" whether she wants to bottle feed or breastfeed. The nurse is concerned because this is Lauren's first baby and she is 37 weeks gestation. The nurse discusses her concerns with the obstetrician using the C.U.S. method of communication.

C: "I am **concerned** about Lauren.

U: I am uncomfortable because she has not started preparing for the birth of her newborn and she is 37 weeks gestation.

S: We have a possible **safety** issue and a warning sign

SAFETY STAT!

During prenatal visits, the fundal height is measured to deter-

---

HEALTH PROMOTION

Parental education is essential because the family must understand the importance of 24-hour-a-day use of the harness and the assessment of the child's skin and circulation around the sites of the straps.

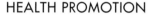

Health Promotion information will help you empower patients to improve their health and the health of their families.

LEARN TO C.U.S.

During a prenatal visit with a Lauren, she acknowledges that she has not prepared any clothes or a crib for her newborn. Lauren "can't decide" whether she wants to bottle feed or breastfeed. The nurse is concerned because this is Lauren's first baby and she is 37 weeks gestation. The nurse discusses her concerns with the obstetrician using the C.U.S. method of communication.

C: "I am **concerned** about Lauren.

U: I am **uncomfortable** because she has not started preparing for the birth of her newborn and she is 37 weeks gestation.

S: We have a possible **safety** issue and a warning sign that she is not coping well with the pregnancy."

Learn to C.U.S. (Concern. Uncomfortable. Safety.) is an effective communication method included in many chapters to help you improve your communication with members of the healthcare team.

Team Works gives you a glimpse into the day and the life of a nurse as part of the healthcare team and how they provide safe, patient care in relation to what you are learning.

TEAM WORKS

Child Life specialists should be involved in the child's presurgical preparation and teaching. They can be instrumental during the highly symptomatic postoperative healing phase by providing distraction, play, and pain adjuncts, such as visualization and guided imagery.

56   **UNIT TWO**   Pregnancy and the Family

- Obtain a thorough past medical history and current health history to detect any potential problems.
- Encourage the woman to ask questions.
- Answer all questions honestly.
- Encourage the patient to obtain all laboratory tests ordered by the healthcare provider.
- Stress the importance of subsequent prenatal visits and care throughout the pregnancy.

Initial Client History

To provide patient-centered care, thorough past medical history, family history, and gynecological and obstetrical histories are very important to obtain. The information in Table 5.1 should be obtained by the health-care provider.

THERAPEUTIC COMMUNICATION

When interviewing a patient for her prenatal visits, remember these points for effective communication:
- Avoid the initial discussion of the patient's gravida or para in front of her partner or family.
- Always provide privacy. The patient may not feel comfortable discussing any health issues with her family, friends, spouse, or a partner who are listening.
- Avoid judgmental comments or behaviors when the patient shares past medical history and obstetrical history.
- Be an active listener in order to recognize patient concerns and educational needs.

CULTURAL CONSIDERATIONS

Cultural questions regarding health care and health beliefs should be part of the initial history for a patient. Every person is an individual and it is important to avoid stereotyping a patient based on her race or ethnicity. However, when a caring nurse asks a patient questions about the patient's cultural background, it may provide valuable information about how cultural, behavioral, and medical factors may influence a pregnant woman's health. (American College of Obstetricians and Gynecologists, 2005).

DRUG FA...

When intervie... medical history, it is imp... that she is currently ta... to the fetus and should ... as soon as possible. Th... list of safe or acceptable... pregnancy.

PRENATAL ASSESSMENT AND CARE

A woman should schedule her first prenatal visit as soon as she knows she is pregnant. The first prenatal visit is important as it is a time for the health-care provider to determine a baseline of the woman's overall health and identify any potential problems that may influence the course of the pregnancy. Laboratory and diagnostic tests will be ordered to obtain a baseline and identify health problems. The woman will also be advised of the need for subsequent visits to monitor her pregnancy for potential complications and to monitor the health of the fetus until labor begins.

Initial Prenatal Assessment

After a detailed health history is obtained, the health-care provider will proceed to a thorough physical examination. During the physical examination, the woman should be provided with privacy and should be made comfortable, both physically and psychologically. Rapport should be established that allows her to ask questions and verbalize any concerns during the examination.

Physical Exam

During the initial visit, the health-care provider should perform a head-to-toe physical examination that covers all major systems. The exam will provide the health-care provider with information regarding current overall health.

In addition to the complete physical examination, a pelvic examination is performed. The patient is draped and placed in the **lithotomy position**. In this position the patient lies on her back, thighs flexed on the abdomen, legs on thighs, thighs abducted (Venes, 2013). This position allows the health care provider a clear view of the external and internal genitalia.

Information obtained during a pelvic examination includes an examination of the external genitalia to detect lesions or discharge. A culture for sexual transmitted infections (STIs) may be done at this time.

Examination of the internal genitalia is done with a vaginal speculum to observe the cervix for the signs of pregnancy (Fig. 5.2). A **Papanicolaou (Pap) test** may be obtained. The Pap test is used to detect cervical cancer. After the speculum is removed, the examiner will perform a **bimanual exam** of the uterus to determine size. During the bimanual exam, the health-care provider places the gloved middle and index fingers into the vagina to identify the cervix. Then the examiner places the other hand midway between the umbilicus and the ...

If a patient-controlled analgesia (PCA) machine is going to be used for postoperative pain control in a child having scoliosis surgery, it will be imperative that the child learns how to use the machine before surgery when learning pain taks place without the distraction of the pain experience.

Nursing Considerations for Scoliosis

The prepubescent and adolescent child is often concerned with body image. Not only does the disorder cause distress, but the bracing and orthotics required can lead to difficulties with adherence to the treatment plan and the consistent use of braces and orthotics. It is important for the pediatric nurse to consistently remind the teen that if the brace is not worn during the greatest growth spurt, the scoliosis may progress, causing further body image concerns.

Postoperative care of the child undergoing surgical correction for significant scoliosis requires meticulous nursing care focused on safety. This care should focus on keeping the child in the immediate postoperative period controlled for pain, free of injury, flat on his or her back, and carefully log-rolled. The pediatric nurse should request assistance from at least one other caregiver and/or a physical therapist (PT) to prevent injury. A PT can be instrumental in motivating and supporting a child in adhering to the treatment plan, as well as in providing safe tips for early mobility (as early as the day after surgery).

TEAM WORKS

Child Life specialists should be involved in the child's presurgical preparation and teaching. They can be instrumental during the highly symptomatic postoperative healing phase by providing distraction, play, and pain adjuncts, such as visualization and guided imagery.

Osteogenesis Imperfecta

A very uncommon disorder with devastating consequences is the genetically linked, autosomal dominant, heterogeneous disease called *osteogenesis imperfecta (OI)*. This disease is commonly known as "brittle bone disease" because the child suffers from fractures and skeletal deformity. This disorder may be so severe that the infant does not live through the birthing process. The child's entire life is affected by this disorder, with a decrease in life expectancy, multiple fractures, and the use of a wheelchair for mobility.

...al Condition...

...a defect in the... Without health... of bone, the... mineralization... architecture, w... not present... ring loss, jo... looseness or increased flexibility), and poor str... bones that support the child's teeth.

Assessments of Osteogenesis Imperfecta

Prenatal screening typically is not performed for... order, so early identification is by death in utero... suffering several fractures during the birthing pr... natal diagnostics are performed and the disease... in utero, then the infant must be born by Cesarea... the greatest chance of safety and survival.

Interventions for Osteogenesis Imperfect...

OI cannot be treated medically. The child and family is offered supportive care and genetic counseling. Research continues in the area of bone marrow transplantation. Goals of supportive care are to reduce the possibility of further fractures, prevent the development of contractures, promote safety, and reduce injury.

Nursing Considerations for Osteogenesis Imperfecta

Newborns, infants, and young children require special physical handling to prevent injury. Very specific guidelines are needed about restricting activities while promoting play, socialization, education, and development. Much education is required for family members to understand the severity of the disease and how it is genetically linked. Families should be encouraged to find further education and support by seeking guidance from the national organizations for OI, including The National Organization for Rare Diseases and the Osteogenesis Imperfecta Foundation.

Juvenile Rheumatoid Arthritis

JRA, also known as *juvenile idiopathic arthritis (JIR)*, is a group of idiopathic chronic inflammatory joint diseases that first manifest during the early childhood period. The disorder may be linked to an autoimmune dysfunction after an exposure to a viral or bacterial infection followed by an acute attack of the joint tissue by the immune system. The rheumatic process leads to the destruction of the child's synovial tissue layers, which line the joints and secrete a lubricating material for ease of joint motion. The chronic nature of the disease leads to very painful joint destruction and fibrosis of the joint cartilage. Joints appear enlarged, abnormally shaped, and larger than normal. They may feel warm during periods of inflammation exacerbation.

Assessments of Juvenile Rheumatoid Arthritis

Upon presentation of a child with painful, swollen joints, confirmation of the disease is by laboratory assay and clinical

THERAPEUTIC COMMUNICATION

When interviewing a patient for her prenatal visits, remember these points for effective communication:
- Avoid the initial discussion of the patient's gravida or para in front of her partner or family.
- Always provide privacy. The patient may not feel comfortable discussing any health issues with her family, friends, spouse, or a partner who are listening.
- Avoid judgmental comments or behaviors when the patient shares past medical history and obstetrical history.
- Be an active listener in order to recognize patient concerns and educational needs.

Therapeutic Communication examples build your foundational knowledge and skills to help you know how to most effectively communicate with patients and their families.

Build your confidence

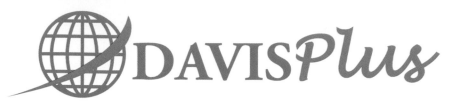

DAVISPlus

Redeem your *Plus* Code on the inside front cover
to access these Davis*Plus* Premium Resources...

- Davis Digital eBook
- Bonus Chapters
- Student Quiz Bank with NCLEX®-style questions and rationales
- Interactive Clinical Scenarios
- Interactive Exercises
- Animations
- Web Links

- Post-Conference Questions and Activities
- Answers to Real-World Case Studies
- Printable Care Plans
- Audio Glossary
- References
- Audio Library
- Pediatric Dosage Calculation Module
- Fetal Heart Monitoring Terminology

Visit **Davis*Plus*.com** today!

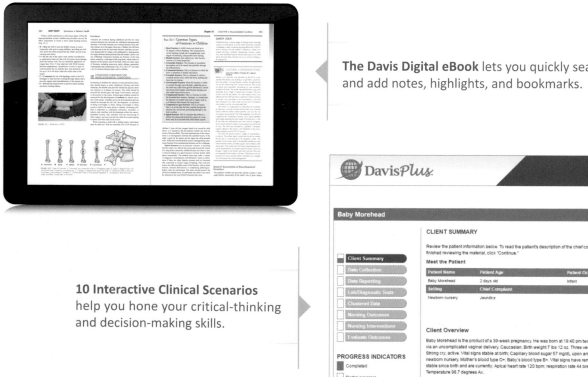

The Davis Digital eBook lets you quickly search and add notes, highlights, and bookmarks.

10 Interactive Clinical Scenarios help you hone your critical-thinking and decision-making skills.

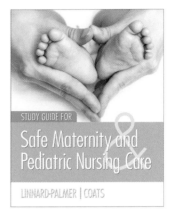
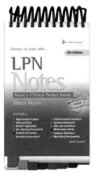

Safe Maternity and Pediatric Nursing Care

Luanne Linnard-Palmer, EdD, MSN, RN, CPN
Nursing Professor
Dominican University of California
San Rafael, California

Gloria Haile Coats, MSN, RN, FNP
Nursing Professor
Modesto Junior College
Modesto, California

 F.A. Davis Company • Philadelphia

F. A. Davis Company
1915 Arch Street
Philadelphia, PA 19103
www.fadavis.com

Copyright © 2017 by F. A. Davis Company

Printed in the United States of America

Last digit indicates print number: 10 9 8 7 6 5 4 3 2 1

Publisher, Nursing: Terri Wood Allen
Manager of Project and eProject Management: Catherine H. Carroll
Senior Content Project Manager: Christine M. Abshire
Art and Design Manager: Carolyn O'Brien
Production Manager: Robert C. Butler
Electronic Project Editor: Sandra Glennie

As new scientific information becomes available through basic and clinical research, recommended treatments and drug therapies undergo changes. The author(s) and publisher have done everything possible to make this book accurate, up to date, and in accord with accepted standards at the time of publication. The author(s), editors, and publisher are not responsible for errors or omissions or for consequences from application of the book, and make no warranty, expressed or implied, in regard to the contents of the book. Any practice described in this book should be applied by the reader in accordance with professional standards of care used in regard to the unique circumstances that may apply in each situation. The reader is advised always to check product information (package inserts) for changes and new information regarding dose and contraindications before administering any drug. Caution is especially urged when using new or infrequently ordered drugs.

Library of Congress Cataloging-in-Publication Data

Names: Linnard-Palmer, Luanne, author. | Coats, Gloria Haile, author.
Title: Safe maternity and pediatric nursing care / Luanne Linnard-Palmer,
  Gloria Haile Coats.
Description: Philadelphia : F.A. Davis Company, [2017] | Includes
  bibliographical references and index.
Identifiers: LCCN 2016032256 | ISBN 9780803624948
Subjects: | MESH: Maternal-Child Nursing—methods | Pediatric Nursing—methods
Classification: LCC RJ245 | NLM WY 157.3 | DDC 618.92/00231—dc23 LC record
available at https://lccn.loc.gov/2016032256

About the Authors

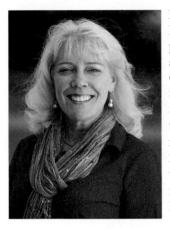 **Luanne Linnard-Palmer, EdD, MSN, RN, CPN** is a professor of pediatric nursing at Dominican University of California located just north of San Francisco in Marin County. She has been teaching in both undergraduate and graduate nursing programs for over 25 years. She currently practices acute care pediatric nursing at Sutter Health's California Pacific Medical Center in San Francisco and works as a Pediatric Oncology Nurse Coordinator for Stanford's Lucille Packard Children's Hospital. Her passion for teaching and clinical practice spans a twenty nine year career. She works closely with a diverse clinical team which includes medical assistants, LVN/LPNs, physicians, medical students and interns, and advance practice nurses. Her goal in writing this book is to provide a foundation of critical information with a focus on safety.

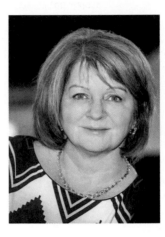 **Gloria Haile Coats, MSN, RN, FNP** is a professor of maternity and pediatric nursing at Modesto Junior College in Modesto, California. She has a diploma from Burge School of Nursing in Springfield, Missouri, a BSN from California State University, Stanislaus; a MSN from California State University, Dominquez Hills; and a Post-Masters family nurse practitioner certificate from Sonoma State University. She has experience in the development, implementation, and evaluation of nursing education and curriculum. Her expertise in nursing education both in the classroom and clinical setting has enabled her to take difficult concepts of nursing education and make them understandable for nursing students. She understands the time constraints in nursing education and her goal for this book is to provide the essential need-to-know information for nurses to provide safe and effective maternity and pediatric care.

This book is dedicated to my father, Howard Warren Linnard and my mother, Bernice Elaine Linnard.
A man whose passion for health, happiness, joy, and love permeated every aspect of his successful life.
A woman whose strength, creativity, work ethic, and love continue to influence the well-being of everyone she encounters.

Luanne Linnard-Palmer

To my husband, Mike, who supported and encouraged me throughout this project. Thank you for graciously giving up sailing weekends so that I could write and meet deadlines.
To my children, Christopher, Melissa, and Logan, you have made me a proud mother. Thank you for tolerating a nurse mom when you were growing up.
And finally, to my students, past and future, I hope that you can see that nursing is my vocation, not a job.

Gloria Haile Coats

Acknowledgments

We would like to express our deepest gratitude to our distinguished Developmental Editor, Julie Scardiglia. Throughout this process, you have been a steadfast pillar of motivation, professionalism, and support. In great appreciation… thank you for seeing us through.

Epigraph

Our very lives, indeed our societies, are enriched by the birth, growth, and development of a child.
Nurses are honored by the trust parents give as we watch over and care for their precious children.

Preface

This text offers the reader a variety of learning experiences that combine the art of nursing care and practice with the foundations of science. It includes essential nursing content from pre-conception to conception, pregnancy, delivery, and neonatal care through adolescent care. The book is organized to present principles and concepts of maternity nursing through the principles and concepts of pediatric nursing—health promotion and health restoration. The contents span pre-conception health through the end of the adolescent developmental stage, and across concepts and systems of illness, injury, recovery, and healing.

Safety

The concept of safety is presented in this text as the overarching framework. In all aspects of maternity and pediatric nursing, safety remains the ultimate responsibility of the nurse in his or her role. Safety is incorporated into one's thinking, actions, skills, and caring practice. Safety-related information is included in multiple places in each chapter, including in the boxed feature Safety STAT!, which provides guidance about essential safety protocols for maternity and pediatric nursing. A succinct introduction to Quality and Safety Education for Nurses (QSEN) is included as an online bonus chapter.

Critical Thinking

Critical thinking is an important and necessary problem-solving process within the profession of nursing. Critical thinking is a systematic way of first identifying the key aspects of a problem and then progressing through a process in which solutions are found and are offered to others. Within the role of the maternity and pediatric nurse, critical thinking is a key process across care. Human variation within conception, bearing children, raising children, and providing for their care influences how a maternity or pediatric nurse assesses families' needs. Providing guidance, education, and care to each unique family is a joy and a challenge. Through the use of critical thinking principles, the nurse can identify the needs of a family and implement caring practices that provide for each individual within the family.

Students will find critical thinking questions in each of the chapters. It is the intent of the authors to challenge the students in their problem-solving skills by providing critical thinking exercises that require the student to find resources, solutions to problems, and answers from clinical settings and diverse practice areas, and then work to solve problems as part of a health-care team.

Themes

The unifying principles of excellent and safe nursing care presented throughout this book include the following:

- Family as the unit of care
- Patient- and family-centered care principles
- Safety across all encounters
- Communication
- Culturally sensitive care

Features

This text provides extensive chapter features to educate students about various aspects of the chapter topic in patient settings and encounters. Each feature will assist the student in learning more about the chapter content by illuminating important topics and ideas. The following features are included in text chapters:

- **Real-World Case Study**: A case study with questions opens each chapter. Students can complete the case study as a "pre-assessment" in order to determine their knowledge level. Alternately, students can use each chapter's case study to challenge themselves to search for answers to the case study questions while reading the chapter, or complete the case study after reading the chapter. Answers to the Real-World Case Study questions are located on the Student Davis*Plus* Web site.
- **Conceptual Cornerstone**: A concept is an organizing principle, a generalization, a classification, or an idea that is used to understand information. A concept in nursing is a way of learning that categorizes relevant information in a way that allows students to apply it to other situations. This type of learning promotes critical thinking because the student is taught to apply a concept and not just memorize facts. Concepts can be applied to understanding disease processes, patient behaviors, family dynamics, and health conditions, and to guide professional practice. Each chapter begins with a Conceptual Cornerstone that can be applied to the information in the chapter.
- **Patient Teaching Guidelines**: Concise guidelines are provided to enable the nurse to answer patient questions and provide or reinforce health care–related teaching specific to each chapter's topic.
- **Health Promotion**: An important task of nursing is to promote health and empower patients to improve their health and the health of their families. Important health promotion information is provided in each chapter to

assist the student nurse to be knowledgeable about health promotion behaviors.

- **Cultural Considerations**: Patient-centered care requires the nurse to be aware of cultural differences and how those differences can impact patient care. This feature addresses cultural considerations in order to promote better nursing care.
- **Labs & Diagnostics**: Laboratory values or diagnostic tests that are pertinent to providing safe maternity and pediatric nursing care are highlighted in this feature.
- **Learn to C.U.S.**: This safety-related feature highlights a method of communication in which the nurse uses the format of C: "I am **c**oncerned," U: "I am **u**ncomfortable," and S: "We have a **s**afety issue" to communicate with members of the health-care team.
- **Therapeutic Communication**: Patient- and family-centered care requires the nurse to be adept at therapeutic communication. Examples of therapeutic communication are included to provide the student nurse with a foundation of skills for effective communication with patients and their families.
- **Team Works**: This feature presents the nurse as part of the health-care team who, with other health-care professionals, provides safe patient care.
- **Drug Facts**: Medications that are relevant to the management of patient care are the focus of this feature. It provides basic need-to-know information regarding medications discussed in the chapter, including information related to safe medication administration.
- **Nursing Care Plan**: Various formats of nursing care plans are provided to allow students to see how the chapter information can be applied in a nursing care plan. Information may include nursing assessments, diagnoses, interventions, and/or expected patient outcomes.
- **Safety STAT!**: The most important safety issues related to safe patient care are highlighted in the Safety STAT! features. Each chapter contains several Safety STAT!s that promote the principles of patient safety.
- **NCLEX®-Style Review Questions**: Each chapter includes NCLEX®-style review questions to assist students with preparing for course and national licensure exams. Answers are located on the Instructor Davis*Plus* Web site.
- **Critical Thinking Questions**: Following the review questions, each chapter includes critical thinking questions that can be used in the classroom or completed by the student to apply the chapter information to a critical thinking situation. Answers are located on the Instructor Davis*Plus* Web site.

▓ AVAILABLE ON 🌐 Davis*Plus*

Bonus Chapters

Safe Maternity and Pediatric Nursing Care focuses on the "need-to-know" content that will allow nurses to achieve safe practice. Faculty is consistently challenged to decide what material is most relevant to present to their students in their packed curriculum. Programs cover OB/Peds content in a variety of course lengths, sometimes taught together and sometimes separate. The authors of this text carefully curated the content so that what is in print is "necessary," and we offer "nice-to-know" content online. The online chapters are fully supported with Active Classroom Instructor's Guide materials, PowerPoint, Instructor and Student Test Banks, and study guide exercises. Bonus chapters include the following:

1: Introduction to QSEN
2: Cultural Competency in Maternity and Pediatric Care
3: Women's Health Promotion Across the Life Span
4: Adapting to Chronic Illness and Supporting the Family Unit
5: Legal Aspects of Pediatric Nursing Care
6: Providing a Safe Environment: Home and School
7: Families Experiencing Stressors

Appendices

The appendices support further learning, classroom activities, and application of text material around the assessment and care of the neonate, child, and adolescent. Appendices include the following:

A. Joint Commission's "Do Not Use" Abbreviations List
B. Thirty Types of Medical Errors and Tips for Preventing Harm: Quality and Safety Imperatives for Nurses Caring for Patients Across the Developmental Period
C. Universal and Standard Precautions for Preventing Disease Transmission
D. Conversion Factors
E. Common Medication Administration Calculations in Pediatrics
F. Normal and Expected Vital Signs for Children
G. Specimen Collection Techniques in Pediatrics
H. Techniques for Effective Change of Shift Report or "Handoffs"
I. Overview of Sex Education and Reproductive Health in Adolescence: Client Teaching Guide
J. Injury Prevention Across Childhood
K. Anticipatory Guidance for New Parents
L. Guidelines for Working With Children Who Are Hospitalized
M. Immunization Schedule

Student Resources

Use your unique Davis*Plus* access code from the inside front cover to access the following premium resources:

- **Davis Digital Version** ebook with full functionality
- **Student Quiz Bank** of NCLEX®-style questions with rationales, including alternate-format questions such as select-all-that-apply
- **Interactive Clinical Scenarios** provide an introduction to ten clinical scenarios that help students hone critical thinking skills and make decisions for patients.

- **Interactive Exercises** such as find the term and quiz show are included for every chapter.
- **Animations** are audio and visual enhancements of topics and concepts.
- **Web links organized by topic** for further research
- **Post-Conference Questions and Activities** ask the student to consider the specific chapter's content related to relevant aspects of clinical care
- **Answers to Real-World Case Studies**
- **Printable Care Plans**
- **Audio Glossary**
- **References**
- **Audio Library** of heart sounds
- **Pediatric Dosage Calculation Module**
- **Fetal Heart Monitoring Terminology**

Instructor Resources

- **Davis Digital Version** ebook with full functionality
- **Electronic Test Bank** of NCLEX®-style questions with rationales for correct and incorrect answers and page references, in ExamView Pro
- **Active Classroom Instructor's Guide** that maps the Student and Instructor Resources and includes Lecture Notes
- **PowerPoint Presentations** of fully customizable slides featuring iClicker student questions
- **Image Bank** includes all of the images from the text.
- **Printable Concept Maps**
- **How to Use the Book in Courses of Varying Lengths** provides suggestions for using the text and online bonus chapters in separate and combined courses.
- **Answers to in-text Review Questions, Critical Thinking Questions, and Post-Conference Questions and Activities**
- **Answers to Study Guide questions and activities**

STUDY GUIDE

This essential companion provides the student with a variety of means to demonstrate knowledge, application, analysis, and evaluation of the material provided throughout the text. There is a study guide chapter for every text chapter, including the Online Bonus Chapters. Each study guide chapter includes exercises that help the learner deepen his or her understanding and demonstrate mastery of the concepts presented in the book.

The study guide includes exercises that address all of the types of text features, including:

- Multiple choice and other NCLEX®-style review questions
- True or false questions
- Matching exercises
- Short-answer questions
- Fill-in-the-blank questions
- Essay questions
- Crossword puzzle
- Concept maps
- Table completion exercises
- Labeling exercises

Answers to the study guide questions are located on Davis*Plus* in the Instructor Resources. This allows instructors to choose whether students should have the answers before completing the study guide exercises.

Contributors

Deborah Vance Beaumont, MSN, RN
Mind Body Nutrition RN
Captain Cook, Hawaii
Chapter 39 Child With a Communicable Disease

Olivia Catolico, PhD, MSN, RN, CNL, BC
Professor of Nursing
Dominican University of California
San Rafael, California
*Bonus Chapter 2 Cultural Competency in Maternity and
Pediatric Care*

Leslie Crane, EdD, MSN, RN
Director of the CNA/HHA Program
Santa Rosa Junior College
Santa Rosa, California
Chapter 32 Child With a Respiratory Condition

Catherine E. Cyr-Roy, RN, BSN, MPA/HSA
RN Instructor
Dominican University of California
San Rafael, California
Solano Community College
Fairfield, California
Bonus Chapter 7 Families Experiencing Stressors

Margaret Fink, EdD, MSN, RN
Professor of Nursing
Dominican University of California
San Rafael, California
*Chapter 1 Healthy People 2020 and Initiatives for Healthy
Families*

**Barbara McCamish, MSN, MPT, RN, PT,
CNL, CHSE**
Clinical Simulation Center Manager
Dominican University of California
San Rafael, California
Bonus Chapter 1 Introduction to QSEN

Natalie (Lu) Sweeney, RN, MSN, CNS
Professor of Nursing
Dominican University of California
San Rafael, California
Chapter 33 Child With a Cardiac Condition

Reviewers

Lori Airth, RN
Practical Nursing Instructor
Northern Lakes College
Valleyview, Alberta, Canada

Mary T. Amundson, RN, MSN
Practical Nursing Faculty
Northland Community and Technical College
East Grand Forks, Minnesota

Janice Ankenmann-Hill, RN, MSN,
    CCRN, FNP-C
Professor and Program Director, Vocational and Associate
    Degree Nursing
Napa Valley College
Napa, California

Darlene Baker, RN, MSN
Director of Health Career Programs
Green Country Technology Center
Okmulgee, Oklahoma

Holli Benge, RN, MSN
Professor/Department Chair
Tyler Junior College
Tyler, Texas

Melanie Benington, RN, MSN
Practical Nursing Training Specialist
Cuyahoga Community College
Cleveland, Ohio

Kristie A. Berkstresser, PhD, RN, CNE, BC
Associate Professor of Nursing
HACC, Central Pennsylvania's Community College
Lancaster, Pennsylvania

Christi Blair, RN, MSN
Nursing Faculty
Holmes Community College
Goodman, Mississippi

Jammie Blankenship, RN, MSN
Practical Nursing Instructor
Kiamichi Technology Centers
Hugo, Oklahoma

Cheryl Bruno-Mofu, RN, ADN
Instructor of Vocational Nursing and Allied Health
Palo Verde College
Blythe, California

Karen Clark, RN, MSN
Instructor of Nursing/Full Time Faculty
Lehigh Carbon Community College
Schnecksville, Pennsylvania

April Cline, RN, CNE, PhD
Practical Nurse Educator, Instructor
Isothermal Community College
Spindale, North Carolina

Michelle Crum, RN, BSN, EJD
Practical Nursing Program Director
Ozarks Technical Community College
Springfield, Missouri

Mary Davis, RN, MSN
Nursing Instructor
Wiregrass Georgia Technical College
Valdosta, Georgia

Natalie Deleonardis, MSN, RN
Coordinator of the North Campus Outreach Practical
    Nursing Program
Pennsylvania College of Technology
Wellsboro, Pennsylvania

Sharon Demers, RN, BN, CAE
Instructor
Assiniboine Community College
Winnipeg, Manitoba, Canada

Sally Flesch, RN, BSN, MA, EdS, PhD
Professor, Coordinator, Practical Nursing Program
Black Hawk College
Moline, Illinois

Tina Forrester, MSN, RN
Practical Nursing Instructor
Bladen Community College
Dublin, North Carolina

Louise S. Frantz, RN, BSN, MHA, Ed
Coordinator Practical Nursing Program
Penn State Berks
Reading, Pennsylvania

Nadra Gibson, RN, BSN
IDNEP
Academy of Medical & Health Science
Pueblo, Colorado

Alice Gilbert, RN, BSN
Director, Instructor
Ukiah Adult School Vocational Nursing Program
Ukiah, California

Linda Griffis, RN
Lead Instructor
Practical Nursing Program
Pearl River Community College
Poplarville, Mississippi

Marie Hedgpeth, RN, MSN, MHA
Practical Nursing Faculty
Robeson Community College
Lumberton, North Carolina

Catherine Krahn Horton, RN, MSN
Nursing Instructor
Madison Area Technical College
Fort Atkinson, Wisconsin

Melody Jaymes, RN, MSN
Practical Nursing Instructor
Huntingdon County Career and Technology Center
Mill Creek, Pennsylvania

Valerie Jenkins, RN, BSN
Quarter 3 Coordinator
Galen College of Nursing
San Antonio, Texas

Kathy A. Johnson, RN, BSN
Practical Nursing Instructor
Greater Lowell Technical School
Tyngsboro, Massachusetts

Robin Kern, RN, MSN
Program Chair, Practical Nursing
Moultrie Technical College
Moultrie, Georgia

Lori A. Koehler, FNP-C, MSN, RN, CEN
Faculty
Northampton Community College
Bethlehem, Pennsylvania

Kelly Kidd, RN, BScN, MN
Professor, Coordinator Practical Nursing Program
Algonquin College
Pembroke, Ontario, Canada

Tracy Lohstroh, MSN
Nursing Faculty/Department Chair for Allied Health
Shawnee Community College
Ullin, Illinois

Nancy Lyons, RN, BSN
Instructor, Coordinator LPN Program
Holy Name Medical Center School of Practical Nursing
Teaneck, New Jersey

Patricia C. Martin, RN, MS
Chair of Nursing, Calmar Campus
Northeast Iowa Community College
Calmar, Iowa

Kathleen J. Maschka, RN, MSN
Nursing Faculty
Minnesota State College – Southeast Technical
Winona, Minnesota

Lynda Matthews, RN, BSN
Coordinator of Practical Nursing Program
Texas County Technical College
Houston, Missouri

Kim McCombs, RN, MSN
Assistant Professor
Black Hawk College
Moline, Illinois

Carolyn McCormick, RN, MSN, CNE
Director Practical Nursing Program
Cape Fear Community College
Wilmington, North Carolina

Judy Melton, RN, MSN
Assistant Director Practical Nurse Education
McDowell Technical Community College
Marion, North Carolina

Barbara Michalski, RN, MSN
Practical Nursing Instructor
Tulsa Technology Center
Tulsa, Oklahoma

Marybeth Millan, BSN, RNC, CCE
Nurse Educator
Ocean City Vocational Technical School
Toms River, New Jersey

Nancy Morris, RN, MSN, Ed
Director/Instructor of Practical Nursing Program
North Georgia Technical College
Toccoa, Georgia

Tracy Moshier, RN, MSN, CCE
Nursing Instructor
Lake Superior College
Duluth, Minnesota

JoAnne M. Pearce, MS, RN
Assistant Professor
Idaho State University
Pocatello, Idaho

Tammy Pehrson, RN, MS
Practical Nursing Program Manager
College of Southern Idaho
Twin Falls, Idaho

Patrice Pierce, RN, MSN
Director of Nursing Program
Central Georgia Technical College
Milledgeville, Georgia

Cheryl Lynn Puckett, MSN, RNC-OB
Associate Professor
Bluegrass Community and Technical College, Danville
    Campus
Danville, Kentucky

Heather (Thomas) Reardon, RN, MS
Associate Professor
College of Southern Idaho
Twin Falls, Idaho

Dana Reece, RN, MSN/Ed
Professor of Nursing
Horry Georgetown Technical College
Georgetown, South Carolina

LuAnn J. Reicks, RN-BC, BSN, MSN
Professor/Practical Nurse Coordinator
Iowa Central Community College
Fort Dodge, Iowa

Ellen Santos, RN, MSN, CNE
Director of Practical Nursing
Assabet Valley Regional Technical School
Marlborough, Massachusetts

Anna Schmidt, RN, MA, PHN
Dean of Health Sciences
Hennepin Technical College
Brooklyn Park, Minnesota

Glynda Renee Sherill, RN, MS
Practical Nursing Instructor
Indian Capital Technology Center
Tahlequah, Oklahoma

Anne Simko, RN, BSN, MS
LPN Department Head
Eli Whitney Technical School
Hamden, Connecticut

Carolyn Slade, AAS
Practical Nursing Instructor
Wiregrass Georgia Technical College
Fitzgerald, Georgia

Rox Ann Sparks, RN, MSN, MICN,
    LNC, ENPC
Assistant Director Vocational Nursing
Merced College – Dr. Lakkireaddy Allied Health Division
Merced, California

Kelly Stone, RN, BSN
PN Program Coordinator
University of Arkansas Community College at Batesville
Batesville, Arkansas

Miranda Stover, RN, BS, MSN
Assistant Professor of Practical Nursing
Iowa Lakes Community College
Emmetsburg, Iowa

Serena Strain, RN, MSN
Nurse Faculty, Lead Instructor
Forsyth Technical Community College
Winston Salem, North Carolina

Sandy Wallace, RN, MS, BA
Professor of Nursing
Kansas City Kansas Community College
Kansas City, Kansas

Resa Yount, RN, BSN
Practical Nursing Senior Instructor
Tennessee College of Applied Technology
Morristown, Tennessee

Contents

UNIT THREE
Birth and the Family   105

UNIT SEVEN
Pediatric Concerns and Considerations   397

The following content can be found online at www.DavisPlus.com:

Appendices

unit ONE

Introduction to Maternity and Pediatric Nursing

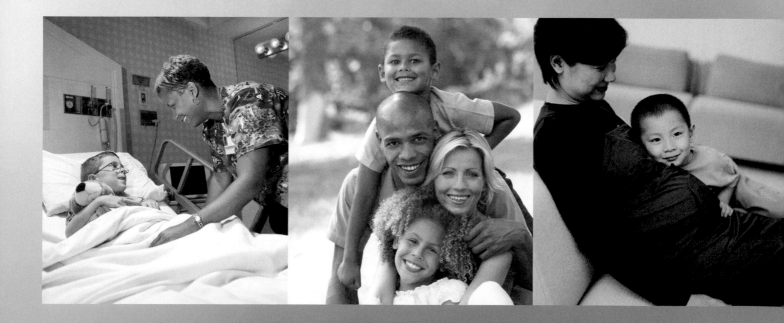

1

Healthy People 2020 and Initiatives for Healthy Families

KEY TERMS

Centers for Disease Control and Prevention (CDC)
genomics
health-care disparity
Healthy People 2020
Leading Health Indicators
social determinants

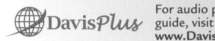 For audio pronunciation guide, visit www.DavisPlus.com

CHAPTER CONCEPTS

Promoting Health

LEARNING OUTCOMES

1. Define the key terms.
2. Describe how the *Healthy People 2020* initiative relates to families, children, and infants.
3. List government agencies that are involved in the *Healthy People 2020* objectives.
4. Describe historical perspectives related to the *Healthy People 2020* initiative.
5. Discuss how the *Healthy People 2020* objectives apply to maternal and child well-being.
6. Explain how maternal and pediatric nurses can be instrumental in promoting *Healthy People 2020* objectives for their clients.
7. Analyze the progress, or lack thereof, for each of the Leading Health Indicators that pertain to families.

REAL-WORLD CASE STUDY

Andrea

■ Andrea, a hard-working financial advisor, and her husband Charles, an assistant professor of English at a nearby private university, became pregnant later in life. Because of their busy work schedules and troubled family histories, they had not planned to have children. Andrea was beyond surprised when she learned that she was pregnant at age 40 while Charles was just turning 50. A few months later, an amniocentesis showed that the couple could expect a healthy baby boy.

Although Andrea and Charles were well educated and enjoyed a social network of middle-class, educated acquaintances, they had few parenting role models. They had no family support because Andrea was an only child who had lost both parents, and Charles had a single mother and siblings who were not in contact. Andrea and Charles set about pending parenthood in a practical manner by purchasing supplies and attending childbirth and parenting classes. Andrea planned to return to work after a 6-week maternity leave, and Charles made plans to teach evening classes so he could be home during the day.

The baby, Andrew, was born by Cesarean section because of failure to progress. Andrea had difficulty initiating breastfeeding, which was unexpected. Charles did not know how to help, and Andrea's nurse was focused on assessing level of sensation and postpartum bleeding. Andrea continued breastfeeding attempts while in the hospital for the next few days. Finally, she asked the nurses to keep Andrew in the nursery and give him a bottle. She just wanted to sleep.

After the family returned home, Andrew cried inconsolably for hours every night. Charles discovered that after giving Andrew a bottle, he would quickly stop crying, allowing the couple to get some much-needed sleep. Andrea continued to attempt breastfeeding, because she wanted to do as the books said was best for her baby.

Upon Andrea's return to work, she struggled to find a time and place where she could pump her milk. She was not comfortable in the women's bathroom and everywhere else she went, she was met with looks or questions. Charles worried about the depleted breast milk supply in the refrigerator, and in an effort to stop Andrew's persistent crying, he began to purchase formula to bottle-feed the baby. Andrew became increasingly interested in these formula feedings. At the same time, Andrea continued to have painful, blistered nipples and difficulty expressing adequate amounts of milk during work hours. The family's pediatrician was concerned about Andrew's inadequate weight gain and suggested more supplemental formula feeding. Andrea began to have serious doubts about continuing to breastfeed.

Questions

1. What are the benefits to breastfeeding that Andrea might have learned?
2. Why did Andrea and baby Andrew have difficulty establishing a breastfeeding relationship?
3. What were the factors involved that made it difficult for Andrea to continue breastfeeding?
4. Keeping in mind the *Healthy People 2020* initiative, how might a nurse assist Andrea during the postpartum period?

CONCEPTUAL CORNERSTONE

Health, Prevention, and Wellness

Health, prevention, and wellness are the three most important concepts to review when reading about and discussing the *Healthy People 2020* initiatives for healthy families. Pediatric nurses can prioritize health promotion activities, improve education for patients and families, and focus care on issues identified on a national basis. Healthy families contribute to productive individuals in society. Preventing illnesses, diseases, and injuries reduces health-care expenses and promotes personal success at school and at work. Wellness relates to a lifestyle of healthy choices that influence how families live, flourish, and grow. Pediatric nurses have a large part in implementing the *Healthy People 2020* initiatives and therefore assisting society in achieving health goals and outcomes.

In 1979, an influential document, a landmark in the history of public health, was published by the Surgeon General to address the health status of Americans and to set goals for improvement. The document titled "Healthy People: The Surgeon General's Report on Health Promotion and Disease Prevention" was created to improve the health of Americans by the year 1990 (Potter and Perry, 2013). The Healthy People program is managed by the Office of Disease Prevention and Health Promotion, U.S. Department of Health and Human Services. The initiative provides science-based, 10-year national objectives for improving the health of all Americans. *Healthy People 2020* comprises 42 topics and hundreds of measurable objectives. Many objectives lack the data to determine a target and are not measurable. These objectives are referred to as *developmental.* Each topic area is overseen by 1 of 18 different federal agencies. For example, maternal, infant, and child health objectives are co-led by two federal agencies: the **Centers for Disease Control and Prevention (CDC)**, and the Health Resources and Services Administration.

Epidemiologists from the U.S. Department of Health and Human Services monitor progress toward these objectives and set targets based on a projected profile of people in the United States and their existing health status (Maurer and Smith, 2013). As this nation moves through in the 21st century, progress has been made in areas such as an increase in physical activity, hypertension management, and homicide rates, but the country is moving away (becoming worse) from the targets in teen suicide, adolescent mental health, and oral health.

HISTORICAL PERSPECTIVE

Since the original 1979 document, updates have been created for each new decade. Table 1.1 provides a historical perspective of initiatives for each decade. Each update was created to reflect health goals for the decade ahead. With each revised initiative, more topic areas and objectives have been added. The focus has moved more than ever toward health promotion and disease prevention. *Healthy People 2020* aligns with the projection that a larger, older, and more diverse U.S. population is on the horizon. The overall goals for the year 2020 are to: (1) increase life expectancy, (2) improve the quality of life, and (3) eliminate health disparities (*Healthy People 2020, 2015*). These goals have not changed since the *Healthy People 2010* document. New topic areas for *Healthy People 2020* include adolescent health; blood disorders; dementia; early and middle childhood; **genomics** (the science of mapping human genes); global health; health-related quality of life; health-care associated infections; lesbian, gay, bisexual, and transgender health; older adults; sleep health; and **social determinants** (conditions in which members of society are born, live, grow, work, and age).

TABLE 1.1 HISTORY OF HEALTHY PEOPLE INITIATIVES

Initiative	Decade for the Initiative Goal
1979 *Healthy People: The Surgeon General's Report on Health Promotion and Disease Prevention* (15 topics)	1980–1990
1990 *Healthy People 2000: National Health Promotion and Disease Prevention Objectives* (22 topics)	1990–2000
2000 *Healthy People 2010: Objectives for Improving Health* (28 topics)	2000–2010
2010 *Healthy People 2020* (42 topics)	2010–2020

Data exist showing progress toward the goals up to 2011. Progress is divided into the categories of target met, improvement occurring, worsening, or no change/unable to tell. Many federal agencies are involved in working toward the proposed objectives of the Healthy People initiative. They include the Agency for Healthcare Research and Quality, the CDC, the National Institutes of Health, the President's Council on Physical Fitness and Sports, and the Food and Drug Administration, among many others. In addition, memorandums of understanding or agreement have been agreed upon with non-federal agencies, such as the American Heart Association and National Recreation and Parks Association. In this way, work is not duplicated and all can share in the goals of promoting quality and quantity of life.

LEADING HEALTH INDICATORS

There are 26 **Leading Health Indicators** that comprise a subset of objectives from the topic areas based on priorities for the decade. Overall life expectancy has increased, showing improvement toward a major Healthy People goal. Morbidity rates from heart disease and stroke, which are among the leading causes of death, have decreased as well, but many public health challenges are still evident. For example, improvements have occurred in four areas: (1) air quality, (2) childhood exposure to secondhand smoke, (3) homicide rates, and (4) increased physical activity for adults. At the same time, increased suicide rates and depression in adolescence are worsening problems. Progress to date on achieving the indicators has been positive, with 14 of the 26 having met their target or are improving. Specifically in the area of pediatric care, progress has been made in meeting the objectives of having less secondhand smoke and fewer teens smoking and using drugs. For adults, physical activity has increased and fewer adults are smoking.

Equitable health care for all has always been a major Healthy People goal. Unfortunately, no significant improvements have occurred in this decade. Table 1.2 gives examples of Leading Health Indicators that affect mothers, babies, children, and teenagers.

TABLE 1.2 LEADING HEALTH INDICATORS THAT PERTAIN TO FAMILIES AND THEIR PROGRESS TOWARD *HEALTHY PEOPLE 2020* TARGETS

Leading Health Indicators	Family-Related Examples	Progress (2008–2012)	Target
Access to health care	All families should have insurance coverage and a consistent primary care provider	Insignificant increase in coverage; needs to increase ~ 20%	100% health insurance coverage
		77.3% of families have primary care provider; insignificant increase	83.9% should have primary care provider
		No change	**No change**
Preventive services	Screening, prevention, immunizations	Millions of children, teens, and adults go without services that would protect them from developing serious diseases	

TABLE 1.2 LEADING HEALTH INDICATORS THAT PERTAIN TO FAMILIES AND THEIR PROGRESS TOWARD *HEALTHY PEOPLE 2020* TARGETS—cont'd

Leading Health Indicators	Family-Related Examples	Progress (2008–2012)	Target
	Diabetes	Diabetes rates are unchanged Immunization rates have improved significantly from 2008–2012 (from 44.3% to 68.4%) **No change**	Prevalence rates of diabetes unchanged 80% of children aged 19–35 months to be vaccinated **No change**
Air quality	Clean land, air, water; free from lead and allergens	Fewer unhealthy air days; exceeding target Between 2009 and 2012, 41.3% of 3–11 year olds exposed to secondhand smoke; this exceeded goal **Achieved target**	Exceeded target for clean air days Fewer than 47% exposed **Achieved target**
Injury and violence	Homicide	In 2010, 5.3 homicides per 100,000 **Achieved target**	Fewer than 5.5 per 100,000 **Achieved target**
	Suicide, child abuse/neglect, domestic violence, car accident	Injury death rate decreased by 4% with 57.1 deaths per 100,000 **Improving**	Fewer than 53.7 per 100,000 **Improving**
Maternal, infant, and child health	Infant death	2006–2009 infant mortality decreased from 6.7 to 6.1 per 1,000	Fewer than 6 per 1,000
	Preterm (less than 37 weeks)	Decreased from 12.7% to 11.5% **Improving**	Fewer than 11.4% **Improving**
Mental health	Suicide	2006-2010 suicide rate increased by 7%—11.3 to 12.1 per 100,000	10.2 per 100,000
	Adolescent depression	8.3% to 9.1% increase in depressive disorder **Worsening**	7.5% or fewer teens with major depressive disorder **Worsening**
Nutrition, physical activity, and obesity		18.2% to 20.6% increase for adults **Achieved Target** Obesity for kids increased from 16.1% to 16.9% **No Change**	20.1% engaging in physical activity **Achieved Target** 14.5% **No Change**
Oral health	Dental visits	Visits to dentist decreased from 44.5% to 41.8% **Worsening**	49% or more to visit dentist each year **Worsening**
Reproductive and sexual health		2006–2010 rate of knowing HIV status increased from 80.9% to 84.2% **Improving**	At least 90% should know their HIV status **Improving**

Continued

TABLE **1.2** **LEADING HEALTH INDICATORS THAT PERTAIN TO FAMILIES AND THEIR PROGRESS TOWARD** *HEALTHY PEOPLE 2020* **TARGETS—cont'd**

Leading Health Indicators	Family-Related Examples	Progress (2008–2012)	Target
Social determinants		Students graduating within 4 years increased from 74.9% in 2007–2008 school year to 78.2% in 2009–2010 **Improving**	82.4% graduated high school within 4 years **Improving**
Substance abuse	Adolescents using alcohol or drugs. ~31% of 16–17 y.o. drink or take drugs	2008–2012 rate of adolescent alcohol or drug use decreased from 18.4% to 17.4% **Improving**	16.6% or fewer using substances **Improving**
Tobacco use for teens	Life expectancy for smokers is at least 10 years less	Smoking rate has decreased from 19.5% to 18.1%; decrease is not significant **No Change**	16% or less should be smoking **No Change**

Source: http://www.healthypeople.gov/2020/leading-health-indicators/Healthy-People-2020-Leading-Health-Indicators%3A-Progress-Update

HEALTHY PEOPLE 2020 LEADS TO HEALTHY FAMILIES

The Healthy People documents do not necessarily discern babies and children from adults; however, one could make the connection that the good health of adults would benefit children. For example, screening for hypertension allows older adults to live longer, higher-quality lives, which leads to a healthier extended family with grandparents. Preventing the spread of HIV leads to healthier parents with longer lives and less likelihood of transmission to infants. Other Healthy People topics pertain to the population at large, such as access to health care, environmental quality, and social determinants. Good nutrition, mental health, increased activity, and injury prevention are examples of topics that pertain to children, teens, and adults. Talking to parents early in pregnancy or before birth may help to promote these topics (Fig. 1.1).

Application: *Healthy People 2020* Objective—Increase the Proportion of Infants Who Are Breastfed

Nurses can be instrumental in helping the population meet Healthy People objectives. A classic example for maternity and pediatric nurses is when assisting a new mother and baby to establish a breastfeeding relationship (Fig. 1.2). Nurses might be called upon to follow the 10 steps of the Baby Friendly Hospital Initiative: "The Baby-Friendly Hospital Initiative (BFHI) is a joint effort of the WHO and the United Nations Children's Fund (UNICEF) to

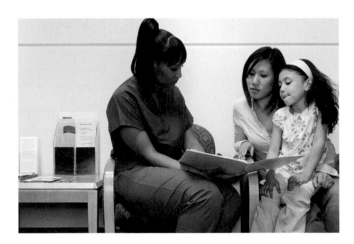

FIGURE **1.1** Education is important to growing families.

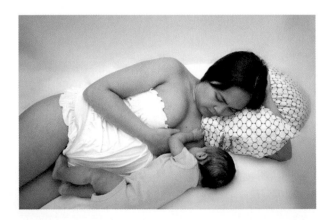

FIGURE **1.2** Encouraging breastfeeding.

encourage, promote, and support breastfeeding as the model for optimum infant nutrition" (Hockenberry, 2013, p. 215).

TEAM WORKS

Team efforts to increase the chance of breastfeeding include teaching parents about the benefits of breastfeeding. A few of the basic benefits of breastfeeding include the following:

- Breast milk is the best source of nutrition for babies because it promotes brain growth and strengthens the newborn's immune system.
- It is best to give exclusively breast milk in the first 6 months of life for safety against choking and improvement of the newborn's health status.
- Babies who receive breast milk have lower rates of infections and other illnesses.
- Mothers who breastfeed have a decreased risk of cancer, anemia, and osteoporosis.
- Families can save money on formula, bottles, and supplies.
- Families do not have to sterilize or wash bottles, thus saving time and money.

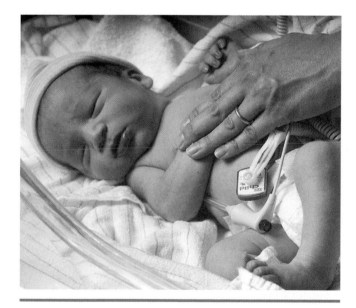

Much of the success in establishing a breastfeeding relationship comes from the will of the mother and support from others. This support can begin with the nurse caring for the mother and newborn immediately after birth. Later on, mothers continue to need support. Nurses can make referrals or provide continued assistance. A handful of nurses become certified as lactation consultants. Nurses are in a natural place to assist mother and newborns with the best form of nutrition. *Healthy People 2020* objectives related to breastfeeding include (Table 1.3):

- Increase the percentage of employers who have worksite lactation programs.
- Decrease the percentage of breastfed newborns who receive formula supplementation within the first 2 days of life.
- Increase the percentage of live births that occur in facilities that provide recommended care for lactating mothers and their babies.

SAFETY *STAT!*

If a mother has difficulty establishing a breastfeeding relationship with her newborn, the pediatric nurse can provide the mother several tips for success despite barriers or roadblocks:

- Mothers who have Cesarean sections might struggle to initiate breastfeeding due to the higher use of pain medication and more difficulty getting into a proper position.
- Receiving support via family role models is helpful, but nurses can provide this type of support as well.
- Infants should be supported and guided to nipple within 1 hour of birth. Nurses can make this early breastfeeding experience a priority.
- As soon as a new mother is brought to the recovery room from the operating room, breastfeeding can begin.
- The new mother will need support and guidance in finding a comfortable position after giving birth or after a surgical Cesarean section.
- Rooming-in and breastfeeding on demand should be promoted, and formula should be avoided.
- Before discharge from the hospital, families need all of their questions to be answered and concerns about breastfeeding addressed. If there are further questions or concerns, a referral for further education and support is warranted. Nurses can make referrals to a Lactation Educator without a physician's order.

TABLE **1.3** *HEALTHY PEOPLE 2020*: **42 TOPIC AREAS WITH MATERNAL–CHILD EXAMPLES**

Objective	Example
1. Improve access to health-care services.	Uninsured pregnant woman does not seek prenatal care because of lack of funding. She has higher likelihood of having a preterm baby. Currently, more children need health insurance coverage to meet the goal.
NEW: 2. Improve the health, safety, and well-being of adolescents and young adults.	Adolescents are at higher risk for homicide, suicide, homelessness, drug use, sexually transmitted infections, unwanted pregnancy, motor vehicle accident, and smoking. Currently, the percentage of violent acts in public schools needs to decrease to meet the goal.
3. Prevent disability related to back conditions, osteoporosis, and arthritis.	*n/a*
NEW: 4. Prevent illness related to blood disorders and blood safety.	Certain blood disorders are specific to childhood, such as sickle cell anemia, thalassemias, and hemophilia. Currently, prevention of complications that result from sickle cell anemia in children needs to increase to meet the goal.
5. Reduce the number of cancer cases and cancer-associated illnesses.	Cancer is the second-leading cause of death in the United States, mostly affecting older persons. Some forms of cancer are specific only to babies and children. Other forms of cancer might affect parents of young children, potentially leaving these children without parents. Cancer screening should begin in adolescence with Pap test and HPV vaccine.
6. Reduce new cases of chronic kidney disease and its effects.	Although not common, children can be afflicted with polycystic kidney disease, autoimmune conditions, or diabetes, which can impair kidney function.
NEW: 7. Reduce morbidity for those with Alzheimer's disease.	*n/a*
8. Improve the quality of life and reduce the economic burden of diabetes.	Most cases of diabetes are for adults with type-2 diabetes. However, 10% of all cases involve children with type-1 diabetes. More women with diabetes are having babies.
9. Promote the health and well-being of persons with disabilities.	Children need equal access in schools and in their environments. Currently, there needs to be an increase in access to early intervention services for children with disabilities to meet the goal.
NEW: 10. Track the well-being of children in early (first 5 years) and middle (6–12 years) childhood.	Experiences in the first years influence the rest of life. There is a need to foster nurturing families, create safe environments, and have access to health care. Currently, there is a need to reduce the proportion of children who have poor quality sleep to meet the goal.
11. Increase quantity and quality of community-based programs that improve health.	Teaching about oral health or prevention of unwanted pregnancy at schools or community health centers. Currently, there is a need to increase the proportion of schools that have a comprehensive health education program to meet the goal.

TABLE **1.3** *HEALTHY PEOPLE 2020*: **42 TOPIC AREAS WITH MATERNAL–CHILD EXAMPLES—cont'd**

Objective	Example
12. Promote health through healthy environment.	Outdoor air quality, water, lead-based paints, and food quality. Eliminating lead poisoning in children is a prominent goal. Currently, blood lead levels in children aged 1–5 need to decrease to meet the goal.
13. Adequate spacing and prevention of unintended pregnancy.	Consequences of intended pregnancy include low birth weight babies, maternal depression, domestic violence, lower income, high school dropout, and sons of single teen mothers more likely to be in jail and daughters more likely to be teen mothers themselves.
14. Reduce food-borne illnesses.	Children less than 4 years of age have the highest rates of campylobacteriosis, cryptosporidiosis, salmonellosis, shigellosis, yersiniosis, and *Escherichia coli* infection.
NEW: 15. Use genomic tools to improve health.	Genetic testing can identify diseases in newborns, allowing for early treatment.
NEW: 16. Improve public health through global disease detection.	Preventing global health threats, such as communicable infections, traffic accidents, obesity, mental illness, and substance use, will benefit the United States.
17. Use health information technology to improve outcomes.	Health information technology can improve the health of families by increasing access to information and support networks.
NEW: 18. Improve health-related quality of life.	Health-related quality of life is improved through participation in physical and social activities.
NEW: 19. Prevent health care–associated infections.	Health care–associated infections are leading causes of death and expense primarily related to invasive lines, surgical sites, and drug-resistant organisms.
20. Reduce the prevalence and severity of communication disorders.	1–3 of every 1,000 children are born with hearing loss, many with autism spectrum disorder. Nearly all states screen for hearing loss in newborns. Currently, there is a need to decrease the occurrence of otitis media in children and adolescents to meet the goal.
21. Improve cardiovascular health.	There is a need to decrease the proportion of children with hypertension to meet the goal.
22. Prevent HIV and its related illness and death.	An estimated 1.1 million people are living with HIV and 75% of them are men. There are fewer new cases than in the past, but more persons are living with HIV. Currently, there is a need to decrease the incidence of perinatally transmitted HIV infection to meet the goal.
23. Increase immunization rates and decrease preventable diseases.	Currently, there is a need to reduce the number of cases of varicella (chicken pox) for those less than 17 years of age to meet the goal.
24. Prevent unintentional injuries and violence.	Most injuries are preventable. Injuries are the leading cause of death for persons aged 1–44.

Continued

TABLE **1.3** *HEALTHY PEOPLE 2020*: **42 TOPIC AREAS WITH MATERNAL–CHILD EXAMPLES—cont'd**

Objective	Example
NEW: 25. Improve the health of lesbian, gay, bisexual, and transgender persons.	Lesbian, gay, bisexual, and transgender persons are more prone to health disparities, higher rates of drinking, obesity for females, and depression.
26. Improve the health of women, infants, and children.	Currently, there is a need to reduce the numbers of neonates with low birth weights and the numbers of preterm deliveries to meet the goal.
27. Ensure the safe use of medical products.	Currently, there is a need to decrease the number of emergency room visits related to medication overdose in children less than 5 years old.
28. Improve mental health through prevention and access to health care.	Disorders can begin early in life and early treatment is essential. Improving family functioning and parenting can help children. Currently, there is a need to increase and improve treatment for children with mental health disorders to meet the goal.
29. Promote health through good nutrition and maintain healthy weight.	Good nutrition is important to growth and development for children. Among children, incidence of obesity is highest among black girls and Hispanics. Currently, there is a need to decrease the numbers of young children who are considered obese to meet the goal.
30. Promote health and safety of people at work.	One-fourth of a lifetime might be spent in the workplace. Young people entering the workforce can be particularly vulnerable to unsafe conditions.
NEW: 31. Improve the health and function of older adults and reduce falls.	
32. Prevent and control oral and craniofacial disease and increase access to dental service.	Oral health is a huge success story over the past 60 years, partly because of water fluoridation. However, there has been an increase in cavities for preschool children. Currently, there is a need to reduce the number of children aged 1–5 who develop caries in their primary teeth to meet the goal.
33. Improve health and fitness through daily activity.	Eighty percent of adolescents do not get enough aerobic and strengthening exercise. Activity for children will improve bone strength, reduce body fat, and improve cardiovascular health, respiratory health, and musculoskeletal condition. Currently, there is a need to increase the proportion of children who watch TV or play video games less than 2 hours per day to decrease sedentary lifestyle to meet the goal.
NEW: 34. Improve the nation's ability to respond to major health incident.	*n/a*
35. Ensure that public health agencies have the necessary infrastructure.	*n/a*
36. Promote respiratory health through better prevention and treatment.	Asthma is on the rise and more common for children living in poverty. Currently, there is a need to reduce the number of hospitalizations related to asthma for children aged 1–5 to meet the goal.

TABLE **1.3** *HEALTHY PEOPLE 2020*: **42 TOPIC AREAS WITH MATERNAL–CHILD EXAMPLES—cont'd**

Objective	Example
37. Promote healthy sexual behaviors and access to prevention services.	There are 25 infectious organisms that can cause sexually transmitted disease. Currently, there is a need to decrease the rates of congenital syphilis to meet the goal.
NEW: 38. Increase public knowledge of how sleep can improve health and quality of life.	*n/a*
NEW: 39. Create environments that promote good health for all.	*n/a*
40. Reduce substance abuse to promote health and safety of all, especially children.	*n/a*
41. Reduce illness and disability related to tobacco and secondhand smoke.	Currently, there is a need to reduce the proportion of children exposed to secondhand smoke to meet the goal.
42. Improve visual health for all through early detection and treatment.	Currently, there is a need to increase the proportion of preschool children who receive vision screening to meet the goal.

Source: http://www.healthypeople.gov/2020/leading-health-indicators/Healthy-People-2020-Leading-Health-Indicators%3A-Progress-Update

Key Points

- The Healthy People initiative was created by the Surgeon General of the U.S. Department of Health and Human Services in 1979. Since then, the initiative has been revised in 1990, 2000, and 2010. The initiative sets objectives for all U.S. citizens to follow over the upcoming decade. Epidemiologists monitor progress toward the targets as the decade progresses.

- *Healthy People 2020* comprises 42 topic areas and hundreds of specific objectives. Some objectives, such as increasing the rate of breastfed babies and decreasing the rate of adolescent depression, are specific to maternal–child care. Other objectives, such as increasing the proportion of those with a usual primary care provider, pertain to individuals across the lifespan but impact growing families.

- Leading Health Indicators contain a subset of 26 priority areas. The *Healthy People 2020* targets have been met in some areas, such as increasing adult physical activity and decreasing childhood exposure to secondhand smoke, but are moving away from targets in other areas, such as decreased adolescent depression and increased visits to the dentist. The target for access to health care is set for 100%.

- Maternal–child nurses should consider the *Healthy People 2020* objectives when providing care. An example of this application occurs with the Baby-Friendly Hospital Initiative. Nurses who work in a baby-friendly hospital must follow 10 steps, including assisting mother and baby to breastfeed within 1 hour of birth, avoiding the use of artificial nipples, caring for mother and baby in the same room, and encouraging breastfeeding on demand.

REVIEW QUESTIONS

1. The *Healthy People 2020* initiative has 42 topic areas with hundreds of objectives. The overall goals of *Healthy People 2020* are to:
   1. Increase life expectancy by at least 10 years
   2. Diminish the numbers of children who are uninsured
   3. Increase life expectancy, improve quality of life, and eliminate health disparities
   4. Build health/fitness clubs and health food stores in every city in the United States

2. Under the topic of maternal, infant, and child health, which of the following constitutes an objective for *Healthy People 2020*?
   1. Increase the rate at which children attend extracurricular activities.
   2. Increase the rate of which infants are breastfed for 2 years.
   3. Increase the rate at which babies are put to bed on their backs.
   4. Increase the rate at which babies are born in the United States.

3. There are 26 Leading Health Indicators that prioritize objectives for the 2010-2020 decade. Which of the following objectives that pertain to children is currently being met?
   1. Increase the rate at which babies are breastfed.
   2. Decrease the number of children who are exposed to secondhand smoke.
   3. Eliminate health-care disparity (differences in access to health care and disease patterns)
   4. Decrease the rate of teen suicide.

4. There are 26 Leading Health Indicators that prioritize objectives for the 2010-2020 decade. Which of the following objectives that pertain to children is currently moving away from the target (worsening)?
   1. The rate of teenage depression
   2. The rate of teenage homicide
   3. The rate of teenage car accidents
   4. The rate of teenage smoking

5. According to the CDC, 75% of mothers start out breastfeeding, but that number diminishes greatly by 6 months, moving away from the Healthy People target of 61% at 6 months. Which of the following would constitute a common barrier for women to continue breastfeeding?
   1. Keeping the baby in the same hospital room with the mother after birth
   2. Having a baby who was born large for gestational age and continues to be overweight
   3. Fear of having the baby's father provide milk to the baby from a bottle
   4. Lack of accommodation to breastfeed or express milk in the workplace

6. One way in which the Healthy People objectives help to increase the rate of breastfed babies is with the establishment of baby-friendly hospitals. Which of the following is a step that the baby-friendly hospital would take on the maternity unit?
   1. Assist the mother to begin breastfeeding within 1 hour of birth
   2. Diminish the amount of newborn crying through use of a pacifier
   3. Provide for maternal sleep by keeping the newborn in the nursery
   4. Maintain a schedule of breastfeeding every 3 hours around the clock

CRITICAL THINKING QUESTIONS

1. Why was the Healthy People initiative created by the Surgeon General in 1979?
2. What changes have occurred since the original document of 1979?
3. What are the Leading Health Indicators?
4. How do the Healthy People objectives apply specifically to the well-being of families?

unit TWO

Pregnancy and the Family

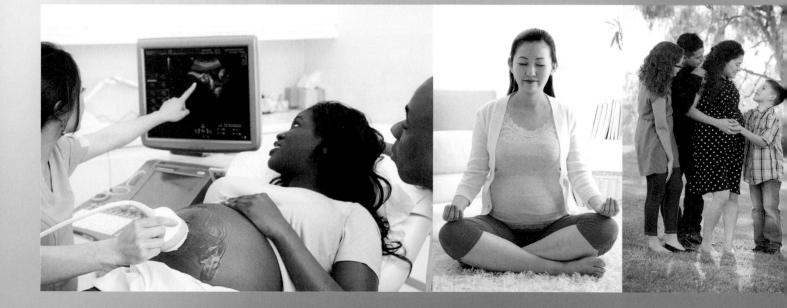

2

Introduction to Maternity Nursing

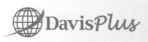 For audio pronunciation guide, visit www.DavisPlus.com

LEARNING OUTCOMES

1. Define the key terms.
2. Write a personal definition of quality health care.
3. Discuss the history of maternity nursing.
4. Compare and contrast the roles of the licensed practical/vocational nurse (LPN/ LVN), registered nurse (RN), nurse practitioner (NP), clinical nurse specialist (CNS), and certified nurse midwife (CNM).
5. Define scope of practice, standards of care, and evidence-based practice.
6. Explain the ethical principles of autonomy, beneficence, nonmaleficence, and justice.
7. Identify possible ethical dilemmas in maternity care.
8. Discuss common fears of nursing students related to maternity nursing.

REAL-WORLD CASE STUDY

Lisa

■ Lisa is a nursing student in her clinical rotation for postpartum care. At the change of shift report, she learned that her assigned patient had a positive drug screen for heroin and that her premature baby is in the neonatal intensive care nursery. Lisa is anxious about providing care for this patient because of her own strong personal beliefs about drugs and pregnancy. Lisa pages her clinical nursing instructor and asks for another assignment. She says to her instructor, "I am uncomfortable with this assignment. It makes me angry to think about what she did to her baby. Can I have another patient instead?"

Questions

1. What do you think the clinical instructor will say?
2. What are Lisa's legal and ethical responsibilities toward this patient?

CONCEPTUAL CORNERSTONE

Health Care Quality

Quality in health care can have many definitions. A nurse manager may view quality as the wise use of resources, a lack of errors in providing care, and positive patient feedback. The nurse at the bedside may view quality as the delivery of safe and effective care. The physician or midwife may view quality as a positive patient response to medications and interventions without complications. The patient may view health care as having good quality only if it meets his own expectations for improvement and recovery. According to the Institute of Medicine (2015), the definition of quality health care is "The degree to which health services for individuals and populations increase the likelihood of desired health outcomes and are consistent with current professional knowledge."

Nurses can improve quality in health care by:

- Providing safe care to patients by working within the scope of practice, utilizing standards of care built on evidence-based practice, and making sound decisions in providing care
- Delivering family- and patient-centered care with attention to the specific needs, values, and expectations of the patient and family
- Improving patient care by identifying errors and hazards and implementing safety principles
- Collaborating with health-care team members to reduce errors and improve care
- Utilizing hospital resources in a cost-effective manner by not wasting materials and time
- Providing equal care to all patients that does not vary in quality based upon gender, ethnicity, culture, or socioeconomic status

(Giddens, 2013; Stevens, 2013; NCQA, 2015)

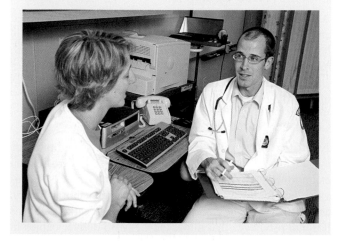

Maternity nursing is an exciting field. Welcoming a new life into the world and supporting the family can be one of the most rewarding aspects of health care. Maternity nursing offers a broad range of nursing opportunities that includes providing care from puberty to menopause. Nurses can specialize in prenatal care, labor and delivery, postpartum care, newborn care, neonatal intensive care, women's health, and infertility care.

HISTORY OF MATERNITY NURSING

For centuries, and before science and medicine, women provided care for women in labor. The laboring woman would be assisted by her sisters, mother, friends, and midwife in a home-centered event. In a community, the woman most experienced with birthing became the midwife, and she would be called upon to assist with births. The midwife would offer pain-relieving herbs and wine, massage, advise, encouragement, and prayer. The midwife learned from experience and did not receive formal training.

Most women survived childbirth with a lay midwife, but death rates from childbirth complications were high. Hypertensive disorders, postpartum hemorrhage, and postpartum infection were the most common causes of death (Klairmont, 2004).

During the 16th and 17th centuries, the study of human anatomy and ancient medical knowledge prompted a renewed interest in human reproduction. The invention of the printing press led to the printing of the first obstetrical texts, which included protocols for labor and deliveries. During this time of renewed interest in reproduction, English surgeons became the birth attendants for the upper classes. Only the commoners and poor used lay midwives.

In the 18th century, surgeons developed methods to recognize and manage abnormal labor. A Scottish surgeon, William Smellie, used forceps for the first time in 1752 (Feldhusen, 2000). Even when a problem arose during labor, midwives and pregnant women were still reluctant to call a surgeon for a delivery; surgeons were associated with death and women were afraid of their virtue being tarnished by a male attendant. Many physicians became interested in assisting with difficult labors and deliveries. Physicians could also offer ether, morphine, and chloroform for pain control. By the end of the 18th century, 50% of births were attended by male physicians.

In the 19th and early 20th centuries, the United States experienced massive immigration from southern and eastern Europe. The immigrants lived in densely populated urban tenements and worked long hours in unsafe conditions. They used midwives for childbirth. Childbirth complications were still common and the death rate for women and newborns was high. The complications and death rates were blamed on the uneducated and unregulated lay midwives. Social and health-care reformers and physicians wanting to improve conditions for the immigrants started a campaign to eliminate the lay midwife. Maternity hospitals for poor women were founded, and obstetrics became a specialty for physicians (Dawley, 2003).

During the early 20th century, physicians offered scopolamine, a drug that produced a "twilight sleep" for pain control. This drug was given in hospitals. It gave the mother an amnesic effect and often she did not remember her labor or delivery. The mother often did not see or hold her baby for hours or a day while waiting for the effects of the medication to subside. Modern women of the times stopped delivering babies at home and births moved into the hospital. Women began to take a more passive role in their childbirth experience, relinquishing control to the physicians. In the hospital setting, the physicians instituted protocols and policies. The nurse's role was to assist the physician and follow the doctor's orders. Coaching by nurses was not valued at that time.

Despite moving birthing into hospitals, the rates of complications and deaths declined very slowly. The government recognized that the complications were because of poor nutrition, poor or no prenatal care, and infectious diseases. Programs were developed to assist pregnant women and improve health care. These programs were helpful, but access to health care for women was a major problem, especially in rural areas. Most physicians practiced in urban areas. Nurses saw an opportunity to expand their roles in advanced practice and provide health care for poor and underserved women. Visiting nurses and professional midwives were used in rural areas to provide prenatal care and to assist with labor and delivery.

In the early 1950s, women became interested in having more control over their birth experience. With the introduction of the Bradley and Lamaze methods for childbirth, women began asking for family-centered care. They also wanted information on child spacing, what to expect during pregnancy, and how to cope with labor and delivery (Feldhusen, 2000). During this time, nurses took on the role of patient advocate and worked with women and their physicians to develop birth plans that were acceptable to both the mothers and the physicians. Their birth plans included participation by the father instead of relegating him to the waiting room. Physicians were reluctant to allow women to have choices in childbirth. Nurses began to expand their role and teach patients self-care and newborn care.

During the 1960s and 1970s, family-centered childbirth became more accepted. Nurses believed in the benefits of early, extended newborn-parent contact and actively changed hospital policies to allow rooming-in and to promote family-centered care.

In the last 50 years, the hospital maternity nurse has assumed many duties that were once assigned to physicians. Labor care, including assessment, administration of medications, inducing labor, and pain management, is the responsibility of the labor and delivery nurse under the protocols established by nurse midwives and physicians. Unless a patient is extremely high risk, most of the care during a hospital delivery will be given by maternity nurses.

ROLES IN MATERNITY NURSING

Maternity nursing focuses on the care of a woman, family, and newborn. Care may begin before conception with planning for pregnancy or infertility problems. Nursing care continues throughout the pregnancy when the role of the nurse may be focused on encouraging a healthy pregnancy or managing complications of pregnancy. During labor and delivery, the nurse has the responsibility to provide labor care until the physician or nurse midwife arrives for the delivery. The focus after delivery is to care for the mother as she recovers and her newborn adjusts to life outside the uterus. A nurse may

provide patient-centered and family-centered care as a licensed practical/vocational nurse, registered nurse, nurse practitioner, clinical nurse specialist, or certified nurse midwife.

Licensed Practical/Vocational Nurse

A licensed practical/vocational nurse (LPN/LVN) is one who has completed a program in a technical school or community college and has passed the National Council Licensure Examination (NCLEX) for LPN/LVNs. The LPN/LVN may provide nursing care in a doctor's office, clinic, or hospital under the direction of a registered nurse, nurse practitioner, physician, or midwife and may assist with preparation of the childbearing female for pregnancy and delivery.

Registered Nurse

A registered nurse (RN) is one who has graduated from an accredited nursing program with either an Associate Degree in Nursing (ADN) or a Bachelor's Degree in Nursing (BSN) and has passed the NCLEX for RNs. The RN can assess the patient, plan and provide care, provide teaching, monitor the progression of the pregnancy through delivery, and provide postpartum and newborn care.

Nurse Practitioner

A nurse practitioner (NP) is an advanced practice nurse who has graduated from an accredited program with either a Master's Degree in Nursing (MSN) or a doctorate of nurse practitioner (DNP) degree and has passed a certification exam. An NP provides advanced care and can prescribe medications. The NP may specialize in women's health throughout the life span, with emphasis on contraception, infertility problems, pre-pregnancy care, pregnancy care, postpartum care, lactation problems, newborn care, and menopause care.

Clinical Nurse Specialist

A clinical nurse specialist (CNS) is an RN who has obtained an advanced degree and clinical preparation at the MSN level, with a focus on education, management, and research roles relative to patient care. The CNS often works in clinics and hospitals alongside nurses to educate and support them in providing excellent patient care.

Certified Nurse Midwife

A certified nurse midwife (CNM) is an advanced practice nurse with a MSN or DNP and who has passed a certification exam in the area of pregnancy and delivery. The CNM provides care for the woman through pregnancy, labor, delivery, and postpartum. The CNM can prescribe medications and has hospital privileges that allow the CNM to deliver babies in the hospital.

TEAM WORKS

Nurses in all capacities, including the LPN/LVN, RN, CNS, NP, and CNM, often work as a team to provide pregnancy and delivery care for a mother and her newborn.

LEGALITIES AND ETHICS

Nurses have guidelines, both legal and ethical, to follow when providing nursing care. Maternity nurses can struggle with ethical and social dilemmas that affect families but have established guidelines that will assist them in providing safe care for patients and their families. This section will discuss the legal guidelines that are in place for which nurses can be held accountable, as well as the ethical guidelines that nurses can use when faced with ethical dilemmas.

Legalities

Every licensed nurse must be aware of the laws of the state in which he or she is licensed regarding the care that they are legally licensed to provide. The nurse must be knowledgeable of the laws applying to practice because when nurses do not meet the standards expected of them, they may be held legally responsible. This section will discuss the scope of practice, standards of care, institutional policies, and evidence-based practice that influences nursing care

Scope of Practice

The nursing scope of practice is determined by the state in which the nurse is licensed. The **scope of practice** is the legal outline of what a nurse can do according to the laws of that state. For example, an LPN/LVN, RN, NP, and nurse midwife all have different levels of legal authority in providing nursing care. In every state, the scope of practice is defined in the nurse practice act (NPA), which is enacted by the state legislature. It is a legal document that clearly outlines the scope of practice from which the Board of Nursing from each state oversees the licensed nurses and their NPA. Every nurse must be familiar with the NPA and the scope of practice in order to remain within the limits of the law and to not risk the loss of licensure for not working within the scope practice.

Standards of Care

Standards of care are a model of established practice that is accepted as the correct way to provide care for a patient; they are guidelines used to determine what a nurse should do. Standards of care provide a guide to the knowledge, skills, attitude, and judgment needed to practice safe nursing care. Nurses who do not follow the standards of care can be found negligent. Nursing negligence is defined as the nurse taking an action or non-action that does not follow the standard of care. For example, nurses can be held accountable for not following standards of care when administering medications, failing to protect a patient or her newborn from harm, and inappropriate delegation to a non-nursing, unlicensed healthcare worker.

Federal and state laws and professional organizations help define standards of care. The American Nurses' Association (ANA) has published standards of professional practice. For maternity nurses, the Association of Women's Health, Obstetric, and Neonatal Nurses (AWHONN) has established standards for the care of women and neonates.

Institution Policies

Nurses are also held accountable for their care through their hospitals' policies. Every hospital has a policy and procedures handbook that clearly outlines how nursing care is to be provided. This handbook might be in paper form or it could be a document available on the hospital electronic medical record system. Hospitals clearly define the chain of command, which is also known as the chain of communication; this is the procedure for reporting problems up the ladder of authority. A nurse is expected to report a problem to the next person up the ladder of authority.

If a nurse is unsure about a policy or a procedure, the policy and procedures handbook will provide specific guidelines. Following the hospital policies and procedures will prevent errors in patient care and promote safe care for the patients.

Evidence-Based Practice

Evidence-based practice is nursing care in which all nursing interventions are based on current valid research evidence. Evidence-based practice takes nursing research and puts it into practice at the patient's bedside. Some hospitals still practice nursing in an "old style" of never updating or changing nursing policies and procedures to match current evidence-based practice. New nurses can embrace evidence-based practice by asking "why" certain nursing conventions are practiced and being open to changes in nursing care when a scientific study indicates that safe and effective nursing care can be provided in a different way.

Ethics

According a Gallup poll (2014), Americans ranked nurses as having the highest honesty and ethical standards of all other professions. Nurses have clear guidance about legal issues in providing nursing care, but ethical decisions may not have clear-cut answers. **Ethics** are defined as moral principles that guide a person's behavior. Ethics are concerned with distinguishing between good and evil and right and wrong. Healthcare ethics are concerned with trying to do the right thing while achieving the best possible outcome for every patient (Chervenak and McCullough, 2012).

Nurses do have guidelines for providing ethical care. The American Nurses Association has a Code of Ethics (2015) that nurses can use to guide their nursing practice. A code of ethics is a formal statement of a group's ideal and values, and it serves as a standard for professional actions. Basic principles of ethical care that address the issues of fairness, honesty, and respect for human beings are:

• *Autonomy:* Patients have the right to have control over their own bodies and make their own decisions. This means that a competent adult can accept or refuse treatment, medications, procedures, diagnostic testing, and surgeries according to their wishes. Autonomy also includes protecting patient confidentiality and informed consent. Nurses can promote autonomy for their patients by providing patients with current evidence-based knowledge about their condition or their child's condition and trust them to make the right decision based on their values and perspective.

- **Beneficence:** This principle refers to acting from a spirit of compassion and kindness to benefit others (Carter, 2015). It also involves balancing the benefits of treatment against the risks and costs involved. Physicians and nurses must view beneficence from the viewpoint of the patient and family. At times, the patient and family may have differing views of the benefits of treatment and disagree with the plan of care. The principle of beneficence guides the health-care team to respect and consider the patient and family viewpoint of the situation. Nurses demonstrate beneficence by helping people reach their highest level of well-being by providing care to patients directly and by assisting to develop health-care policies that promote health for a large population.

- **Nonmaleficence:** This principle means "do no harm." It means to do no harm or to inflict the least possible harm to reach a beneficial outcome. Nurses carefully administer medication and double-check dosages in order to "do no harm" to the patient by making a medication error. Nurses do have to perform procedures that may be uncomfortable for patients. Nurses demonstrate nonmaleficence when administering an injection to relieve pain; the injection may be painful. However, the intent of the nurse is not to harm the patient but to provide relief from pain.

- **Justice:** This ethical principle refers to acting out of fairness for individuals, groups, organizations, and communities (Sundean and McGrath, 2013). It also refers to the fair allocation of services and resources. Nurses can demonstrate justice by joining committees and having a voice in making health-care policy decisions.

In providing nursing care to mothers and their newborns, nurses will see that, in the case of ethical problems, it can be challenging. There are no answers that fit every situation and every patient. Nurses might be frustrated with the lack of guidance about how to manage ethical dilemmas in the work place. Hospitals have ethics committees that can provide guidance in clinical situations in which clear-cut answers are not obtainable. Nurses who encounter ethical dilemmas should report through the chain of command to receive assistance. There are many ethical issues that a nurse may encounter when providing care to women and babies. Some of the ethical issues may include:

- Abortion
- An addicted mother using drugs during pregnancy
- A patient who wants an elective Cesarean birth because she does not want to deliver vaginally
- Provision of futile care for a premature newborn
- A young adolescent with no family support leaving the hospital with a newborn
- A homeless or drug-addicted mother who leaves the hospital with her newborn
- Infertility treatment that is expensive and not successful

A nurse is obligated to provide care that meets the legalities and standards of practice, regardless of feelings about a patient or a patient's decisions. Nurses must evaluate their own values about health care, illness, life, and death and avoid imposing their own values onto the patient. Understanding the cultural and ethical differences will help reduce conflicts in providing care. Finally, a nurse who stays current on evidence-based practice and current treatment options can offer the best information to patients and families during ethical discussions.

THERAPEUTIC COMMUNICATION

When a nurse is supporting patient autonomy, the nurse may need to identify the patient's values as they relate to the health-care situation. The nurse rarely offers an opinion. Nurses support autonomy by allowing patients to make their own decisions. Therapeutic phrases that might assist the nurse to understand the patient's values and viewpoint are:

- "Are you considering another course of action? Tell me about it."
- "How will you discuss this with your family?"
- "Will it be difficult for you to discuss this with your family?"
- "Now that you have made a decision, how do you feel?"
- "What information do you need to make a decision?"
- "How can I help you with this decision?"

THE MATERNITY NURSING STUDENT

Sometimes students are anxious and fearful about studying maternity nursing and participating in the clinical experience. A nursing student in the maternity unit is given the privilege of caring for a woman during one of the most exciting and personal events of her life. Many students are apprehensive about the clinical rotation of maternity care. The fears may be due to:

- **Being childless:** A student does not have to have children or have been pregnant to provide safe care. As with any topic in nursing education, personal experience is not required in order to provide appropriate care. The student should present in a professional manner and not appear embarrassed or uncomfortable.
- **Being a male student:** Many male students feel uncomfortable in maternity nursing. They feel as if they are alone in a women's world. Women are accustomed to having male care providers. Often, their obstetricians are males. A male student does not have to apologize for being a male, but the male student must appear confident and maintain a professional demeanor at all times.
- **Insufficient knowledge:** Students may feel anxious on the first clinical day due to lack of knowledge. A student does not have to know everything on the first day. However, some students do not study the maternity content because "I have kids, I've been through this." Having children does give the student an understanding of the patient's perspective, but now the student needs to perceive

the childbirth experience as a nursing professional. The student needs to be prepared, complete the assigned reading, and ask the instructor for clarification. Every student has basic skills that will allow the student to provide safe care. If the patient asks a question that the student cannot answer, the student should inform the patient that he or she will find out and return with an answer. Patients like their caregivers to be authentic, and it is acceptable to say you are a student and do not know the answer.

Finally, remember that this is the patient's experience, not the student's experience. The patient does not need or want to hear about the student's own labor and birth. The patient should be encouraged to talk about her labor and birth; talking about her birth experience is therapeutic as she intellectually and emotionally processes this important event in her life.

SAFETY *STAT!*

Even if it is your first day in postpartum or labor and delivery, you can still promote patient safety by closely observing possible safety risks whenever you enter a patient's room. For example: Are the side rails up? Is there a spill on the floor? Is the correct IV fluid hanging? Are visitors washing their hands? Is the newborn wrapped warmly and lying in a safe location?

Key Points

- Nurses can improve quality in health care by working within the scope of practice and using standards of care based on scientific study.
- Throughout history, the role of nurses in maternity care has evolved from following only the physicians' orders to becoming a patient advocate and providing the majority of patient care.
- There are many roles and capacities available for nurses in providing maternity care.
- The nursing scope of practice is the legal outline of what a nurse can do according to the laws of the state in which the nurse is licensed.

- Standards of care should be built on evidence-based practice and are guidelines for the correct way to care for a patient.
- Medical ethics provide guidelines for providing ethical care to patients.
- Autonomy, beneficence, nonmaleficence, and justice are principles that guide medical ethics.
- Nursing students can be successful in maternity nursing by being prepared and maintaining a professional demeanor.

REVIEW QUESTIONS

1. The nursing scope of practice is:
   1. Regulated by the nurse's employer
   2. Regulated by state laws
   3. Regulated by physicians
   4. Regulated by professional organizations

2. The ethical term *justice* means that:
   1. Nurses do no harm to a patient.
   2. Nurses follow all the legal requirements of their jobs.
   3. Nurses treat a patient with kindness.
   4. Nurses are fair in utilizing resources for patients.

3. Nurses can contribute to quality health care by: (*select all that apply*)
   1. Following standards of care
   2. Delivering patient-centered care
   3. Using aggressive behaviors to get physicians to listen
   4. Providing equal care to all patients
   5. Refusing to follow evidence-based practice

4. A nursing student was just asked by his patient if she could take a medication from home for her headache. The nursing student is unsure of the answer. What should the nursing student do?
   1. Tell the patient it is alright to take the medication.
   2. Tell the patient to wait and he will find out.
   3. Admit that he does not know.
   4. Act like he did not hear the patient.

5. Which nursing roles have the legal authority to prescribe medication? (*select all that apply*)
   1. LVN/LPN
   2. RN
   3. NP
   4. CNM
   5. CNS

CRITICAL THINKING QUESTION

Write about an ethical dilemma that you have experienced or
have observed in the clinical setting.

For additional resources and information, visit
www.DavisPlus.com.
Post-Conference Questions and Activities,
Answers, and References can be found on
Davis*Plus*.

Human Reproduction and Fetal Development

3

LEARNING OUTCOMES

1. Define the key terms.
2. Identify the structures and functions of the female reproductive system.
3. Identify the structures and functions of the male reproductive system.
4. Summarize the actions of the hormones that affect reproductive functioning.
5. Discuss the female and male reproductive cycles.
6. Describe the fertilization process.
7. Discuss the stages of embryonic development.
8. Describe fetal circulation.
9. Identify significant developmental changes of the fetus at various gestations.
10. Describe the functions of the placenta, umbilical cord, amniotic membranes, and amniotic fluid.
11. Contrast the differences between monozygotic twins and dizygotic twins.
12. Explain the FDA Pregnancy Category system for safe medication use in pregnancy.
13. Discuss possible risks to safe fetal development due to possible teratogens in medications, street drugs, foods, and environment.

REAL-WORLD CASE STUDY

Layla

■ Layla, aged 28, just confirmed with a home pregnancy test that she is 6 weeks pregnant with her first baby. She is employed at a plant and floral nursery in a rural agricultural area. Layla has an active job that provides physical exercise. She is of average weight, eats healthy food, and takes her lunch daily to work. At her first visit to the obstetrician's office, she is curious about fetal development and is concerned about having a healthy pregnancy and baby.

continued on page 22

KEY TERMS

amniotic fluid
amniotic membrane
blastocyst
cervix
chorion
colostrum
corpus luteum
dizygotic twins
ductus arteriosus
ductus venosus
embryo
endometrium
epimetrium
estrogen
follicle-stimulating hormone (FSH)
foramen ovale
human chorionic gonadotropin (hCG)
human placental lactogen
luteinizing hormone (LH)
microencephaly
monozygotic twins
myometrium
placenta
progesterone
relaxin
teratogen
testosterone
umbilical cord
villi
Wharton's jelly

DavisPlus　For audio pronunciation guide, visit www.DavisPlus.com

CHAPTER CONCEPTS

Female Reproduction
Male Reproduction
Pregnancy
Safety

Questions

1. What information can the nurse provide Layla about the development of a 6-week gestation fetus?
2. What information should the nurse provide to promote a safe pregnancy for Layla regarding possible teratogens in her work environment?
3. What dietary advice regarding safe food choices should the nurse give Layla?

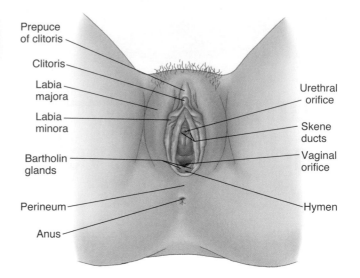

FIGURE 3.1 Female external genitalia.

CONCEPTUAL CORNERSTONE

Reproduction

The concept of reproduction is a foundational concept in the biological sciences. This chapter begins the discussion of this concept of the reproduction of humans. Pregnancy is usually an expected event for couples who engage in consensual sex without contraceptive measures. Unplanned pregnancies occur when couples engage in consensual sex and lack education regarding contraception, do not choose to use contraception, when intercourse is not consensual, or when contraceptives fail. The scope of the concept of reproduction ranges from normal reproductive health to problems associated with reproduction.

The nurse must be familiar with the structures and functions that make childbearing possible. This chapter presents a brief summary of the male and female reproductive cycles, organs, and functions. The process of fertilization, embryonic development, and fetal development are discussed along with possible teratogenic risks to the developing fetus.

FEMALE REPRODUCTIVE SYSTEM

The female reproductive system consists of external organs, internal organs, the female pelvis, breasts, and the female reproductive cycle.

External Organs

The external genital organs in women are the mons pubis, the labia majora and minora, the clitoris, the vestibule of the vagina, and the glands (Fig. 3.1).

- The mons pubis is a pad of fat that lies over the symphysis pubis. After puberty, it is covered with hair. The labia majora are two folds of tissue that extend from the mons pubis to either side of the vulva. They develop during puberty and are covered with hair. After menopause, hormonal decline causes some atrophy of the labia.
- The labia minora are two smaller folds of tissue that form a hood-like structure, called the prepuce, which

surrounds the clitoris. The labia minora have sweat and sebaceous glands to lubricate the surface.
- The clitoris is a small sensitive organ containing erectile tissue. It lies in front of the vulva and below the mons pubis.
- The vestibule of the vagina is the area between the labia minora, and where the urethra and vagina open.
- The Bartholin glands are located on either side of the vagina under the labia majora. Their ducts open to secrete lubricating fluids to moisten the vulva and to facilitate sexual intercourse.
- In addition, the perineum is the skin from the vaginal opening to the anus. It lies over muscles and fibrous tissue that separate the vagina and rectum.

Internal Organs

The internal organs of reproduction are the ovaries, the fallopian tubes, the uterus, and the vagina (Fig. 3.2). The ovaries are two small glands located on either side of the uterus slightly behind and below the Fallopian tubes. The ovaries are attached to the broad ligament, a suspensory ligament, and the ends of the fallopian tubes. The ovaries are about the size and shape of almonds. The pair of ovaries store approximately one-half million eggs. The ovaries also secrete the hormones estrogen and progesterone during each reproductive cycle.

The fallopian tubes are attached to the uterus at one end, and at the opposite end they curve over the ovaries with fringe-like ends. The function of the fallopian tubes is to provide a channel for the sperm to travel and to transport the egg into the uterus.

The uterus is a muscular triangle-shaped organ located between the rectum and bladder. The function of the uterus is to provide the environment for the growth of a fetus (Fig. 3.3).

The top portion of the uterus is called the *fundus*. The lower portion of the uterus that projects into the vagina is called the **cervix**. It provides a protective entrance to the uterus. This portion of the cervix is surrounded and supported

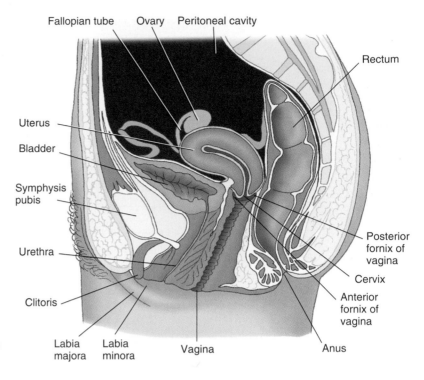

FIGURE 3.2 Internal female genitalia and cross section of the rectum.

by the uterosacral ligaments, the transverse ligaments, and the pubocervical ligaments. The cervix is very elastic and has the ability to stretch to allow for childbirth. The elasticity is due to the high fibrous and collagenous content of the supportive tissue and the large number of folds in the cervical lining. The cervical canal contains mucus-secreting glands. The functions of the cervical mucus are to:

- Act as a bacteriostatic agent
- Lubricate the vaginal canal
- Provide an alkaline environment to protect sperm from the acidic vaginal secretions

The uterus has two coats: a muscular coat with longitudinal and circular fibers and an inner lining mucous membrane which is in folds also known as rugae. The uterus has three layers:

- The **endometrium** is a mucous membrane that lines the cavity of the uterus. It is the site where the embryo implants after arriving in the uterus.
- The **myometrium** is the middle layer of smooth muscle. The function of this layer is to contract and expel the fetus during childbirth.
- The **epimetrium** is a serous membrane that lines most of the external surface.

The uterus is supported by several suspensory ligaments. These ligaments provide support and stabilize the reproductive organs:

- The broad ligament keeps the uterus centrally placed and provides stability. It is located on each side of the uterus and attaches to the pelvic sidewall (Fig. 3.3).
- The round ligaments are situated between the broad ligaments anterior and inferior to the fallopian tubes.

- The cardinal ligaments arise superiorly and laterally from the uterus and inferiorly from the vagina to provide the primary support for the uterus.
- The uterosacral ligaments attach the uterus to the sacrum.

The vagina is a 4- to 6-inch elastic muscular tube that extends from the cervix to the external vaginal introitus. Vaginal tissue is composed of smooth muscle, elastic connective tissue, and is lined with stratified squamous epithelium, which is similar to skin. It lies behind the bladder and urethra and in front of the rectum. The vagina begins at the vulva and ends at the cervix. Its two main functions are for sexual intercourse and childbirth.

Female Pelvis

The bones of the female pelvis are formed posteriorly by the sacrum and coccyx, and on the sides and front by the hip bones. The hip bones consist of three sections: the ilium, the ischium, and the pubis. The female pelvis is shorter, wider, and more circular than the male pelvis, which makes the female pelvis the right shape for childbearing. The ischial spines are the narrowest diameter the fetus must pass through during childbirth (Fig. 3.4).

Breasts

The breasts are two glands that secrete milk. In the center of the surface is the nipple, which projects outward beyond the skin level. The nipple is pink until pregnancy and then it becomes darker. Inside the breasts are ducts that lead to the nipple. The tissue of the gland is similar to a sebaceous gland but is more highly developed to produce milk instead of sebum. The gland is divided into lobes by fibrous tissue. The lobes are subdivided into lobules. The breasts develop during puberty and further development occurs during pregnancy

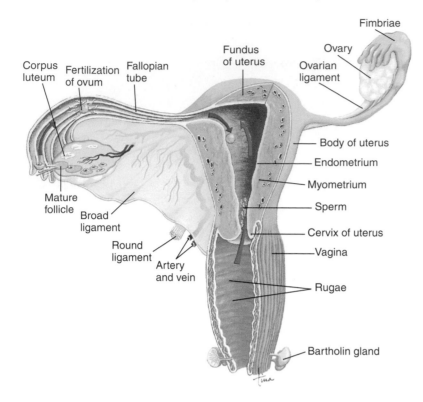

FIGURE 3.3 Female reproductive system shown in anterior view. The left ovary has been sectioned to show the developing follicles. The left fallopian tube has been sectioned to show fertilization. The uterus and vagina have been sectioned to show internal structures. Arrows indicate the movement of the ovum toward the uterus and the movement of sperm from the vagina toward the fallopian tube.

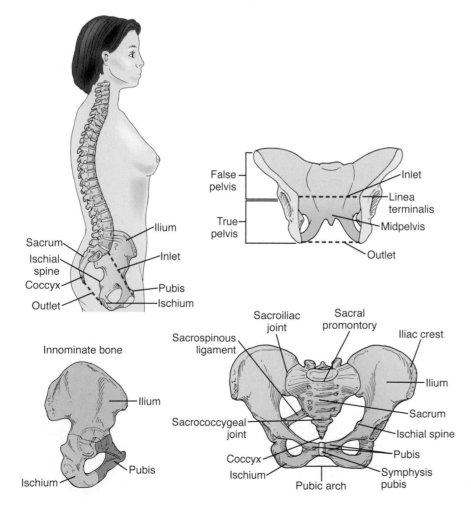

FIGURE 3.4 Female bony pelvis.

due to the effects of hormones from the pituitary and ovaries. **Colostrum**, a fluid rich with antibodies, may be secreted in small amounts during pregnancy and prior to milk production. Milk production begins 2 to 3 days after childbirth (Fig. 3.5).

Female Reproductive Cycle

The menstrual cycle begins at the first day of menstrual bleeding and ends on the first day that menstrual bleeding begins again (Fig. 3.6). The follicle-stimulating hormone, luteinizing hormone, estrogen, and progesterone are involved in the female reproductive cycle.

Follicular Phase

During the follicular phase, the anterior lobe of the pituitary secretes **follicle-stimulating hormone (FSH)**. This hormone stimulates the development of a follicle in the ovary. The follicle consists of cells that surround an egg in one of the ovaries. As the egg follicle matures, it begins to secrete estrogen, which causes the endometrium in the uterus to begin thickening and preparing for the fertilized egg to implant. When the level of estrogen increases, it prevents FSH from further secretion. The pituitary gland responds to the decrease in FSH and begins to release luteinizing hormone (LH).

Luteal Phase

The luteal phase begins on the day the egg is released. The increased levels of **luteinizing hormone** (LH) gradually peak approximately day 14 of the cycle, causing ovulation or the release of the egg from the follicle. After the follicle on the ovary releases an egg, LH converts the ruptured follicle into the **corpus luteum**, which secretes the hormone progesterone. **Progesterone** completes the development of the uterine lining in preparation for a fertilized egg. If the egg is not fertilized, the corpus luteum begins to degenerate, causing the levels of progesterone and estrogen to decrease, which leads to the shedding of the uterine lining. The menstrual cycle then begins again. If fertilization and implantation

occur, the endometrium does not degenerate. When implantation occurs, the woman is pregnant (Fig. 3.6).

HEALTH PROMOTION
Preconception Health
Women should prepare for pregnancy before actually becoming pregnant. The most important things a woman can do for preconception health are:
- Stop smoking and drinking alcohol.
- Take 400 to 800 mcg of folic acid to lower the risk of defects of the brain and spine.
- Obtain an optimal weight.
- If the woman has a medical condition, such as diabetes, epilepsy, or asthma, she should make an appointment to discuss her pregnancy with her health-care provider.
- Avoid contact with toxic substances at home or work.
- Discuss over-the-counter and prescription medications with her health-care provider.
- Make sure vaccinations are up to date.

MALE REPRODUCTIVE SYSTEM

The male reproductive system consists of the scrotum, penis, and testicles in which the sperm are produced.

External Organs

The external male reproductive organs are the scrotum and the penis. The scrotum is made of two sacs separated by a septum. Within each sac are a testicle, the epididymis, and the beginning of a spermatic cord.

The penis contains cavernous tissue. This tissue has spaces that fill with blood, causing the penis to become erect. The arteries that supply blood to this region become dilated and filled with blood, which produces an erection. Semen is expelled, or ejaculated, through the end of the penis when a male reaches sexual climax (Fig. 3.7).

Internal Organs

The testicles are located in the scrotum. They are the reproductive glands of the male. They are suspended in the scrotum by the spermatic cords. Each testicle consists of 200 to 300 lobules. Each lobule contains tiny tubules called the *convoluted seminiferous tubules*. The lining of the tubular walls contains cells that develop into spermatozoa. The tubules are supported by loose connective tissue. This connective tissue contains groups of interstitial cells, which secrete the hormone testosterone. **Testosterone** promotes the development of male reproductive organs and the secondary male characteristics, such as hair growth and the deeper voice that occurs during puberty.

The epididymis is a tightly coiled tube attached to the back of the testis. The seminiferous tubules of the testis open into the epididymis. The epididymis transports sperm and brings the sperm to maturity, as they are immature when they leave

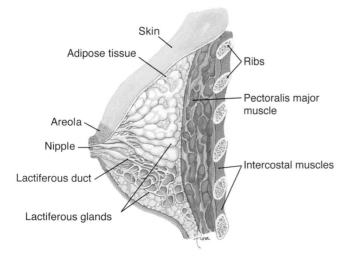

FIGURE 3.5 Mammary gland shown in a midsagittal section.

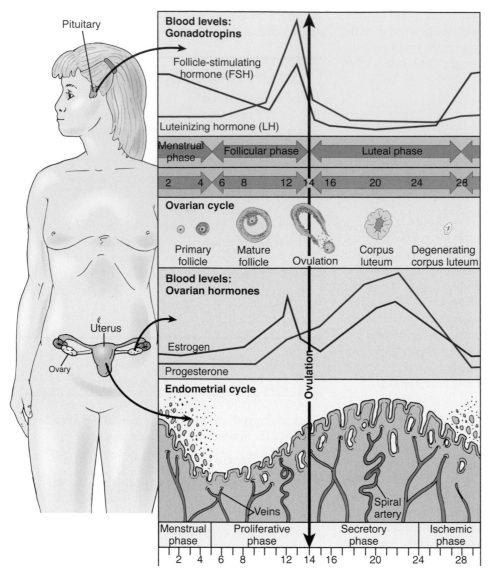

FIGURE 3.6 The female reproductive cycle. Levels of the hormones secreted from the anterior pituitary are shown relative to one another and throughout the cycle. Changes in the ovarian follicle are depicted. The relative thickness of the endometrium is also shown.

the testis. The sperm gain motility in the epididymis and have the ability to move after 18 to 24 hours. The epididymis leads to the deferent duct. During sexual arousal, contractions force the mature sperm into the vas deferens. The sperm are stored there until ejaculation. This duct is a continuation of the duct of the epididymis; it passes through the inguinal canal and runs between the base of the bladder and the rectum to the prostate gland. At the prostate gland, it is joined by the duct of the seminal vesicle. The prostate gland is located below the bladder and in front of the rectum. The urethra runs through the center of the prostate gland. The prostate gland provides additional fluid to support the sperm.

The seminal vesicles are two pouch-like sacs that attach to the vas deferens near the bladder. The vas deferens transports mature sperm to the urethra. The seminal vesicles create a sugar-rich fluid that provides energy to the sperm. The fluid from the seminal vesicles composes most of the volume of the ejaculate. Ejaculatory ducts are formed by the fusion of the vas deferens and the seminal vesicles. The ejaculatory ducts empty into the urethra.

The urethra is the tube that carries urine out of the body. It also has the function of carrying sperm when the male reaches climax. When the penis is erect, the flow of urine is blocked from the bladder and only semen is ejaculated.

The Male Reproductive Cycle

Hormones are responsible for the correct functioning of the male reproductive system. The FSH and LH are responsible for regulating the production of sperm. Both hormones are released from the anterior pituitary gland. FSH stimulates sperm production in the testes and LH stimulates the production of testosterone. Testosterone influences immature spermatozoa to develop and become mature sperm cells. It takes 72 days for immature sperm to become mature sperm.

SAFETY *STAT!*

For couples planning a pregnancy, the male should be aware that fever, exposure to excessive heat, such as hot tubs

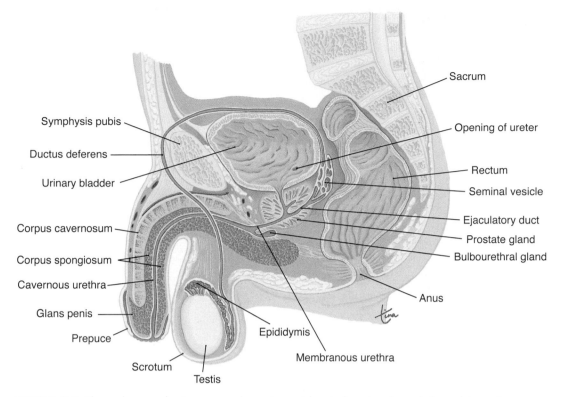

FIGURE 3.7 The male reproductive system shown in a midsagittal section through the pelvic cavity.

and saunas, cigarette smoking, and heavy alcohol use may reduce semen production (Mayo Clinic, 2012).

FERTILIZATION

For fertilization to occur without medical assistance, sexual intercourse must take place. For the male, sexual excitement leads to erection of the penis. Erection is caused by increased blood flow to the penis, which causes it to increase in length and girth. After erection, it is possible for the male to insert the penis into the vagina and ejaculate seminal fluid.

The female sexual response includes erection of the clitoris, enlargement of the breasts, and erection of the nipples. Before and during intercourse, the walls of the vagina release fluid to lubricate during intercourse. Sexual climax may occur before or during intercourse.

The male sperm and the female egg, called *gametes*, meet in the fallopian tubes, where fertilization occurs. Of 14 million deposited into the vagina, only 1 to 10 sperm reach the fallopian tube. One sperm will penetrate the outer layer of the ovum, and then fertilization occurs. Each gamete brings one set of 23 single chromosomes, and when fused, the total of 46 chromosomes produces a cell, the zygote (Fig. 3.8).

The sex of the embryo is determined at fertilization. The female brings two sex chromosomes, XX, and the male contributes two sex chromosomes, XY. At the moment of fertilization, if the zygote has an X chromosome from the mother and an X chromosome from the father, it will be a girl (XX); if the zygote has an X chromosome from the mother and a Y chromosome from the father, it will be a boy (XY).

If fertilization occurs, the lining of the uterus does not begin to degenerate and provides a place for the zygote to implant. Estrogen and progesterone levels remain high. An additional hormone, **human chorionic gonadotropin (**hCG**),** is produced to support the development of the embryo. This hormone is produced by the fertilized egg. It is made by the cells that will form the placenta. Elevated levels of hCG can be first detected by a blood test about 11 days after conception and in urine tests about 12 to 14 days after conception.

LABS & DIAGNOSTICS

Women who want to become pregnant can monitor their hormone levels at home with an over-the-counter ovulation test. The test detects the changes in estrogen and in the LH that triggers ovulation. The home test indicates the peak fertility days in a woman's menstrual cycle.

The zygote begins to divide immediately by mitosis. Mitosis is the process by which cells divide. During mitosis, the cell replicates each of the chromosomes, and then separates the chromosomes in the cell nucleus into two identical sets of chromosomes, each with a new nucleus that produces two complete cells. Then the zygote continues to grow, from two cells to four cells to eight cells to 16 cells and to 32 cells to produce an **embryo**. An embryo is the stage of development between the fertilized ovum and the fetus. At the 32-cell

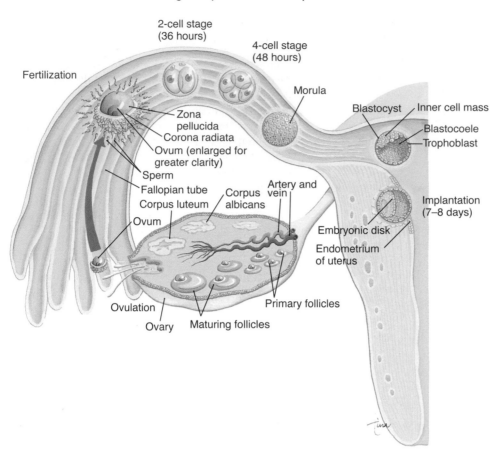

FIGURE 3.8 Ovulation, fertilization, and early embryonic development.

stage, the embryo has progressed to a morula, from which a blastocyst develops. A **blastocyst** is a maturing embryo in which some cell differentiation has occurred. In the blastocyst stage, the embryo will implant 7-10 days after fertilization into the thickened, vascular uterine endometrium.

The placenta develops at the site of implantation. The placenta is an organ that provides the fetus with oxygen and nourishment from the maternal blood during intrauterine life, the gestation period.

STAGES OF FETAL DEVELOPMENT

The embryo changes from a hollow ball of cells through two processes: morphogenesis and cell differentiation. During morphogenesis, the cells are moving and maturing to complete a human form. Cell differentiation means that the cells specialize into different kinds of cells needed to build a human body, such as nerve cells, muscle cells, skin cells, etc. The circulatory system for the fetus develops differently than normal human circulation because of the unique way that blood circulates in the placenta and fetal unit during pregnancy.

Fetal Circulation

During fetal development, the fetal circulation is different from after birth. While in the uterus, the fetus does not need as much blood to circulate through the liver or lungs; the placenta provides oxygenation and filtration that the lungs and liver perform after the birth.

Fetal circulation begins when oxygenated blood from the placenta enters the fetus through the umbilical vein. The oxygenated blood bypasses the liver through the **ductus venosus** and combines with deoxygenated blood in the inferior vena cava. Blood then rejoins deoxygenated blood from the superior vena cava and empties into the right atrium. Pressure is greater in the right atrium than the left atrium, so most blood will move through the **foramen ovale.** A small amount of blood does travel from the right atrium to the right ventricle into the pulmonary system but most bypasses the pulmonary arteries and moves directly into the aorta through the **ductus arteriosus** and out to the rest of the body. Deoxygenated blood returns to the placenta through the umbilical arteries (Fig. 3.9).

 LEARN TO C.U.S.

A nurse is working in the emergency department and providing care to Anna, a 16-year-old patient. Anna is being treated for a urinary tract infection. The physician has ordered ciprofloxacin 250 mg bid. As the nurse prepares to administer the first dose of the medication, the patient confides

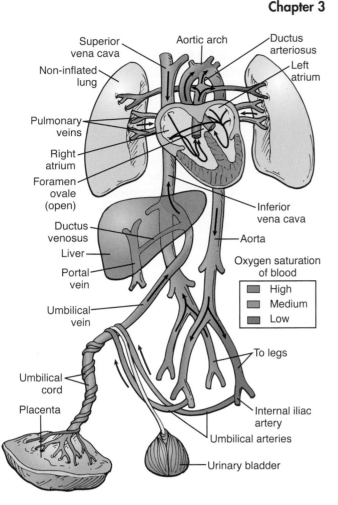

FIGURE 3.9 Fetal circulation.

three layers are the foundation for the tissues and organs of the body (Figs. 3.10 and 3.11).

- ***Ectoderm:*** The cells of the ectoderm, or outer layer, become the nervous system, the epidermis of the skin, tooth enamel, and the lens and cornea of the eye.
- ***Mesoderm:*** The middle layer, the mesoderm, becomes the connective tissue, skeleton, skeletal muscles, the circulatory system, and the dermis of the skin.
- ***Endoderm:*** The inner layer, the endoderm, becomes the digestive tract and accessory organs, the respiratory tract, kidney nephrons, the bladder, and endocrine glands.

Table 3.1 notes significant events that occur during the development of the embryo through the third month.

Second Trimester

During the second trimester, the organs and structures continue to develop as a woman becomes more aware of her growing fetus. Table 3.2 notes significant events that occur during the development of the embryo in months 4 through 6.

Third Trimester

The third trimester is a time for the fetus to gain weight, mature, and prepare for life outside the uterus. Table 3.3 notes significant events that occur during the development of the embryo in months 7 through 9.

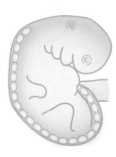

FIGURE 3.10 Embryo at 4 weeks' gestation (28 postovulatory days). All four limb buds are present. *Source:* Smith, 2013. *The multidimensional human embryo, Carnegie Stages.* Retrieved from http://embryo.soad.umich.edu/carnStages/carnStages.html.

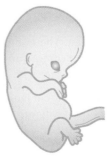

FIGURE 3.11 The embryo at 8 weeks (56 to 57 postovulatory days) has a human appearance. *Source:* Smith, 2013. *The multidimensional human embryo, Carnegie Stages.* Retrieved from http://embryo.soad.umich.edu/carnStages/carnStages.html.

that she may be pregnant. Her menstrual period is ~2 weeks late. The nurse calls the physician and uses the C.U.S. communication strategy.

C: "Hello, doctor. I am **concerned** about administering this medication to Anna."

U: I am **uncomfortable** about it because she has confided that she may be pregnant.

S: Ciprofloxacin is a Category C medication for pregnancy. This is a **safety** issue for the fetus. Can I have an order for a pregnancy test before administering the medication?"

Significant events that occur during fetal development are noted below by trimester.

First Trimester

Even before a woman is aware that she is pregnant, the first trimester is a critical time of rapid changes to the fertilized cell and the development of major organs and structures. Morphogenesis and cell differentiation establish three germ layers in the embryo within 2 weeks after fertilization. The

TABLE 3.1 FETAL GROWTH AND DEVELOPMENT IN THE FIRST TRIMESTER

Gestational Age	Developmental Milestones
Week 3	• 2-mm length, crown to rump (C-R) • A membrane called the *amnion* that is filled with fluid surrounds the embryo. • The placenta begins to develop.
Week 4	• 4- to 6-mm length C-R, 0.4-g weight • The heart beats and is pumping blood. • The limb buds are formed. • The placenta is developed and working.
Week 6	• 12-mm length C-R, 0.8-g weight • The limb buds develop digits. • A skeleton of cartilage forms. • The liver is functioning.
Week 8	• 2.5- to 3-cm length C-R, 2-g weight • All internal organs are produced. • Heart development is complete. • The embryo has a humanlike appearance.
Week 10	• 5- to 6-cm length C-R, 14-g weight • Fingers and toes begin nail growth. • The eyelids are fused. • Fingerprints are apparent in the skin.
Month 3	• 8-cm length C-R, 45-g weight • Large head • Two distinct eyes • The sex can be determined by examining the external organs. • Bone tissue is replacing cartilage.

TABLE 3.2 FETAL GROWTH AND DEVELOPMENT IN THE SECOND TRIMESTER

Gestational Age	Developmental Milestones
Month 4	• 13.5-mm length crown to heel (C-H), 200-g weight • The skeleton is established. • The appearance of scalp hair and lanugo begins. • The skeletal muscles contract and produce body movement.
Month 5	• 19-cm length C-H, 435-g weight • The internal organs continue to develop. • The fetus reacts to loud noises. • Brown fat and vernix begin to form. • The fetus actively sucks and swallows amniotic fluid.
Month 6	• 23-cm length C-H, 780-g weight • Fused eyelids begin to open. • Hand grip and startle reflex have developed. • Respiratory movements occur. • Alveoli appear in lungs.

CULTURAL CONSIDERATIONS

Cultural beliefs influence how a woman and her family may respond to pregnancy. There are many variations in the ways that culture influences a pregnant woman. The nurse should recognize that each woman is different regardless of her ethnic background. She may be acculturated to the United States or may follow the traditional beliefs of her culture. Culturally competent care is basically patient-centered care. The nurse should ask the right questions to obtain the patient's point-of-view of pregnancy and to open discussion regarding her fears or cultural taboos of pregnancy.

There are common taboos in pregnancy that are culturally based. A common taboo is that if the pregnant woman reaches her arms over her head, it will cause the umbilical cord to wrap around the fetal neck. This belief is common among African Americans, Anglo Americans, Asians, and Hispanics. Another pregnancy taboo common in the Mexican culture is to avoid lunar eclipses. The belief is that an eclipse could cause a congenial deformity (Galanti, 2015).

Understanding the pregnant woman's fears in pregnancy leads the nurse to include education and reassurance in the nursing care plan.

TABLE 3.3 FETAL GROWTH AND DEVELOPMENT IN THE THIRD TRIMESTER

Gestational Age	Developmental Milestones
Month 7	• 27-cm length C-H, 1200-g weight • Internal organs are maturing. • Body fat increases. • The fetus uses the senses of vision and hearing. • Hiccups may occur.
Month 8	• 31- to 35-cm length C-H, 2,000- to 2,700-g weight • Active periods are more noticeable by the mother. • A few sole creases form on the bottom of the feet. • Earlobes are soft, with little cartilage. • A layer of fat begins to be stored for insulation and nourishment.
Month 9	• 48- to 52-cm length C-H, 3,200+g weight • The fetus matures and becomes prepared for birth. • The fetus has smooth, pink skin with vernix present in skin folds. • Lanugo is present on the fetus' shoulders and upper back. • The fetus' earlobes are firmer due to increased cartilage.

Source: Sadler, 2012; Moore, 2013

PATIENT TEACHING GUIDELINES

Reducing the Risks of Birth Defects
• Avoid all medications, even over-the-counter medications, unless directed by your health-care provider.
• Avoid alcohol, tobacco products, and street drugs.
• Notify any dentist or health-care provider that you are pregnant.
• Eat a variety of healthy foods from all food groups.
• Follow safe food-handling practices.
• Avoid exposure to environmental substances that can have a harmful effect on the fetus.

ACCESSORY STRUCTURES OF PREGNANCY

The accessory structures of pregnancy include the placenta, the umbilical cord, placental membranes, and amniotic fluid.

Placenta

The **placenta** provides the fetus with oxygen and nourishment. It begins to grow when cells from the fetus, called *trophoblasts*, attach to the uterus wall and then grow into the tissues of the uterus. The cells grow deep into the uterine wall and connect indirectly with the mother's blood vessels. At the same time, the fetal circulatory system is developing as

NURSING CARE PLAN for the Pregnant Patient

Nursing Diagnosis: Deficient knowledge related to fetal development.
Interventions:
• Provide a month-by-month guide to fetal development.
• Provide a Web site to explore fetal development photographs.

Nursing Diagnosis: Deficient knowledge related to environmental teratogens.
Interventions:
• Discuss potential teratogens and provide written material to review at home.
• Provide a Web site that includes information pertaining to teratogens.

Nursing Diagnosis: Anxiety related to concerns about possible birth defects.
Interventions:
• Encourage a healthy lifestyle with avoidance of possible teratogens.
• Allow the pregnant woman to verbalize her fears and provide appropriate reassurance.

the fetal blood vessels form in the placental villi. These vessels connect back to the fetus through the umbilical cord. The umbilical cord attaches the fetus to the placenta. As the placenta continues to grow, villi are formed. **Villi** are finger-like projections that are surrounded by the mother's blood. The mother's blood enters the space around the villi in the placenta through arteries that form out of the uterine arteries. Blood flows around the villi and transfers to the fetal blood supply occur. Gas, nutrient exchange, antibodies, and waste removal take place across the villi walls. The walls also keep the fetus' blood from mixing with the mother's blood. The placenta provides for all fetal oxygenation and nutritional needs while in the uterus (Fig. 3.12). The mature placenta is 15 to 18 cm and weighs approximately 1 pound (Venes, 2013).

The placenta also functions as an endocrine organ because it produces hormones that support the pregnancy. The hormones produced are:

• **Progesterone**
  • Supports the endometrium to support the developing embryo.
  • Calms and quiets the uterine muscle to allow for successful implantation.
• **Estrogen**
  • Stimulates growth of the myometrium and improves blood flow to the placenta and fetus.
  • Stimulates breast development to prepare for breastfeeding.
• **Human Chorionic Gonadotropin**
  • Stimulates the corpus luteum to produce estrogen and progesterone during the first 10 weeks after conception.
  • The hormone tested to determine pregnancy either by urine or blood test.

• **Human Placental Lactogen**
  • Assists with milk preparation.
  • Increases the mother's metabolism during pregnancy.
• **Relaxin**
  • Works with progesterone to maintain the pregnancy.
  • Causes relaxation of pelvic ligaments to aid in birthing (acts as a source for hormone information).

After the safe delivery of the baby, the placenta is delivered. Often, the placenta is referred to as the *afterbirth*. The umbilical cord is clamped and cut, and the site of the attachment on the baby is commonly known as the *umbilicus*, *navel*, or *belly-button*.

Umbilical Cord

The **umbilical cord** is formed by the fifth week of gestation. It joins the fetus to the placenta. The umbilical cord is composed of two arteries and one vein. The vein carries oxygenated blood to the fetus and the two arteries carry blood away from the placenta. The vessels are surrounded by Wharton's jelly. **Wharton's jelly** is a gelatinous substance that provides support and protection for the vessels inside the cord. The umbilical cord at full-term is about 20 inches long and 0.75 inches in diameter.

Membranes and Amniotic Fluid

The chorionic membrane supports the embryo as it grows. The **chorion** is a thick membrane that develops from the trophoblast and becomes part of the placenta villi. The chorionic villi can be used for genetic testing at 8 to 11 weeks gestation. After 12 weeks, the chorion degenerates except for the portion that has become part of the placenta villi.

The **amniotic membrane** is a thin membrane formed from the ectoderm layer. It contains the **amniotic fluid**, also

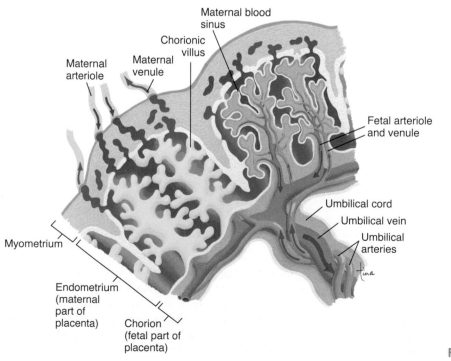

FIGURE 3.12 Placenta and umbilical cord.

known as the *bag of waters* (BOW) and the growing fetus. The functions of the amniotic fluid are:

- Cushions the fetus.
- Provides buoyancy, which allows movement, symmetrical growth, and muscle development.
- Prevents the amniotic membrane from adhering to the fetus.
- Prevents compression of the umbilical cord.
- Protects the fetus from bacteria from the vagina.
- Provides fluid for the analysis of fetal health and maturity.

The average volume of amniotic fluid is 700 to 800 mL. Variations in the amount of fluid can indicate potential health problems of the fetus.

MULTIPLE PREGNANCY

A **multiple pregnancy** means that a woman has two or more embryos in her uterus. These embryos can come from the same egg or different eggs. Babies born from the same egg are termed *identical* and babies born from two or more eggs are termed *fraternal*.

In the case of twins, **monozygotic twins** form when a single fertilized egg splits. The split occurs most often in the blastocyst stage and each embryo will have its own amniotic sac but will share a placenta. They both implant in the uterus and develop as two babies. They are always the same sex.

When two eggs are fertilized by two separate sperm, it is termed *dizygotic* twins. Each zygote develops separately and implants into the uterus. Each embryo will have its own amniotic sac and placenta. There will be genetic similarities because they are siblings but they will not have the exact same genetic origin (Fig. 3.13).

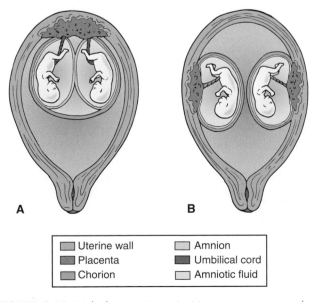

Uterine wall	Amnion
Placenta	Umbilical cord
Chorion	Amniotic fluid

FIGURE 3.13 Multiple gestations. A, Monozygotic twins with one placenta, one chorion, and two amnions. B, Dizygotic twins with two placentas, two chorions, and two amnions.

A woman is more likely to have a multiple pregnancy if she:

- Is older than age 35.
- Is of African-American descent.
- Has a family history of twins.
- Has undergone fertility treatment to become pregnant.
- Has given birth to multiples previously.

EFFECTS OF TERATOGENS ON FETAL DEVELOPMENT

Many medications and substances can be a risk for the developing fetus, so the safest approach to medications in pregnancy is to use as little as possible. A **teratogen** is any substance that may cause a birth defect. Most substances have the ability to cross the placenta from the mother and the fetus and possibly cause abnormalities. The fetal susceptibility depends on the period of development. For example, the brain and skeleton are at risk for damage by teratogens from the third week of gestation to the end of the pregnancy. The heart is most susceptible to injury during the third and fourth weeks of gestation. The genitalia are more sensitive to injury during the eighth and ninth weeks (Draper, 2011).

SAFETY *STAT!*

The fetus is very vulnerable to the effects of medications during the first trimester. Before administering any medication to a woman of childbearing age, the nurse should verify that the date of her last menstrual period is in the woman's health record.

DRUG FACTS

If a woman is currently taking medication for depression, asthma, diabetes, seizures, HIV, or other health problems, she should talk to her health-care provider. Abruptly stopping medications may be more harmful for her than her fetus. She needs to discuss the benefits and risks of the medications during pregnancy with her health-care provider.

Medications

The Federal Drug Administration provides a Pregnancy Category System for medication use in pregnancy (FDA, 2013).

- *Category A medications.* In adequate, well-controlled studies in pregnant woman, these medications have not shown an increased risk of fetal abnormalities.
- *Category B medications.* In animal studies, these medications have revealed no evidence of harm to the fetus; however, there are no adequate and well-controlled studies in pregnant woman. In some animal studies, Category B medications have shown an adverse effect, but adequate and well-controlled studies in pregnant women have failed to demonstrate a risk to the fetus.

• *Category C medications.* In animal studies, these medications have shown an adverse effect and there are no adequate and well-controlled studies in pregnant women.
• *Category D medications.* In adequate, well-controlled studies and in observation in pregnant women, these medications have demonstrated a risk to the fetus. However, the benefits of therapy may outweigh the risks.
• *Category X medications.* In adequate, well-controlled studies and by observation in animals or pregnant women, these medications have demonstrated positive evidence of fetal abnormalities. The use of Category X medications is contraindicated in women who are or may become pregnant.

SAFETY *STAT!*

A pregnant woman should be cautioned that over-the-counter medications may not be safe in pregnancy. She should always check with her health-care provider before taking any medications, even over-the-counter.

Tobacco

Smoking is one of the most important modifiable causes of poor pregnancy outcomes (ACOG, 2012). Smoking causes vasoconstriction, which leads to a smaller placenta. A smaller placenta decreases the nourishment and oxygenation that the fetus receives. This can lead to a small baby with delayed development. The adverse effects of smoking in pregnancy and excessive exposure to secondhand smoke are:

• Low birth weight.
• Premature rupture of membranes.
• Placenta previa.
• Placenta abruption.
• Preterm labor.
• Ectopic pregnancy.

The American College of Obstetricians and Gynecologists (ACOG, 2011) suggest that the nurse use the Five As Model to address smoking in pregnancy:

1. Ask about tobacco use.
2. Advise her to quit.
3. Assess willingness to make an attempt to quit.
4. Assist in a quit attempt.
5. Arrange for follow-up.

Smoking interventions may provide a tool to assist the pregnant woman to stop smoking and promote a healthy pregnancy and fetus.

SAFETY *STAT!*

A pregnant woman who does not smoke but breathes secondhand smoke is more likely to have lower birth-weight babies than women that are not exposed to secondhand smoke. After birth, babies that are around secondhand smoke have more ear infections, asthma, respiratory infections, and more likely to die from Sudden Infant Death Syndrome (U.S. Department of Health and Human Services, 2014).

Alcohol

The American Academy of Obstetrician and Gynecologist's policy is that the pregnant woman should avoid alcohol throughout the pregnancy to prevent lifelong problems for the child. Children born with the most serious problems caused by alcohol consumption during pregnancy have a syndrome called *fetal alcohol syndrome* (FAD). The child may exhibit the following symptoms:

• Small for gestational age at birth.
• Vision and hearing problems.
• Facial abnormalities, such as a small head, flat face, and narrow eye openings.
• Trouble with concentration and learning in school.
• Trouble controlling behavior.

Caffeine

High usage of caffeine has been linked with miscarriage and preterm birth. The American College of Obstetricians and Gynecologists Committee Opinion (2010) states that light and moderate use of caffeine (less than 200 mg per day) are not likely to cause miscarriage or preterm birth.

Marijuana

Marijuana usage affects the trophoblast cells as they are implanting into the uterine wall, which affects placental development and implantation (Chen et al., 2011) Research has shown that intrauterine exposure to tetrahydrocannabinol (THC), the chemical responsible for most of marijuana's psychological effects, can affect the neurological development of the newborn.

Cocaine

Cocaine use during pregnancy has been studied for many years with the conclusions that use during pregnancy leads to growth retardation and microencephaly. **Microencephaly** is the term for a small brain and head. Depending upon usage during the gestational week, the genitals, kidneys, and brain may have abnormalities. Cocaine use during pregnancy has been associated with:

• An increased number of placenta abruptions.
• Neurobehavioral abnormalities that are exhibited after birth (Hudak and Tan, 2012).

Heroin

Heroin in pregnancy and its associated lack of prenatal care have been associated with adverse outcomes in pregnancy. It crosses the placenta and often leads to neonatal addiction. Other effects include:

- Increased risk of premature birth
- Low birth weight
- Hypoglycemia
- Intracranial hemorrhage in the uterus

Methamphetamines

According to the National Institute of Drug Abuse (2011), less than 1% of pregnant women used methamphetamines in the past year. Any use during pregnancy is of concern. Research is limited, but methamphetamine use in pregnancy has been associated with:

- Elevation in the heart rate of the mother and fetus.
- Increased risk of preterm labor.
- Increased risk of placental abruption (American Pregnancy Organization, 2013).

THERAPEUTIC COMMUNICATION

Nurses play an important role in providing support and education during pregnancy. Authenticity and truthfulness are essential for developing a therapeutic relationship with a pregnant woman and her partner. Nurses need to be open and honest with women and their partners as they discuss sensitive lifestyle issues, such as tobacco, drugs, and alcohol use that could cause birth defects. Techniques that encourage communication include the use of non-judgmental open-ended questions, conveying acceptance, and focusing on patient concerns.

Environmental Toxins

Exposure to substances in the home or outdoor environment can have harmful effects on pregnancy. The pregnant woman will want to be aware of the following potential hazards:

- To prevent exposure to chemicals, cleaning products, or heavy metals, follow safety guidelines at work.
- Avoid exposure to lead. It is toxic to the brain and nervous system of the fetus. Lead is found in toys, costume jewelry, pottery, and some folk remedies.
- Avoid exposure to mercury by avoiding fish that contain mercury. Mercury affects brain development in the fetus.

Fish that contain mercury are marline sea bass, orange roughy, swordfish, and tuna.

- Avoid foods that may harbor listeria. It is a type of bacteria found in water and soil. It has been found in uncooked meats, uncooked vegetables, unpasteurized milk, and food made from unpasteurized milk. Deli meats have the potential to be contaminated after cooking and before packaging.
- Avoid exposure to paint. It is a mix of chemicals that can lead to birth defects and developmental disabilities.
- Avoid exposure to pesticides used to control weeds, insects, and cockroaches (March of Dimes, 2011).
- To reduce the risk of potential problems for the developing fetus, the pregnant woman should look for BPA-free plastic products. According to the *National Report on Human Exposure to Environmental Chemicals* by the Centers for Disease Control and Prevention, the BPA in plastic bottles was shown to have hormone-like effects on the developing reproductive system and neurobehavioral changes in the offspring in animal testing.
- Avoid hot tubs and saunas. Maternal hyperthermia has been linked to possible central nervous system defects (Moore, 2013).
- Avoid contamination with toxoplasma. It is acquired three ways: food contamination, pet-to-human through feces, and mother-to-fetus. Pregnant woman should avoid eating undercooked pork, lamb, and venison, and should avoid emptying the cat litter box. Toxoplasmosis is a serious illness that can be transmitted from the mother through the placenta to the fetus. It can cause blindness and central nervous system problems for the fetus.
- Avoid travel to countries with active Zika virus transmission. Zika virus has been linked to fetal anomalies.

TEAM WORKS

Some women become pregnant during times of living an unhealthy lifestyle, such as alcohol or drug addiction. Women who have these problems and want to deliver a healthy baby will require a team approach to assist them with living drug and alcohol free during the pregnancy. The team approach to assisting these women includes nurses, obstetricians, mental health workers, social workers, self-help groups such as Alcoholics Anonymous (AA) and Narcotics Anonymous (NA), and the patient's family or significant other.

Key Points

- The female external reproductive organs include the mons pubis, the labia minora, the labia majora, the clitoris, the vestibule of the vagina, and the glands.
- The female internal organs of reproduction are the ovaries, the fallopian tubes, the uterus, and the vagina.
- The female pelvis is shorter, wider, and more circular than a male pelvis, which makes it the right shape for childbearing.
- The menstrual cycle, which occurs due to the influence of the hormones estrogen and progesterone, prepares the uterus for a fertilized egg to implant. If fertilization does not occur, menses begin.
- The male reproductive system is composed of the scrotum, penis, and testicles.
- Testosterone promotes the development of male reproductive organs and secondary male characteristics.

- Fertilization takes place in the outer third portion of the fallopian tube leading to the formation of a zygote that begins dividing and travelling down the fallopian tube to implant in the uterus.
- There are three embryonic layers of cells that differentiate. The ectoderm layer becomes the central nervous system, skin, and glands. The mesoderm layer becomes the skeletal, urinary, reproductive, and circulatory systems. The endoderm layer develops into the respiratory system, liver, digestive system, and pancreas.
- The placenta provides oxygenation and nutrition and removes waste products for the fetus. It also produces hormones: progesterone, estrogen, human chorionic gonadotropin, human placental lactogen, and relaxin, all of which support the pregnancy.
- The amniotic fluid surrounds the fetus to provide buoyancy, protection, movement, and can be studied to monitor fetal health.

- Fetal circulation transports blood to the heart and brain and shunts away from the lungs and liver. The placenta is functioning for the lungs and liver.
- The first trimester is the most critical time for organ development in the fetus when the cells are differentiating and forming the foundation for the tissues and organs of the body.
- Pregnant women should avoid medications unless directed by her health-care provider.
- The FDA has a pregnancy category system, A, B, C, D, and X, for determining safety of medications during pregnancy and lactation.
- Teratogenic substances such as lead, mercury, pesticides, bacteria, and street drugs can adversely affect the growth and development of the fetus.

REVIEW QUESTIONS

1. The ovaries secrete the following hormones during the menstrual cycle. (*select all that apply*)
   1. Estrogen
   2. Testosterone
   3. Thyroxine
   4. Progesterone
   5. Oxytocin
   6. Follicle-stimulating

2. The usual location of fertilization is:
   1. the uterus.
   2. the vagina.
   3. the fallopian tube.
   4. the ovary.

3. The fertilized ovum usually implants in the:
   1. endometrium of the uterus.
   2. upper portion of the fallopian tube.
   3. inside the cervix.
   4. near the ovary.

4. The hormone first detected by a blood test about 11 days after conception and in urine tests about 12 to 14 days after conception is:
   1. estrogen.
   2. hCG.
   3. progesterone.
   4. placental lactogen.

5. The major male hormone of reproduction, testosterone, is produced in the:
   1. pituitary.
   2. thyroid.
   3. adrenal glands.
   4. testicles.

6. The functions of the placenta are to: (*select all that apply*)
   1. supply oxygen to the fetus.
   2. supply nourishment to the fetus.
   3. produce hormones.
   4. provide protection from infection.
   5. provide cushioning protection for the fetus.

7. The substance that provides support and protection for the vessels inside the umbilical cord is:
   1. Wharton's jelly
   2. Progesterone
   3. Colostrum
   4. Amniotic fluid

8. According to the FDA, medications in this category are contraindicated for use in pregnancy.
   1. Category A
   2. Category C
   3. Category D
   4. Category X

9. Heroin use during pregnancy has been associated with the following adverse outcomes: (*select all that apply*)
   1. Neonatal addiction
   2. Increased risk of premature birth
   3. Low birth weight
   4. Hypoglycemia
   5. Intracranial hemorrhage in the uterus

10. Twins that share the same placenta in the uterus are:
    1. Dizygotic
    2. Amniotic
    3. Monozygotic
    4. Chorionic

CRITICAL THINKING QUESTIONS

1. At birth, the nurse notices that the umbilical cord has one vein and one artery. Which body system is at risk for a congenital anomaly?

2. Is it safe for a pregnant patient to use a nicotine patch to stop smoking?

3. If the pregnant patient has a low level of amniotic fluid, what problems could occur for the fetus?

DavisPlus

For additional resources and information, visit **www.DavisPlus.com.** Post-Conference Questions and Activities, Answers, and References can be found on Davis*Plus.*

4 Physical and Psychological Changes of Pregnancy

KEY TERMS

amenorrhea
anemia
ballottement
Chadwick's sign
Couvade syndrome
dysuria
Goodell's sign
Hegar's sign
hemorrhoids
Kegel exercise
linea nigra
melasma
pruritic urticarial papules and plaque of pregnancy (PUPP)
quickening
striae gravidarum
varicose veins
vena caval syndrome

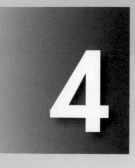 **DavisPlus** For audio pronunciation guide, visit www.DavisPlus.com

CHAPTER CONCEPTS

Female Reproduction
Pregnancy
Promoting Health
Self

LEARNING OUTCOMES

1. Define the key terms.
2. Differentiate presumptive, probable, and positive signs of pregnancy.
3. Describe the physiological changes in each body system occurring during pregnancy.
4. Plan safe and effective nursing interventions that address the common physiologic discomforts of pregnancy.
5. Identify physiologic discomfort symptoms that should be reported to the health-care provider.
6. Identify normal laboratory values for the pregnant woman.
7. Discuss Reva Rubin's four maternal tasks that the woman accomplishes during pregnancy.
8. Discuss the psychosocial changes occurring during pregnancy for the woman, her partner, and family.
9. Identify psychosocial issues of the pregnant adolescent.
10. Discuss possible cultural differences in viewing a normal pregnancy.

REAL-WORLD CASE STUDY

Lisa

■ Lisa, aged 23, is pregnant with her first baby and is at 32 weeks gestation. She has had an uncomplicated pregnancy and is eagerly awaiting her due date. Today she is at the office of her health-care provider for her routine prenatal checkup. She reports that her nose is "always congested." "Can I take a cold medicine from the drug store?" she asks.

Questions

1. What explanation can the nurse provide for this physiologic change of pregnancy?
2. What are some appropriate nursing interventions for this patient?

CONCEPTUAL CORNERSTONE

Patient Education

Some pregnant women are curious about pregnancy changes. They read pregnancy literature, surf the web, and attend classes. Other pregnant women only rely on the advice of family, friends, and health-care providers for pregnancy concerns. The nurse will encounter a variety of patients who will have diverse learning needs. The nurse can take a patient-centered approach to teaching by assessing the educational needs of the patient and then plan personalized teaching appropriate for that patient. It is important to keep in mind some principles of adult learning. Adults learn best when the learning is related to an immediate need, and is person-centered and problem-centered (Bastable et al., 2011). Education empowers the pregnant patient to make changes in her life to improve her health and to promote a safe pregnancy and healthy fetal outcome.

Pregnancy is a state that causes considerable physical and psychological changes in the woman. In addition to the obvious changes in the reproductive system, virtually every system is affected, and changes occur to adapt to the pregnancy and the growing fetus. Even before the woman suspects she is pregnant, changes are occurring.

DIAGNOSIS OF PREGNANCY

Every woman is different, and pregnancy symptoms can vary from one woman to the next and from pregnancy to pregnancy in the same woman. The signs and symptoms of pregnancy are generally grouped into three categories: presumptive, probable, and positive.

Presumptive Signs of Pregnancy

Presumptive signs of pregnancy are the subjective signs that a woman notices occurring in her body. These signs are the least reliable because they can sometimes be caused by health conditions not related to pregnancy. Many of the early signs are due to the rapid rise in hormone levels that begin at implantation of the trophoblast. Usually within 2 weeks after missing a menstrual period, she will begin to experience some of these presumptive signs:

- Nausea and vomiting.
- Fatigue.
- Urinary frequency.
- Breast enlargement and tenderness.
- **Amenorrhea**: absence of the menstrual period.
- **Quickening**: fetal movement felt by the mother after 18 to 20 weeks.

Probable Signs of Pregnancy

Probable signs of pregnancy are objective signs. They can be detected by a health-care provider during a physical exam or can be evaluated by a laboratory test or an in-home pregnancy test.

- **Goodell's sign**: softening of the cervix.
- **Chadwick's sign**: a bluish-purple coloration of the vaginal mucosa and cervix.
- **Hegar's sign**: softening of the lower uterine segment.
- **Ballottement**: a technique in which the health-care provider pushes against the woman's cervix and then can feel the fetus floating away from the cervix.
- Positive pregnancy test : a test in which human chorionic gonadotropin (hCG) is detectable in more than 98% of patients by day 11 of gestation (Shields, 2012).

Positive Signs of Pregnancy

Positive signs of pregnancy can only be attributed to the presence of a fetus. An experienced health-care provider can confirm that a fetus is growing inside the uterus.

- Fetal heart auscultation by Doppler.
- Fetal movement felt by an experienced practitioner.
- Ultrasound: a means of testing used to verify an embryo or fetus.

After a pregnancy has been confirmed, the health-care provider will arrange a schedule of visits with the pregnant woman to provide prenatal care to ensure the health of the mother and baby, and to prepare for the upcoming birth.

NORMAL PHYSIOLOGICAL CHANGES IN PREGNANCY

Maternal physiology undergoes many changes throughout gestation. Most changes occur as the result of the effects of progesterone, estrogen, and the growing fetus. Each body system changes to adjust to the increasing demands of the growing fetus. The nurse can provide patient teaching and anticipatory guidance to the pregnant patient and her family on how to manage the physiologic changes of pregnancy.

The normal physiology changes in pregnancy are presented in seven body system tables:

- Table 4.1. Reproductive System Changes in Pregnancy
- Table 4.2. Respiratory System Changes in Pregnancy
- Table 4.3. Cardiovascular System Changes in Pregnancy
- Table 4.4. Gastrointestinal System Changes in Pregnancy
- Table 4.5. Urinary System Changes in Pregnancy
- Table 4.6. Integumentary System Changes in Pregnancy
- Table 4.7. Musculoskeletal System Changes in Pregnancy

Each table notes the types of changes experienced by patient observations, and the nursing implications for care.

Reproductive System Changes

The types of reproductive system changes in pregnancy, what the patient observes, and the related nursing care implications are found in Table 4.1. See also Figure 4.1.

TABLE 4.1 REPRODUCTIVE SYSTEM CHANGES IN PREGNANCY

Types of Changes	Patient Observations	Nursing Implications
Uterine: • Length from 6.5 to 32 cm • Width from 2.5 to 24 cm • Depth from 2.5 to 22 cm • Weight from 50 to 1,000 g • Wall thickness from 1 to 0.5 cm	• The uterus expands to accommodate a fetus, placenta, umbilical cord, 50–100 mL of amniotic fluid and fetal membranes.	• Growth occurs at a predictable pace. • At 12 weeks gestation, the uterus can be palpated above the symphysis pubis. • At 20 weeks gestation it is located at the umbilicus (Fig. 4.1)
Cervix: • Estrogen causes the cervix to become congested with blood, causing a bluish purple color to the cervix, vagina, and labia. (*Chadwick's sign*) • Softening of the lower uterine segment (*Hegar's sign*) • Estrogen and progesterone cause cervical softening by decreasing collagen fibers, increased vascularity, and edema (*Goodell's sign*). The soft cervix is preparing for dilation during labor and childbirth. • Cervical mucus forms a plug in the cervical canal. The closed cervix with the mucous plug prevents bacteria from entering the uterus.	• "Bloody show" may be evident during early labor as the congested cervix starts to dilate and the mucous plug is released.	• Loss of the mucous plug and "bloody show" are early signs of labor.
Vagina and Vulva: • Increased vascularity causes the vagina and vulva to appear bluish. • Vaginal mucosa thickens and the vaginal folds become more noticeable. A softening of the collagen fibers occurs due to hormonal influences. • Increased levels of glycogen are present in vaginal cells. An acidic vaginal environment develops due to the effect of *Lactobacillus acidophilus* on glycogen in the vaginal cells. • Softening of the connective tissue allows the vagina to distend during childbirth. This causes rapid sloughing of cells and an increase in vaginal discharge. • The acidic environment prevents growth of bacteria normally found in the vagina. • The glycogen rich environment favors the growth of *Candida albicans*.	• Increased vaginal discharge is noted by the patient. • Increased vascular congestion of the vulva and decreased venous blood return from the lower extremities will cause edema of the vulva. • Yeast infections are common in pregnant women.	• Reassure the patient that the increased vaginal discharge is normal and may increase as the due date arrives. • Discuss vulvar hygiene of gentle external cleansing with nonperfumed soap and water. • Teach patient the signs and symptoms of vaginal yeast infection, such as increased vaginal discharge that is white, thick, cottage-cheese-like, and vaginal itching. These symptoms should be reported to the health-care provider.
Ovaries: • After ovulation, luteinizing hormone stimulates the corpus luteum and it produces progesterone for 6–7 weeks. The corpus luteum continues to increase in size during this period of time and sometimes the cyst can rupture.	• The corpus luteum may rupture and cause pain and vaginal bleeding in some women.	• Advise the woman to contact her health-care provider if pain or bleeding occurs.

TABLE 4.1   REPRODUCTIVE SYSTEM CHANGES IN PREGNANCY–cont'd

Types of Changes	Patient Observations	Nursing Implications
Breasts: • There is increased blood volume in the breast tissue. Estrogen and progesterone cause breast enlargement, tingling, and increased sensitivity. During the second trimester, colostrum develops from the acini cells in the milk glands.	• Breasts feel engorged with a feeling of heat and tingling. • Breast tenderness and enlargement. Colostrum may leak from the nipples.	• Reassure the woman that leaking colostrum is a normal process of the breasts preparing for lactation. • To promote comfort, advise the woman to wear a supportive bra.
Sexual Activity • During pregnancy, there is an increase in vaginal lubrication and an increase in blood flow to the genital area.	• Many pregnant women feel that during the first trimester libido decreases due to nausea, fatigue, sore breasts, and anxieties about miscarriage. • During the second trimester, women generally feel more energetic and have an increase in libido. • By the third trimester, physical discomfort can make traditional sexual acts more difficult and less frequent. Fatigue is a major predictor to sexual frequency during pregnancy (Murtagh, 2010).	• Reassure the woman and her partner that sexual intercourse will not harm the fetus. • Sexual needs can be met in a variety of ways. Positions such as side by side, woman on top, and hands and knees can be used during pregnancy. • The literature does not support an association between sexual intercourse and increased risk of preterm labor and delivery (Murtagh, 2010).

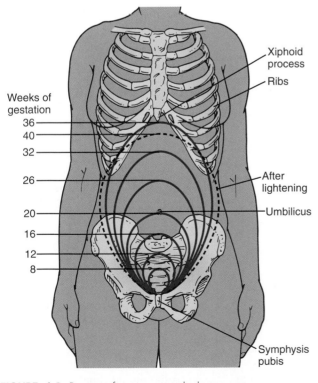

Weeks of gestation
36
40
32
26
20
16
12
8

Xiphoid process
Ribs
After lightening
Umbilicus
Symphysis pubis

FIGURE 4.1 Pattern of uterine growth during pregnancy.

PATIENT TEACHING GUIDELINES

Kegel Exercises

Kegel exercises will help the patient to strengthen her perineal muscles.

Instructions:

• Rapidly contract and relax the muscles of the perineum and vagina for 10 sec.
• Relax for 20 sec.
• Repeat the routine.
• The number of repetitions should be increased gradually to between 50 and 150 per day.

SAFETY *STAT!*

Preventing Vena Cava Syndrome

Supine hypotension, also known as **vena caval syndrome**, is a safety issue in pregnancy. As the pregnancy advances and the woman lies supine, the weight of the uterus can compress the inferior vena cava, which reduces blood return to the heart and cardiac output. This decrease in cardiac output causes the blood pressure to drop and the perfusion of blood in the placenta decreases. Early symptoms that the woman may experience are:

- Tachycardia
- Dizziness
- Feelings of light-headedness or fainting
- Nausea
- Sweating

  If not corrected by having the mother turn to her left side, the fetus may begin to show signs of distress with deceleration of the heart rate.

Respiratory System Changes

The types of respiratory system changes in pregnancy, what the patient observes, and the related nursing care implications are found in Table 4.2.

Cardiovascular System Changes

The types of cardiovascular system changes in pregnancy, what the patient observes, and the related nursing care implications are found in Table 4.3. See also Figure 4.2.

TABLE 4.2 RESPIRATORY SYSTEM CHANGES IN PREGNANCY

Types of Changes	Patient Observations	Nursing Implications
• The respiratory rate increases to 18–20 respirations per minute (RPM). • Oxygen consumption increases by 20% and the tidal volume (amount of air breathed in each minute) increases. This provides for the extra oxygen demands of the uterus, placenta, and fetus.	• Pregnant women may feel short of breath easily when lying down and with mild exertion.	• To reduce the feeling of shortness of breath, encourage the woman to elevate her head on an extra pillow at night and to walk up stairs more slowly.
• Estrogen causes hypertrophy and increased vascularity of nasal and lung tissue, and progesterone causes relaxation of the smooth muscle of the bronchi, bronchioles, and alveoli. These hormonal changes cause an increase in oxygen consumption. The effects of the hormones also cause increased mucous production.	• A pregnant woman breathes faster and more deeply. The increased vascularity causes a feeling of nasal and lung congestion (Alexander et al., 2010). • Rhinitis and nosebleeds can occur.	• The pregnant woman needs education regarding these normal changes and reassurance. • The woman should use gentle nose-blowing, use a cool mist humidifier, drink fluids, and avoid overuse of nasal spray decongestants due to the rebound effect of prolonged use. • If frequent nosebleeds occur, she should notify her health-care provider.
• The enlarging uterus causes upward pressure and elevation of the diaphragm. • Cartilage and muscles relax and the chest broadens, to allow room for the enlarging uterus.	• Chest circumference may increase as much as 6 cm.	• Educate the pregnant woman of this normal physiologic change of pregnancy.

TABLE 4.3 CARDIOVASCULAR SYSTEM CHANGES IN PREGNANCY

Types of Changes	Patient Observations	Nursing Implications
General Cardiovascular System Changes: • An increase in circulatory blood volume begins by week 6 and will reach 50% more than the pre-pregnancy volume. • 500 mL of blood is needed to provide for increased oxygen consumption of the	• Pregnant women have warm hands and feet. • Nasal blood flow is increased, causing nasal congestion. • The weight of the uterus obstructs blood return from	• On assessment, slight cardiac hypertrophy may be identified, as well as an asymptomatic systolic murmur. • Inform the pregnant woman that she should avoid the supine

TABLE **4.3** CARDIOVASCULAR SYSTEM CHANGES IN PREGNANCY–cont'd

Types of Changes	Patient Observations	Nursing Implications
growing fetus, the enlarging uterus, and the breasts. • Increased volume also supports the mother's weight gain of 10–15 kg and protects the woman from blood loss at delivery (Hornstein and Schwein 2012). • Heart rate increases 10–20 beats greater than pre-pregnancy levels. • Blood volume increases causing veins to enlarge. • The increase in blood volume correlates with the increase in fetal weight. • 30% more blood circulates through the kidneys to remove waste from mother and fetus. • Cardiac output increases up to 50% during the first half of pregnancy. • Blood pressure remains stable even though there is an increase in blood volume. There may be a slight decrease in systolic pressure and increase in diastolic pressure.	the veins in the legs. This may result in varicose veins of the legs, vulva, and rectum. • **Varicose veins** are swollen veins raised above the surface of the skin. They may be twisted or bulging and are dark purple or blue in color. They are located most often on the backs of the calves or on the inside of the leg. • When the pregnant woman is supine, the weight of the uterus may cause hypotension when the uterus partially occludes the vena cava and aorta.	position. Lying on her back can cause feelings of light-headedness and cause her blood pressure to drop. This is called supine hypotension or *vena caval syndrome*. Side-lying provides for better brain and placental profusion (Fig. 4.2).
Blood Components: • Red blood cell mass increases by 40%. This provides increased oxygen carrying capacity to the mother and growing fetus. • More red blood cells also give the mother some protection from hemorrhage in childbirth. • Hemodilution occurs due to increased volume causing physiological anemia of pregnancy. **Anemia** is a reduction of red blood cells. • Leukocytes increase during pregnancy ranging from 5,000 to 15,000. The cause is unknown but may be due to physical stress of pregnancy and hormonal changes. • Fibrinogen levels rise by 50%. • Increased risk for thrombophlebitis and thrombus formation.	• The anemic pregnant woman may experience fatigue, hair loss, or pica. • *Pica* is an abnormal craving for a nonfood substance, such as ice, dirt, paint, or clay. • If a venous thrombus occurs, the woman may notice erythema, hot or warm skin, painful area on the leg and swelling of the surrounding area of the calf.	• Iron supplement is usually prescribed to pregnant women by the 2nd semester to prevent anemia. • The woman should be instructed to include iron-rich foods in her diet, such as red meat, spinach, kale, broccoli, and raisins. • It may be difficult to determine whether infection is occurring during the pregnancy. Any possible signs of infection should be reported to the health-care provider. • Inform the woman that if she develops signs of a venous thrombus, such as warmth, redness, or swelling of her calf, she should notify her health-care provider. • Instruct the pregnant woman to avoid standing or sitting for prolonged periods of time to prevent venous stasis.

LABS & DIAGNOSTICS: COMMON LABORATORY BLOOD VALUES

Common Laboratory Blood Values	Non-pregnant Woman	Pregnant
Hemoglobin (HGB)	11.7–15.5 g/dL	11.5–13 g/dL
Hematocrit (HCT)	33–45%	31.5–41%
Red blood cells (RBCs)	3.91–5.11	No change
White blood cells (WBCs)	4.5–11.1	5.9–14
Serum creatinine	0.51–1.1 mg/dL	0.49–0.9 mg/dL
Serum blood urea nitrogen (BUN)	8–21 mg/dL	8–10 mg/dL
Serum uric acid	2.5–7 mg/dL	2–5.8 mg/dL
Urine creatinine clearance	75–115 mL/min	150–200 mL/min
Urine uric acid	250–750 mg/24 hr	Increases
serum glucose	<100 mg/dL	Gradual decrease of 10%
Alanine transaminase (ALT)	7–35 units/L	Unchanged
Aspartate aminotransferase (AST)	15–30 units/L	Unchanged
Alkaline phosphatase (ALP)	25–125 units/L	Up to 2–4 times due to placental tissue and fetal bone growth
Lactate dihydrogenase (LDH)	100–330 units/L	Upper end of normal to 700 units/L
Fibrinogen (factor I)	200–400 mg/dL	Progressive increase of 1–2g/L
Platelets	150,000–450,000 per mm³	Less than 150,000 per mm³
Fibrin split products (FSPs); also known as fibrin degradation products (FDPs)	Less than 10 mcg/mL	Increased greater than 10 mcg/mL
D-dimer	0–0.5 mcg/mL	Greater than 0.5 mcg/mL

Van Leeuwen et al., 2013

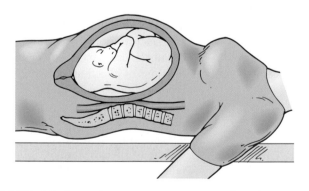

FIGURE 4.2 Supine hypotension, or vena caval syndrome, may occur if the pregnant woman lies on her back. This causes compression of the vena cava.

Gastrointestinal System Changes

The types of gastrointestinal system changes in pregnancy, what the patient observes, and the related nursing care implications are found in Table 4.4.

 LEARN TO C.U.S.

Marta is 14 weeks pregnant and arrives for her prenatal visit. She has only gained 1 pound since her last visit, which was 1 month ago. She states that she is still experiencing nausea and vomiting "practically all day." "I mentioned it to my doctor last month, but he said it would stop when I entered my second trimester. I really feel like he thought I was overly concerned about it and acting like a baby over a little nausea. I don't feel like he was listening to me." Concerned, the nurse discusses the issue with the physician using the C.U.S. method of communication.

C: "I am **concerned** about Marta.

U: I am **uncomfortable** with this situation because she is still experiencing nausea and vomiting and is not gaining adequate weight.

S: We have a **safety** issue regarding her health and the health of the fetus."

TABLE 4.4 GASTROINTESTINAL SYSTEM CHANGES IN PREGNANCY

Types of Changes	Patient Observations	Nursing Implications
• Advancing maternal age, high levels of hCG, estrogen, and prostaglandin, reduced tone of the GI system, and reduced stomach acidity are all thought to contribute to nausea and vomiting, also known as morning sickness. (Shrim et al., 2010)	• Usually occurs between 6 and 12 weeks gestation. • Nausea may occur in the mornings or may occur as a result of strong aromas.	Instruct the patient to: • Eat several small meals instead of three large meals to keep her stomach from being empty. • Eat dry toast, saltines, or dry cereals before getting out of bed in the morning. • Sip on water, weak tea, or clear soft drinks. • Avoid smells that upset her stomach.
• Progesterone causes smooth muscle relaxation, which affects the esophageal sphincter and allows gastric contents to reflux into the esophagus causing heartburn.	• The woman may experience heartburn or epigastric discomfort after eating a large meal or if she lies down right after eating.	• If experiencing heartburn, eat bland foods that are low in fat and easy to digest, such as cereal, rice, and bananas. • Avoid lying down after a meal. • Avoid overeating. • Smaller frequent meals may eliminate heartburn.
• The increased levels of hormones slow down digestion and relax the smooth muscles in the intestines causing constipation for many women. • In addition, the pressure of the expanding uterus on the intestinal tract can contribute to constipation.	• Signs of constipation include having hard, dry stools; less than three bowel movements per week; and painful bowel movements.	Educate the patient to: • Drink 8–10 glasses of water daily. • Eat fiber-rich foods, such as fresh or dried fruit, raw vegetables, and whole-grain cereals. • Increase mild physical activity, such as walking. • Avoid straining for a bowel movement. • Notify health-care provider if constipation is severe.
• The gallbladder becomes hypotonic due to the effects of progesterone on smooth muscle. • This causes a delay in emptying, which can predispose to the development of gallstones.	• The woman may develop upper right quadrant pain after fatty meal.	• Instruct the woman to notify her health-care provider of any abdominal pain.
• Up to 50% of pregnant women get hemorrhoids (Shields, 2012). • Hemorrhoids are common for many reasons. The increase in blood volume causes veins to enlarge. • The expanding uterus also puts pressure on the veins in the rectum. • Constipation can worsen hemorrhoids if the woman strains to have a bowel movement.	• **Hemorrhoids** are swollen and bulging veins in the rectum. They can cause itching, pain, and bleeding.	• Educate the woman to notify her health-care provider if the hemorrhoids are painful and/or bleeding. • Increase fiber and fluid intake to avoid straining for a bowel movement. • Reassure the woman that hemorrhoids usually improve after delivery.

PATIENT TEACHING GUIDELINES

Foods High in Fiber
Patients who increase fiber intake can reduce or avoid the discomforts of constipation and hemorrhoids. Foods high in fiber include:
- Prunes
- Pears
- Mangos
- Apples
- Whole-grain breads
- Beans
- Lentils
- Nuts
- Broccoli
- Cabbage

 DRUG FACTS

Iron Supplements
May be prescribed to prevent or treat iron-deficiency anemia.

Nursing Implications:
- For best absorption, the patient should take the medication 1 hour before or 2 hours after a meal.
- Absorption is improved if taken with orange juice.
- If gastric irritation occurs, it can be taken with meals.
- Advise the patient that the stool may become dark green or black.

- Constipation is the major side effect, so encourage the patient to drink adequate amounts of water.

Vallerand et al., 2011

Urinary System

The types of urinary system changes in pregnancy, what the patient observes, and the related nursing care implications are found in Table 4.5. See also Figure 4.3.

Integumentary System

The types of integumentary system changes in pregnancy, what the patient observes, and the related nursing care implications are found in Table 4.6. See also Figure 4.4.

HEALTH PROMOTION

Skin Care during Pregnancy
There are varieties of skin changes that occur during pregnancy. To promote good skin care during pregnancy, encourage the patient to:
- Wear sunscreen every day and avoid prolonged exposure to the sun. This will prevent or minimize the appearance of melasma on the face.
- Use moisturizing lotion to decrease dry skin and minimize itching of the abdominal skin.
- To control acne, use gentle face wash and scrubs.
- Read package labels carefully and avoid retinoids, benzyl peroxide, or salicylic acid ingredients in skin products.

TABLE 4.5 URINARY SYSTEM CHANGES IN PREGNANCY

Types of Changes	Patient Observations	Nursing Implications
• Kidney work load increases due to increased blood volume and cardiac output. • The increase in blood flow is necessary to remove metabolic wastes from the mother and fetus. • The glomerular filtration rate increases, but the ability of the renal tubules to reabsorb glucose does not increase and therefore, mild glycosuria is common in pregnancy. • Mild proteinuria is also common. • The effect of progesterone on the renal pelvis causes dilation and the distention can lead to urinary stasis and possible urinary tract infection.	• If the patient develops a urinary tract infection, she may experience urinary urgency, frequency, and dysuria. **Dysuria** is painful urination.	• The nurse should monitor the kidney function tests, creatinine, BUN, etc, for abnormalities and report them to the health-care provider. • The woman has an increased risk of urinary tract infections and should be educated on the signs and symptoms. Signs and symptoms of a urinary tract infection are urinary urgency, frequency, and dysuria.

TABLE 4.5 URINARY SYSTEM CHANGES IN PREGNANCY—cont'd

Types of Changes	Patient Observations	Nursing Implications
• Temporary bladder control problems are common in pregnancy. The enlarged uterus and fetus push down on the bladder, urethra, and pelvic floor muscles (Fig. 4.3).	• Increased pressure on the bladder can lead to a more frequent need to urinate, as well as leaking of urine when sneezing, coughing, or laughing.	Educate the woman to: • Take frequent bathroom breaks. • Increase consumption of fluids to avoid dehydration. Instruct the patient on performing Kegel exercises. See Patient Teaching Guidelines for Kegel exercises. Inform the woman that if she experiences burning along with frequency of urination, it may be an infection and she should notify her health-care provider.

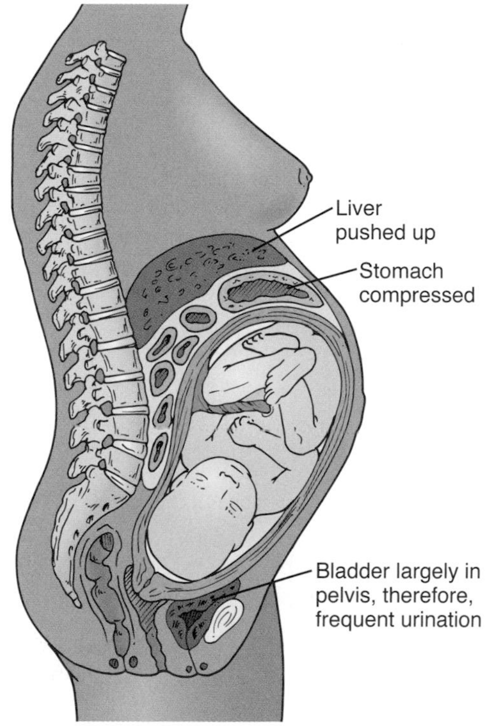

FIGURE 4.3 Compression of the bladder results from the growing uterus.

Labels: Liver pushed up; Stomach compressed; Bladder largely in pelvis, therefore, frequent urination

Musculoskeletal System

The types of musculoskeletal system changes in pregnancy, what the patient observes, and the related nursing care implications are found in Table 4.7.

PSYCHOLOGICAL ADAPTATION TO PREGNANCY

Pregnancy and childbirth is considered a life transition also known as a *maturational crisis*. Even a woman and her partner who planned and wanted a pregnancy may experience ambivalent feelings and worries about the pregnancy, impending parenthood, and integrating a child into the family. The nurse should keep in mind that there are many factors that influence how a pregnant woman, the baby's father, siblings, and grandparents react to the news of a new baby entering their lives. Examples of factors may include access to health care, financial issues, lack of family support, availability of day care, transportation problems, and previous experiences with childbirth and childrearing. The nurse who observes problems with adaptation to pregnancy can make appropriate referrals and provide assistance to ensure that the adaptation to this maturational crisis is smooth.

The Mother

The physical and psychological changes that occur during pregnancy and the experience of labor and birth influence the transition to motherhood. The psychological journey to the role of motherhood is described by Rubin (1984) and Mercer (1995) in their classic theories of maternal role attainment.

According to Reva Rubin, four maternal tasks the woman accomplishes during pregnancy lead to maternal identity. These tasks include:

1. Seeking safe passage for herself and her fetus.
2. Securing acceptance of herself as a mother and for her fetus.
3. Learning to give up self and to accept herself as mother to the infant.
4. Committing herself to the child as she progresses through pregnancy.

Ensuring Safe Passage for Herself and the Fetus

During the first trimester, the woman expresses concern for her own health and her pregnancy symptoms. Even women profoundly happy about the pregnancy are surprised to experience emotions that rapidly change from tears to irritability and to joy without provocation, all due to the hormonal

TABLE 4.6 INTEGUMENTARY SYSTEM CHANGES IN PREGNANCY

Types of Changes	Patient Observations	Nursing Implications
• Hyperpigmentation occurs due to elevated levels of estrogen, progesterone, and melanocyte-stimulating hormone.	• **Melasma**, also called the *mask of pregnancy*, are brownish patches on the forehead, cheeks, and nose. • **Linea nigra**, a hyperpigmented line, may extend from the symphysis pubis to the fundus. • On the breasts, the areola may darken.	• Educate the pregnant woman that melasma increases with exposure to the sun. Sunscreen may reduce the severity. • Reassure the woman that the hyperpigmentation usually disappears after childbirth.
• **Striae gravidarum**, also known as *stretch-marks*, occur due to separation of collagen fibers of the connective tissue as the skin expands. See Figure 4.4 for skin changes in pregnancy.	• Striae gravidarum occur on the abdomen, hips, thighs, and breasts. They may be red and itch.	• There is no documented proof that creams prevent striae; however, creams may sooth the itchiness.
• **Pruritic urticarial papules and plaques of pregnancy** (PUPP) is the most common pregnancy-specific dermatosis, occurring in 1 of 130 to 300 pregnancies. The disorder is more common with first pregnancies and multiple gestations, and familial occurrences have been reported (Tunzi and Gray, 2007).	• The rash appears on the abdomen and occasionally involves extremities. The face usually is not affected. • PUPP are itchy plaques and papules with erythematous patches of papules and vesicles.	• Usually develops in the third trimester. • Oral antihistamines and topical corticosteroids may be administered for pruritus. For extreme symptoms, oral corticosteroids may be prescribed. • Reassure the woman that the rash will disappear after childbirth.

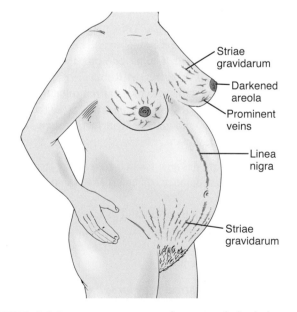

FIGURE 4.4 Integumentary system changes include darkening of the areolae, appearance of the linea nigra, and striae gravidarum.

Striae gravidarum — Darkened areola — Prominent veins — Linea nigra — Striae gravidarum

shifts that are occurring physically. She seeks information by observing mothers and other pregnant women, and from literature or information acquired on the Internet.

Some women may experience ambivalence about pregnancy, but still seek competent prenatal care and engage in healthy self-care, such as avoiding alcohol consumption and eating healthy. The reality of pregnancy often causes introspection during the first trimester as she adapts to the physical changes and the changes in her life and lifestyle.

TEAM WORKS

Carla is a new certified nursing assistant working on the antenatal floor of the Obstetric Unit. She is assigned to Liza, a pregnant patient, 8 weeks gestation, admitted for treatment of severe nausea and vomiting. Carla mentions to the nurse that Liza is "so self-centered. She is irritable and all she talks about is how bad she feels." The nurse uses this opportunity to educate Carla about the tasks of pregnancy. The nurse explains to Carla that Liza is in her first trimester and that it is normal for her to be concerned about her health as she

TABLE 4.7 MUSCULOSKELETAL SYSTEM CHANGES IN PREGNANCY

Types of Changes	Patient Observations	Nursing Implications
• Postural changes: the upper spine extends to support the enlarging uterus. This gives the pregnant woman a "swayback" appearance and leads to backache. • Her center of gravity shifts forward placing more strain on the lower back.	• Increased backache as the uterus enlarges and the woman gains weight.	• Teach the woman to practice good posture, wear low-heeled shoes, sleep on her side, and try heat, cold, or massage to manage backache.
• Loose joints: the effects of relaxin, a pregnancy-related hormone, affects the sacroiliac joints and the symphysis pubis causing them to soften and stretch to allow more room in the pelvis to make birth easier.	• She may feel clumsy and may experience "waddling" due to the laxity of her joints.	• Teach her to lift with good body mechanics and to wear low-heeled shoes, and exercise caution when walking on unlevel surfaces.

adjusts to pregnancy. The hormones of pregnancy also cause irritability and unstable emotions. The nurse encourages Carla to be an empathetic listener and to be patient with Liza's self-centeredness.

Seeking Acceptance of the Child by Others

In this task, support and acceptance of the pregnancy by the woman's partner and family are most important. She desires their acceptance of the pregnancy and her developing maternal identity. If there are other children in the family, the woman works to build acceptance of the new baby. This may involve adjustments of psychological, social, and physical space within the family to make a place for the coming child.

Mercer (1995) states that a pregnant woman's relationship with her own mother is significant in adapting to pregnancy. Her mother's reaction to the pregnancy indicates acceptance of the grandchild. As the pregnant woman's mother reminisces about her pregnancy and her daughter's early childhood, it helps the daughter to anticipate and prepare for pregnancy, labor, and motherhood.

Bonding With the Infant

While completing this developmental task, the mother begins to develop bonds of attachment and feelings of love for the infant. She feels fetal movement and feels an intimate connection with the unborn fetus. She may fantasize about the ideal child. This strong emotional "binding-in" process motivates the woman to be a good mother. The woman observes women mothering their children and reflects on her own style of mothering.

The woman's own mother was identified by Rubin as the strongest model. If the pregnant woman's mother was perceived as a good mother, the woman takes on her mothering style. If the woman's own mother was a poor role model, the pregnant woman adjusts her thinking to prepare herself to be a better mother.

Committing Herself to the Child Through Pregnancy

Next, the woman begins to develop the ability for self-denial and learns to meet the needs of another being before herself. She begins to prepare for the baby by preparing a nursery and accumulating clothing and baby-care items. At this time, some women begin reading books on newborn care and parenting and attend childbirth classes.

According to Rubin and Mercer, the pregnant woman undergoes psychosocial changes throughout the pregnancy. Unsuccessful resolution of these changes has been associated with difficulties in pregnancy, delivery, child abuse, and neglect.

 CULTURAL CONSIDERATIONS

Pregnant Chinese women may assume a "sick role" in which they depend on others for assistance. They also believe that pregnancy disrupts the cultural belief regarding the need to balance "hot" and "cold" which is vital for sound health. To manage the disruption in balance, the pregnant woman may eat special soups and chicken broth.

Indian women view pregnancy as a normal process that does not require any intervention by health-care professionals.

Some Indian women believe that it is the responsibility of others to satisfy a woman's cravings. There is a belief that if the newborn baby drools excessively, the mother's cravings were not met during the pregnancy. There are no restrictions of physical activity and women may continue their daily activities, including carrying heavy loads, until labor begins.

The pregnant Japanese woman does not discuss morning sickness even within the family. They are usually advised to avoid activities that require concentration because they believe the epinephrine released with mental stress may harm the newborn. A Japanese tradition is for the woman to move to her parents' home in the eighth month to prepare for delivery.

Hispanic woman are encouraged to stay active during the pregnancy because it is believed that this will lead to a healthier baby with a better temperament. As the culture is very respectful of its elders, women will often look to mothers, aunts, and grandmothers for advice on pregnancy and childbirth (Queensland Health, 2012; Galanti, 2015).

The Pregnant Adolescent

The pregnant adolescent has many psychosocial issues to manage. She will be completing the developmental tasks of adolescence, as well as the developmental tasks of becoming a mother. Priorities typical for her age are the importance of appearance, the importance of the peer group, and a focus on one's own needs.

Most teens do not plan on becoming pregnant and may keep the pregnancy a secret as long as possible. Denial of the pregnancy until late in gestation is common. The young woman will experience anxiety related to informing her parents, the baby's father, and her friends about her pregnancy. Ambivalence, resistance, and inconsistency can be expected with the pregnant adolescent. The nurse will need to assess the developmental level and the young woman's support system when planning physical and psychological care for this patient.

THERAPEUTIC COMMUNICATION

Elizabeth, aged 17, is in her second trimester of her pregnancy. She is visibly upset as she arrives for her prenatal appointment. The nurse can use therapeutic communication to inquire about Elizabeth's mood.

Nurse: "Elizabeth, you seem upset." Technique: making an observation.

Elizabeth: "I am so mad at my mother. I hope I am not like her with my child."

Nurse: "What's the problem?" Technique: clarifying.

Elizabeth: "She is just so bossy."

Nurse: "You feel like she tells you what to do, too much?" Technique: reflecting.

The Father

The most important person to the pregnant woman is usually the father of the baby. The mother has a need for the father to accept the child. The father's role is important in the couple's and the family's adjustment to the new baby. Some men do experience the physical changes called **Couvade syndrome**, which is a sympathetic response to the pregnancy. He may gain weight and even experience nausea.

The father may not exhibit many physical changes, but he does undergo psychological changes throughout the pregnancy. He experiences psychological changes during each trimester, just as the woman experiences psychological adjustments. In the first trimester, he may feel ambivalence about becoming a father, or have strong protective feelings of nurturing and protecting the woman. As the pregnancy progresses, he may be concerned about his ability to be a good father and may examine his own father–child relationship to determine the type of father he will be.

If the pregnancy is unplanned or unwanted, some fathers may not readily accept changes in lifestyles or life plans. The father-to-be may feel left out and unsure of his position in the relationship after the baby is born. Many men eventually adjust to the unwanted pregnancy and begin to look forward to fatherhood. However, some men may engage in extramarital affairs for the first time during a pregnancy and some men express their disappointment and frustration with violence. Some women are battered by their partner for the first time during a pregnancy. Domestic violence has become an issue during pregnancy and the American College of Obstetricians and Gynecologists (2012) suggests that screening for domestic violence be done at each prenatal visit.

The father may also be concerned about his ability to be the only emotional support during childbirth in a "woman's world" of giving birth. Fathers-to-be may not discuss their fears and worries but often cope with their uncertainties by finding concrete tasks to do, such as preparing the baby's room, painting furniture, shopping for baby furniture, assembling car seats, and attending childbirth classes. Toward the end of the pregnancy, most fathers are preparing for parenthood with thoughtful contemplation of being a loving, nurturing, supportive father.

Siblings

For the siblings, a new baby is a major crisis. The sibling's response is influenced by the child's age, the parents' attitudes, and how well prepared the child is for the upcoming birth. Parents can prepare siblings by encouraging their participation in preparing the baby's room, taking them on a tour of the hospital, reading books on babies, visiting friends with infants, and promoting a positive attitude about the coming addition to the family.

Toddlers may notice physical changes in the mother and may sense that there are changes coming, which often lead them to be clingy and irritable. Older children take an

NURSING CARE PLAN   Body Image in Pregnancy

Nadia is 28 years old and pregnant with her first baby. She is in the 28th week of her uncomplicated pregnancy. Nadia has been an athlete and very active physically for her entire life. She ran a marathon when she was 4 weeks pregnant, and has continued to run until the last 2 weeks. At that time, it became too uncomfortable to continue running. She states that she feels "slow and fat. I hate the way I look." She is at her health-care provider's office for a routine prenatal visit.

Nursing Diagnosis: Body image disturbance
Expected Outcome: By the next prenatal visit, Nadia will express acceptance of her body size.
Interventions:
  • Acknowledge her feelings. Listen to her concerns emphatically.
  • Encourage Nadia to discuss her feelings with her husband.
  • Explore other methods of exercise that are safe during pregnancy, such as swimming and walking.
  • Encourage moderate daily exercise.
  • Encourage healthy nutritional intake to decrease excessive weight gain.
  • Educate Nadia on expected weight gain pattern during pregnancy to promote a safe pregnancy and healthy fetus.
  • Explain that weight loss after pregnancy is gradual.
  • Assist Nadia to consider a realistic plan for weight loss after childbirth.
Evaluation: The nurse notes that at her subsequent prenatal visits, Nadia has healthy weight gain and expresses pride in her growing uterus and healthy pregnancy.

interest in the physical changes occurring in the mother and may ask questions about conception, pregnancy, and childbirth. Older children and teenagers may feel embarrassed by the sexuality of their parents and may express embarrassment about the pregnancy but be pleased about the arrival of a new sibling.

The parents need to introduce the news that a new baby is coming at an appropriate time for the child. For an older sibling, the earlier he or she can be given the news is best. A toddler who has a limited concept of time will begin to think that a new baby is only a "story" and not a reality if informed too early of the new baby's arrival. Toddlers have difficulty sharing the parent with another child. The preschool child may feel a sense of loss, a feeling of being "replaced," or may feel jealous of the baby. Older school-aged children will contemplate and plan for ways to be helpful with a new baby in the home.

Grandparents

With the news of the impending arrival of a grandchild, most expectant grandparents are pleased with the possibility of a new baby in the family. The news of a new baby causes them to remember their own experiences of pregnancy and raising children. They begin to recall the "firsts" of their child, like the first steps or first words. These memories are shared in the family, and the grandparents use them to as a way of providing a link between the generations. The grandparent's support and presence strengthens the family and provides nurturing support to the parents-to-be as they attain their parenting roles.

Expectant grandparents have to face the reality of aging when they realize that their child will become a mother or father. They may react negatively to the news and state "they are too young to be grandparents." Nonsupport of the pregnancy adds stress and decreases the self-esteem of the parents-to-be.

Key Points

■ This chapter has outlined the physiological, anatomical, and psychological changes that develop during the course of pregnancy.

■ There are presumptive, probable, and positive signs of pregnancy.

■ Early physical changes are due to the increasing levels of estrogen and progesterone, which rise in response

to the demands brought on by the fetus, placenta, and uterus.

■ Physiological changes that occur later in the pregnancy are more anatomical and are caused by the expanding uterus.

■ When a woman becomes pregnant, she expects to see an expanding abdomen, but does not often expect the other changes occurring in her body in response to the growing fetus.

■ There are major psychosocial changes that occur as the woman makes the transition to motherhood.

■ The father of the baby and the grandparents will also have psychosocial issues to address.

■ The pregnant adolescent has special needs during the pregnancy.

■ There are cultural differences in how a normal pregnancy is viewed, and in the physical and psychological changes that occur.

REVIEW QUESTIONS

1. The nurse is discussing pregnancy care with a woman who just had her pregnancy confirmed by her health-care provider. She is 8 weeks pregnant. Which of the following topics should be discussed with the pregnant woman at this time? (*select all that apply*)
   1. Nutrition for a healthy pregnancy
   2. Her feelings about being pregnant
   3. Managing nausea
   4. Her birth plan

2. A woman states that she is feeling a "little confused or uncertain about being pregnant." A therapeutic response by the nurse would be:
   1. "Don't worry, everything will be all right."
   2. "There are plenty of women that would be happy to be pregnant."
   3. "It's not unusual to have ambivalent feelings about pregnancy."
   4. "As long as you take care of yourself, you will be just fine."

3. A pregnant woman, 37 weeks gestation, is lying on her back. She is experiencing light-headedness and states, "I feel like I'm going to faint." The nurse should:
   1. Reassure her that she is OK.
   2. Turn her to her side immediately.
   3. Administer oxygen at 4 L/min.
   4. Call the health-care provider immediately.

4. A woman 36 weeks gestation states that she does not understand why her ankles are swelling by the end of the day. The best response by the nurse is:
   1. "You may need to pay more attention to your dietary intake of salt."
   2. "Your circulation in your legs is compromised by the weight of the uterus."
   3. "You may be developing a complication; you should contact your health-care provider."
   4. "Every pregnant woman experiences swollen ankles."

5. A woman states that she "thinks she is pregnant." Which of the following presumptive signs of pregnancy may she be experiencing? (*select all that apply*)
   1. Absence of menstruation
   2. Fetal heart heard by Doppler
   3. Nausea
   4. Sore tender breasts
   5. Positive pregnancy test

6. A pregnant patient, 9 weeks gestation, arrives at the clinic for a routine pregnancy visit. She comments on the morning sickness that she experiences "every day." The nurse knows that morning sickness is due to: (*select all that apply*)
   1. High levels of hCG, estrogen, prostaglandin
   2. Reduced tone of the GI system
   3. Reduced stomach acidity
   4. Overeating at meals
   5. The enlarging uterus pressing on the stomach

CRITICAL THINKING QUESTIONS

1. A woman 8 weeks pregnant complains that she is "so nauseated in the morning that she can't really eat breakfast." How would you explain the nausea of pregnancy and what nursing interventions could you offer this patient?

2. What strategies can the nurse suggest to a pregnant woman to assist her to prepare her other children, ages 2 and 8, for the new addition to the family?

For additional resources and information, visit **www.DavisPlus.com.** Post-Conference Questions and Activities, Answers, and References can be found on Davis*Plus*.

Antepartal Nursing Assessment

LEARNING OUTCOMES

1. Define the key terms.
2. Discuss diagnostic testing to confirm pregnancy.
3. Explain the GTPAL system.
4. Explain scopes of practice and roles of the family practice physician, an obstetrician, and a certified nurse midwife on the health-care team.
5. Determine the estimated date of delivery using Naegele's rule.
6. Describe how patient-centered care is dependent on a thorough past medical history, cultural history, social history, and pregnancy history.
7. Explain the purpose and procedure of the complete physical exam and pelvic exam.
8. Define the common laboratory tests utilized during pregnancy.
9. Explain the commonly used screening tests for fetal abnormalities.
10. List the usual pattern of prenatal visits to the health-care provider.
11. Discuss nursing care provided during subsequent visits to the health-care provider.
12. Communicate effectively with the patient regarding domestic violence.
13. Discuss the monitoring of fetal growth and development.

REAL-WORLD CASE STUDY

Jean

■ Jean is 40 years old. She arrives for her first prenatal visit with the obstetrician. This is her sixth pregnancy and thinks she is 6 weeks gestation. Her past medical history reveals that she had a therapeutic abortion at age 15 and one spontaneous abortion at 22 years old. She has three living children, aged 15, 12, and 8 at home. Her last child was born at 32 weeks gestation and spent 2 weeks in the hospital neonatal intensive care unit.

continued on page 54

KEY TERMS

amniocentesis
antepartal
bimanual exam
diagonal conjugate
gravida
ischial tuberosity diameter
lithotomy position
Naegele's rule
obstetric conjugate
papanicolaou (Pap) test
para
viability

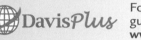 **DavisPlus** For audio pronunciation guide, visit www.DavisPlus.com

CHAPTER CONCEPTS

Assessment
Pregnancy
Promoting Health
Violence

Questions

1. What is Jean's GTPAL?
2. What would be the frequency of prenatal visits for Jean?
3. What screening tests for fetal health would be recommended for Jean?

CONCEPTUAL CORNERSTONE

Change

A common feature of everyone's life is change. A human undergoes change that begins with conception and ends with death. The concept of development refers to the physical and psychological changes that occur over the lifespan. Several theorists, such as Freud, Erikson, Piaget, and Kohlberg, have developed theories of human development. The common theme of their research is that humans move through physical and psychological development in a predictable way. Developmental milestones are tasks that are completed at a certain age range. Some psychological changes occur due to developmental crises, such as pregnancy. To provide patient-centered care, a nurse must be able to assess the patient's developmental level and provide appropriate care for that level (Giddens, 2013).

For a pregnant woman, the **antepartal** period begins with conception and ends with the onset of labor. As she begins her prenatal care, the nurse frequently answers questions and provides support to the pregnant woman. The nurse should have an understanding of the elements of antepartum assessment and the usual plan of care to promote a healthy pregnancy. Assessment involves history, examination, and diagnostic testing. This chapter discusses the selection of a health-care provider, the initial prenatal interview and examination with the health-care provider, and subsequent prenatal care. Commonly used laboratory tests and screening tests for health of the mother and fetus are also covered.

INITIAL PRENATAL ASSESSMENT

The initial prenatal assessment begins with the woman's suspicions of pregnancy, such as a missed menstrual period and other physical signs. This section discusses the diagnosis of pregnancy, the selection of a health-care provider, terminology specific to pregnancy, and the components of a prenatal history.

Diagnosis of Pregnancy

The diagnosis of pregnancy can be made by several methods. Amenorrhea, which is the absence of a menstrual period, is usually the first sign that a woman notices. Amenorrhea can be caused by other medical reasons such as thyroid abnormalities, poor nutrition, hormonal imbalances, anorexia, obesity, fad diets, stress, medications, and viral infections.

- *Pregnancy Testing of Human Chorionic Gonadotropin (hCG) Levels*: this can be done at home. This hormone is produced by the trophoblast after conception. This is the first hormone to rise with pregnancy. There are at least 25 home pregnancy tests marketed in the United States. The test is generally used in the week after the missed menstrual period. Urine hCG is variable at that time but can be detected with a home test (Shields, 2012).

PATIENT TEACHING GUIDELINES

How to Use a Home Pregnancy Test

- Purchase a home pregnancy test kit. The store brand kits are produced at the same place as the more expensive kits are manufactured and they will generate reliable results. Check the expiration date on the box.
- The test measures the levels of the hormone hCG in the urine. Drinking too much water prior to the test may dilute the urine too much for a clear result.
- Most brands of kits suggest waiting at least 1 day after a missed menstrual period, but 1 week is considered best.
- Read the instructions carefully. Each test is specific for method of collecting urine, the length of time of the test, and the symbols used to indicate positive or negative.
- Allow time and reduce distractions so that you can perform the test correctly.
- Wash your hands with soap and water, and then remove the testing stick from the wrapper.
- Urinate in the cup provided or directly on the test stick. Try to obtain a midstream specimen, which means urinate a little into the toilet, and then catch the rest in the cup or directly on the test stick.
- For the plastic cup method, a dropper is used to place urine on the test stick.
- Wait the stated amount of time.
- Check the results. The symbols used to indicate pregnancy vary among brands. If unsure of the interpretation, re-read the instructions.

- *Abdominal ultrasonography*: this may be done to confirm pregnancy at 6 to 8 weeks gestation It may also be done at 18 to 20 weeks and again later in the pregnancy to confirm the age of the fetus and to monitor for any problems with the internal organs and body systems. Ultrasound waves create a picture of the fetus on a monitor. The mother needs to have a full bladder and must be able to lie still for several minutes for the exam.
- *Transvaginal ultrasonography* (*TVUS*): this method can detect a pregnancy at 4 to 5 weeks gestation, which is 1 week sooner than traditional abdominal ultrasonography. With TVUS, the patient is not required to have a full bladder or endure uncomfortable abdominal pressure on

the abdominal wall (Shields, 2012). Some women may object to insertion of the vaginal probe.

Pregnancy Terminology

The terms *gravida* and *para* are used to describe pregnancies, not the number of fetuses. **Gravida** refers to the number of times a woman has been pregnant. For example, a woman pregnant for the second time is a gravida 2. **Para** refers to a woman who has produced a viable infant regardless of whether the fetus was alive at birth. **Viability** is defined as a newborn weighing at least 500 g or greater than 20 weeks gestation.

A multiple birth is considered to be a single parous experience (Venes, 2013). The gravida and para system does not provide enough detail regarding the pregnancy and childbirth experience. Most health-care providers use the GTPAL acronym to give data that are more comprehensive in order to provide appropriate care:

- G: the number pregnancies regardless of the outcome or number of fetuses (G represents **gravida**).
- T: the number of **term** infants born at 37 weeks gestation and beyond.
- P: the number of **preterm** infants born after 20 weeks gestation and before 37 weeks gestation.
- A: the number of pregnancies that ended in a spontaneous or therapeutic **abortion**.
- L: the number of **living** children.

For example, Maria is pregnant for the third time and she had a spontaneous abortion 2 years ago. She has a 5-year-old daughter who was born at 39 weeks gestation. Maria's GTPAL is G3, T1, P0, A1, and L1.

Selection of a Health-care Provider

There are options available for the pregnant woman as she selects a health-care provider to give medical care during her pregnancy and birth.

- *Family physicians*: provide health care for the complete life span. Their medical education qualifies family physicians to manage most uncomplicated pregnancies, including minor surgical procedures for vaginal delivery. Some family physicians perform Cesarean sections, but may need to refer a patient to an obstetrician for that procedure.
- *Obstetrician-gynecologists (OB-GYNs)*: provide health care for all phases of pregnancy, from preconception planning to postpartum recovery. Women with pre-existing medical conditions or at risk to develop complications, such as diabetes or pre-eclampsia, should select an OB-GYN.
- *Certified nurse midwives (CNMs)*: provide preconception, maternity, and postpartum care for women at low risk of complications during pregnancy. Midwives generally offer a low-technology approach to the birthing process. Midwives cannot perform Cesarean sections and will need to transfer care to an OB-GYN if complications occur.

Determining the Estimated Date of Delivery

Most women do not deliver on their due date. However, the establishment of a due date or the estimated date of delivery (EDD) is important. It allows the health-care provider to monitor the growth and progress of the pregnancy. The method for determining the EDD is based on **Naegele's rule**. The formula is to subtract 3 months from the first day of the last menstrual period and then add 7 days, which will indicate the approximate date of delivery (Venes, 2013).

For example, if the first day of the woman's last menstrual period was January 1, subtracting 3 months is equal to October 1. Next, add 7 days. The EDD would be October 8.

A pregnancy wheel can also be used to determine the estimated due date or date of delivery. The wheel is based on Naegele's rule. The pregnancy wheel works by adding 40 weeks to the date of the last menstrual period. It provides approximate conception date, gestation week, and due date (Fig. 5.1).

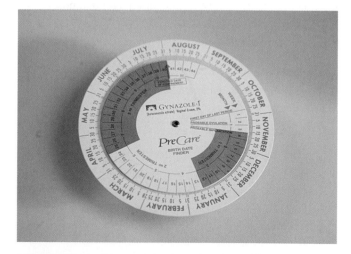

FIGURE 5.1 A gestation wheel is a handy tool for determining the gestational age. The arrow labeled "first day of LMP" is placed on the date of the last menstrual period (LMP). The date at the arrow labeled "expected delivery" is then noted.

- Obtain a thorough past medical history and current health history to detect any potential problems.
- Encourage the woman to ask questions.
- Answer all questions honestly.
- Encourage the patient to obtain all laboratory tests ordered by the health-care provider.
- Stress the importance of subsequent prenatal visits and care throughout the pregnancy.

Initial Client History

To provide patient-centered care, thorough past medical history, family history, and gynecological and obstetrical histories are very important to obtain. The information in Table 5.1 should be obtained by the health-care provider.

THERAPEUTIC COMMUNICATION

When interviewing a patient for her prenatal visits, remember these points for effective communication:

- Avoid the initial discussion of the patient's gravida or para in front of her partner or family.
- Always provide privacy. The patient may not feel comfortable discussing any health issues with her family, friends, spouse, or a partner who are listening.
- Avoid judgmental comments or behaviors when the patient shares past medical history and obstetrical history.
- Be an active listener in order to recognize patient concerns and educational needs.

CULTURAL CONSIDERATIONS

Cultural questions regarding health care and health beliefs should be part of the initial history for a patient. Every person is an individual and it is important to avoid stereotyping a patient based on her race or ethnicity. However, when a caring nurse asks pertinent questions about the patient's cultural background, it may provide valuable information about how cultural, behavioral, and medical factors may influence a pregnant woman's health (American College of Obstetricians and Gynecologists, 2005).

DRUG FACTS

When interviewing the patient for past and current medical history, it is important to develop a list of medications that she is currently taking. Some medications pose a hazard to the fetus and should be reported to the health-care provider as soon as possible. The woman should be provided with a list of safe or acceptable over-the-counter medications during pregnancy.

PRENATAL ASSESSMENT AND CARE

A woman should schedule her first prenatal visit as soon as she knows she is pregnant. The first prenatal visit is important as it is a time for the health-care provider to determine a baseline of the woman's overall health and identify any potential problems that may influence the course of the pregnancy. Laboratory and diagnostic tests will be ordered to obtain a baseline and identify health problems. The woman will also be advised of the need for subsequent visits to monitor her pregnancy for potential complications and to monitor the health of the fetus until labor begins.

Initial Prenatal Assessment

After a detailed health history is obtained, the health-care provider will proceed to a thorough physical examination. During the physical examination, the woman should be provided with privacy and should be made comfortable, both physically and psychologically. Rapport should be established that allows her to ask questions and verbalize any concerns during the examination.

Physical Exam

During the initial visit, the health-care provider should perform a head-to-toe physical examination that covers all major systems. The exam will provide the health-care provider with information regarding current overall health.

In addition to the complete physical examination, a pelvic examination is performed. The patient is draped and placed in the **lithotomy position**. In this position the patient lies on her back, thighs flexed on the abdomen, legs on thighs, thighs abducted (Venes, 2013). This position allows the health care provider a clear view of the external and internal genitalia.

Information obtained during a pelvic examination includes an examination of the external genitalia to detect lesions or discharge. A culture for sexual transmitted infections (STIs) may be done at this time.

Examination of the internal genitalia is done with a vaginal speculum to observe the cervix for the signs of pregnancy (Fig. 5.2). A **Papanicolaou (Pap) test** may be obtained. The Pap test is used to detect cervical cancer. After the speculum is removed, the examiner will perform a **bimanual exam** of the uterus to determine size. During the bimanual exam, the health-care provider places the gloved middle and index fingers into the vagina to identify the cervix. Then the examiner places the other hand midway between the umbilicus and the symphysis pubis and presses downward toward the pelvic hand. Using the fingers, the examiner palpates for the uterine fundus to determine size, position, tenderness, and consistency. The ovaries are also palpated for size, position, and tenderness (Fig. 5.3).

The pelvic bones are assessed to determine size and adequacy for a vaginal birth. The pelvic assessment measurements are featured in Figure 5.4.

- **Diagonal conjugate**: the distance from the lower posterior border of the symphysis pubis to the sacral promontory.

TABLE 5.1 INITIAL CLIENT HISTORY

Personal Information	Past Medical History	Family History	Cultural, Religious, and Spiritual History	Gynecological and Obstetrical History	Partner's History	Current Medical History	Current Pregnancy
• Age • Relationship status • Support systems • Race or ethnic background • Occupation • Economic level • Educational level • Any history of emotional or physical abuse in her current relationship. Does the patient feel safe in her current living situation?	• Surgical procedures • Hospitalizations • Childhood diseases	• Occurrence of multiple births • History of birth defects • History of chromosomal abnormalities, such as Down's syndrome. • History of diabetes, hypertension, cardiovascular, bleeding disorders, thyroid, respiratory, or renal diseases. • Causes of death of deceased parents or siblings. • History of genetic disorders, such as cystic fibrosis or sickle cell disease.	• Any religious or spiritual beliefs that may influence the acceptance of medical treatment or care • Determine whether the patient or family have any attitudes about the sex of the fetus. • Cultural preferences that may influence obstetrical care and the childbirth experience • Would the patient prefer a religious preference on the char?.	• Age of menses onset • Menstrual cycle: frequency and duration of menstrual flow • History of dysmenorrhea • History of infertility and any fertility treatment • Previous STIs • Date of last Pap test • Contraception history • No. of past pregnancies • No. of spontaneous or elective abortions • No. of living children • Loss of a child (miscarriage, SIDS, accident, relinquishment) • Complications with previous pregnancy or childbirth • Prenatal education	• Age • Use of alcohol, tobacco, illicit drug use • Occupation • Blood type and Rh • Thoughts and feelings about the pregnancy	• Height, weight, and current BMI • Blood type and Rh if known • Current medications • Allergies to foods or medications • Chronic diseases such as diabetes, hypertension, cardiovascular, bleeding disorders, thyroid, respiratory, or renal. • Illicit drug use • Tobacco use • Alcohol use • Immunization record, especially rubella. • History of mental health problems, such as depression and anxiety	• First day of last menstrual period (LMP) • Planned or unplanned pregnancy? • Results of pregnancy tests, if completed • Thoughts and feelings about the pregnancy • Any pregnancy discomforts noted • Any personal preferences regarding the birth • Any educational needs regarding pregnancy and childbirth

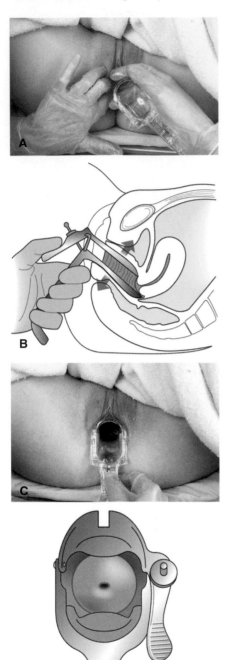

FIGURE 5.2 Pelvic exam. *A,* Inserting the speculum. *B,* Proper position of speculum in the vagina. *C,* Opening the speculum. *D,* View through the speculum.

- **Obstetric conjugate**: this diameter extends from the sacral promontory to the upper inner border of the symphysis pubis and measures ~ 11 cm. It is the most important of the pelvic measurements, because it is the first boney strait through which the fetus has to pass during the birth process.
- **Ischial tuberosity diameter**: the smallest dimension of the pelvis. It should be at least 10 cm to allow the fetus' head to pass through the pelvis. The examiner will note whether the ischial spines are blunt or prominent.

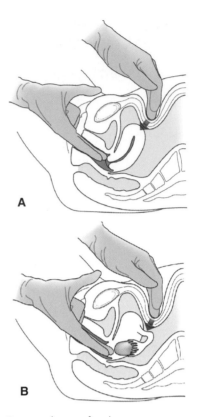

FIGURE 5.3 Bimanual exam for determining uterine size, position, tenderness, and consistency. *A,* Palpating the uterus. *B,* Palpating the ovaries.

Laboratory Tests

The National Institutes of Health (2013) recommend the following laboratory testing for all pregnant women:

- **Complete blood count (CBC)** to determine overall health and to detect anemias.
- **Antibody screen** to determine whether the mother has been exposed to fetal blood.
- **Blood typing and Rh** to identify which blood type: A, B, AB, or O, and Rh status
- **Rubella titer** to determine whether patient has immunity or will need the immunization after giving birth.
- **Varicella titer** to determine immunity to varicella or need to vaccinate after childbirth.
- **Hepatitis B** to determine presence of the antigen and to detect infection.
- **HIV** and **STI screen** to detect HIV status and any sexually transmitted diseases that may require treatment.
- **Pap test** for detecting cervical cancer.
- **Urinalysis** to detect bacteria, ketones, glucose, and protein in the urine.
- **Glucose challenge test** to screen for gestational diabetes. It is usually done between 24 and 28 weeks gestation unless the mother is high risk for diabetes. If she is high risk, the test is usually ordered by the health-care provider to be done after the initial prenatal visit. For the 1-hour test, the patient is given 50 g of oral glucose. After 1 hour, the

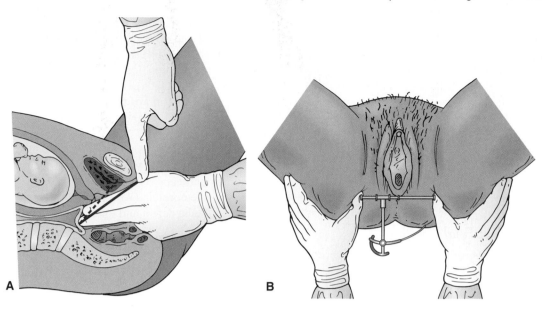

FIGURE 5.4 Pelvic measurements to determine adequacy for vaginal delivery. *A,* The diagonal conjugate and the true conjugate (conjugate vera). *B,* Use of a pelvimeter to measure the ischial tuberosity diameter.

blood glucose level is checked. Normal is less than 140 mg/dL. If greater than 140, a 3-hour screening test is done (Van Leeumen et al., 2011).

SAFETY *STAT!*

Pregnant women are tested for rubella immunity with a rubella titer early in the pregnancy. Rubella is a virus that can cause congenital defects of the heart, hearing, and vision, especially if she contracts the virus during the first trimester. If the pregnant woman is not immune to rubella,

she cannot have the vaccine during pregnancy. Rubella outbreaks have been documented in many countries around the world. A pregnant woman who is not immune should be careful about foreign travel, especially during the first trimester, when the fetus is at the highest risk for problems associated with the virus.

LABS & DIAGNOSTICS

An antibody screen is a test done to find antibodies that attack red blood cells. The most common problems with

NURSING CARE PLAN for Prenatal Care

Nursing Diagnosis: Knowledge deficit regarding pelvic exam and first prenatal visit
Interventions:
- Provide positive feedback to the patient for scheduling the prenatal appointment with the health-care provider.
- Explain the importance of prenatal visits.
- Explain the reason for the pelvic examination.
- Explain to the patient what to expect during the procedure.
- Provide for privacy to answer questions.
- Offer to stay with the patient during the procedure to allay anxiety.

Nursing Diagnosis: Anxiety related to fear of chromosomal abnormalities and birth defects
Interventions:
- Acknowledge her fear and allow her to verbalize concerns.
- Provide information regarding diagnostic tests that can be completed during early pregnancy, such as chorionic villi sampling, nuchal translucency testing, quadruple screen blood test, and amniocentesis.

antibodies are related to the Rhesus (Rh) factor. For example, if an Rh-negative woman is pregnant and the fetus has Rh-positive blood, and if tiny amounts of the fetal blood enters the mother's circulation, her body may make antibodies to attack the red blood cells of the fetus. This is called Rh sensitization. There are other more rare blood factors that can cause problems for the fetus if the mother is sensitized and begins making antibodies. Regardless of the cause, the mother begins making antibodies that destroy red blood cells during future pregnancies. The antibody screen is usually repeated at 28 and 36 weeks gestation.

Screening Tests for Fetal Health

The American Congress of Obstetricians and Gynecologists (ACOG) recommends that all women be offered screening for Down's syndrome, trisomy 13, trisomy 18, and Turner's syndrome. Accurate gestational age should be determined when using these screening methods to increase the reliability of the tests.

• *Chorionic villi sampling* (*CVS*) is done between 11 and 13 weeks gestation. With ultrasound guidance, a thin tube is inserted into the chorionic villi via the cervix or abdomen. Cells are obtained for karyotyping for genetic disorders (Fig. 5.5). Possible complications following CVS are spontaneous abortion and infection.

LABS & DIAGNOSTICS

CVS is considered a safe procedure; however, it is an invasive diagnostic test with potential risks. Spontaneous abortion is the primary risk and it occurs in 1 of every 100 procedures (American Pregnancy Association, 2013). This diagnostic test is not recommended for a woman with an infection, who is pregnant with twins, or who is experiencing vaginal bleeding. Following the procedure, the woman may experience cramping or spotting.

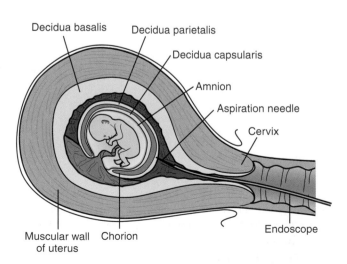

FIGURE 5.5 CVS (chorionic villi sampling) test done for genetic disorders.

• *Nuchal translucency testing* (*NTT*) is performed between 11 and 13 weeks gestation to screen for chromosomal abnormalities. An ultrasound exam is used to measure the translucent area on the back of the fetal neck. Fetuses with genetic disorders often have excessive accumulation of fluid in this area that can be seen by the end of the first trimester (Fetal Medicine Foundation, 2015).

• *Quadruple screen* is performed on the mother's serum between 15 and 20 weeks to detect levels of specific serum markers:
  • Alpha-fetoprotein (AFP): high levels may indicate fetal neural tube defect and lower levels could indicate risk for Down's syndrome or trisomy 18.
  • Human chorionic gonadotropin (hCG): higher levels indicate risk for Down's syndrome.
  • Unconjugated estriol (UE): lower levels indicate a risk for Down's syndrome.
  • Inhibin-A: higher levels indicate a risk for Down's syndrome.

• *Amniocentesis* may be performed to diagnose Down's syndrome, cystic fibrosis, spina bifida, and other genetic disorders. Under ultrasound guidance, a thin needle is used to remove amniotic fluid and cells from the amniotic sac surrounding the fetus. Possible complications after amniocentesis are:
  • Spontaneous abortion
  • Infection
  • Needle injury to the fetus
  • Leaking of amniotic fluid
  • Rh sensitization
  • Infection transmission; if the mother is HIV-positive or has hepatitis C or toxoplasmosis (Fig. 5.6).

SAFETY *STAT!*

Following an amniocentesis, the woman should not leak fluid from the abdominal puncture site. The amniotic sac should seal over after the needle is removed. Instruct the patient to immediately call her health-care provider if she notices any leaking of fluid from the abdominal puncture site. Leaking fluid could lead to infection of the uterus.

Subsequent Prenatal Visits

The pregnant woman will usually visit her health-care provider with the following schedule:

• Monthly for the first 28 weeks gestation
• Every 2 weeks until 36 weeks gestation
• Weekly after 36 weeks until childbirth

Care During Subsequent Prenatal Visits

It is important for the pregnant woman to obtain regular care during her pregnancy in order for the health-care provider to identify complications early and implement

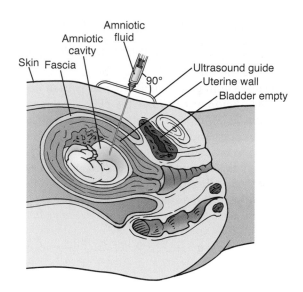

FIGURE 5.6 Amniocentesis testing for genetic disorders.

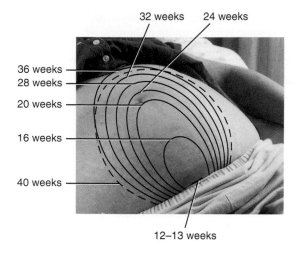

FIGURE 5.7 Fundal height measurements as the pregnancy progresses. Fundal measurement should approximately equal the number of weeks of gestation.

appropriate care. During each visit, the health-care provider and nurse will:

- Evaluate any physical or psychological patient concerns and answer questions.
- Weigh the patient to monitor for appropriate weight gain.
- Monitor vital signs for increasing blood pressure.
- Perform urinalysis to monitor for:
  - Glucose: may indicate gestational diabetes.
  - Ketones: produced when the body is breaking down fat for energy.
  - Protein: may be a sign of pre-eclampsia, kidney damage, or urinary infection.
  - Nitrates: indicates urinary tract infection.
- Measure fundal height:
  - The distance between the top of the pubic bone to the top of the uterus.
  - The fundus reaches the level of the umbilicus at ~20 weeks and measures ~20 cm (Fig. 5.7).
  - Each subsequent visit to the health-care provider should indicate growth of the uterus.

SAFETY *STAT!*

During prenatal visits, the fundal height is measured to determine appropriate fetal growth. The pregnant patient should not be placed flat on her back any longer than necessary to complete an accurate measurement. In the supine position, the large uterus can compress the vena cava and cause a drop in blood pressure and cardiac output. This causes her to feel faint and dizzy. She should be encouraged to lie on her side to prevent supine hypotensive syndrome.

- Monitor fetal heart rate.
  - A handheld device called a Doppler is used to listen to the fetal heart rate (FHR). It may be

heard as early as 8 weeks, but more commonly at 10 to 12 weeks.
- Perform a psychological assessment.
  - Warning Signs:
    - Increasing anxiety about the pregnancy
    - Inappropriate responses or preoccupations about the pregnancy
    - Failure to acknowledge quickening
    - Signs of substance abuse
    - Inability to cope with stress
    - Failure to prepare for the baby, such as preparing clothing and selecting feeding method

 LEARN TO C.U.S.

During a prenatal visit with a Lauren, she acknowledges that she has not prepared any clothes or a crib for her newborn. Lauren "can't decide" whether she wants to bottle feed or breastfeed. The nurse is concerned because this is Lauren's first baby and she is 37 weeks gestation. The nurse discusses her concerns with the obstetrician using the C.U.S. method of communication.

C: "I am **concerned** about Lauren.

U: I am **uncomfortable** because she has not started preparing for the birth of her newborn and she is 37 weeks gestation.

S: We have a possible **safety** issue and a warning sign that she is not coping well with the pregnancy."

- Provide education.
  - Address topics appropriate to gestational age.
  - Include warning signs of pregnancy.
- Screen for domestic violence. Pregnancy often triggers domestic violence or exacerbates the problem (Bacchus et al., 2011).
  - Screening Questions:
    - "Do you feel safe?"
    - "Do you and your partner fight?"

• "Does the fighting become physical?"
• "Have you ever been hit or hurt?"

SAFETY *STAT!*

Warning Signs of Domestic Violence

• Late or absent for prenatal appointments
• Injuries to the face, head, neck, chest, or abdomen
• Vaginal bleeding
• Genitourinary infections
• Signs of anxiety, depression, and self-harm
• Signs of alcohol or substance abuse
• Document all information and report using the established agency policy.

Assessment of Fetal Development

The assessment of fetal development most commonly includes fetal heartbeat and quickening.

• Fetal heartbeat: the ultrasound Doppler is used in the prenatal setting to evaluate the FHR. The normal FHR is 110 to 160 bpm. If unable to hear the FHR by 12 weeks gestation, an ultrasound exam may be completed to evaluate the fetal development.
• Quickening: this is expected between 16 and 22 weeks gestation. A first-time pregnant woman usually notices quickening later than an experienced mother.

Key Points

■ Family practice physicians, obstetricians-gynecologists, and certified nurse midwives can provide prenatal and delivery care for the patient.

■ A complete and thorough past medical history, family history, spiritual history, cultural history, gynecological history, and pregnancy history are required to provide patient-centered care.

■ A complete head-to-toe assessment with a pelvic examination is required to assess the overall health of the mother and the adequacy of the pelvis for childbirth.

■ Laboratory tests, including a CBC, rubella screen, varicella screen, antibody screen, HIV, STI panel, Pap

test, urinalysis, Rh, and blood type, provide baseline information about the patient's health status.

■ Prenatal visits are planned throughout the pregnancy to continually monitor mother and fetal health.

■ The GTPAL system is used to provide data on pregnancy history.

■ Screening tests, such as CVS, NTT, and quadruple screen, are performed for early diagnosis of genetic abnormalities.

■ Domestic violence often begins during pregnancy. Screening questions should be asked at each prenatal visit.

■ Fetal heart rate and quickening are two early assessments of fetal development.

REVIEW QUESTIONS

1. Quickening is usually noticed first:
   1. Between 8 and 12 weeks gestation.
   2. Between 12 and 16 weeks gestation.
   3. Between 16 and 20 weeks gestation.
   4. Between 20 and 24 weeks gestation.

2. A pregnant patient asks why the quadruple screen test is done. The nurse answers that the test is performed:
   1. Between 8 and 12 weeks to detect spina bifida.
   2. Between 8 and 12 weeks to detect cardiac and renal abnormalities.
   3. Between 15 and 20 weeks to detect central nervous system abnormalities.
   4. Between 15 and 20 weeks to detect Down's syndrome or trisomy 18.

3. A pregnant patient 8 weeks gestation is at a prenatal visit. Most likely, if no complications have developed, her next visit would be scheduled in _____ weeks.
   1. 4
   2. 6
   3. 8
   4. 10

4. A urinalysis is performed at each prenatal visit to screen for: (*select all that apply*)
   1. Ketones
   2. Glucose
   3. Bacteria
   4. Protein
   5. Drugs
   6. Anemia

5. Mary, aged 24, is pregnant with her second baby. She is 20 weeks gestation. The nurse is concerned that Mary may be experiencing psychological stress. A sign that she may be experiencing psychological stress could be that:
   1. She has not started preparing the baby's room.
   2. She is excited about her upcoming baby shower.
   3. She frequently misses her prenatal appointments.
   4. She has not selected a name for the baby.

6. The nurse is concerned that a patient may be experiencing domestic violence. Signs of domestic violence include: (*select all that apply*)
   1. Late or absent for prenatal appointments
   2. Signs of injuries to the face, neck, chest, or abdomen
   3. Complaints of backache after working all day
   4. Shortness of breath when climbing stairs
   5. Signs of anxiety and self-harm
   6. Vaginal bleeding

7. The height of the uterine fundus is measured to:
   1. Determine appropriate fetal growth.
   2. Detect genetic abnormalities.
   3. Reassure the mother.
   4. Estimate the date of delivery.

8. What is the frequency of prenatal visits for a pregnant woman at 38 weeks gestation?
   1. Daily
   2. Weekly
   3. Every 2 weeks
   4. Every 3 weeks

9. The health-care provider would be very concerned if a fetal heart rate was not detected with a Doppler at _____ weeks gestation.
   1. 6
   2. 8
   3. 10
   4. 12

CRITICAL THINKING QUESTIONS

1. Martha is 39 years old and pregnant for the first time. She is a type 1 diabetic, takes medication for hypertension, and is very concerned about delivering a healthy baby. Which type of health-care professional would be the best choice to provide prenatal and delivery care for Martha?

2. Jennie, aged 45, is pregnant and 8 weeks gestation. She is concerned about potential genetic problems of the fetus due to her age. Which screening tests would you recommend?

3. Estelle, aged 36, is 32 weeks pregnant with her third child. She works as a hairdresser and stands for long periods of time during her work day. What questions should the nurse or health-care provider ask Estelle about her occupation history to assist her with maintaining a healthy pregnancy?

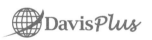

For additional resources and information, visit **www.DavisPlus.com**. Post-Conference Questions and Activities, Answers, and References can be found on Davis*Plus*.

KEY TERMS

chorioretinitis
hydrocephalus
hyperthermia
leukorrhea
morbidity
mortality
neural tube defects
nocturia
oligohydramnios
pica
pneumonitis
polyhydramnios
thrombosis

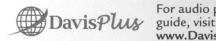 **DavisPlus** For audio pronunciation guide, visit www.DavisPlus.com

CHAPTER CONCEPTS

Infection
Nursing
Nutrition
Promoting Health
Safety

LEARNING OUTCOMES

1. Define the key terms.
2. Provide guidance to the pregnant patient on managing the common discomforts of pregnancy.
3. Promote safe and effective self-care practices during pregnancy.
4. Discuss the nutritional needs of the pregnant patient.
5. Define pica and the dangers for the pregnant patient.
6. Discuss the dangers and prevention of viral infections in pregnancy.
7. Teach the pregnant patient about the recommended weight gain in pregnancy.
8. Plan appropriate prenatal care for the pregnant adolescent.
9. Discuss the additional nutritional needs of the pregnant adolescent.
10. Identify risks for the pregnant patient over the age of 35.
11. Explain the tests used to monitor fetal well-being during the pregnancy.
12. Compare and contrast the Bradley method and Lamaze method of childbirth education.
13. Discuss the components of a birth plan.

REAL-WORLD CASE STUDY

Ruby

■ Ruby is 25 years old at 34 weeks gestation of her first pregnancy. She has experienced no complications with her pregnancy and is in good health. Her pre-pregnancy body mass index (BMI) was 19.0 and she has gained 15 pounds during the pregnancy. She reports an increase in heartburn and states, "I don't even want to eat because I know I will get heartburn afterward. I am also very constipated."

Questions

1. Based on Ruby's BMI of 19.0, has she gained enough weight in the pregnancy?
2. What advice can the nurse give Ruby to manage the heartburn?
3. What advice can the nurse give Ruby to manage the problem of constipation?

CONCEPTUAL CORNERSTONE

Health Promotion

The concept of health promotion can be defined as the improvement of health and the prevention of disease. The focus of health promotion includes nutrition, exercise, hygiene, vaccinations, protection from environmental hazards, avoidance of harmful substances, protection from accidents, and stress reduction. Health promotion usually requires most people to change behaviors, and change is not easy. Pregnant women are usually very motivated to change behaviors to improve their health and to promote a healthy fetus and pregnancy. When providing care, a nurse has many opportunities to teach and support the pregnant patient in health promotion.

The focus of this chapter is on nursing care during pregnancy. The patient will undergo profound changes to her body and will experience discomforts that are a natural part of pregnancy. Nurses caring for pregnant patients need a clear understanding of care that will promote a healthy and safe pregnancy, and that will prepare the woman for her eventual delivery.

FOCUS ON THE PATIENT

Nearly every body system is affected in pregnancy. As hormones change and the fetus grows, she will experience changes in her body that produce physical discomforts. As the pregnancy progresses, the pregnant woman will have questions about maintaining her health, managing the discomforts of pregnancy, self-care, and safety for herself and her fetus.

Relief of Common Discomforts of Pregnancy

The common discomforts of pregnancy are caused by the hormonal and physiological changes of pregnancy. The nurse can provide anticipatory guidance and teaching to provide strategies for managing the common discomforts (Table 6.1).

TABLE 6.1 RELIEVING THE COMMON DISCOMFORTS OF PREGNANCY

Discomfort	Methods of Relief
Nausea and Vomiting	• Eat crackers first thing when arising. • Avoid foods with strong odors. • Consume peppermint candies. • Use relaxation techniques with slow breathing to decrease nausea. • Eat small, frequent meals. • Avoid spicy foods.
Nasal Stuffiness, Discharge, and Obstruction	• Increase fluid intake. • Use nasal saline drops. • Use a humidifier in the home.
Urinary Frequency, Urgency, and **Nocturia** (urination during the night)	• Perform Kegel exercises to improve the muscle tone of the perineum. • Maintain adequate hydration during the day, but decrease fluids 2 hr before bedtime.
Increased **Leukorrhea** (vaginal discharge)	• Avoid tight-fitting clothing. • Wear cotton underwear. • Wear a pad or panty-liner to absorb moisture. • Perform daily perineal hygiene to prevent infection.
Increased Fatigue	• Schedule rest periods throughout the day. • Maintain a regular consistent bedtime with adequate sleep.
Heartburn	• Avoid overeating and eat small, frequent meals. • Do not eat less than 3 hr before bedtime. • Avoid spicy and greasy foods. • Elevate the head with an extra pillow at night. • Consume milk products, as doing so may be helpful.
Constipation	• Increase fluid intake. • Increase fiber intake to 35 g per day. • Exercise daily. • Use only bulk-forming laxatives or mineral oil after increasing fluids, fiber, and exercise.

Continued

TABLE **6.1**   **RELIEVING THE COMMON DISCOMFORTS OF PREGNANCY**—cont'd

Discomfort	Methods of Relief
Hemorrhoids	• Avoid straining at defecation. • Increase fluid intake. • Increase fiber intake. • Avoid standing for long periods of time.
Backache	• Maintain good posture. • Use correct body mechanics when lifting: bend at the knees, not the waist. • Wear low-heeled shoes. • Support the uterus with a pillow underneath when lying on the side to sleep.
Leg Cramps	• Avoid constrictive clothing. • Elevate the legs periodically. • Dorsiflex the foot to stop the cramp. • Include adequate amounts of calcium and phosphorus in the diet. (Youngkin and Davis, 2004)
Shortness of Breath	• Avoid constrictive clothing. • Sleep with an extra pillow to elevate the head. • Allow extra time for stair climbing and walking.
Ankle Edema	• Elevate the legs periodically to increase venous return. • Rest in a side-lying position to promote placental circulation and to increase venous return.
Round Ligament Pain	• Support the uterus with a pillow or pregnancy support garment. • Take a warm bath. • Apply warmth to the ligament area. • Avoid standing for long periods of time.

 DRUG FACTS

Many pregnant women experience nasal stuffiness and congestion. Nasal decongestants are contraindicated in pregnancy. Some women may purchase nasal decongestants for short-term use. The prolonged use of nasal decongestants can cause rebound congestion. The nasal congestion worsens and the intervals between uses of the decongestant must be shortened. Decongestants can cause vasoconstriction of the uterine arteries, which reduces the fetal blood supply. Teach the pregnant woman to manage the problem by using nonpharmacologic methods of reducing nasal congestion, such as saline nasal spray and humidification.

SAFETY *STAT!*

Remind the patient that over-the-counter medications, for example, omeprazole, are category C medications, which are not safe for pregnancy.

PROMOTION OF SELF-CARE DURING PREGNANCY

Self-care is personal, medical care performed voluntarily by the patient. Most pregnant women are motivated to learn about self-care and learn about it through reading books and Internet searches. Some of the information may be helpful and some may be inaccurate. For the pregnant woman, the nurse can support self-care with accurate information. Self-care during pregnancy instruction empowers her to make healthy lifestyle choices in order to maintain or improve her health and the health of her fetus.

Personal Hygiene

An increase in vaginal discharge and perspiration during pregnancy makes personal hygiene very important. Showers are safe throughout pregnancy. Tub baths are permitted throughout pregnancy except after the amniotic membranes rupture. It is important to remember that the pregnant woman should avoid excessively hot showers and baths due to the detrimental effects of **hyperthermia**. Hyperthermia is elevated body heat caused by either fever or artificially with hot tubs, saunas, or sunshine. Hyperthermia has been linked to neural tube defects. **Neural tube defects** affect the spinal cord, spine, or brain.

SAFETY *STAT!*

Women should be cautioned about tub baths during the last trimester. The pregnant woman is at risk for falling and should ask for help when exiting the tub.

Breast Care

A daily shower or bath usually provides for breast cleanliness. During late pregnancy, colostrum may crust on the nipple. Colostrum is a yellowish fluid secreted by the breasts during late pregnancy and precedes the production of milk. It is rich in antibodies and minerals. It can be removed with a washcloth and warm water. The pregnant woman should avoid the excessive use of strong soaps on the nipple because of its drying effect.

During pregnancy, breast support is necessary. Support of the breasts prevents back strain and retains breast shape. Whether she plans to breastfeed or bottle feed, support from a well-fitting bra is essential. Tips for bra selection include:

• The breast tissue should fit entirely inside the cup.
• The straps should be wide and not too tight.
• The bra should have sufficient hooks to allow it to expand as needed.

Clothing

Maternity clothing has changed over the years from large, loose clothing that hides the pregnant abdomen to tighter-fitting clothing. Maternity clothing can be expensive and is worn for only a short time. Many women improvise with their pre-pregnant clothes and only buy a few essential items. The most important points to remember are comfort and safety. The clothes need to be loose enough to allow for movement and circulation. High-heeled shoes are not recommended due to the potential for falls as the abdomen expands and the pregnant woman's center of gravity shifts.

Exercise

According to the American Pregnancy Association guidelines (2013), 30 minutes of exercise per day is recommended for pregnant women (Fig. 6.1). Table 6.2 provides information about the benefits of exercise, forms of safe exercise, forms of exercise that are not appropriate during pregnancy, and safety tips for exercising during pregnancy.

PATIENT TEACHING GUIDELINES

Patient Exercise
Teach patients to stop exercising if they feel the following warning signs:
• Dizziness or feeling faint
• Fluid leaking from the vagina

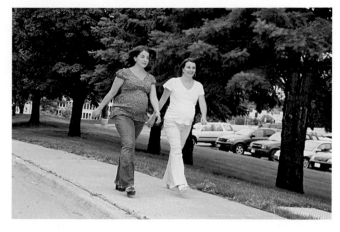

FIGURE 6.1 Exercise during pregnancy has many benefits and enhances the woman's sense of well-being.

TABLE 6.2 EXERCISING DURING PREGNANCY

Benefits of Exercise	• Reduction of backaches and constipation • Potential prevention of gestational diabetes • Improved muscle tone, strength, and endurance • Improvement in sleep
Forms of Safe Exercise	• Walking • Swimming • Cycling • Aerobics • Running, if the pregnant woman was a runner before pregnancy
Forms of Exercise Not Appropriate During Pregnancy	• Skiing, gymnastics, and other sports that include a risk of falling • Contact sports such as hockey, basketball, and soccer • Scuba diving as decompression sickness can affect the fetus
Safety Tips for Exercising During Pregnancy	• Maintaining adequate hydration • Avoiding overheating • Wearing a supportive bra and well-fitting shoes • After the first trimester, avoid exercising on the back; the supine position restricts blood flow, causing vena cava syndrome

- Vaginal bleeding
- Chest pain
- Headache
- Increased shortness of breath
- Decreased fetal movement

SAFETY *STAT!*

Many women practice yoga as exercise. Many health clubs offer prenatal yoga classes.

Yoga can be continued throughout the pregnancy with some modifications to promote a safe pregnancy.

- Increased body heat is never recommended during pregnancy. Avoid "hot yoga" classes.
- Avoid yoga poses that involve lying flat on the stomach or back.
- Avoid poses that involve twisting, hopping, and jumping.
- Maintain adequate hydration during exercise.

Sleep and Rest

Pregnant women experience fatigue and will need more rest; fatigue increases as the fetus gets larger. She should incorporate rest periods into her day to decrease fatigue and allow for 8 hours of sleep at night. At times, sleep may be difficult due to backaches and the growing fetus. She may need to use additional pillows to support her uterus and take the strain off the lower back when lying down.

Employment

According to the American Congress of Obstetricians and Gynecologists (2012) and the Centers for Disease Control and Prevention (CDC, 2014), pregnant women without complications can continue to work throughout the pregnancy. Hazards to fetal well-being need to be considered when the pregnant woman is employed outside the home. Prolonged standing may increase maternal fatigue. The pregnant woman should contact her industry nurse for information about environmental hazards and research environmental hazards related to her employment.

Seatbelts

Seatbelts should be worn to protect the mother and the fetus. It should be placed low, across the abdomen and across the hipbones. The shoulder strap should be placed between the breasts and over the clavicle (Fig. 6.2). Pregnant women should try to keep the abdomen 10 in. from the air bag (IIHS, 2013).

Travel Restrictions

The second trimester is considered to be the safest time to travel. Prolonged sitting during pregnancy increases the risk of venous stasis, which leads to thrombosis. **Thrombosis** is a blood clot, usually in the lower extremities, that restricts blood flow. Ambulation every 2 hours will help to decrease the risk of developing a venous thrombus.

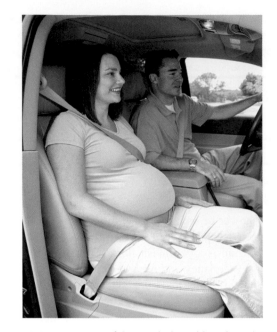

FIGURE 6.2 Proper use of the seatbelt and headrest during pregnancy.

Air travel can cause dehydration due to low oxygen tension, low humidity, and recirculated air. Drinking water and avoiding caffeine are important to prevent dehydration when traveling.

Dental Care

Overall, good health includes sufficient dental care. During pregnancy, the gums are commonly edematous and may bleed easily because of the effects of hormones and increased blood supply. If treatment for cavities or infection is required, the dentist should be informed of the pregnancy. X-rays should be done only if necessary, with appropriate abdominal shielding utilized to protect the fetus.

Sexual Activity

Sexual intercourse during pregnancy is safe unless the amniotic membrane has ruptured or vaginal bleeding is occurring. The American College of Obstetricians and Gynecologist (ACOG, 2013) states that sexual activity during pregnancy is safe for most women unless there is a specific contraindication. The women should limit or avoid sex if she has preterm labor, more than one miscarriage, placenta previa, infection, bleeding, and/or breaking of the amniotic membranes. ACOG recommends that the couple try different positions for comfort as the pregnancy advances.

THERAPEUTIC COMMUNICATION

A patient may feel uncomfortable asking questions of a personal nature about sexual activity during pregnancy. The pregnant couple usually has concerns and needs education regarding safe sexuality in pregnancy. The nurse needs to initiate the conversation with open-ended questions and use a matter-of-fact approach such as "Your body is going through many changes right now. Some of the changes can affect your sexual activity. What questions do have about that?"

PATIENT TEACHING GUIDELINES

Pregnancy Warning Signs

These warning signs must be reported to the health-care provider:

- Abdominal pain
- Vaginal bleeding
- Infection
- Severe headaches
- Swelling of the hands and face
- Premature rupture of membranes
- Preterm labor
- Absence of fetal movement

AVOIDING VIRAL INFECTIONS

Viral infections in pregnancy are major causes of maternal and fetal morbidity and mortality. The medical definition of **morbidity** is a disease state and **mortality** refers to death (Venes, 2013). The usual way that the fetus is infected is by transmission through the placenta when the virus circulates through the maternal blood. Infections known to cause congenital defects (present at birth) have been described with the acronym TORCH (toxoplasma, others, rubella, cytomegalovirus, and herpes). Other viruses include those known to cause congenital infections. The additional viruses are parvovirus B19, varicella-zoster virus (VZV), measles virus, and HIV. Evidence such as physical signs and symptoms of viral disease may be apparent in the newborn at birth or may not be evident until years later.

HEALTH PROMOTION

Prevention of viral infections in pregnancy is important. Some general instructions for the pregnant woman to prevent viral infections should include:

- Practice good hand washing techniques.
- Avoid young children with colds and infections.
- Avoid raw or undercooked meat.
- Avoid cleaning the cat litter box.
- Avoid yard work that may cause exposure to cat feces.
- Avoid sharing drinks and eating utensils with small children.
- Make sure vaccinations are current before becoming pregnant again.
- Get a yearly flu vaccine.

Toxoplasmosis

Toxoplasmosis is frequently acquired by eating raw meat or through exposure to cat feces. The symptoms are vague and the pregnant woman may experience body aches, headache, fatigue, and a sore throat. When the woman becomes infected, the parasite invades the placenta and the fetus is infected for life. The disease is transmitted more frequently during the third trimester. The signs of infection may not be present at birth, but 70% to 90% of those infected will develop clinical illness by young adulthood (Mariano, 2012). Infected infants develop **chorioretinitis,** inflammation of the choroid and retina of the eye that can lead to blindness, obstructive hydrocephalus, mental retardation, seizures, motor delays, and developmental delays.

Patient Teaching:
- Avoid raw or undercooked meat.
- Avoid cleaning the cat litter box.
- Avoid yard work that may cause exposure to cat feces.

Cytomegalovirus

Cytomegalovirus (CMV) is a herpes virus that is acquired through intimate contact with saliva, urine, and other body fluids. It can be acquired through sexual contact, organ transplantation, transmission through the placenta, and breast milk. Maternal CMV infection may cause no symptoms or may be noticeable by fever, mild depression, and muscle aches. Infection of the fetus can cause intrauterine growth retardation, hearing loss, vision loss, microencephaly (small brain), and **hydrocephalus** (increased fluid in the brain), and delayed motor development. The most important risk factor for CMV infection for the pregnant woman is exposure to young children. Approximately 20% of young children shed CMV in their saliva or urine even if they never had symptoms (Cannon, 2010).

Patient Teaching:
- Use good hand washing technique after changing diapers or wiping children's noses.
- Do not share food, drinks, or eating utensils with young children.

Herpes Simplex Virus

Infection with herpes simplex virus (HSV) is one of the most common sexually transmitted infections. Symptoms of herpes simplex virus typically appear as a blister or as multiple blisters on or around affected areas such as the mouth, genitals, or rectum. The greatest risk is to the fetus if the mother becomes initially infected with HSV during the third trimester. Neonatal herpes infection occurs more frequently in babies from mothers who acquired HSV during the pregnancy (Straface et al., 2012). Most neonatal infections result from exposure to genital HSV during the delivery. Most obstetricians will schedule a Cesarean birth if the woman has a history of frequent outbreaks of herpes or an active case at the due date. The newborn infected with HSV may have skin, eye, or mouth lesions, encephalitis, or dysfunctions of the liver, lungs, central nervous system, and brain (Straface et al., 2012).

Patient Teaching
- Inform the health-care provider of any past history of herpes outbreaks.
- Inform the health-care provider of any new herpes outbreaks during the pregnancy so that antiviral therapy can be started.
- Practice safe sex with a new partner by using condoms and avoiding sexual contact with anyone with an open sore on the genitals.

Rubella

Rubella is very dangerous to the developing fetus. It is spread by airborne secretions. Signs and symptoms of maternal infection are a rash starting on the face or neck, enlarged lymph nodes, joint pain, fever, and cough. The fetus is infected through placental transmission, and the most dangerous time for the fetus is the first 12 weeks of the pregnancy. Congenital rubella syndrome is associated with four common abnormalities: deafness, central nervous system abnormalities, eye defects, and cardiac malformations.

Patient Teaching:
- Know your immunization history.
- Avoid exposure to young children, especially during the first trimester.
- Report any rash or illness to the health-care provider.
- Obtain the rubella vaccine after delivery.

Parvovirus B19

Parvovirus B19 (B19V) is the virus that causes erythema infectiosum, also known as fifth disease. Fifth disease is a childhood disease characterized by the "slapped face" rash that appears along with a fever. It is transmitted by the respiratory route, through blood products, and by placenta transmission during pregnancy. Approximately 40% of pregnant women do not have antibodies for this virus and are at risk for infection (Marino, 2012). If the pregnant woman acquires the virus, it is often asymptomatic. This is a disease that causes the fetus to have anemia and be unable to manage fluid. The fluid builds up in the fetal lungs or heart. The neonate may be born with liver swelling, heart failure, jaundice, and edema of the body.

Patient Teaching:
- Avoid young children exhibiting viral symptoms, such as a fever or rash.
- Practice frequent hand washing.
- There is no vaccine available for prevention.

Varicella-Zoster Virus

Primary varicella infection, also known as *chickenpox*, is considered a medical emergency during pregnancy. Varicella-zoster virus (VZV) is transmitted as an airborne virus. It causes fever, anorexia, and itchy vesicles. The person is contagious until the last vesicle crusts over. **Pneumonitis**, which is inflammation of the lungs, is a complication that is likely to occur with the adult pregnant patient. The risk for life-threatening respiratory complications is significant (Marino, 2012). If the fetus acquires the virus, it can result in spontaneous abortion, chorioretinitis, cataracts, limb malformations, and brain dysfunctions.

Patient Teaching:
- Avoid any person known to have the disease.
- Follow vaccination guidelines for children in the home.
- Obtain the vaccine after delivery to provide protection for subsequent pregnancies.

Measles Virus

Measles, also known as *rubeola*, can have severe consequences for the pregnant woman. It is transmitted by the airborne route of coughing and sneezing. The symptoms are fever, cough, conjunctivitis, and rash. Pregnant women are also at risk to develop pneumonitis with this disease. Most pregnant women have been vaccinated. However, measles are not eradicated worldwide and visitors to the United States can bring the virus. Travel outside of North America can also increase the risk of exposure to measles (CDC, 2013). Rubeola is not known to cause specific birth defects but has been associated with spontaneous abortion, premature labor, and low birth weight (Mariano, 2012).

Patient Teaching:
- When planning travel during pregnancy, be aware that measles are a common disease of Europe, Asia, Africa, and the Pacific.
- Avoid any person known to have the disease.
- Follow vaccination guidelines for children.
- Obtain the vaccine after delivery to provide protection for subsequent pregnancies.

HIV

According to The Joint United Nations Programme on HIV/AIDS (2013), there were an estimated 35.3 million people living in the world with HIV in 2012. Most countries have placed an emphasis on prenatal treatment to prevent mother-to-fetus transmission with 900,000 pregnant women receiving antiretroviral treatment.

Approximately 30% of women in the United States are not tested for HIV during pregnancy (Mariano, 2012). The CDC recommends routine third trimester screening for women with high-risk behaviors or who have symptoms of the disease.

Before becoming pregnant, women diagnosed with HIV should be counseled about the ability to decrease mother-to-fetus transmission with highly active antiretroviral therapy (HAART). The risk of transmission to the fetus is linked to viral load, which is the amount of active virus in the system. Zidovudine (ZVD) is the most common medication used to reduce viral load. This drug also crosses the placenta and provides fetal prophylaxis. Antiretroviral therapy has not been shown to cause any negative effects on pregnancy and should be started as early as possible during the pregnancy to reduce the risk of transmission to the fetus to less than 2% (Mariano, 2012).

Patient Teaching
- Notify the health-care provider if HIV-positive.
- Consider HIV testing.
- Take all antiretroviral medications as prescribed.
- Avoid a high-risk lifestyle, such as IV drug use, and practice safe sex with untested partners.

LABS & DIAGNOSTICS

Types of HIV Tests
- Antibody tests look for HIV antibodies in the patient's blood:
  - Enzyme immunoassay (EIA) tests use blood, saliva, or urine to detect HIV antibodies. Results can take up to 2 weeks.
  - Rapid HIV antibody tests also use blood, saliva, or urine to detect HIV antibodies. These results take 10 to 20 minutes.
  - A positive result from either test requires a follow-up test called a Western blot to confirm the result.
- Antigen tests require a blood sample and detect HIV earlier than an antibody test.
- The PCR test detects the genetic material of the HIV and identifies HIV in the blood within 2 to 3 weeks of infection. Babies born to HIV-infected mothers are tested using this method because the baby may have the HIV antibodies from the mother for several months and would test positive on a standard antibody test (AIDS.gov, 2013).

NUTRITION IN PREGNANCY

Healthy eating in pregnancy enables optimal weight gain for the fetus and reduces complications. The requirement for many nutrients is increased; the mother should take a multivitamin with iron during the pregnancy. During pregnancy, the basic principles of healthy eating remain the same. There are a few nutrients in pregnancy that the woman may want to pay special attention to when choosing foods. General guidelines for nutrition include:

- The pregnant woman should avoid empty calories such as soft drinks, desserts, and fried foods.
- Folate is a B vitamin that helps prevent neural tube defects in the developing fetus. A lack of folic acid in the diet during pregnancy can also increase the risk of low birth weight and preterm delivery. Foods high in folic acid include cereal, beans, spinach, kale, broccoli, romaine, asparagus, and peanuts.
- Calcium and vitamin D are needed for bones and teeth. Dairy products are the best sources of these nutrients.
- Protein is important for fetal growth, especially during the second and third trimesters. Good sources of protein are lean meat, poultry, eggs, dried beans, tofu, dairy products, and peanut butter.
- Iron needs are increased in pregnancy as the woman's blood volume expands to meet the needs of the fetus. Iron is also needed to make hemoglobin, which carries oxygen to the tissues. Good sources of iron include lean red meat, poultry, iron-fortified cereals, green leafy vegetables, and dried fruit.

During early pregnancy, most women experience an increase in appetite with extra caloric needs of 200 kcal/day (Trupin, 2012).

 CULTURAL CONSIDERATIONS
Some Asian and Hispanic cultures practice a system of hot and cold body balance. Pregnancy is considered a "hot" condition. Therefore, foods considered "hot," such as protein, might be restricted. A culturally competent nurse and health-care provider should assess the pregnant woman's diet to determine whether she is obtaining adequate protein to promote fetal growth and development (Galanti, 2015).

Pica

Pica is an eating disorder that can occur with pregnant women. **Pica** is the practice of eating non-nutritive foods. It involves craving followed by the ingestion of nonfood substances. There are three common forms of pica:

- Geophagy: the ingestion of soil, clay, or similar substances.
- Amylophagy: the ingestion of raw starch or similar substances.
- Pagophagy: the ingestion of ice or freezer frost (Hong, 2012).

The cause of pica is not known, but the American Dietetic Association (2013) believes that it is due to an imbalance or deficiency of vitamins or minerals, usually iron.

Common substances craved during pregnancy are dirt, clay, laundry starch, charcoal, ice, toothpaste, coffee grounds, baking soda, and cigarette ashes (American Pregnancy Association, 2013). If the mother eats nonfood substances instead of a healthy diet, it could be harmful to the fetus. It is also possible that the nonfood substances could be toxic or contain parasitic ingredients.

Management of Pica

The nurse or health-care provider should question the woman in a nonjudgmental way about pica practices. She may be embarrassed to admit that she is eating non-nutritive substances. The management of pica practices can include:

- Encouraging her to eat a balanced diet with sufficient iron, vitamins, and minerals.
- Recommending that she select a close friend, family member, or spouse to be her support person that can assist her with avoiding harmful substances.

• Limiting her access to the non-nutritive substances that she is craving.
• Substituting chewing gum or healthy, low-calorie snacks for the substance that she is craving.
• Using distraction, such as taking a walk, calling a friend, or reading a book, until the craving disappears.

Recommended Weight Gain

The American College of Obstetricians and Gynecologists (2013) has developed guidelines for weight gain in pregnancy. Excessive weight gain is associated with an increased risk for gestational diabetes, pregnancy-associated hypertension, and the delivery of infants who are large for their gestational age (Trupin, 2012). The guidelines for weight gain for a woman pregnant with one fetus are:

• BMI less than 18.5 is considered underweight and she should gain 28 to 40 pounds.
• BMI between 18.5 and 24.9 is considered normal weight and she should gain 25 to 35 pounds.
• BMI between 25 and 29.9 is considered overweight and she should gain 15 to 25 pounds.
• BMI greater than 30 is considered obese and she should gain 11 to 20 pounds.

The weight gained in pregnancy is due to changes in the mother's body and the growth of the uterus and fetus. The breakdown for weight gain is:

• Breasts: 1 to 2 pounds
• Blood volume: 3 to 4 pounds
• Fat: 6 to 9 pounds
• Body fluid: 2 to 3 pounds
• Uterus growth: 2 to 3 pounds
• Placenta: 2 to 3 pounds
• Amniotic fluid: 2 to 3 pounds

TEAM WORKS

Providing safe care for the morbidly obese pregnant woman may require a team approach. She is at risk for gestational diabetes, hypertension, and for a Cesarean birth. An appropriate team to provide care for this woman would be an obstetrician, an endocrinologist, a neonatologist, a nurse, a dietician, and a physical therapist to assist with exercise.

CARE OF THE PREGNANT ADOLESCENT

Adolescence is a period of transition between childhood and adulthood. Developmental issues need to be considered when planning care for the pregnant adolescent. When the nurse is working with a pregnant adolescent, keeping in mind the developmental tasks can impact care and compliance with planned prenatal care. Normal adolescent development has

implications for the ways in which teens experience pregnancy and prenatal care.

The emerging ability to think abstractly may enable the teen to see the relationship between her behavior and the health of the fetus. The nurse should use direct concrete communication with the adolescent and provide information about the positive effects of healthy behaviors and fetal health. The adolescent may need more frequent prenatal visits or follow-up phone calls to encourage compliance with physician visits and nutrition guidelines.

Body image is a major issue for the adolescent. She may resist gaining weight, which could lead to complications of the pregnancy. The nurse should stress the relationship between healthy nutrition and exercise with good physical appearance.

Adolescents experience egocentric thinking in which everyone is focused on their behavior or that their feelings, fears, and experiences are unique. She may think that the normal pregnancy discomforts are unique to her situation. Addressing discomforts of pregnancy in a group teaching session may help her to see that pregnancy discomforts are normal and common among pregnant women.

The nurse should remember that the adolescent is establishing emotional independence from her parents and is becoming more emotionally reliant on friends. Peer groups are an important part of her identity. Peers may supply support for pregnancy needs. She may view the pregnancy as a way to strengthen her relationship with the father of the baby. Parents and other family members should be encouraged to allow the pregnant adolescent to take responsibility for her own pregnancy-related care, yet allow her time to be a "regular teenager."

Experimentation with risk-taking behaviors is common in adolescents. The pregnant adolescent may experiment with alcohol or smoking during the pregnancy. The health-care provider and nurse need to be clear on the dangers of risk-taking behaviors and pregnancy.

Nutritional Needs of the Pregnant Adolescent

Adolescents often do not have good eating habits. They enjoy convenience foods and fast food that is high in fat and low in nutritional value. The lifestyle of the adolescent contributes to their poor nutritional status. They often do not like to get up early enough for a healthy breakfast before school, and they may have jobs, extracurricular activities, and prefer to hang out with friends after school and on the weekends. This type of schedule does not leave time for healthy family meals.

Most adolescents who desire to maintain the pregnancy want to have a healthy baby. This goal can be used to assist the adolescent to eat healthy.

Weight gain is a major issue for the pregnant adolescent. She does not like to see the changes in her body and may resist gaining weight. This is detrimental to her own physical growth that is occurring during pregnancy and has a negative impact on the body and brain development of the fetus.

The inadequate consumption of calcium is a problem for the pregnant adolescent. Her own bones are still growing but she loses calcium from her bones to the fetus during the third trimester.

Poor nutrition choices often cause the pregnant adolescent to consume a diet low in iron. This can cause her to feel fatigued, short of breath, and unable to concentrate.

Inadequate weight gain and poor nutritional choices can lead to delivery of a small-for-gestational-age newborn.

Suggestions to improve adolescent nutrition can include:

- Encouraging her to consume a minimum of 2,000 calories per day (Stang & Story, 2012), choosing foods from all food groups.
- Keeping a daily food diary to record or check off protein, vegetables, dairy products, and fruit consumed.
- Replacing soft drinks and juices with milk or yogurt.
- Taking calcium supplements with food to increase absorption.
- Taking iron supplements with water or orange juice between meals to increase absorption.
- Avoiding anemia by eating meat, beans, and dark, leafy green vegetables.
- Avoiding eating too much convenience or fast food.
- Teaching her the healthy food choices available at fast-food restaurants.
- Providing positive reinforcement for healthy food choices.
- Providing a referral to a dietician if needed.

CARE OF THE EXPECTANT COUPLE OLDER THAN AGE 35

Advanced maternal age for childbearing has been traditionally set at 35 years old although the average age for a first pregnancy in the United States has been increasing in recent years (Mathew and Hamilton, 2009). Some of the reasons women delay pregnancy are that they want to be in a stable relationship, they have fertility problems, or they want to be established in their careers. An advanced maternal age for childbearing is seen by health-care professionals to be correlated with poorer outcomes in pregnancy. This may be because of a higher incidence of chronic medical conditions among older women.

Risks for Pregnancy in Patients Older Than Age 35

Women older than age 35 have an increased risk for pregnancy complications. These include the following:

- It may take longer for the woman older than age 35 to conceive. An older woman may not ovulate each month even if she is still having regular menstrual periods.
- Fathers older than age 45 have an increased risk of fathering children with neural tube defects, autism spectrum disorders, schizophrenia, and bipolar disorder (Wiener-Megnazi et al, 2012).
- The chance of having twins increases with age. Assisted reproductive technologies such as in vitro fertilization or fertility medications contribute to the risk of a multiple pregnancy.
- There is an increased risk of miscarriage. This may be because of the higher likelihood of chromosomal abnormalities.
- The risk of chromosome abnormalities is higher due to the aging of the eggs.
- There is a higher risk for complications of pregnancy such as gestational diabetes, placenta previa, and high blood pressure.
- There is an increased risk for developing labor complications that may lead to a Cesarean birth.

Women older than age 35 can have healthy pregnancies. They may be overwhelmed with the information available. The nurse should be sensitive to the feelings and experiences of the older patient to meet her health-care educational needs and to provide emotional support. To improve pregnancy outcomes, a patient at an advanced maternal age should:

- Meet with a health-care provider for preconception counseling, especially if the mother-to-be has chronic health-care problems.
- Obtain early prenatal care and regular prenatal follow-up care.
- Receive education regarding testing for chromosomal abnormalities.
- Follow all prenatal care recommendations regarding nutrition, medications, and self-care as with any younger pregnant patient.

FOCUS ON THE FETUS

During pregnancy visits to the health-care provider, maternal and fetal well-being are monitored. Sometimes simple non-invasive tests are conducted to determine fetal well-being or if complications arise, more invasive tests may be ordered by the health-care provider to evaluate the health of the fetus. Table 6.3 provides information about tests that may be performed to determine fetal well-being.

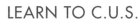 **LEARN TO C.U.S.**

The nurse is preparing a woman for a nonstress test (NST) in the labor and delivery unit. The patient is 36 weeks gestation. The woman states, "The baby doesn't move around as much as he did a week or so ago." During the NST, the nurse notes that the fetal heart rate only accelerates for 10 seconds and there is minimal fetal movement. The nurse calls the health-care provider using the C.U.S. method of communication.

"Hello, doctor. I am **concerned** about the patient's NST today. I am **uncomfortable** because it was not entirely normal. I wanted to notify you as soon as possible because I feel that we have a patient **safety** issue."

(Text continued on page 78)

NURSING CARE PLAN for Self-Care and Disease Prevention in Pregnancy

Nursing Diagnosis: Knowledge deficit related to management of nausea in early pregnancy.
Interventions:
- Eating crackers first thing when arising
- Avoiding foods with strong odors
- Consuming peppermint candies
- Using relaxation techniques with slow breathing to decrease nausea
- Eating small, frequent meals
- Avoiding spicy foods

Nursing Diagnosis: Pain related to low backache.
Interventions:
- Maintaining good posture
- Using correct body mechanics when lifting: bend at the knees, not the waist
- Wearing low-heeled shoes
- Supporting the uterus with a pillow underneath when lying on the side to sleep

Nursing Diagnosis: Knowledge deficit related to the prevention of toxoplasmosis.
Interventions:
- Avoiding raw or undercooked meat
- Avoid cleaning the cat litter box
- Avoiding yard work that may cause exposure to cat feces

TABLE 6.3 TESTS PERFORMED TO DETERMINE FETAL WELL-BEING

Fetal Measure	Procedure	Explanation	Nursing Care	Patient Teaching
Fundal Height Measurement	A tape measure is used to measure the distance from the symphysis pubis to the top of the fundus at each prenatal visit.	• Growth is expected at each visit to determine normal fetal growth.	N/A	When the fetus is growing appropriately, there will be an increase in fundal height at each prenatal visit.
Fetal Kick Counts	This count is done to monitor fetal well-being.	• Four fetal movements in 1 hr are considered reassuring for fetal well-being. • If fetal movements are decreased, she should eat, rest, and refocus on fetal movement. • Decreased fetal movement should be reported to the health-care provider.	• Teach the pregnant woman how to do a fetal kick count. • Teach her when to report her findings to the health-care provider.	• The mother is to palpate and note fetal movement daily for 1 hr.

TABLE **6.3**   **TESTS PERFORMED TO DETERMINE FETAL WELL-BEING—cont'd**

Fetal Measure	Procedure	Explanation	Nursing Care	Patient Teaching

Amniocentesis	A thin needle is used to remove amniotic fluid and cells from the amniotic sac surrounding the fetus (Fig. 5.6). Amniocentesis later in pregnancy can indicate fetal well-being, and the amniotic fluid will indicate whether the fetus is mature enough for delivery.	• Bilirubin levels can be obtained to determine whether the fetus is experiencing hemolytic disease.
		• Fluid can be cultured to determine whether infection is present.
		• Fetal lung maturity can be determined by testing the lecithin/sphingomyelin (L/S) ratio, phosphatidyl glycerol (PG), and lamellar body count (LBC).
		  • L/S ratio greater than 2:1 indicates mature fetal lungs.
		  • L/S ratio less than 2:1 indicates immature fetal lungs and risk for respiratory distress at birth.
		  • Positive PG indicates mature fetal lungs.
		  • Lamellar bodies present indicate fetal lung maturity.
			• Explain the procedure to the woman.
			• Explain that the fetus will be monitored, and ultrasound guidance is used for needle placement.
			• Provide comfort and emotional support.
			• Label specimens and send to the laboratory for analysis.
			• Administer Rh-immune globulin (RhoGAM) to Rh-negative women after the procedure to decrease the risk of antibody formation.
				• Report any decrease in fetal movement, bleeding, cramping, leaking of fluid, or fever to the health-care provider.

Nonstress Test (NST)	This test is performed after 28 weeks to monitor for fetal distress. A fetal monitor is attached to the mother's abdomen and the fetus is monitored for several minutes. Every time the woman perceives fetal movement, it is noted on the fetal monitor. A healthy fetal response is a rise in the heart rate with fetal movement.	• For a fetus at greater than 32 weeks gestation, the NST is considered reactive when the fetal heart rate (FHR) increases 15 beats above baseline for 15 sec twice in 20 min. • For a fetus at fewer than 32 weeks, accelerations of at least 10 beats per min and lasting 10 sec is considered reactive.	• Apply the fetal monitor. • Interpret the FHR and accelerations, and report to the health-care provider. • Provide comfort and emotional support.	• Explain the procedure. • Explain the interpretation and the need for follow-up tests if indicated.

Continued

TABLE 6.3 TESTS PERFORMED TO DETERMINE FETAL WELL-BEING—cont'd

Fetal Measure	Procedure	Explanation	Nursing Care	Patient Teaching
		• A nonreactive NST is a test without sufficient accelerations of heart rate with movement in 40 min of testing (ACOG, 2012)		
Contraction Stress Test (CST)	The purpose is to evaluate the well-being of a fetus by observing the fetal response to the stress of contractions. An external fetal monitor is applied and IV oxytocin is administered until there are three uterine contractions in 10 to 20 min lasting 40 sec or longer.	• The CST is considered negative or normal when there are no late or variable decelerations of FHR noted on the fetal monitor. A negative CST is associated with good fetal outcomes. • The CST is considered positive if there are late or variable decelerations of FHR with 50% of the contractions. Further testing with a Biophysical Profile is recommended.	• Apply the fetal monitor. • Start the IV access and safely administer the oxytocin. • Provide comfort and emotional support. • Monitor the patient throughout the procedure • Report interpretation of the test to the health-care provider.	• Explain the procedure. • Explain that the uterine contractions will not be severe and should stop when the test is over and the oxytocin is discontinued. • Teach the patient to report any increase in contractions or decrease in fetal movement after she returns home.
Amniotic Fluid Index (AFI)	Ultrasound is used to measure the depth of the pockets of amniotic fluid in four quadrants of the uterus. Amniotic fluid amount is based on fetal urine production, which depends upon fetal renal function. If the fetus is not obtaining enough oxygenation through the placenta, blood is shunted from the kidneys to other vital organs and, therefore, fetal urine is decreased.	• The average measurement of amniotic fluid pockets is greater than 2 cm and less than 8 cm per pocket (Perinatology, 2010). • Abnormal AFI is less than 5-cm total measurement and is called **oligohydramnios**, which is the state of low amniotic fluid. • Oligohydramnios is associated with poor fetal outcomes. • If the AFI is greater than 24-cm total measurements, it is considered to be	• Explain the procedure to the patient. • Provide comfort and emotional support.	• This test in noninvasive and requires only that the patient lay quietly. • There are no needles involved and no risk to the fetus.

TABLE 6.3 TESTS PERFORMED TO DETERMINE FETAL WELL-BEING—cont'd

Fetal Measure	Procedure	Explanation	Nursing Care	Patient Teaching
		polyhydramnios, which is excessive amniotic fluid. This condition is associated with congenital anomalies, such as neural tube defects and gastrointestinal defects.		
Biophysical Profile (BPP)	This test is done in the third trimester to monitor the overall health of the fetus. This test involves an abdominal ultrasound along with a stress test. The BPP monitors the fetal movement, breathing movements, heart rate, and the amount of amniotic fluid. The BPP test consists of a nonstress test with an additional 30 min of ultrasound observation. A score of 0 (absent) to 2 (present) is given to each component of the test.	• One or more episodes of fetal breathing movements of 30 sec or more within the 30 min of observation is expected. • Three or more body limb movements are expected in 30 min. • One or more fetal extremity extension with return to fetal flexion or an opening and closing of the hand is expected. • An amniotic fluid depth of 2 cm or more in two pockets of fluid perpendicular (at a 90° angle) is expected. • An overall score of 8 to 10 is reassuring of fetal well-being. • A score of 6 may indicate a need to deliver the fetus early, depending upon the gestational age. • Special training is required to interpret the results.	• Explain the procedure. • Apply the external fetal monitor.	• Explain any required follow-up and assist the patient to understand the results.

Continued

TABLE 6.3 TESTS PERFORMED TO DETERMINE FETAL WELL-BEING—cont'd

Fetal Measure	Procedure	Explanation	Nursing Care	Patient Teaching
Group B Streptococcus Screen	This test is done at 36 to 37 weeks to screen for group B streptococcus, which can be a danger to the fetus. Group B streptococcus, also known as *group B strep*, is a common bacteria carried in the genital tract and intestines. It does not usually cause problems for adults, but a fetus could pick up the bacteria during delivery and become ill. The health-care provider swabs the vagina and rectum during the third trimester and sends the samples to the laboratory.	• If the test is negative, no action is needed. • A positive strep B test requires antibiotics to be given during labor to decrease the risk of group B strep disease in the newborn.	• Administer IV antibiotics as ordered during labor if necessary.	• Administer IV antibiotics as ordered during labor if necessary. • Explain the need for antibiotics to prevent disease in the newborn.

LABS & DIAGNOSTICS

The CDC recommends that all pregnant women be screened for group B streptococcus (GBS) at 35 to 37 weeks gestation. Rapid GBS test kits can provide results within minutes on vaginal or rectal fluid swab specimens submitted in a sterile redtop tube. Optimally, when sending a specimen for a culture, it should be sent before any antibiotics are started (Van-Leeuwen et al., 2013).

FOCUS ON FAMILY

In the months leading up to the birth, many couples prepare for the birth by attending childbirth classes and by developing a birth plan. There are a variety of childbirth classes available, and many options for childbirth that the woman and her partner can consider. This section highlights common childbirth preparation methods and choices available when planning a birth. The patient should be encouraged to discuss her birth plan with her family, health-care providers, and the nurses providing labor care.

Childbirth Preparation

Many couples prepare for the upcoming birth by attending childbirth preparation classes. Most begin approximately 30 to 32 weeks gestation. There is a variety of classes available. The two most popular are Lamaze techniques and the Bradley method of childbirth preparation. The classes are usually taken with a partner, friend, or relative to be the birth coach and assist the woman throughout her labor (Fig. 6.3).

Lamaze

Lamaze classes are the most widely used method in the United States. This method of preparation is named after a French doctor and was introduced in the United States in the 1950s. The method provides women with techniques to assist her with coping with the pain of labor. It centers on breathing patterns with a focal point and relaxation techniques that conserve energy for the pushing stage of labor. The Lamaze method does not support or discourage medications in labor, but views medications as an option if needed. Lamaze classes educate the mother-to-be on the birth process and options available for managing the pain and making decisions during the labor and delivery process.

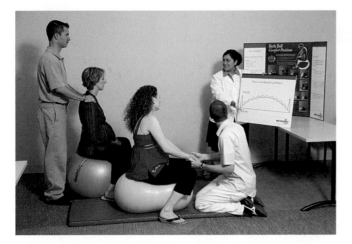

FIGURE 6.3 Childbirth education classes help to prepare the expectant couple for many aspects of the childbearing year.

The Bradley Method

The Bradley method became popular in the 1990s when a book was published by Dr. Bradley titled "The Husband-Coached Childbirth." It prepares the woman to deliver without medications. The husband is prepared to coach his wife through a birth experience without medications or unnecessary medical interventions. The Bradley method does not emphasize breathing techniques; its focus is on muscle control. Muscle tension increases the pain of labor and active relaxation during labor reduces pain.

Childbirth Class Topics

Topics typically covered in childbirth classes include:

• Normal labor, birth, and postpartum care
• Relaxation techniques
• Breathing techniques
• Comfort measures during labor
• Medical procedures
• Breastfeeding
• Tour of the hospital labor and delivery
• Developing a birth plan

Birth Plan

Some women prefer to develop a birth plan that allows her to communicate her desires for the labor and delivery with her health-care provider and the labor and delivery nurses. A birth plan may be very detailed or it may be brief. Some topics typically included in a birth plan are provided in Table 6.4.

TABLE 6.4   BIRTH PLANNING

Topics Related to Birth Planning	Items to Consider in Birth Planning
Before Labor or Early Labor	• Induction preferences • Laboring at home • Hospital admittance
Induction of Labor	• Timing of the induction • Choice of induction techniques
Environment During Labor	• Birthing bed or chair • Music and television • Shower and birthing tub • Comfort measures
Medical Interventions	• Fetal monitoring • Epidural • IV fluids • Vaginal exams
Second Stage of Labor	• Pushing positions • Pushing methods
Delivery	• Inclusion of family and friends • Episiotomy • Cord cutting • Placenta delivery
The Newborn	• Medications • Initiating breastfeeding • Separation from the mother

Key Points

▪ A nurse can provide anticipatory guidance for managing physical discomforts due to the hormonal and physiological changes of pregnancy.

▪ The patient should be educated on self-care during pregnancy to promote a safe, healthy pregnancy.

▪ Viral infections are major causes of morbidity and mortality in pregnancy. The nurse should be aware of common viral infections and teach the patient methods to avoid the viruses.

▪ Healthy nutrition and appropriate weight gain in pregnancy promote optimal health for the fetus and mother-to-be.

▪ Pregnant adolescents have additional nutritional needs because of their own growth and development.

▪ The developmental needs of the pregnant adolescent must be considered when planning care during pregnancy.

▪ There are pregnancy risks for women older than age 35, but a healthy pregnancy and fetus are possible.

▪ There are many tests outlined in the chapter that are available to monitor fetal well-being during pregnancy.

▪ The Bradley method and Lamaze method are two childbirth education programs that assist pregnant couples to prepare for childbirth.

▪ Some women prepare a birth plan to communicate her desires for labor and delivery.

REVIEW QUESTIONS

1. The pregnant patient states that she has a low iron level. Which foods can the nurse suggest to increase patient dietary intake of iron? (*select all that apply*)
   1. Milk
   2. Spinach
   3. Beef steak
   4. Carrots
   5. Kale
   6. White bread

2. Which statement made by the patient indicates understanding of the amniocentesis procedure?
   1. "I will need to avoid food and water for 8 hours before the procedure."
   2. "The test is only done in the third trimester."
   3. "A long needle is placed through my abdomen to obtain amniotic fluid."
   4. "The procedure requires 48 hours of bed rest afterward."

3. Which statement made by a pregnant adolescent indicates that more teaching is needed regarding her understanding of pregnancy nutrition?
   1. "I should eat at least 2,000 calories a day from all food groups."
   2. "I can drink diet soft drinks because they have no calories."
   3. "I can make healthy food choices at a fast-food restaurant."
   4. "I need extra calcium for my bones and for fetal development."

4. The risks of pregnancy over the age of 35 include: (*select all that apply*)
   1. Miscarriage
   2. Twins
   3. Leg cramps
   4. Anemia
   5. Gestational diabetes
   6. Cesarean birth

5. The biophysical profile of the fetus evaluates: (*select all that apply*)
   1. Fetal movement
   2. Fetal position
   3. Placenta location
   4. Fetal heart rate
   5. Fetal breathing movements
   6. Amount of amniotic fluid
   7. Cervical changes

6. The nurse is preparing a discussion with pregnant women about seatbelt use during pregnancy. The nurse should include which statement in the discussion?
   1. The shoulder belt is not safe; just use the lap belt.
   2. Place the lap portion of the belt low across the abdomen and hipbones.
   3. The abdomen should be 5 inches from the steering wheel.
   4. Loosen the seat belt so that it will not be too tight.

7. To prevent venous thrombosis formation during travel, the pregnant woman should: (*select all that apply*)
   1. Change position frequently.
   2. Walk around every 2 hours.
   3. Restrict fluid intake.
   4. Take aspirin daily.
   5. Elevate the legs whenever possible.

8. Patient teaching to decrease the risk of developing hemorrhoids includes:
   1. Daily laxative use
   2. Increasing fiber intake
   3. Decreasing fluid intake
   4. Decreasing exercise

CRITICAL THINKING QUESTION

Allison is 15 years old and pregnant with her first baby. She is 8 weeks pregnant and voicing concern about gaining too much weight in the pregnancy. What approach can the nurse use to educate her about nutrition and weight gain in pregnancy?

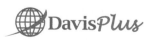

For additional resources and information, visit **www.DavisPlus.com.** Post-Conference Questions and Activities, Answers, and References can be found on Davis*Plus.*

Nursing Care of the Woman With Complications During Pregnancy

7

LEARNING OUTCOMES

1. Identify the key terms.
2. Discuss the nursing care of a patient experiencing hyperemesis gravidarum.
3. Identify bleeding complications of early and late pregnancy.
4. Recognize signs of complications following a spontaneous abortion.
5. Discuss the nursing care for the patient following a ruptured ectopic pregnancy.
6. Compare and contrast the abnormalities of placenta abruptio, placenta accreta, and placenta previa.
7. Define hydatidiform mole and explain usual medical treatment and nursing care.
8. Provide safe and effective nursing care for patients experiencing a placental abnormality such as placenta abruptio, placenta accreta, and placenta previa.
9. Identify signs of hypovolemic shock caused by blood loss from bleeding complications of pregnancy.
10. Summarize the management of patients with Rh incompatibility.
11. Develop a plan of care for women with multiple gestational pregnancy.
12. Develop a plan of care for a patient experiencing pregnancy-related hypertensive disorders.
13. Outline the nurse's role in assessment, managing care, and patient teaching for a patient with gestational diabetes.

KEY TERMS

abortion
choriocarcinoma
dilation and curettage (D&C)
eclampsia
ectopic pregnancy
hydatidiform mole
hyperemesis gravidarum
hysterectomy
insulin resistance
isoimmunization
ketones
perfusion
placenta abruptio
placenta accreta
placenta previa
pre-eclampsia
salpingectomy
salpingostomy
viable

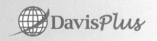 **DavisPlus** For audio pronunciation guide, visit **www.DavisPlus.com**

CHAPTER CONCEPTS

Communication
Grief and Loss
Medication
Perfusion
Promoting Health

REAL-WORLD CASE STUDY

Tonya

■ Tonya is a 30-year-old patient pregnant with her first baby. She is in gestational week 41 and has had no previous complications during her pregnancy. Tonya arrived in the labor and delivery unit experiencing severe abdominal pain and vaginal bleeding. As the nurse assists her into bed, Tonya says: "I used cocaine this afternoon. I haven't used drugs my entire pregnancy, but because it was my birthday and I was overdue, I used the cocaine. I thought the only risk to using drugs was during the first trimester. Did I cause this bleeding? Is my baby in danger?"

1. What bleeding complication of late pregnancy is Tonya experiencing?
2. What nursing interventions are appropriate for this situation?
3. How would you answer Tonya's questions of "Did I cause this bleeding? Is my baby in danger?"

CONCEPTUAL CORNERSTONE

Adherence

The concept of adherence can be defined as the extent to which a patient follows the health-care provider's instructions for prescribed treatments to promote health or to manage a condition (Giddens, 2013). Nurses have an opportunity to work with patients undergoing life-changing events such as pregnancy. When working with a pregnant patient, the nurse has the chance to educate the patient about preventive health-care measures to promote a safe and health pregnancy.

When a patient experiences pregnancy complications such as the conditions discussed in this chapter, the nurse can reinforce the treatment plan of the health-care provider and suggest actions to improve the chance of a good outcome for the patient and her fetus. Nurses play a major role in assisting patients to accept and maintain needed changes during a crisis such as a complicated pregnancy. While planning patient-centered care, nurses should recognize that the patient's willingness and ability to adhere to a treatment plan is influenced by the patient's own personal experience, attitudes, motivation, and culture.

Complications can occur during pregnancy that can threaten the fetus and the expectant mother. This chapter discusses the care of the woman with complications of hyperemesis gravidarum, bleeding disorders of early and late pregnancy, maternal-fetal blood incompatibility, hypertensive disorders of pregnancy, and gestational diabetes.

CULTURAL CONSIDERATIONS

Medical professionals value prenatal care. Americans generally view pregnancy and birth as medical conditions and seek early prenatal care. Some cultures, such as the Hispanic culture, view pregnancy as a normal condition, not a medical condition, and rely on the older women in the family to educate pregnant women about pregnancy and prenatal care. In providing culturally competent and patient-centered care, the nurse should not mistake the patient's absence of early prenatal care as a lack of interest or concern for a healthy pregnancy.

CARE OF THE WOMAN WITH HYPEREMESIS GRAVIDARUM

Nausea and vomiting, also known as *morning sickness*, are common during the first trimester of pregnancy for many women. If the nausea and vomiting interfere with an adequate intake of fluid and food, and/or persists past 20 weeks of gestation, it is termed **hyperemesis gravidarum**.

Incidence and Risk Factors

Hyperemesis gravidarum occurs in 0.5% to 2% of all pregnancies (Ogunyemi, 2014). The cause is unknown, but elevated hormone levels and the relaxation of smooth muscle, which results in delayed gastric emptying, are believed to contribute to this condition (Puscheck, 2014). Hyperemesis can cause problems for the mother and fetus. Severe hyperemesis gravidarum can result in preterm labor. The dehydration that occurs may lead to poor placental perfusion and inadequate oxygenation to the fetus. Fetal growth can be compromised, leading to an infant who is small for gestational age. In addition, women with hyperemesis gravidarum in the second trimester have an increased risk for preterm labor, **pre-eclampsia** (ie, an increase in blood pressure, protein in the urine, and edema), and placental abruption (Moussa, 2014).

Signs and Symptoms

Signs and symptoms of hyperemesis gravidarum include:

- Vomiting multiple times throughout the day
- Poor appetite
- Weight loss (greater than 5% of prepregnancy weight)
- Dehydration
  - Dry mouth and skin
  - Poor skin turgor
  - Concentrated urine
  - Decreased urine output
  - Elevated heart rate
  - Alkalosis from loss of hydrochloric acid

Medical Care

Most care may be provided at home, but some women will require hospitalization for IV fluid administration and antiemetics. Metoclopramide, domperidone, and cyclizine are considered safe for pregnancy (Vallerand, Sanoski, and Deglin, 2013) Research studies have determined that acupuncture and acupressure are effective as modes of treatment to avoid the use of medications in the critical first trimester of pregnancy (Wilcox, 2013). In severe cases, the health-care provider will also investigate other possible causes of nausea and vomiting, such as gastroenteritis, pancreatitis, hepatitis, ulcers, and kidney disorders (Puscheck, 2014).

The health-care provider may order the following laboratory studies to monitor the patient's health status:

- Complete blood cell count (CBC) to monitor for signs of infection and dehydration
- Electrolytes to monitor for imbalances caused by dehydration
- **Ketones** to monitor the use of fat stores to provide energy to the mother and her fetus
- Liver enzymes to monitor liver inflammation

Nursing Care

Nursing care of the pregnant patient with hyperemesis gravidarum includes:

- Administering IV fluids and antiemetics
- Monitoring laboratory results and reporting any abnormalities to the health-care provider
- Monitoring for weight loss
- Providing for psychosocial needs by referral to appropriate resources and by allowing time to therapeutically listen to the patient's concerns

Patient Teaching

Teach patients with hyperemesis gravidarum to do the following:

- Eat small, frequent meals.
- Avoid spicy and fatty foods.
- Identify and avoid odors or foods that may trigger nausea.
- Maintain fluid intake by sipping throughout the day to avoid dehydration.
- Monitor for signs of dehydration. Teach the patient these signs if she does not already know them.
- Notify her health-care provider if she notices the following warning signs:
  - Dark urine
  - Bloody vomitus
  - Abdominal pain
  - Dehydration
  - Lack of urine output for 8 hours
  - Inability to keep food down for 24 hours
  - Ketones in the urine (Instruct the patient on use of urine dipsticks to monitor for ketones at home.)

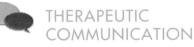

THERAPEUTIC
COMMUNICATION

Nonadherence

Margarita is a Hispanic primigravida patient who had her initial prenatal appointment with the nurse midwife at 8 weeks

of gestation but has missed her appointments since that time. Now, she is at 22 weeks of gestation and the nurse calls to discuss the missed prenatal appointments. In this situation, the communication approach by the nurse should not shame or scold Margarita for missing her prenatal visits.

Nurse: "Hello, Margarita, we would like to schedule a prenatal appointment with you. We haven't seen you for a while."

Margarita: "Well, I didn't really need an appointment, I have been feeling fine."

Nurse: "Sometimes pregnant women have questions that we can answer during your appointment."

Margarita: "My grandmother has answered my questions. I am really doing fine."

Nurse: "Could we make an appointment just to check that everything is progressing well with the pregnancy and your baby? We can also talk about future appointments at that time."

Margarita: "Sure, let me check my work schedule."

CARE OF THE WOMAN WITH BLEEDING DISORDERS OF EARLY PREGNANCY

Bleeding during pregnancy is always an abnormality and, especially in the first trimester, threatens the viability of the pregnancy. Bleeding disorders of early pregnancy include abortion, ectopic pregnancy, and gestational trophoblastic disease (GTD).

Abortion

The term *abortion* is used to describe a pregnancy loss or termination prior to the fetus being viable. The term *viable* describes a fetus that is able to live outside the uterus. Medically, fetus viability is defined as attaining an age greater than 20 weeks of gestation or a fetal weight greater than 500 g (Derricott, 2014).

Incidence and Risk Factors

Spontaneous abortion, also known as *miscarriage*, is the most common type of pregnancy loss. It occurs in 10% to 20% of all clinically recognized pregnancies (Puscheck, 2014). A spontaneous abortion can be caused by chromosomal abnormalities, uncontrolled diabetes, hypothyroidism, maternal infection, reproductive abnormalities, or maternal injury. Spontaneous abortions are classified according to symptoms and the outcome:

- **Threatened abortions** are diagnosed when vaginal bleeding occurs, possibly accompanied by abdominal cramping. The woman may or may not lose the fetus.
- **Inevitable abortions** happen when the cervix dilates and the amniotic membranes rupture. The fetus and placenta are expelled unless a health-care provider intervenes.
- **Incomplete abortions** occur when some of the uterine contents of pregnancy are expelled, but not all. This

retention of products of conception leads to uterine bleeding and cramping.
- **Complete abortions** occur when all uterine contents are expelled. When this occurs, uterine cramping and bleeding stops without interventions.
- **Missed abortions** occur when the fetus dies during the first half of the pregnancy. The fetus is not expelled and the woman carries the fetus until spontaneous abortion occurs.

Signs and Symptoms

The signs and symptoms of a spontaneous abortion include lower abdominal cramping and vaginal bleeding.

Medical Care

If bleeding does not stop after a spontaneous abortion, a **dilation and curettage (D&C)** may be necessary. A D&C is a surgical procedure in which the cervix is dilated and the physician gently scrapes the lining of the uterus to remove the products of conception. Another common procedure is vacuum extraction; a cannula is attached to a suction device. These procedures will usually stop the bleeding. Also, to control bleeding, some patients may require medications such as oxytocin (Pitocin) or methylergonovine (Methergine). These medications cause uterine contraction and therefore slow uterine bleeding.

After an abortion, serious complications may occur. The patient should be observed for signs of infection and hemorrhage because they may occur, especially after or during a missed abortion.

Nursing Care

Nursing care of the pregnant patient who has had either a planned or spontaneous abortion includes the following:

- For a threatened abortion, instructing the patient to avoid sexual activity, tampons, douches, and strenuous exercise
- Instructing the patient to notify her health-care provider of any bleeding during a pregnancy
- Monitoring vital signs, intake and output, oxygen saturation, and laboratory test results
- Recognizing the signs of hypovolemic shock, which include decreased blood pressure, increased heart rate, clammy skin, lightheadedness, and confusion
- Anticipating the need for IV fluids and oxygen therapy
- Administering medications, such as oxytocin or methylergonovine, ordered by the health-care provider to control bleeding
- Possibly alerting the laboratory to blood type; crossmatching the patient for a possible blood transfusion
- Administering Rh$_o$(D) immune globulin (RhoGAM) to Rh-negative woman within 72 hours to prevent isoimmunization
- Assisting the patient to discuss her feelings of loss; some patients have feelings of guilt and need an opportunity to ask questions and talk about the experience

Patient Teaching

Teach the patient who has had either a planned or spontaneous abortion the following:

- Teach the patient the warning signs of complications after an abortion. The following warning signs should be reported to the health-care provider:
  - Heavy, bright-red bleeding
  - Foul-smelling vaginal discharge
  - Fever
  - Pelvic pain
- Do not resume sexual activity or use of tampons or douches until advised by the health-care provider.
- If there was significant blood loss, the patient may need iron supplements.
- Encourage adding liver, green leafy vegetables, and eggs to the diet to provide iron.
- Instruct the patient that it is normal to go through a grieving process that may last 6 to 12 months.
- Encourage the patient to allow her body to rest and recover before attempting another pregnancy and to discuss another pregnancy with her health-care provider.

Ectopic Pregnancy

An **ectopic pregnancy** occurs when the fertilized ovum implants outside the uterus. Most ectopic pregnancies occur in the fallopian tubes, but they can occur anywhere outside the uterus (Fig. 7.1).

Incidence and Risk Factors

Ectopic pregnancies occur in 2 out of 100 pregnancies (Derricott, 2014). Risk factors for ectopic pregnancies include scarring of the fallopian tubes or blocks in the tubes, which can slow down the movement of the fertilized ovum; advanced maternal age; reproductive anomalies; a history of fallopian tube surgery; a history of pelvic inflammatory disease; repeated induced abortions; repeated sexually transmitted infections; intrauterine devices (IUD); a history of assisted reproductive technology (ART); women who douche regularly; and women who smoke (Sepilian, 2014).

Signs and Symptoms

Signs and symptoms of ectopic pregnancy include vaginal bleeding and abdominal pain.

If the fallopian tube ruptures, the following additional symptoms may occur:

- Severe abdominal pain
- Shoulder or neck pain from blood leaking out of the fallopian tube into the abdomen and irritating the diaphragm
- Weakness
- Dizziness
- Decreased blood pressure
- Increased heart rate

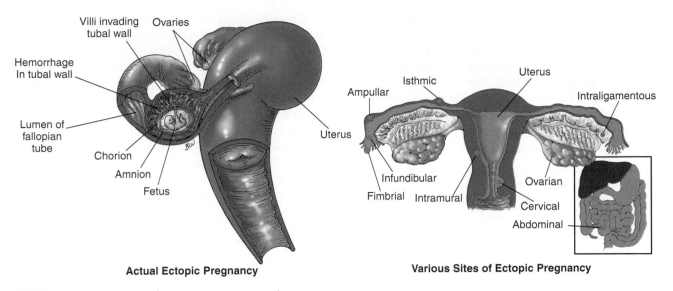

FIGURE 7.1 Various sites of ectopic pregnancy implantation.

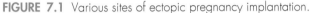

 DRUG FACTS

Methotrexate

If methotrexate is used to treat an ectopic pregnancy, the patient should avoid foods and vitamins with folic acid and alcohol. These can all decrease the effectiveness of methotrexate.

Medical Care

If the fallopian tube has not ruptured, methotrexate may be administered. Methotrexate is an antineoplastic drug. It is a folic acid antagonist that interferes with DNA synthesis. Methotrexate interferes with the cell multiplication. It will cause the embryo to stop growing and reduce the chance of fallopian tube rupture. Certain criteria must exist to use this drug: The fetus is less than 3.5 cm long, the fetus is not alive, and the patient is stable hemodynamically.

If a ruptured fallopian tube has occurred, a linear salpingostomy is performed to save the tube. A **salpingostomy** is a small linear incision made into the fallopian tube to remove the products of conception. The tube is allowed to heal without suture to prevent scarring (Derricott, 2014). If the fallopian tube is ruptured and is not able to be saved or the patient does not desire a future pregnancy, the tube may be removed by a laparoscopic salpingectomy. A **salpingectomy** is surgical removal of the fallopian tube.

Nursing Care

Nursing care of the pregnant patient who has had an ectopic pregnancy includes the following:

- Monitoring the patient for signs of hypovolemic shock caused by hemorrhage, including:
  - Decreased blood pressure
  - Increased heart rate

- Restlessness
- Confusion
- If the patient undergoes a salpingostomy or salpingectomy, monitoring postoperative vital signs, oxygen saturation, intake and output, and vaginal bleeding according to institutional policies
- Assessing and controlling pain
- Administering RhoGAM within 72 hours to prevent isoimmunization
- Assisting the patient with emotions such as anger, sadness, or guilt, which are a part of coping with pregnancy loss

Patient Teaching

Teach the patient who has had an ectopic pregnancy the following:

- Notify the health-care provider if fever, chills, or significant bleeding occurs.
- If methotrexate was administered, educate the patient about the common side effects: nausea and vomiting.
- Discuss with the patient that grieving after a pregnancy loss is normal and may last for 6 to 12 months.
- Encourage the patient to discuss the timing of another pregnancy attempt with her health-care provider.

Gestational Trophoblastic Disease

GTD, also known as *hydatidiform mole* or *molar pregnancy,* is a genetic abnormality that occurs during early placental attachment and fetal development. The trophoblast cells, which would normally attach the ovum to the uterine wall, develop abnormally. The abnormal development causes the placenta, but not the fetus, to grow and develop. The chorionic villi of the placenta swell, forming fluid-filled sacs. The sacs appear like tiny clusters of grapes inside the uterus. The fluid-filled villi may grow large enough to fill the uterus to the size of an advanced pregnancy (Fig. 7.2).

The molar pregnancy is classified as complete or partial. A complete molar pregnancy completely fills the uterus. In a partial molar pregnancy, a fetus or amniotic sac is present along with the fluid-filled sacs. The fetus is not viable in a molar pregnancy.

Incidence and Risk Factors

GTD pregnancies occur in 1 out of 1,000 pregnancies in the United States and Europe (Derricott, 2014). Women of Asian descent, women of advanced maternal age, and women with a previous molar pregnancy are at an increased risk of having a molar pregnancy.

Signs and Symptoms

Signs and symptoms of GTD include:

- Light-to-heavy bleeding with blood that may be brown or bright red
- Uterine growth that is larger than expected for gestational age
- Absent fetal heart tones and movement
- Serum hCG levels that are increased
- Hyperemesis
- Gestational hypertension

Medical Care

Medical treatment for molar pregnancy may include the drug methotrexate. This drug interferes with cell multiplication. It stops the hydatidiform mole from continuing to grow and may prevent the patient from needing surgery to stop the growth of the molar pregnancy.

The abnormal tissues are removed by vacuum aspiration or by surgical curettage to entirely empty the uterus. Hemorrhage is a frequent complication after the evacuation of a molar pregnancy (Moore, 2014). IV oxytocin is administered after the procedure to contract the uterus and prevent hemorrhage.

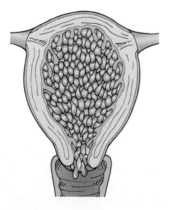

FIGURE 7.2 Hydatidiform mole, a pregnancy in which the chorionic villi break down into fluid-filled clusters inside the uterus.

A possible complication of a molar pregnancy is a **choriocarcinoma**: A fast-growing cancer that can develop in the uterus following a molar pregnancy. This type of cancer develops from germ cells, which are cells that ordinarily turn into sperm or eggs. Choriocarcinomas resemble the cells that surround an embryo in the uterus. To monitor for malignancies, the patient will need follow-up care with serially monitored hCG levels for 9 to 12 months and must avoid pregnancy during this time. Gestational trophoblastic malignancies are almost 100% curable; however, pregnancy makes it difficult to monitor for abnormalities.

Nursing Care

Nursing care of the pregnant patient who has had GTD includes the following:

- Assessing for signs and symptoms of shock:
  - Decreased blood pressure
  - Increased heart rate
  - Restlessness
  - Confusion
- Ensuring pre-operative patient preparation:
  - CBC
  - Blood type and crossmatching
- Administering RhoGAM to Rh-negative women to prevent isoimmunization
- Monitoring postoperative vital signs, oxygen saturation, intake and output, and vaginal bleeding according to institutional policies
- Supporting the patient in her reaction to grief and loss
- Emphasizing the importance of consistent follow-up; there is a small, but real, risk of developing malignant disease (Moore, 2014)

Patient Teaching

- Teach the patient to report to her health-care provider if she experiences any of the signs and symptoms of complications:
  - Excessive bleeding
  - Foul-smelling vaginal discharge
  - Fever
- The patient should be instructed to avoid tampons, douches, and sexual activity until the health-care provider indicates that it is safe to resume these activities.
- Teach the patient the need for regular follow-up appointments to monitor serum hCG levels because of the risk of choriocarcinoma.
- Educate the patient about the need to delay another pregnancy to monitor the hCG levels without the interference of hCG from pregnancy.
- Instruct the patient that it is normal to go through a grieving process that may last 6 to 12 months.
- Future pregnancies should be monitored by early sonographic evaluation because of the increased risk of the recurrence of hydatidiform mole.

CONCEPTUAL CORNERSTONE

Perfusion

Concepts integrate thinking and assist with transferring knowledge from one patient problem to another patient with a similar condition. The concept of perfusion is applicable in this chapter because of the complications of pregnancy that may result in blood loss. **Perfusion** is blood circulating through the body and oxygenating the tissues. Impaired central perfusion occurs in conditions that decrease cardiac output or cause shock. If adequately oxygenated blood cannot freely travel to all parts of the body, a state of inadequate tissue perfusion exists. The bleeding disorders of pregnancy all relate to the concept of perfusion. Regardless of the cause of poor perfusion, whether it is caused by blood loss from a spontaneous abortion, placenta previa, or placental abruption, the basic nursing care is similar. Immediate nursing interventions include monitoring vital signs; noting capillary refill time; noting peripheral pulses; inspecting perineal pads, noting the color and amount of blood; and administering IV fluids and blood products as ordered by the health-care provider.

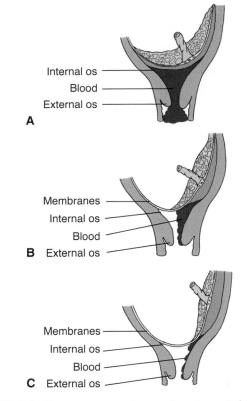

FIGURE 7.3 Placenta previa: A, complete, B, partial, C, marginal

CARE OF THE WOMAN WITH BLEEDING DISORDERS OF LATE PREGNANCY

Bleeding in late pregnancy can be a potential emergency because it usually indicates placenta attachment problems and the fetus may not be receiving sufficient nourishment. Bleeding disorders of late pregnancy include placenta previa, placenta abruptio, and placenta accreta.

Placenta Previa

Placenta previa is a placenta that is implanted near the opening of the cervix. As the pregnancy nears term and the cervix begins to dilate, bleeding occurs because the placenta is becoming unattached to the uterus. This bleeding puts the unborn child at risk because the placenta is supplying oxygen to the fetus until after birth, when the baby begins to breathe.

There are different forms of placenta previa (Fig. 7.3):

1. *Marginal*: The placenta is next to the cervix but does not cover the opening.
2. *Partial*: The placenta covers part of the cervical opening.
3. *Complete*: The placenta covers all of the cervical opening.

Incidence and Risk Factors

Placenta previa occurs in 1 out of 200 pregnancies (Derricott, 2014). There are several risk factors for placenta previa:

• Previous Cesarean section
• Recreational cocaine use (Derricott, 2014)
• Previous placenta previa

• Uterine scarring from endometriosis
• Previous spontaneous abortion

Signs and Symptoms

The characteristic symptom of placenta previa is painless, bright-red bleeding. Spotting may occur throughout the second and third trimesters. Painless hemorrhaging may occur in late pregnancy or when labor begins.

Medical Care

A placenta previa can be diagnosed by transabdominal ultrasound. Vaginal cervical examination must be avoided if a patient has painless bleeding. A vaginal cervical examination may result in hemorrhage if the health-care provider further disrupts the implantation of the placenta.

Medical management will depend on the type of placenta previa, the gestational age, the amount of bleeding, and fetal status. Bedrest may be required to reduce the pressure of the uterus and fetus on the cervix and placenta. The patient will also be advised to avoid exercise, sexual intercourse, tampons, and douching. Nonstress tests (NSTs) may be done during bleeding episodes to evaluate fetal status.

A Cesarean delivery is necessary for a complete placenta previa. It may also be necessary for the other types as well, depending upon the exact location of the placenta previa and the amount of blood loss occurring during labor. The fetus is monitored closely, and any signs of fetal distress will indicate the need for an emergency Cesarean birth.

Nursing Care

Nursing care of the pregnant patient with placenta previa includes the following:

- Instructing the patient to avoid vaginal cervical examinations to prevent perforation of the cervix
- Monitoring fetal heart tones with external monitoring; reporting nonreassuring or abnormal heart rate patterns to the health-care provider immediately
- Monitoring fetal heart rate and movement
- Obtaining venous access for the prompt administration of fluids or blood products that may be ordered by the health-care provider
- Instituting medical orders of blood typing and cross-matching to prepare for possible blood transfusion

Patient Teaching

Teach the patient with placenta previa the following:

- Teach the importance of maintaining bedrest to reduce pressure on the placenta and cervix.
- The patient should abstain from sexual intercourse, douching, and tampons.
- The patient must notify the health-care provider of any increase in vaginal bleeding.
- The patient should perform a daily fetal kick count and report to her health-care provider if fewer than 10 kicks are counted in one hour (ACOG, 2013).

PATIENT TEACHING GUIDELINES

Kick Counts

The mother lies on her side and counts distinct fetal movements daily; 10 movements in a 2-hour period are reassuring. After counting 10 movements, the count is discontinued. Fewer than 10 movements should be reported to the physician.

Placenta Abruptio

Placenta abruptio is the premature separation of the placenta from the wall of the uterus. Bleeding occurs between the uterine wall and the placenta. An abruption can be partial or complete. An abruption is partial if the margins of the placenta remain attached and a section detaches from the uterine wall (Fig. 7.4). With a complete abruption, the entire placenta separates from the uterine wall. A placenta abruptio is a life-threatening event for the fetus and the patient. A patient experiencing an abruption is at risk for severe hemorrhaging resulting in hypovolemic shock, disseminated intravascular coagulation (DIC), and death (Cunningham, Levino, Bloom). The placenta provides oxygenation to the fetus, so an abruption of the placenta can lead to fetal hypoxia and death.

Incidence and Risk Factors

Placental abruption occurs in 1 out of 200 deliveries (Cunningham, Levino, Bloom, et al 2014). Risk factors for placenta abruptio include the following:

- Abdominal trauma
- Hypertension
- Cocaine use (Deering, 2014)
- Alcohol abuse
- Cigarette smoking
- Multiple pregnancy
- Short umbilical cord
- Diabetes mellitus
- Advanced maternal age
- History of placental abruption

Signs and Symptoms

Signs and symptoms of placenta abruptio include:

- Vaginal bleeding that may be light or heavy, depending upon the size of the abruption
- Severe uterine tenderness
- A firm, boardlike abdomen, which is caused by irritation of the abdominal muscle by bleeding (Deering, 2014)
- Pain in the abdomen or lower back
- Uterine irritability and poor uterine resting tone, as indicated by the fetal monitor

Medical Care

The diagnosis is made based on the symptoms and by abdominal ultrasound. Treatment is determined by the severity of

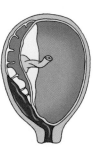

Partial separation (concealed hemorrhage)   Partial separation (apparent hemorrhage)   Complete separation (concealed hemorrhage)

FIGURE 7.4 Placenta abruptio.

the abruption. An emergency Cesarean section may be required to save the fetus. A vaginal delivery may be attempted if the abruption is small, and the mother and fetus are stable (Cunningham, Levino, Bloom, et al, 2014).

Nursing Care

Nursing care of the pregnant patient with placenta abruptio should include monitoring the status of the patient and the fetus.

- Frequently assess vital signs and fetal heart tones, reporting abnormal results to the health-care provider immediately.
- Notify the health-care provider and document any nonreassuring fetal heart patterns.
- Monitor for blood loss.
- Assess and document the patient's pain levels.
- Inform the patient of the status of the fetus.
- Provide emotional support to the patient and her family.

Patient Teaching

Patient teaching for the patient with a placenta abruptio includes the following:

- Instruct the patient to report any bleeding or abdominal pain to her health-care provider.
- Inform the patient that a Cesarean birth may be required.
- Answer questions with clear and honest information.

Placenta Accreta

Placenta accreta occurs when the placenta is attached too deeply into the wall of the uterus, causing complications with removal. After childbirth, the placenta normally releases easily from the uterine wall. However, a patient with placenta accreta encounters a difficult removal, with possible complications of hemorrhage and hysterectomy.

Incidence and Risk Factors

There are three types of placenta accreta: placenta accreta, placenta increta, and placenta percreta. Combined, they occur in approximately 1 out of 533 pregnancies. A sharp increase in recent years parallels the increase of Cesarean delivery (ACOG, 2012). Risk factors include:

- Abnormalities of the uterine wall, such as scarring after a Cesarean delivery or uterine surgery
- Low implanted placenta
- Women more than 35 years old
- Previous Cesarean delivery
- Risk increases with each pregnancy

Signs and Symptoms

Signs and symptoms of placenta accreta include the following:

- Third trimester vaginal bleeding may be the only symptom observed.
- An unexplained rise in the level of alpha-fetoprotein has been linked to placenta accreta.

Medical Care

An extensive placenta accreta usually requires a Cesarean birth followed by a hysterectomy. A **hysterectomy** is a surgical procedure to remove the uterus. This procedure prevents severe hemorrhage, which could be life-threatening.

Nursing Care

Nursing care of the pregnant patient with placenta accreta includes the following:

- Preparing the patient for a Cesarean birth
- Providing emotional support for the patient who is coping with a hysterectomy at a young age

Patient Teaching

Teach the patient who has placenta accreta the following:

- Explain to the patient that there is nothing she can do to prevent placenta accreta.
- A Cesarean birth may be scheduled as early as 35 weeks of gestation to avoid an unscheduled delivery.
- Encourage the patient to discuss surgical options with her physician.
- Explain that after the hysterectomy she will no longer have menstrual periods or be able to become pregnant again.

CARE OF THE WOMAN WITH RH INCOMPATIBILITY BETWEEN MATERNAL AND FETAL BLOOD

Rh incompatibility can occur during pregnancy if the woman has been exposed to fetal blood cells that are Rh positive. Rh factor is a surface antigen on a red blood cell. An antigen is any substance that causes the immune system to produce antibodies against it. Rh incompatibility occurs when a woman who does not have the surface antigen (ie, Rh negative), is exposed to blood that has the antigen (ie, Rh positive). When the Rh-negative woman is exposed to Rh-positive blood, her immune system produces antibodies against the Rh factor. This is called *isoimmunization*. The antibodies will attack any Rh-positive blood cells. This will not cause a problem for the mother. However, the antibodies can pass to the developing baby and destroy some of the baby's blood cells.

Exposure to the Rh-positive blood may occur during a spontaneous abortion, trauma, invasive obstetric procedures, or normal childbirth (Salem, 2014). In 90% of cases, sensitization occurs at delivery (Salem, 2014). Blood from an Rh-positive fetus may enter in small amounts during any of these events and sensitize the woman, causing her to produce antibodies. The fetus during the first pregnancy is rarely affected and not at risk. When a subsequent pregnancy occurs, the sensitized woman's immune system produces Rh antibodies that cross from the placenta to the fetal circulation. Once the antibodies cross over the placenta into the fetus's circulation, they form antigen-antibody

NURSING CARE PLAN Bleeding in Pregnancy

Nursing Diagnosis: Knowledge deficit regarding effects of bleeding in pregnancy
Interventions and Rationales:

- Inform the patient and her significant other of the effect bleeding can have on the mother, the course of the pregnancy, and the fetus. *Patients that are knowledgeable about their condition are more likely to be cooperative with the treatment plan and understand the consequences of their condition.*
- Teach the patient the signs and symptoms of bleeding. *Patients will understand that vaginal bleeding or abdominal pain in the presence of amenorrhea or a positive pregnancy test requires evaluation. Bleeding with or without abdominal pain or cramping should be reported to the health-care provider.*
- Explain that a spontaneous abortion (ie, miscarriage) can rarely be prevented. *Understanding that spontaneous abortion cannot be prevented may alleviate some feelings of anguish or guilt.*
- Teach fetal movement counts. Directions: Beginning at 28 weeks of gestation: The mother lies on her side and counts distinct fetal movements daily; 10 movements in a 2-hour period are reassuring. After counting 10 movements, the count is discontinued. Fewer than 10 movements should be reported to the physician. *Fetal movement counting indicates fetal well-being. Fewer than 10 movements in a 2-hour period indicates a need for fetal NSTs.*
- Teach signs and symptoms of maternal complications with vaginal bleeding. *The mother should contact her health-care provider if she begins to experience bleeding accompanied by dizziness, lightheadedness, passing of clots, rapid heart rate, and shortness of breath.*
- For patients in the second and third trimesters, explain home management of placenta previa and placenta abruptio. *The patient should avoid heavy lifting, intercourse, the use of tampons, or any increased activity that could increase the risk of placental separation from the uterus.*
- Educate the patient about any medications that may be prescribed, including name, purpose, possible side effects, and correct administration. *A knowledgeable patient is more likely to be compliant with the planned care. Also, the patient will understand correct administration and side effects of medications, optimizing a positive outcome for the pregnancy.*

Nursing Diagnosis: Anticipatory grieving related to the potential loss of pregnancy
Interventions and Rationales:

- Encourage the patient and her significant other to verbalize their concerns, feelings, and fears regarding the potential loss. *This will assure the patient that grief is a normal reaction to the potential loss.*
- Observe the patient's behavioral response. *Responses such as guilt, anger, denial, and depression are normal reactions to grief.*
- Clarify any misconceptions about possible fetal loss caused by vaginal bleeding. *Vaginal bleeding does not always result in fetal loss. The nurse can educate the patient and family about factual information without providing false hope.*
- Collaborate with Social Services in the care of the patient. *The social worker can evaluate the patient for concerns that can be addressed through social services and support groups.*

Nursing Diagnosis: Acute pain related to uterine cramping and backache associated with vaginal bleeding
Interventions and Rationales:

- Evaluate pain severity using a scale of 0–10, with 10 being the most severe pain. *A baseline evaluation of pain will assist in subsequent assessments of pain and will assist the nurse and health-care provider to determine the appropriate analgesia for the situation.*
- Evaluate the location and duration of pain. *The location and duration of pain can provide information about the cause of the pain.*
- Administer pain medication if appropriate for the condition causing the pain. *This intervention will provide pain relief. If medication is not appropriate for the situation, offer nonpharmacological methods of pain relief.*
- Provide emotional support. *Emotional support by the nurse can relieve stress and anxiety, which can decrease the level of pain that patient is experiencing.*

complexes with the fetal Rh-positive red blood cells. These complexes destroy the fetal red blood cells, causing the fetus to have a condition known as *alloimmune-induced hemolytic anemia* (Fig. 7.5).

Incidence and Risk Factors

The incidence of Rh-negative blood type is 15% to 20% for Caucasians and 5% to 10% for African Americans. For individuals of Chinese and American Indian descent, the incidence of Rh-negative blood type is less than 5% (Salem, 2014).

Signs and Symptoms

The woman will not physically notice any symptoms of Rh incompatibility. The disorder will only be detected by a routine prenatal laboratory test, the indirect Coombs' test, ordered by the health-care provider.

Medical Care

All pregnant women should have a blood test to determine Rh and blood type. Rh-negative women should have an antibody titer test (ie, indirect Coombs' test) to determine if they are sensitized and have developed antibodies against Rh-positive blood. If the indirect Coombs' test is negative, the health-care provider will repeat the test at 28 weeks of gestation. A negative indirect Coombs' test indicates that the fetus is not at risk of developing hemolytic disease.

If the woman has a positive indirect Coombs' test, she will be evaluated at intervals to determine the level of antibodies and to monitor the condition of the fetus. To prevent hemolytic disease in the Rh-positive fetus, RhoGAM is administered at 28 weeks of gestation. RhoGAM prevents the formation of antibodies against Rh-positive blood and helps to prevent the fetus from developing complications of hemolytic anemia. As the antibodies attack the Rh-positive fetal blood cells, the fetus compensates by producing extra red blood cells. Amniocentesis may be performed to evaluate the amount of bilirubin from the destroyed red blood cells that is in the amniotic fluid. Amniocentesis is a procedure in which amniotic fluid is taken from the uterus and the cells are analyzed to provide information on the health of the fetus. A rise in the bilirubin in the amniotic fluid indicates that the fetus is losing too many red blood cells because of the antibodies crossing the placenta from the mother and destroying the fetal blood cells. The health of the fetus may be in danger.

Nursing Care

Nursing care of the woman with Rh incompatibility with the fetal blood includes the following:

• Encouraging the Rh-negative mother to be compliant with all requests by the health-care provider for blood tests to determine antibody titers
• Providing emotional support for the Rh-negative woman with a positive antibody titer as she undergoes testing throughout the remainder of the pregnancy
• Administering RhoGAM after abortion, chorionic villus sampling, amniocentesis, trauma, and at 28 weeks of gestation
• Sending the umbilical cord blood to the laboratory at the time of birth to determine the baby's blood type, Rh, and antibody titer (ie, direct Coombs' test); RhoGAM should be administered within 72 hours of childbirth if the baby is Rh-positive

Patient Teaching

Teach the patient who has Rh incompatibility with the fetal blood the following:

• Explain Rh incompatibility to the woman and reassure her that the antibodies do not harm her, but are a potential problem for the fetus.
• Explain that if RhoGAM is not administered, antibodies may develop that can cross the placenta and destroy the erythrocytes of the fetus.
• Explain the purpose of RhoGAM and the importance of receiving it at 28 weeks of gestation and possibly within 72 hours of childbirth.

CARE OF THE WOMAN WITH MULTIPLE GESTATIONS

Multiple gestations are becoming more common as women with fertility issues are receiving treatment that can result in multiple gestations. They are monitored closely and multiples are detected early. In the past, multiple pregnancies were

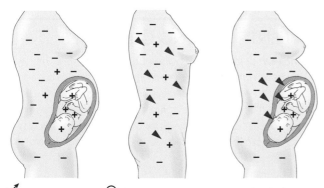

♂ Rh+ father   ♀ Rh− mother   ◣ Anti-Rh(O) antibodies

FIGURE 7.5 Isoimmunization occurring with an Rh+ father and Rh− mother. The fetus is Rh+; at childbirth, a small amount of blood enters the mother's bloodstream. The mother's immune system produces antibodies against the Rh+ blood. In subsequent pregnancies, if the fetus is Rh+, the mother's immune system sends the antibodies through the placenta to attack the fetal red blood cells.

often a surprise. Women who receive adequate prenatal care are rarely surprised at the time of birth by twins, triplets, or other multiple births.

Incidence and Risk Factors

According to the Centers for Disease Control and Prevention (CDC) (2013), the U.S. twin birth rate is 33.7 per 1,000 live births. The triplet or higher birth rate for the United States is 137.6 per 100,000 live births (2010). There is an increased risk for twins if the mother used fertility drugs, is older, has a family history of multiples, or used assisted reproductive technologies to become pregnant.

Signs and Symptoms

Possible signs that may indicate a multiple pregnancy are:

- Rapid weight gain in the first trimester
- Intense nausea and vomiting because of hormone increases
- Extreme breast tenderness because of hormone increases

Medical Management

Management of multiple pregnancies may include the following:

- *Increased calories and well-balanced nutrition:* The American College of Obstetricians and Gynecologists (2012) recommends women carrying twins gain at least 35 to 45 pounds. Mothers of multiples need more calories, protein, and other nutrients, including iron.
- *Frequent prenatal visits:* Multiple pregnancy increases the risk for complications. Frequent visits to the health-care provider may help detect complications early enough for effective management. The mother's nutritional status and weight should also be monitored more closely.
- *Increased rest:* Some women may need increased rest or even bedrest if complications develop. Multiple pregnancies often require bedrest beginning in the middle of the second trimester.
- *Referrals:* Referral to a perinatologist for special testing and evaluations and to coordinate care of complications may be necessary.
- *Maternal and fetal testing:* Testing may be needed to monitor the health of the fetuses, especially if there are pregnancy complications. Ultrasound biophysical profiles may be required to monitor the health of the fetuses.
- *Monitoring for complications*:
  - Incompetent cervix
  - Preterm labor
  - Pre-eclampsia
  - Gestational diabetes
  - Placental abruption
- Infants small for gestational age
- Increased risk for Cesarean birth

Nursing Care

Nursing care of the patient with multiple gestations includes the following:

- Prenatally, providing information about nutrition, an increased need for rest, and signs and symptoms of complications
- Encouraging the patient to verbalize her fears and ask questions
- During labor, monitoring fetal heart rates continually
- Preparing the woman for a possible Cesarean birth
- Ensuring that extra nurses and physicians are available at the birth for any newborn complications

Patient Teaching

Teach the patient who has multiple gestations the following:

- Provide written instructions for a healthy pregnancy diet.
- Instruct the woman to be alert for signs of preterm labor:
  - Contractions
  - Cramping
  - Low back ache
  - Increase in vaginal discharge
  - Loss of mucous plug
  - Pelvic pressure
- Encourage the woman to be compliant with office visits to monitor for pregnancy complications.
- Encourage her to schedule rest periods daily.
- Report any increase in edema, headaches, and visual disturbances to her health-care provider. These could be signs of hypertension.
- Report any vaginal bleeding to her health-care provider.

PATIENT TEACHING GUIDELINES

Urinalysis

During each prenatal visit, the patient is asked to give a clean-catch urine specimen for analysis. This analysis provides early information about possible complications of pregnancy. This urinalysis checks for high levels of sugars, proteins, ketones, and white blood cells, and bacteria, leukocytes, and nitrates related to:

- Bladder or kidney infections
- Diabetes
- Dehydration
- Pre-eclampsia

  Protein: Higher levels of protein may indicate a possible urinary tract infection or kidney disease. Pre-eclampsia may be a concern if high levels of protein are found later in pregnancy, combined with high blood pressure.

  Sugar: During pregnancy, it is normal for the kidneys to leak some sugar from the blood into the urine. However, high levels of sugar could indicate gestational diabetes.

Ketones: When the body is breaking down fats instead of carbohydrates for energy, ketones are found in the urine. High levels of ketones indicate that the patient is not getting enough to eat or may be dehydrated.

Bacteria, leukocytes, and nitrites: The presence of these items indicate that there may be a urinary tract infection.

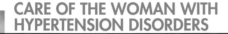

CARE OF THE WOMAN WITH HYPERTENSION DISORDERS

There are a range of hypertensive disorders that can complicate a pregnancy. The hypertension disorders fall under the umbrella term of *pregnancy-induced hypertension (PIH)*. These disorders of blood pressure are:

- Gestational hypertension
- Chronic hypertension
- Pre-eclampsia and eclampsia
- Superimposed pre-eclampsia

Pathophysiology

A pregnant patient can experience any hypertensive disorder alone, but these disorders are thought to be an evolving manifestation of a single pathological process and share a common origin.

The exact cause of hypertensive disorders, especially pre-eclampsia and eclampsia, remains unknown, despite much research. Pre-eclampsia, eclampsia, and HELLP syndrome (hemolytic anemia, elevated liver enzymes, and low platelet count) are the most serious disorders of hypertension in pregnancy. Pre-eclampsia manifests as an increase in blood pressure, protein in the urine (ie, proteinuria), and edema. If untreated, seizures begin and it is termed *eclampsia*. HELLP syndrome is considered a variation of pre-eclampsia, and causes a breakdown of red blood cells, elevated liver enzymes, and a low platelet count in addition to the symptoms of pre-eclampsia.

These disorders are multisystem diseases that are specific to the second half of pregnancy. The main target organs are the brain, kidney, liver, lungs, and heart.

Placenta

Current thinking is that the primary pathophysiology of pregnancy hypertension disorders is related to the placenta. Pre-eclampsia occurs in women who have an intrauterine pregnancy and in those with a hydatidiform mole, indicating that the placenta is playing a role in the pathophysiology (Carlson, 2015). The problem has been identified as abnormal trophoblastic implantation, which causes reduced placental perfusion. During implantation, the tiny villi in the placenta that eventually form arteries do not develop, and the placenta does not receive the blood supply that it should. The restriction of placental blood flow leads to hypoxia of the placental environment, which causes a release of factors called *antiangiogenic proteins* that enter the mother's circulation and act on endothelial cells, causing injury to the cells and producing vasospasm. Decreased blood flow to the placenta can also cause infarctions of the placenta tissue that lead to increased risk for placenta abruptio and a fetus with intrauterine growth retardation.

Blood Pressure and the Cardiovascular System

Hypertension in pre-eclampsia is caused by vasoconstriction. Also, if the placenta does not develop normally, the increased blood supply that should be going from the mother to the placenta does not occur, causing hypertension and edema.

Endothelial cell damage, which causes arteriolar vasospasm, may contribute to an increased capillary permeability. This increases edema and further decreases intravascular volume, predisposing the woman with pre-eclampsia to pulmonary edema. Women with pre-eclampsia also exhibit a hyperresponse to angiotensin-II and epinephrine, both of which elevate the blood pressure.

Kidney

The endothelial cell injury, which results in vasospasm, causes poor renal perfusion. This leads to a loss of protein, which reduces the colloid osmotic pressure. This will cause the woman with pre-eclampsia to have protein in her urine. The poor renal perfusion allows fluid to shift to interstitial spaces, resulting in edema. There is also a rise in blood urea nitrogen (BUN), creatinine, and uric acid levels.

Liver

Vasospasm in the liver impairs liver function. This causes hepatic edema and bleeding, which lead to necrosis of liver tissue. The necrosis causes an elevation in liver enzymes. A report of epigastric pain by the patient may indicate liver damage. The liver damage also activates the coagulation cascade with thrombocytopenia. The thrombocytes are increased in activation and size, but have a shorter lifespan. When HELLP syndrome develops, the hemolysis that occurs produces red blood cell fragments that leave fibrin in the blood vessels. The fibrin causes decreased blood flow to the liver and leads to liver impairment.

LABS & DIAGNOSTICS

Liver Enzymes

The liver performs many biochemical functions such as eliminating toxins, managing the breakdown of red blood cells, and detoxifying drugs, alcohol, and environmental toxins. Liver enzymes help the liver to do its job. They are substances that speed the rate of chemical or metabolic reactions. Enzymes utilized by the liver primarily exist in the cells of the liver. Under normal circumstances, these enzymes are also present in the bloodstream in low concentrations. However, when the liver is not working as it should, either because of inflammation or injury, these enzymes spill over into the bloodstream. In obstetrics, liver enzyme tests are used to assess liver disease that may occur with hypertension disorders of pregnancy:

- Alanine aminotransferase (ALT): Normal range less than 40 units/L; found in liver cells and in muscle and kidney cells; released with tissue damage
- Aspartate aminotransferase (AST): Normal range less than 40 units/L; found in liver cells and in muscle and kidney cells; released with tissue damage
- Alkaline phosphatase: Normal range 44 to 147 units/L; if found, it will be in the liver, biliary tract, bone, intestine, and placenta

Immune System

Immunologic factors may play a role in the development of pre-eclampsia. The presence of a foreign protein, for example, the placenta or fetus, may be identified by the mother's immune system as an antigen. This may then trigger an abnormal response by the immune system (Carson, 2015). This theory is supported by the increased incidence of pre-eclampsia or eclampsia in first-time mothers or to multiparous women pregnant by new partners (Moussa, 2014). Pre-eclampsia may be an immune disease in which the maternal antibody system is overwhelmed from excessive fetal antigens in the maternal circulation.

Brain and Central Nervous System

Cerebral edema, vasoconstriction from vasospasm, and damage to capillary linings may lead to seizures or hemorrhage. Cerebral vasospasm in the pregnant woman may be observed as a frontal throbbing headache. She may also experience vision symptoms associated with central nervous system irritation, or an indication of cerebral edema. Vision changes include a temporary loss of vision, flashing lights, auras, light sensitivity, and blurry vision or spots.

Effects on the fetus because of poor placenta perfusion include:

- Intrauterine growth retardation
- Premature separation of the placenta (ie, placenta abruptio)
- Persistent fetal hypoxia

Chronic Hypertension

Chronic hypertension refers to patients who are hypertensive before pregnancy or who become hypertensive during the early pregnancy. Frequently, the hypertension is related to obesity or a strong family history of hypertension. Many young women do not receive routine health care until they become pregnant and so may be diagnosed with hypertension at the first prenatal visit.

Signs and Symptoms

Signs and symptoms of chronic hypertension include BP of 140/90 mm Hg or greater before pregnancy or that occurs before 20 weeks of gestation.

Medical Care

Medical care of the pregnant patient who has chronic hypertension includes the following:

- Increasing the frequency of prenatal checkups
- Periods of rest to improve placental perfusion and promote diuresis to decrease blood pressure
- Low-sodium diet
- Administration of antihypertensive medications preferable for pregnancy: methyldopa or nifedipine (Moussa, 2014)

Nursing Care

Nursing care of the pregnant patient who has chronic hypertension includes the following:

- Monitoring blood pressure and reporting elevations to the health-care provider
- Administering antihypertensive medication and monitoring for side effects

Patient Teaching

Teach the patient who has chronic hypertension the following:

- Rest on the left side to increase placenta blood flow and promote diuresis.
- Drink eight glasses of water a day to prevent dehydration.
- Eat a low-sodium diet: do not add table salt, avoid canned foods, read labels carefully, and eat fresh high-fiber foods.
- Consume a daily diet of high-protein and high-fiber foods.
- Correctly administer antihypertensive medications and recognize any possible side effects.
- Schedule regular prenatal checkups with the health-care provider.
- Check blood pressure and urine for protein.
- Check daily for fetal kick counts.
- Record weight daily.
- Instruct the patient about the signs and symptoms of pre-eclampsia and report to the health-care provider if any of these signs occur:
  - Increase in blood pressure
  - Protein in the urine
  - Excessive heartburn
  - Increase in weight of more than one pound per week
  - Frontal headache
  - Decrease in fetal movement noted by a fetal kick count
  - Nausea and vomiting
  - Abdominal pain
  - Uterine contractions
  - Low back pain

LEARN TO C.U.S.

Lucille, aged 17, has arrived at the emergency department complaining of a severe headache and seeing dark spots in front of her eyes. She admits that she missed her last prenatal visit because she had "a test at school." She is at 36 weeks of gestation. On physical assessment, the nurse notes that she has a blood pressure of 160/94 mm Hg, the fetal heart rate is 160 bpm, and she has swollen feet and hands. The emergency room is very busy; there are several patients to be seen before it will be Lucille's turn to be evaluated by a physician. The nurse locates the doctor in the busy emergency unit and uses the C.U.S. method of communication.

C: "Doctor, I am **concerned** about Lucille. She is 17 years old and at 36 weeks of gestation.

U: I am **uncomfortable** because she is complaining of a severe headache and vision disturbance, and I noted swelling of her hands and feet. Her blood pressure is 160/90 mm Hg.

S: We have a **safety** issue because she may get worse before you have a chance to assess her and provide orders for her care."

Gestational Hypertension

Gestational hypertension is a condition of elevated blood pressure that begins in pregnancy and can lead to pre-eclampsia if not treated. Typically, the blood pressure returns to normal after delivery.

Signs and Symptoms

Signs and symptoms of gestational hypertension include:

- BP of 140/90 mm Hg or greater for the first time during pregnancy
- BP returns to normal less than 12 weeks postpartum
- No proteinuria

Medical Care

Medical care of gestational hypertension includes:

- Increase in the frequency of prenatal checkups
- Conservative treatment with a sodium restriction to 1,500 mg daily
- Resting on the left side to improve placenta blood flow, promote dieresis, and reduce blood pressure
- Antihypertensive medication if the patient's blood pressure remains elevated despite a low-sodium diet; methyldopa and nifedipine are preferable antihypertensive medications for pregnancy (Moussa, 2014)

Nursing Care

Nursing care of gestational hypertension includes:

- Monitoring blood pressure
- Teaching the patient the signs and symptoms of pre-eclampsia
- Teaching the patient correct administration of antihypertensive medication

Patient Teaching

Teach the patient who has gestational hypertension the following:

- Rest on the left side to increase placenta blood flow.
- Drink eight glasses of water a day to prevent dehydration.
- Eat a low-sodium diet: do not add table salt, avoid canned foods, read labels carefully, and eat fresh high-fiber foods.

Pre-eclampsia

Pre-eclampsia is defined as hypertension and proteinuria after 20 weeks of gestation. Edema is commonly present also but not necessary for a diagnosis of pre-eclampsia.

Incidence and Risk Factors

The incidence of pre-eclampsia is estimated to range from 2% to 6% in healthy nulliparous women (Kee-Hak, 2014).

Risk factors for pre-eclampsia include:

- Primigravida
- Maternal age more than 35 years
- Previous history of pre-eclampsia
- Chronic hypertension
- Multiple gestations
- Chronic renal disease
- Chronic hypertension
- Obesity
- Hydatidiform mole
- Egg donation or donor insemination
- Urinary tract infection

Signs and Symptoms

Signs and symptoms of pre-eclampsia are organized into categories of mild pre-eclampsia and severe pre-eclampsia.

MILD PREECLAMPSIA. Signs and symptoms of mild pre-eclampsia include hypertension (ie, BP greater than or equal to 140/90 mm Hg) on two occasions at least 6 hours apart.

SEVERE PREECLAMPSIA. Signs and symptoms of severe pre-eclampsia include:

- Systolic BP (SBP) of 160 mm Hg or higher, or diastolic BP (DBP) of 110 mm Hg or higher, on two occasions at least 6 hours apart
- Proteinuria of more than 5 g in a 24-hour collection OR more than 3+ on two random samples collected at least 4 hours apart
- Pulmonary edema or cyanosis
- Oliguria (ie, 400 mL or less in 24 hours)
- Persistent headaches
- Epigastric pain
- Impaired liver function
- Thrombocytopenia
- Visual disturbances (eg, blurred vision, dark spots in the visual field)
- Edema

Medical Care

The treatment for each patient with severe pre-eclampsia is individualized, but it must be treated aggressively. Severe hypertension is a threat to the mother and fetus. The goal of management is to control hypertension, prevent seizures, prevent long-term complications, and prevent maternal or fetal death. Childbirth is the treatment for pre-eclampsia. The symptoms start to decrease soon after birth. The fetus should be monitored for maturity, and labor induced as soon as appropriate for the fetus.

Medical care includes:

- Prescribe home bedrest for mild pre-eclampsia symptoms.
- Order diagnostic tests: CBC, liver function tests (LFTs), and platelet levels.
- Hospitalize the patient with severe pre-eclampsia.
- Conduct daily urinalysis to detect protein in the urine.
- Measure weight daily.
- Administer antihypertensive medications.
- If hospitalized, magnesium sulfate is given to prevent seizure activity. It is given IV with an infusion pump. An initial loading dose of 4 to 6 g is given over 5 min (Vallerand, Sanoski, and Deglin, 2013). That dose is followed with a maintenance dose of 2 g/hour. The patient is observed closely for magnesium toxicity.
- Prostaglandin gel may be given to prepare the cervix for labor.
- Oxytocin may be given to induce labor. A vaginal delivery is preferred to reduce risks associated with surgical births.

Nursing Care

Nursing care of pre-eclampsia includes:

- Monitoring blood pressure at least every two hours
- Monitoring urine output hourly and checking for protein
- Taking a daily weight measurement
- Administering antihypertensive medications
- Assessing the patient's level of consciousness (LOC) and vision
- Monitoring for nervous system irritability by testing for ankle clonus: Ankle clonus is a series of abnormal reflex movements of the foot induced by quick dorsiflexion of the patient's foot. Normally, no movement or clonus is present. The nurse should record the number of beats noted and report to the health-care provider. Hyperreflexia could indicate an impending seizure (Fig. 7.6).
- Reporting any changes in LOC or vision

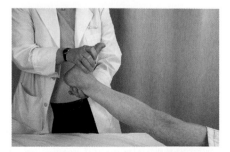

FIGURE 7.6 Testing for clonus.

- Monitoring laboratory results for signs of liver impairment
- Auscultating the lungs for signs of pulmonary edema, such as crackles and dyspnea
- Monitoring the fetus for well-being
- Providing a quiet environment for the patient
- Administering magnesium sulfate as ordered
- Checking brachial, radial, and patellar reflexes (ie, deep tendon reflexes [DTRs]) for hyperreflexia, which indicates brain irritability
- Monitoring for signs of magnesium toxicity; hyporeflexia and depressed respirations are associated with magnesium toxicity
- Providing emotional support for the patient and her family
- Postpartum management:
  - Continue to monitor blood pressure, hyperreflexia, urine output, and proteinuria. Eclampsia can occur up to 48 hours after delivery.
  - Signs of improvement include a return of blood pressure to a normal range, increased urinary output, and decreasing edema.

Patient Teaching

Teach the patient who has pre-eclampsia the following:

- If being treated at home, instruct the patient about how to check her own blood pressure and urine for protein.
- Teach her how to check for fetal kick counts daily.
- Instruct her to rest daily on her left side to improve placental blood flow.
- Instruct her to record her weight daily.
- Instruct the patient about the signs and symptoms of severe pre-eclampsia and to report to the health-care provider immediately if any of these signs occur:
  - Increase in blood pressure
  - Excessive heartburn
  - Sudden increase of weight
  - Frontal headache
  - Decrease in fetal movement
  - Severe nausea and vomiting
  - Abdominal pain
  - Vision changes
- Instruct the patient about the importance of magnesium sulfate administration and possible side effects.

DRUG FACTS

Magnesium Sulfate Therapy

Pharmacological Effects: Magnesium sulfate blocks neuromuscular transmission. Effects include a minor to moderate neurological depression manifested by diminished reflexes and somnolence (ie, drowsiness) (Vallerand, 2013).

Indications: It is prescribed to depress the central nervous system to prevent seizures.

Dose: A typical dose is 4 to 6 g in 100 mL of fluid given IV over 15 to 20 minutes followed by a maintenance dose of 2 g as a continuous infusion. Calcium gluconate is the antidote for magnesium sulfate toxicity.

Nursing Implications:

- Before administering this medication, assess the patient for a respiratory rate of at least 12 breaths per minute, an oxygen saturation of 95% or higher, urine output of at least 30 mL/hr, and the presence of DTRs.
- Monitor reflexes; if a response is absent, no additional doses should be given.
- Administer on time and with the correct dosage.
- Have a second practitioner independently double-check the original order, dose calculations, and infusion pump settings. Accidental overdose can result in serious harm to the patient.
- Monitor for signs of toxicity, such as hypotension, depressed DTRs, flushing, drowsiness, and decreased respirations.

LABS & DIAGNOSTICS

Assessing Deep Tendon Reflexes

- *Brachial reflex*: Support the woman's arm by laying it on your forearm. Instruct her to relax and let her arm go limp. Place your thumb over the tendon. Strike your thumb with the small end of the reflex hammer. A normal response is a slight flexion of the forearm.
- *Patellar reflex*: Dangle the patient's legs over the side of the bed. Place your hand on the patient's thigh and strike the distal patellar tendon just below the kneecap. If the patient is supine, flex each leg to a 45-degree angle and place your dominant hand behind her knee to support it. The normal response is contraction of the quadriceps muscle with extension of the knee.

  The reflexes are graded on the DTR rating scale:
- Reflex absent = 0
- Hypoactive reflex = +1
- Normal reflex = +2
- Slightly above average reflex = +3
- Hyperactive reflex = +4
  1. Report and document 0, +3, and +4 reflexes.
  2. Assess for clonus. Support the patient's lower leg with your hand. The foot is dorsiflexed to stretch the Achilles's tendon. Hold the flexion. If clonus is present, you will observe a rapid tapping motion of the foot. This indicates hyperreflexia.
  3. Report and document hyperreflexia.

Eclampsia

Pre-eclampsia becomes **eclampsia** with the onset of a seizure. Most cases of eclampsia occur in the third trimester, in the first 48 hours of the postpartum period. Although early detection of pre-eclampsia is possible, there are no tests that can indicate pre-eclampsia will progress to eclampsia (Ross, 2014).

Incidence and Risk Factors

Eclampsia occurs in about 1 in 2,000 pregnancies. The risk factors for eclampsia are:

- Primigravida
- Family history of pre-eclampsia
- Multifetal gestations
- Chronic hypertension
- Gestational diabetes
- Obesity
- Lower socioeconomic status
- Vascular and connective tissue disorders (Ross, 2014)

Signs and Symptoms

Signs and symptoms of eclampsia are:

- The same symptoms as pre-eclampsia, including:
  - SBP of 160 mm Hg or higher, or DBP of 110 mm Hg or higher, on two occasions at least 6 hours apart
  - Proteinuria of more than 5 g in a 24-hour collection OR more than 3+ on two random samples collected at least 4 hours apart
  - Pulmonary edema or cyanosis
  - Oliguria (ie, 400 mL or less in 24 hours)
  - Persistent headaches
  - Epigastric pain
  - Impaired liver function
  - Thrombocytopenia
  - Visual disturbances (eg, blurred vision, dark spots in the visual field)
  - Edema
- Seizures that may occur before or during labor, or during or after delivery

Medical Care

Medical care of the patient who has eclampsia includes the following:

- Continuing magnesium sulfate, as well as IV fluids and antihypertensive medications
- Planning either a vaginal or Cesarean birth after the seizures are controlled and she is stable

Nursing Care

Nursing care of the patient who has eclampsia includes the following:

- During a seizure, clearing the airway, administering oxygen, and providing for patient safety
- Documenting a description of the seizure, the length of the seizure, and the nursing care provided during a seizure
- Following a seizure, reorienting the patient
- Providing emotional support for the patient and her family
- Postpartum management includes:
  - Continuing to monitor blood pressure, hyperreflexia, urine output, and proteinuria; eclampsia can occur up to 48 hours after delivery

Patient Teaching

Teach the patient who has eclampsia the following:

- Explain the importance of preventing another seizure.
- Explain that the main treatment for eclampsia is delivery of the fetus. After delivery, her blood pressure will return to normal and the seizures will discontinue.
- Reassure the patient that she will never be alone during a seizure.

HELLP Syndrome

HELLP syndrome is named for the three main features of the disease: hemolysis, elevated liver enzyme levels, and low platelet counts:

H = hemolysis of red blood cells
EL = elevated liver enzymes
LP = low platelet count

The breakdown of red blood cells can cause oxygenation and perfusion problems for the woman and her fetus; for example, the placenta may not receive enough oxygenated blood to supply the fetus. The inflammation in the liver manifested by the elevated liver enzymes can cause right-upper-quadrant abdominal pain. The inflamed liver is unable to detoxify the blood as usual. The low platelet count will cause bleeding and clotting problems for the patient. HELLP is considered by most physicians to be a variant of pre-eclampsia and eclampsia that can be life-threatening. This hypertension disorder affects the liver and blood cells significantly, and the symptoms are sometimes mistaken for gastritis, gall bladder disease, hepatitis, or the flu. The mortality rate for women diagnosed with HELLP syndrome is about 25%. The cause of HELLP syndrome is unknown and there is no preventive management (Khan, 2013).

Incidence and Risk Factors

HELLP syndrome occurs in 10% to 20% of pregnant women with severe pre-eclampsia and eclampsia. It occurs most often before 37 weeks of gestation or after the baby is born (Khan, 2013).

Risk factors for HELLP syndrome include the following:

- Caucasian
- Age greater than 25 years
- History of hypertension
- Previous history of HELLP syndrome

Signs and Symptoms

Diagnosis is based upon symptoms of pre-eclampsia and/or eclampsia with the following laboratory test results:

- Elevated lactate dehydrogenase (LDH), AST, ALT, BUN, and bilirubin level because of liver damage
- Elevated uric acid level and creatinine counts because of renal damage
- Low platelet count

Signs and symptoms of HELLP syndrome include:

- Fatigue
- Fluid retention
- Pain in the upper right quadrant of the abdomen
- Blurry vision
- Nosebleeds or other bleeding that is difficult to stop
- Jaundice

Medical Management

Medical management of the patient with HELLP syndrome includes the following:

- Delivery of the baby as soon as possible
- Corticosteroid treatment to help the fetus' lungs mature faster
- Blood transfusions if required
- Antihypertensive medications
- Magnesium sulfate to prevent seizures

POSSIBLE COMPLICATIONS. Possible complications include:

- DIC, a clotting disorder that can lead to excessive blood loss
- Pulmonary edema; excessive fluid in the lungs
- Kidney failure
- Liver failure
- Placenta abruptio

Nursing Care

Nursing care of the patient with HELLP syndrome includes the following:

- Monitoring blood pressure at least every two hours
- Monitoring urine output hourly and checking for protein
- Administering medications such as antihypertensive medications, corticosteroids, and magnesium sulfate, if ordered by the health-care provider
- Monitoring for signs of bleeding
- Administering platelets or packed red blood cells, if ordered
- Assessing and reporting any changes in the patient's LOC and vision
- Monitoring for nervous system irritability by testing for ankle clonus
- Monitoring laboratory results, as well as LFTs, for signs of liver impairment
- Auscultating the lungs for signs of pulmonary edema, such as crackles and dyspnea
- Monitoring the fetus for well-being
- Providing a quiet environment for the patient
- Checking brachial, radial, and patellar reflexes (DTRs) for hyperreflexia, which indicates brain irritability
- Monitoring for signs of magnesium toxicity; hyporeflexia and depressed respirations
- Providing emotional support for the patient and her family

Patient Teaching

Teach the patient who has HELLP syndrome the following:

- Instruct the patient about medications and possible side effects.

- Instruct the patient to immediately report bleeding from the gums, nose, or venipuncture site, and any unusual bruising.
- Educate patient about the need to deliver the fetus to stop the progression of HELLP syndrome.

CARE OF THE WOMAN WITH GESTATIONAL DIABETES

Gestational diabetes is defined as a condition in which the blood glucose level is elevated during pregnancy in a woman not previously diagnosed as diabetic. Like other types of diabetes, gestational diabetes affects how cells use glucose.

When a pregnant woman eats a meal, a rise in blood glucose occurs and a series of hormonal actions begin. The secretion of insulin stabilizes her blood sugar and ensures that there is a supply of glucose available to the growing fetus. Glucose is absorbed into the bloodstream, which elevates blood glucose levels. This rise in glucose stimulates the secretion of insulin from the beta cells of the pancreas. Insulin binds to cell receptors and facilitates the entry of glucose into the cell, which uses the glucose for energy. The increased insulin secretion from the pancreas and the subsequent cellular utilization of glucose results in lower blood glucose levels. Lower glucose levels then result in decreased insulin secretion.

If insulin production and secretion are altered by disease, blood glucose is affected. If insulin production is decreased, glucose entry into cells is inhibited, resulting in hyperglycemia. The same effect will be seen if insulin is secreted from the pancreas but is not used properly by target cells. If insulin secretion is increased, blood glucose levels may become very low (ie, hypoglycemia) as large amounts of glucose enter tissue cells and little remains in the bloodstream. Pregnant women tend to develop hypoglycemia between meals and during sleep because the fetus continues to draw glucose across the placenta from the maternal bloodstream.

The placenta provides the growing fetus with nutrients and produces hormones to maintain the pregnancy. The hormones of pregnancy produced by the placenta include estrogen, cortisol, and human placental lactogen, all of which can have a blocking effect on insulin. Unlike other types of diabetes, gestational diabetes is not caused by a lack of insulin, but by the blocking effects of other hormones on the insulin that is produced. This condition is referred to as ***insulin resistance,*** a condition in which the body produces insulin but does not use it effectively. When people have insulin resistance, glucose builds up in the blood instead of being absorbed by the cells and used by the body. As the placenta grows, more of these hormones are produced, and insulin resistance becomes greater. Normally, the pancreas is able to make additional insulin to overcome insulin resistance, but when the production of insulin is not enough to overcome the effect of the placental hormones, gestational diabetes results. Gestational diabetes usually starts halfway through the pregnancy, at about 20 to 24 gestational weeks.

Incidence and Risk Factors

Gestational diabetes occurs in 3% to 10% of all pregnancies (Moore, 2014). Risk factors for a woman to develop gestational diabetes include:

- Age greater than 25 years
- Physical inactivity
- Being overweight, with a BMI of 30 or higher
- Gestational diabetes with a previous pregnancy
- Previous birth of a baby weighing more than 9 pounds
- Unexplained stillbirth
- African American, Native American, Hispanic, or Asian
- Having prediabetes, a condition in which blood glucose is higher than normal but is not high enough for a diagnosis of diabetes
- Having a parent or sibling with type 2 diabetes
- History of polycystic ovary syndrome (PCOS)

Signs and Symptoms

Some women will have no noticeable symptoms. Of those who do, signs and symptoms of gestational diabetes include:

- Increased thirst
- Feeling hungrier and eating more than usual
- Increased urination
- Fatigue
- Frequent infections of the bladder, vagina, and skin
- Blurred vision

Medical Management

Current recommendations by the American Diabetes Association are that high-risk women should be identified at the first prenatal visit and screened at that time with a two-step glucose tolerance test (GTT). All pregnant women should receive an oral GTT between the 24th and 28th weeks of pregnancy to screen for the condition, regardless of whether she tested nondiabetic at a previous screening.

The woman with gestational diabetes requires careful medical management and nursing care to prevent complications for her and her fetus. In addition to routine pregnancy laboratory tests, the gestational diabetic should also have the following tests to monitor for possible complications: hemoglobin A1c (HbA1c), BUN, serum creatinine, thyrotropin (TSH), free thyroxine (FT4), and capillary blood sugar levels two to four times daily.

The woman will also need to be monitored for ketoacidosis. Diabetic ketoacidosis (DKA) is an accumulation of ketones in the blood because of high glucose levels. In pregnancy, there is a state of accelerated starvation, especially in the second and third trimesters. The fetus and the placenta use large amounts of maternal glucose as a major source of energy, which leads to decreased maternal fasting glucose. This increased use of glucose, along with insulin deficiency, leads to an increase in free fatty acids, which are then converted to ketones in the liver. In gestational diabetes, DKA can occur at blood sugar levels of 200 mg/dL as compared with 350 mg/dL with nonpregnant diabetics. This condition requires immediate management to prevent complications for the mother such as coma and possible death of the fetus.

Signs and symptoms of DKA are:

- Increased urine production
- Increased thirst
- Nausea
- Vomiting
- Abdominal pain
- Weakness
- Weight loss
- Hyperventilation
- Ketone breath (ie, sweet-smelling breath)
- Tachycardia
- Hypotension
- Dry mucous membranes
- Disorientation
- Coma

Complications

Complications for the mother include diabetic retinopathy, which is damage to the retina and vision of the pregnant woman from elevated glucose levels. Hypertension complicates 10% of diabetic pregnancies (Moore, 2014). Hypertension can lead to pre-eclampsia and stroke.

The fetus can experience accelerated growth and become large for gestational age (LGA). The large fetus develops a condition called *macrosomia,* or overgrowth and deposits of fat in the abdominal and shoulder areas. If the mother gains excessive weight during the pregnancy, it increases the chance for preterm delivery, an LGA baby, and a Cesarean birth. Birth injuries are more common in infants of diabetic mothers because of the infant's size. Injuries that can occur are brachial plexus injury, facial nerve injury, and cephalohematoma. After birth, the infant is at risk for hypoglycemia, which can lead to neonatal seizures, coma, and brain damage. Infants of diabetic mothers also have an increased risk for respiratory distress syndrome.

PREVENTING FETAL COMPLICATIONS. Throughout the pregnancy, the goal is to prevent complications relating to the diabetes. Periodic testing for fetal well-being is part of the management of care. The recommended tests are:

- Fetal movement counting performed every night from 28 weeks of gestation until birth
  - A reassuring result is 10 movements in less than 2 hours.
- NSTs to begin at 28 to 34 weeks for insulin-dependent diabetics and at 36 weeks for diet-controlled diabetics
  - Reassuring results are two heart rate accelerations in 20 minutes.
- Contraction stress test done weekly, beginning at 28 to 34 weeks for insulin-dependent diabetics and at 36 weeks for diet-controlled diabetics
  - Reassuring results are no heart rate decelerations in response to three contractions in 10 minutes.

- Ultrasonic biophysical profile starting at 34 weeks of gestation
  - A reassuring result is a score of 8 in 30 minutes.

TEAM WORKS

Care of the Gestational Diabetic

The gestational diabetic can have a healthy fetus and avoid complications. Often, to provide optimal care, a team approach is used. The patient may be referred to the following health-care professionals:

- Dietician to educate her about calories, carbohydrates, and selecting healthy meals
- Diabetic educator nurse to teach her how to administer her medications
- Endocrinologist to provide medical management of her diabetes
- Neonatologist if complications have occurred during the pregnancy
- Obstetrical nurse to educate her about how to perform fetal kick counts, and explain normal pregnancy discomforts and warning signs of pregnancy

---

Recommended Therapies

The woman should check her blood sugar with a finger stick when she awakes in the morning, just before meals, and either 1 or 2 hours after meals.

As the pregnancy progresses there will be increased fetal demand for glucose, which can cause the woman to experience episodes of hypoglycemia. Also, as she progresses into each trimester, insulin resistance rises. The increase in insulin resistance prevents its proper use at the cellular level. Glucose cannot enter cells and accumulates in the bloodstream, resulting in hyperglycemia.

Dietary therapy is the first line of treatment for the gestational diabetic. Guidelines include:

- Preferably six meals per day, with three major meals and three snacks
- Complex carbohydrates with cellulose, such whole grains and legumes
- Carbohydrates making up 50% or less of the meal

Insulin or oral medications may be prescribed to achieve optimal glucose levels if diet alone cannot keep the glucose levels acceptable. The goal of insulin therapy is to achieve glucose profiles similar to the nondiabetic woman. The blood sugar range for the nondiabetic woman is 70 to 120 mg/dL. See Table 7.1 for target blood glucose ranges for the gestational diabetic. Obtaining these blood sugar levels will require the woman and her health-care provider to pay meticulous attention to her care. Lispro, aspart, regular (also known as *Humulin R*), and NPH insulins (neutral protamine Hagedorn, also known as *Humulin N* and *Novolin N*) are well-studied in pregnancy and are considered safe (Moore, 2014). An insulin regimen for the gestational diabetic requires frequent adjustments in the amount, type, and timing of insulin injections.

TABLE 7.1 TARGET BLOOD GLUCOSE LEVELS FOR WOMEN WITH GESTATIONAL DIABETES

Time of Day	Target
When patient awakes and before meals	95 mg/dL
1 hour after a meal	140 mg/dL or lower
2 hours after a meal	120 mg/dL or lower

SAFETY *STAT!*

As the health-care provider adjusts insulin doses, there is a risk of low blood sugar occurring. If the blood sugar drops below 70 mg/dL, the patient will usually have symptoms. The symptoms of low blood sugar include sweating, nervousness, sleepiness, dizziness, nausea, headache, and confusion. If the patient exhibits these symptoms, the patient's blood sugar should be checked and the patient given a snack that contains sugar.

Insulin is considered the standard treatment for the management of diabetes and pregnancy. However, oral medications such as glyburide and metformin can also be prescribed. Clinical trials have shown these drugs to be effective and not harmful to the fetus (Moore, 2014). Glyburide readily crosses the placenta and cannot be used during the first trimester because the risk to the embryo is unknown. This drug has been shown to be safe for lactation because it does not transfer to breast milk.

Nursing Care

Nursing care of the woman with gestational diabetes includes the following:

- Assessing the patient's understanding of gestational diabetes and providing additional teaching and reference materials
- Referring the patient to a registered dietician and reinforcing the dietary plan
- Monitoring blood sugar levels and adjusting care based on orders from the health-care provider
- Administering insulin or oral hypoglycemic medications as prescribed by the health-care provider
- Teaching the patient how to perform a capillary finger stick for glucose monitoring
- Monitoring for signs of hyperglycemia and DKA
- Monitoring fetal growth and well-being by performing NSTs as ordered by the health-care provider

HEALTH PROMOTION

How to Prevent Health Problems Related to Gestational Diabetes

A pregnant woman with gestational diabetes can prevent problems or complications during her pregnancy and have a safe pregnancy and healthy newborn. Guidelines she should follow are:

- Keep all prenatal appointments. She may need to see her health-care provider more often than someone without gestational diabetes.
- Check her blood sugar daily and keep a log to take to her prenatal appointments.
- If medications are prescribed, she should take them as directed and on time.
- Follow a healthy diet, choosing foods from all food groups.
- Get regular daily exercise to use the excess sugar in the bloodstream.
- Know the symptoms of low blood sugar: sleepiness, perspiration, tremors, rapid heart rate, cool clammy skin, blurred vision, and confusion.
- Treat low blood sugar quickly. Keep glucose tablets or gel nearby at all times.
- Notify the health-care provider if she is not able to maintain her blood sugars within the parameters that are expected by her health-care provider.

Patient Teaching

Teach the patient with gestational diabetes the following:

- Demonstrate the capillary finger stick blood glucose procedure for home glucose monitoring. Encourage the patient to perform a return demonstration to monitor for understanding.
- Review the health-care provider's preferred schedule for monitoring blood sugars at home.
- Explain and demonstrate insulin administration and encourage the patient to perform a return demonstration.
- Teach the patient the signs of hyperglycemia and hypoglycemia.
- Encourage the patient to engage in at least 30 minutes of exercise daily.
- Teach the patient to monitor fetal well-being with daily kick counts beginning at 28 weeks of gestation.
- Encourage the patient to keep a daily log of blood sugar levels, diet, and exercise to monitor her progress and to provide information to her health-care provider at her visits.

Key Points

- Pregnancy is usually a natural process that ends with a healthy baby and mother. There are many possible complications that threaten the positive outcome. The nurse is essential in assisting the health-care provider to manage the care of women with complications of pregnancy.
- Hyperemesis gravidarum can cause complications for the mother and fetus, such as fluid and electrolyte disturbances and preterm labor.
- Abortion is a pregnancy loss prior to the fetus being a viable size. There are several types of spontaneous abortions: threatened, inevitable, incomplete, and complete. All have the potential for excessive blood loss and infection.
- An ectopic pregnancy occurs when a fertilized ovum implants outside the uterus. This condition can be life-threatening to the woman and may require surgical treatment.
- GTD, also known as *hydatidiform mole*, is a genetic abnormality that results in abnormal growth of the placenta without fetal growth occurring. This condition requires aggressive treatment and follow-up for one year to monitor for cancer.

- Bleeding disorders of late pregnancy include placenta previa, placenta abruptio, and placenta accreta. They all have the potential to cause maternal hemorrhage and possible fetal loss if not identified and managed appropriately when diagnosed.
- The Rh-negative woman requires monitoring throughout pregnancy and after delivery to prevent isoimmunization.
- Multiple gestations are becoming more common, and women pregnant with multiples require careful monitoring throughout pregnancy to prevent complications, and preterm delivery.
- There is a range of hypertensive disorders of pregnancy that can complicate a pregnancy. Women with hypertensive disorders such as gestational hypertension, chronic hypertension, pre-eclampsia, eclampsia, and HELLP syndrome require close monitoring to prevent adverse outcomes for the mother and fetus.
- Women with gestational diabetes may require a team approach to manage the condition and prevent complications such as an infant that is LGA, requiring a Cesarean birth.

REVIEW QUESTIONS

1. A 30-year-old pregnant woman, gravida 1, para 0 is 30 weeks pregnant. She reports at her regularly scheduled office visit that she is experiencing vaginal bleeding that began "about three days ago." She also states, "I didn't call because I am not having any pain and I can feel the baby moving." The appropriate diagnostic procedure for her would be:
   1. A vaginal cervical examination
   2. A contraction stress test
   3. Abdominal ultrasound
   4. Internal fetal monitoring

2. A nurse is caring for a patient who just experienced a first trimester spontaneous abortion. Which comment by the nurse is considered appropriate? (*select all that apply*)
   1. "It must have been God's will."
   2. "You can try getting pregnant again soon."
   3. "If you have any questions, I am available to talk."
   4. "At least you weren't very far along."
   5. "There must have been something wrong with the fetus."
   6. "Is there anyone I could call for you—a friend, pastor, or rabbi?"

3. A priority nursing intervention for a patient with a ruptured ectopic pregnancy is to:
   1. Obtain IV access and begin infusing IV fluids.
   2. Reassure her that "everything will be okay."
   3. Provide pain medication.
   4. Infuse IV antibiotics.

4. The purpose of RhoGAM is to:
   1. Prevent the mother from developing Rh antibodies.
   2. Prevent the fetus from developing Rh antibodies.
   3. Change the mother's Rh factor from negative to positive.
   4. Change the baby's Rh factor to negative.

5. A woman at 38 weeks of gestation was involved in a car accident. She has numerous abrasions but no broken bones or head injury. The emergency department nurse knows that the most common complication that may occur for this woman is:
   1. HELLP syndrome
   2. Placenta previa
   3. Placenta abruptio
   4. Pre-eclampsia

6. A major risk factor for gestational diabetes is:
   1. Anemia
   2. Hypertension
   3. Obesity
   4. Asthma

7. The most serious complication of a hydatidiform mole pregnancy is the development of:
   1. Cancer
   2. Diabetes
   3. Infertility
   4. Hypertension

8. Patient teaching for the patient with pre-eclampsia should include:
   1. Continue normal activities, including daily exercise.
   2. Monitor blood pressure twice daily.
   3. Limit fluid intake to 320 mL per day.
   4. Monitor weight monthly.

9. Magnesium sulfate is administered to the pregnant patient with pre-eclampsia to:
   1. Prevent nausea and vomiting.
   2. Decrease the pain of labor contractions.
   3. Reduce central nervous system irritability to prevent seizures.
   4. Replace magnesium in a patient with a low magnesium level.

10. Immediately after birth, the infant born to a mother with gestational diabetes should be monitored for:
    1. Seizures
    2. Hypoglycemia
    3. Respiratory distress
    4. Jaundice

CRITICAL THINKING QUESTIONS

Ectopic Pregnancy

1. What is an ectopic pregnancy?

2. What are the various implantation sites?

3. Explain the treatment options and nursing care.

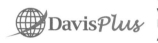

For additional resources and information, visit **www.DavisPlus.com**. Post-Conference Questions and Activities, Answers, and References can be found on Davis*Plus*.

unit THREE

Birth and the Family

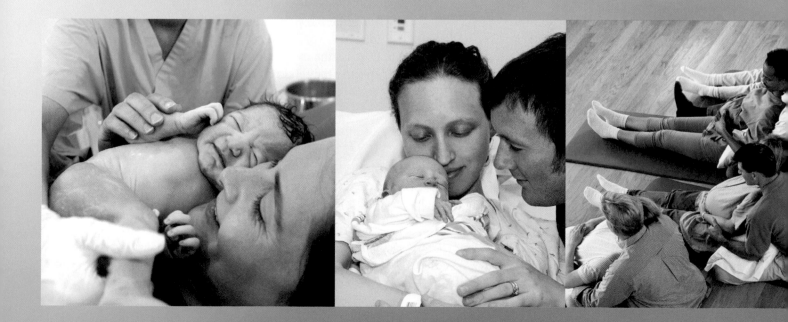

KEY TERMS

acme
attitude
Braxton Hicks contractions
decrement
dilation
duration
effacement
engagement
estriol
fetal lie
fetal presentation
fetal station
frequency
increment
intensity
lightening
oxytocin
prostaglandins

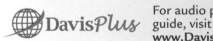 **DavisPlus**   For audio pronunciation guide, visit www.DavisPlus.com

CHAPTER CONCEPTS

Communication
Female Reproduction
Management
Pregnancy

LEARNING OUTCOMES

1. Define the key terms.
2. Discuss the theories related to the factors that cause the onset of labor.
3. List the signs of labor.
4. Describe the process of effacement and dilation that occurs in the cervix during labor.
5. Distinguish between true and false labor.
6. List and describe the "Seven Ps" of labor.
7. Distinguish between fetal lie, presentation, and position.
8. Teach a patient how to time uterine contractions.
9. Discuss the factors that contribute to patient satisfaction with the birth experience.
10. Discuss the *Healthy People 2020* goal of reducing Cesarean births.
11. Recognize the characteristics of a normal labor so as to provide knowledgeable care to the laboring patient.
12. Describe the stages of labor.
13. Discuss the three phases of the first stage of labor.
14. Explain the positional movements that occur as the fetus exits the birth canal.
15. Describe the signs of placental separation from the uterus.
16. Discuss the maternal systemic responses to labor.
17. Discuss the fetal response to labor.

REAL-WORLD CASE STUDY

Nadia

■ Nadia is pregnant with her first baby. She is in her 37th week of gestation and has noticed an occasional episode of a few mild uterine contractions. They seem to stop after a few minutes and are not really painful. Nadia calls the labor and delivery unit of her local hospital and asks to speak to the nurse. She has questions about labor contractions.

REAL-WORLD CASE STUDY *continued*

"Are these mild contractions that I am having preterm labor? How do I know if I am having true labor contractions?"

1. If the contractions are real labor, would Nadia be considered to be in preterm labor?
2. What information can the nurse give Nadia about the differences between true and false labor?
3. What are some other signs of impending labor?

Childbirth is a natural process. The focus of this chapter is on normal labor and delivery. Topics discussed in this chapter include the physiology of labor, signs of labor, true versus false labor, critical factors that influence labor, the stages of labor, maternal systemic response to labor, and fetal response to labor.

CONCEPTUAL CORNERSTONE

Professionalism

In nursing, professionalism refers to the characteristics and actions of a nurse representing the profession. There are many requirements to assume the role of the professional nurse. Among the requirements are the knowledge, skills, and attitudes to provide safe and effective care (Giddens, 2013). Knowledge is the foundation of nursing practice. Nurses who provide care for women in labor and childbirth need a solid understanding of the normal labor and birth process to provide effective care and to identify potential problems that may arise during the labor and delivery.

THE PHYSIOLOGY OF LABOR

Labor is a physiological process during which the fetus, umbilical cord, placenta, and amniotic membranes are expelled from the uterus. This process of expelling the uterine contents is accomplished through uterine contractions and cervical effacement and dilation. This section will discuss the theories of the causes of labor; the uterine and pelvic musculature; changes in the cervix during labor; and signs of labor.

THERAPEUTIC COMMUNICATION

Lenora, aged 17, is pregnant with her first baby. The nurse discussed childbirth education classes with Lenora using therapeutic communication.
Nurse: "Are you signed up for a childbirth class?"
Lenora: "No."
Nurse: "The classes fill up quickly; you don't want to miss it."
Lenora: "I don't think I'll go to one."
Nurse: "What are your concerns about it?"
Lenora: "I don't have the money and they aren't at the right time."
Nurse: "Let's work together to find one that works for you. We have several options available in this area."

Possible Causes of Labor Onset

Labor usually begins between 38 weeks and 42 weeks of gestation. The exact cause of labor onset is not clearly understood but there are several theories that are currently being studied that may contribute to the onset of labor. It is believed that a combination of factors leads to the onset of labor:

- Increased levels of **oxytocin:** a pituitary hormone that is secreted into the bloodstream and stimulates the uterine muscle. Oxytocin is also produced in uterine tissues in late pregnancy, with concentrations increasing at the onset of labor. Oxytocin receptors in the uterus also increase at the end of pregnancy. This leads to an increased sensitivity of the uterine tissues to oxytocin, and subsequent myometrial (ie, uterine muscle) activity.
- Oxytocin also helps in stimulating increased prostaglandin production through receptors in the decidua (ie, the lining of the uterus). **Prostaglandins** are hormonelike substances with a variety of effects on tissues, including contraction and relaxation of smooth muscle. Prostaglandins produce cervical softening and increase uterine muscle sensitivity. Oxytocin and prostaglandins are thought to be the most important biochemical factors in stimulating contractions.
- During pregnancy, progesterone is produced by the placenta. It relaxes uterine smooth muscle by hindering the conduction of impulses from one cell to the next. Toward the end of pregnancy, progesterone levels decline, which allows estrogen to stimulate contractions.
- The *corticotropin-releasing hormone hypothesis* is that the maturing fetus produces cortisol from the adrenal glands. The cortisol is detected in the fetal blood and then the placenta converts the hormone into estriol. **Estriol** is one of three types of estrogens that occur naturally in the body. The rising level of estriol produces an imbalance with estradiol, another estrogen, which triggers labor.
- The *uterine stretch theory* is that the large, hollow organ becomes overstretched, leading to a natural expulsion of the contents.

Uterine Muscle

The musculature of the pregnant uterus is arranged in three layers.

- An external layer arches over the fundus and extends to the ligaments that support the uterus.
- An internal layer has fibers that act as sphincters around the openings of the tubes and internal opening of the cervix.

• Between the external layer and internal layer is a middle layer that is composed of a dense network of fibers perforated by blood vessels. This network of muscle fibers and blood vessels contracts after placenta delivery to control blood loss (Templin, 2011).

Musculature Changes in the Pelvic Floor

The muscles of the pelvic floor, the levator ani muscle and the fascia, pull the vagina and rectum upward and forward with each contraction. The pressure of the fetal head progressing through the birth canal causes these muscles to thin from approximately 5 cm to 1 cm at the time of birth (American College of Obstetricians and Gynecologists, 2014).

Signs of Labor

Although every woman's experience is unique, most primigravidas and multiparas experience the following signs of the onset of labor.

Bloody Show

Bloody show is evident when the mucus from inside the cervix is released. This blood-tinged mucus is sometimes referred to as the *mucous plug,* and may be noted any time before or during labor.

Burst of Energy

Some women experience a burst of energy, which is also called *nesting,* about 24 to 48 hours before labor begins. She may experience the desire to complete many projects before her baby arrives.

Rupture of Membranes

Rupture of membranes (ROM) is also referred to as the *water breaking.* The rupture of the membranes surrounding the fetus and amniotic fluid often signals that labor is beginning. The membranes can rupture any time during labor. The fluid should be clear with no offensive odor. The rupture can manifest as a large gush or a small trickle of fluid.

SAFETY *STAT!*

Amniotic fluid that is not clear, such as yellow or green, should be reported immediately to the health-care provider. It could indicate an unhealthy fetus.

Lightening

Lightening is usually noticed by the mother after the 38th week of pregnancy as the fetus descends or drops into the pelvis. The mother notices this because the drop of the fetus into the pelvis allows her to have more room in her upper abdomen and makes breathing easier. After lightening takes place, she will notice that she has to urinate more often because of pressure of the fetal head on her urinary bladder and she may experience an increase in leg cramps from the increased pressure on the nerves and blood vessels in her pelvis and legs.

Contractions

During pregnancy, women often experience contractions. One type, Braxton Hicks contractions, begins sometime during the second trimester. They can be uncomfortable but do not produce cervical dilation or effacement. The second type of contraction causes cervical dilation and effacement and indicates true labor.

• Uterine contractions that occur regularly and become more intense as time passes indicate true labor. Contractions are sometimes described as pressure or aching in the lower back or pelvis that then spreads around to the abdomen. The contraction starts mildly, gets stronger, progresses to a peak, and then fades away.
• **Braxton Hicks contractions** are irregular, mild contractions that occur in late pregnancy and do not produce cervical effacement and dilation. Braxton Hicks contractions are described by women as feeling like menstrual cramps.

Cervical Changes

During most of pregnancy, the cervix is approximately 3 to 4 cm thick and closed. Toward the end of the pregnancy, the cervix starts to soften and begins to open as collagen fibers in the cervix are broken down by collagenase and elastase. During labor, the cervix continues to dilate to 10 cm or large enough to accommodate the fetal head.

Effacement is the cervix-thinning process that may begin toward the end of pregnancy. Each uterine contraction causes the muscles of the upper uterine segment to shorten and cause a longitudinal traction on the cervix, causing this thinning effect. Effacement is measured in percentages. A thick, uneffaced cervix is defined as 0% effaced and a fully thinned or effaced cervix is 100% effaced. This measurement is subjective depending upon the skill and opinion of the practitioner performing the cervical examination. The cervix of the primipara effaces slowly before significant dilation occurs. With the multipara, effacement and dilation usually occur simultaneously (Fig. 8.1).

Dilation is the opening of the closed cervix to approximately 10 cm or large enough to accommodate the fetal head.

SAFETY *STAT!*

For second and subsequent labors, the cervix usually dilates and effaces faster. Patients should be instructed to come to the hospital sooner with a second or subsequent delivery to avoid an unplanned birth outside the hospital.

Differences Between True and False Labor

When labor begins, it may not be easy for the nurse or the patient to determine if it is real or false labor. There are some

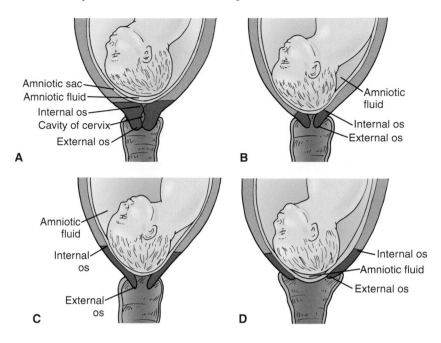

FIGURE 8.1 Cervical effacement and dilation. The membranes are intact. A, Before labor. B, Early effacement. C, Complete (ie, 100%) effacement. The fetal head contacts the cervix. D, Complete dilation (ie, 10 cm).

points to remember when evaluating a patient for signs of true labor:

- True labor contractions:
  - Come at regular intervals
  - Become increasingly more intense as labor progresses
  - Increase in duration over time
  - Include discomfort that usually begins in the back and radiates to the front
  - Cause effacement and dilation to occur
  - May intensify with walking
  - Do not diminish with a warm shower or rest
- False labor contractions:
  - Are irregular
  - Do not increase in duration
  - Do not cause cervical effacement and dilation to occur
  - May cease with rest or a warm shower
  - Do not intensify with a walk

CRITICAL FACTORS IN LABOR

Traditionally, educators and health-care providers have used the "Seven Ps" to describe the significant factors in the process of labor: *passage, passenger, powers, position, psyche, pain management,* and *patience* are critical factors in labor.

Passage

The passage is the route through which the fetus must pass to be delivered vaginally. The passage consists of the pelvis and the soft tissues. The soft tissues yield to the pressure of the fetal presenting part, which is usually the head. The pelvis is most important to the outcome of labor because bones and joints do not yield easily to the fetal head. The pelvis is usually measured by the health-care provider at the first prenatal

visit to determine if the woman's pelvis is adequately sized for a vaginal delivery.

During late pregnancy, concentration of the hormone relaxin increases, causing a softening of the cartilage that connects the pelvic bones. This softening of cartilage allows the pelvis to stretch somewhat to allow for passage of the fetus through the pelvis.

SAFETY *STAT!*

The hormone relaxin affects all joints of the body. A term pregnant patient is at risk of falling because of the loosening of her pelvic joints, knees, and ankles.

The pelvis has three subdivisions important for childbirth:

- ***The inlet:*** This area consists of the area from the symphysis pubis (the anterior), the sacral promontory, and the linea terminalis. The transverse diameter is approximately 13.5 cm and the anteroposterior (AP; ie, diagonal conjugate) is 11.5 cm or greater. The inlet is surrounded by bone, except for the cartilage at the sacroiliac joint and symphysis pubis, and cannot enlarge much to take in the fetus.
- ***The midpelvis:*** This area is the narrowest part of the pelvis that the fetus must pass through during childbirth. The midpelvis diameter is measured at the level of the ischial spines. The transverse diameter of the midpelvis averages 10.5 cm.
- ***The outlet:*** This area has three measured diameters. The AP diameter ranges from 9.6 to 11.5 cm, varying with the curve between the sacrococcygeal joint and the coccyx. This diameter can increase if the coccyx is moveable. The transverse diameter measures the ischial tuberosities and averages 11 cm. The third diameter is the posterior

sagittal diameter, measuring the distance from the sacro-coccygeal joint to the middle of the transverse diameter, and is normally at least 7.5 cm. The angle of the pubic arch is also important because it must be at least 90 degrees to allow passage of the fetus (Watson, 2011).

Passenger

The passenger is the fetus with the placenta. When providing labor care, the health-care provider and the nurses determine the fetal lie, presentation, position, attitude, and station and continue to monitor fetal changes as labor progresses.

Fetal Head

The fetal head is an important factor in labor and birth. The frontal, parietal, and occipital bones are not fused in the fetus. These bones are soft and pliable with gaps between them known as *suture lines*. This allows the bones to overlap as the head progresses through the pelvis from the force of the uterine contractions. This overlapping process causes an elongation shape of the skull and is called *molding*.

The diameter of the fetal skull is important to consider during the labor process. The biparietal diameter measures the largest transverse diameter of the fetal skull, which is the distance between the two parietal bones. The optimal position for the fetal head at birth is fully flexed with the chin on the chest, which produces the smallest fetal head dimension.

Fetal Lie

Fetal lie refers to the alignment of the fetus with the mother:

- *Longitudinal lie* refers to a fetus that is lying parallel with the mother.
- *Transverse lie* refers to a fetus that is lying perpendicular to the mother's body.
- *Oblique lie* refers to a fetus that is lying at an angle between the transverse lie and the longitudinal lie (Fig. 8.2).

Fetal Presentation

Fetal presentation refers to the part of the fetus that is first to enter the pelvis.

- Cephalic presentation: The head is the presenting part.
- Breech presentation: The buttocks are the presenting part (Fig. 8.3A and B).

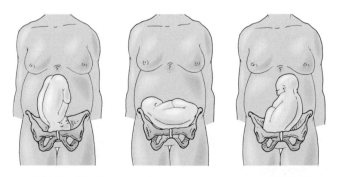

FIGURE 8.2 The fetal lie refers to the relationship of the long axis of the woman to the long axis of the fetus. A, Longitudinal lie. B, Transverse lie. C, Oblique lie.

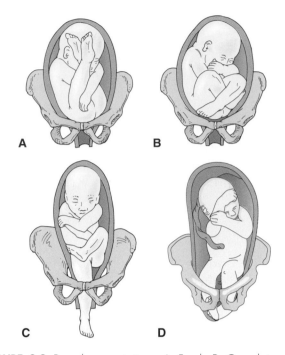

FIGURE 8.3 Breech presentations. A, Frank. B, Complete or full. C, Footling (single). D, Footling (double).

- Shoulder presentation: The shoulder is the presenting part.
- Footling breech presentation: The feet are the presenting part (Fig. 8.3C and D).

Fetal Position

Fetal position refers to the relationship of a given point on the fetus' presenting part with the mother's pelvis. The landmark for the head or cephalic presenting part is the occipital bone (indicated by the letter *O*). For a breech presentation, the landmark is the sacrum (indicated by the letter *S*). The maternal pelvis is divided into four quadrants: left anterior, right anterior, left posterior, and right posterior. The fetal position is determined by noting the presenting part and the maternal pelvis quadrant that the fetus is facing. The position is indicated by a three-letter abbreviation:

- The first letter indicates whether the presenting part is tilted toward the left (*L*) or right (*R*) of the maternal pelvis.
- The second letter indicates the presenting part of the fetus (eg, *O* for occipital or *S* for sacrum).
- The third letter indicates the location of the presenting part in relationship to the anterior, transverse, or posterior part of the maternal pelvis.

The most common fetal position in labor is *LOA* (the left occiput anterior position), which means that the fetus occipital bone (ie, the back of the head) is facing the left anterior quadrant of the pelvis (Fig. 8.4).

Fetal Attitude

The fetal **attitude** refers to the positioning of the fetus' body parts. The most common fetal attitude and the most successful

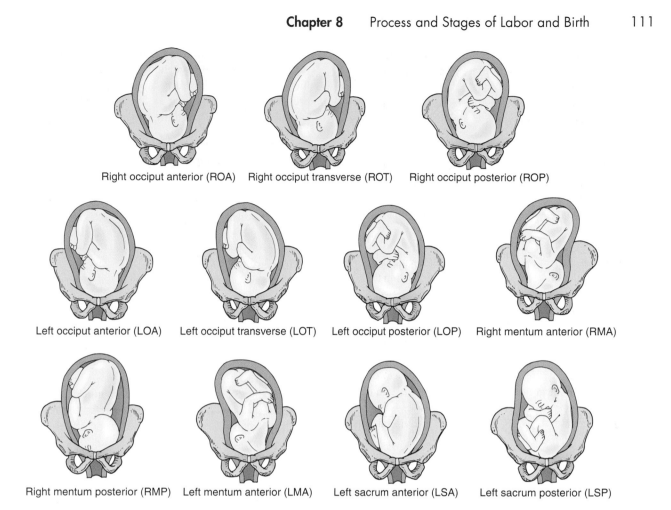

FIGURE 8.4 Fetal presentations and positions. The position refers to how the presenting fetal part is positioned in relationship to the maternal pelvis: front (ie, anterior), back (ie, posterior), or side (ie, transverse).

for a vaginal delivery is when the fetus is in a fully flexed position with the chin on the chest, the back rounded, the thighs flexed on the abdomen, and the legs flexed at the knees. A fetus that is not fully flexed exhibits changes in the presenting part diameter as passage through the pelvis occurs, leading to birthing difficulty (Fig. 8.5).

Fetal Station

Fetal station is the measurement in centimeters of the fetal head in relationship to the maternal ischial spines in the

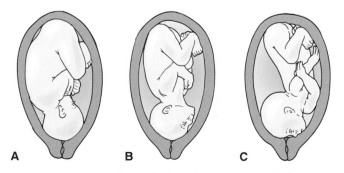

FIGURE 8.5 The fetal attitude describes the relationship of the fetal body parts to one another. A, Flexion (cephalic or vertex). B, Moderate flexion. C, Extension.

pelvis. Station measurements provide information on the descent of the fetus through the birth canal.

- The measurement ranges from –5 cm to +5 cm.
- When the head is above the ischial spines, a negative number is applied. When the head is 1 cm above the ischial spines, the measurement is –1.
- When the fetal head is at the level of the ischial spines it is measured as 0 station.
- When the head is 1 cm through the ischial spines, it is termed *+1 station* (Fig. 8.6).

Powers

During labor, the power of the uterine contractions and the woman's ability to push are critical factors of labor. At the onset of labor, the patient and her support person will be timing contractions at home. After arrival at the hospital, the health-care provider and labor and delivery nurses will time and evaluate contractions with the use of the fetal monitor or manually by palpating contractions. Uterine contractions in labor occur in a regular rhythmic fashion. Each contraction has three phases:

1. The **increment,** which can be described as the onset and buildup of intensity of the contraction

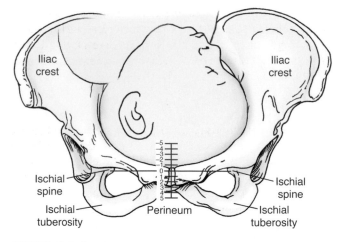

FIGURE 8.6 Station.

2. The **acme**, which is the peak of the contraction
3. The **decrement,** which is the subsiding of the contraction (Fig. 8.7)

To describe contractions, the following terms are used:

- **Onset:** The exact time that a contraction begins
- **Duration:** The actual time that a contraction lasts from beginning to end
- **Frequency:** The time between contractions, which is measured from the beginning of one contraction to the beginning of the next contraction
- **Intensity:** The strength of the contraction at the peak or acme of the contraction; can be measured by palpation by an experienced practitioner and by internal fetal monitoring

At the peak of a strong contraction, uteroplacental blood flow is decreased and the fetus receives no fresh oxygenated blood supply. Between each contraction is a period of relaxation.

During the second stage of labor the woman will be required to push along with contractions to continue to move the fetus through the birth canal. Her pushing efforts can prevent interventions such as forceps or vacuum extraction assistance during the birthing process.

PATIENT TEACHING GUIDELINES

How to Time Uterine Contractions

An informed woman who knows how to time contractions will have valid information to provide the health-care provider if she thinks she is starting labor. Such knowledge will also help the patient to distinguish between true and false labor. The steps for timing contractions are:

- Note the exact time that a contraction begins. This is the *onset* of the contraction.
- Note the exact time that the contraction stops. From the onset to this point is the *duration,* or length, of the contraction.
- Note the exact time that the next contraction begins. From the first onset to this point is the *frequency* of the contractions.

Teach your patient that contraction frequency is the time from the beginning of one contraction to the beginning of the next. Duration of the contraction is the actual length of time the contraction was noticeable.

Position

Maternal position changes in labor can influence the length of the labor. Upright positions of standing, sitting, kneeling, or walking have been shown to reduce the length of labor by approximately one hour and are associated with less epidural anesthesia (Berghella, 2012). Women should be encouraged to choose a position that is comfortable for them; an exception is the supine position, which can produce blood flow problems for the woman and the placenta.

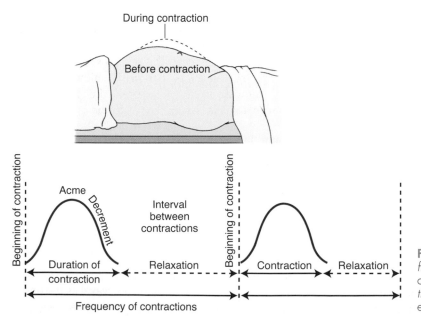

FIGURE 8.7 Counting contractions. *Contraction frequency* is the time from the beginning of one contraction to the beginning of the next. *Contraction duration* is the time from the beginning to the end of the same contraction.

Studies have shown that an upright, lateral, or squatting position during the second stage for pushing and delivery reduces the need for assisted delivery. These positions have been shown to reduce reports of severe pain during this stage, as well as a reduction in abnormal fetal heart rate patterns (Berghella, 2012). Women without an epidural should be encouraged to deliver in an upright position.

Psyche

Childbirth is a life-altering experience that women never forget. Physical and mental preparation for labor and delivery are very important aspects of managing the labor process. It is generally noticed by nurses in the labor and delivery unit that women who lack confidence in their ability to manage and cope with labor seem to have longer labors with more interventions and a higher rate of Cesarean births. The woman's state of mind (ie, psyche) during the process is important to create a positive outcome for her and her family. Factors that contribute to a positive birth experience include:

- Childbirth education, which prepares the woman for labor and delivery; patients with childbirth education tend to arrive at the labor and delivery unit in active labor and are confident of their ability to manage labor (Berghella, 2012)
- Trust in the health-care provider and the staff who care for her
- Nurses who integrate the patient's birth philosophy, cultural beliefs, and religious values and beliefs into the plan of care
- Information updates provided about labor progress
- Clear, concise information given on necessary procedures during the labor and birth process
- Nurses, the health-care provider, and the support person giving reassurance and praise for managing labor and offering advice regarding coping techniques
- Continuous one-on-one support throughout labor and birth by someone who can advocate for the woman's desires or plans
- Assisting the laboring woman to maintain her sense of control of herself and the labor situation

Pain Management

Labor and delivery is a normal physiological process, but it is painful. Every woman perceives and reacts to pain differently. Women who are anxious during labor have high levels of the stress hormone epinephrine in the blood, which can lead to abnormal fetal heart rate patterns, decreased uterine contractility, and a longer active labor phase (Berghella, 2012). The challenge of the team (ie, woman, support person, nurse, anesthesiologist, and health-care provider) is to find the right combination of pain management methods to promote a positive experience for the woman in labor as well as a safe delivery for the fetus.

There is a range of pain management methods used by women during childbirth. There are nonpharmacological measures, such as such as massage, warm baths, and relaxation techniques, as well as pharmacological methods used to manage pain. Chapter 10, Nursing Care During Labor, presents a full discussion of pain management during labor and birth.

Patience

The process of labor takes time. There are many obstetric interventions that are widely used, such as the induction of labor, the augmentation of labor with oxytocin, and regional anesthesia (ie, epidural) that influence the length of the labor process. Delaying these types of interventions and allowing labor to progress naturally may decrease medical interventions and decrease the Cesarean birth rate. *Healthy People 2020* has two goals related to Cesarean birth in the United States:

1. Reduce the rate of Cesarean birth among low-risk women to 23.9% of live births from a baseline of 26.5%
2. Reduce the rate of Cesarean births among women who have had a prior Cesarean birth to 81.7% of live births from a baseline of 90.8%

To achieve these goals, patience during labor is required. Methods to increase patience include:

- Educate the woman and her family that every labor is different and it is difficult to predict how long a labor will last.
- Avoid interventions such as epidural anesthesia that reduce the woman's ability to push and her participation in delivery of the fetus (Barclay, 2014).
- Avoid induction of labor when the cervix has not softened sufficiently to make it receptive to induction methods.
- Avoid the induction of labor for convenience. Women induced have a significantly longer time in labor (Simpson, 2012).
- Provide reassurance to the mother of fetal well-being during the labor process.
- Provide nonpharmacological pain interventions as well as pharmacological support for pain during labor.
- If the fetal monitor indicates that the fetus is healthy, do not place pressure on the obstetrician or midwife to rush the birth. Allow a longer pushing phase. Longer pushing has not been associated with poor outcomes.

STAGES OF LABOR AND BIRTH

Obstetricians have divided labor into three stages that outline labor progress in a continuous progression.

TEAM WORKS

Women with an understanding of normal labor and delivery process will experience less stress during labor (Berghella, 2012). A team approach to educating her and her partner about the labor experience would include the following team members:

- The office nurse during prenatal visits
- The childbirth educator who provides childbirth education classes
- The nurse in labor and delivery who assesses the immediate learning needs of the patient
- The doula providing labor support
- The nurse-midwife or obstetrician providing care and delivering the fetus

First Stage

The first stage of labor begins with regular uterine contractions and ends with complete cervical dilation at 10 cm. The first stage is divided into three phases: the latent, active, and transition phases.

Latent Phase

The latent phase is the early phase of labor. The length of latent phase can be unpredictable from woman to woman and from labor to labor. Typically for the primipara, it may last close to 20 hours. The latent phase for a multipara is usually around 10 to 12 hours. The amniotic membranes may spontaneously rupture in the early-to-midportion of the first stage of labor. If they rupture, the labor process usually speeds up because the presenting part is able to apply pressure to the cervix during contractions.

Characteristics of latent labor are:

- Uterine contractions are generally mild and erratic before becoming regular and stronger. The contractions may range from 5 to 20 minutes apart and last 20 to 40 seconds.
- Most of the cervical effacement occurs.
- Cervical dilation increases to 3 centimeters.
- The woman and her partner may feel excited and relieved that labor has started but anxious about the birth process.
- The woman usually can cope with the pain of contractions by using relaxation and breathing techniques.

HEALTH PROMOTION

Hydration During Labor

Hydration is important during labor. The woman in early labor at home should be encouraged to consume liquids to maintain hydration. However, it is common for the laboring woman to experience some nausea and vomiting, especially during the transition phase of active labor. With this in mind, the woman should be encouraged to hydrate with clear liquids and to avoid large spicy meals during early labor.

Active Phase

The next part of the first stage of labor is the active phase, which is the phase of the most rapid cervical dilation. The active phase is the most predictable, lasting an average of 5 hours in primiparas and 2 hours in mothers who have birthed before.

Characteristics of active labor:

- Uterine contractions become more frequent, have a longer duration, and increase in intensity. Generally, the contractions are 2 to 3 minutes apart and the duration is around 60 seconds.
- Dilation increases from 3 to 4 cm to 8 cm.
- Cervical dilation averages 1.2 cm/hr for primiparas and 1.5 cm/hr for multiparas (Cheng, 2014).
- Fetal descent is progressing.
- The woman becomes labor-focused and may require more assistance to cope with the increasing intensity of the uterine contractions.

Transition Phase

The transition phase is the most intense phase of labor, leading to complete dilation. The characteristics of transition are:

- Painful uterine contractions that are 2 to 3 minutes apart and last 60 to 90 seconds.
- The cervix is 100% effaced.
- The woman may feel pelvic or rectal pressure caused by fetal descent into the pelvis.
- She may have more trouble with concentration and coping and may become irritable.
- Nausea and vomiting are common.
- For the primipara, this stage can last 3.5 hours; for multiparas, it varies, but is generally shorter.

Anytime during labor, an unexpected problem may occur that can lead to a Cesarean birth. Possible causes of a Cesarean birth are:

- Fetal distress
- Abnormal position of the fetus
- Disproportion between the fetus and the mother's pelvis
- Umbilical cord prolapse
- Failure of labor to progress
- Medical conditions such as pre-eclampsia
- Placenta previa or placental abruption

If a Cesarean birth becomes the safest choice for the mother and fetus, the obstetrician and the nurse will continue to provide patient-centered care by including the patient in the decision making and preparation for the surgical birth. Chapter 12, Birth-Related Procedures, discusses Cesarean births and nursing care in detail.

SAFETY STAT!

A patient in the transitional phase of labor should never be left alone. She could be close to delivery. The nurse should be at the bedside monitoring patient progress.

Second Stage

The second stage of labor begins with full cervical dilation (ie, 10 cm) and ends with delivery of the fetus. Characteristics of the second stage of labor are:

- Uterine contractions occur every 2 to 3 minutes and last 60 to 80 seconds.
- There is increased bloody show.
- The woman feels the urge to bear down and push.
- The duration of this stage varies, with an average duration of 30 to 90 minutes for a primipara and 15 to 30 minutes for a multipara.

CULTURAL CONSIDERATIONS

Various research studies have been done to determine if there were differences in the length of labor among different racial and ethnic groups. No significant differences in the first stage of labor have been identified. There were differences identified in the length of the second stage of labor. The second stage was shorter for African American women and Hispanic women compared to a longer second stage for Caucasian women. Asian women were determined to have the longest second stage of labor (Greenburg, Cheng, and Hopkins, 2006).

Pushing

Pushing time for primiparas can be up to 3 hours, and for multiparas it varies from 1 to 30 minutes. Different techniques are used in labor to move the fetus through the pelvis. Two common methods of pushing are the open glottis and closed glottis methods:

- In closed glottis pushing, the woman is directed to take a deep breath during a contraction and push with all her energy for at least 10 seconds or more.
- In open glottis pushing, the woman is allowed to experience involuntary pushing when she feels the desire. She instinctively will hold her breath and push for about 6 seconds. She will follow pushing by taking several deep breaths and pushing again when she feels the urge to bear down.

SAFETY *STAT!*

The Association of Women's Health, Obstetric, and Neonatal Nurses (AWHONN) has made a statement that discourages closed glottis pushing for a prolonged time. Closed glottis pushing has been associated with decreased placental blood flow, leading to hypoxemia for the fetus and possible fetal distress. Open glottis pushing has not been associated with these complications and has been associated with a shorter second stage of labor.

Positional Changes of the Fetus

In order for the fetus to pass through the birth canal, the fetal head and body must adjust to the passage and go through positional changes. These positional changes are referred to as *cardinal movements*. The positional changes are discussed in the order in which they occur (Fig. 8.8).

- **Engagement** occurs when the widest diameter of the presenting part, which is most often the fetal head, enters the mother's pelvis to a level of the maternal ischial spines.
- *Descent* is the downward passage of the fetus through the pelvis. Downward movement occurs in small increments during a contraction.
- *Flexion* occurs as the fetal head encounters resistance from the pelvic bones and soft tissues of the pelvic floor, causing the fetus to flex the head. The chin is brought into contact with the chest and changes the diameter of the presenting part from 11 cm to 9.5 cm, which is optimal for passage through the pelvis (Cheng, 2014).

Internal Rotation

Internal rotation occurs as the head, which is usually in the transverse position, rotates 45 degrees to an AP position under the symphysis pubis of the pelvis.

- *Extension* follows descent and flexion of the head when the occiput comes into contact with inferior margin of the symphysis pubis and the force of uterine contractions causes the occiput to extend and rotate around the symphysis.
- *Restitution* and *external rotation* occur as the fetus head untwists to the left or right, returning the head to original anatomical position.
- *Expulsion* is the final step; the fetal head is delivered and the anterior shoulder is rotated under the symphysis, followed by the posterior shoulder and the rest of the fetus' body (Fig. 8.9).

Third Stage

The third stage begins with the birth of the newborn and ends with the delivery of the placenta.

Placental Separation

After the baby is born, the uterus will continue to contract and will decrease in size. The delivery of the placenta is expected within 30 minutes of the delivery of the baby. Signs that the placenta is separating from the uterus are:

- The umbilical cord lengthens.
- A sudden trickle of blood is noted at the vaginal opening.
- The uterus rises upward.

Placental Expulsion

After separation, some practitioners will exert gentle traction to guide the placenta out of the birth canal. The umbilical cord should never be pulled to remove the placenta. The placenta will be expelled with either the fetal side (shiny gray)

NURSING CARE PLAN for the Patient Preparing for Labor

Nursing Process: Assessment
- Assess the patient's level of knowledge.
- Encourage questions from the woman and her support person.

Nursing Goal: The patient will have an understanding of the labor and birth process.

Nursing Diagnosis: There is a knowledge deficit related to the normal labor process.

Interventions:
- Briefly review the normal labor process.
- Answer questions at the level of the patient's understanding.
- Provide pictures and diagrams of the birth process.

Evaluation:
- The patient will verbalize understanding of the birth process.

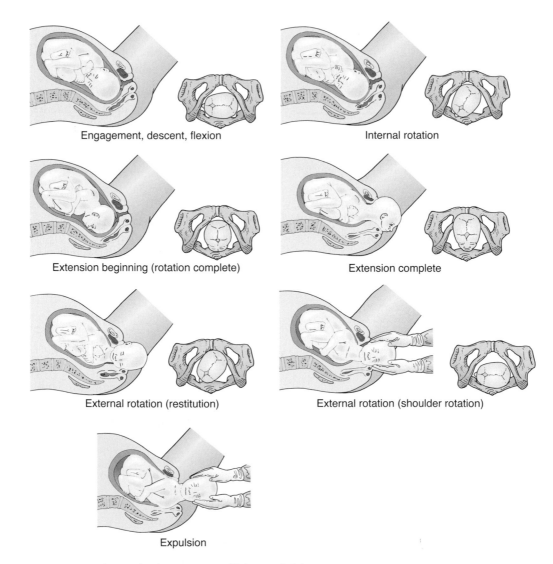

Engagement, descent, flexion

Internal rotation

Extension beginning (rotation complete)

Extension complete

External rotation (restitution)

External rotation (shoulder rotation)

Expulsion

FIGURE 8.8 The cardinal movements of labor and delivery.

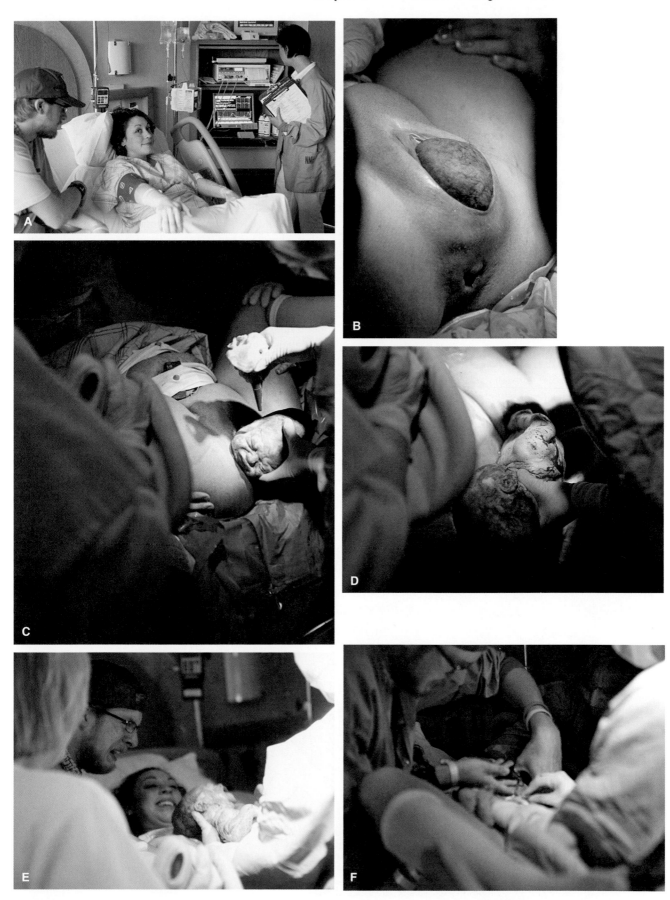

FIGURE 8.9 Vaginal birth sequence. A, Pushing in an upright position allows gravity to assist with fetal descent. B, Crowning. C, Birth of the head. D, Expulsion. E, The infant is shown to the parents. F, The baby's father cuts the umbilical cord.

or the maternal side (red, raw appearance) presenting first. The health-care provider will inspect the placenta to determine if the entire placenta has been delivered. Undelivered fragments or sections left in the uterus can cause hemorrhage or infection to occur (Fig. 8.10).

If the placenta does not separate spontaneously, the health-care provider may need to use manual extraction to deliver the placenta. If the placenta does not separate easily with gentle manual extraction, a surgical procedure of a dilation and curettage may be required.

Upon delivery of the placenta, the nurse should massage the uterus to minimize blood loss. Usual blood loss for a vaginal delivery is 500 mL and for a Cesarean birth 1,000 mL.

CULTURAL CONSIDERATIONS

The placenta has a role in some cultural rituals. Some cultural groups such as the Navajos, Cambodians, and Costa Ricans bury the placenta to protect and ensure the health of the mother and baby. The Hmong culture believes that the placenta is a "jacket" that the soul must don at death to avoid wandering alone and naked for eternity (Galanti, 2015). In providing patient-centered care, the nurse should assist the patient and her family if there is a desire to take the placenta from the hospital.

LABS & DIAGNOSTICS

Pregnant women are at risk of anemia because of the demands of the growing fetus in late pregnancy. Because of the potential problem of blood loss at delivery, the nurse should be aware of the hemoglobin and hematocrit of the patient admitted in labor. Hemoglobin reflects the oxygen-carrying capacity of the blood, which is important in the case of blood loss. Normal hemoglobin for an adult female is 11.7 to 15.5 g/dL.

A hematocrit provides information on the percentage of red blood cells. The hematocrit is usually tested with the hemoglobin, and these levels parallel each other to provide more information on the severity of the anemia. A normal hematocrit for an adult female is 33% to 45%. Any low values should be reported to the health-care provider. Critical values for hemoglobin are less than 6.6 g/dL and a hematocrit less than 19.8% (Van Leeuwen, Poelhuis-Leth, and Bladh, 2013).

Fourth Stage

The fourth stage of labor begins with the delivery of the placenta and ends with the physiological stabilization of the mother. This stage can last from 1 to 4 hours. Expected physical findings during this stage include:

- The uterus is firm and the fundus is located midline, halfway between the symphysis pubis and the umbilicus.
- Lochia (ie, vaginal discharge) is heavy, with bright red blood mixed with clots.
- Mild uterine cramping (ie, afterpains) may be noted as the uterus contracts to return to prepregnancy size.

MATERNAL SYSTEMIC RESPONSE TO LABOR

The most significant response during labor occurs in the reproductive system. However, the cardiovascular, respiratory, renal, gastrointestinal, and hematopoietic systems are also affected during labor.

Cardiovascular System

At the peak of a contraction, blood flow to the placenta from the mother is decreased. This decrease of blood to the placenta causes the woman's blood volume to increase. An increase in blood volume will cause a rise in blood pressure and a decrease in the pulse rate. Supine hypotension may

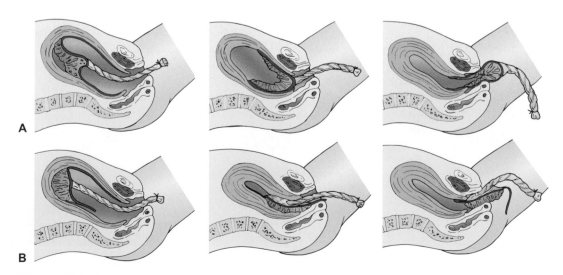

FIGURE 8.10 Separation and expulsion of the placenta.

occur if the woman is allowed to lie on her back during labor. The mother should be encouraged to labor in a side position or slightly upright to avoid hypotension.

Respiratory System

Anxiety and pain will cause an increase in the rate and depth of respirations. If the woman is allowed to breathe too deeply and too fast, hyperventilation can occur because of her exhalation of too much carbon dioxide.

Urinary System

The position of the fetus in the uterus places pressure on the urinary bladder. The woman adjusts physically to the constant feeling of pelvic pressure and may not notice a full bladder. A full bladder can impede labor process and fetal descent; therefore she should be encouraged to urinate throughout labor.

Gastrointestinal System

During labor, gastric motility slows down. Nausea and vomiting can occur during labor, so large quantities of food and liquids are usually not advisable during labor. It is common for the woman to experience thirst and dry mouth from the increased respiratory rate.

Hematopoietic System

Blood loss at delivery is expected. Expected blood loss for a vaginal delivery is 500 mL. Because of the increased blood volume during pregnancy, most women have no adverse effects from this amount of blood loss. A hemoglobin of 11 g/dL and a hematocrit of 33% or higher further indicates that the woman can handle the blood loss without problems (Van Leeuwen, 2013). The leukocyte count for a pregnant woman at term is usually higher than a nonpregnant woman, averaging 14,000 to 16,000 per mm^3. Fibrinogen is elevated throughout pregnancy and continues to remain elevated during labor. Although there is an increase in clotting factors, fibrinolysis (ie, clot breakdown) actually slows down, which promotes coagulation when the placenta separates from the uterus.

FETAL RESPONSE TO LABOR

The fetus experiences labor along with the mother. If the fetus is healthy, the stress of labor does not produce adverse effects for the fetus. Fetal responses to labor include:

- Heart rate changes with accelerations related to fetal movement and decelerations related to head compression as the fetus moves through the birth canal
- A decrease in circulation and perfusion during the peak of a contraction
- An increase in arterial carbon dioxide pressure (P_{CO_2})
- A decrease in fetal oxygen pressure (P_{O_2})
- A decrease in fetal breathing movements (Gardner, et al, 2015)

Key Points

- The professional nurse is knowledgeable about the normal labor process.
- There are several theories related to the possible causes of the onset of labor. These theories focus on oxytocin, prostaglandins, progesterone, cortisol, estriol, and the overstretched uterus.
- Every woman is unique, but common signs of labor are lightening, contractions, cervical changes, ROM, bloody show, and a burst of energy.
- During labor, the cervix must efface and dilate to allow the fetus to leave the uterus.
- There are seven critical factors, the "Seven Ps," that are involved in labor. These factors are *passage, passenger, powers, position, psyche, pain,* and *patience.*
- There are four stages of childbirth:
  - The first stage of labor ends with complete dilation of the cervix.
  - The second stage of labor ends with the birth of the newborn.
  - The third stage ends with the delivery of the placenta.
  - The fourth stage ends when the woman is physiologically stable.
- During the second stage, the fetus must move through positional changes to fit through the pelvis.
- During labor, the woman experiences changes in the following body systems: cardiovascular, respiratory, urinary, gastrointestinal, and hematopoietic.
- Labor is stressful for the fetus also, and there are noticeable physiological responses during labor.

REVIEW QUESTIONS

1. The nurse is describing true and false labor to a patient. Which of the following statements made by the patient indicates that she understands the difference?
   1. "A false labor contraction usually starts in the back and radiates around to the front of my abdomen."
   2. "True labor contractions cause cervical changes."
   3. "True labor contractions will go away with a warm shower."
   4. "False labor contractions get stronger if I take a walk."

2. The shortest phase of labor is usually the:
   1. Pushing phase
   2. Transition phase
   3. Active phase
   4. Latent phase

3. Which maternal positions are considered appropriate for labor? (*select all that apply*)
   1. Side-lying
   2. Supine
   3. Sitting
   4. Standing
   5. Walking

4. Powers, as one of the "Seven Ps," refers to:
   1. The fetal descent in the pelvis
   2. The uterine contractions and pushing efforts
   3. The fetus and placenta
   4. The pelvis and soft tissues

5. Signs that the placenta is separating from the uterus are: (*select all that apply*)
   1. A trickle of blood comes from the uterus.
   2. The uterus stops contracting.
   3. The maternal pulse slows.
   4. The umbilical cord lengthens.
   5. The uterus rises upward.

6. The abbreviation *LOA* means that the fetal occiput is:
   1. On the examiner's left side
   2. Facing the mother's left side of her pelvis
   3. Facing the mother's pubic bone
   4. Facing the mother's right side of her pelvis

7. The stage of labor when it is most appropriate to push is
   1. The first stage
   2. The second stage
   3. The third stage
   4. The fourth stage

8. A station of –1 means that:
   1. The fetus is very close to delivery.
   2. The fetal head has passed through the ischial spines by 1 cm.
   3. The fetal head is 1 cm above the ischial spines.
   4. The fetus is unlikely to be born vaginally.

9. A woman is admitted in labor. Her hemoglobin is 12.6 g/dL. The nurse knows that:
   1. The patient has an infection.
   2. The patient may have problems with excessive blood loss.
   3. The patient has a normal hemoglobin level.
   4. The patient is anemic.

10. A contraction began at 11:00:00 and ended at 11:00:30. The next contraction began at 11:05:00. How far apart were the two contractions?
    1. 30 seconds
    2. 5 minutes and 30 seconds
    3. 4 minutes and 30 seconds
    4. 5 minutes

CRITICAL THINKING QUESTIONS

1. The *Healthy People 2020* goal is to reduce the number of Cesarean births in the United States. Explore ways that nurses can contribute to achieving that goal.

2. A laboring patient's mother comes to the nurse's station and insists on speaking to the charge nurse. The mother states, "I want the doctor called! She has been in labor too long. I can't stand to see her suffer. She needs a C-section." How should the nurse respond to this request?

Davis*Plus*

For additional resources and information, visit **www.DavisPlus.com**. Post-Conference Questions and Activities, Answers, and References can be found on Davis*Plus*.

Nursing Assessment During Labor

9

LEARNING OUTCOMES

1. Define the key terms.
2. Compare and contrast the advantages and disadvantages of a hospital birth, birthing center birth, and home birth.
3. Summarize admission procedures in the labor and delivery unit.
4. Review the initial maternal assessment in the labor and delivery unit.
5. Describe the process of a cervical examination and discuss the information obtained during the cervical examination.
6. Demonstrate Leopold's maneuvers and discuss the purpose of the maneuvers.
7. Describe continuing assessment of the woman and fetus during labor.
8. Identify maternal and fetal conditions that indicate fetal monitoring is necessary for promotion of a safe birth.
9. Differentiate internal and external monitoring.
10. Analyze a fetal monitor strip.
11. Identify unsafe or nonreassuring fetal heart decelerations.
12. Choose appropriate nursing interventions for nonreassuring fetal heart patterns.
13. Define the three categories of the fetal heart rate (FHR) classification system.

REAL-WORLD CASE STUDY

Jenna

■ Jenna has just been admitted to the labor and delivery unit. This is her first baby. She is dilated 2 cm and is in early labor with contractions that are 5 minutes apart and lasting 50 to 60 seconds. Jenna attended childbirth classes, prepared a birth plan, and states that she is not sure she likes the idea of continuous fetal monitoring.

1. How can the nurse explore Jenna's concerns regarding continuous fetal monitoring?
2. How can the nurse provide patient-centered care and use electronic fetal monitoring during Jenna's labor?

KEY TERMS

acceleration
amnioinfusion
cephalic
certified nurse midwife (CNM)
deceleration
early decelerations
episodic decelerations
intrauterine pressure catheter (IUPC)
late decelerations
Leopold's maneuvers
meconium
nadir
periodic decelerations
tachysystole
tocolytic medications
variability
variable decelerations

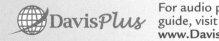 For audio pronunciation guide, visit www.DavisPlus.com

CHAPTER CONCEPTS

Assessment
Collaboration
Oxygenation
Pregnancy

CONCEPTUAL CORNERSTONE

Oxygenation

Fetal monitoring is an important assessment tool that is used in labor and delivery to monitor the health of the fetus. Fetal monitoring gives information regarding the oxygenation status of the fetus while coping with the stress of labor. The fetus receives oxygen that comes from the maternal lungs, heart, and blood vessels to the uterus, placenta, and umbilical cord. Any disruption of the path of oxygen from the mother to the fetus will cause a deceleration of the fetal heart rate (FHR) and possible hypoxia for the fetus. Regardless of the type of abnormal fetal heart deceleration, whether it is a variable deceleration or a late deceleration, it is caused by a disruption in oxygenation to the fetus. Nursing observation of abnormal decelerations followed by prompt interventions can promote oxygenation of the fetus and prevent a brain injury caused by hypoxia.

Most babies in the United States are born in hospitals. However, there are other options available, such as birthing centers and homes. This chapter provides information about birth setting options for patients to consider. In the hospital setting, nurses provide most of the care during labor. The nurse caring for a patient in labor has the major responsibility of careful assessment of the mother and fetus. This chapter provides information on initial assessment of the woman and fetus and ongoing assessments throughout labor. Fetal monitoring is a crucial part of the assessment of the health of the fetus; the chapter concludes with detailed information about analyzing a fetal monitoring strip and nursing interventions for nonreassuring fetal heart patterns.

SETTINGS FOR CHILDBIRTH

Pregnancy and childbirth are normal life events for most women and their newborns. For women with uncomplicated pregnancies, there are a variety of settings that may be utilized for childbirth: the hospital, the birthing center, and the home.

Hospital

In the United States, 98.6% of babies are born in hospitals (Martin, Hamilton, Ventura, et al, 2014). Table 9.1 notes the advantages and disadvantages of using a hospital to give birth.

Birthing Center

A birthing center is a homelike setting where **certified nurse midwives (CNMs)** provide family-centered care. Birthing centers are typically located in large urban areas; many women may not have access to a birthing center. Table 9.2 notes the advantages and disadvantages of using a birthing center to give birth.

Home

According to the Centers for Disease Control (CDC, 2013), 1.4% of births in the United States occur outside a hospital. Some women with an uncomplicated pregnancy select a

TABLE 9.1   ADVANTAGES AND DISADVANTAGES OF USING A HOSPITAL TO GIVE BIRTH

Advantages of a Hospital Birth	Disadvantages of a Hospital Birth
• It is the safest environment for high-risk patients. • Emergency equipment and personnel are available at all times. • The pediatrician can be present for the delivery if a problem is anticipated. • It is the only option if a Cesarean delivery is required. • Until discharge, the woman has 24-hour support from nurses.	• Many women giving birth for the first time have never been in a hospital and find the environment intimidating. • The father may be less actively involved with the process. • The birth is managed by experts who may not agree with the mother's birth plan. • Hospitals can be noisy and the new mother may not receive much rest.

TABLE 9.2   ADVANTAGES AND DISADVANTAGES OF USING A BIRTHING CENTER TO GIVE BIRTH

Advantages of a Birthing Center Birth	Disadvantages of a Birthing Center Birth
• The facility is dedicated to providing labor and delivery care only. • The woman is encouraged to make her own decisions regarding comfort measures, eating, and moving during labor. • The woman can give birth in any position she prefers. • The woman can invite family and friends to participate in the birth process. • A birthing center is usually affiliated with a hospital in the event that an emergency occurs and the woman needs to be transported.	• Most centers have rigid screening criteria and high-risk mothers are not allowed to use the center for labor and birth. • Discharge is usually within 24 hours. • Transfer to a hospital may be required if a complication occurs. • There are no pediatricians present at the birth.

home birth. Home births may be attended by a licensed certified midwife or by lay midwives who have varying degrees of formal education. The American Academy of Pediatrics (AAP) supports the woman's right to make a medically informed decision about delivery and has published a position paper informing mothers-to-be about standards of care for a newborn. The AAP recommends that there be a person dedicated to the care of the newborn at every home delivery. This person would provide resuscitation, warmth, and assign Apgar scores (Pullen, 2013). Table 9.3 notes the advantages and disadvantages of having a home birth.

PATIENT TEACHING GUIDELINES

When to Go to the Hospital or Birthing Center

The patient should always follow the directions of the obstetrician or nurse midwife about monitoring early labor at home. However, there are some general guidelines that nurses can provide the patient for when to arrive at the hospital or birthing center. She should come to the hospital if:

• The amniotic membranes rupture
• The contractions are 5 minutes apart for an hour and increasing in intensity and duration

TABLE **9.3** ADVANTAGES AND DISADVANTAGES OF HAVING A HOME BIRTH

Advantages of Having a Home Birth	Disadvantages of a Having a Home Birth
• The mother is able to relax in her home environment and have more privacy. • Continuous one-on-one care is given. • The caregivers are invited into the home and will not leave because their shifts are over or another patient needs care. • Labor is allowed to progress normally, without interventions. • The cost of a home birth is less than a birthing center or hospital. • Bonding is enhanced because the mother and baby are not separated.	• The patient has to accept the consequences of medical and health decisions made during labor and birth. • Medication for pain is usually not available. • The laboring woman must be moved to the hospital in the event of an emergency. • Home deliveries are ten times more likely to result in an Apgar score of 0 than hospital deliveries (Grimebaum, Sapra, and Chervenak, 2014).

• Her previous labor was rapid; she should come in if contractions are 7 to 10 minutes apart
• Any vaginal bleeding occurs, even if it is painless
• She feels any urge to push or bear down during contractions

ADMISSION TO THE HOSPITAL OR BIRTHING CENTER

Patients can often fill out hospital or birthing center paperwork and supply medical insurance and payment information prior to arriving in labor. This will streamline the process when she arrives in labor and may be unable to focus on completing hospital forms.

On arrival, the hospital will ask the patient to sign consent for admission and medical and nursing care. This process places the patient information into the hospital computer system and allows the ordering of laboratory tests and medications.

Upon arrival in the labor and delivery unit, the patient and her support person should be greeted by a registered nurse and admission data obtained. Most obstetricians forward prenatal care records to the hospital prior to the patient's due date. The nurse has two patients to assess: the woman and her fetus.

 ## CULTURAL CONSIDERATIONS

Cultural Influences on Birth Practices

It is common practice in the United States for a laboring woman to be accompanied by the baby's father during labor and birth. This is not common practice in all cultures. The labor and delivery nurse needs to be sensitive to the cultural practices of the patient. For example, an Orthodox Jewish husband may see his wife as "unclean" during childbirth; he may remain in the room but not touch her during labor. Another example is the Mexican culture. In Mexico, a husband usually does not attend the birth; he is present in the hospital, but not in the labor and delivery room. The woman will be accompanied by another female and the male provides his support from the waiting room (Galanti, 2015).

Admission Data Collection

The nurse should review the records to identify any potential problems and high-risk patients. A medication history should be obtained, including information about current medications, vitamins, supplements, or alternative therapies.

Maternal Assessment

Every patient who comes under the care of a nurse must be assessed to obtain a baseline of the patient's condition. This baseline provides information that will assist the nurse to monitor progress of labor and to notice early signs of potential problems and possible safety issues for the patient and fetus. The nurse should prioritize the admission assessment process in the event that the labor is progressing quickly. The nurse may need to assess the contractions, cervical dilation, and fetus quickly to notify the obstetrician or nurse midwife of an impending delivery. A complete admission assessment usually includes:

- Vital signs (eg, temperature, respiratory rate, pulse, and blood pressure)
- Documentation of allergies to food and medications
- Documentation of the last food intake
- A complete head-to-toe assessment
- Skin assessment
- Falls risk assessment
- Pain assessment
- Cultural needs assessment
- Documentation of the time labor began, including the frequency and duration of contractions
- The presence or absence of bloody show
- Cervical examination

Cervical Examination

The nurse will perform a cervical examination to determine cervical dilation, effacement, and fetal position. The cervical examination provides the woman with a progress report and gives the nurse needed data for anticipating the birth and reporting progress to the health-care provider. Vaginal examinations can be uncomfortable for the woman and the nurse must be gentle. If there is any frank bright-red bleeding coming from the vagina, the nurse must not perform a vaginal examination. There is a possibility that the bleeding is caused by a placenta previa, a condition in which the placenta covers the cervix. The nurse may cause hemorrhage if the placenta is perforated by the examiner's fingers. The steps to perform a vaginal cervical examination are:

1. The nurse should perform hand hygiene and provide for privacy.
2. The nurse positions the woman onto her back with her knees flexed.
3. The nurse applies sterile gloves and places a drop of lubricant on the dominant hand.
4. With the nondominant hand, while gently opening the labia, the nurse inspects the labia and notes any bleeding or fluid leaking from the vagina. The nurse will also note any ulcerated lesions or vesicles that should be reported to the health-care provider.
5. With the dominant hand, the nurse introduces the index and middle fingers into the vagina toward the posterior vaginal wall.
6. The nurse touches the cervix and notes the position and the amount of effacement and dilation present. At the same time, the nurse will confirm the presenting part and rate the station in the pelvis. As dilation increases, the nurse can determine fetal position by palpating the posterior fontanelle.
7. The examiner withdraws the hand and removes lubricant from the labia by wiping from front to back to avoid rectal contamination in the vaginal area.

8. The nurse assists the woman to sit up or lie on her side.
9. The nurse documents findings and reports progress, if needed, to the health-care provider (Fig. 9.1).

SAFETY *STAT!*

A vaginal cervical examination must never be attempted if the woman is bleeding from the vagina. The bleeding may be caused by placenta previa and a nurse could puncture the placenta and cause hemorrhage.

Assessment of Amniotic Membranes

If the amniotic membranes have ruptured prior to admission, the nurse should obtain the time of rupture and characteristics of the fluid (eg, color, odor, amount) from the patient. The membranes can rupture as a gush or a slow leak. The amniotic fluid should be clear.

Yellow-stained fluid can indicate a blood incompatibility between the mother and fetus. The breakdown of red blood cells that occurs because of the incompatibility produces the yellow tint.

Greenish amniotic fluid can indicate fetal distress, which causes the fetus to pass meconium into the fluid. **Meconium** is usually the first bowel movement, but is expelled from the intestines of the fetus when stress or hypoxia (ie, decreased oxygen) is experienced in the uterus. Any abnormal color should be reported to the health-care provider immediately.

Amniotic fluid is alkaline and can be tested with Nitrazine paper. The nurse takes a small piece of Nitrazine paper and touches it to any fluid around the perineum. If amniotic fluid is present, the alkaline fluid will produce a deep blue color on the Nitrazine paper.

SAFETY *STAT!*

It is extremely important for the nurse to determine when the amniotic membranes ruptured. If the fetus is not delivered within 24 hours of the rupture of membranes, there is an increased risk of infection.

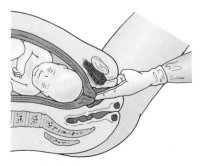

FIGURE 9.1 Vaginal examination to assess cervical dilation.

Laboratory Tests

Admission laboratory tests are completed to assess the health of the woman. Although it varies among hospitals and health-care providers, the following laboratory tests are commonly ordered on admission:

- **Complete blood cell count (CBC):** This test evaluates the red blood cells, white blood cells, and platelets. The results provide diagnostic information regarding the general health of the patient.
- **Blood type and screen:** This test evaluates the blood type and Rh in the event of a need for a blood transfusion. Generally, the health-care provider will ask the laboratory to hold the specimen for 72 hours in the event a blood transfusion is required.
- **Urinalysis:** This test screens for infection, glucose, bilirubin, nitrates, and proteins, and provides information about the overall health of the patient.
- **Group B streptococcus (GBS) screen:** This test determines if the organism is present in the genital canal tract. Some obstetricians screen patients for GBS at 37 weeks of gestation. If no screening has occurred, a rapid GBS test kit can provide results in minutes on a vaginal or rectal fluid swab. Women who have a positive screen usually do not have symptoms. However, the fetus can be exposed to the organism during the birth process and it can cause pneumonia and sepsis in the newborn (Van Leeuwen, Poelhuis-Leth, and Bladh, 2013).

LABS & DIAGNOSTICS

Because of the blood loss of delivery, it is important to know if the laboring patient has a low hemoglobin and hematocrit prior to giving birth. Often the woman is screened for anemia at the initial prenatal appointment and then again at 24 to 28 weeks of gestation. Screening at admission will provide important information for planning care in the event that she has become anemic during the last weeks of pregnancy.

Additional Assessment Data

The nurse who wants to provide patient-centered care will also collect information regarding the patient's desires and needs for support in labor. Additional information that should be collected includes:

- **Birth plan:** If the woman arrives with a birth plan, the nurse should review it with the patient and make sincere efforts to follow the plan as long as it does not interfere with a safe birth.
- **Support person:** The nurse should determine who the main support person is and reassure that person that the labor and delivery staff will also provide any needed support during labor.
- **Childbirth classes:** If the patient attended Lamaze or Bradley childbirth classes, the nurse should be prepared to support and assist with breathing and relaxation techniques.

If childbirth classes were not attended, the nurse should be prepared to teach relaxation and breathing techniques as labor progresses.

THERAPEUTIC COMMUNICATION

Many patients arrive in labor and delivery with a birth plan. The woman and her support person may be anxious and fearful that the nurse will not listen or implement her birth plan. The nurse should use open-ended questions and, with an open mind, gently explore options that may be agreeable to the patient and the nurse if the nurse cannot safely adhere to the complete birth plan.

Fetal Assessment

During labor, the nurse is responsible for the well-being of two patients: the mother and the fetus. On admission, to assess the health status of the fetus, the nurse should:

- Perform **Leopold's maneuvers**, a method of uterus palpation to determine fetal position and presentation. This provides information about possible complications in labor and makes it easier to position electronic fetal monitoring equipment. The steps for performing Leopold's maneuvers are:
  1. The examiner should perform hand hygiene and provide privacy for the patient.
  2. The nurse positions the woman supine with a small rolled towel or pillow under her left side to tilt the uterus to the side, which helps to avoid orthostatic hypotension.
  3. The nurse observes the abdomen for fetal movement.
  4. For the first maneuver, the nurse stands at the foot of the woman, facing her, and places both hands flat on her abdomen (Fig. 9.2). Palpation is performed on the uterus fundus to determine the shape, consistency, and mobility. This palpation will determine if the fetal head (will feel firm) or buttocks (will feel soft) is located in the fundus.
  5. For the second maneuver, the nurse places the left hand on the left side of the uterus and holds it still while palpating the right side of the uterus with the right hand (Fig 9.3). The process is repeated on the left side. This palpation locates the back of the fetus. The fetal back feels firm and smooth. The side of the uterus with arms and legs will feel bumpy.
  6. For the third maneuver, the nurse grasps the lower portion of the abdomen above the symphysis pubis and gently presses the thumb and fingers together (Fig. 9.4). This palpation determines which part of the fetus is at the inlet of the pelvis. A head presentation will be firm, and buttocks will feel soft to the examiner. If the presenting part is upwardly moveable, it is not engaged in the pelvis.
  7. The fourth maneuver is only completed if the fetus is in a cephalic presentation. **Cephalic** is a medical

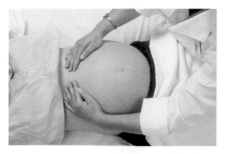

FIGURE 9.2 Leopold's first maneuver assesses whether the fetal head or buttocks is in the fundus.

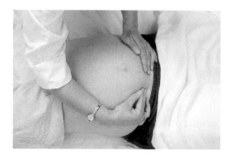

FIGURE 9.3 Leopold's second maneuver determines on which side of the uterus the fetal back is.

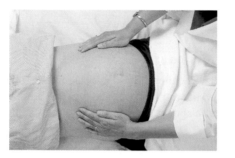

FIGURE 9.4 Leopold's third maneuver shows whether the fetal head or buttocks is at the inlet of the pelvis.

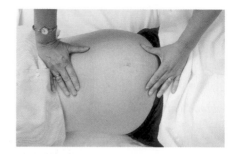

FIGURE 9.5 Leopold's fourth maneuver is used only for cephalic presentation to determine fetal attitude and position in the pelvis.

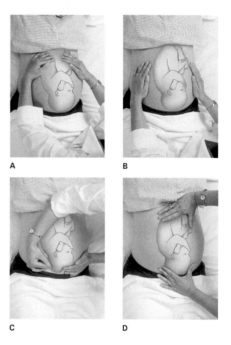

A   **B**

C   **D**

FIGURE 9.6 Assessing fetal presentation and position utilizing Leopold's maneuvers. A, Leopold's first maneuver. B, Leopold's second maneuver. C, Leopold's third maneuver. D, Leopold's fourth maneuver.

term of Latin origin that means *head.* The nurse places her fingers on both sides of the uterus about two inches above the inguinal ligaments and presses downward and inward in the direction of the birth canal (Fig. 9.5). This palpation provides information of the fetal attitude and extension into the pelvis (Fig. 9.6).

- The nurse performs a baseline FHR assessment using a handheld Doppler device. All patients arriving in labor should be monitored to evaluate the status of the fetus. The patient should be monitored for a minimum of 20 minutes to determine fetal well-being and to establish baseline information (Menihan and Kopel, 2014).
- After the baseline is determined, the health-care provider, nurse, and patient can discuss a plan to intermittently or continually monitor fetal well-being.

SAFETY *STAT!*

To prevent vena cava syndrome, the nurse must make sure the woman has a small rolled towel or pillow under her buttocks to tilt the uterus off the vena cava. Failure to prevent vena cava syndrome can cause hypotension in the mother and potentially a drop in FHR.

After completing the admission assessment, the nurse should notify the health-care provider of the admission assessment data and report any of the following signs or symptoms that can indicate a problem:

- Temperature greater than 38°C
- Blood pressure greater than 140/90 mm Hg or less than 90/60 mm Hg
- Maternal heart rate greater than 110 bpm

- Respiratory rate greater than 24 breaths per minute
- Uterine bleeding
- An abnormal FHR pattern
- Uterine contractions lasting 2 minutes or longer or contractions of normal duration but occurring within 1 minute of each other
- Any abnormal finding from physical assessment
- Impending delivery
  - Some women arrive at the hospital with an impending delivery. The health-care provider should be notified immediately if the patient is advanced in her cervical dilation.

Procedures

Admission procedures vary but most hospitals no longer require perineal shaving and enemas, which was common practice for years.

IV infusions are still commonly ordered to provide fluids and prevent dehydration. IV access can also be utilized to administer pain medication or blood products in the event of an emergency. Some nurse midwives will allow a saline or heparin lock to be placed in the vein without attached fluids, giving the woman more mobility.

CONTINUAL ASSESSMENT OF THE LABORING WOMAN

The labor and delivery nurse must provide continual assessment and monitoring of the patient's health and progress during labor. The obstetrician traditionally does not provide the majority of the assessment in labor. Instead, the labor and delivery nurse manages the patient's care, and any delays in cervical dilation, fetal descent, and labor progress should be reported to the health-care provider immediately. The obstetrician relies on the nurse to report any problems and to notify the obstetrician to arrive in time for the delivery.

Vital Signs

During latent labor, the blood pressure, pulse, and respirations are assessed every hour. The temperature is assessed every 4 hours unless abnormal. When labor has progressed to the active and transition phases, vital signs are assessed every 30 minutes. The temperature is assessed every 2 hours during active and transition labor.

Contractions

During the latent phase of labor, uterine contractions are monitored for frequency, duration, and intensity every 30 to 60 minutes. During the active and transition phases, contractions should be monitored every 15 to 30 minutes because labor progresses faster during these phases (AWHONN, 2012).

Cervical Examinations

Vaginal cervical examinations are performed periodically. There are no rules about timing for the vaginal examinations. The patient is usually eager for labor progress updates, but the nurse needs to educate the patient that frequent cervical examinations can lead to an increased risk for infection. The experienced nurse takes into consideration the woman's parity, past labor length, contraction pattern, and the woman's response to labor to determine the frequency of the vaginal cervical examinations. The information about dilation, effacement, and station provide the woman and her family with a progress report on the labor process.

Amniotic Fluid

The amniotic membranes may rupture spontaneously or the health-care provider may use an amniohook to break the bag of fluids. An amniohook is a sterile, long, thin plastic hook that slides through the cervix to rupture the amniotic sac. After rupture, the nurse should assess the fluid for color, odor, and amount. The FHR should be assessed immediately, followed by a vaginal cervical examination if the fetal heart rate drops. There is always a possibility of cord compression at the cervix if the presenting part was not engaged in the pelvis when the membranes rupture. The sudden gush of fluid can cause the umbilical cord to be washed out of the cervix and when the presenting part settles down against the cervix, compression can occur.

SAFETY *STAT!*

The FHR must be assessed immediately when the amniotic membranes rupture in case the umbilical cord becomes compressed with the sudden loss of the cushioning amniotic fluid. The nurse should listen to the fetal heart rate with a Doppler as soon as possible after rupture of the amniotic membranes. The health-care provider must be immediately notified of any drop in fetal heart rate.

Progress of Labor

The labor and delivery nurse will monitor the patient's progress in labor, taking into consideration the frequency, duration, and strength of the contractions. It is generally accepted that the primipara patient will have a longer labor and cervical dilation will take longer. It is expected that the primipara will dilate approximately 0.5 to 1.0 cm per hour and the multipara will dilate slightly faster (Tuuli, Keegan, Odibo, et al, 2013).

TEAM WORKS

The nurse in the labor and delivery unit usually has routine standing orders and protocols to follow when managing the care of a patient in labor. If the nurse notices through assessment that there are potential problems, the nurse is expected to notify the health-care provider immediately to collaborate on care.

FETAL MONITORING

Fetal monitoring can help detect signs that the fetus is not tolerating the stress of labor. Changes in FHR and contraction patterns can help the nurses and health-care providers to intervene to prevent injury or death of the fetus. Nurses who provide bed-side care in labor and delivery receive additional education to become experts on reading fetal monitoring strips and to learn appropriate interventions based on the FHR pattern.

Intermittent Fetal Monitoring

Intermittent fetal monitoring can be done with a handheld Doppler device. A handheld Doppler uses ultrasound waves that bounce off the fetal heart, producing echoes that reflect the FHR. This device is used in hospitals, birthing centers, and clinics to monitor the FHR. Intermittent monitoring can also be accomplished by applying the fetal monitor, obtaining a 20-minute evaluation, and then removing the monitor. Intermittent monitoring allows the woman to move around and change position easily. A disadvantage of intermittent monitoring is that if done with a Doppler, the nurse cannot evaluate **variability** (ie, beat-to-beat intervals of the fetal heart that represent a healthy sympathetic and parasympathetic nervous system in the fetus) and types of **decelerations** (ie, drops in the FHR from the baseline). Another disadvantage of intermittent fetal monitoring is that if the fetal condition changes between scheduled monitoring sessions, early signs of deterioration of the fetal health may not be detected.

Continual Fetal Monitoring

Continual monitoring can be done with a fetal monitor applied externally or internally. Continuous fetal monitoring during labor should be considered for high-risk women. Maternal or fetal conditions that indicate continuous fetal monitoring is necessary to provide safe and effective care include:

- Hypertensive disorders
- Preterm pregnancy
- Post-term pregnancy
- Maternal cardiac disease
- Oligohydramnios, which is a condition of decreased amniotic fluid
- Polyhydramnios, which is a condition of increased amniotic fluid
- Multiple gestation
- Induction of labor
- Administration of epidural anesthesia
- Vaginal birth after Cesarean (VBAC)
- Diabetes

Procedure for Applying the Fetal Monitor

The process of fetal monitoring must be explained to the patient and her family prior to application. Explain to the woman that fetal monitoring will detect changes in heart rate patterns during labor. If problems are detected, the nurse can initiate interventions to prevent problems for the fetus.

External Monitoring

The procedure for external monitoring is the following:

1. The nurse should start with hand hygiene and perform Leopold's maneuvers to determine the position of the fetus.

2. Ultrasound gel is applied to the ultrasound transducer and the transducer is placed over the area where the fetal back is located. This is the best location to obtain a clear signal of the heart rate. The transducer is then secured with a belt around the woman's abdomen.
3. External monitoring of the FHR provides information about heart rate baseline, variability, **accelerations** (ie, short increases in the FHR above the baseline), and decelerations.
4. A tocodynamometer is used to measure the frequency and duration of uterine contractions. It is placed on the fundus of the uterus and secured with a belt.
5. The fetal heart transducer and the tocodynamometer send a signal to the fetal monitor and it is recorded on monitor paper. In the United States, the standard paper speed for fetal monitoring is 3 cm per minute. On the fetal monitoring paper, each dark vertical line represents one minute and each lighter color line represents ten seconds (Fig. 9.7).

Table 9.4 notes the advantages and disadvantages of using external monitoring for the fetus.

Internal Monitoring

Internal monitoring for the fetus requires the application of a fetal scalp electrode (FSE) to directly monitor the fetal heart. A vaginal examination is performed, and an experienced nurse advances the electrode through the vagina and attaches it to the presenting part. Internal monitoring may be initiated by the nurse if the external method does not provide reliable information regarding the condition of the fetus.

Contractions can be monitored with an **intrauterine pressure catheter (IUPC)**, a small flexible tube inserted into the uterus along the uterine wall that provides exact measurement of contraction length and intensity. Most hospitals require the obstetrician or the nurse-midwife to insert the IUPC (O'Connell, 2014).

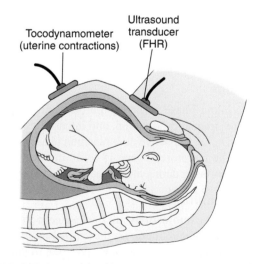

FIGURE 9.7 External fetal heart rate (FHR) monitor and tocodynamometer.

TABLE 9.4 ADVANTAGES AND DISADVANTAGES OF USING EXTERNAL MONITORING FOR THE FETUS

Advantages of External Monitoring	Disadvantages of External Monitoring
• The transducers are easy to apply quickly. • External monitoring does not require that the membranes be ruptured and is considered noninvasive.	• The woman may find the belts across her abdomen uncomfortable. • External monitoring cannot measure the pressure or intensity of the contractions. • FHR recordings may have gaps or artifacts caused by movement of the fetus and poor conduction through the maternal tissues. • Uterine contractions may not be monitored correctly if the tocodynamometer slides off the uterus with maternal position changes.

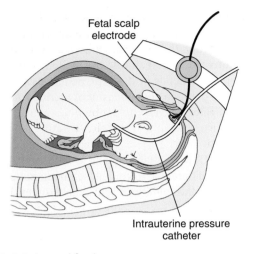

FIGURE 9.8 Internal fetal monitor.

A vaginal examination is performed and the IUPC is inserted through a guide tube through the cervix and into the uterus. IUPC monitoring may be initiated if more information is required regarding uterine activity, especially the intensity of the contractions (Fig. 9.8). Table 9.5 notes the advantages and disadvantages of using internal monitoring for the fetus.

Interpretation of Fetal Monitoring

The nurse in labor and delivery who evaluates the information provided with fetal heart monitoring must have clinical judgment skills and expertise in fetal monitoring. Initiation of fetal monitoring must only be performed and evaluated by licensed experienced health-care professionals (AWHONN, 2012).

The purpose of fetal monitoring in labor is to assess the fetal oxygenation. Fetal oxygenation occurs by the transfer of oxygen to the fetus and the physiological response if the transfer is interrupted. According to Menihan and Kopel (2014), there are principles that can be applied to FHR interpretation:

1. Oxygen is transported to the fetus along a path that includes the maternal lungs, heart, blood vessels, uterus, placenta, and umbilical cord. Interruption of blood flow at any place in the path can result in an FHR deceleration. Therefore all significant decelerations indicate an interruption in oxygen to the fetus.
2. A disruption in fetal oxygenation can result in hypoxia for the fetus. The first step that occurs is hypoxemia, which is decreased oxygen in the blood. Hypoxemia, if not corrected, leads to hypoxia, which is a state of decreased oxygen levels in the tissues. Tissue hypoxemia can lead to metabolic acidosis in the fetus. An acidotic fetus will show signs of minimal or absent variability and absent accelerations.
3. Fetal neurological injury will not occur if hypoxemia is corrected and significant fetal acidemia does not occur.

TABLE 9.5 ADVANTAGES AND DISADVANTAGES OF USING INTERNAL MONITORING FOR THE FETUS

Advantages of Internal Monitoring	Disadvantages of Internal Monitoring
• Internal monitoring does not require belts around the abdomen and continual readjustment. • Accurate information is available about FHR, variability, accelerations, and decelerations, regardless of fetal activity. • The IUPC detects the frequency, duration, resting tone, and strength of the uterine contractions. • The internal scalp electrode can be combined with external contraction monitoring.	• Internal monitoring is invasive and increases the risk of uterine infection. • Internal monitoring requires extensive training for safe application.

The interpretation of the FHR should follow a systematic approach, starting with the baseline FHR, the interpretation of FHR variability, the presence of accelerations, **periodic decelerations** (ie, decelerations associated with contractions), changes or trends in the FHR pattern over time, and the frequency, duration, and intensity of uterine contractions (Cahill and Spain, 2015).

Baseline

The normal FHR during labor is 110 to 160 bpm. The baseline is evaluated during a 10-minute segment, not including periods of marked variability and episodic changes (Fig. 9.9).

- An FHR below 110 bpm is considered bradycardia and may be caused by an occiput posterior or transverse position of the fetus or severe deterioration of the health of the fetus (Cahill and Spain, 2015).
- An FHR greater than 160 bpm is considered tachycardia. However, if the FHR indicates good variability, it is not a sign of fetal distress. Tachycardia may be caused by maternal fever, medications, early fetal hypoxia, or fetal heart failure.

DRUG FACTS

If the FHR baseline indicates tachycardia or bradycardia, obtain a history of current medications from the patient. Medications used to slow or stop preterm labor such as terbutaline sulfate (Brethine) can cause fetal tachycardia. Magnesium sulfate used to treat pre-eclampsia can sedate the fetus, leading to bradycardia.

Variability

FHR variability is defined as fluctuations in the baseline that are irregular in frequency and amplitude. Variability is caused by an interaction between the sympathetic nervous system, which causes accelerations of the FHR, and the parasympathetic nervous system, which causes decelerations. This communication between the two systems results in beat-to-beat changes, which are called *variability*. A moderate variability reveals a complete pathway through the cerebral cortex, medulla oblongata, vagus nerve, and heart. Moderate variability is considered normal and indicates a functioning central nervous system in the fetus. Conditions that affect the communication between the two systems, such as low blood oxygen, can cause a loss of heart rate variability. Marked variability is a less common sign of fetal hypoxia. Therefore variability is an indicator of fetal oxygenation and reserve during labor (Menihan and Kopel, 2014).

Variability is graded as follows:

- Absent variability = fluctuations are undetectable
- Minimal variability = less than 5 bpm
- Moderate variability = 6 to 25 bpm
- Marked variability = greater than 25 bpm

Persistently absent or minimal variability is the most significant sign of fetal distress in labor. Causes of absent or minimal variability are:

- Fetal metabolic acidosis
- Fetal sleep cycles
- Prematurity
- Congenital anomalies
- Central nervous system depressant medications
- Betamethasone: a medication used to prepare the preterm fetal lungs for delivery

Table 9.6 notes the medical management and nursing interventions related to treating FHR variability.

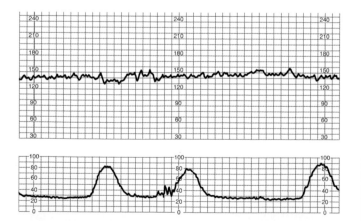

FIGURE 9.9 Fetal heart rate (FHR) baseline. The normal baseline FHR is 110 to 160 bpm. *Top,* FHR. *Bottom,* Uterine contractions.

TABLE 9.6 MEDICAL MANAGEMENT AND NURSING INTERVENTIONS RELATED TO TREATING FETAL HEART RATE VARIABILITY

Medical Management	Nursing Interventions
- The health-care provider may elect to rupture the membranes to allow initiation of internal fetal monitoring. - If known, treat the cause of the minimal or absent variability.	- Change the maternal position to promote fetal oxygenation. - Provide fetal scalp stimulation. - Apply an FSE for more accurate information regarding variability. - Increase IV fluids to promote maternal hydration and increase uterine perfusion. - Notify the health-care provider about minimal or absent variability.

Accelerations

Accelerations are an abrupt increase in FHR above the baseline, with the onset to peak of the acceleration being less than 30 seconds and the acceleration lasting less than 2 minutes in duration (Fig. 9.10). Accelerations predict adequate fetal oxygenation. Fetal movement usually results in accelerations. Expected accelerations are defined as:

- For a fetus less than 32 weeks of gestation, there should be accelerations of 10 or more bpm above the baseline for 10 or more seconds.
- For a fetus more than 32 weeks of gestation, there should be accelerations of 15 or more bpm above the baseline for 15 or more seconds.

An absence of accelerations for more than 80 minutes has been associated with increased neonatal morbidity (Cahill and Spain, 2015).

Table 9.7 notes the medical management and nursing interventions related to treating FHR accelerations.

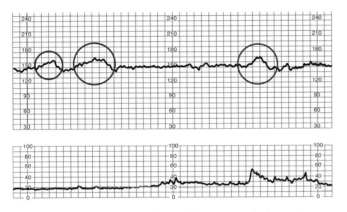

FIGURE 9.10 *Top,* FHR, with accelerations circled in red. *Bottom,* Uterine contractions.

TABLE 9.7 MEDICAL MANAGEMENT AND NURSING INTERVENTIONS RELATED TO TREATING FETAL HEART RATE ACCELERATIONS

Medical Management	Nursing Interventions
• If no accelerations are noted, the health-care provider should assess fetal oxygenation.	• If accelerations are not noted, the nurse can stimulate the fetal scalp to cause accelerations. • Change the maternal position to awaken a sleeping fetus and observe for accelerations. • Notify the health-care provider of an absence of accelerations.

Decelerations

A deceleration is a decrease in FHR from the baseline. **Episodic decelerations** are drops in the FHR not associated with uterine contractions, and periodic decelerations are drops in the FHR that are associated with uterine contractions.

Early Decelerations

Early decelerations are a gradual decrease in the FHR with the onset of deceleration to **nadir** (ie, lowest point) equal to or less than 30 seconds. The nadir occurs at the same time as the peak of the contraction. Early decelerations are caused by the compression of the fetal head in the pelvis and are not considered to be dangerous for the fetus. No nursing interventions are required, excepting observation and documentation (Fig. 9.11).

Late Decelerations

Late decelerations occur after the uterine contraction begins, and the nadir is noted after the peak of the contraction. Late decelerations can be caused by maternal hypotension, uterine hyperactivity, or placental insufficiency, leading to a decrease in oxygen to the fetus and causing a possible hypoxic state (Fig. 9.12). Table 9.8 notes the medical management and nursing interventions related to treating late FHR decelerations.

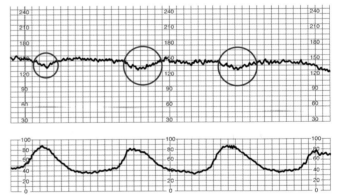

FIGURE 9.11 *Top,* FHR, with early decelerations circled in red. *Bottom,* Uterine contractions.

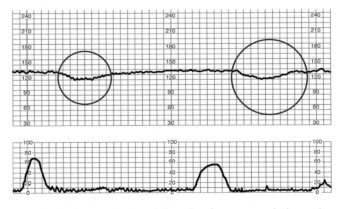

FIGURE 9.12 *Top,* FHR, with late decelerations circled in red. *Bottom,* Uterine contractions.

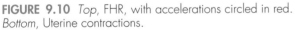

TABLE 9.8 MEDICAL MANAGEMENT AND NURSING INTERVENTIONS RELATED TO TREATING LATE FETAL HEART RATE DECELERATIONS

Medical Management	Interventions
• Determine the cause of the decelerations and treat. • If caused by uterine hyperactivity, **tocolytic medications** that suppress uterine activity may be prescribed. • Cesarean delivery should be considered for recurrent late decelerations with minimal or absent variability.	• Place the patient on her side to promote optimal placenta perfusion. • Discontinue oxytocin to decrease uterine activity, if applicable. • Correct maternal hypotension by changing her position and increasing the rate of IV fluids. • Administer oxygen by tight face mask at 10 L/min. • Assess maternal hydration and increase IV fluids if appropriate • Notify the physician or nurse midwife. • Consider an internal FSE for more accurate data about the fetal condition. • Provide support to the patient and her family to manage anxiety.

Variable Decelerations

Variable decelerations are an abrupt decrease in FHR of 15 beats or more. The onset to nadir is less than 30 seconds. This type of deceleration can be periodic or episodic and can vary in duration, length, and timing with the uterine contractions. On the fetal monitor, the variable deceleration can resemble a U, W, or V in appearance. Variable decelerations can be caused by cord compression, which disrupts the oxygenation of the fetus (Fig. 9.13). Table 9.9 notes the medical management and nursing interventions related to treating variable FHR decelerations.

Fetal Heart Rate Classification System

In 2008, three categories of classification were created to assist health-care providers and nurses with defining FHR patterns, identifying risks, and promoting a common standard of care in labor and delivery (AWHONN, 2012; Gittinger, 2015). Table 9.10 provides the FHR classification system.

Contraction Evaluation

Uterine activity is also important in evaluating the fetus and the progress of labor. Contractions can be evaluated by palpation of the fundus and by monitoring. Contraction evaluation includes:

• *Frequency of contractions:* The time from the beginning of a contraction to the beginning of the next contraction; it is recorded in minutes
• *Duration:* The actual time that a contraction is palpated or measured by the monitor; it is usually recorded in seconds
• *Intensity:* The strength of a contraction measured by internal monitoring or palpation. The most reliable method of determining strength is with internal monitoring. Mild contractions have an average strength of 33-35mg Hg, moderate contractions 35-45mg Hg, and strong contractions >45mm Hg.
• *Resting tone:* When the uterus is relaxed between contractions; it is measured by internal monitoring or palpation only

Normal contraction frequency has been defined by the American College of Obstetricians and Gynecologists (ACOG) as five or fewer contractions in a 10-minute window, averaged over 30 minutes (Menihan and Kopel, 2014). The term for contractions that occur more often is *tachysystole.* Tachysystole can be caused by overstimulation from oxytocin or can occur spontaneously without a known cause. Table 9.11 notes the medical management and nursing interventions related to treating tachysystole.

NURSING CARE PLAN For the Patient with Fetal Distress

Sophie is a patient in labor and delivery. Her labor is being induced because she is 2 weeks overdue with her third child. The nurse has applied the external fetal monitor and Sophie is receiving IV oxytocin (Pitocin) to start her labor contractions. The nurse has noticed that Sophie is now having contractions 3 minutes apart with a duration of 60 seconds. Observing the fetal monitor, the nurse notes that the fetus has had two late decelerations.

Nursing Diagnosis: The fetus is experiencing impaired gas exchange.
Goal: The late decelerations will resolve and the FHR will be within the normal range of 120-160bpm.
Nursing Interventions:
   • Turn the patient to her side to promote maximal placental perfusion.
   • Apply oxygen via face mask to increase fetal oxygenation.
   • Stop oxytocin (Pitocin) to decrease uterine tone.
   • Notify the physician of late decelerations.

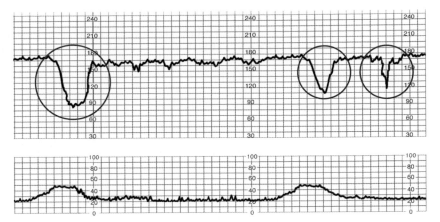

FIGURE 9.13 *Top,* FHR, with variable decelerations circled in red. *Bottom,* Uterine contractions.

TABLE 9.9 MEDICAL MANAGEMENT AND NURSING INTERVENTIONS RELATED TO TREATING VARIABLE FETAL HEART RATE DECELERATIONS

Medical Management	Nursing Interventions
• Administer tocolytic medications to stop preterm labor by decreasing uterine activity. • Perform **amnioinfusion**, which is a procedure in which room temperature normal saline is infused into the uterus through an IUPC to increase the volume of fluid in the uterus. The increase in fluid may relieve the compression of the fetal body on the umbilical cord. • Consider delivery if the fetal condition is deteriorating.	• Change the patient's position to decrease cord compression. • Discontinue oxytocin to decrease uterine activity, if applicable. • Administer oxygen by tight face mask at 10 L/min. • Assess maternal hydration and increase IV fluids if appropriate. • Notify the physician or nurse midwife. • Consider an internal FSE for more accurate data about the fetal condition. • Perform amnioinfusion, if ordered, to correct umbilical cord compression. • Provide support to the patient and her family to manage anxiety.

TABLE 9.10 FHR CLASSIFICATION SYSTEM

Category I	Category II	Category III
• Considered to be normal or reassuring	• Considered to be indeterminate • Includes FHR tracings that do not match Categories I or III	• Considered abnormal or nonreassuring
• FHR between 110 and 160 bpm • Baseline FHR variability is moderate • Accelerations are present or absent • Late or variable decelerations are absent • Early decelerations are present or absent	• Tachycardia • Minimal baseline variability OR • Absent baseline variability not accompanied by decelerations OR • Marked baseline variability • Prolonged decelerations lasting longer than 2 minutes but less than 10 minutes OR • Recurrent variable decelerations with minimal or moderate variability OR • Variable decelerations with slow return to baseline, or "overshoots" (ie, goes over the baseline) when returning to baseline	• Absent baseline variability along with: • Recurring late decelerations • Recurring variable decelerations • Bradycardia • Sinusoidal pattern, which is a smooth undulating (ie, up and down, wavelike) pattern that varies from 10–15 bpm and occurs in three to five cycles per minute. It is considered an ominous sign of fetal distress.

TABLE 9.11 MEDICAL MANAGEMENT AND NURSING INTERVENTIONS RELATED TO TREATING TACHYSYSTOLE

Medical Management	Nursing Interventions
• Treat the cause, such as by decreasing or stopping the infusion of oxytocin.	• Decrease or stop oxytocin if applicable. • Change the maternal position. • Administer a tocolytic medication if ordered. • Increase the IV rate to improve hydration. • Support the laboring woman and her family. • Evaluate fetal oxygenation.

Key Points

- Hospital births are considered to be the safest for the woman and the fetus. A woman may arrive at the hospital in any phase of labor.
- Some women prepare a birth plan and bring it to the hospital. The nurse must be sensitive to the needs and desires of the patient.
- Most women are accompanied by a support person to assist her in coping with labor.
- Initial assessment includes a complete physical examination along with contraction, cervical, and pain assessments.
- Leopold's maneuvers assist the nurse to determine fetal position.
- The nurse will perform a cervical examination to determine cervical dilation, effacement, and fetal position. There are no rules about examination frequency, but the nurse is aware that frequent examinations can cause uterine infections.
- Uterine contractions are monitored for frequency, duration, and intensity every 30 to 60 minutes during the latent phase of labor.
- During the active and transition phases, contractions should be monitored every 15 to 30 minutes because labor progresses faster during these phases.
- Intermittent fetal monitoring can be done with a handheld Doppler device or by applying the fetal monitor for 20 minute periods to evaluate the fetus.
- High-risk women should receive continual fetal monitoring.
- External fetal monitoring is less invasive and provides basic information regarding the FHR baseline, variability, accelerations, and decelerations.

- Internal fetal monitoring is more invasive but provides accurate information about FHR, variability, accelerations, and decelerations, regardless of fetal activity.
- Early decelerations are caused by head compression as the fetus moves through the maternal pelvis.
- Late decelerations are caused by insufficient blood flow through the placenta that decreases oxygenation of the fetus.
- Variable decelerations are caused by cord compression, which decreases blood flow and therefore decreases oxygenation of the fetus.
- A Category I FHR pattern is considered normal or reassuring and is defined by a FHR between 110 and 160 bpm, moderate baseline variability with accelerations present, and no late or variable decelerations.
- A Category II FHR pattern is considered indeterminate. It is defined by FHR tracings that do not match Categories I or III, which include tachycardia, minimal baseline variability, absent baseline variability not accompanied by decelerations, prolonged decelerations lasting longer than 2 minutes but less than 10 minutes, or variable decelerations with slow return to baseline or "overshooting" when returning to baseline.
- A Category III FHR pattern is considered abnormal or nonreassuring and is defined as including absent baseline variability along with recurring late decelerations, recurring variable decelerations, and bradycardia.

REVIEW QUESTIONS

1. A laboring patient reports to the nurse that "I think my water just broke!" The first action the nurse should take is:
   1. Assess the FHR.
   2. Check the fluid with Nitrazine paper.
   3. Notify the health-care provider.
   4. Note the color of the fluid.

2. A patient arrives in the labor and delivery unit with painless vaginal bleeding. The nurse knows that a vaginal examination is contraindicated because:
   1. It may cause an infection.
   2. It may stimulate labor contractions.
   3. It may tear a low implanted placenta.
   4. It may rupture the membranes.

3. The nurse notes on the fetal monitor that the fetus is experiencing a late deceleration. Which nursing actions are appropriate in this situation? (*select all that apply*)
   1. Continue to observe the fetal monitor for three more contractions.
   2. Turn the patient to her side.
   3. Apply oxygen via face mask.
   4. Increase the oxytocin to speed up labor.
   5. Assist the patient into a pushing position.

4. A patient is concerned about why the nurse is screening her for GBS. The nurse explains that:
   1. "Group B strep is sexually contracted, and we don't want the baby to catch a sexually transmitted infection."
   2. "Group B strep can cause you to become very ill during labor."
   3. "Group B strep is contagious and we may need to isolate you after delivery."
   4. "Group B strep can cause health problems for the newborn."

5. During the initial assessment in labor and delivery, the health-care provider must be notified *immediately* if: (*select all that apply*)
   1. The patient's blood pressure is greater than 140/90 mm Hg.
   2. The patient is accompanied by five family members.
   3. The patient has brought a detailed birth plan to the hospital.
   4. An abnormal or nonreassuring FHR pattern is noted.
   5. Vaginal bleeding is observed.

6. A CBC is ordered for a newly admitted labor patient. The nurse knows that this laboratory test provides information regarding: (*select all that apply*)
   1. The status of the patient's immune system
   2. If the patient has an infection
   3. The patient's blood sugar
   4. The patient's blood type and Rh
   5. If the patient is anemic

7. The nurse is having difficulty obtaining information on the fetal monitor regarding the variability of the FHR. The nurse knows that the best plan of action is to:
   1. Turn the woman to her side.
   2. Apply an FSE.
   3. Apply oxygen via face mask.
   4. Prepare the woman for delivery.

8. Leopold's maneuvers are performed to:
   1. Determine the position of the fetus.
   2. Determine the size of the woman's pelvis.
   3. Determine the size of the fetus.
   4. Determine the fundal height.

9. Which of the following patients should receive continual fetal monitoring in labor? (*select all that apply*)
   1. A patient with a hypertensive disorder
   2. A patient delivering her first baby
   3. A patient with a post-term pregnancy
   4. A patient with a preterm pregnancy
   5. A patient with a positive GBS test

10. A disadvantage of internal fetal monitoring is:
    1. Accurate information regarding FHR variability is not possible.
    2. An artifact on the printout is very common.
    3. It is invasive and increases the risk of uterine infection.
    4. It cannot provide data about the uterine resting tone.

CRITICAL THINKING QUESTION

Prepare a discussion on the pros and cons of hospital and home births for a prenatal class.

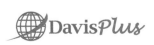

For additional resources and information, visit **www.DavisPlus.com.**
Post-Conference Questions and Activities, Answers, and References can be found on DavisPlus.

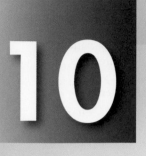

10

Nursing Care During Labor

DavisPlus For audio pronunciation guide, visit www.DavisPlus.com

CHAPTER CONCEPTS

Comfort
Nursing Roles
Pregnancy
Stress

LEARNING OUTCOMES

1. Define the key terms.
2. Explain medical interventions that may occur during each stage of labor.
3. Plan safe and effective patient-centered nursing care for each stage of labor.
4. Prepare patient teaching appropriate for each stage of labor.
5. Discuss immediate postdelivery care for the woman.
6. Complete an Apgar score on a newborn.
7. Explain the immediate needs and goals of care for the newborn.
8. Explain the physiological causes of labor pain.
9. Identify nursing interventions that provide nonpharmacological pain relief.
10. Discuss the advantages and disadvantages of analgesia and anesthesia options for pain control in labor.
11. Compare and contrast epidural anesthesia and spinal anesthesia.
12. Describe nursing responsibilities for the patient receiving analgesic and anesthetic drugs during labor.
13. Identify safety issues that may arise when the patient receives analgesic and anesthetic drugs for pain control in labor.

REAL-WORLD CASE STUDY

Claire

■ Claire arrives at the labor and delivery unit in early labor with her first baby. She is accompanied by her husband, Steven, and her sister, Lydia. Claire attended childbirth classes with her sister. Steven is a college student and must work in the evenings, making it difficult for him to attend childbirth preparation classes. Steven

REAL-WORLD CASE STUDY *continued*

is very interested in being supportive and helpful to Claire during labor.

1. How should the nurse inquire about Steven's learning needs related to labor and delivery?
2. How can the nurse provide patient-centered care for Claire?
3. What actions can the nurse take to include Steven in providing labor support for Claire?

CONCEPTUAL CORNERSTONE

Pain

Labor and childbirth involves pain. The pain is an acute pain that is short-lived and diminishes with healing. Every woman has a different pain tolerance and response to pain. The nurse should conduct a thorough pain assessment and should avoid making assumptions about the patient's pain experience. A complete pain assessment requires questioning the patient about the location, intensity, quality, onset, and duration of the pain. The nurse in labor and delivery has a key role in managing the patient's pain. The patient should be educated about safe, pharmacological strategies available for pain management, as well as nonpharmacological strategies. Nonpharmacological techniques may be effective alone for mild to moderate pain and give comfort to the patient (Giddens, 2013). Unrelieved pain can interfere with the patient's ability to relax and participate in her birth experience. Every labor patient will be unique in her response to pain. The nurse must complete a thorough pain assessment and individualize the plan of care.

The nurse has a major role in managing the pain of labor and childbirth. This chapter includes medical interventions and appropriate nursing interventions to provide safe and effective care for each stage of labor. The physiology of labor pain and pain management options include nonpharmacological techniques, systemic analgesia, and regional anesthetics.

The labor and delivery nurse has the opportunity to participate in one of life's major milestones. Women never forget their childbirth experience. The nurse can be instrumental in assisting the woman in coping with the pain of labor and promoting self-esteem and positive memories about her childbirth experience.

NURSING CARE DURING LABOR AND BIRTH

Many women prepare for labor and the birth by reading, attending childbirth classes, and talking to other women.

Most young women have never faced pain of the same intensity of labor and childbirth and are anxious when they arrive at the hospital. Many women do not really know how they will cope with labor contractions until labor actually begins. The role of the labor and delivery nurse is to manage the stages of labor and assist the patient to manage her pain.

Labor is divided into stages and phases. The labor and delivery nurse manages the care of the labor under the direction of the obstetrician's or nurse midwife's orders. The nurse will have medical interventions to carry out for each stage of labor, as well as nursing interventions individualized for the patient.

The labor and delivery nurse is aware that no two laboring patients or labors are the same. To provide patient-centered care during labor and delivery, the nurse assesses the patient and her fetus, plans interventions to meet the needs of the patient, assists the patient with managing pain, and then evaluates and makes changes to the interventions to attain the goal of a safe delivery for the mother and fetus.

This section discusses the stages of labor with the standard medical interventions and nursing interventions for each stage.

HEALTH PROMOTION

Packing List for Labor

Many couples have prepared for labor either by formal childbirth classes or by reading and self-study. The patient may benefit from packing the following items to promote comfort during labor:

*   Socks or slippers
*   Hair ties or clips
*   Lip balm or moisturizer
*   Flip-flops or shower shoes
*   Toothbrush and toothpaste
*   Massage oil or lotion
*   A comforting picture to focus on during contractions
*   A relaxing music playlist on a phone, iPod, or MP3 player
*   Robe
*   Gum for dry mouth
*   Snacks for the labor coach

Stage 1, Phase 1: Early or Latent Phase of Labor

Latent labor is accompanied by generally mild and erratic contractions that range from 5 to 20 min apart and last 20 to 60 sec. The cervix is effacing and slowly dilating to 3 cm. The woman is usually excited and relieved that labor has begun but is also ambivalent about facing labor pain. She may be making phone calls, texting her friends, or watching television for distraction and to manage her excitement. A woman usually describes the pain as feeling like strong menstrual cramps, and she can usually cope with the pain using relaxation and breathing techniques.

Medical Interventions

Medical interventions that are commonly ordered during early labor are:

- Complete blood cell count (CBC), blood type, Rh, and urinalysis
  - Sexually transmitted infection screen, depending on state laws
- IV infusion of lactated Ringer's solution or normal saline to prevent dehydration in labor
- Intermittent or continual fetal monitoring

Nursing Care

After completing the initial assessments of physical examination, cervical examination, and pain assessment, appropriate nursing care for latent labor includes:

- Admission to the labor and delivery unit and orientation of the patient and her support person to the labor room
- Establishing a therapeutic relationship with the woman by spending time with her and demonstrating a willingness to answer questions
- Inquiring about concerns or questions
- Reassuring the support person that the nurse will be assisting with providing comfort measures and support for both of them during labor
- Reinforcing relaxation techniques learned in childbirth classes or teaching simple relaxation techniques
- Inserting the IV or saline lock, if ordered, for fluid maintenance or medication administration
- Reviewing laboratory results and notifying the physician, if necessary
- Administering penicillin G IV, if indicated, for group B streptococcus (GBS)
- Encouraging fluid intake with clear fluid and ice chips; food may or may not be permitted by the health-care provider
- Explaining the fetal monitor and applying it for intermittent or continual monitoring
- Providing ongoing assessment of the vital signs, cervical dilation and effacement, fetal heart rate (FHR), and contractions

Patient Teaching

Preparing the patient for early labor should include the following information:

- Inform her that the contractions are mild at the beginning of labor but will get progressively stronger and last longer.
- She should try to stay relaxed. There are a variety of ways that women can stay relaxed, such as listening to music, receiving a massage, or engaging in a distraction such as television or conversation.
- Position changes are encouraged, and walking is safe in labor.
- She should drink clear liquids to avoid dehydration. If the health-care provider consents, she can eat light, easily-digested food.
- Instruct her to notify the nurse if her water breaks or any bleeding is noted.

DRUG FACTS

For GBS prophylaxis, penicillin G is usually given at an initial dose of 5 million units IV, then followed with 2.5 million units every 4 hours until delivery. Ampicillin is used as an alternative choice and is given with an initial dose of 2 g IV followed with 1 g IV every 4 hours until delivery. For women allergic to penicillin, cefazolin, erythromycin, or clindamycin may be prescribed (Vallerand, Sanoski, et al, 2013).

TEAM WORKS

Some laboring women have a doula at the hospital to assist with labor support. The word *doula* comes from Greek, meaning a trained and experienced professional who provides physical, emotional, and informational support to the laboring woman. Doulas are not usually nurses, but are trained to assist the woman during labor and act as an advocate for carrying out the patient's birth plan. Some doulas are certified by DONA International.

Stage 1, Phase 2: Active Phase of Labor

The next part of the first stage of labor is the active phase, which is the phase of the most rapid cervical dilation. Active labor is characterized by contractions that are 2 to 3 min apart with a duration of about 60 sec. Dilation increases from 3 to 4 cm to 8 cm of dilation. Fetal descent progresses, which causes feelings of pelvic pressure.

The patient is no longer talkative or interested in conversation. She becomes labor focused and may require more assistance to cope with the increasing intensity of the uterine contractions. Pain management and comfort measures become more important during this phase of labor.

During the active phase, the contractions become stronger and more difficult for the woman to manage. **Hyperventilation** can occur if the woman breathes too fast and too deep in response to pain in labor. Hyperventilation causes a decrease in carbon dioxide in the blood. Signs of hyperventilation include feelings of anxiety, a feeling that she cannot get enough air, an elevated heart rate, lightheadedness or vertigo, numbness or tingling of the fingers, and chest tightness. Management of hyperventilation can be done by encouraging the patient to do one of the following: (1) slow down breathing and breathe through pursed lips, as if blowing out a candle, (2) close her mouth and one nostril and breathe through one nostril only, or (3) cover her nose and mouth with a paper bag and breathe in and out into the bag for a few breaths only or for about 15 seconds. These interventions will raise the level of carbon dioxide in the blood and decrease symptoms.

Medical Interventions

Medical interventions that may occur during active labor are:

- Performing an **amniotomy,** which is the artificial rupture of the uterine membranes with an amniohook
- Orders for pain medication or **epidural** anesthesia, which is the injection of drugs through a catheter placed in the epidural space around the vertebral bones
- Evaluation of the maternal condition and progression of labor
- Evaluation of the fetal condition

Nursing Care

Nursing care appropriate for the active phase of labor includes:

- Doing a complete pain assessment, including the description, location, radiation, and degree of discomfort
- Performing vaginal examinations to monitor cervical dilation, fetal position, and descent
- Giving the woman and her support person frequent updates on progress
- Providing emotional support in the form of praise, reassurance, listening, and physical presence
- Assisting the woman's support person to provide comfort and encouraging the support person to take a break as needed
- Encouraging clear liquids
- Monitoring vital signs every 30 min
- Monitoring the FHR and contractions every 15 to 30 min, adjusting the transducers as needed
- Providing nonpharmacological pain relief and comfort measures (See the Nonpharmacological Pain Management section later in chapter.)

- Administering pain medication as ordered and per patient requests
- Evaluating the effectiveness of pharmacological and nonpharmacological pain relief
- Changing the disposable pad underneath the patient as she continues to leak fluid and mucus from the vagina
- Encouraging position changes and allowing her to walk if her membranes are intact
- Assisting with elimination; for example, a full bladder can slow down the descent of the fetus into the pelvis
- Reviewing and reinforcing relaxation and breathing techniques using a calm, soothing voice and touch

Patient Teaching

When preparing the patient for active labor, the nurse should include the following information:

- The contractions will be getting stronger and last longer as the fetus is moving down through the pelvis.
- She should use breathing and relaxation techniques with every contraction.
- Encourage her to ask for what she needs to promote relaxation, such as massage, music, or a cool cloth for her forehead.
- If relaxation and breathing techniques are not keeping her comfortable, it would be an appropriate time to consider IV or epidural medication.
- She should change positions often and avoid lying on her back unless the head of the bed is raised 30 to 45 degrees. See Figure 10.1 for labor positions.
- It is important to urinate at least every 2 hours. A full bladder can make it more difficult for the baby to descend through the pelvis.

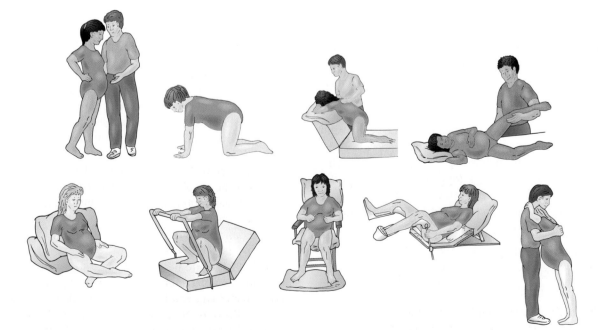

FIGURE 10.1 Various positions for labor and birth.

• She may notice more pressure in the pelvis area and may not even notice the need to urinate.
• Instruct her to call the nurse when the membranes rupture.

Stage 1, Phase 3: Transition Phase of Labor

This is the most intense phase of labor; it leads to complete effacement and dilation of the cervix to 10 cm. The transition phase is characterized by painful contractions that peak abruptly, are 2-3 min apart, and last 60 to 90 sec. The transition phase may last 1 to 3 hours for a first-time mother and only a few minutes to an hour for a subsequent labor and delivery.

The use of pain medication in the transition phase of labor should be done with caution. Commonly used medications are meperidine, fentanyl, nalbuphine, butorphanol, and morphine. These medications cross the placenta and circulate into the fetal system. In the fetal system, these medications affect the central nervous system and can subdue the respiratory center. This is not a problem as long as the fetus is in the uterus because the fetus is receiving oxygen through the umbilical cord. At birth, the respiratory center must function correctly and a sedated baby will have respiratory difficulties because of a depressed respiratory center. To avoid this problem, small doses of pain medication are administered and the timing is controlled by the nurse to allow the peak effect of the medication to have left the mother's system before the fetus is born. A woman experiencing a fast-moving transition phase may not receive pain medication if it is not safe for the fetus (Yarnell, 2013).

The woman may feel pelvic or rectal pressure because of fetal descent into the pelvis. She may have more trouble with concentration and coping and may become irritable. Nausea and vomiting commonly accompany this phase of labor. If the patient becomes nauseated, the nurse needs to assist her to a safe position, such as sitting up or elevating her head, to prevent aspiration if she vomits. The health-care provider may order antinausea medication if the nausea is severe.

During this phase she may have the urge to push. The patient and the support person should be taught by the nurse to immediately call the nurse if the patient begins to push or bear down. A nurse should assess the patient to determine if she is fully dilated. Pushing too early can cause the cervix to swell and slow down dilation of the cervix.

Assisting a patient in labor, especially during the transition phase, requires teamwork. The health-care provider, labor and delivery nurse, the labor support person or coach, a doula, and friends can all work together to provide positive support and comfort measures for the laboring woman. Continuous support has a more beneficial effect for reducing anxiety and pain than intermittent support (Iliadou, 2012).

Medical Interventions

Medical interventions that may be ordered during this phase are:

• Amniotomy if not previously performed
• Pain medication if safe, depending upon the labor progress

Nursing Care

Nursing care appropriate for the transition phase of labor care includes:

• Assessing FHR and contractions every 15 min
• Assessing cervical dilation
• Communicating labor progress to the health-care provider
• Assisting with breathing techniques, particularly if she loses focus or has a strong desire to push
• Providing comfort measures
• Continuing to remind her to urinate
• Providing for personal hygiene such as perineal care and changing disposable pads frequently
• Preparing the patient and the room for delivery
• Cautiously administering pain medication, if desired by the patient
• Remaining in the room with the patient and family
• Providing encouragement to the woman and her support person

Patient Teaching

Patient teaching for this phase of labor should include the following information:

• The contractions will be stronger and closer together. She may feel as if there is no break and no chance to relax between contractions. This is the hardest but shortest phase of labor.
• She may notice strong pressure in the lower back and rectum. If she notices a desire to push, she must notify the nurse. Pushing too early can cause the cervix to become edematous (ie, swollen) and slow down dilation of the cervix.
• She may want to use pant-blow breathing to prevent early pushing. The nurse may instruct or assist her in this breathing technique. Pant-blow breathing is quick breathing in and out of the mouth. After every 3 to 5 quick breaths (ie, panting), the patient should do a longer exhale (ie, blowing).
• Nausea and vomiting may occur. She should notify the nurse for assistance.
• She may notice more blood-tinged vaginal mucus as the capillaries in the cervix rupture.
• She may feel impatient, overwhelmed, and irritable during this phase. It will be more difficult to maintain focus and concentration, but the nurse will be available to assist her.
• Even if an epidural has been administered, she may experience nausea, vomiting, leg shakiness, and alternating chills and sweats. Report these signs of transition to the nurse.

DRUG FACTS

Promethazine (Phenergan) 25 to 75 mg intramuscularly (IM) or 25 to 50 mg IV may be given for nausea and vomiting in labor. It does not cause respiratory depression but it does increase the effectiveness of narcotic analgesics (Vallerand and Sanoski, 2013).

PATIENT TEACHING GUIDELINES

Relaxation

The nurse can suggest any of the following relaxation methods for the patient to try:

• Display an item that she brought for the baby, such as a blanket or going home outfit, to look at when labor is hard. It will help her to focus on the goal.
• Listen to relaxing music.
• Dim the lights.
• Visualize a favorite location or holding the baby in her arms.
• Scan her body and notice any areas of tension and then focus on relaxing that area of her body.

  In addition, the support person can use gentle pressure on the patient's lower back or massage her back.

PATIENT TEACHING GUIDELINES

Breathing Techniques

If the patient did not attend childbirth classes or does not remember relaxation breathing techniques, the nurse can teach simple relaxation breathing to the patient.

• At the beginning of the contraction, instruct her to take a long, slow, deep breath, breathing in through the nose and out through the mouth. Have her continue breathing slowly and easily, about half as deep as the first breath, throughout the contraction. At the end of the contraction, have her take another slow, long, deep breath.
• As the contractions become stronger, encourage the patient to breathe light and shallow in and out through her mouth, increasing the number of breaths per contraction.
• Pant-blow breathing is effective to avoid pushing. She should quickly pant three to four times, then blow out.
• Between contractions, encourage her to rest and breathe normally to avoid hyperventilation.

Stage 2: Pushing and Birth

As soon as the cervix is completely dilated, the woman enters the second stage of labor, which ends with the birth of the baby. The contractions during this phase may be 2 to 3 min apart and last about 60 sec. Generally, the contractions are not as intense as during the transition phase of labor. She may experience the urge to push at this time. Women who have chosen epidural anesthesia may not experience the urge to push and may be unable to actively push. If so, the medication may be decreased to allow her to feel and use the muscles required for pushing. The nurses may instruct her to rest and wait for the effects of the epidural to diminish enough to allow her to push. The fetus will move slowly through the birth canal with the pressure from the contractions. This method is commonly called *laboring down*. The woman may have felt tired and discouraged during the transition phase but often gets a renewed sense of energy. For the first time

throughout labor, she can have some control of the birth as she begins pushing.

SAFETY *STAT!*

The Urge to Push

Pushing without a nurse or health-care provider present could result in an unattended birth and lead to complications for the woman and her baby.

Medical Interventions

Medical interventions that may occur during this stage include providing perineal anesthesia administration. **Anesthesia** administered to this area causes partial or complete loss of sensation to the perineal area. The fetal head places intense pressure on the perineal nerves and serves as natural anesthesia. To provide perineal anesthesia, an injection of an anesthetic into the perineal area between the vagina and rectum is administered. An **episiotomy,** which is an incision into the perineum, can be done without the injection of an anesthetic, but anesthesia is necessary for repair. An episiotomy is performed to enlarge the vaginal outlet. Two types of episiotomies are done: (1) a midline episiotomy is an incision between the vagina and rectum and (2) a mediolateral episiotomy is an incision from the vagina diagonally to the left or right (Fig. 10.2).

Cleansing of the perineum is ongoing as the woman pushes. Occasionally, some fecal matter emerges as she pushes and this is wiped away. Some health-care providers massage the perineum as the head descends to assist with gentle stretching and to avoid large tears in the perineum. As the woman pushes, the health-care provider will determine if an episiotomy is necessary to allow more room for the fetal head and to prevent large tears in the perineal area.

As the head emerges from the birth canal, the health-care provider will check for a tight cord around the neck. If there

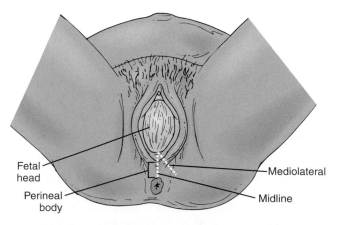

FIGURE 10.2 An episiotomy is a surgical incision of the perineum performed to allow more room for the birth. The most common method is the midline episiotomy: an incision made from the vaginal opening toward the rectum.

is a tight cord, it may need to be clamped and cut before the entire body can emerge from the birth canal. Next, the health-care provider will suction the mouth and airway thoroughly before the chest emerges from the birth canal and the baby is born.

After the baby is born, the umbilical cord is clamped and cut. Early clamping may be necessary to evaluate the baby, but rushing to clamp the cord is not necessary. Delaying clamping of the cord results in higher hemoglobin and hematocrit values and possibly allows greater iron stores for the newborn (Smith, 2012). The parents may have a preference regarding the timing of the cord cutting and may wish to participate in it.

A cord blood specimen may be sent to the laboratory. Practices vary but the specimen may be sent to the laboratory for a complete blood count (CBC), blood type, Rh, and antibody screen.

After the cord is cut, the infant should be thoroughly dried and may be placed skin-to-skin with the mother to promote bonding. If the support person wishes to hold the infant, he or she should be wrapped in a warm blanket with the head covered with a cap to maintain warmth.

Nursing Care

Nursing care appropriate for this stage of labor may include:

- Monitoring the FHR every 5 to 15 min
- Providing comfort measures and remaining with the patient
- Giving encouragement and praising for pushing efforts
- Providing for perineal hygiene; as she pushes, she may pass fecal material
- Being an advocate for the patient's desires regarding her birth plan
- Assuming care for the baby after the cord is cut

Patient Teaching

Patient teaching regarding pushing should include:

- Instructing the patient to notify the nurse of the urge to push
- Instructing her to avoid pushing until the nurse gives instructions
- Encouraging her to use an upright position, which is effective for pushing
- Encouraging her to rest and relax between contractions

Assist the patient to push effectively with either closed glottis pushing or open glottis pushing:

- With closed glottis pushing, the woman is directed to take a deep breath during a contraction and push with all her energy for 10 sec or more.
- With open glottis pushing, the woman is allowed to experience involuntary pushing when she feels the desire. She instinctively will hold her breath and push for about 6 sec. She will follow pushing by taking several deep breaths and pushing again when she feels the urge to bear down.

LEARN TO C.U.S.

The labor nurse has the important role of monitoring labor progress and alerting the health-care provider to arrive in time for the delivery. Using the C.U.S. method can be helpful when communicating with the health-care provider.

C: "Dr. Smith, I know that your orders state that I should call you to come to the hospital when the patient is 8 cm dilated, but I am **concerned**. Her labor is progressing very quickly, and

U: I am **uncomfortable** with that order. She is 6 cm dilated but has progressed from 3 cm to 6 cm in one hour.

S: We have a **safety** issue. I would like you to come to the hospital now so that you won't miss the delivery."

Stage 3: Birth Through Delivery of the Placenta

The third stage of labor is from the birth of the baby until the completed delivery of the placenta and the attached membranes. The length of this stage of labor is typically 5 to 15 min (Smith, 2012). The mother and her support person are usually very excited about the birth, and she may not notice the delivery of the placenta. Following delivery of the baby, uterine contractions continue, causing the release of the placenta. The patient may describe the contractions as a cramping sensation. As the placenta detaches, it moves into the lower uterine segment. When the placenta detaches, it leaves arteries exposed; this could lead to hemorrhage if not for the anatomy of the uterine muscle and the contractions applying pressure on the vessels. The health-care provider will notice signs that the placenta is detaching. These signs are:

- The umbilical cord lengthens.
- The uterine shape becomes firmer, rounder, and moves up in the abdomen.
- A gush of blood occurs because of the separation from the uterus (Smith, 2012).

Some health-care providers order a bolus of oxytocin given IV or IM to promote strong uterine contractions, leading to a faster placenta delivery.

When the placenta delivers, it usually presents with the fetal side facing the health-care provider. The physician or nurse midwife usually turns the placenta over to inspect the maternal side to determine if any pieces are torn or missing (Fig. 10.3). Missing pieces should be identified because they can lead to hemorrhage or infection if left inside the uterus.

Medical Interventions

Medical interventions for this stage of labor may include:

- Clamping the cord with two hemostats and cutting the umbilical cord about 8 to 10 inches from the infant's umbilicus
- Obtaining a cord blood specimen for the lab
- Ordering oxytocin infusion or IM injection
- Managing the delivery of the placenta
- Inspection of the cervix, vagina, and perineum for tears

that medical or nursing interventions may be needed to improve the newborn's cardiorespiratory status. If the 5-min Apgar score is below 7, the newborn should be assessed every 5 min until the score is 7 or above (Vennes, 2013) (Table 10.1).

SAFETY *STAT!*

Naloxone

Naloxone (Narcan) should be available at every delivery. This drug can be administered to a newborn to reverse the effects of opioid pain medication administered too close to delivery. For newborns, 0.01 mg/kg is given IM. The dose may be repeated every 2 to 3 min until a response is obtained (Vallerand and Sanoski, 2013).

Nursing Care

Nursing care during stage 3 includes:

• Administering oxytocin if ordered
• Providing assistance to the health-care provider
• Assuming care for the newborn with an emphasis on assessing the airway and providing warmth
• Assessing the umbilical cord for the normal two arteries and one vein
• Performing a 5-min Apgar assessment

DRUG FACTS

Oxytocin

Oxytocin (Pitocin) acts on the smooth muscle of the uterus, causing uterine contractions. In the third and fourth stage of labor it is used to control postpartum bleeding. For control of postpartum bleeding, dilute 10 to 40 units in one liter of IV fluid and infuse at a rate of 20 to 40 milliunits/min to control uterine **atony**, which is a lack of normal uterine muscle tone (Vallerand and Sanoski, 2013).

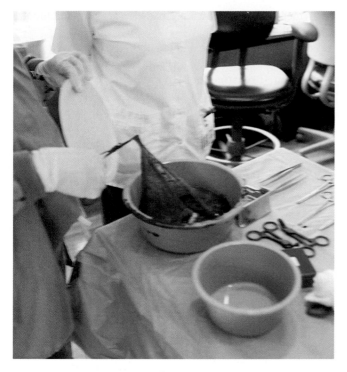

FIGURE 10.3 Examination of the placenta.

• Suturing of any tears or an episiotomy repair
• Completing a 1-minute Apgar score

Apgar Score

Apgar score was developed by Virginia Apgar, an American obstetrical anesthesiologist, as a quick, systematic method of assessing a newborn's physical condition at birth (Tabers, 2013). Apgar method is used to assess the newborn's heart rate, muscle tone, response to stimuli, and color rating by assigning a score of 0 to 2 to each category. The newborn is assessed at 1 min after birth and again at 5 min after birth. A 1-min Apgar assessment that scores between 7 and 10 indicates that the newborn is adjusting to extrauterine life. A score below 7 indicates

TABLE 10.1 APGAR SCORE

Physiological Parameter	0	1	2
Heart Rate	Absent	Slow: below 100	Above 100
Respiratory Effort	Absent	Slow: irregular, weak cry	Good; strong cry
Muscle Tone	Flaccid	Some flexion of extremities	Well-flexed
Reflex Irritability	No response	Grimace	Vigorous cry
Color	Blue, pale	Pink body, blue extremities	Completely pink

Range of Apgar Score: from 0 to 10

A 5-minute Apgar score of 7 to 10 is considered normal. Scores of 4, 5, and 6 are intermediate and not markers of increased risk of neurological dysfunction because such scores may be the result of physiological immaturity, maternal medications, the presence of congenital malformations, and other factors (ACOG, 2006).

Stage 4: After Birth

The first hour after birth is a critical time for the mother and infant. Bleeding problems can occur in the mother. The delivery of the placenta does not indicate the end of the threat for heavy bleeding. The uterus tends to relax after the delivery of the placenta, and the first hour after birth requires close observation of the mother. The infant is also making the transition from intrauterine life to extrauterine life and requires frequent assessments.

Nursing Care of the Mother

The goals of nursing care for the first hour are to provide safe care for the mother and to promote bonding with the infant. Appropriate nursing care for this period includes:

- **Providing a warm blanket:** Immediately after delivery, hormones begin dropping, endorphins are released, and the adrenaline level decreases, causing some women to shiver. The shivering is not harmful to the woman and will pass, but most women appreciate a warm blanket during this time.
- **Monitoring blood pressure and pulse every 15 min:** Notify the health-care provider if there are significant changes in the vital signs.
- **Assessing the uterus for firmness every 15 min or more often if needed:** The uterus should be round, firm, and located between the umbilicus and the symphysis pubis during the first hour.
- **Massaging the uterus:** Perform gentle massage of the uterus with the palm of the hand on the fundus and the other hand supporting the lower uterine segment (Fig. 10.4).
- **Monitoring vaginal discharge:** Monitor the vaginal discharge, known as lochia, every 15 min for the amount, clots, color, and odor. Usual blood loss in the first hour requires no more than two saturated obstetrical peripads and has only a few small clots. Alert the health-care

provider if more than two peripads are soaked with blood during the first hour.
- **Promoting bonding:** Promote bonding by allowing the new family time alone to get acquainted with the baby.
- **Promoting breastfeeding:** To promote breastfeeding, assist the mother to latch-on the infant.
- **Providing perineal comfort:** Provide perineal comfort with an ice pack.

SAFETY *STAT!*

The newborn has been immersed in body fluids. Standard safety precautions must be followed. Therefore until the first bath, the nurse should wear gloves when touching the newborn.

Nursing Care of the Infant

The immediate goals of newborn care are to monitor the infant's transition to extrauterine life, to complete required nursing care, and to promote bonding and attachment with the parents. Appropriate nursing care for the newborn in the first hour of life includes:

- **Maintaining the infant's warmth:** Maintain thermoregulation by wrapping the infant in warm blankets, covering the head with a cap, or placing the infant skin-to-skin with the mother (Fig. 10.5). The infant should be placed under a warmer for any procedures.
- **Maintaining the infant's airway:** Maintain a clear airway in the infant by gently suctioning excess secretions with a bulb syringe.
- **Providing umbilicus care:** Apply the umbilical clamp closer to the umbilicus and trim off excess cord.
- **Properly identifying the infant:** Follow hospital procedures for identifying the infant and attach hospital security mechanisms to the infant.
- **Administering vitamin K:** Administer vitamin K IM in the vastus lateralis muscle. Vitamin K is necessary for blood clotting.

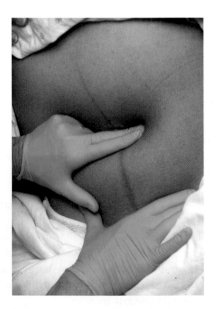

FIGURE 10.4 The nurse massaging the fundus.

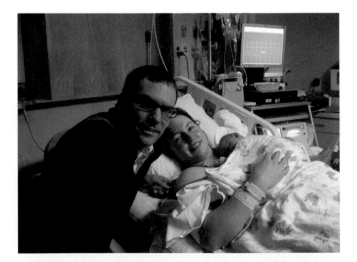

FIGURE 10.5 Newborn and mother with skin-to-skin contact.

- **Administering erythromycin:** Administer erythromycin 0.5% ophthalmic ointment within 2 hours of birth to prevent eye infections known as *ophthalmia neonatorum* from untreated sexually transmitted infections.
- **Encouraging infant/mother bonding:** Allow the mother to hold and bond with the infant as much as possible.

DRUG FACTS

Vitamin K

Vitamin K is a fat-soluble vitamin that promotes blood clotting. It is generally synthesized in the intestines. A newborn cannot produce vitamin K until after microorganisms are introduced with feedings. Administration of 0.5 to 1 mg IM of vitamin K at birth is the standard of care (Vallerand and Sanoski, 2013).

PAIN MANAGEMENT IN LABOR AND BIRTH

Laboring women report a wide range of pain levels. Every patient reacts differently to pain during labor. There are physical and psychosocial factors that may influence the woman's response to pain. The laboring patient's pain level is influenced by the following:

- Women who have supportive care in labor cope with pain more successfully (Iliadou, 2012).
- Anxiety related to labor has an important role. Women who do not believe they can deliver a baby vaginally will most likely have a Cesarean birth (Iliadou, 2012).
- Past pain experiences influence current perceptions of pain.
- Cultural concepts of childbirth and pain vary.
- Past birth experiences, either positive or negative, have an influence.
- A long labor can lead to exhaustion and poor coping.
- A woman who does not understand labor may be fearful of her experience.
- A large fetus and a fetus in the posterior presentation can lead to an increase in pain perception.

Patients need to be educated about the different methods of labor analgesia available. **Analgesia** is the absence of a normal sense of pain that is achieved by the administration of pain relievers. Health professionals can support the woman in labor by providing up-to-date, objective, and evidence-based information on the advantages and disadvantages of the various methods of pain relief.

There are many nonpharmacological and pharmacological methods that have been used over the years. No method, either nonpharmacological or pharmacological, should be forced upon a patient. The nurse should make it clear from the onset of labor that the patient has a choice in pain management and she should ask for whatever she needs during labor and childbirth. The nurse will support her choice and provide appropriate nursing care.

The Physiology of Pain

Pain in the first stage of labor, particularly during the active and transition phases, consists of visceral pain from the stretching and dilation of the cervix, and uterine pain from a decrease in blood supply during contractions. ***Visceral pain*** refers to pain in internal organs and is caused by activation of receptors in the chest, abdomen, or pelvic area that send signals to the spinal cord and on to the brain. During labor, fibers from the uterus come together near the cervix and send out afferent (ie, nerve fibers carrying information to the spinal cord and brain) and efferent (ie, nerve fibers carrying information from the brain and spinal cord to the muscles and tissues) impulses to and from the spinal cord through the dorsal nerve roots at T10 to L1 (Yarnell, 2013).

Toward the end of the first stage of labor, when the fetal head begins to descend, and throughout the birth as stretching of the perineum occurs, somatic pain is activated through the pudendal nerve, which originates through the second to fourth sacral nerves. **Somatic pain** is caused by activation of pain receptors in the body surface or musculoskeletal tissues. At this point in labor, the patient is experiencing visceral and somatic pain (Norwitz and Schorge, 2013).

Pain sensation and transmission are illustrated by the gate control theory of pain. The foundation of the gate control theory is that different types of nerve fibers are involved in pain transmission and these join together in an area of the spine called the *substantia gelatinosa,* where there is a "gate" for the transmission of pain to the brain. There are thick and thin fibers. If the contribution from thin fibers is greater than that of thick fibers, then pain is experienced because the gate is open. If input from the thick fibers is stronger than the thin fibers, no pain is experienced because the gate is closed. The gate can be closed by descending pathways from the brain; this may explain the actions of analgesics and nonpharmacological methods that cause the release of endorphins in the brain, which act as natural analgesics (Yarnell, 2013).

Nonpharmacological Pain Management

There are a variety of childbirth preparation methods that a woman may use in labor. These methods have the goal of making labor a positive experience, with the woman actively participating in managing her pain. They are very effective for the first stage of labor.

- **Dick-Read method:** This method emphasizes relaxation during labor and childbirth using hypnosis. The theme of this method is childbirth without fear. Women using hypnosis report feeling relaxed, calm, and in control during labor. This method is not widely used in the United States.
- **Bradley method:** This method is taught in an intense 12-week class that emphasizes preparation through relaxation and breathing techniques. These techniques assist the laboring woman to manage her pain and avoid pain medication and interventions during labor. This method also puts emphasis on training the partner to assist her during labor and childbirth.

• **Lamaze method:** This method of childbirth education has the goal of increasing a woman's confidence in her ability to give birth (Lamaze International, 2013). Women and their coaches are taught a variety of coping strategies for labor, including breathing and relaxation techniques.

All methods of childbirth preparation include nonpharmacological techniques that promote relaxation and the release of endorphins to close the gate for pain recognition. Not all nonpharmacological techniques work with every woman. Nonpharmacological techniques that the nurse can provide or assist the support person to implement for the patient in labor include:

• Creating a relaxing environment with low lighting, warmth, and quiet
• Displaying a picture of a relaxing scene or baby's first outfit for the woman to view during labor
• Playing relaxing music or sounds, such as a bubbling stream or birds
• Using aromatherapy with lavender, sage, or jasmine
• Stimulating the skin with massage to the lower back, or light fingertip massage of the abdomen; stroking of the arm to shoulder or knee to thigh is also relaxing
• Talking the woman through progressive relaxation by having her focus on relaxing her neck and shoulders, and then progressing the relaxation throughout her body
• Positioning pillows under the uterus to relieve some of the strain on the lower back during labor
• Walking, swaying, or rolling on a birthing ball to help her to relax and to ease labor pain
• Using diversion and distraction methods, such as counting or focusing on a task during a contraction
• Applying a cool washcloth to the forehead, which is comforting when she is tired and hot from the work of labor
• Providing ice chips or clear liquids, if permitted by the health-care provider, to soothe her dry mouth and throat
• Assisting her to use breathing techniques, which are a tool that promotes relaxation and diversion in labor

Pharmacological Pain Management

Various methods of pain management are available to women in labor. These methods include systemic analgesics, regional analgesics and anesthetics, local anesthesia, and general anesthesia. The patient needs to be involved in choosing the method that will be effective for her.

Systemic Analgesics

Systemic analgesics commonly used in labor include butorphanol (Stadol), meperidine (Demerol), morphine, fentanyl, and nalbuphine hydrochloride (Nubain). Table 10.2 provides the types and dosages of medications used in labor.

These medications may be given IM but are most commonly given IV. Analgesics given in labor do not totally eliminate the pain, but they do make the woman more comfortable and able to use relaxation and breathing techniques to cope with labor. The advantages of IV administration of analgesics are a prompt onset and the ability to use smaller doses of medication to control pain (Yarnell, 2013).

TABLE 10.2 MEDICATION DOSAGES IN LABOR

Medication	Dose
Butorphanol (Stadol)	2–4 mg IM or 0.5–2 mg IV
Meperidine (Demerol)	50–100 mg IM or 25–50 mg IV
Morphine	5–10 mg IM or 2–5 mg IV
Nalbuphine hydrochloride (Nubain)	10 mg IM or IV
Fentanyl	50–100 mcg IV

Source: Vallerand and Sanoski, 2013.

Side effects that may occur are:

• Nausea and vomiting
• Drowsiness
• Sedation
• Respiratory depression with meperidine, morphine, and fentanyl
• Neonatal respiratory depression

NURSING CARE. Nursing responsibilities for managing pain and systemic analgesics include:

• Reviewing the patient's drug allergies prior to administration
• Assessing pain with the 1 to 10 pain scale, as well as obtaining information regarding the location, radiation, pattern, and description of pain
• Ensuring that labor is well-established before administering analgesics, or the labor may slow down
• Not administering narcotic analgesics within 1 hour of delivery because they may cause neonatal respiratory depression
• Providing a higher dose of medication to women with a history of drug abuse to provide pain relief

Regional Analgesics and Anesthetics

Regional anesthesia has become a very popular method of pain management in labor. In the United States, approximately 60% of laboring women choose regional analgesia for labor pain (Satpathy, 2013). Regional analgesic techniques include **pudendal block** (ie, injection into the pudendal nerve) analgesia, epidural analgesia, spinal analgesia, or a combination of epidural and spinal analgesia (Fig. 10.6). These methods of analgesia and anesthesia are provided by a physician or nurse anesthetist. The nurse caring for the patient is responsible for assisting the health-care provider and monitoring the patient's care before, during, and after administration of these types of analgesia and anesthesia.

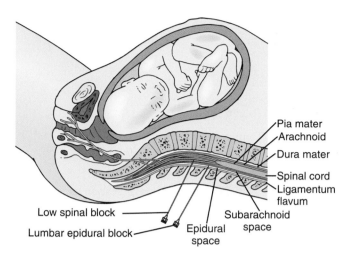

FIGURE 10.6 The spinal canal: injection sites for regional anesthesia.

PUDENDAL BLOCK. With a pudendal block, anesthetic is injected into the pudendal nerve, which anesthetizes the vulva and perineum. It is typically injected in the second stage of labor right before the birth. The advantages of pudendal block are:

• Control of pain from perineal stretching
• Fast administration for a forceps delivery
• Continuous anesthesia for episiotomy repair

Nursing Care. Nursing care for the patient with pudendal anesthesia includes:

• Monitoring for urinary retention
• Monitoring for signs of infection

EPIDURAL ANESTHESIA. The epidural is an effective form of pain relief in labor. An epidural is administered with a small needle and catheter between the fourth and fifth vertebrae into the epidural space. An anesthetic drug, analgesic drug, or a combination of both are injected or infused into the epidural to decrease pain and perception. The epidural space surrounds the spinal cord where the nerves branch off. The sensation of pain is blocked in that area. There are four types of epidural analgesia and anesthesia that may be used (Satpathy, 2013):

1. A single epidural injection with a small needle; no catheter is inserted into the epidural space.
2. An intermittent bolus of medication is inserted into the epidural space when the patient requires pain control.
3. A continuous infusion epidural with a small catheter inserted into the epidural space; the infusion is adjusted to individualize the analgesia and anesthesia.
4. A patient-controlled epidural anesthesia in which the patient controls her own analgesic therapy. A basal rate is continually infused and the patient can administer additional doses if needed (Satpathy, 2013).

The advantages of epidural analgesia and anesthesia are:

• Complete pain relief
• Does not produce respiratory depression for the fetus

Disadvantages of epidural analgesia and anesthesia are:

• Labor may slow down for about an hour after administration.
• A drop in blood pressure commonly occurs immediately after medication infusion begins.
• A urinary catheter is frequently required because of lack of feeling in the bladder area.
• The patient's legs and feet may be numb or tingly.
• Some patients are given a lighter epidural and may be able to walk, but most cannot.
• Epidural anesthesia prolongs stage 2 of labor (Yarnell, 2013).
• Fever and itchiness are common side effects.
• Pushing is difficult. Often, the epidural is allowed to wear off before the woman feels the urge to push.
• If the epidural needle goes in too deep, it can penetrate the dura and cause a small leak of spinal fluid, leading to a spinal headache.
• Women with epidural anesthesia have a higher rate of vacuum extraction or forceps delivery of the baby (Yarnell, 2013).

Nursing Care. Nursing care prior to administration of epidural analgesia and anesthesia includes:

• Assessing her knowledge of epidural anesthesia and obtaining consent
• Obtaining a baseline temperature, heart rate, respiratory rate, blood pressure, and FHR, and confirming the FHR pattern
• Administering a bolus of IV fluids, if ordered, to decrease the risk of hypotension

Nursing care during the administration of the epidural includes:

• Providing verbal support and encouragement to the patient
• Assisting with the administration by assisting the patient to maintain a lateral position with the head and chin flexed onto the chest, or sitting with the head flexed, knees bent, and feet supported on a stool (Satpathy, 2013) (Fig. 10.7).

Nursing care after administration of an epidural includes:

• Monitoring the blood pressure and FHR every 5 min for 15 min (AWHONN, 2012) to detect hypotension
• If patient-controlled anesthesia is used, assessing the patient's understanding about how to use the device
• Positioning the patient in the lateral or upright position with uterus displacement to avoid hypotension
• Monitoring for urinary retention and catheterizing if needed
• Monitoring for **pruritus** (ie, itching) and notifying the health-care provider for a medication order to treat the itching
• Assessing the effectiveness of the epidural and pain relief

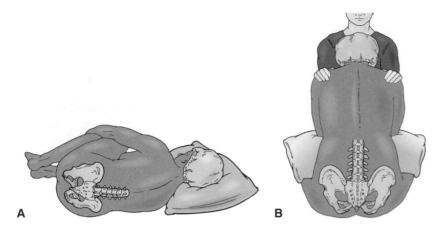

A   **B**

FIGURE 10.7 A, Lateral position for spinal and epidural administration. B, Sitting position for spinal or epidural administration.

SAFETY *STAT!*

A major complication that can occur is the inadvertent infusion of the anesthetic into the intravascular space instead of the epidural space. If this occurs, the patient will exhibit signs of tachycardia or bradycardia, hypertension, tinnitus (ie, ringing in the ears), dizziness, a metallic taste in the mouth, and cardiac arrest. If any of these signs are noted, the health-care provider must be notified immediately (Yarnell, 2013).

SPINAL ANESTHESIA. Spinal anesthesia is used less often than an epidural because it is fast-acting but short-lasting. **Spinal anesthesia** involves placing a needle into the **intrathecal space** (ie, within the spinal canal), injecting medication, and removing the needle. Spinal anesthesia has the increased risk of spinal headache because of the possible leakage of spinal fluid. The leaking of spinal fluid causes cerebral irritability, which leads to a severe headache. This can be prevented by requiring the patient to lie flat for 8 hours after the injection and providing adequate IV hydration to assist the body in replacing the missing cerebral spinal fluid (Satpathy, 2013).

COMBINED SPINAL-EPIDURAL ANESTHESIA (CSE). It is possible to combine the fast-acting spinal anesthesia with the duration of the epidural. This technique involves placing the epidural needle, and then a spinal needle is advanced through the epidural needle into the intrathecal space, where a small amount of medication is injected. Then the spinal needle is removed and the epidural catheter remains for continual infusion of medication (Yarnell, 2013). Nursing care appropriate for the epidural patient is also appropriate for patient receiving spinal anesthesia or CSE.

Local Anesthesia

Local anesthesia is injected into the perineum between the vagina and rectum for fast, temporary relief of the stretching pain during delivery, repair of any tears, or an episiotomy. The medication is commonly injected while the woman is pushing. It numbs the area that is infused by the needle but provides no relief of pain from the contractions. Local anesthesia does not harm the baby. The medication commonly used by the physician or nurse midwife is lidocaine, procaine, or tetracaine (ACOG, 2014).

General Anesthesia

General anesthesia is used when an emergency situation arises and the woman needs a Cesarean birth quickly, leaving insufficient time to start an epidural or spinal anesthesia. Medication is given IV to cause the patient to lose consciousness, and then an endotracheal tube is placed in the trachea to allow the administration of oxygen and gas to keep her unconscious until the birth is over.

Disadvantages to general anesthesia are:

- The anesthesia affects the baby and he or she may be less alert when born.
- A rare complication is aspiration of foods or liquids from the woman's stomach if she ate or drank within 8 hours of the Cesarean. The aspiration can lead to pneumonia (ACOG, 2014).

CULTURAL CONSIDERATIONS

There are cultural differences in response to pain. Some patients come from cultures that encourage expressive responses to pain. Other cultures promote a quieter, more tolerant expression of pain. It is important that nurses be aware of their own cultural beliefs and response to pain, and avoid making judgments about the patient's pain. Some nurses may find it difficult to care for expressive patients and may perceive them to be difficult and ignore them. If the nurse believes that pain is part of childbirth, the patient may not receive interventions that manage the pain to the patient's satisfaction. To provide patient-centered care, the nurse must not base pain assessment on the patient's expression of pain but be careful to perform a complete pain assessment and avoid stereotyping patients (Galanti, 2015).

NURSING CARE PLAN for the Unprepared Adolescent Patient

Angie is a 15-year-old with a term pregnancy who arrives in early labor with mild contractions at the labor and delivery unit. She is accompanied by her father, Bill. The baby's father is not involved in Angie's life. Angie is an only child, lives alone with her father, and, because she is obese, she was able to hide her pregnancy from her father until she was in her seventh month. Because of her denial of the pregnancy, Angie's prenatal care began late in the pregnancy and she did not attend childbirth classes. She has never been in a hospital. Angie and her father are anxious about labor and Angie asks, "Can you knock me out until it's over?"

Nursing Diagnosis: Angie is experiencing pain related to labor contractions.
Expected Outcome: Angie will state that her pain is at an acceptable level.
Nursing Interventions:
- Discuss safe pain management options with Angie.
- Provide nonpharmacological pain control and comfort measures.
- Teach Bill nonpharmacological comfort measures to use with Angie.
- Teach Angie simple breathing techniques.
- Assess for the appropriateness of an epidural for pain management.
- Provide praise and encouragement.

Nursing Diagnosis: Angie is experiencing powerlessness related to an inability to cope with contractions.
Expected Outcome: Angie will demonstrate the ability to make choices for her labor and delivery care.
Nursing Interventions:
- Provide Angie with options regarding her care whenever possible.
- Give positive feedback regarding her choices.

Nursing Diagnosis: Angie is experiencing fear related to an unfamiliar environment.
Expected Outcome: Angie will demonstrate decreased fear, evidenced by her ability to ask questions, cooperate with care, and relax.
Nursing Interventions:
- Explain procedures and expectations to Angie in nonmedical terms.
- Encourage questions.
- Provide reassurance in a nonjudgmental manner.

Nursing Diagnosis: There is a knowledge deficit related to age and a lack of childbirth preparation.
Expected Outcome: Angie will have an understanding of the birth process.
Nursing Interventions:
- Provide patient teaching regarding each stage of labor.
- Show her nonthreatening pictures of the birth process.
- Encourage questions.

Key Points

- Medical interventions for early labor include a CBC, blood type, Rh, urinalysis, IV infusion, and fetal monitoring.
- Nursing interventions in early labor focus on admission procedures, establishing rapport with the patient and her family, and explaining procedures.
- Medical interventions in active and transition phases of labor may include an amniotomy to rupture membranes and orders for IV pain medication or epidural anesthesia.
- Nursing interventions in active and transition labor focus on pain management. The nurse should assist the patient

and her support person by using nonpharmacological comfort measures and educating the patient about her options for pharmacological strategies for relieving pain.
- Immediate postdelivery care of the patient involves the assessment of uterine tone, monitoring the amount of bleeding, and promoting bonding with the infant.
- Apgar score is a systemic method to determine the physical status of the newborn.
- The placenta should separate from the uterus within 5 to 15 min after the birth. Signs of placental separation are a sudden gush of blood, cord lengthening, and the uterine

shape becoming firmer and rounder and moving up in the abdomen.

■ Care for the newborn immediately after birth includes thermoregulation, maintaining a clear airway, administration of eye prophylaxis and vitamin K, identifying the newborn, and applying hospital safety measures.

■ Every woman reacts to pain in labor differently. There are a variety of factors that influence pain response, including support in labor, length of labor, past experiences with pain, and cultural responses to pain.

■ Many women prepare for labor by attending childbirth classes that teach Dick-Read method, the Bradley method, or the Lamaze method.

■ Systemic analgesics can be given IM or IV. Small doses are given to prevent respiratory depression of the mother. The nurse has the responsibility to manage labor pain with systemic analgesics by avoiding administration too close to delivery to prevent newborn breathing problems.

■ Regional anesthesia includes epidural, spinal, or a CSE.

REVIEW QUESTIONS

1. A patient in the active phase of labor begins to experience nausea and has become very irritable. The nurse suspects that the patient is:
   1. Going to have a long labor
   2. Moving into the transition phase of labor
   3. Not satisfied with the nonpharmacological comfort measures
   4. Going to require more pain medication

2. A patient's membranes ruptured and the contractions have become more intense over the last few minutes. Her blood pressure is 122/80 mm Hg and respiratory rate is 32 bpm. She is 6 cm dilated. She reports a feeling of numbness and tingling of her fingers. Which nursing action is appropriate for this situation?
   1. Check the FHR.
   2. Turn her to her left side.
   3. Ask her to breathe into a paper bag.
   4. Recheck her blood pressure.

3. The nurse notices that the patient's husband is very engrossed in watching the football game on the television. The patient has progressed into the active phase of labor. Which approach by the nurse is the most appropriate for involving the husband in the labor care?
   1. "You need to turn that TV off and help your wife."
   2. "Did you ask your wife if she wants to watch the game?"
   3. "Did you take childbirth classes together?"
   4. "I would like to show you how to help her relax."

4. A patient has a doula to support her in labor and immediately after the birth. Which actions are appropriate for the doula? *(select all that apply)*
   1. Assessment of the FHR on the monitor
   2. Massaging the patient's back
   3. Discussing the patient's birth plan with the nurse
   4. Checking for cervical dilation
   5. Notifying the health-care provider of labor progress
   6. Assisting the patient with breastfeeding
   7. Monitoring uterine tone and the amount of bleeding after delivery

5. A woman had a normal vaginal delivery 7 min ago. The nurse notes that there is a sudden lengthening of the umbilical cord and a gush of blood leaves the vagina. The nurse is aware that:
   1. The placenta has probably just separated from the uterus.
   2. The woman is beginning to hemorrhage.
   3. The woman may have a cervical laceration.
   4. The episiotomy requires suturing to stop the bleeding.

6. A patient is returned to her side-lying position after sitting on the side of the bed for the administration of an epidural. The *priority* assessment at this time is:
   1. Assess for cervical dilation.
   2. Assess for numbness of her feet.
   3. Assess her blood pressure.
   4. Assess her oxygen saturation status.

7. During the transition phase of labor, a patient complains of thirst and dry lips and mouth. Appropriate nursing interventions include: *(select all that apply)*
   1. Offer ice chips.
   2. Offer a wet washcloth for her lips.
   3. Order a liquid meal tray.
   4. Offer lip balm.
   5. Inform her that she is about to deliver and afterward she can drink fluids.

8. A patient arrives at the labor and delivery unit in early labor. The nurse expects the following statement from the patient:
   1. "I can't stand this pain!"
   2. "Leave me alone!"
   3. "I need to call my sister and tell her I'm here."
   4. "I need the epidural now."

9. The nurse is aware that a common side effect(s) of IV opioid anesthesia is (are): *(select all that apply)*
   1. Nausea
   2. Unable to urinate
   3. Drowsiness
   4. Unable to feel the urge to push
   5. Decreased respiratory rate

10. The laboring patient wants medication for pain management. The health-care provider has ordered butorphanol (Stadol) 1 mg IV. The patient asks the nurse if it is safe for the baby. The best response by the nurse is:
    1. "Of course it is, trust me! I have been working in this department for 20 years. You'll be glad you took it."
    2. "It's such a small dose, I could give it to a 10-year-old. The baby is getting his oxygen through the umbilical cord."
    3. "Don't worry, the baby will be fine. My goal is help you have a safe labor and I am watching out for your baby."
    4. "I am giving you a small dose so that the peak effect wears off before the baby is born. That reduces the risk of harm to the baby."

CRITICAL THINKING QUESTIONS

A young primigravida is in labor and is accompanied by her grandmother. She states that her grandmother attends all the family births. The nurse notices that every time the patient has a contraction, the grandmother encourages her to push. The patient is experiencing contractions every 3 min with a duration of 60 sec. Her cervix is 90% effaced and she dilated to 6 cm.

1. What stage and phase of labor is she in?
2. Should she be pushing?
3. How should the nurse communicate with the grandmother?

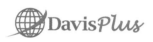

For additional resources and information, visit **www.DavisPlus.com.** Post-Conference Questions and Activities, Answers, and References can be found on Davis*Plus.*

11

Nursing Care of the Woman With Complications During Labor and Birth

KEY TERMS

amniotic band syndrome
cephalopelvic disproportion (CPD)
cerclage
cervical incompetence
chorioamnionitis
disseminated intravascular coagulation (DIC)
external version
fetal demise
fetal fibronectin (fFN)
fibromyomas
macrosomia
nuchal cord
precipitous delivery
premature rupture of membranes (PROM)
preterm premature rupture of the membranes
    (PPROM)
retained placenta
shoulder dystocia
uterine inversion
uterine rupture

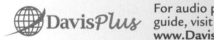 **DavisPlus**   For audio pronunciation guide, visit www.DavisPlus.com

CHAPTER CONCEPTS

Critical Thinking
Female Reproduction
Nursing
Perfusion
Stress

LEARNING OUTCOMES

1. Define the key terms.
2. Discuss the medical interventions and nursing care for the patient with an incompetent cervix.
3. Identify 10 risk factors associated with preterm labor.
4. Discuss nursing care and the common tocolytic medications used to manage preterm labor.
5. Identify the major complication of PROM.
6. Define post-term pregnancy and the possible fetal consequences of post-term pregnancy.
7. Differentiate between oligohydramnios and polyhydramnios and describe potential complications.
8. Describe the variations in the passage, passenger, powers, position, psyche, pain management, or patience that can contribute to complications in labor.
9. Discuss the risks of a vaginal breech delivery.
10. Define macrosomia and describe nursing care for the patient and fetus.
11. Describe umbilical cord prolapse and the potential risk to the fetus.
12. Identify risk factors, symptoms, and management of the patient with a placental abruption.
13. Define precipitous labor and delivery and state nursing care that promotes safety for the woman and her fetus.
14. Identify risk factors for shoulder dystocia.
15. Formulate an emergency nursing care plan for a patient experiencing uterine rupture.
16. Discuss the causes of a uterine inversion.
17. Compare and contrast retained placenta and placenta accreta.
18. Identify signs and symptoms of amniotic fluid embolism (AFE) and discuss medical interventions.

19. Using the nursing process plan, formulate a plan of care with appropriate nursing diagnoses for a patient experiencing a complication of labor and birth.
20. Discuss the grieving process and patient-centered nursing care of the family experiencing perinatal loss.

REAL-WORLD CASE STUDY

Colette

■ Colette is 16 years old and pregnant with her first baby at 30 weeks' gestation. She kept the pregnancy a secret from her mother until recently and just began prenatal care 3 weeks ago. Colette's mother brought her to the hospital because she has been experiencing mild uterine contractions for a few hours. Colette has been admitted to the labor and delivery unit for evaluation. During the admission interview, Colette admits that she smokes and has had an occasional beer.

1. What risk factors for preterm labor can you identify?
2. How is preterm labor diagnosed?
3. List one medication that may be ordered by the health-care provider to slow or stop preterm labor.
4. What patient teaching is appropriate for Colette before she is discharged home?

CONCEPTUAL CORNERSTONE

Anxiety

Complications during labor and delivery cause anxiety for the patient and her family. Fear of the unknown, a feeling of loss of control, and concern of possible risks to the fetus or patient increase anxiety. The patient may verbalize anxiety and difficulty with coping. She may cry, exhibit clinging behaviors, and be unable to problem-solve or make decisions. The nurse may note physical signs of anxiety such as increased blood pressure, pulse, and respirations, as well as increased perspiration, nausea, and diarrhea.

Anxiety can be contagious. The nurses must be aware of their feelings of anxiety and observe how the patient reacts to the nurse's behavior and communication. The nurse's use of therapeutic communication can assist the patient to control anxiety. During stressful situations, the nurse must remain calm. Communication with the patient should be simple, honest, direct, and concrete, with reassurance of the safety of the woman and the fetus.

Labor and delivery is a life event that often proceeds without complications or deviations from the norm. During labor, the nurse is the primary care provider and plays a vital role in making labor and delivery safe for the patient and her fetus by being alert for possible complications. Nurses must be aware of the signs and symptoms of complications that can occur. The earlier the complication is identified and the health-care provider notified, the better the chance the complication can be addressed and treated to protect the pregnant woman and her fetus from a poor outcome. This chapter discusses prelabor complications, labor-related complications, emergencies during birth, and care of the family experiencing perinatal loss.

PRELABOR COMPLICATIONS

After the first trimester, a majority of pregnancies continue to term without complications. However, there are complications that can occur before labor that may significantly affect the outcome of the pregnancy and the woman's plans for labor and birth. This section of the chapter discusses complications that occur before labor.

Care of the Woman With an Incompetent Cervix

Cervical insufficiency, also known as **cervical incompetence,** is defined by the American College of Obstetricians and Gynecologists as the inability of the uterine cervix to retain a pregnancy in the second trimester in the absence of uterine contractions. The diagnosis is based on a history of a previous second trimester loss with the absence of uterine contractions, preterm premature rupture of membranes (PPROM), painless dilation of the cervix, and a rapid delivery of the fetus (Norwitz, 2014).

Causes and Symptoms

Cervical insufficiency may occur because of anatomical abnormality of the uterus or from obstetric trauma such as a cervical laceration from a previous delivery. Treatment for cervical dysplasia and cancer has been associated with cervical incompetence, as well as multiple pregnancy terminations. For many women with cervical insufficiency, the cause is unknown (Norwitz, 2014).

Most patients have no obvious symptoms of cervical insufficiency, but pelvic pressure, back pain, increased vaginal discharge, and mild cramping may be noticed. Women with a previous history of cervical incompetency should be screened with a diagnostic ultrasound and physical examination during the late first trimester.

Medical Interventions

Medical intervention for an incompetent cervix is surgical cerclage. **Cerclage** is the use of sutures around the cervix to prevent the opening of the cervix (Fig. 11.1). It is usually performed at 12 to 14 weeks' gestation and removed after 37 weeks' gestation or the onset of labor.

The procedure is usually performed as an outpatient procedure and the patient will return home a few hours after the

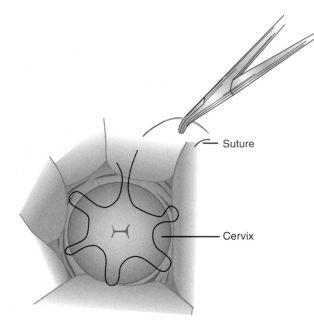

FIGURE 11.1 Cerclage.

procedure. Nursing care for the patient after cerclage is performed includes:

• Monitoring for signs of infection
• Monitoring for signs of ruptured membranes
• Monitoring for signs of bleeding
• Monitoring for signs of uterine activity
• Teaching the patient signs of ruptured membranes, signs of infection, and signs of preterm labor; see the Patient Teaching Guidelines box
• Providing emotional support to the patient and her family

PATIENT TEACHING GUIDELINES

Ruptured Amniotic Membranes

Points to review with patients about ruptured membranes should include the following:

• Amniotic fluid is usually clear or may have white flecks in it.
• The fluid has a distinct musty odor; it does not smell like urine.
• The membranes may rupture and cause a large gush, or there may be a slow leak.
• When the membranes rupture, the patient should note the time, color, and amount, and notify her health-care provider.

Care of the Woman at Risk of Preterm Labor

Preterm labor is defined as the presence of uterine contractions with enough frequency and intensity to cause effacement and dilation of the cervix prior to 37 weeks gestation. Preterm birth is the leading cause of neonatal mortality in the United States (Ross, 2013).

The exact causes of preterm labor are unknown, but the following risk factors have been identified:

• Late or no prenatal care
• Previous preterm birth
• Aged younger than 17 and older than 35
• Domestic violence
• Placenta abruptio
• Overdistention of the uterus because of multiple gestations or polyhydramnios
• An incompetent cervix because of multiple traumas (eg, abortions) or cone biopsy for diagnosis and treatment of cervical dysplasia or cancer
• Cervical inflammation because of bacterial vaginosis or trichomonas
• Maternal inflammation because of an infection, such as a urinary tract infection
• TORCH infections (toxoplasmosis, other [syphilis, varicella-zoster, parvovirus], rubella, cytomegalovirus, and herpes infections)
• Hormonal changes because of maternal or fetal stress
• Uteroplacental insufficiency because of hypertension, diabetes, smoking, drug abuse, or alcohol use
• A short cervix length of less than 25 mm during the second trimester

Medical Interventions

Medical interventions start with verification of the gestational age of the fetus by reviewing the date of the last menstrual period and obtaining ultrasound verification of fetal size. The medical management focus is to delay delivery for several days to allow the fetal lungs to mature.

True diagnosis occurs after monitoring labor contractions, assessing for changes in effacement and dilation of the cervix, and confirming the presence of **fetal fibronectin (fFN)** in vaginal fluid. fFN is a protein that helps the amniotic sac to adhere to the uterine wall. It is detected before 22 weeks' gestation and after 37 weeks' gestation. If the protein is not detected, it is a sign that delivery is not imminent; detection between 22 weeks and 37 weeks indicates preterm labor (Rigby, 2014). Medical interventions of preterm labor include the following:

• Progesterone supplementation has been shown to reduce preterm birth in patients at high risk for preterm delivery, particularly women with a short cervix (less than 15 mm) and prior history of preterm birth (Ross, 2013).
• Treat any infections, such as group B strep (GBS) or urinary tract infections, that may be the cause of the onset of premature labor.
• IV hydration increases vascular volume and may decrease uterine contractions.
• Bedrest may be ordered to decrease uterine stimulation.
• Tocolytic drugs, which are medications that suppress uterine contractions, may be ordered by the health-care provider (Table 11.1). Current management of preterm labor utilizes tocolytic drugs for short-term use only while waiting for the fetal lungs to mature (Kirkpatrick, 2012).
• Corticosteroid therapy accelerates fetal lung maturity. These medications stimulate the production of mature surfactant in the fetal lungs, which decreases the risk of respiratory distress syndrome in the newborn.

TABLE 11.1 TOCOLYTIC DRUGS

Drug	Action	Dose	Maternal Effects	Fetal Effects	Nursing Considerations
Magnesium sulfate	Relaxes smooth muscle; therefore decreases uterine activity	IV infusion of loading dose of 4–6 g IV over 20 min followed by a maintenance dose of 1–4 g/hr depending upon uterine response and urine output	Flushing, headache, drowsiness, blurred vision, respiratory depression	Duration of longer than 5–7 days may cause hypocalcemia in the neonate and possible skeletal abnormalities related to osteopenia.	Obtain a magnesium level 1 hour after loading dose and then every 6 hours to monitor for magnesium overdose. Serum level of 4–8 mg/dL is acceptable. Monitor for signs of toxicity: respiratory rate less than 14 breaths per minute; hypotension; absent or minimal deep tendon reflexes
Indomethacin	Prostaglandin inhibitor that stops the production of cytokines that initiate labor	50 mg loading dose followed by 25–50 mg every 6 hours for 48 hours	GI upset	Can cause oligohydramnios because of a decrease in fetal renal blood flow. Can constrict the patent ductus arteriosus if used after 32 weeks' gestation.	Monitor contractions and treat GI upset.
Nifedipine	Calcium channel blocker that inhibits smooth muscle contractions of the uterus	10–20 mg PO every 4–6 hours	Hypotension and tachycardia	May decrease uteroplacental blood flow	Monitor maternal blood pressure and fetal heart rate.

Sources: Vallerand and Sanoski, 2014; Ross, 2013.

DRUG FACTS

Progesterone may be given to high-risk women to prevent preterm labor. The dose is 250 mg intramuscularly (IM) weekly, started between 16 and 21 weeks' gestation and continuing until 37 weeks' gestation (Ross, 2013).

Nursing Care

The nurse has the role of implementing the health-care provider's orders, coordinating care, stabilizing the patient, providing patient teaching, and offering emotional support to the patient and her family. Nursing care for the preterm labor patient includes:

- Assessing the patient for signs of infection and rupture of membranes
- Assessing cervical effacement and dilation
- Assessing fetal heart rate (FHR) and uterine contraction activity, and notifying the health-care provider of any nonreassuring patterns
- Obtaining fluid for fFN if ordered by the health-care provider
- Providing oral and/or IV hydration
- Administering antibiotics if ordered
- Administering tocolytics as ordered and monitoring for effectiveness and side effects (also see Box 11.1 for contraindications for the use of tocolytics):
  - Assessing vital signs according to hospital protocol, which is usually every 15 min
  - Notifying the health-care provider if systolic blood pressure is greater than 140 mm Hg or less than 90 mm Hg
  - Notifying the health-care provider if diastolic blood pressure is greater than 90 mm Hg or less than 50 mm Hg
  - Assessing for presence of deep tendon reflexes (DTRs)
  - Assessing urine output every hour; notify health-care provider if less than 30 mL/hr (ACOG, 2012).

- Administering corticosteroids as ordered
- Providing emotional support to the woman and her family, including allowing her to verbalize fear, anger, and frustrations
- Answering questions directly and honestly
- Explaining all medications and diagnostic tests to the patient
- Determining if the patient and her family understand the plan of care
- Monitoring the patient's response to treatment
- Providing diversional activities
- Providing hygiene and self-care, depending upon activity restrictions
- If preterm birth is imminent, notifying the neonatologist and intensive care nursery
- If the patient will be sent home, preparing discharge instructions and determining the patient's understanding of discharge instructions

HEALTH PROMOTION

Prevention of Preterm Labor

The pregnant patient can promote a healthy pregnancy and prevent preterm labor by following these guidelines:

- Seek early and regular prenatal care.
- Eat a healthy diet.
- Avoid smoking, alcohol, and illicit drugs.
- Get the health-care provider's advice before taking any medications, even over-the-counter medications.
- Get immediate medical care for any infections.
- Work closely with the health-care provider to manage any chronic conditions such as diabetes and hypertension.

SAFETY STAT!

Calcium gluconate, 1 g administered by slow IV push, is the antidote for magnesium toxicity that could occur if magnesium sulfate is used to stop preterm labor.

Box 11.1 Contraindications for the Use of Tocolytic Drugs

- Severe pre-eclampsia
- Placental abruption
- Intrauterine infection
- Fatal fetal chromosomal abnormalities
- Advanced cervical dilation
- Evidence of placental insufficiency
- Signs of fetal distress

Source: Kirkpatrick, 2012.

PATIENT TEACHING GUIDELINES

Home Care for Preterm Labor

Teach the patient to do the following:

- Follow activity restrictions imposed by the health-care provider.
- Drink eight glasses of fluid each day.
- Eat a healthy, balanced diet.
- Follow the medication schedule.
- Perform a daily kick count and notify the health-care provider if less than 10 kicks or fetal movements are noticed in 2 hours.
- Place fingers on the fundus of the uterus and note any tightening of the uterine muscle. Notify the health-care provider if more than five contractions are noted in an hour.

- Notify the health-care provider if she experiences any of the following:
  - Membranes rupture
  - Low backache
  - Cramping or pelvic pressure
  - Fever higher than 38°C

DRUG FACTS

Betamethasone is a corticosteroid used to stimulate the production of mature surfactant in the fetal lungs. Its use before birth reduces the risk of respiratory distress in the newborn. The usual dose is 12 mg IM every 24 hours for two doses (Vallerand and Sanoski, 2014).

Care of the Woman With Premature Rupture of Membranes

The term **premature rupture of membranes (PROM)** refers to the patient that is at least 37 weeks' gestation before the onset of labor. **Preterm premature rupture of the membranes (PPROM)** is the rupture of membranes before 37 weeks' gestation (Jazayeri, 2013).

Patients experiencing PROM will have a leakage of fluid, vaginal discharge, and pelvic pressure but no contractions. A vaginal speculum is used to examine the cervix and to observe for leaking or pooling of fluid in the vagina. To verify that the fluid is amniotic fluid, Nitrazine paper and microscopic observation of a ferning pattern of the dried fluid confirm the diagnosis. Nitrazine paper turns a dark purple color because of the pH of the amniotic fluid.

SAFETY *STAT!*

All patients, regardless of due date, should notify the health-care provider if the amniotic membranes rupture. After 24 hours, there is an increased risk of infection for the mother and the fetus.

Medical Interventions

Medical interventions of PROM may include expectant management or the induction of labor. Expectant management is waiting for the woman to begin labor without additional interventions. If the mother or fetus demonstrates instability, expectant management is followed by the induction of labor or Cesarean birth to deliver the fetus. PPROM is more difficult to manage than PROM at term because the premature fetus faces more potential problems.

Expectant management of PPROM and PROM includes:

- Ultrasonic evaluation of the fetal weight, presentation, gestational age, and amniotic fluid index
- Procuring informed consent from the patient regarding the plan of care and risks of PPROM

- Monitoring the FHR and contractions for 24 to 48 hours
  - If the FHR is reassuring, the patient will be placed on bedrest and monitored at least once a day.
- Monitoring for maternal signs of tachycardia and fever, which indicate possible **chorioamnionitis** (ie, infection of the amniotic and chorionic membranes), requiring antibiotics and a plan for delivery of the fetus
- For the patient with PPROM who is managed expectantly, providing seven days of antibiotics (Kumar, 2012)
- If needed, ordering corticosteroids to accelerate fetal lung maturation

Nursing Care

Nursing care for the patient with PROM includes:

- Providing emotional support and education to the patient and her support person
- Avoiding vaginal cervical examinations, which increase the risk of infection
- Monitoring FHR and uterine activity, and notifying the health-care provider of any nonreassuring FHR patterns
- Monitoring maternal vital signs every 4 hours
- Administering antibiotics and corticosteroids if ordered by the health-care provider
- Notifying the health-care provider of any signs of maternal infection or bleeding

Chorioamnionitis

Infection is the most serious complication associated with PROM. The risk of chorioamnionitis, which is infection of the fetal amnion and chorion membranes, increases after 24 hours. With the onset of chorioamnionitis, the mother is also at risk for endometritis, sepsis, and death. After 24 hours the neonate is at increased risk of fetal distress and infection.

The clinical signs and symptoms of chorioamnionitis are:

- Fever greater than 38°C
- Maternal tachycardia (greater than 120 bpm)
- Fetal tachycardia (greater than 160 bpm)
- Purulent or foul-smelling amniotic fluid or discharge
- Uterine tenderness
- Increased white blood count (greater than 15,000 cells/mm³) (Sherman, 2014)

MEDICAL INTERVENTIONS. Medical interventions include delivery of the fetus as soon as possible, supportive care, and antibiotic administration. Antibiotics most commonly ordered for the patient with chorioamnionitis are penicillin, clindamycin, ampicillin, cefotaxime, or gentamicin.

NURSING CARE. Nursing care for the patient with chorioamnionitis includes:

- Recognizing and reporting abnormal vital signs and signs of infection
- Administering ordered antibiotics
- Providing an explanation of the infection and plan of care to the patient
- Continuing vigilant monitoring of maternal and fetal vital signs and response to treatment

• Providing emotional support to the patient and her support person
• Notifying the neonatologist of the impending birth of the fetus, which could be infected because of maternal infection

---

PATIENT TEACHING GUIDELINES

Signs of Premature Rupture of Membrane Infection
Signs of infection from ruptured membranes include:
• Elevated temperature greater than 37.6°C
• Offensive odor of the amniotic fluid
• Rapid heart rate
• Flulike symptoms

Care of the Woman With a Post-Term Pregnancy

A post-term pregnancy is defined as a pregnancy that extends past 42 weeks (Caughey, 2013). Risk factors for a post-term pregnancy are:

• Family history of post-term births
• Obesity

The fetal consequences of a post-term pregnancy are:

• Placental insufficiency, which causes fetal distress and a risk for meconium aspiration
• Increased risk of a stillborn newborn
• Increased fetal mortality
• **Macrosomia** (ie, excessive newborn weight), which leads to complications such as **cephalopelvic disproportion (CPD)** (ie, the fetal head is too large for the maternal pelvis), prolonged labor, and **shoulder dystocia** (ie, fetal shoulders are wedged or stuck in the maternal pelvis)

Maternal risks of post-term pregnancy are:

• Increased labor dystocia
• Increased perineal injury because of the larger size of the fetus
• Increased rate of Cesarean delivery (Caughey, 2013)

Medical Interventions

Medical interventions for the post-term pregnancy begin with the correct identification of the fetal due date. The date of the last menstrual period will be compared with the ultrasound dating to estimate the fetal age. Ultrasound dating during the first trimester is the most accurate; however, ultrasound dating later in pregnancy has a margin of error of plus or minus 10 days (Bingham and Spong, 2014).

If the health-care provider considers the fetus to be post-term, there are three current theories for medical management:

1. Elective induction of labor
2. Expectant management of the pregnancy, allowing labor to begin spontaneously
3. Monitoring of fetal well-being with testing such as stress tests, nonstress tests, and biophysical profile

The mother should be fully informed of the risks of a post-term pregnancy, and the medical intervention should be selected with her health-care provider.

Nursing Care

Nursing care for the woman with a post-term pregnancy includes:

• Assisting with any ordered testing to determine fetal well-being
• Notifying the health-care provider of any nonreassuring test results
• Providing patient teaching regarding the risks of post-term pregnancy
• Answering patient questions regarding testing
• Providing emotional support to the patient and her support person

Care of the Woman With Abnormal Amniotic Fluid Volume

Amniotic fluid cushions the fetus, allows lung growth, contributes to pulmonary development, allows fetal movement, and provides a barrier against infection. Before 8 weeks' gestation, amniotic fluid is produced by the passage of fluid across the amnion membrane. Around 8 weeks' gestation, the fetus begins to urinate into the uterine cavity and fetal urine becomes the source of amniotic fluid production (Norwitz and Schorge, 2013). Amniotic fluid volume varies, with the volume increasing with gestational age. The peak amount is 800 to 1,000 mL around the 37th week of gestation (Carter, 2012). Amniotic fluid volume is an indication of fetal well-being. An abnormally high level of fluid is termed *polyhydramnios* and an abnormally low level of amniotic fluid is termed *oligohydramnios.*

During a normal pregnancy, the fetus swallows amniotic fluid, which reduces the amount of fluid to balance the normal production by the fetal kidneys. If the fetus does not swallow or has a gastrointestinal (GI) blockage, it can lead to polyhydramnios.

The most common cause of oligohydramnios is rupture of the membranes surrounding the fetus. Because the fetal urine produces the majority of the amniotic fluid, a fetal renal anomaly or urinary tract obstruction can lead to oligohydramnios.

Diagnosis of abnormal amniotic fluid volume is usually noticed by alterations in fundus growth during the pregnancy and by ultrasound evaluation. The patient with oligohydramnios may have slower uterine growth and a small-for-gestational-age fetus, and the patient with polyhydramnios demonstrates rapidly enlarging uterine growth. Ultrasound evaluation of the amount of fluid present, as well as visualization of the internal organs of the fetus, can identify potential causes of the abnormal amniotic fluid volume, such as lung, kidney, and GI anomalies.

Medical Interventions

Medical interventions of abnormal amniotic fluid volume include the following:

- Bedrest to reduce the chance of preterm labor
- Maternal oral hydration of 2 liters of fluid per day, which increases amniotic fluid volume (Carter, 2012)
- Removal of fluid via amniocentesis, which may provide abdominal comfort
- Serial ultrasonography to monitor fetal growth and the amount of amniotic fluid
- Administration of indomethacin, a medication that inhibits prostaglandin
- Administration of steroids to enhance fetal lung maturity if preterm delivery is expected
- Consultation with a maternal-fetal medicine specialist when significant abnormal amniotic fluid volume is diagnosed
- Plan for delivery if the biophysical profile is nonreassuring
- During labor, potentially utilizing amnioinfusion to provide fluid in the uterine cavity to prevent cord compression (See Chapter 12, Birth-Related Procedures, for more information about amnioinfusion.)
- After the birth, referral to a neonatologist, pediatric surgeon, pediatric cardiologist, or pediatric nephrologist if required

DRUG FACTS

Indomethacin (Indocin)

Indomethacin is a prostaglandin inhibitor that reduces fetal urine output and therefore reduces the amount of amniotic fluid. The usual dose is 25 mg orally every 6 hours (Abou-Ghannon, Usta, et al, 2012). It should be administered with food to decrease GI irritation.

SAFETY *STAT!*

Indomethacin is an NSAID. Patients who have an aspirin allergy are at increased risk for developing a hypersensitivity reaction. Monitor for urticaria and respiratory distress (Vallerand and Sanoski, 2014).

Potential complications of abnormal amniotic fluid volume include:

- Oligohydramnios
  - Preterm labor
  - Fetal distress because of cord compression
  - **Amniotic band syndrome,** a condition in which adhesions between the amnion and fetus occur, causing deformities such as limb amputation
  - Musculoskeletal deformities such as club foot because of compression (Norwitz and Schorge, 2013)
- Polyhydramnios
  - Preterm labor because of increased uterine size
  - amniotic fluid embolism (AFE)
  - Maternal hemorrhage because of uterine atony from overdistended uterus

Nursing Care

Nursing care for the patient with abnormal amniotic fluid volume includes:

- Providing emotional support to the patient and her family
- Answering questions with terms that the patient will understand
- Monitoring maternal vital signs and FHR, and notifying the health-care provider of any abnormal results
- Teaching the patient signs of preterm labor
- Teaching the patient signs of ruptured membranes
- Assisting with amniocentesis if indicated
- Administering indomethacin if ordered
- Assisting with amnioinfusion if ordered by the health-care provider

LABOR-RELATED COMPLICATIONS

A pregnancy that has gone smoothly can still develop an unexpected complication in labor. A complication that develops can have a devastating effect on the outcome of the pregnancy. The nurse must be alert to signs of a complication and must intervene to promote a safe outcome for the woman and her fetus.

Care of the Woman With Dysfunctional Labor

Dysfunctional labor is defined as difficult labor or an abnormally slow progress of labor. Other terms that are often used interchangeably in the obstetrical literature are *dystocia*, *failure to progress* (ie, lack of cervical dilation) and *cephalopelvic disproportion* (Joy, 2013).

Abnormal labor constitutes any labor pattern that falls outside the normal labor curve. Friedman's curve was a classic obstetrical study published in 1955 in which Dr. Friedman studied and described the average amount of time it took women to dilate during labor. He plotted the labors on a graph and then determined the average time it took a woman to dilate each centimeter. He determined that normal nulliparous active labor should progress at 1.2 cm per hour and multiparous labor should progress at 1.5 cm per hour. From his research, a labor graph or curve was developed and utilized by obstetricians for years.

Researchers, such as Zang (2010) and Laughon (2012), have questioned whether Friedman's labor curve is applicable to women of the 21st century. Zang and Laughon have come to the conclusion that labors are longer than they were 60 years ago because of women being older, having higher body mass indices (BMI), using epidurals, and having labor induced.

Dysfunctional labor can usually be attributed to one of the **Ps** of labor: passage, passenger, powers, position, psyche, pain management, and patience.

Passage

The passage, which is the birth canal through the pelvis, may contribute to dysfunctional labor because the pelvic bones may be too narrow to allow the passage of the fetus through the birth canal. Also, the obese patient has more tissue for the fetus to pass through for delivery.

MEDICAL INTERVENTIONS. Medical interventions of dysfunctional labor will depend upon the suspected cause. Medical interventions for problems with the passage may include:

- Allowing a trial labor to evaluate labor progression
- X-ray pelvimetry to determine the size of the anterior-posterior diameter through which the fetus must pass for vaginal delivery
- Possible forceps or vacuum extraction for delivery

NURSING CARE. Nursing care for a laboring patient with problems with the passage includes:

- Monitoring labor progress and reporting slow dilation to the health-care provider
- Evaluating bowel and bladder status to reduce soft-tissue obstruction in the pelvic area

Passenger

The passenger, or the fetus, may contribute to dysfunctional labor because of macrosomia. A large fetus can cause labor to progress more slowly and may be too large to pass through the pelvis for a vaginal delivery. This is termed *disproportion*. Women who have a larger second baby may have a longer labor than their first pregnancy.

MEDICAL INTERVENTIONS. Medical interventions for problems related to the passenger may include:

- Leopold's maneuvers to estimate fetal weight and position
- Ultrasound examination to determine fetal size
- Allowing trial labor and, if fetal descent and engagement do not occur, scheduling a Cesarean birth

NURSING CARE. Nursing care for a laboring patient with problems with the passenger includes:

- Monitoring fetal descent through vaginal examination and reporting slow progress
- Anticipating possible forceps or vacuum-assisted delivery
- Emotionally supporting the patient through a long labor and pushing stage
- Preparing the woman for a Cesarean birth if determined necessary by the health-care provider

Powers

The term *powers* refers to labor contractions. A woman may experience hypotonic labor contractions that are too mild to produce cervical dilation. Another problem could be that the uterine muscle may not contract in a coordinated manner because of the disruption of communication between uterine segments from scarring or fibroids (Joy, 2013).

MEDICAL INTERVENTIONS. Medical interventions for problems related to the powers may include:

- Rupture of amniotic membranes to stimulate labor contractions
- Augmentation of labor with oxytocin (Pitocin) to stimulate effective labor contractions

- Planning a Cesarean birth if the amniotomy and oxytocin are not successful in producing effective uterine contractions

NURSING CARE. Nursing care for a laboring patient with problems with the powers of labor includes:

- Assessing for poor or ineffective uterine contractions and reporting them to the health-care provider
- Administering IV oxytocin per the health-care provider's order to augment labor (See Chapter 12.)

Position

The term *position* refers to fetal presentation. A posterior, brow, shoulder, or breech presentation will cause slower cervical dilation and labor progression. Most women cannot deliver a posterior, brow, or shoulder presentation vaginally because of the size and shape of the female pelvis.

MEDICAL INTERVENTIONS. Medical interventions for problems related to the position may include the following:

- For a posterior presentation, the mother will be informed that labor will progress slowly until the fetus rotates to an anterior presentation. Failure to rotate may lead to a Cesarean birth.
- For a breech and brow presentation, an external version may be attempted. **External version** is a procedure in which the health-care provider attempts to change the fetal position externally. If the version is not successful, a Cesarean birth is scheduled.

NURSING CARE. Nursing care for a laboring patient with a fetus in posterior position includes:

- Anticipating severe back pain until the fetus rotates to the anterior position
  - Providing comfort measures, such as sacral massage and the application of low back counter pressure during contractions
- Encouraging position changes to promote fetal rotation, such as the side-lying position; sitting, kneeling, or standing while leaning forward to move the fetus away from the posterior pelvis; and squatting while pushing
- Explaining the fetal position to the patient and her support person
- Providing ongoing positive reinforcement of the patient's coping mechanisms
- Providing nonpharmacological comfort measures
- Administering pain medication as ordered by the health-care provider
- If the patient requests an epidural, notifying the anesthesiologist and assisting with epidural administration

Nursing care for a laboring patient with a fetus in breech or brow positions includes:

- Assisting with external version if attempted by the health-care provider
- Explaining the fetal position to the patient and her support person

- Preparing the patient for a Cesarean birth if the version is not attempted or unsuccessful

Psyche

The woman's psyche contributes to labor progression and can contribute to dysfunction. Some women may have extreme anxiety because of past birthing experiences or a lack of knowledge of the birth process. Extreme anxiety contributes to a release of stress hormones, resulting in decreased utero-placental perfusion, which puts the fetus at risk for hypoxia (Guardino and Schetter, 2014).

MEDICAL INTERVENTIONS. Medical interventions for problems related to the psyche may include:

- Reassuring the patient that she will be well cared for during labor
- Emphasizing to the patient that a team of nurses and the health-care provider will monitor her care and the well-being of the fetus

NURSING CARE. Nursing care for a laboring patient with problems related to the psyche may include:

- Providing nonpharmacological comfort measures
- Encouraging her support person to participate in providing encouragement and comfort measures
- Providing positive encouragement and reassurance to increase her self-esteem and her ability to manage her labor and delivery
- Assisting with relaxation techniques
- Providing appropriate pharmacological pain control
- Monitoring fetal well-being and reporting any nonreassuring FHR patterns
- Listening to the concerns of the patient regarding her labor and delivery

Pain Management

Pain management can contribute to a dysfunctional labor. IV narcotic medication given too early in latent labor may slow down the contractions and labor progress. Epidural anesthesia during labor contributes to slower dilation and a longer labor (Laughon, 2012). Women with an epidural experience a longer second stage of labor because of their inability to push effectively.

MEDICAL INTERVENTIONS. Medical interventions for problems related to pain management may include:

- Providing clear guidelines to the nurses for the use of narcotics in labor and the appropriate timing of epidural administration
- Allowing the effects of epidural anesthesia to decrease before encouraging pushing during the second stage of labor

NURSING CARE. Nursing care for a laboring patient with pain management problems includes:

- Implementing nonpharmacological comfort measures to delay the need for narcotics and epidural anesthesia (Fig. 11.2)

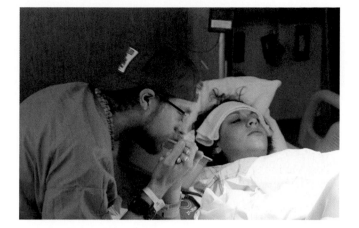

FIGURE 11.2 A cool washcloth provides comfort in labor.

- Ensuring that the patient is well-established in active labor before administering narcotic medication or the initiation of epidural anesthesia

Patience

Patience by the patient, nurses, and health-care providers is important if labor is progressing slowly. Health-care providers no longer strictly adhere to Friedman's curve for diagnoses of dysfunctional labor. Newer evidence shows that labor progresses more slowly than was thought in the past. Women may need more time to labor and deliver vaginally instead of being rushed to a Cesarean delivery (Barclay, 2014). Health-care providers should closely monitor the fetus and mother and allow labor to progress slowly without interventions, such as a Cesarean, as long as the mother and fetus show no signs of distress.

MEDICAL INTERVENTIONS. Medical interventions for problems related to patience may include:

- Monitoring the patient and her fetus for well-being and, if no problems are evident, allowing labor to progress without medical interventions
- Reassuring the woman that even though her labor is progressing slowly, the fetus is stable with no signs of distress

NURSING CARE. Nursing care for a laboring patient with problems with patience includes:

- Providing the woman with updates on labor progress
- Providing positive encouragement to the patient and her support person as she manages a long labor
- Monitoring the fetus for distress and reporting any nonreassuring FHR patterns

Care of the Woman and Fetus at Risk Because of Breech Presentation

Breech presentation occurs in 3% to 4% of all pregnancies and is defined as a fetus in a longitudinal lie with the buttocks or feet closest to the cervix (Fischer, 2012). There are three types of breech presentations:

1. **Frank breech:** the hips are flexed and the knees are extended

2. **Complete breech:** the hips are flexed and the knees are flexed
3. **Footling or incomplete breech:** one or both hips are extended and the foot presents (Fig. 11.3)

Vaginal breech deliveries were common until 1959, when it was proposed that Cesarean delivery would reduce complications (Fisher, 2012). The current practice is that prior to 36 weeks' gestation, a vaginal delivery may be possible (Fig. 11.4). However, the parents should be informed about the risks of breech delivery and decide with the health-care provider whether to proceed with a vaginal delivery. After

37 weeks, the current practice is to plan a Cesarean delivery for a breech presentation (ACOG, 2012).
    The risks of a vaginal breech delivery are:

• Low Apgar scores because of cord compression
• Cord prolapse
• Fetal head entrapment because the fetal head does not have time to mold in the maternal pelvis
• Neonatal trauma because of malposition of the fetal arms

Medical Interventions

Medical interventions of the breech presentation begin with ultrasonography to confirm fetal position, age, and size. Some health-care providers attempt a cephalic version procedure to reposition the fetus. This procedure is discussed in Chapter 12. Most breech presentations are delivered by Cesarean delivery; however, vaginal deliveries do occur when a second twin is breech or a **precipitous delivery** (ie, rapid delivery) occurs.

Nursing Care

Nursing care for the woman with a breech fetus includes:

• Notifying the health-care provider as soon as a breech presentation is suspected based on physical assessment of the mother

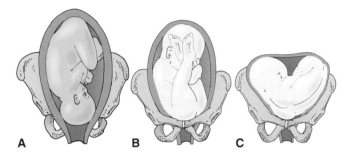

FIGURE 11.3 Breech presentations. A, normal cephalic. B, complete breech. C. transverse.

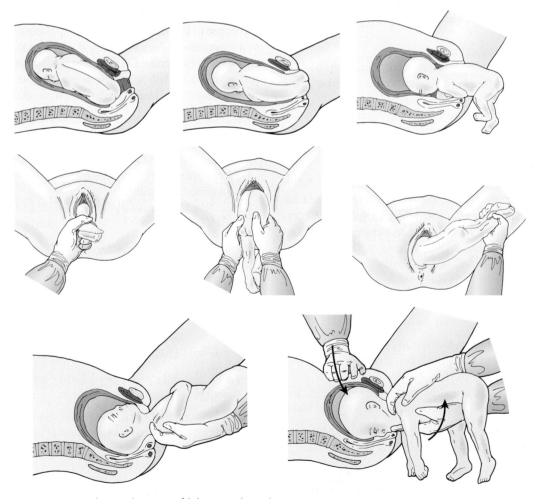

FIGURE 11.4 The mechanisms of labor in a breech presentation.

- Monitoring the mother's vital signs and the FHR
- Assisting with a cephalic version if attempted by the health-care provider
- Preparing the woman for a Cesarean birth (See Chapter 12 for nursing care related to Cesarean birth.)
- Reassuring and providing emotional support to the woman and her support person

Care of the Woman and Fetus at Risk for Macrosomia

Macrosomia refers to a newborn with excessive weight. The diagnosis of fetal macrosomia can only be made by weighing the newborn to confirm the weight. Fetal macrosomia is defined as a birth weight greater than 4,000 to 4,500 g and occurs in 1% to 10% of pregnancies (Jazayeri, 2012). Macrosomia is associated with an increased risk for neonatal morbidity, neonatal injury, maternal injury, and Cesarean birth.

Contributing Factors

Factors that are associated with macrosomia include:

- Genetics
- Maternal obesity
- Excessive maternal weight gain
- Postmaturity
- Gestational diabetes, which stimulates insulin and growth factors, leading to fetal growth and the storage of fat and glycogen
- Male newborns
- Hispanic women, who have a higher risk factor than other ethnicities (Jazayeri, 2012)

Medical Interventions

Medical interventions to avoid macrosomia focus on decreasing risk factors by monitoring maternal gestational diabetes and excessive weight gain, and avoiding postmaturity by inducing labor before the fetus becomes too large.

During labor, the health-care provider will monitor for labor progress and descent of the fetus into the pelvis. Indications that the fetus may be not descending may lead to Cesarean delivery.

Nursing Care

Nursing care for the woman and fetus at risk for macrosomia include:

- Monitoring dilation, effacement, and station during labor
- Monitoring FHR for nonreassuring patterns and reporting them to the health-care provider
- Preparing the woman for a Cesarean delivery (See Chapter 12 for nursing care related to Cesarean birth.)
- Providing emotional support, comfort measures, and pain control to the patient as she labors

Care of the Woman With a Prolapsed Umbilical Cord

An umbilical cord prolapse is an obstetrical emergency that occurs when the umbilical cord passes through the cervix at the same time or before the presenting part. The prolapse is termed *occult* when the cord passes through the cervix at the same time as the presenting part but cannot be seen or felt by an examiner. With an overt prolapsed cord, the cord is in front of the fetus and is visible or palpable in the birth canal or visibly extruding from the vagina.

The diagnosis of an overt umbilical cord prolapse is made during a vaginal examination when the examiner notices a soft, pulsating mass in the vagina. The diagnosis of a covert cord prolapse is more difficult and may be suspected based on the FHR tracing. Prolapse of the cord becomes an emergency because it leads to compression of the cord by the fetal presenting part (Fig. 11.5). Compression of the umbilical cord causes a decrease in blood flow and oxygen to the fetus. Severe, sudden FHR decelerations with prolonged bradycardia or variable decelerations are observed on the fetal monitor (Fig. 11.6).

The main event leading to a cord prolapse is the rupture of membranes, either spontaneously or artificially by the health-care provider. The risk factors for a prolapsed cord are:

- Fetal malposition, such as breech or brow presentation
- Rupture of membranes when the head is not engaged in the pelvis
- Prematurity
- Small-for-gestational-age fetus

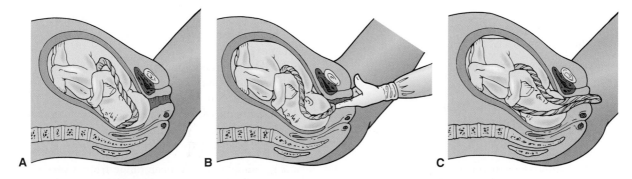

FIGURE 11.5 Umbilical cord prolapse. A, Occult; the cord cannot be seen or felt during a vaginal examination. B, Complete; the cord is felt as a pulsating mass. C, Frank; the cord precedes the fetal head or feet and can be seen protruding from the vagina.

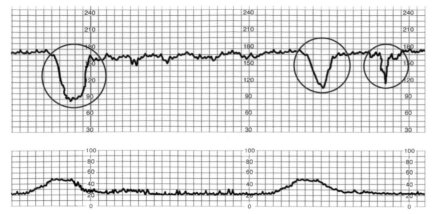

FIGURE 11.6 Variable decelerations from umbilical cord compression (circled in red).

- Polyhydramnios
- Multiple gestation
- PROM
- Grand multiparity
- Placement of an intrauterine pressure catheter or fetal scalp electrode
- Attempted rotation of the fetal head
- Placement of a cervical ripening balloon catheter
- External cephalic version (Phelen and Holbrook, 2013)

Medical Interventions

Medical interventions for an umbilical cord prolapse include:

- Arrange for an immediate Cesarean delivery.
- Place two fingers into the vagina to elevate the presenting part off the cord.
  - Care is taken to avoid palpating the cord, which could lead to vasospasm. The person manually elevating the fetus will maintain this position until the uterine incision is made.
- Position the mother in the knee-chest or Trendelenburg's position to allow gravity to assist with elevation of the fetal presenting part (Fig. 11.7).
- Some health-care providers fill the bladder with 500 to 750 mL of fluid to assist with elevation of the fetal presenting part.
- If the cord is outside the mother's body, cover it with wet gauze and replace it gently in the vagina.
- Provide oxygen via face mask to increase the oxygen levels for the fetus (Fig. 11.8).

Nursing care for the patient with a prolapsed umbilical cord includes:

- Elevating the presenting part if diagnosed by the nurse during a vaginal examination
- Repositioning the woman into knee-chest or Trendelenburg's position
- Applying high-flow oxygen via face mask
- Notifying up the chain of command and the health-care provider of the cord prolapse and the impending Cesarean birth

- Preparing the mother for a Cesarean birth
- Notifying the pediatrician or neonatologist of the impending Cesarean birth
- Monitoring the FHR pattern and reporting nonreassuring heart rate patterns
- Assisting the health-care provider as needed
- Providing emotional support to the woman and her family

There is the potential for a poor outcome for the fetus with an umbilical cord prolapse. However, prompt intervention, especially if delivery is achieved within 30 min of diagnosis, leads to good outcomes for the fetus (Phelen and Holbrook, 2013).

Uterine Bleeding

Placenta abruption (ie, placenta abruptio) is defined as the premature separation of the placenta from the uterus. This can cause the mother to lose blood and can cause fetal hypoxia or death because of a decrease of oxygenated blood transferring from the mother to the placenta to the fetus. Risk factors for placenta abruption are:

- Maternal hypertension, which is the most common cause (Deering, 2013)
- Maternal trauma from domestic violence, motor vehicle accidents, and falls
- Smoking
- Alcohol consumption
- Maternal age over 35 years or younger than 20 years
- Substance abuse, particularly cocaine (Deering, 2013)
- Amniocentesis
- PROM (24 hours or longer)
- Prolonged rupture of membranes (Gaufberg, 2013)
- Uterine infection
- Uterine **fibromyomas** (ie, benign uterine tumor) located behind the placenta (Deering, 2013)
- Previous placental abruption

A placental abruption can range from a very small separation of the placenta from the uterus (class 1), to a partial separation from the uterus (class 2), to a severe complete separation of the placenta from the uterus (class 3) in which

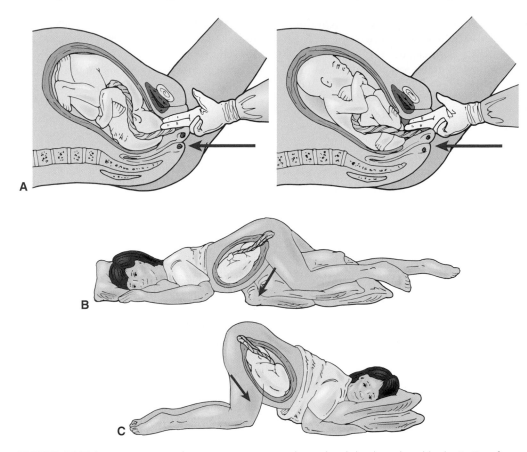

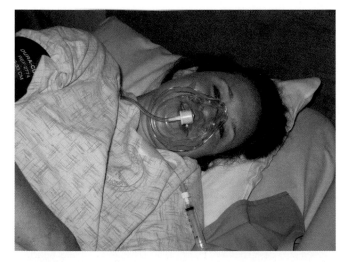

FIGURE 11.7 Interventions to relieve pressure on a prolapsed umbilical cord until birth. A, Two fingers of a gloved hand are placed in the vagina to lift the presenting part off the cord. B, The maternal hips are elevated with two pillows; this intervention is often combined with Trendelenburg's position. C, The knee-chest position uses gravity to shift the fetus out of the maternal pelvis.

FIGURE 11.8 A laboring patient receiving oxygen through a face mask.

fetal death may occur. The classic symptoms of an abruption are:

- No, mild, moderate, or heavy vaginal bleeding
- Mild to severe uterine tenderness
- Back or abdominal pain

- Maternal tachycardia
- Maternal hypotension
- Fetal distress

Medical Interventions

Medical interventions of a placental abruption include:

- Treatment of hemorrhagic shock with IV fluids with normal saline (NS) or lactated Ringer's (LR) solution, and blood transfusions if needed
- Continuous high-flow oxygen
- Amniotomy, which is artificial rupture of the amniotic sac, to decrease intrauterine pressure from blood inside the amniotic membranes
- Continuous fetal monitoring
- Delivering the fetus by Cesarean delivery if fetal distress occurs or the mother becomes hemodynamically unstable

Nursing Care

Nursing care for the patient experiencing a placenta abruptio includes:

- Closely observing the patient and reporting any signs of possible abruption
- Monitoring the FHR and reporting any signs of distress or nonreassuring FHR patterns

- Placing an oxygen face mask on the patient with high flow
- Administering IV fluids or blood as ordered
- Preparing the patient for a Cesarean delivery
- Providing emotional support to the patient and her family

THERAPEUTIC COMMUNICATION

How to Provide Emotional Support

When unexpected complications arise, the nurse can provide emotional support to the patient and her family in the following ways:

- Explain what is happening in nonmedical terminology.
- Explain why procedures are done.
- Reassure the patient that everyone is working as a team to provide the best care for her and her baby.
- Use therapeutic touch by holding her hand or placing a hand on her shoulder.
- Stay with her as much as possible.
- Provide updates to the waiting family members.

Care of the Woman Experiencing Precipitous Labor and Birth

A *precipitous delivery* refers to an unusually rapid labor of less than 3 hours and ending with a rapid spontaneous delivery of the infant (Smith, 2012). A precipitous labor can occur in the labor and delivery suite of the hospital or may occur in the home or car on the way to the hospital. Factors that may predispose a woman to a precipitous delivery include:

- A multipara with relaxed perineal floor muscles
- A multipara with unusually strong and forceful contractions
- A woman with a high pain threshold
- A multipara with a history of short labors

A precipitous labor and birth can cause complications for the woman and the infant. Possible complications for the woman include lacerations to the cervix, vagina, and perineum, and hemorrhage because of uterine atony. The infant is at risk for intracranial hemorrhage because of rapid expulsion of the head, aspiration of amniotic fluid, and infection as a result of unsterile delivery.

Nursing Care

Nursing care for a precipitous labor includes:

- Obtaining a thorough history of previous labor lengths and complications to identify a woman at risk for precipitous labor and delivery
- Assessing the patient for an impending delivery:
  - Complaints of a sudden desire to push
  - Sudden increase in bloody show
  - Sudden bulging of the perineum or crowning of the fetal head
- Remaining calm and notifying health-care provider
- Not leaving the patient alone

- Obtaining a precipitous delivery pack, which contains towels, scissors, cord clamp, gloves, and a bulb syringe for suction
- Washing hands and applying gloves
- Cleansing the perineum if time permits
- Giving clear directions to the woman and available assistants
- Checking for the amniotic sac; if it is still intact, it must be ruptured before the head emerges and the infant's first breath occurs
- Supporting the perineum and the infant's head as it emerges; instructing the mother to pant-blow to avoid forceful pushing of the head out the birth canal
- After the head emerges, using the bulb syringe to suction the mouth and nose of the infant
- Allowing the infant to spontaneously complete the birth movement of external rotation
- Checking for a **nuchal cord** (ie, fetal umbilical cord around the neck)
  - If present and tightly around the neck, clamping and cutting the cord before the shoulders emerge
  - Assisting the patient to pant-blow while allowing a controlled delivery of the shoulders; the infant will be expelled rapidly after the posterior shoulder emerges
- After delivery, thoroughly suctioning the infant's mouth and nose
- Preventing hypothermia of the infant by drying the infant and placing the infant skin-to-skin with the mother
- Determining the 1- and 5-min Apgar scores
- Assessing the placenta for intactness after delivery (should occur within 30 min; never pull or tug on the cord)
- Massaging the uterus immediately after the delivery of the placenta
- Placing the infant to breastfeed to promote the release of oxytocin to enhance uterine involution
- Documenting the following:
  - Fetal presentation and position
  - Presence of nuchal cord and management
  - Color of amniotic fluid
  - Time of delivery
  - Sex of infant
  - Apgar scores
  - Time of placenta delivery and appearance of placenta
  - Maternal condition

SAFETY *STAT!*

If a delivery is imminent, never leave the patient alone and never attempt to delay delivery by applying pressure to the fetal head.

EMERGENCIES AND COMPLICATIONS DURING BIRTH

Emergencies or complications that occur during the birth can be stressful and dangerous for the patient or the fetus. The nurse, with a calm manner, will need to quickly assist the health-care provider with interventions and provide emotional support for the patient during the situation.

Shoulder Dystocia

A **shoulder dystocia** occurs when one or both shoulders become wedged in the maternal pelvis after the head has been delivered. When the fetus begins the cardinal movements of descent, flexion, and internal rotation, the shoulders reach the pelvic inlet. After the fetal head is delivered, the shoulders need to rotate within the pelvis in a winding manner to leave the pelvis. If the shoulders are too large or the maternal pelvis is too small, the anterior shoulder can become wedged behind the symphysis pubis or the posterior shoulder can become wedged at the sacral promontory.

Risk factors for shoulder dystocia are:

• History of shoulder dystocia in a previous delivery
• Fetal macrosomia
• Diabetes
• Excessive weight gain
• Obesity
• Post-term pregnancy
• Precipitous second stage of labor
• Prolonged second stage of labor
• Induction of labor for potential macrosomia

Possible complications of shoulder dystocia are:

• Postpartum hemorrhage from uterine atony because of fetal macrosomia
• Third- or fourth-degree perineal laceration
• Neonatal clavicle fracture
• Neonatal fractured humerus
• Brachial plexus (ie, nerve supply to the upper extremities) injury

Medical Interventions

Medical interventions for shoulder dystocia involve repositioning the laboring patient and the fetus. McRoberts' maneuver is the usual first-line maneuver for shoulder dystocia used in the United States (Allen, 2014). To perform this maneuver, the health-care provider requires two assistants to hyperflex the mother's thighs against her abdomen. This movement raises the symphysis pubis about 9 mm, which may provide enough room to release the shoulder from the pelvis. The flattening of the lumbar spine may help with advancing the posterior shoulder (Fig. 11.9).

Along with the McRoberts maneuver, the health-care provider may request that the nurse provide firm downward pressure to the maternal abdomen just above the symphysis pubis. The suprapubic pressure compresses the soft tissue that may be making the situation worse and helps to rotate the anterior shoulder away from the symphysis pubis.

Nursing Care

Nursing care for a shoulder dystocia includes:

• Assisting the patient into positions requested by the health-care provider

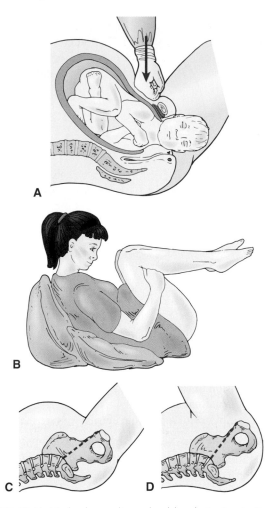

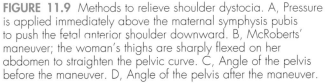

FIGURE 11.9 Methods to relieve shoulder dystocia. A, Pressure is applied immediately above the maternal symphysis pubis to push the fetal anterior shoulder downward. B, McRoberts' maneuver; the woman's thighs are sharply flexed on her abdomen to straighten the pelvic curve. C, Angle of the pelvis before the maneuver. D, Angle of the pelvis after the maneuver.

• Providing suprapubic pressure as directed by the health-care provider
• Providing encouragement and support to the patient
• Assessing the newborn for complications of shoulder dystocia and notifying the pediatrician or pediatric nurse practitioner

Uterine Rupture

Uterine rupture is the nonsurgical opening of the uterus (Fig. 11.10). A complete rupture includes all of the layers of the uterine muscle: the endometrium, myometrium, and serosa. A partial or incomplete rupture happens when one or two layers separate. Risk factors for uterine rupture include:

• Uterine manipulation for a version
• Abdominal trauma
• Previous Cesarean birth
• A birth interval of less than 18 months

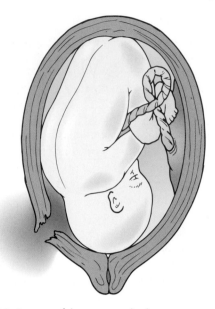

FIGURE 11.10 Rupture of the uterus in the lower uterine segment.

Diagnosis and Symptoms

A uterine rupture can only be definitively diagnosed with a surgical incision to view the uterus. Suspected uterine rupture is based on maternal and fetal symptoms.

Fetal symptoms of a possible uterine rupture include:

• Nonreassuring FHR pattern with variable and late decelerations
• Bradycardia

Maternal symptoms of a possible uterine rupture include:

• Change in uterine shape
• Constant abdominal pain
• Uterine tenderness

If a uterine rupture is suspected, the health-care provider must be notified immediately. In the operating room, the physician will assess the degree of rupture and repair if possible. If the rupture is large, a hysterectomy may be performed.

Nursing Care

After notifying the health-care provider of the suspected uterine rupture, the nursing care for the patient includes:

• Notifying the anesthesiologist, neonatologist, and intensive care nursery of the impending birth
• Monitoring fetal and maternal vital signs
• Preparing the patient for a Cesarean birth
• Reassuring and providing emotional support to the patient and her support person
• Performing blood type and crossmatch for a possible transfusion
• If no IV line is started, inserting an 18-gauge line for possible blood transfusion

Uterine Inversion

Uterine inversion is a rare complication but can lead to hemorrhage, shock, and death if unrecognized and not treated promptly. During a uterine inversion, the uterus inverts and the uterine fundus prolapses to or through the dilated cervix. The inverted uterine wall may extend to or through the cervix. In severe cases, the entire uterus and vagina may invert and prolapse out of the patient's body. In about 60% to 70% of cases, the placenta remains attached at the moment of inversion (O'Grady, 2013). The patient will experience uterine bleeding that varies depending upon the severity of the inversion.

Acute inversions occur within 24 hours of delivery and subacute inversions occur more than 24 hours after delivery but before the 30th postpartum day. Possible causes of uterine inversion are a flaccid uterus, excessive pressure on the fundus during delivery of the placenta, a placenta accreta, and the application of too much traction on the umbilical cord in an attempt to deliver the placenta (O'Grady, 2013).

The signs of a uterine inversion are:

• Postpartum hemorrhage
• Sudden appearance of a vaginal mass
• Signs of shock (ie, hypotension and tachycardia)

Medical Interventions

Medical interventions of an inverted uterus include:

• Rapid diagnosis and aggressive management to reduce blood loss and return the uterus to its correct position
• Moving the patient to the operating room
• Infusing IV fluids and possibly blood products to manage the hypotension
• Attempting transvaginal replacement after the woman has been given uterine tocolytics to relax the uterine muscle
• If manual transvaginal replacement is not successful, administering anesthesia and preparing the woman for a surgical procedure to repair and replace the uterus
• After the uterus is replaced, administering medications that cause uterine contractions, such as oxytocin or methylergonovine maleate (Methergine), to assist the uterus to stay in position
• Some physicians place a Rusch balloon catheter into the uterus for 12 hours after replacement to exert pressure on the placental site and therefore control postpartum hemorrhage and maintain uterine position (Kerialos and Chaudhuri, 2011).

Nursing Care

Nursing care for the patient experiencing a uterine inversion includes:

• Calling for assistance immediately
• If the health-care provider is not present, notifying her or him immediately
• Monitoring vital signs and blood loss
• Assisting with notification and coordination of care with the operating room and anesthesiologist
• Administering fluids and blood products as ordered by the health-care provider
• Assisting with transfer to the operating room
• Providing emotional support to the patient and her family

Retained Placenta

After delivery, the placenta should deliver within 30 min. Occasionally, after a vaginal delivery, a **retained placenta** occurs. The entire placenta may not detach from the wall of the uterus or, as the placenta separates from the uterus, small pieces or fragments of the placenta may be left attached to the uterus. Risk factors for retained placenta include mismanagement of the third stage of labor with excessive pulling of the umbilical cord before a complete separation of the placenta, entrapment of the placenta by a constricting ring of uterine muscle, or abnormally adherent placenta tissue (Smith, 2012). A retained placenta prevents the uterus from contracting, causing uterine atony. This can lead to complications of hemorrhage and infection. The health-care provider should carefully inspect the placenta after delivery to notice if any placenta lobules or pieces of tissue are missing from the placenta and are possibly adhered to the uterine wall.

Medical Interventions

Medical interventions of a retained placenta include:

- Oxytocin or methylergonovine maleate may be ordered, which produce uterine contractions to assist the uterus to expel the placenta.
- The health-care provider may attempt manual removal of the placenta. A gloved hand and lower forearm is inserted in the uterus and the health-care provider gently separates the placenta from the wall of the uterus.
  - IV pain medication, or spinal or epidural anesthesia, may be ordered because of the pain associated with this method of placenta removal.
- If manual removal is unsuccessful, a dilation and curettage (D&C) will be performed with the patient under general anesthesia or epidural anesthesia.
- A blood transfusion may be ordered if bleeding is excessive.
- Rarely, a hysterectomy may be required.

Nursing Care

Nursing care for the patient with a retained placenta may include:

- Administering oxytocin or methylergonovine maleate as ordered by the health-care provider
- Administering pain medication if ordered by the health-care provider
- Administering tocolytics to relax the uterus if oxytocics are not effective
- Monitoring vital signs and blood loss
- Ordering blood type and crossmatch of packed red blood cells if ordered by the health-care provider
- Anticipating surgical interventions if manual removal is not successful
- Explaining the situation to the patient and her support person
- Providing emotional support and reassurance to the patient and her support person

Placenta Accreta

If the placenta has actually invaded and grown into the uterine wall, it is termed a *placenta accreta*. Placenta accreta can lead to massive hemorrhage and possibly DIC. **Disseminated intravascular coagulation (DIC)** is a life-threatening disorder in which the body responds to hemorrhage by overproducing clotting factors that can cause clots that cut off the blood supply to major organs. The patient may require a hysterectomy to save her life. The average blood loss at delivery for a woman with a placenta accreta is 3,000 to 5,000 mL; 90% of patients with placenta accreta require a blood transfusion (ACOG, 2014).

The incidence of placenta accreta has increased and corresponds to the increased Cesarean delivery rate (ACOG, 2014). Women at risk for placenta accreta are those with scarring in the uterus caused by a Cesarean delivery; with a subsequent pregnancy, the placenta can attach anteriorly or posteriorly over the previous Cesarean scar. Placenta accreta may be diagnosed in some cases by ultrasonography during the pregnancy.

MEDICAL INTERVENTIONS. Medical interventions for a placenta accreta may include the following:

- If diagnosed before labor, a planned Cesarean hysterectomy may be scheduled with a team of obstetricians, obstetrical surgeons, an anesthesiologist, a neonatologist, a hematologist, and nurses to ensure a safe outcome for the mother and fetus. If the woman has a strong desire to maintain her fertility, the delivery plan will be individualized, with the woman having been advised of complications that may occur while trying to save the uterus.
- If diagnosed after delivery, management of hemorrhage is the priority while transporting the patient to an operating room for operative interventions.

NURSING CARE. Nursing care for a placenta accreta may include:

- Providing support to the health-care provider
- Following the institution's protocol for postpartum hemorrhage
- Providing emotional support to the patient and her support person

---

LABS & DIAGNOSTICS

Coagulation Tests

There is no single laboratory test that is used to diagnose an impending DIC. The following tests are often performed and repeated at intervals to monitor the patient's status. These tests indicate if the patient's blood is clotting normally:

- PT (prothrombin time): measures the extrinsic coagulation pathway; is usually prolonged with DIC
- PTT (partial thromboplastin time): measures the intrinsic coagulation pathway; is usually prolonged with DIC
- Fibrinogen: A clotting factor that is low with DIC
- D-dimer: A test that measures protein resulting from clot breakdown; usually elevated with DIC

Amniotic Fluid Embolism

AFE is a rare obstetric emergency in which maternal mortality is near 80%, with 50% of the patients dying within the first hour of the onset of symptoms (Moore, 2012). The exact pathophysiology of AFE is poorly understood. The current theory is that during labor or other procedure, amniotic fluid and fetal debris enters the maternal circulation, triggering a massive anaphylactic reaction. The disorder progresses in two phases:

1. In phase one, hypoxia is the major problem. It is caused by pulmonary artery vasospasm with pulmonary hypertension and elevated right ventricular pressure. The patient may progress into left-sided heart failure and respiratory distress.
2. Women who survive phase one enter into phase two. The primary problem in phase two is massive hemorrhage with uterine atony and DIC (Moore, 2012).

The signs and symptoms of AFE are:

- Dyspnea with labored breathing
- Altered mental status and confusion
- Severe hypotension
- Seizures
- Cyanosis around the mouth and peripherally
- Fetal bradycardia because of maternal hypoxia
- Pulmonary edema seen on chest x-ray
- Uterine atony that does not respond to bimanual massage after delivery
- Severe hemorrhage
- Cardiac arrest

Medical Interventions

Medical interventions of AFE include:

1. Administering oxygen to keep oxygen saturation normal
2. Initiating cardiopulmonary resuscitation (CPR) if the patient arrests
3. Treating hypotension with crystalloids and blood products
4. Continually monitoring the fetus
5. Arranging Cesarean birth if the mother is unresponsive to resuscitation, remains severely hypotensive, or FHR analysis indicates a nonreassuring pattern
6. Ordering arterial blood gas analysis, complete blood cell count (CBC), and coagulation tests
7. Admitting the patient to the intensive care unit (ICU)

Nursing Care

Nursing care for the patient with AFE includes:

- Promptly recognizing symptoms and calling for assistance from the health-care provider and the hospital rapid response team if available
- Initiating CPR if the patient arrests
- Arranging for assistance from laboratory personnel and the respiratory therapy department
- Initiating orders from the health-care provider for fluids and blood products

- Arranging transfer to the ICU
- Providing emotional support for the patient and her family

CARE OF THE FAMILY EXPERIENCING PERINATAL LOSS

Perinatal loss is also called *pregnancy loss* and includes ectopic pregnancy, spontaneous abortion, late-pregnancy loss, stillbirth, or newborn death up to the 28th day of life (ACOG, 2009). The death of a fetus at any stage is a **fetal demise**. A fetal demise is traumatic and unexpected in this age of medical advances and technology. Perinatal loss is devastating because it occurs at a time that is usually associated with joy and celebration. The parents' dreams and hopes for their child and the future suddenly disappear, and the loss is significant.

In most patients, the only symptom of a fetal demise is a decrease or loss of fetal movement. The nurse may be unable to obtain fetal heart tones, but this alone is not diagnostic of a fetal demise. An ultrasound examination can confirm fetal loss by direct visualization of the fetal heart with the absence of cardiac activity (Hugin, 2014).

If the diagnosis of fetal demise occurs before labor begins, termination of the pregnancy will be offered to the patient. Early fetal loss can be managed by cervical dilation and surgical evacuation. Late pregnancy loss requires cervical ripening and the induction of labor.

Causes of Perinatal Loss

The cause of fetal demise is unknown in 60% of all cases (Hugin, 2014). In cases in which a cause is clearly identified, it is usually because of maternal, fetal, or placenta pathology:

- Prolonged pregnancy beyond 42 weeks
- Poorly controlled diabetes
- Hypertension
- Pre-eclampsia
- Eclampsia
- Uterine rupture
- Maternal trauma or death
- Infection
- Multiple gestations
- Congenital abnormality
- Genetic abnormality
- Intrauterine growth restriction
- Listeria and cytomegalovirus
- Umbilical cord accident, such as a cord that is prolapsed or wrapped around the fetus
- Placenta abruptio
- Fetomaternal hemorrhage
- PROM

After the fetal demise, the health-care provider will want to investigate the cause if it is not readily identifiable. A careful maternal history should be obtained along with antibody screens and a CBC. The placenta and membranes should be inspected and an autopsy and chromosomal analysis should be completed on the fetus.

NURSING CARE PLAN for the Woman With a Labor Complication

Nursing Diagnosis: The woman has fear related to uncertainty about the pregnancy outcome.
Interventions:
- Allow the woman to verbalize fears and anxiety.
- Ask her what is helpful to her in managing anxiety.
- Provide a quiet environment.
- Monitor vital signs and report abnormalities.
- Promote relaxation with music, lighting, and massage.
- Encourage the participation of the support person in providing care.

Nursing Diagnosis: The woman has anxiety related to medical procedures.
Interventions:
- Explain any procedures in simple nonmedical terminology.
- Provide written and verbal information regarding the procedure.
- After the health-care provider has explained the risks and benefits of a procedure, reinforce the health-care provider's teaching and answer questions.

Nursing Diagnosis: The woman displays ineffective coping related to a lack of knowledge.
Interventions:
- Explain the complication to the woman and her support person in easy-to-understand terminology.
- Answer all questions in a direct manner.
- Reassure the patient that her safety and that of the fetus are a priority.

Nursing Diagnosis: There is a risk for injury of the woman and fetus because of the labor complication.
Interventions:
- Monitor the woman for any adverse signs and symptoms and report to health-care provider.
- Monitor the fetus for nonreassuring FHR patterns and report to health-care provider.
Evaluation of Outcome:
- The patient verbalizes a decrease in anxiety and fear.
- The patient's vital signs remain within normal limits.
- The FHR pattern does not demonstrate any problems with the fetal status.
- The patient verbalizes that she is able to cope with the complication and understands the plan of care.

The Grieving Process

The parents and family that suffer a perinatal loss often undergo a range of emotions. Family and friends may not understand the intensity of the grief and the behavior of the parents while they work through their grief. *Grief* is the response to loss of someone or something. Everyone grieves differently. The grief process is highly personal and there is no specific timeline for mourning and healing after the devastation of a perinatal loss.

The couple who suffered the loss will grieve in different ways. Men and women have different patterns of managing grief. The range of emotions that are often experienced includes:

- **Denial:** The woman and her family may express disbelief and are unable to grasp the reality of the circumstances. The parents may react with numbness and an inability to acknowledge the death or impending death of their baby. In the event of fetal demise, the mother may request repeated confirmation of an absence of FHR or may question the nurse's or health-care provider's accuracy or skill in assessment. Denial will diminish as the parents slowly acknowledge the loss.
- **Guilt:** The woman may wonder if she did anything to cause the fetal death. She may review her pregnancy in her mind, searching for the possible cause and her share of any blame. The parents may become preoccupied with identifying activities or choices that could have contributed to the death. The mother may feel as if her body failed her. Self-blame may prolong the grieving process, especially if the mother was ambivalent about the pregnancy (Kerstig and Wagner, 2012).
- **Anger:** The parents may experience anger toward each other, the health-care provider, the nurses, or a higher power. They may feel resentful about the unfairness of their loss.
- **Depression:** The parents may experience a loss of sleep, appetite disturbances, a loss of energy, or crying spells, and may be unable to concentrate. During a depressive state, the parents lack joy in any pleasure of life and may feel lonely and empty. These are normal feelings and, for many people, this phase must occur before acceptance and adjustment can begin.

- **Acceptance:** When the parents and family accept the loss as a part of their lives, healing occurs. They are then able to function normally and experience joy in life's events. Even when they have achieved acceptance, individuals will typically return to earlier feelings for a short time throughout their own lifetime. Those feelings will be triggered by holidays such as Mother's Day or Father's Day, the date the fetus was due or died, or observing families with babies.

Nursing Care for the Family Experiencing Perinatal Loss

Support provided by nurses can have a positive effect on the long-term adjustment of couples coping with perinatal loss (Moore, Parrish, et al, 2011). Interventions vary, depending upon the gestational age at the time of loss. Cultural needs should be considered as the nurse plans interventions for the family. Nurses can assist parents who experience a stillbirth or newborn death while in the hospital by:

- Providing privacy
- Acknowledging the family's grief
- Providing a quiet environment by minimizing interruptions and turning off alarms and monitors if possible
- Remaining present with nonverbal behaviors that communicate that the nurse is willing to sit, listen, and support the patient and her family
- Honoring cultural beliefs and rituals
- Facilitating spiritual support if requested by the family
- Allowing the family members to gather significant others such as grandparents and siblings
- Cleaning, dressing, and wrapping the baby in a clean blanket or allowing the parents to care for the baby
- Allowing the family to hold the infant as long as needed
  - Encouraging the mother to touch and hold the baby just as she would a live child; this assists the parents to create memories of the baby, which facilitates the grief process (Hugin, 2014)
- Encouraging the family to talk about their experience
- Connecting the family to a social worker, grief counselor, or support group before discharge
- Creating a memory package for the parents; items that may be included for parents are:
  - A lock of hair
  - A photo
  - ID bracelets
  - Footprints and/or handprints
- Providing information regarding grief support, such as community support groups, for after the mother leaves the hospital

TEAM WORKS

Teamwork is important when assisting a family to cope with perinatal loss. In addition to the nurses and health-care provider providing direct care to the grieving family, other health-care team members should be included in the plan of care. A pastor or spiritual leader, grief counselor, and social worker should be invited to participate in caring for the grieving family.

THERAPEUTIC COMMUNICATION

A Grieving Family

- Allow the family to express their feelings without judgment.
- Listen to the patient and family. They need to talk about their loss and the emotions that accompany that loss.
- Be patient.
- Do not use medical terms such as *products of conception*, *dead fetus*, or *stillbirth*. These terms do not describe the "baby" or the human experience of the parents.
- Therapeutic responses:
  - "I am so sorry."
  - "Your baby is beautiful." (If true and appropriate for the circumstance of the loss)
  - "This is not what you expected…"
  - "Is there someone you would like me to call for you?"
- Nontherapeutic responses:
  - "It was for the best."
  - "It was God's will."
  - "In time you will forget."

CULTURAL CONSIDERATIONS

Nurses who deal with culturally diverse populations and immigrant women need to modify interventions to meet the patient's needs. Everyone grieves differently, and cultures may have differing rituals or grieving practices. The woman and her family should be asked what would bring comfort and significance to this difficult situation. Any ritual practices and mourning should be respected and implemented if possible. For example, a Native American family may focus on rituals to release the spirit, an Amish family may not want a picture of the infant, and a Jewish family may request to bury the infant within 24 hours (Callister, 2014).

Key Points

- Prelabor complications such as incompetent cervix and preterm labor that are diagnosed early can be managed with medical and nursing care to prevent preterm birth and possible perinatal loss.

- Nursing care for the preterm labor patient includes monitoring of contractions and the fetus, bedrest, administration of tocolytic medications, hydration, and corticosteroids to accelerate fetal lung maturity.

- The most serious complication of premature rupture of the membranes is chorioamnionitis.

- Post-term pregnancy is linked to increased fetal mortality and an increase in Cesarean deliveries.

- Abnormal amniotic fluid volume is usually first noticed by alterations in fundal height during the pregnancy. Poly-hydramnios and oligohydramnios are both associated with possible fetal anomalies of the lung, kidney, and GI tract.

- Dysfunctional labor can usually be attributed to one of the Ps of labor: passage, passenger, powers, position, psyche, pain management, and patience.

- Breech presentations increase the risk for umbilical cord prolapse and difficulty delivering the fetal head. Most breech presentations are delivered via Cesarean birth.

- A prolapsed umbilical cord is an emergency because of the risk of fetal hypoxia.

- Fetal distress, maternal abdominal pain, and uterine tenderness with or without vaginal bleeding are the classic signs of placental abruption.

- A precipitous labor occurs with less than 3 hours of labor and a rapid spontaneous delivery of the infant. A precipitous labor can result in vaginal, cervical, and perineal lacerations for the mother and intracranial hemorrhage and amniotic fluid aspiration for the newborn.

- Shoulder dystocia is a complication that occurs when the fetal shoulders are wedged in the pelvis after the delivery of the head. The nurse may assist the health-care provider with maneuvers to produce delivery of the shoulders.

- Women with previous Cesarean delivery, abdominal trauma, or closely spaced births are more at risk for uterine rupture. Uterine rupture is the nonsurgical opening of the uterus.

- Uterine inversion is a rare complication in which the uterus inverts and the fundus prolapses through the dilated cervix.

- A placenta that is not delivered within 30 min of the birth is a retained placenta. A retained placenta can lead to hemorrhage and infection.

- AFE is a rare emergency with a high mortality rate. The early signs of amniotic embolism are dyspnea, hypotension, altered mental status, and cyanosis. It can quickly progress to seizures, hemorrhage, and cardiac arrest.

- Fetal demise is a death of the fetus at any stage of pregnancy. Nurses can assist the family with coping with the traumatic and devastating loss. The family will experience a range of emotions as they work through the grieving process.

REVIEW QUESTIONS

1. Which of the following are risk factors for preterm labor? *(select all that apply)*
   1. Multiple gestation
   2. Urinary tract infection
   3. Rh negative mother
   4. Bacterial vaginosis
   5. A previous spontaneous abortion (ie, miscarriage)

2. A patient at 37 weeks' gestation is admitted to labor and delivery. Her membranes ruptured 12 hours ago at home. The monitor indicates that the FHR is 150 bpm with moderate variability, no variable or late decelerations, and no uterine contractions. The patient asks the nurse, "Why can't I stay at home until my labor begins?" The best reply by the nurse would be:
   1. "It looks like the baby may be experiencing some distress."
   2. "We want to monitor you for signs of infection."
   3. "Your doctor wants you here."
   4. "We can keep you comfortable until labor starts."

3. Which of the following statements regarding oligohy-dramnios is true?
   1. There will be at least 1,500 mL of amniotic fluid.
   2. Throughout the pregnancy, the placenta is the chief source of amniotic fluid.
   3. The patient may experience a post-term pregnancy.
   4. The fetus may be small for gestational age.

4. Which of the following patients will the nurse monitor carefully for signs of placental abruption?
   1. The multigravida, giving birth for the fifth time
   2. The multigravida who is 30 weeks' gestation
   3. The primigravida who abuses cocaine
   4. The primigravida who is 22 years old

5. Nursing care for patient with PROM includes: *(select all that apply)*
   1. Monitoring FHR and contractions
   2. Frequent vaginal cervical examinations
   3. Administration of antibiotics if ordered
   4. Monitoring the patient's vital signs
   5. Placing the patient in knee-chest position

6. Which of the following are signs of an imminent precipitous delivery? *(select all that apply)*
   1. A bulging perineum
   2. The mother stating a desire to push
   3. Nausea and vomiting
   4. Increase in bloody show and mucus
   5. Contractions that are 3 min apart and strong

7. Which pregnant patient is at greatest risk for macrosomia?
   1. The primigravida who is a diabetic
   2. The multigravida who is Rh negative
   3. The primigravida who abuses alcohol
   4. The multigravida who worked as a hair stylist

8. After a patient's membranes ruptured, the nurse performs a vaginal examination and notices that the umbilical cord has fallen through the cervix into the vagina. The nurse should: *(select all that apply)*
   1. Manually elevate the fetal head off the cord.
   2. Leave the patient and immediately call the doctor.
   3. Place the patient in knee-chest position.
   4. Ask the woman to empty her bladder.
   5. Apply oxygen via facemask.

9. A patient is experiencing vaginal bleeding and severe abdominal pain. The nurse suspects that the patient is experiencing a:
   1. Placenta previa
   2. Placenta accreta
   3. Placental abruption
   4. Placental inversion

10. Which of the following patients is at highest risk for uterine rupture?
    1. A 15-year-old primigravida with a large fetus
    2. A multigravida, scheduled for her fourth Cesarean birth
    3. A primigravida pregnant with triplets
    4. A multigravida delivering her second child in 2 years

CRITICAL THINKING QUESTIONS

1. A woman at 32 weeks' gestation is in preterm labor. Efforts to slow labor have failed and significant cervical dilation has occurred. The woman states, "What is happening? I don't understand labor. I was supposed to start childbirth classes tonight!" Formulate a nursing plan for preparing this patient for labor.

2. Discuss the fetal and maternal risks because of a post-term pregnancy.

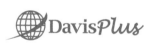

For additional resources and information, visit **www.DavisPlus.com.** Post-Conference Questions and Activities, Answers, and References can be found on Davis*Plus*.

Birth-Related Procedures

12

LEARNING OUTCOMES

1. Define the key terms.
2. Describe the amniotomy procedure and discuss nursing responsibilities.
3. Explain the purpose of an amnioinfusion.
4. Prepare patient teaching for the patient undergoing an external cephalic version.
5. Describe how a Bishop's score is calculated and explain the significance of the score.
6. Discuss methods used to ripen a cervix and induce contractions.
7. Prepare a patient-centered nursing care plan for the woman undergoing labor induction or augmentation.
8. Differentiate between vacuum extractor–assisted and forceps-assisted vaginal delivery.
9. List common indications for a Cesarean delivery.
10. Discuss nursing responsibilities when preparing a patient for a Cesarean birth.
11. Plan patient teaching for a Cesarean birth.
12. Identify the factors that indicate a patient is a good candidate for a VBAC.
13. Plan nursing care for the patient undergoing a TOLAC.

KEY TERMS

augmentation
Bishop's score
collaboration
external cephalic version
forceps
labor induction
Pfannenstiel's incision
trial of labor after Cesarean (TOLAC)
vacuum extraction
vaginal birth after Cesarean (VBAC)

DavisPlus For audio pronunciation guide, visit www.DavisPlus.com

CHAPTER CONCEPTS

Assessment
Nursing Roles
Perioperative
Stress

REAL-WORLD CASE STUDY

Wendy

■ Wendy is a gravida two, para one. She is 41 weeks gestation. Wendy is obese and has gestational diabetes that is controlled with medication. She is admitted to the labor and delivery unit for labor induction with oxytocin. During cervical examination, the nurse notes that Wendy is dilated 2 cm and the cervix is soft, in a midposition, and 50% effaced. The fetal head is at 0 station.

1. What is Wendy's Bishop's score?
2. Is Wendy a good candidate for a labor induction?
3. How would the nurse explain oxytocin induction to Wendy?
4. What additional concerns may the nurse have regarding safe care for Wendy?

The nurse caring for a patient in labor and delivery may be collaborating with the health-care provider or performing various procedures to assist with a safe labor and delivery. Before, during, and after the procedure, the nurse will need to be alert for possible complications and be prepared to provide safe and effective nursing care for the patient. Therapeutic procedures covered in this chapter include external cephalic version, amniotomy, amnioinfusion, cervical ripening, induction/augmentation of labor, vacuum-assisted delivery, forceps-assisted delivery, Cesarean birth, and vaginal birth after Cesarean (VBAC).

AMNIOTOMY

Amniotomy is the artificial rupture of the amniotic membranes (AROM). Amniotomy usually stimulates labor or starts labor in the term patient within 12 hours after rupture of the membranes (Norwitz and Schorge, 2013). AROM may

be indicated if labor is progressing slowly. Once the cushion of amniotic fluid is gone, the fetal head will press directly on the cervix, causing faster effacement and dilation and promoting labor progress.

Amniotomy is considered by many health professionals to be safe and harmless. However, it should not be attempted when the fetal head is not engaged in the pelvis or if in a breech presentation because of the risk of umbilical cord prolapse when the amniotic fluid flows out of the uterus. In addition, women with prolonged time between rupture of membranes and delivery are at increased risk of infection.

The health-care provider uses a disposable plastic hook (ie, amniohook) to perforate the amniotic sac. The nurse midwife or the physician will perform a vaginal examination to determine cervical dilation, effacement, fetal station, and fetal presentation. The hook is passed through the cervix and then perforates the sac, causing a release of the amniotic fluid (Fig. 12.1). The hole may be enlarged with a finger.

Nursing Care

Nursing care for an amniotomy includes the following:

• Explaining the procedure to the patient and her support person
• Providing sterile gloves, sterile lubricant, and a sterile amniohook to the health-care provider
• Placing disposable pads underneath the patient to absorb the fluid
• Monitoring the fetal heart rate (FHR) and pattern for one full minute after membranes rupture
• Notifying the health-care provider of any abnormal or nonreassuring FHR patterns

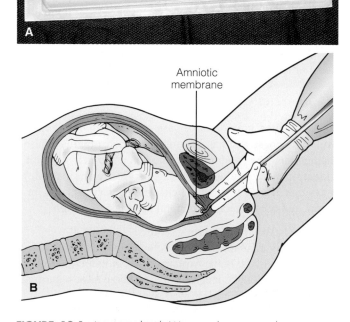

FIGURE 12.1 An amniohook (A) is used to rupture the membranes in an amniotomy (B).

- Documenting the time of the amniotomy and the color, quantity, and odor of the amniotic fluid
- Changing the pads regularly as they become saturated
- Monitoring the woman's temperature every 2 hours; report elevations greater than 38°C

AMNIOINFUSION

Amnioinfusion is the procedure of infusing 0.9% normal saline into the uterus through a catheter placed through the cervix into the amniotic cavity. The purpose of an amnioinfusion is to add fluid to the uterus to relieve cord compression, which causes variable decelerations, or to add fluid because of oligohydramnios. Oligohydramnios can be caused by premature rupture of membranes, postmaturity of the fetus, or uteroplacental insufficiency (ie, the placenta does not provide enough blood supply to the fetus).

Amnioinfusion may also be used to dilute meconium-stained fluid. Meconium-stained fluid occurs when the fetus experiences hypoxia and releases the contents of the intestinal tract (ie, fecal material, or meconium) into the amniotic fluid. If the fetus inhales the meconium fluid, it could cause aspiration pneumonia.

Possible Complications

Possible complications of amnioinfusion include:

- Overfilling the uterus, causing high intrauterine pressure
- Prolapsed cord
- Placenta abruptio
- Uterine infection
- Maternal chilling if cold solution is used
- Fetal bradycardia if cold solution is used
- Fetal tachycardia if hot solution is used

Nursing Care

The nursing care for a patient undergoing an amnioinfusion procedure includes the following:

- Explain the procedure to the patient and her support person.
- Connect the IV solution to IV tubing and flush.
- If the fetus is preterm, the solution should be warmed with an infusion warmer before and during the infusion. For term pregnancies, room temperature solution is acceptable.
- Assist the health-care provider to insert the intrauterine pressure catheter (IUPC).
- After insertion, note uterine resting tone with the patient on her left side, right side, and back. Record the findings.
- Attach the IV tubing to the amnioport on the IUPC. Bolus with 250 to 600 mL as ordered by the health-care provider.
- Place the tubing in the infusion pump and set at the ordered rate. Commonly, the maintenance rate is from 120 to 180 mL/hr (Norwitz & Schorge, 2013)
- Document the procedure in the medical record.
- Assess and record uterine resting tone every 30 min. A resting baseline of less than 25 mm Hg should be maintained (Norwitz & Schorge, 2013)

- Monitor the FHR pattern and notify the health-care provider of any nonreassuring patterns.
- Assess and record the amount, color, and odor of fluid on the patient's under pad every 30 min.
- Discontinue infusion before delivery.

EXTERNAL CEPHALIC VERSION

An **external cephalic version** is the attempt by the health-care provider to move a malpositioned fetus, such as a breech or transverse lie, into a vertex cephalic presentation after 37 weeks' gestation. The health-care provider manipulates through the abdominal wall to reposition the fetus. See Box 12.1 for contraindications for an external cephalic version.

Fetal position will first be confirmed with ultrasound imagery. The health-care provider will locate the umbilical cord, assess the placental location, determine the amount of amniotic fluid, evaluate the fetal age, and assess for any fetal anomalies. External fetal monitoring is conducted to confirm a healthy FHR pattern.

Next, tocolytic medications are administered to relax the uterus. Once the uterus is relaxed, the health-care provider will use two hands on the surface of the abdomen. One hand is placed on the fetal head and the other is placed on the fetal buttocks (Fig. 12.2). The health-care provider will push and roll the fetus into a head-down position (Ehrenberg-Buchner, 2013).

External cephalic version has a success rate of 58% and is more likely to be successful if the mother has had at least one pregnancy and childbirth, there is normal amniotic fluid volume, and the procedure is done after 36 weeks and before labor begins (ACOG, 2012). If the first attempt is not successful, a second attempt with epidural anesthesia to improve uterine relaxation and reduce pain may be scheduled.

Risks and Complications

Potential risks or complications of an external cephalic version include:

- Twisting of the umbilical cord, causing decreased oxygenation to the fetus

Box 12.1 Contraindications for an External Cephalic Version

- Uterine abnormalities
- Multiple gestation
- Oligohydramnios
- Previous Cesarean birth
- Cephlopelvic disproportion
- Nonreassuring FHR occurring
- Hyperextended neck in the fetus
- Placenta previa

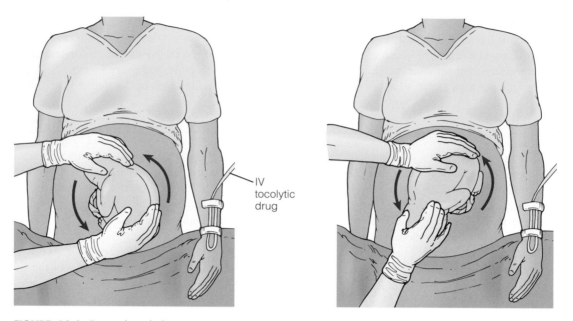

FIGURE 12.2 External cephalic version is a maneuver performed through the maternal abdominal wall in an attempt to change the fetal position from a breech to a cephalic presentation.

- Rupture of amniotic membranes, causing the onset of labor
- Placenta abruptio
- Rupture of the uterus
- Bleeding that could lead to a mixing of maternal and fetal blood

Nursing Care Before and During the Procedure

Nursing care for the patient undergoing an external cephalic version includes the following:

- Obtaining informed consent from the patient
- Providing emotional support and answering patient questions
- Confirming that RhoGAM was given at 28 weeks' gestation to prevent isoimmunization if the patient is Rh-negative
- Performing a nonstress test to evaluate the fetus
- Administering IV tocolytics to relax the uterus
- Continuously monitoring FHR patterns to detect bradycardia and variable decelerations
- Monitoring maternal vital signs and pain

SAFETY *STAT!*

During an external cephalic version, the patient is usually supine. Carefully monitor the blood pressure for signs of vena cava compression. Alert the physician of hypotension and reposition the patient to correct the problem.

Nursing Care After the Procedure

After the procedure, the patient and fetus should be observed for at least 1 hour. Labor may be induced or the patient may be discharged to wait for spontaneous labor to begin. Nursing care after the external version includes:

- Monitoring for contraction frequency, duration, and intensity
- Monitoring for a decrease in fetal activity
- Monitoring the FHR for abnormalities
- Monitoring for rupture of amniotic membranes
- Assessing for pain and discomfort
  - Notifying the health-care provider if the patient complains of increased abdominal pain; could be a sign of a placental abruptio, because pain should diminish after the procedure
- For Rh-negative patients, obtaining an order for a Kleihauer-Betke test to detect the presence of fetal blood in the circulation
  - Administering RhoGAM if more than 15 mL of fetal blood is present to suppress the patient's immune response to Rh-positive blood
- Reviewing signs of labor and ruptured membranes, including guidelines for returning to the hospital, before discharging the patient
- Providing information to the patient to promote safety and health for the patient and her fetus if the patient does not remain in the hospital

Teaching points should include the following:

- An external version is not always successful; sometimes the fetus returns to the position before the version.
- If vaginal bleeding begins or fetal movement decreases, contact the health-care provider immediately.
- An external version may stimulate labor or rupture membranes.
- If contractions begin, time them from the beginning of one contraction to the beginning of the next. If they

become regular for an hour, contact the health-care provider.
- Signs of ruptured membranes include:
  - A sudden gush of fluid from the vagina
  - A slow leak or dripping of fluid from the vagina

LABS & DIAGNOSTICS

Kleihauer-Betke's Test

Kleihauer-Betke's test is a blood test that measures the amount of fetal hemoglobin transferred from the fetus to the mother's bloodstream. This test is usually ordered for Rh-negative mothers who have suffered a traumatic injury or procedure that could cause bleeding. Normal values are less than 1% of fetal cells present. If more than 15 mL of fetal blood is detected, RhoGAM is usually administered to the patient (Van Leeuwen, Poelhuis-Leth, et al, 2015).

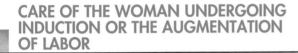

CARE OF THE WOMAN UNDERGOING INDUCTION OR THE AUGMENTATION OF LABOR

Induction and augmentation of labor use artificial methods to stimulate uterine contractions. The process of **labor induction** uses chemical or mechanical methods to start cervical effacement, dilation, and contractions. **Augmentation** is the stimulation of hypotonic uterine contractions if labor has begun but the contractions are ineffective in producing dilation and labor progression.

Indications

Indications for the induction or augmentation of labor include the following:

- Post-term pregnancy
- Prolonged rupture of membranes
- Pregnancy-induced hypertension
- Diabetes
- Chorioamnionitis
- Fetal demise
- Hypotonic contractions that do not produce dilation and labor progression

Labor cannot be successfully induced if the cervix is not ready or "ripe" enough to respond to methods, either chemical or mechanical, to start labor. The **Bishop's score** is a tool used by many health-care providers to evaluate cervical ripening and is predictive of readiness for the induction of labor (Goldberg, 2015). The score is based upon the findings of a cervical examination. Points are given for cervical dilation, cervical effacement, station of the fetus, consistency (soft to firm), and position of the cervix. A Bishop's score of 5 or more is significant for successful induction of labor. Table 12.1 provides details for calculating the Bishop's score.

TABLE 12.1 CALCULATING THE BISHOP'S SCORE

Criteria	Score
Dilation of the cervix	• 0 cm = 0 points • 1–2 cm = 1 point • 3–4 cm = 2 points • 5–6 cm = 3 points
Effacement of the cervix	• 0%–30% = 0 points • 40%–50% = 1 point • 60%–70% = 2 points • 80%+ = 3 points
Station of the fetal head	• –3 = 0 points • –2 = 1 point • –1 and 0 = 2 points • +1 and +2 = 3 points
Consistency of the cervix tissue	• Firm = 0 points • Medium = 1 point • Soft = 2 points
Position of the cervix	• Posterior position = 0 points • Midposition = 1 point • Anterior position = 2 points

Cervical Ripening

Cervical ripening refers to the softening of the cervix before the onset of labor and is necessary for cervical dilation and giving birth. The softening is due to physiological changes to the collagen fibers caused by enzymes and hormones. Cervical ripening by mechanical or chemical means are methods of inducing and augmenting labor.

Contraindications

Contraindications to cervical ripening include the following:

- Fetal malpresentation, such as breech or transverse lie
- Active herpes infection
- Regular uterine contractions
- Nonreassuring FHR pattern
- Placenta previa
- Unexplained uterine bleeding
- Previous Cesarean delivery (Goldberg, 2015)

Foley's Catheter

The most commonly used mechanical method of cervical ripening and inducing labor is the use of a Foley's balloon catheter. This is a safe and cost-effective method of cervical ripening; most women deliver within 24 hours of the insertion of a Foley's balloon (Kilpatrick and Esacoff, 2013). Using aseptic technique, the health-care provider inserts a 16F transcervical Foley's catheter balloon to or past the internal os of the cervix. The balloon is filled with 30 to 80 mL of sterile water. Gentle traction is applied and the catheter is taped to the inner thigh. Direct pressure is applied to the lower uterine segment of the uterus and cervix. The direct pressure on the lower uterine segment tissues causes the release of prostaglandins that result in cervical softening (Goldberg, 2015).

COMPLICATIONS. Complications of a transcervical Foley's catheter for cervical ripening and labor induction are rare. Reported complications have included infection, vaginal bleeding, acute transient febrile reaction, nonreassuring FHR pattern, and pain (Kilpatrick and Esacoff, 2013).

NURSING CARE. Nursing care of a transcervical Foley's catheter includes the following:

- Explaining the procedure to the patient and her support person
- Assisting the health-care provider with insertion of the Foley's catheter
- Monitoring the mother's vital signs and the FHR pattern as ordered by the health-care provider or hospital policy; report any abnormalities immediately

Prostaglandin Gel

The chemical method of applying prostaglandin gel around the cervix has been shown to be as effective as mechanical methods of cervical ripening and labor induction. Prostaglandin gel works on the fibers of the cervix to relax, soften, and dilate it. The gel also causes an increase in intracellular calcium levels, causing contraction of the uterine muscle.

The room temperature gel is placed in and around the cervix with an applicator. The patient should remain in the lateral recumbent position for 15 to 30 min after insertion of the gel to prevent leakage from the vagina.

SIDE EFFECTS AND COMPLICATIONS. Side effects and complications of prostaglandin gel include the following:

- Fever
- Nausea and vomiting
- Headache
- Diarrhea
- Tachysystole (ie, uterine hyperstimulation), which is five or more uterine contractions in 10 min (Fig. 12.3)
- Fetal decelerations in response to the tachysystole

NURSING CARE. Nursing care for the patient receiving prostaglandin for cervical ripening and labor inducement includes the following:

- Obtaining a baseline FHR pattern and uterine contraction activity before insertion
- Obtaining baseline maternal vital signs before insertion
- Informing the patient that she will need to lie on her side for 15 to 30 min after the insertion to prevent leakage of the gel and that she may notice a feeling of warmth in her vagina
- Monitoring the FHR pattern, uterine contractions, and maternal vital signs every 30 min
- Obtaining orders for medication to control nausea and vomiting if occurring
- Providing comfort measures and emotional support to the patient and her support person
- Repeating the dose in 6 hours if no uterine or cervical response occurs

---

🔵 DRUG FACTS

Dinoprostone (Prepidil Endocervical Gel)
Action: Initiates softening, effacement, and dilation of the cervix and stimulates the myometrium to cause contractions
   Dose: 0.5 mg (ie, contents of preloaded syringe) inserted around and in the cervical os. The dose may be repeated 6 hours later if needed. The maximum dose is 1.5 mg per 24 hrs.

Oxytocin Infusion

Oxytocin (Pitocin) infusion is a chemical method of inducing labor. Nursing care for the patient with an oxytocin infusion involves close monitoring and a thorough understanding of the procedure of infusing IV oxytocin to ensure a safe labor induction or augmentation of labor. The oxytocin is diluted in 1,000 mL of lactated Ringer's solution or normal saline and infused by IV (Fig. 12.4).

NURSING CARE. Nursing care includes the following:

- Obtaining a Bishop's score rating before starting oxytocin infusion
- Connecting the oxytocin infusion piggyback to the main IV line and administering it via an infusion pump

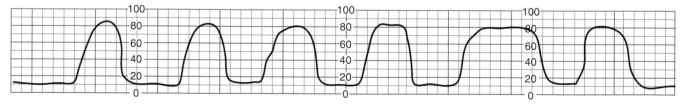

Tachysystole

FIGURE 12.3 Uterine tachysystole.

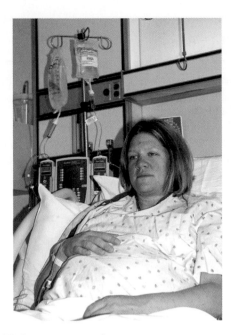

FIGURE 12.4 IV oxytocin administration.

• Monitoring maternal blood pressure, pulse, and respirations every 30 min and every time an increase in dosage occurs
• Monitoring the FHR and contraction patterns every 15 min and every time the dose is increased
• Increasing oxytocin as prescribed and then maintaining the dose if there is:
  • Reassuring FHR between 110 and 160 bpm
  • Cervical dilation of 1 cm/hr
  • Contraction frequency of every 2 to 3 min
  • Contraction duration of 60 to 90 sec
  • Contraction intensity of 40 to 90 mm Hg (if a IUPC is inserted)
  • Uterine resting tone of 10 to 15 mm Hg (if a IUPC is inserted)

SAFETY *STAT!*

Oxytocin would be immediately discontinued if hyperstimulation of the uterus occurs. Signs of uterine hyperstimulation include:
• Contractions that occur more frequently than every 2 min
• Contractions that last longer than 90 sec
• Contraction intensity greater than 90 mm Hg as shown by IUPC
• Uterine resting tone over 20 mm Hg between contractions as shown by IUPC
• No relaxation of the uterus between contractions
• A nonreassuring FHR pattern

DRUG FACTS

Oxytocin

Oxytocin acts on the uterine fibers to produce contractions. For labor induction, the recommended dose is 1 to 2 milliunits/min,

increased by 1 to 2 milliunits every 15 to 60 min until an effective labor pattern is established. Oxytocin has a short half-life of 3 to 12 min; therefore when the medication dosage is reduced or stopped, the nurse will see a very quick reduction in the strength, duration, and frequency of uterine contractions.

ASSISTED VAGINAL BIRTH

The term *assisted vaginal birth* refers to surgical procedures, such as **vacuum extraction** (ie, a cuplike device is used to assist with delivery of the infant) and **forceps** (ie, a metal instrument is used to assist with delivery of the infant's head) to expedite a vaginal delivery. There is controversy among health-care providers regarding if and when assisted vaginal deliveries should be performed and which instrument is the best to use (O'Grady, 2015). Vacuum extractor delivery and forceps delivery are used in modern obstetric management for approximately 5% of vaginal deliveries (Ross, 2013). However, the vacuum extractor has become the instrument of use by most practitioners.

Indications and Prerequisites

Indications for assisted vaginal delivery include the following:

• Maternal exhaustion
• Inadequate maternal expulsive efforts, such as those caused by a spinal cord injury or neuromuscular disease
• Fetal distress or a nonreassuring FHR pattern
• A prolonged second stage of labor

Prerequisites for an assisted delivery include the following:

• The fetal head must be engaged and the position known to the practitioner to promote safe placement of the forceps or cup device.
• The cervix must be fully dilated.
• Amniotic membranes must be ruptured.
• The pelvis must be an adequate size for delivery.
• The patient must have adequate analgesia to manage the discomfort of the procedure.
• The patient must be in the lithotomy position.
• The patient's bladder should be empty to allow more room for application of the device.
• Verbal consent, if possible, should be obtained from the patient (Ross and Beall, 2014).

Vacuum Extraction–Assisted Birth

A **vacuum extraction**–assisted delivery involves the use of a cuplike device that attaches to the fetal head with suction. The cup is lubricated with sterile lubricant or surgical soap, the labia are spread, and the cup is attached to the fetal head. Vacuum suction at 450 to 600 mm Hg is applied, and the health-care provider applies traction to assist with delivery of the fetal head. Traction is timed with uterine contractions and the patient assists by pushing during the contraction (Fig. 12.5) (O'Grady, 2015).

NURSING CARE PLAN for Induction of Labor

Monica is 20 years old. This is her first pregnancy and she is 41 weeks' gestation. She is admitted to the labor and delivery department for induction of labor with oxytocin. She is accompanied by her boyfriend. They are anxious and have many questions about induction.

Nursing Diagnosis: There is a knowledge deficit regarding induction of labor.
Interventions:
- Orient the patient and her boyfriend to the room and unit.
- Discuss the need for an induction of labor.
- Explain how to calculate the Bishop's score.
- Explain the expected procedure of IV oxytocin to start labor.
- Explain the purpose of the vaginal cervical examination.
- Explain fetal monitoring.
- Encourage questions from Monica and her boyfriend.

Expected Outcome: Monica and her boyfriend will verbalize understanding of the process of labor induction.

Nursing Diagnosis: Monica is experiencing fear and anxiety.
Interventions:
- Assess Monica's psychological and emotional status.
- Encourage verbalization of fears and feelings.
- Answer questions clearly and honestly.
- Provide opportunities for Monica to participate in decisions.
- Use therapeutic communication, verbally and nonverbally.

Expected Outcome: Monica will demonstrate and verbalize reduced anxiety regarding the induction of labor.

Nursing Diagnosis: There is a risk for injury.
Interventions:
- Perform a focused physical assessment on the patient that includes respiratory, cardiac, skin, and fundal height assessments.
- Perform a cervical examination to determine the Bishop's score and readiness for labor induction.
- Apply electronic fetal monitoring and obtain a 20-min record of the FHR to establish a baseline and to determine fetal well-being before beginning the induction of labor. Notify the health-care provider of any abnormalities.
- Obtain baseline vital signs of the patient including temperature, pulse, respirations, and blood pressure. Notify the health-care provider of any abnormalities.
- Insert an IV catheter in the nondominant arm, if possible.
- Obtain the premixed oxytocin solution ordered by the health-care provider from the pharmacy.
- Place the oxytocin solution in an infusion pump to run as an IV piggyback.
- Begin the infusion as ordered by the health-care provider, usually 1 to 2 milliunits/min.
- Gradually increase oxytocin by 1 milliunit/min every 30 min until contractions are 2 to 3 min apart.
- Once adequate labor is established, oxytocin may be slowly decreased, if possible.
- Continue to monitor the FHR and contraction pattern every 15 min while infusing oxytocin.
- Monitor the maternal heart rate and blood pressure every hour.
- Monitor the maternal temperature every 2 hours.

Expected Outcome: Develop and maintain a good labor pattern with contractions every 2 to 3 min, lasting 40 to 60 sec, with uterine tone relaxing between contractions and the FHR pattern demonstrating a reassuring pattern.

SAFETY *STAT!*

When using a vacuum extraction device, the nurse and the health-care provider must follow the manufacturer's instructions and hospital policy on the amount of suction pressure to be used for the extraction to avoid injury to the fetus or patient.

Possible Complications

Possible complications that can occur with a vacuum-assisted birth include:

- Fetal scalp bruising and lacerations
- Fetal scalp injuries that cause either a cephalohematoma or, rarely, a hematoma

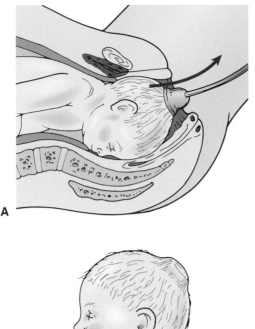

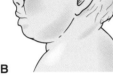

FIGURE 12.5 Vacuum extraction facilitates the delivery of the fetal head and is associated with fewer lacerations of the maternal birth canal. A, The vacuum extractor is applied with a downward and outward traction. B, A caput succedaneum is formed from the suction cup.

• Maternal lacerations of the cervix, vagina, or perineum (O'Grady, 2015)

Nursing Care

Nursing care for the patient undergoing vacuum-assisted delivery includes:

• Explaining the procedure to the patient and her support person
• Assisting the health-care provider by setting up the vacuum extraction device correctly and according to the manufacturer and hospital policies
• Assisting the patient into the lithotomy position
• Assessing for bladder distention and catheterizing if needed; a full bladder can impede fetal descent
• Monitoring FHR before and during the procedure
• Observing the newborn for any signs of complications

Forceps-Assisted Birth

A forceps-assisted delivery involves the use of a metal instrument that has two curved spoonlike blades with locking handles that fit on either side of the fetal head and assist with delivery of the head. The health-care provider applies the blades to each side of the fetal head and then gently applies traction during contractions (Fig. 12.6).

Possible Complications

Possible complications of a forceps-assisted delivery include the following:

• Lacerations of the vagina and perineum, with an increased risk of incontinence of flatus and feces (Ross, 2013)
• An increase in pelvic floor disorders such as bladder and rectal prolapse (Ross, 2013)
• Bruising of the fetal head
• Brachial plexus injury and facial nerve injury to the fetus

Nursing Care

Nursing care for the patient undergoing a forceps-assisted birth includes:

• Explaining the procedure to the patient and her support person
• Providing the health-care provider with the requested forceps
• Assisting the patient into the lithotomy position
• Assessing for bladder distention and catheterizing if needed; a full bladder can impede fetal descent
• Monitoring the FHR before and during the procedure:
  • Observing for decelerating FHR occurring from compression of the cord between the fetal head and forceps
  • Notifying the health-care provider to remove the forceps if variable decelerations or bradycardia occurs
• Observing the newborn for bruising and abrasions at the site of forceps application
• Monitoring the woman postpartum for possible lacerations of the cervix, vagina, and perineum

CESAREAN BIRTH

In 2014, the Cesarean delivery rate in the United States was 32.2% of all births. This is a decline from 32.8% in 2012. The Cesarean rate increased approximately 60% from 1996 to 2009 (Hamilton, Martin, et al, 2014). Approximately 50% of Cesarean births are repeat Cesareans. Lowering the Cesarean rate in the United States is a goal of *Healthy People 2020.* The target is to reduce the primary rate to 23.9% and the repeat Cesarean rate from 90% to 81.7% for women at low risk for complications.

Indications

A Cesarean birth is usually performed when complications arise during labor in which a vaginal birth could compromise the health of the mother or fetus. Common indications for a Cesarean birth are:

• Labor dystocia
• Persistent nonreassuring FHR patterns
• Breech or transverse lie presentation
• Fetal macrosomia
• Cephalopelvic disproportion
• Occiput posterior and occiput transverse positions of the fetus
• Maternal obesity

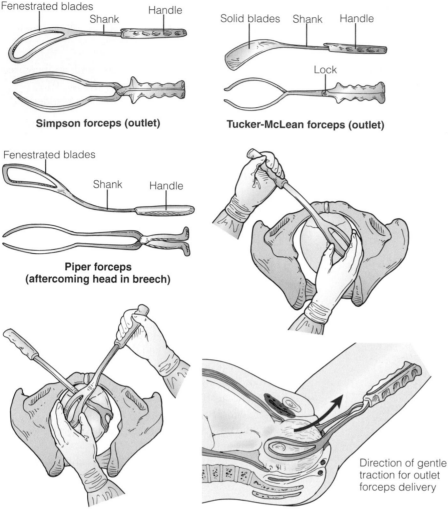

Simpson forceps (outlet)

Fenestrated blades
Shank
Handle

Tucker-McLean forceps (outlet)

Solid blades   Shank   Handle
Lock

**Piper forceps
(aftercoming head in breech)**

Fenestrated blades
Shank
Handle

Direction of gentle
traction for outlet
forceps delivery

FIGURE 12.6 Forceps are instruments with curved blades that are used to facilitate the birth of the fetal head.

- Multiple gestations
- Active genital herpes at the time of birth
- Prolapsed umbilical cord
- Placenta previa
- Placental abruptio (ACOG, 2014)

HEALTH PROMOTION

Preparing for a Scheduled Cesarean Birth

Women who have a scheduled repeat Cesarean birth can prepare for the birth by:

- Discussing the desired birth plan with the health-care provider, such as anesthesia, lighting, music, support person, skin-to-skin contact with the baby, and early breastfeeding
- Obtaining preoperative laboratory work
- Completing preregistration with the hospital
- Packing for 3 to 5 days in the hospital
- Arranging for help at home after discharge

The Procedure for a Cesarean Birth

After the decision has been made for a Cesarean delivery, the patient will sign an operative consent agreeing to the surgical delivery. Some hospitals have an operating room for Cesarean delivery within the labor and delivery department and other hospitals use the general hospital operating rooms. The nurse will usually make the call to the operating room or notify the charge nurse of an impending Cesarean delivery. The usual sequence of events for a Cesarean delivery includes the following:

- The patient must sign a consent form for a Cesarean delivery.
- An indwelling catheter is inserted to keep the bladder empty and urine away from the surgical site. In most cases, this procedure may be done in the labor and delivery department before moving the patient to the operating room.
- Preoperative medications may be ordered by the physician.
- Administration of an epidural or combined spinal-epidural (CSE), unless the birth is an emergency; in that case, general anesthesia may be the fastest option.
- After administration of the epidural, the support person is usually allowed to enter the operating room.
- The patient is positioned on her back with a wedge under the hip, tilting the uterus off the vena cava to prevent maternal hypotension and decreased placental perfusion.

- Intermittent monitoring of the fetal status is continued until the Cesarean begins.
- The patient's lower abdominal hair near the incision site may be clipped.
- A grounding pad is placed on her thigh to prevent shock from the electrocautery used to manage bleeding during the procedure.
- A sterile abdominal prep to kill organisms that may cause infection will be done before application of the sterile drapes.
- Two incisions are made by the surgeon. In the abdominal wall, the surgeon may make a vertical midline incision between the umbilicus and symphysis pubis (ie, **Pfannenstiel's incision**, also called a *bikini cut*) above the symphysis pubis. In the uterus, a low vertical incision is the most common location, unless the fetus is large or in distress, in which case the surgeon may opt for a midline incision. The uterus incision does not always match the skin incision. For example, a woman may have a midline abdominal incision and a low vertical incision on the uterus (Fig. 12.7).
- After the incision, the amniotic fluid is suctioned out and the baby is quickly removed from the uterus. Then the newborn's airway is suctioned and the umbilical cord is clamped and cut.
- The baby is placed under a warmer and the nurse assumes care for the newborn.
- The placenta will be removed and the incisions sutured.
- The patient will be transported to the recovery room for monitoring (Joy, 2014).
- To promote patient-centered care, the nurse should encourage the mother to see and touch the newborn before the baby is taken from the operating room to the newborn nursery; the nurse should also reunite the mother and baby in the recovery room for bonding and breastfeeding, if possible (Fig. 12.8).

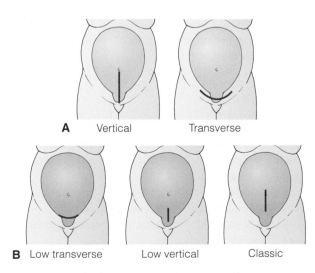

FIGURE 12.7 Abdominal and uterine incisions. A, Skin (ie, abdominal wall) incisions. Vertical and transverse (ie, Pfannenstiel's incision). B, Uterine wall incisions: low transverse, low vertical, and classic.

A Vertical   Transverse

B Low transverse   Low vertical   Classic

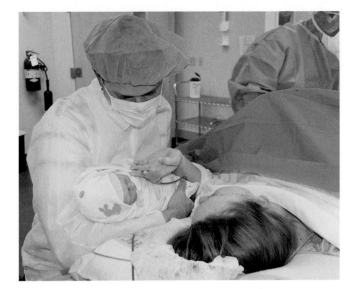

FIGURE 12.8 A family in a Cesarean birth.

SAFETY *STAT!*

Most women who deliver by Cesarean are given spinal or epidural anesthesia. The nurse should be aware that general anesthesia may be required. The nurse should obtain a diet history for the previous 8 hours before delivery and report this information to the anesthesiologist to prevent aspiration during the procedure.

Risks

The risks of a Cesarean delivery include:

- Hemorrhage
- Anesthesia complications
- Venous thromboembolism
- Shock
- Cardiac arrest

Long-term risks associated with Cesarean delivery include:

- Placenta previa or accreta in future pregnancies
- Uterine rupture

Nursing Care

Nursing care for the patient before a Cesarean birth includes the following:

- Alerting the operating room team of an impending Cesarean birth
- Obtaining the signed operative consent from the patient
- Continuing to monitor the fetus throughout preparations for the operating room
- Providing emotional support to the patient and her support person
- Administering any ordered preoperative medications
- Inserting an indwelling urinary catheter
- Inserting an IV catheter of sufficient size to allow a blood transfusion, if required

- Preparing the support person for the operating room
  - If it is hospital policy, informing the support person that he or she is not allowed into the operating room until the epidural or spinal anesthesia is complete

DRUG FACTS

Preoperative Medications

The pregnant patient does not receive a sedative before surgery because of the risk of the medication causing respiratory depression in the newborn. However, the nurse will usually administer an antacid such as famotidine (Pepcid) 20 mg IV or citric acid-sodium citrate solution (Bicitra) 30 mL orally to reduce gastric acid and decrease the risk of nausea, vomiting, and possible aspiration when anesthesia is administered. An antibiotic such as cefazolin (Ancef) 1 g IV is frequently ordered to reduce the risk of infection.

CULTURAL CONSIDERATIONS

Some non-Christian, rural, southeast Asians may refuse or be reluctant to agree to a Cesarean birth. They believe that the soul is attached to different parts of the body and that during surgery, the soul may leave the body, causing illness or death (Galanti, 2014).

Vaginal Birth After Cesarean

A **vaginal birth after Cesarean (VBAC)** may be an option for some women. The decision to try for a vaginal birth is based upon a careful physical examination and a thorough obstetrical history. The health-care provider gives the patient an estimate of her chance of a successful vaginal birth and advises her of the major complication of a VBAC, which is a ruptured uterus.

Indications and Contraindications

The woman desiring a VBAC has an increased chance of success if she has:

- Had a prior vaginal delivery
- Had a prior VBAC

- Spontaneous labor
- Cephalic presentation of the fetus

Contraindications for a VBAC include (Caughey, 2013):

- A large-for-gestational-age fetus
- Malpresentation, such as a breech, brow, or transverse lie
- Cephalopelvic disproportion
- More than two prior Cesarean births
- Gestational age greater than 41 weeks
- Gestational diabetes
- Macrosomia
- Maternal obesity
- Short interpregnancy interval

Nursing Care

A woman desiring a VBAC will be allowed to begin spontaneous labor. This is termed a ***trial of labor after Cesarean (TOLAC).*** She and the fetus will be closely monitored for signs of a ruptured uterus or fetal distress during the TOLAC. Hospitals typically require the health-care provider to be onsite and a team on call for a Cesarean delivery in the event of an emergency. If the labor progresses normally and the FHR pattern is reassuring, she will continue to a vaginal delivery.

Nursing care for the patient undergoing a TOLAC for a VBAC includes:

- The usual routine care of a laboring patient with careful monitoring of the FHR, contraction pattern, and maternal vital signs
- Vaginal cervical examinations, reporting a lack of progress to a health-care provider
- Observe closely for signs of uterine rupture and report any of the following findings:
  - Acute abdominal pain
  - The patient reports a "popping" sensation
  - Palpation of fetal parts outside the uterus
  - Repetitive or prolonged FHR deceleration
  - Vaginal bleeding

Key Points

- Maternal stress during procedures can lead to fetal distress. The nurse needs to provide emotional support to reduce stress for the patient.
- Collaboration is important because the nurse works together with other health-care team members and the patient to provide safe and effective patient-centered care.
- The nurse must be familiar with obstetric procedures and be ready to assist the health-care provider or, in some cases, perform the procedures. The nurse must be able to provide emotional support and monitor the patient for complications.

- Amniotomy is AROM to stimulate labor. After an amniotomy, contractions usually become more intense and labor progresses faster.
- Amnioinfusion is the procedure of infusing fluid into the amniotic cavity to relieve cord compression.
- An external cephalic version is a procedure to manipulate the fetus into a head-down presentation.
- The induction of labor is a process that can involve mechanical or chemical means to soften and dilate the cervix and stimulate uterine contractions.

- The labor and delivery nurse takes an active role in initiating the induction of labor and needs to have an understanding of the safe administration of oxytocin.
- Augmentation of labor is the stimulation of hypotonic uterine contractions if labor has begun but the contractions are ineffective in producing dilation.
- The Bishop's score is a tool used by health-care providers to determine if the cervix is ready or "ripe" for labor.
- A vacuum extraction device attaches to the fetal head with suction to allow the health-care provider to apply traction and assist with the delivery.

- Forceps are metal, spoonlike instruments that fit around the fetal head to allow the health-care provider to assist with the delivery.
- A Cesarean birth is usually performed when complications arise during labor.
- A VBAC is possible for many patients. A TOLAC is allowed and, if no complications occur, she is allowed to deliver vaginally.

REVIEW QUESTIONS

1. A patient is admitted to labor and delivery. She had poor prenatal care, is pregnant with her second child, and is Rh negative. She is prepared for an external cephalic version. The nurse expects the health-care provider to order which of the following medications?
   1. Prostaglandin gel
   2. Oxytocin (Pitocin)
   3. Magnesium sulfate
   4. RhoGAM

2. Nursing care following an amniotomy would include which of the following? *(select all that apply)*
   1. Observe the color and amount of fluid.
   2. Observe the FHR pattern.
   3. Monitor the patient's temperature every 8 hours.
   4. Change pads underneath the patient.
   5. Administer IV antibiotics.

3. The nurse explains to the patient that the purpose of the Bishop's score is to:
   1. Determine the well-being of the fetus.
   2. Determine progress during labor.
   3. Determine the readiness of the cervix for labor.
   4. Determine maternal well-being.

4. A patient asks what a "trial of labor" means. The *best* response by the nurse is:
   1. "You need to make progress in the next hours or a Cesarean will be scheduled."
   2. "The doctor is giving you time to make progress in labor before considering a Cesarean delivery."
   3. "Your pelvis is a little small but we are going to let you labor and see if you make it."
   4. "A Cesarean delivery will be done, but we are going to let you experience labor first."

5. The patient having her labor augmented asks, "What do you mean by hypotonic contractions?" The nurse's best response is:
   1. "Your contractions are infrequent and have decreased in intensity."
   2. "Your contractions are not hard enough."
   3. "Your labor is not progressing as it should."
   4. "Don't worry about that, we'll get your contractions going."

6. A patient is receiving oxytocin to induce her labor. The nurse notes that the patient has had two contractions 90 sec apart and each contraction lasted 90 sec. The FHR has dropped to 100 bpm following the second contraction. Select the appropriate nursing interventions. *(select all that apply)*
   1. Reduce the dose of oxytocin that is infusing.
   2. Apply oxygen via facemask to the patient.
   3. Place the patient on her left side.
   4. Stop the infusion of oxytocin.
   5. Notify the physician or nurse midwife.

7. Which of the following are contraindications for a VBAC? *(select all that apply)*
   1. One prior Cesarean delivery
   2. Maternal obesity
   3. Macrosomic fetus
   4. A prior vaginal delivery
   5. Gestation of 41 weeks

8. The nurse is preparing to assist the nurse midwife with an amnioinfusion. The patient asks, "Why do I need this?" The best response by the nurse is:
   1. "You need extra fluid in your uterus to allow the baby to move around."
   2. "The decreased fluid in the uterus is causing the baby to lie on the umbilical cord."
   3. "You need extra amniotic fluid to prevent a dry birth."
   4. "This will replace fluid in your uterus to prevent an infection."

9. The nurse knows that a possible side effect of prostaglandin gel is:
   1. Frequent urination
   2. Leg cramps
   3. Nausea
   4. Backache

10. A major responsibility of the nurse caring for a patient receiving oxytocin for labor induction is to:
    1. Monitor the IV site.
    2. Monitor the patient's urinary output.
    3. Monitor the patient's coping mechanisms for labor.
    4. Monitor for tachysystole.

CRITICAL THINKING QUESTIONS

1. A good friend who is pregnant and 38 weeks' gestation tells you that she is planning to have her labor induced "a little early" because her doctor is going on vacation. What is your best response, as a nurse, to your friend?

2. A patient is having her labor induced with oxytocin. She is obese and the nurse must palpate contractions because the external fetal monitor is not effective in recording the contractions. The nurse notes that the patient's cervix is 5 cm dilated, and the contractions are every 3 min and last 90 sec. With palpation, the nurse notes that the uterus does not seem to fully relax between contractions.

   a. What additional information does the nurse need in this situation?

   b. What interventions are appropriate?

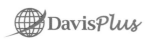

For additional resources and information, visit **www.DavisPlus.com**. Post-Conference Questions and Activities, Answers, and References can be found on Davis*Plus*.

Postpartum Period and the Family

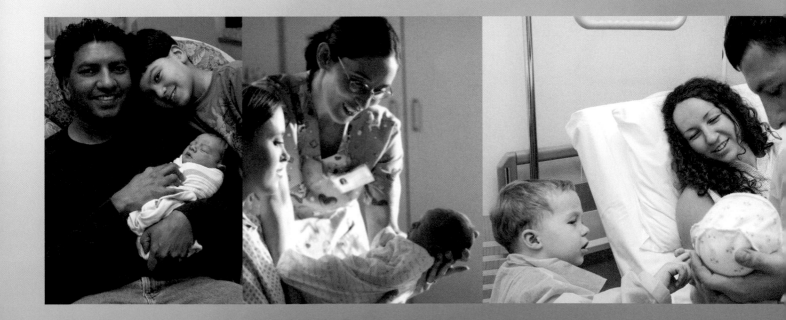

13

Physiological and Behavioral Adaptations During the Postpartum Period

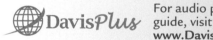
DavisPlus

For audio pronunciation guide, visit www.DavisPlus.com

LEARNING OUTCOMES

1. Define the key terms.
2. Identify the normal physiological changes following childbirth in the reproductive, integumentary, gastrointestinal, cardiovascular, respiratory, urinary, and musculoskeletal systems.
3. Explain the process of involution of the uterus after delivery.
4. Discuss the effect of a full bladder on uterine involution.
5. Explain afterpains to a multiparous patient.
6. Describe the phases of lochia progression.
7. Prepare patient teaching regarding the resumption of menses after childbirth.
8. Describe the postpartum psychological adaptations including the taking-in phase, the taking-hold phase, and the letting-go phase.
9. Identify signs that the mother is bonding with her newborn.
10. Distinguish between bonding and attachment.
11. Plan nursing interventions that can facilitate family-centered care and family attachment.

REAL-WORLD CASE STUDY

Camila

■ Camila is 23 years old and gave birth to her first child, Javier, after a long labor and vacuum extraction assistance for the delivery. It has been 4 hours since the birth and Camila complains of perineal pain and fatigue. The nurse observes Camila talking quietly to her infant as she strokes his body with her fingertips. After a short visit in her room, she sends Javier to the nursery.

1. What phase of Rubin's maternal role attachment is Camila in?
2. What nursing care is appropriate for this situation?

CONCEPTUAL CORNERSTONE

Family Dynamics

Nurses today emphasize family-centered care, particularly in the areas of labor and delivery, postpartum, and the nursery. A family can consist of married parents and their children, cohabiting parents, single parents, same-sex parents, and grandparents raising children. The birth of a new family member causes relationships and the interactions (ie, dynamics) between the family members to change. The word *dynamics* in this context means change or growth. When two people add a third person, a child, to the relationship, the family dynamics become more complicated. The complexity of the family dynamics changes with each child who is born and by the relationships that exist with the grandparents and other extended family members.

The nurse caring for a patient in the postpartum unit can support the change in the family dynamics by including family members in caring for the newborn and in teaching about newborn care and breastfeeding. The nurse can provide information for the parents about sibling rivalry and can encourage the siblings to visit the mother and to meet the new baby in the family. The nurse can also observe interactions between family members, identify problems, and make recommendations or appropriate referrals if needed to facilitate the change in family dynamics (Giddens, 2013).

The postpartum period, also known as the **puerperium,** is the 6-week period following the delivery of the placenta and lasts until the reproductive organs return to a nonpregnant state. Nurses need to be aware of normal physiological and psychological changes that take place during this period to provide safe and effective care.

POSTPARTUM PHYSICAL ADAPTATIONS

Immediately after delivery, the woman's body begins to change anatomically and physiologically to return to a nonpregnant state. A postpartum shivering occurs in 25% to 50% of women. The shivering is noticeable and may frighten the woman. It may occur anytime from 1 to 30 min after delivery and lasts for 2 to 60 min. The exact cause of the shivering is not known, but is thought to be related to a fetal-maternal transfusion that occurred when the placenta was delivered and maternal and fetal blood have the opportunity to mix (Posner, Dy, et al, 2013). Providing the patient with a warm blanket and reassurance that the shivering will pass is all that is required to provide for patient comfort.

The Reproductive System and Associated Structures

The reproductive system has the most changes immediately after the delivery and requires the knowledge and attention of the nurse to differentiate normal from abnormal adaptations after childbirth.

Uterus Involution

Immediately after the placenta is delivered, estrogen and progesterone levels drop quickly and oxytocin continues to be released, which causes the uterus to contract and begin the process of shrinking down to a nonpregnant size. This process is called *involution.* The uterus weighs 1,000 to 1,200 g immediately after birth; this decreases to 500 g by day 7, and to 50 g by 6 weeks, because of the decrease in size of the myometrial cells (Posner, Dy, et al, 2013).

After delivery, the uterus is the size of a grapefruit; the top portion, known as the *fundus,* is located midline and halfway between the umbilicus and symphysis pubis. Within approximately 1 hour, the fundus is firm and even with the umbilicus. The uterus continues to descend approximately 1 cm (ie, a fingerbreadth) per day. Usually, by day 10, the uterus is not palpable above the symphysis pubis (Fig. 13.1) (Derricot, 2013).

The intermittent contractions that some women describe as cramping are called *afterpains.* Afterpains are caused by the release of oxytocin. Afterpains are more noticeable for multiparous women because the uterus has been stretched

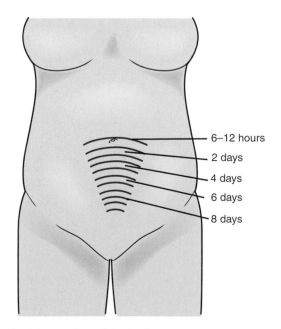

FIGURE 13.1 Location of the fundus at 6 to 12 hours postpartum and at 2, 4, 6, and 8 days postpartum.

before and must work harder to regain tone and return to a nonpregnant size.

Immediately after the delivery of the placenta, the interlacing uterine muscles contract the blood vessels that were attached to the placenta to prevent hemorrhage. In addition, the large blood vessels at the site where the placenta was attached thrombose, which means that blood clots close the vessels, preventing hemorrhage from the placental attachment site. At the placental site, the process of **exfoliation** begins. Exfoliation is the sloughing of dead tissue at the placental site, leaving the site smooth and without scar tissue. This allows the successful implantation of a fertilized ovum in subsequent pregnancies.

PATIENT TEACHING GUIDELINES

Afterpains

Afterpains can be quite intense and painful for women who have given birth previously because of a decrease in uterine muscle tone. Afterpains can also be noticed while breastfeeding as a result of nipple stimulation, which causes the release of oxytocin. The afterpains usually last for a few days and can be alleviated with ibuprofen or acetaminophen.

 DRUG FACTS

Ibuprofen (Advil) inhibits prostaglandins, which cause the afterpains. Prostaglandins are produced as part of the inflammatory process. The patient receives the pain relief as well as the anti-inflammatory properties from this medication. The most common side effect is gastrointestinal discomfort. It should be given with food.

Lochia

The inner lining, which is the endometrial surface of the uterus, begins to slough off, resulting in a vaginal discharge made up of blood and necrotic decidua. The discharge is known as *lochia.* The total volume of postpartum lochia is approximately 200 to 500 mL, and the process of discharging it may last up to 6 weeks. The lochia gradually gets lighter in color and amount over time. The types of lochia are:

- **Lochia rubra** is bright red and it lasts for 1 to 3 days.
- **Lochia serosa** is pink or brown in color and lasts for 4 to 9 days.
- **Lochia alba** is the final stage of uterine sloughing. The discharge is yellow-white and may continue up to 6 weeks after delivery.

Cervix

After delivery, the cervix is open and lacks tone. The cervical os (ie, opening) closes slowly and by day 14 is usually barely dilated. A parous cervix will have a slitlike opening instead of the small round opening of a nonparous cervix.

Vagina

After delivery, the vagina lacks tone. Gradually, over the next 4 weeks, the edema decreases and the vaginal folds, known as *rugae,* appear. The vaginal tissue may not lubricate easily until hormone balance is restored. The vagina will never return to a pre-pregnant size, but does decrease in size and return to near–pre-pregnancy size as recovery continues.

Perineum

The area between the vagina and anus stretches and thins to allow the birth. Perineal lacerations may occur during delivery or an episiotomy may be performed to enlarge the birth canal. After delivery, the perineum is usually bruised and edematous and the muscle tone is weak. The tone will gradually be restored over the next 4 to 6 weeks. Kegel exercises can promote the return of tone to the perineal and vaginal areas. Kegel exercises are easy to do, and every patient should receive information about how to perform Kegel exercises to improve perineal tone.

HEALTH PROMOTION

Kegel Exercises

Patient instructions for Kegel exercises are as follows:
- Find the muscles that you use for stopping urination.
- Squeeze these muscles for 3 sec, relax 3 sec, and then squeeze again for 3 sec.
- Do not tighten the stomach and thigh muscles—just the muscles in the vagina and perineum.
- Repeat the exercise 10 to 15 times each session and do three sessions daily.
- Add 1 sec each week until you are able to squeeze for 10 sec.
- Kegel exercises work better if done on a regular basis (WebMD, 2013).

Ovaries and Ovulation

The resumption of normal function of the ovaries is variable and influenced by breastfeeding. Menstruation is usually delayed and may not resume for weeks or months for breastfeeding women, and that depends on how much and how often the infant is breastfed. The delay is caused by the suppression of ovulation by the hormone prolactin.

The mother who does not breastfeed may ovulate as early as 27 days after delivery. In general, menstruation, which marks the beginning of ovulation, begins in 6 to 12 weeks for bottle feeding women (Spiliopouolos, 2013).

PATIENT TEACHING GUIDELINES

Postpartum Menstruation

The first menstrual period for a postpartum woman can occur anytime from 6 to 12 weeks after childbirth or even longer if the patient is breastfeeding. Ovulation occurs before menses, so it is important for the nurse to discuss birth control and family planning with patients before discharge from the hospital.

Breasts

Before milk production begins, the breasts secrete colostrum—a thin, yellowish fluid that provides nutrition and antibodies to the breastfeeding infant. The nipple stimulation provided by the infant causes a release of prolactin from the anterior pituitary. The hormone prolactin initiates milk production, and between the second and fourth day, the breasts become engorged with milk. The breasts may feel warm and tender. Mothers refer to this as having their milk "come in." Women who choose not to breastfeed will also experience the milk coming in.

HEALTH PROMOTION

Suppression of Breast Milk

Women who choose not to breastfeed their infants will still experience milk production. The production of breast milk can be suppressed by the following:

- Avoiding nipple stimulation
- Wearing a tight-fitting bra that provides compression to the breast
- Using ice packs on the breasts to promote comfort
- Avoiding applying heat to the breasts, such as from a warm or hot shower
- Not expressing milk from the breasts; expressing milk triggers the body to produce more milk

  Women who choose not to breastfeed their infants will find that milk production will usually cease in 5 to 7 days (Derricott, 2013).

Integumentary System

The abdominal skin will resume its pre-pregnancy state with the exception of abdominal striae (ie, stretch marks), which may take weeks to fade to a silvery color. The linea nigra down the middle of the abdomen will fade but may never completely go away. The effects of melanocyte-stimulating hormones, which cause skin hyperpigmentation called *melasma* on the face, will fade away over a period of days and weeks. Hair loss over the postpartum period is also common but usually resolves without medical intervention (Derricott, 2013).

Gastrointestinal System

After delivery, most women are hungry and thirsty because of the amount of energy exerted during the birthing process. Food and fluids may have been restricted during labor. The combined effects of restricted intake, elevated progesterone levels during pregnancy, and anesthesia often lead to sluggish intestinal peristalsis and constipation. Internal and external hemorrhoids caused by the weight of the uterus and by pushing during childbirth can cause pain with defecation.

 DRUG FACTS

Stool Softeners

A stool softener, such as docusate, may be prescribed to the postpartum patient to prevent straining. The onset for oral stool softeners is usually 12 to 72 hours. This medication is safe to use for breastfeeding women. The most common side effects are diarrhea and abdominal cramps (Vallerand and Sanoski, 2013).

Cardiovascular System

Expected blood loss from a vaginal delivery is 250 to 500 mL; from a Cesarean birth, it is 800 to 1,000 mL. Immediately after the birth, fluid changes occur that allow the body to adjust to postpartum blood loss and to prevent hypovolemia. A 60% to 80% increase in cardiac output occurs immediately after delivery and decreases to nearly normal by 1 hour postdelivery. The high output state is caused by the following circumstances:

- After the placenta is delivered, 500 to 700 mL of blood enters the circulation.
- The uterus becomes smaller, which causes more blood to enter the circulation.
- There is improved blood flow to the vena cava because of the reduction in the size and weight of the uterus.
- There is rapid mobilization of extracellular fluid by the body.

After delivery, there is a loss of plasma volume that is greater than that of red blood cells, which causes a temporary rise in the hemoglobin and hematocrit. An accurate determination of these two levels may be difficult to obtain (Ouzounian and Elkayam, 2012). Along with the increase of circulating blood volume, fibrinogen levels increase and remain increased for several days after delivery.

SAFETY *STAT!*

Because of increased levels of fibrinogen, the postpartum patient is more susceptible to blood clots. Therefore ambulation is important for the patient to prevent venous stasis in the legs.

The postpartum patient's body begins to remove excess fluid stored during the pregnancy by the process of **diuresis,** which is the secretion and passage of large amounts of urine. The woman may excrete up to 3,000 mL of fluid per day for the first few days (Derricott, 2013). Fluid is also lost through **diaphoresis,** which is excessive perspiration.

LABS & DIAGNOSTICS

An increase in neutrophils, which are white blood cells that fight infection, is normal in the postpartum period. This is because of inflammation, pain, and the stress of birth. The white blood cell count may increase to levels as high as 30,000 cells/mm³.

Respiratory System

The elevated diaphragm in late pregnancy will return to its normal position, reducing shortness of breath and making breathing easier. The postpartum patient's respiratory rate will return to the pre-pregnancy level. Pregnancy nasal congestion also disappears quickly.

Urinary System

The urinary bladder and urethra are edematous after delivery because of the effects of the fetus passing through the birth canal. The bladder tone decreases and the woman may not feel the urge to urinate. Therefore the bladder can become distended and push the uterus upward and to the side. Displacing the uterus can interfere with involution and can lead to hemorrhage for the postpartum patient.

SAFETY *STAT!*

A distended bladder can displace the uterus and interfere with the ability of the uterus to contract and control bleeding. The nurse must monitor for a distended bladder to prevent postpartum hemorrhage.

SAFETY *STAT!*

Poor bladder tone and poor emptying of the bladder can lead to urinary tract infections. The nurse must monitor the patient for signs of a urinary tract infection, including dysuria (ie, painful urination), urinary urgency and frequency, fever, and tenderness over the costovertebral angle.

Musculoskeletal System

The hormone relaxin, which is responsible for relaxing the pelvis ligaments and joints during pregnancy in anticipation of delivery, begins to subside. The woman may feel hip pain for a few days as the hips recover from over-flexion during pushing and as she experiences the effects of the tightening of her pelvis to the pre-pregnant state.

The abdominal muscles lack tone right after delivery. Some women experience a separation of the abdominal wall muscles called ***diastasis recti*** (Fig. 13.2). In some cases, this can be corrected with abdominal exercises. For some women, surgical correction may be needed if exercises are not effective to tighten and bring the muscles close together again.

HEALTH PROMOTION

Abdominal Exercises
Abdominal exercises to regain abdominal muscle tone can generally be started at 4 weeks postpartum for vaginal deliveries and 6 weeks postpartum for a Cesarean delivery.

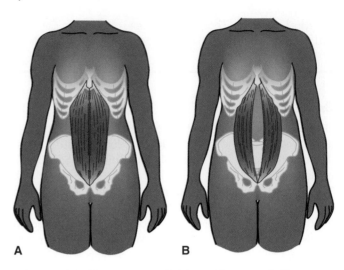

A   **B**

FIGURE 13.2 Diastasis recti. A, Normal location. B, Diastasis recti: a separation of the rectus muscles.

POSTPARTUM PSYCHOLOGICAL ADAPTATIONS

Even though the new mother may have known the sex of her baby and saw his "picture" via ultrasound prior to delivery, she is faced with a change in her life and the new role of motherhood. This new role may be overwhelming for some women, while others seem to step into their new role without hesitation. Reva Rubin's (1977) classic research on maternal role attainment divided the postpartum adjustment to motherhood into three phases: (1) the taking-in phase, (2) the taking-hold phase, and (3) the letting-go phase.

Taking-In Phase

In the taking-in phase, the mother is centered on her own needs, such as rest, pain relief, sleeping, and eating. She feels dependent at this time and she needs mothering. During this phase, the new mother often wants to review her labor and delivery experience. This review helps her to integrate it with the reality of her baby being born and the reality of motherhood.

She may not initiate interaction with the newborn, but when handed the newborn to hold, she will stroke the baby with her fingertips and may position the baby facing her so that she can explore the baby's face. This is known as the *en face position.* Fingertip touching and the en face position are signs of positive bonding behaviors. This taking-in of information allows her to identify her infant and begin the **bonding** process. Bonding is the start of a lifelong relationship with the newborn (Fig. 13.3). The mother begins to feel a closeness and a love for the baby. Bonding may occur instantaneously for some women, but for others it is a slower process that grows over a few days or weeks. The taking-in phase may last a day or two.

Taking-Hold Phase

In the taking-hold phase, the mother initiates care of the baby. She wants to be more independent and make her own decisions,

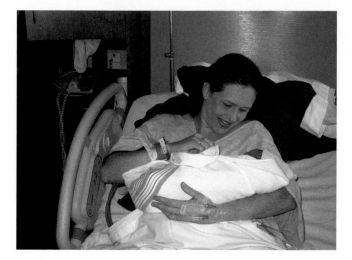

FIGURE 13.3 A new mother bonding with her infant.

but is concerned and anxious about her own physical care, breastfeeding, and baby care. The new mother requires praise and positive reinforcement for the things that she does well, such as supporting the baby's head or correct positioning for breastfeeding. She is open to learning about self-care, newborn care, and bonding, and so this is the right time to begin teaching her about these elements. Reassurance of her abilities to be a good mother is important during this time. This phase may last up to 10 or more days.

During the taking-hold phase, many women experience the postpartum blues. This phenomenon is thought to be caused by the decrease in estrogen and progesterone that occurred with the delivery of the placenta, as well as the exhaustion of motherhood that occurs from lack of uninterrupted sleep and demands of breastfeeding every 2 to 2½ hours. The woman may feel sad, irritable, or spontaneously erupt into tears for reasons she cannot explain. Usually this sadness passes after a good cry or in a day or two. Anticipatory guidance for the woman and her support person is important so that they will know that the postpartum blues are common and self-limiting. Occasionally the blues do not subside and the woman experiences postpartum depression. Postpartum depression is a serious disorder and the woman needs medical treatment. Postpartum depression is discussed in Chapter 14: Assessment and Care of the Family After Birth.

Letting-Go Phase

In this phase, the new mother is adjusting or "letting-go" of her previous childless, more independent role. She must adjust to the responsibility of having her baby dependent on her for everything, as well as the lifestyle changes that go along with parenthood. Women who already have children will experience this stage but will go through it more quickly as they adjust to resuming infant care and dividing attention between their children. During this phase, attachment with the newborn occurs. **Attachment** is the establishment of an emotionally positive and rewarding relationship between an infant and the parent. The mother learns to understand her infant's

cries and body language and receives positive feedback from the infant when the infant's needs are met. The mother learns to trust herself and her instincts when caring for the child and feels confidence in her ability to mother the infant.

THERAPEUTIC COMMUNICATION

When the new mother expresses anxiety regarding her ability to care for the newborn, the nurse has an important role in providing positive reinforcement, praise, and reassurance to the new mother. Phrases that may be helpful include:
- "You are holding him perfectly."
- "Look, he's looking right into your eyes."
- "Yes, that's the right position for breastfeeding."

HEALTH PROMOTION

Promoting Bonding with the Newborn
The following nursing interventions can promote bonding after childbirth:
- Promote skin-to-skin contact between the parents and the newborn.
- Encourage breastfeeding.
- Encourage eye contact.
- Allow the baby to stay with the parents as much as possible; avoid unnecessary trips to the nursery.

DEVELOPMENT OF FAMILY ATTACHMENT

Postpartum is a time of change for the family unit. A new baby is a major change for a family; family attachment, the integration of the newborn into the family unit, takes time.

Many fathers begin bonding with the fetus before the birth by attending health-care appointments, ultrasound appointments, and childbirth classes. He is often involved in preparing the baby's room and planning for the trip to the hospital. After the birth, the father should be encouraged to room-in and stay as much as possible with the mother and newborn at the hospital. New fathers are often observed staring at the newborn for extended periods of time. This behavior is known as **engrossment** and is comparable to the en face bonding that is observed with the mother and infant (Fig. 13.4).

He should be encouraged to hold the infant and assist with newborn care. The nurses should include the father in newborn care teaching before discharge.

Sibling bonding and attachment can be promoted by allowing the sibling to visit in the hospital. Current phone and video technology allow a child to have easy contact with his or her mother when she is hospitalized, but a visit with her in the hospital will reduce separation anxiety and feelings that the new baby is more important. A visit with mom, dad, and the new baby will promote family bonding faster.

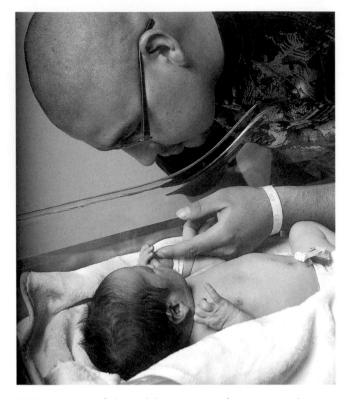

FIGURE 13.4 A father exhibiting a sign of engrossment by gazing at his newborn son.

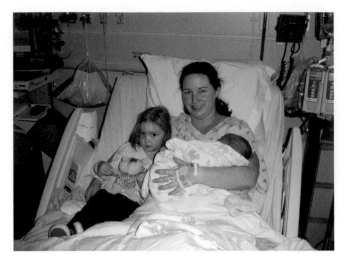

FIGURE 13.5 A new mother with the newborn and an older child in bed.

The parents need to be cautioned that the older child may exhibit signs of jealously and may regress in his or her behavior. For example, a three-year-old who was potty-trained may begin wetting his pants. Even if older siblings are prepared for the birth and the new family member, their behavior may be unpredictable. The child may also express uncomplimentary opinions about the new baby. Often, the sibling vacillates between protective, loving feelings and dislike for the new family member (Fig. 13.5).

CULTURAL CONSIDERATIONS

Postpartum and nursery nurses closely watch the new mother for signs of successful bonding with her newborn. The nurses may become concerned if cultural practices and beliefs appear to reflect poor bonding. For example, the rural Vietnamese may believe in spirits that are attracted to infants and may attempt to "steal" the infant by inducing illness or death. To protect their infant, the family may provide only required care, such as feeding and diaper changing, but may not "show off" the baby to reduce attention on the newborn. Their apparent lack of attention is actually a demonstration of their love for the newborn. Nurses who are not culturally competent can cause distress for a family if the nurse insists that the new parents bond and care for an infant in a way that conflicts with their cultural beliefs (Galanti, 2015).

Key Points

- The reproductive system undergoes the most changes immediately after birth, but all body systems are affected.
- The process of the uterus returning to its pre-pregnant state is called *involution.*
- The vaginal discharge following childbirth is called *lochia* and it may last for up to 6 weeks after delivery.
- There are three types of lochia: rubra, serosa, and alba.
- The breasts secrete colostrum first, followed by milk in 2 to 4 days.
- Abdominal striae and the linea nigra will fade but usually do not completely disappear.
- Constipation and hemorrhoids are common after delivery.
- To balance fluids in the body, diuresis and diaphoresis occur for the first few days after delivery.

- Lack of bladder tone can lead to an overdistended bladder, which can prevent uterine involution and cause excessive bleeding.
- Joint and muscle pain is common after delivery as the woman recovers and adjusts to the decrease in relaxin hormone.
- Rubin's classic research identified three phases of maternal role attainment: the taking-in, taking-hold, and letting-go phases.
- Nursing interventions can facilitate family attachment and changes in family dynamics.

REVIEW QUESTIONS

1. The process of the uterus returning to its pre-pregnant state is known as:
   1. Exfoliation
   2. Involution
   3. Evolution
   4. Intonation

2. A multiparous patient asks the nurse, "Why am I cramping? Is something wrong?" The best response by the nurse is:
   1. "The cramping is called *afterpains* and it will go away soon."
   2. "I can get you pain medication, if you'd like it."
   3. "The cramping is called *afterpains* and they are normal contractions of the uterus as it goes through the involution process."
   4. "Let's get your mind off that. Would you like to hold your new baby?"

3. A woman who does not want to breastfeed can suppress milk production by: *(select all that apply)*
   1. Wearing a tight-fitting bra
   2. Applying ice packs to the breasts
   3. Allowing the baby to nurse for short times only
   4. Standing in the shower and allowing warm water to soften the breasts
   5. Asking for medication to dry up the milk supply

4. A postpartum woman calls the nurse because she just woke up and her gown and sheets are soaked with perspiration. The nurse knows that:
   1. The patient's body is ridding itself of excess fluid through diaphoresis.
   2. The patient has a fever and has probably developed an infection.
   3. The room temperature is too hot for the patient.
   4. The postpartum hormone changes have given her a hot flash.

5. The nurse can promote maternal-infant bonding by:
   1. Allowing the mother uninterrupted rest by caring for the baby in the nursery
   2. Encouraging the grandmother to care for the newborn
   3. Providing all the newborn care
   4. Encouraging skin-to-skin contact between the newborn and the mother

6. In 12 hours after delivery, the nurse expects the fundus to be located:
   1. At the level of the umbilicus
   2. Two finger-breadths below the umbilicus
   3. Three finger-breadths below the umbilicus
   4. Right above the symphysis pubis

7. A new mother is very interested in caring for her newborn but is concerned about her ability to be a good mother. According to Rubin's phases on role attainment, the new mother is in which of the following phases?
   1. Taking-in phase
   2. Taking-hold phase
   3. Letting-go phase
   4. Attachment phase

8. At 2 weeks after delivery, a patient arrives at the obstetrician's office for a checkup. The nurse expects to see: *(select all that apply)*
   1. Lochia alba
   2. Edema of the ankles
   3. Abdominal striae
   4. Diaphoresis
   5. Fundus halfway between the umbilicus and symphysis pubis

9. A patient who is 1 day postpartum asks the nurse, "Do you think I have a urinary tract infection? I keep making trips to the bathroom." Which of the following actions is correct? *(select all that apply)*
   1. Obtain an order for a urinalysis and culture.
   2. Assess the patient for pain with urination.
   3. Assure her that frequent urination is normal.
   4. Call the doctor or midwife.

10. The patient asks the nurse why she is receiving a stool softener. The best response by the nurse is:
    1. "It is ordered by your midwife."
    2. "This medication will make your first bowel movement easier."
    3. "Breastfeeding women often have constipation."
    4. "You haven't been drinking enough fluids."

CRITICAL THINKING QUESTIONS

1. How can a mother assist her 4-year-old child to bond with the new family member?

2. A new mother is being discharged home. She is accompanied by the baby's father and her mother, who is a new grandmother. The grandmother intends to provide help at home. How can the nurse advise the grandmother about helping the new parents at home?

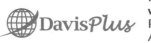

For additional resources and information, visit
www.DavisPlus.com.
Post-Conference Questions and Activities, Answers, and References can be found on Davis*Plus*.

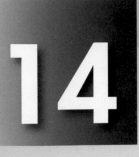

14

Assessment and Care of the Family After Birth

DavisPlus For audio pronunciation guide, visit www.DavisPlus.com

CHAPTER CONCEPTS

Assessment
Infection
Mood
Nursing Roles
Perfusion

LEARNING OUTCOMES

1. Define the key terms.
2. Demonstrate the correct method of uterine massage for postpartum assessment.
3. Discuss possible causes of uterine atony.
4. Outline postpartum care in the first hour after delivery.
5. Demonstrate a focal postpartum assessment using the BUBBLE LE mnemonic.
6. Plan patient-centered care that addresses the special needs of the adolescent postpartum patient.
7. Describe a therapeutic approach for managing the psychosocial needs of a patient who is relinquishing her infant for adoption.
8. Plan discharge teaching for the postpartum patient.
9. Identify the signs and symptoms of postpartum hemorrhage (PPH) and review appropriate management of PPH.
10. Discuss the causes, signs and symptoms, and management of a patient with a hematoma.
11. Recognize signs and symptoms of a postpartum infection and discuss appropriate management of the infection.
12. Identify women at risk for thrombophlebitis, as well as nursing interventions to prevent thromboembolism in the postpartum patient.
13. Differentiate between postpartum depression and postpartum psychosis and identity appropriate nursing interventions for each disorder.

REAL-WORLD CASE STUDY

Alice

■ Alice delivered her fourth child, a baby boy weighing 10 pounds and 2 ounces, 1 hour ago and has been transferred to the postpartum unit. The nurse reports that Alice was 42 weeks gestation and had her labor induced with oxytocin. She had a long second stage, pushed

REAL-WORLD CASE
STUDY *continued*

for 2 hours, and then required an assisted delivery with forceps. Her uterus became soft and boggy between assessments and has required massage and an increase in the rate of the IV oxytocin to maintain a firm fundus. The postpartum nurse begins the physical assessment and notes that the uterus is boggy and her peripad is saturated with blood.

1. What risk factors does Alice have for PPH?
2. What additional information should the postpartum nurse collect about Alice?
3. What actions should the nurse take at this time?

CONCEPTUAL CORNERSTONE

Infection

An infection occurs when a host is invaded by microorganisms that enter the body, multiply, and cause illness or even death. When an infection occurs, it can be acute or chronic. It can be a localized infection in one area of the body, such as in a wound, or it can become systemic, which means the infection affects the entire body. In postpartum, infections are usually localized and can occur in uterine tissue, wound tissue, the urinary tract, and the breast. However, a localized infection that is not identified and treated early can progress into a systemic infection, which could have debilitating effects for the patient.

The nurse needs to be alert for patients with risk factors that predispose them to infection in the postpartum period. Regardless of the location of the infection, there are similarities in the signs and symptoms of an infection, such as fever, redness, ecchymosis, and drainage. Prompt recognition of signs of infection and initiation of antimicrobials, fluids, and nutrition can change the course of the infection and the length of stay for the patient.

Assessment and care of the postpartum patient and her family begins immediately after the birth. The nurse who provides care during this phase of recovery needs to have knowledge about the physiological and psychosocial aspects of recovering from pregnancy and childbirth to provide safe and effective nursing care.

NURSING CARE DURING THE EARLY POSTPARTUM PERIOD

Immediate postpartum care most often occurs in a hospital. Most women remain in the hospital for 2 days after a vaginal delivery and 3 to 5 days after a Cesarean delivery. During this time, women are recovering from childbirth and assuming care for their newborns. Nurses use this time in the hospital

to provide physical care and to monitor for complications. Nurses also teach the woman about self-care before discharge.

Uterine Assessment

After delivery and expulsion of the placenta, the uterus is about the size of a grapefruit and is located midline in the abdomen, halfway between the umbilicus and symphysis pubis. Slowly, over the next several hours, the fundus (ie, the top portion of the uterus) will rise on the midline of the abdomen to the level of or slightly above the umbilicus. Thereafter, the height of the fundus decreases by at least 1 cm or 1 fingerbreadth daily as the uterus goes through the process of involution. By the 10th day, the fundus is usually not palpable.

To palpate the fundus, the nurse should position one hand at the base of the uterus just above the symphysis pubis and the other hand at the umbilicus. The nurse should press downward with the hand at the umbilicus until the fundus is palpated as a firm, hard, globular mass in the abdomen (Fig. 14.1). The nurse will note the position of the fundus and document the location.

SAFETY *STAT!*

Never palpate a uterus without supporting the lower segment because the uterus could invert if not stabilized.

Next, the nurse will assess the consistency of the mass. If it is soft or "boggy," the nurse will support the lower uterine segment and gently massage in a circular pattern with the other hand until the uterus becomes firm. If massage is not effective, there may be a large blood clot in the uterus or extreme uterine atony. *Atony* refers to a lack of muscle tone, which could lead to PPH. Many women receive oxytocin after delivery to promote uterine contractions. If the uterus does not remain firm with the administration of oxytocin and massage, the health-care provider should be notified.

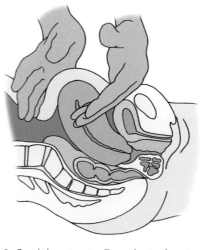

FIGURE 14.1 Fundal massage. To palpate the uterus, the upper hand is cupped over the fundus; the lower hand stabilizes the uterus at the symphysis pubis.

Another problem that could lead to uterine atony is a full bladder, which can displace the uterus and make involution difficult. A full bladder can push the uterus to the side and interfere with uterine contractions that attempt to produce involution to control bleeding from the placenta site. The nurse should assess the patient's bladder. If bladder distention is noted, the nurse should assist the patient to urinate and then reassess the uterus to determine if it is firm and has returned to the midline of the abdomen.

SAFETY *STAT!*

The first time a postpartum patient wants to get out of bed, the nurse should assist her in the event that she experiences **orthostatic hypotension** (ie, a drop in the blood pressure when standing) because of blood loss and physiological changes in the cardiovascular system that cause her to be at risk for fainting.

Lochia Assessment

Immediately after delivery of the placenta, a large amount of dark red blood flows from the uterus. The uterus begins to contract to control bleeding and then the volume of vaginal discharge slows. The vaginal discharge after birth is referred to as *lochia*. This first discharge of dark red blood is termed *lochia rubra*. The lochia progressively changes to a brownish red and then a lighter color called *lochia serosa* around the 3rd to 4th day. Over a period of 1 to 2 weeks, the lochia becomes even lighter and more of a yellowish color, called *lochia alba*. The period of time that the woman will experience lochia may last from 3 to 6 weeks (Spiliopoulos, 2013).

While the nurse is assessing for uterine tone, the lochia can be observed (Fig. 14.2). The peripad (ie, similar to a menstrual pad) is viewed to inspect the amount and character of the lochia. The amount of discharge is determined by the amount of lochia on a peripad after 1 hour (Ward, 2015). Nurses document the amount of lochia by using the following terms (in. refer to the diameter of the spot where the lochia has been absorbed into the pad):

• *Scant* is less than 1 in. of lochia on the pad.
• *Light* is less than 4 in. of lochia on the pad.
• *Moderate* is less than 6 in. of lochia on the pad.
• *Heavy* is when the pad is saturated within an hour.

The character of the lochia refers to the color (ie, rubra, serosa, or alba) and the presence of clots. It is common for small clots to be present because of blood pooling in the lower uterine segment. The patient should be turned to her side to make sure that blood is not pooling under her thighs instead of being absorbed by the peripad. Small clots can just be documented, but large clots can interfere with involution or indicate signs of hemorrhage and should be reported.

During the first hour after delivery, it is common for two peripads to be saturated. After the first hour, bleeding is considered excessive if the patient saturates more than one pad per hour.

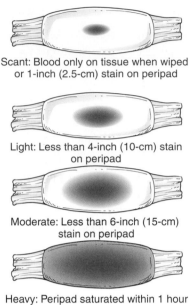

Scant: Blood only on tissue when wiped or 1-inch (2.5-cm) stain on peripad

Light: Less than 4-inch (10-cm) stain on peripad

Moderate: Less than 6-inch (15-cm) stain on peripad

Heavy: Peripad saturated within 1 hour

FIGURE 14.2 Assessment of lochia flow in 1 hour.

Nursing Care During the First Hour After Delivery

The newly delivered patient will remain in the labor and delivery area for a minimum of 1 hour after delivery. The first hour after delivery is the most dangerous hour in childbearing because of the risk of hemorrhage after delivery. During this first hour, the following nursing interventions should take place:

• Check vital signs, including pulse and blood pressure, every 15 min.
• Palpate the fundus of the uterus for firmness and location every 15 min.
• While assessing the uterine tone, the nurse will note the amount of vaginal bleeding. Observe the peripads for the amount of lochia, color, odor, and the presence of clots.

When the labor and delivery nurse is confident that the patient is stable and exhibiting no signs of hemorrhage, the patient is transferred to the postpartum unit. Upon arrival at the postpartum unit, the nurse will assess the patient and continue close monitoring according to hospital protocol.

Postpartum Assessment and Nursing Interventions

The postpartum nurse will perform an appropriate physical assessment for the postpartum patient with the focus on the reproductive system. A mnemonic for remembering the postpartum focal assessment is BUBBLE LE: **b**reasts, **u**terus, **b**ladder, **b**owels, **l**ochia, **e**pisiotomy/laceration, **l**egs, and **e**motions.

Breasts

The nurse should inquire about breast and nipple pain. The breast should be lightly palpated to assess for engorgement and the nipples inspected for redness, irritation, blisters, or bleeding.

Nursing interventions include the following:

- Suggest that the woman wear a bra with good support to promote comfort as the milk comes in.
- If nipple soreness is present, observe the woman breastfeed and correct latch-on problems.
- Provide pain relief such as Tylenol for sore nipples before breastfeeding.
- Assess her knowledge of breastfeeding and provide appropriate teaching if needed.
- Remind her that frequent breastfeeding every 2 to 2½ hours will help prevent engorgement when her milk comes in (Fig. 14.3).

PATIENT TEACHING GUIDELINES

Managing Engorgement for the Nonbreastfeeding Patient

Women who do not plan to breastfeed will still produce breast milk and become engorged. Patient teaching to promote comfort and reduce milk production includes:

- Wear a supportive bra 24 hours a day until engorgement subsides.
- Apply ice packs to the breasts for 20 min several times a day.
- Avoid any stimulation of the nipple; for example, do not stand in a warm shower and let the water run over the breasts.
- Do not pump or hand-express milk; the breast will replace the milk, which will exacerbate the engorgement.
- Take an analgesic, such as Tylenol, for the pain.
- Engorgement usually subsides within 48 hours.

Uterus

The fundus is palpated for location and consistency. It should be firm and in the midline. The nurse will document the location of the fundus in relationship to the umbilicus (see Fig. 13.1). For example, if the fundus is 1 cm or 1 finger-breadth beneath the umbilicus, it is documented as U-1 in the medical record. The nurse should inquire about cramping and abdominal pain.

Nursing interventions include the following:

- Some cramping is expected, but abdominal pain or tenderness should be reported to the health-care provider.
- If the uterus is not involuting as expected, note lack of tone, signs of bladder distension, or signs of infection and report findings.
- Have the patient feel her fundus as the nurse explains the process of involution.

Bladder

The nurse should palpate the bladder when assessing the fundus. Bladder distention should not be present. If the bladder is distended, the nurse will note a raised area over the bladder area.

Nursing interventions include the following:

- If bladder distention is noted, assist the patient to the bathroom to urinate before completing the assessment.
- If the patient cannot urinate because of bladder distention, an order must be obtained for a catheterization.
- Question the patient about frequency and amount of urination.
- Instruct the patient to drink at least eight glasses of water a day to decrease the risk of a urinary tract infection (UTI).
- Teach the patient about the normal diuresis process after childbirth.
- Teach the patient about proper perineal care of wiping from front to back after urination and defecation. Many health-care providers order a peri-bottle for cleansing the perineum. The bottle is filled with warm water and squirted over the perineum after urination and defecation to cleanse the perineum before applying a clean peripad.
- Remind the patient to change her peripad after each urination and defecation.

Bowels

Bowels are assessed by the auscultation of bowel sounds. The patient who experienced a Cesarean birth may not have audible bowel sounds for several hours because of the effects of anesthesia on peristalsis.

Nursing interventions include:

- Asking the patient if she has had a bowel movement; the bowels tend to be sluggish because of the effects of prenatal iron and the decrease in peristalsis from labor
- Encouraging the patient to drink extra fluids and to select fruits and vegetables from her hospital menu
- Administering stool softeners if ordered by the health-care provider
- Encouraging walking to promote an increase in peristalsis

Lochia

The nurse will assess the amount and type of lochia. The amount and color (ie, rubra, serosa, or alba) will be documented.

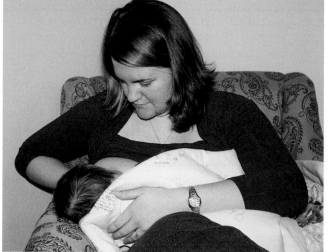

FIGURE 14.3 A new mother breastfeeding her newborn. The infant should feed at each breast for at least 15 to 20 min.

Nursing interventions include the following:

- Ask the patient when her pad was changed. This provides a better indication of the amount of lochia noted.
- Report any abnormal amount, color, or foul odor.
- Teach the woman about the progression of lochia.

Episiotomy/Laceration

The episiotomy is best viewed by having the patient turn to her side and bring her upper knee forward. While the patient is on her side, gently lift the upper buttock and inspect the perineum for bruising, erythema, edema, **hematoma** (ie, a collection of blood in the subcutaneous space), and for intactness of the episiotomy or the repaired laceration. Note if hemorrhoids are present and notify the health-care provider if they are large and painful.

Nursing interventions include the following:

- Ask the patient her level of perineal or rectal pain and medicate appropriately according to the health-care provider orders.
- Report any abnormal findings to the health-care provider.
- Offer an ice pack for the first 24 hours to reduce pain and swelling.
- After 24 hours, warm water soaking (ie, sitz bath) may relieve episiotomy and hemorrhoid pain and aid in healing (Fig. 14.4).

PATIENT TEACHING GUIDELINES

Preparing a Sitz Bath at Home

Some patients obtain episiotomy pain relief with a warm **sitz bath**. The word "sitz" comes from German and means *to sit* (Todd, 2014). Some hospitals provide the patient with a round plastic basin that is placed on the toilet seat. It comes with a bag that can be filled with warm water. As the woman sits on the basin, warm water flows from the bag through long tubing into the basin and around her perineum and then into the toilet.

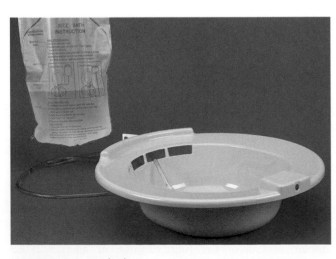

FIGURE 14.4 Sitz bath.

A home sitz bath can be prepared by filling a clean bath tub with 2 to 3 in. of warm water. For added comfort, a clean towel can be placed in the tub for her to sit on. No soap, shower gels, or bubble bath should be added. The woman can sit on the soft wet towel in the warm water for 10 to 15 min 3 times a day.

Legs

After questioning the patient about leg pain, the nurse should assess the legs for adequate circulation by checking the pedal pulses and noting the temperature of the legs. Pedal edema may last for a few days after delivery as body fluids shift (Derricott, 2013). The legs should be inspected for any red, warm, or tender areas.

Nursing interventions include the following:

- Report any abnormal findings immediately.
- Encourage the patient to ambulate frequently.
- Teach the patient to avoid crossing the legs.
- Encourage the patient to keep her legs elevated when sitting.
- Encourage high-risk patients to wear compression hose or apply sequential compression devices to the legs.

Emotions

Throughout the assessment process, the nurse is noticing the patient's emotions. Emotions change as the patient moves through the stages of role attainment. Emotionally, the patient may range from excited to apprehensive to exhibiting signs of the "postpartum blues," with tearfulness and irritability.

Nursing interventions include the following:

- Explain to the patient that the "postpartum blues" are a normal part of postpartum recovery. Reassure her and her family that it usually passes within a few days.
- Encourage the patient to rest frequently, verbalize her needs, and allow her family and friends to assist during the recovery time.

SAFETY *STAT!*

Teach the patient to report any feelings of depression or a desire to harm herself to her health-care provider immediately. She may be developing a postpartum depression or postpartum psychosis. Interventions may be needed to protect the woman and her baby.

LABS & DIAGNOSTICS

- Nonpathological leukocytosis occurs during labor and in the immediate postpartum period. The white blood cell (WBC) count can be as high as 25,000 to 30,000 cells/mm³ because of inflammation (ie, not from infection). The WBC returns to normal by the end of the first postpartum week (Van Leeuwen and Bladh, 2015).

- Platelet levels fall after the placenta separates from the uterus and then begins to increase by the 4th postpartum day, returning to normal by the 6th postpartum week.
- The hemoglobin and hematocrit are difficult to interpret because of changing blood volume and the natural diuresis that occurs to normalize fluid balance. Right after birth, the hemoglobin and hematocrit will decease because of blood loss. The diuresis and movement of extracellular fluid causes hemoconcentration, leading to an increase in the hematocrit.

Nursing Care After a Cesarean Birth

The woman who experienced a Cesarean birth requires the same monitoring for uterine involution and lochia as the patient who experienced a vaginal birth, with the addition of monitoring the Cesarean incision for signs of infection. In addition, she usually does not experience pain in the perineal area, but instead from her abdominal incision.

She will require postoperative care to prevent complications of bedrest, such as atelectasis, thrombosis, and infection. In addition to normal postpartum monitoring, nursing care for a Cesarean delivery patient includes the following:

- Assessing and medicating for pain according the health-care provider's orders
- Monitoring the incision for signs of infection: redness, edema, ecchymosis, drainage, and approximation of wound edges
- Encouraging ambulation to prevent venous thrombosis
- Discontinuing the urinary catheter as ordered and monitoring the patient for resumption of a normal voiding pattern
- Applying elastic stockings or sequential compression devices to prevent sluggish blood flow
- Encouraging turning, coughing, and deep breathing every 2 hours, along with use of an incentive spirometer, to prevent atelectasis, which could lead to hospital-acquired pneumonia

Nursing Care of the Adolescent

The postpartum adolescent receives the same assessment and physical care as any other postpartum patient. The nurse needs to provide support and education regardless of the nurse's personal philosophy about teen parenthood. The postpartum adolescent requires more structured teaching about the care of the newborn and herself. She may have limited or no prior contact with babies. The adolescent should be treated as an adult, and the nurse should not talk down to her and should be careful with the tone of the interactions. Tone of voice can indicate emotion, such as anger, irritability, or disapproval. A teenager will be sensitive to the nurse's tone and attitude when receiving teaching about her newborn. The nurse should encourage questions and never make the adolescent patient feel embarrassed about any lack of knowledge. The teaching should be directed to the teenager, not to her parents or to the support persons who may accompany her.

If the father is present, he should be included in the teaching. Teaching in small segments with demonstrations, videos, and written material is appreciated by teenagers. Providing her with periods of rest between teaching sessions and infant care may prevent her from becoming overwhelmed.

The nurse can role-model infant care and encourage bonding between the new mother and her infant. During the taking-in phase, the patient will be very centered on her own needs. She will require more mothering from the nurse and her family than an older patient. Her fears of being able to take on the maternal role require that she receive positive reinforcement from the nurses about her attempts at newborn care. Encouragement and praise will increase her self-confidence and self-esteem as she takes on the role of motherhood.

Some adolescents who have had little or no exposure to newborns have unrealistic expectations. For example, she may expect her baby to look like the perfect baby from infant food commercials on television or she may be surprised that newborns must be fed around the clock. She may not be prepared for the amount of time that breastfeeding and infant care requires. The nurse should encourage verbalization of her fears and needs during the postpartum recovery in the hospital and should provide education, emotional support, and appropriate referrals.

Teen mothers are at higher risk for postpartum depression. The patient should be taught the signs and symptoms of depression and should be instructed to report them to her health-care provider. She and the father should be referred to support groups for teen parents for ongoing support (Joy, 2014).

TEAM WORKS

Postpartum Care of the Pregnant Adolescent

A team approach to providing patient-centered care for the postpartum adolescent includes the following:

- The physician or nurse-midwife provides physical care before and after the birth.
- The nurse provides assessment, physical care, and teaching about self-care and newborn care.
- The social worker evaluates family support and provides community referrals, such as support groups for the adolescent mother.
- The lactation specialist assists her with initiating successful breastfeeding.
- The dietician provides her with information about her nutritional needs.

Nursing Care for the Woman Who Relinquishes Her Infant for Adoption

A woman who intends to relinquish or "give up" her baby for adoption usually arrives in the labor and delivery department with a birth plan. There are a variety of scenarios that may occur. The woman may want the adoptive parents present at the birth or want them called afterward. The mother may request to hold her infant only at delivery and then ask that the infant be kept in the nursery. She may not want to hold or see the infant at all. Some women choose to keep the infant in the room until the baby is turned over to the new parents or to the social worker at discharge. The nurse needs to respect and support the decisions the woman has made about her infant.

The nurse needs to provide empathetic care to the woman who relinquishes her infant for adoption. The nurse should avoid the phrase, "giving up the baby" and instead use the phrase "plan for adoption." The nurse should also encourage the patient to talk by using the following phrases:

• "What can I do to help you?"
• "Share with me your plan for the baby."
• "Tell me how you're feeling today."

Some women have arranged for an open adoption in which she selected the adoptive parents and will stay in contact with the adoptive parents, receiving pictures and updates as the child grows. Other women may choose a closed adoption, in which there is no identifying information between the mother and the adoptive parents. After the adoption is finalized, the records are sealed and may not be available until the child is 18 years old. If a woman decides to relinquish the infant and does not have a plan in place, the nurse should consult the hospital policy manual for the correct procedure for assisting the woman with her decision.

She will require the same physical care and self-care teaching as any postpartum patient. A woman who relinquishes her newborn will experience grief and loss. Women who relinquish their infants have a higher incidence of postpartum depression (Foli, Schweitzer, et al, 2013) and need to be educated about the signs and symptoms to report to her health-care provider. Appropriate referrals for counseling and support should also be part of the nursing care plan.

Preparation for Discharge

At discharge time, the new mother is too excited to focus on teaching. Ideally, teaching should occur in small segments and not be left until the patient is packed and ready to leave her room.

Preparing for discharge requires educating the patient about self-care. Written instructions should be provided along with the verbal teaching.

Self-care instructions should include the following information:

• The stitches used for lacerations and the episiotomy repair will dissolve over time.
• At first, the perineum may be sore and painful. Use acetaminophen and warm sitz baths to control pain.
• As the perineum heals, it is normal for itching to occur.
• Continue to change the peripad after each urination or defecation.
• Cleanse the perineum with warm water in the peri-bottle.
• Do not use tampons or douche until after the follow-up appointment with the obstetrician.
• Continue to wear a supportive bra as the breasts adjust to milk production.

• Wash hands before breastfeeding and after every diaper change.
• It is important to keep the 6-week follow-up appointment with the health-care provider to make sure that postpartum recovery is complete.
• Continue prenatal vitamins and iron until the 6-week follow-up appointment with the health-care provider.
• Exercise can be started according to the health-care provider. Walking and stretching is safe starting at 2 weeks postpartum. Vigorous exercise should be started after the 6-week checkup.
• Call the health-care provider if she experiences:
  • A fever of 38.0°C or greater
  • Increasing pain, redness, swelling, or discharge from a Cesarean incision or episiotomy
  • An increase in vaginal bleeding and a return to lochia rubra after transition to serosa or alba
  • An increase in vaginal bleeding and passing clots larger than a quarter
  • Foul lochia odor
  • Increasing abdominal pain or tenderness

Women usually have questions about sexual activity and contraception but may be too shy to ask. The nurse should introduce the topic in an open matter-of-fact manner that makes her comfortable to ask questions.

Most health-care providers believe that sexual intercourse can resume when bright red bleeding has ceased, the vagina and vulva are healed, and the woman is physically comfortable and emotionally ready (Spiliopoulos, 2013). The woman needs to be cautioned that ovulation may resume at any time and that she could become pregnant. Suggest that condoms be used until she can discuss birth control options with her health-care provider at the 6-week checkup.

HEALTH PROMOTION

Benefits of Exercise After Pregnancy

Exercise after pregnancy has many benefits, including:

• Restoring muscle tone, especially the abdominal muscles
• Aiding in weight loss if combined with reduced calorie intake
• Improving mood and relieving stress
• Improving cardiovascular fitness
• Allowing the new mother to take time for herself

SAFETY *STAT!*

Rh$_o$(D) immune globulin (RhoGAM) is administered intramuscularly (IM) within 72 hours of birth to prevent sensitization to the Rh factor in an Rh-negative woman with an infant who is Rh-positive. This injection will prevent hemolytic disease in subsequent pregnancies. Each vial of RhoGAM is crossmatched to a specific woman. The nurse must do all appropriate checks for patient identification to prevent an error in administration.

POSTPARTUM COMPLICATIONS

Pregnancy and childbirth are considered common events in life. Most women are healthy and their labor and delivery course is without incident. They spend a short time in the hospital and return home with the new baby, but complications can arise that can have harmful effects on the postpartum patient. It is important that the nurse be alert for signs of complications after childbirth and report them immediately to prevent life-threatening events.

Care of the Woman With Postpartum Hemorrhage

PPH is the leading cause of maternal mortality in the world (Smith, 2014). PPH is defined as a blood loss of more than 500 mL for a vaginal delivery and more than 1,000 mL for a Cesarean delivery. PPH that occurs during the first 24 hours after birth is called *early hemorrhage.* The most likely time for PPH is the first 4 hours after birth (Ward, 2015). Late hemorrhage occurs after 24 hours and before 6 weeks postpartum (Yiadom, 2014). Risk factors for PPH include:

- Obesity
- Retained placenta
- Failure to progress during the second stage of labor
- Placenta accreta
- Lacerations
- Large for gestational age (LGA) newborn
- Instrumental delivery
- Hypertensive disorders
- Induction of labor
- Augmentation of labor with oxytocin
- Overdistension of the uterus
- Previous PPH (Smith, 2014)

Many sources suggest the use of the Four Ts as a mnemonic to remember the causes of PPH: **t**one, **t**issue, **t**rauma, and **t**hrombosis (Smith, 2014, Cunningham, et al, 2014).

Tone

Uterine atony is the most common cause of PPH. The uterus loses tone when the muscles fail to contract after delivery of the placenta. When the muscles do not contract, the blood vessels that connected the placenta to the uterine muscle remain open, causing a rapid blood loss that can lead to hypovolemic shock. The uterine muscles may not contract because of fatigue caused by prolonged labor or forceful labor with oxytocin induction or augmentation. Sometimes, the uterine muscles may not respond and contract because they have been overstretched from distension from multiple fetuses or polyhydramnios (Smith, 2014, Cunningham, et al, 2014). A common cause of late PPH is **subinvolution,** which is the failure of the uterus to follow the pattern of normal involution; it remains large instead of returning to its pre-pregnancy size.

Tissue

After delivery of the fetus, the uterus contracts to release the placenta. If a portion of the placenta remains attached to the uterine wall, the uterus cannot compress the open vessels and control bleeding. Retained placental fragments are the most common cause of late PPH. Women with abnormal implantation of the placenta, such as placenta accreta and previa, are at high risk for retained tissue.

Trauma

Trauma to the uterus, cervix, and vagina can cause hemorrhage. Forceps delivery is the most common cause of cervical and vaginal lacerations. Lacerations can also occur from manipulation of a shoulder dystocia and by abnormal presentations of the fetus.

Thrombin

Immediately after the birth, disorders of coagulation and platelets do not result in excessive bleeding because of the work of the uterus in contracting and controlling bleeding (Smith, 2014). In the days afterward, fibrin deposits over the placental site, and clots within the vessels that supplied the placenta with blood flow are needed to control bleeding. Any pre-existing condition such as thrombocytopenia, underlying clotting disorder, or sepsis could interfere with clotting and cause a late PPH.

Signs and symptoms of PPH include:

- Peripad saturation in 15 min or less
- Heavy vaginal bleeding
- Constant trickling or oozing of blood from the vagina
- Uterine atony
- Passing of blood clots from the vagina larger than a quarter
- Return of lochia rubra after the lochia has progressed to serosa or alba
- Cool, clammy, pale skin
- Tachycardia and decreased blood pressure: late signs that may not change until a significant amount of blood is lost (Smith, 2014)

SAFETY *STAT!*

Rapid recognition of signs of PPH is essential for successful management. Routine nursing assessment and documentation of uterine tone, vaginal blood loss, and vital signs must be performed during the immediate postpartum period.

Care for the woman experiencing a PPH is a collaborative process of the health-care team. The nurse is usually the first person to identify excessive bleeding. Most obstetrical units have an emergency protocol for managing PPH, which may include notifying a rapid response team to assist during the crisis. Management for the woman experiencing PPH includes:

- A nurse stays with the patient and continues fundal massage with continual lower segment support, vital signs measurement, assessment of the patient's level of consciousness, and assessment of amount of vaginal bleeding.
- When excessive vaginal blood loss is observed, the nurse's initial action is to begin fundal massage. The

lower uterine segment is supported to prevent uterine prolapse. It is important **not** to express clots by over massage and by applying too much pressure on the uterus if it remains boggy. The clots may be providing pressure at the placental site and reducing blood loss.

- Another team member can notify the physician or nurse midwife of the suspected hemorrhage.
- Weigh peripads and linens on a gram scale to obtain an accurate measurement of the amount of blood lost.
- Assess the patient's bladder and, if distended, insert an indwelling Foley's catheter to empty the bladder and to assess urinary output and kidney status.
- Maintain or initiate IV fluids. Appropriate fluids are isotonic fluids, albumin, and packed red blood cells to maintain blood volume.
- Monitor oxygen saturation with a pulse oximeter and apply oxygen at 2 to 3 L via nasal cannula to increase red

blood cell saturation. If the PPH continues uncontrolled, increase the oxygen liter flow as needed to increase the oxygen saturation.

- Elevate the patient's legs to a 20- to 30-degree angle to improve venous blood return.
- Provide psychosocial support to the patient and her family.
- The health-care provider may order oxytocic drugs. See Table 14.1 for more information about these drugs.
- The health-care provider may perform a bimanual compression of the uterus by placing one hand on the abdomen and the other hand as a fist inside the vagina (Fig. 14.5).
- If massage, compression, and medications are not successful in slowing bleeding, the patient may be moved to the operating room for an invasive procedure to occlude the vessel with a clot, uterine artery ligation,

TABLE 14.1 MEDICATIONS FOR POSTPARTUM HEMORRHAGE

Medication	Action	Dose	Nursing Implications
Oxytocin (Pitocin)	Stimulates uterine smooth muscle to produce contractions. Also has a diuretic effect and vasopressor effect (ie, constriction of blood vessels and rise of blood pressure).	10–40 units in 1,000 mL of IV fluids infused at 20–40 milliunits per min or 10 units IM	• Infuse with pump for accurate infusion rate. • This drug can cause water intoxication. Monitor for signs and symptoms such as drowsiness, confusion, and headache. • Medicate for uterine cramping if needed.
Methylergonovine (Methergine)	Directly stimulates uterine and vascular smooth muscle.	0.1–0.2 mg IM, then oral 0.2 mg q4–6h × 24 hours	• This drug is not effective if the patient has hypocalcemia. • This medication is usually refrigerated and only stable at room temperature for 60 days. • Use only if clear, colorless, and has no precipitate.
Carboprost (Hemabate)	Stimulates the smooth muscle of the uterus and the gastrointestinal tract.	250 mcg deep IM, repeat prn q15–90min, no more than 2,000 mcg or eight doses	• This drug is used after oxytocin and/or methylergonovine have been tried to control PPH. • In addition to cramping, major side effects include nausea and vomiting. Consider an antiemetic if needed. • Keep refrigerated. • This medication is very expensive.
Misoprostol (Cytotec)	Acts as a prostaglandin analogue (similar to prostaglandin) to stimulate contractions.	400–1,000 mcg rectally	• This drug is effective to control PPH but is an off-label use, which means it is not marketed by the manufacturer for this purpose.

uterine packing, dilation and curettage (D&C), or a hysterectomy.

• If the health-care provider suspects laceration or retained placental fragments, the patient may be taken to the operating room for sedation and visualization of the vagina and uterus for repair, or for a D&C.

After the emergency is over, the team should debrief and discuss the management of care for this patient as a way to improve patient care in the future. The patient and her family should be encouraged to ask questions and express their feelings about the emergency. As soon as the woman is stabilized, she should be encouraged to resume bonding and breastfeeding.

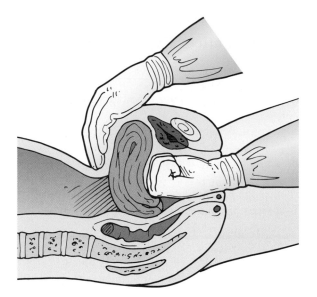

FIGURE 14.5 Bimanual compression.

LABS & DIAGNOSTICS

If a patient with PPH requires an emergency blood transfusion, O-negative blood is ordered while the laboratory completes a type and crossmatch of the patient's blood, and obtains the correct blood type and Rh. O-negative blood is the universal donor because it will not cause a blood transfusion reaction.

NURSING CARE PLAN for the Postpartum Patient Experiencing Hemorrhage

Nursing Diagnosis: The patient has a fluid volume deficit related to uterine atony and evidenced by vaginal bleeding
Expected Outcome: Stop excessive bleeding and improve fluid volume.
Interventions and Rationale:
1. Perform uterine fundal massage with one hand while the other hand supports the lower uterine segment. Uterine massage stimulates uterine contractions and correct hand placement prevents uterine prolapse.
2. Change peripads and weigh them on a gram scale to determine the amount of blood loss. Observing blood loss on a peripad is subjective. Weighing will give an accurate assessment of blood loss.
3. Monitor vital signs. Changes in vital signs are late signs of excessive blood loss, so the nurse needs to be alert to subtle changes.
4. Evaluate the urinary bladder. A full urinary bladder prevents uterine involution.
5. Infuse isotonic IV fluids per hospital protocol. Isotonic fluids will increase fluid volume.
6. Infuse oxytocic medications per the health-care provider's orders. Oxytocic medications such as oxytocin, methylergonovine, and carboprost (Hemabate) are effective in improving uterine muscle tone.

Nursing Diagnosis: Patient exhibits ineffective tissue perfusion related to vaginal bleeding.
Expected Outcome: Bring vital signs and blood gases within normal limits.
Interventions and Rationale:
1. Monitor vital signs and oxygen saturation levels every 5 to 10 min. Changes in tissue perfusion will cause changes in vital signs and oxygen saturation levels.
2. Note the discoloration of the nail, lip mucosa, gums, and tongue, and note the skin temperature. With blood being shunted to vital organs, vasoconstriction occurs in peripheral tissues, causing cyanosis and cold skin temperature.
3. Monitor blood gas levels and pH per hospital hemorrhage protocol; changes in blood gases and pH levels are a sign of tissue hypoxia.
4. Administer oxygen via nasal cannula to increase oxygen in the red blood cells.

Continued

NURSING CARE PLAN for the Postpartum Patient Experiencing Hemorrhage—cont'd

Nursing Diagnosis: The patient is experiencing anxiety and fear related to excessive blood loss and the threat of death.

Expected Outcome: The client can verbalize her anxiety; anxiety is under control for the patient.

Interventions and Rationale:

1. Assess the client's psychological response to the post-childbirth bleeding. The patient's perceptions of the situation influence the intensity of her anxiety.
2. Explain the treatments and rationale. Anxiety is reduced when the patient understands the treatment plan.
3. Remain calm, empathetic, and supportive. If the nurse is anxious, the patient will become more anxious.

Care of the Woman With a Hematoma

A hematoma is a collection of blood outside a blood vessel. The blood accumulates because the wall of an artery, vein, or capillary has been damaged and blood leaks into tissues surrounding the vessel. The hematoma can be small or large and can cause significant swelling and pain. During childbirth, there is pressure and trauma to the genital tract. Common locations for hematomas are in the vaginal wall or the vulvar area (Figs. 14.6 and 14.7). Risk factors for hematoma formation during or after childbirth are episiotomy, lacerations to the genital tract, delivery using forceps or vacuum extraction, nulliparity, and a difficult or prolonged second stage of labor. The signs and symptoms of a hematoma are:

- Constant pain and pressure in the vagina or rectal area
- Discoloration (ie, bruising) and bulging of the tissue
- Tenderness of the tissue
- A feeling of needing to defecate because of pressure on the rectum
- Inability to urinate because of pressure on the urethra
- Possible signs of shock if the hematoma is large

If the signs and symptoms indicate a possible hematoma, the nurse should carefully observe the perineal area by having the patient turn to her side and gently lift the buttock to inspect for swelling and discoloration. Any abnormal findings should be reported immediately to the health-care provider. Medical management of a hematoma includes:

- If the hematoma is less than 3 cm to 5 cm in size, ice is applied for 20 minutes every 2 hours for about 12 hours, then warm sitz baths are prescribed. The sitz bath will provide comfort and assist with reabsorption of the clot (Ward, 2013).
- Pain medication is ordered.
- If the hematoma is larger than 5 cm, the woman may be taken to the operating room for sedation so that the hematoma can be drained.
- If significant blood loss has occurred, the patient is managed as having a PPH.

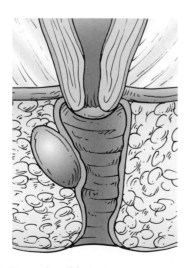

FIGURE 14.6 Vaginal wall hematoma.

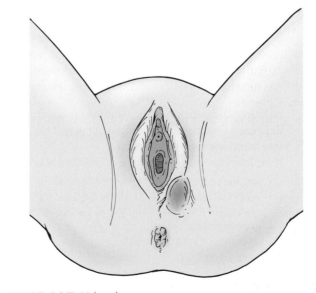

FIGURE 14.7 Vulvar hematoma.

Nursing care for the patient with a hematoma includes the following:

- Assessing pain and administering pain medication
- Applying an ice pack for 20 minutes, followed in 12 hours by a warm sitz bath
- If the hematoma is visible externally, frequently assessing it to determine if the hematoma is changing in size
- Monitoring vital signs for signs of shock
- Explaining each treatment and the rationale to the patient

Care of the Woman With a Uterine Infection

Women who experience a prolonged labor, experience a prolonged rupture of membranes, undergo internal monitoring, experience a Cesarean delivery, or have frequent vaginal infections are at risk for a uterine infection, also known as *endometritis.* Bacteria normally present in the vagina and cervix, such as *Escherichia coli* and group B streptococcus (GBS), can enter the uterus and infect the lining of the uterus after the rupture of membranes. The signs and symptoms of endometritis are:

- Elevated temperature greater than 38.3°C for 2 or more consecutive days
- Foul-smelling lochia
- Scanty, odorless lochia may be noted when the infection is caused by group A β-hemolytic streptococci (Wong, 2014).
- Lower abdominal tenderness on one or both sides of the abdomen

Medical management for endometritis may include:

- Pelvic examination to obtain specimens for culture
- Complete blood cell count (CBC)
- Blood cultures, if severe infection is suspected
- Pelvic ultrasound to detect retained placenta, abscess, or infected hematoma
- Administration of IV fluids and antibiotics (Wong, 2015); see Table 14.2 for information about commonly prescribed antibiotics for postpartum infections

Nursing care for the patient with endometritis includes the following:

- Administering IV fluids and antibiotics
- Administering pain medication and antipyretics for the fever as ordered
- Encouraging fluid intake
- Explaining each treatment and rationale to the patient
- Supporting her with bonding and breastfeeding

Care of the Woman With a Wound Infection

For the postpartum patient, wound infections can occur in the episiotomy incision, perineal lacerations, and in Cesarean incisions. Signs and symptoms of a wound infection for postpartum patients include:

- Redness
- Warmth
- Poor wound approximation
- Tenderness
- Pain
- Fever and malaise if wound is untreated (Derricott, 2013)

Medical management of a postpartum wound infection usually includes laboratory studies, such as a CBC and wound culture, and the administration of antibiotics.

Nursing care for the patient with a wound infection includes the following:

- Obtaining a wound culture if ordered
- Administering antibiotics as ordered
- Encouraging adequate fluid intake and protein intake to aid in healing
- Assessing for pain and medicating as ordered
- Teaching the patient proper hand washing to prevent the spread of bacteria

Care of the Woman With Urinary Tract Infection (UTI)

UTIs are common in the immediate postpartum phase. The urethra and bladder can be traumatized as the baby moves through the birth canal for delivery. Women who have a Foley's catheter during labor and women with prolonged labors are at higher risk for a UTI. The most common organisms causing a UTI are the normal bowel flora, including *E coli* and *Klebsiella, Proteus,* and *Enterobacter* species (Wong, 2011). Signs and symptoms of a UTI are:

- Urgency of urination
- Dysuria (ie, painful urination)
- Increased frequency of urination
- Urination of small amounts
- Fever
- Flank pain
- **Hematuria** (ie, blood in the urine)

Medical management for the patient with a UTI is largely based on patient symptoms. It may include a urine specimen sent to the laboratory for a urinalysis, culture and sensitivity test, and oral antibiotics. See Table 14.2 for more information about appropriate antibiotics.

Nursing care for the patient with a UTI includes the following:

- Administering antibiotics
- Encouraging fluid intake to assist with flushing the bacteria out of the urinary tract
- Teaching the patient to clean the perineum from front to back and to use the peri-bottle provided for cleaning after urination and defecation

HEALTH PROMOTION

Preventing a UTI is a priority during the postpartum period. Studies have shown that the placement of a urinary catheter for more than 2 days has been found to increase the risk of infection. Catheters should be removed as soon as possible after an epidural or Cesarean birth to prevent UTI infection in the postpartum patient (SUNA, 2014).

TABLE 14.2 ANTIBIOTICS FOR POSTPARTUM INFECTIONS

Antibiotic and Dosing	Infection Type	Nursing Implications
Cefoxitin (Mefoxin) 1 g every 6–8 hours IM or IV	Endometritis Wound	• Obtain a history of previous use of cephalosporins and allergic reactions to penicillins. • Observe the patient for signs and symptoms of allergic reaction, such as rash, shortness of breath, or wheezing, and report immediately. • Monitor bowel function. Immediately report diarrhea, abdominal pain, fever, or bloody stools.
Gentamicin (Garamycin) 1–2 mg/kg every 8 hours IV	Endometritis	• Obtain a history of allergies and a previous use of aminoglycosides. • Monitor for injury to the eighth cranial nerve, such as tinnitus and hearing loss. Report immediately.
Clindamycin (Cleocin) 300–600 mg every 6–8 hours IV	Endometritis Mastitis	• Obtain a history of previous allergies and use of clindamycin. • Monitor bowel function. Immediately report diarrhea, abdominal pain, fever, or bloody stools.
Dicloxacillin (Dynapen) 125–250 mg every 6 hours PO	Mastitis UTI	• Obtain a history of allergies and previous use of penicillins. • Monitor for the side effects of diarrhea, nausea, and vomiting.
Cephalexin (Keflex) 500 mg every 6 hours PO	Mastitis UTI Wound	• Obtain a history of allergies and the previous use of cephalosporins and penicillins. • Observe the patient for signs and symptoms of allergic reaction, such as rash, shortness of breath, or wheezing, and report immediately.
Cefazolin (Ancef) 500 mg–2 g every 6–8 hours IV	Wound	• Obtain a history of allergies and previous use of cephalosporins and penicillins. • Observe the patient for signs and symptoms of allergic reaction, such as rash, shortness of breath, or wheezing, and report immediately.
Ciprofloxacin (Cipro) 500–750 mg every 12 hours PO	UTI	• Obtain a history of allergies and previous use of fluoroquinolones. • Monitor bowel function. Immediately report diarrhea, abdominal pain, fever, or bloody stools.

Source: Vallerand, A. and Sanoski, C (2014) *Davis's Drug Guide.14th ed.* FA Davis: Philadelphia, PA

Care of the Woman With Mastitis

Mastitis is an infection of the breast tissue. The most common organism to cause mastitis is *Staphylococcus aureus,* which is transmitted from the breastfeeding infant's mouth or throat. *S aureus* is also present on the woman's hands. The bacteria can enter the mother's breast through cracked nipples caused by improper latch-on of the infant or by the mother touching her own breasts. Mastitis can also develop from blocked milk ducts and milk stasis, also caused by improper latch-on of the infant (Fig. 14.8) (Derricott, 2013). Mastitis usually occurs in one breast with a sudden onset of symptoms. Signs and symptoms of mastitis are:

• Red swollen area or mass in the breast
• Fever of 38.3°C or higher

• Pain or a burning sensation while breastfeeding
• Skin redness, often in a wedge-shaped pattern
• Malaise

Medical management for mastitis is based upon a breast examination and consideration of symptoms. The health-care provider will determine if a breast abscess has developed, which is a possible serious complication of mastitis. Antibiotics and pain relievers, such as acetaminophen or ibuprofen, are usually ordered.

Nursing care for the patient with mastitis includes the following:

• Teaching the mother to wash her hands before handling her breasts for breastfeeding
• Observing latch-on of her infant and teaching the correct method of latch-on

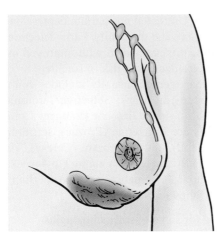

FIGURE 14.8 Mastitis usually occurs several weeks after childbirth. The axillary lymph nodes are enlarged and there is a warm, tender, hardened area on the affected breast.

- Teaching the woman to feed the infant regularly to decrease the risk of milk stasis and blocked milk ducts caused by engorgement
- Administering antibiotics as ordered
- Assessing pain and administering analgesics as ordered
- Reassuring the patient that she can continue to breastfeed while undergoing treatment
- Applying warmth to the breast to cause vasodilation and opening of the milk ducts
- Teaching every breastfeeding patient the signs of mastitis because it can happen anytime while a woman is breastfeeding

Care of the Woman With Postpartum Thromboembolic Disease

Thromboembolic disorders are the leading cause of maternal mortality in the United States (Springel, 2014). **Thromboembolism** is a condition in which the blood vessel becomes inflamed and a blood clot develops. A postpartum patient's risk for venous thromboembolism (VTE) is highest in the first 12 weeks after delivery. This is because of the pregnancy-related hypercoagulability caused by hormones, and by sluggish blood flow to the legs during pregnancy and delivery (MacReady, 2014; Hughes, 2014). The major causes of thrombosis are venous stasis, hypercoagulable blood, and injury to the endothelial surface of a blood vessel. A pregnant woman experiences compression of the large vessels in the leg and pelvis due to the weight of the uterus, causing venous stasis. During pregnancy, the fibrin levels are elevated, which can promote clot formation during pregnancy and during the postpartum recovery period. Blood vessels can be damaged by lower extremity trauma and prolonged labor and pushing. All of these factors that occur during pregnancy greatly increase the risk of thromboembolic disorders. About 1 in 1,000 pregnancies and deliveries are complicated by VTE. This condition includes deep vein thrombosis (DVT) and pulmonary embolism (PE).

A **thrombus** is a clot made up of platelets and fibrin that develops on a vessel wall. A thrombus can form whenever the flow of blood is impeded. The vessel wall becomes inflamed because of the presence of the thrombus, and this is termed *thrombophlebitis*. A DVT is a blood clot that develops in a deep vein of the leg or pelvic region. The clot can become dislodged from the vein and travel to the lungs, causing a PE. A PE leads to extreme respiratory distress and is frequently fatal.

Risk factors for VTE are:

- Obesity
- Prolonged bedrest
- Advanced maternal age
- Stillbirth
- Premature birth
- Gestational diabetes
- Cesarean delivery
- Multiparity
- Varicose veins
- Smoking (Waknine, 2013)

The nurse can prevent venous thromboembolic disorders by:

- Encouraging all postpartum patients to ambulate frequently
- Carefully assessing the legs for signs of thromboembolic problems and promptly reporting any abnormal assessment findings
- Identifying high-risk women and obtaining orders for compression stockings or sequential devices to prevent venous stasis

Signs and symptoms of VTE are:

- Swelling
- Pain or tenderness
- Erythema
- Pain on ambulation
- Stiffness of the leg
- Large, hard, cordlike vein
- No signs for some patients

To definitively diagnose a VTE, the health-care provider will usually order a Doppler ultrasound of the leg or pelvis to identify a clot. If the ultrasound is unclear, magnetic resonance imaging (MRI) is recommended (ACOG, 2014). Medical management of VTE includes:

- IV heparin therapy (Springel, 2014) is used until the international normalized ratio (INR) has been at therapeutic levels for 2 days followed by transition to oral warfarin (Coumadin) for at least 6 to 12 weeks postpartum.
- Low-molecular weight heparin, such as enoxaparin (Lovenox), may be used instead of heparin.
- Compression stockings are used to improve blood flow in the legs.
- The woman is placed on bedrest with the affected leg elevated.
- Analgesics may be prescribed to control pain.
- Moist heat may be applied to reduce pain and increase circulation.

LABS & DIAGNOSTICS

The prothrombin time (PT) and/or the INR should be monitored when the patient is receiving anticoagulant therapy. The desired PT with anticoagulant therapy is 1.5 to 2 times the control PT in sec. The desired INR is 2 to 3 (Venes, 2013).

Nursing care for the woman with thromboembolic disorders includes the following:

- Administering heparin or enoxaparin as ordered
- Monitoring the INR and PT and notifying the health-care provider of results
- Applying compression stockings correctly; improper application impedes blood flow, causing venous stasis
- Maintaining bedrest for the patient, with the affected leg elevated
- Administering analgesics as ordered
- Applying moist heat per hospital policy
- Monitoring for complications such as pulmonary emboli. The symptoms are shortness of breath, chest pain, and cough.

Care of the Woman With Postpartum Depression

Postpartum depression is more serious and incapacitating than postpartum blues. It can interfere with a woman's ability to care for herself and her newborn. Postpartum depression occurs in 10% to 15% of women and usually develops during the first 4 months postpartum but can occur anytime in the first year after childbirth (Joy, 2014).

Women at highest risk of developing postpartum depression are those with a personal history of depression or postpartum depression with a previous birth. Other risk factors that have been identified are recent stressful life events, lack of social support, unintended pregnancy, and financial factors (Joy, 2014).

Recognition of and prompt intervention for postpartum depression are important for maternal and infant well-being. Signs and symptoms of postpartum depression include:

- Intense sadness
- Anxiety
- Feelings of guilt or inadequacy
- Ambivalence toward the baby and family
- Lack of motivation for self-care or infant care
- **Anhedonia** (ie, lack of pleasure)
- Appetite disturbances
- Insomnia
- Fatigue
- Suicidal thoughts and preoccupation with death

Postpartum depression is usually first noticed by the patient's significant other and family. The health-care provider can use screening tools such as the Edinburgh Postnatal Depression Scale, a 10-item questionnaire used to detect postpartum depression. Postpartum depression can range from mild to severe. Untreated postpartum depression affects the mother, the infant, and the family. Early detection and initiation of treatment is associated with improved mother-baby attachment and a decreased risk of suicide.

Medical management usually includes counseling and antidepressant medications. Selective serotonin reuptake inhibitors (SSRIs) are the first-line treatment. Commonly prescribed SSRIs are fluoxetine (Prozac), sertraline (Zoloft), paroxetine (Paxil), and citalopram (Celexa). The patient's symptoms usually start improving in 2 to 4 weeks.

Nursing care for the patient with postpartum depression includes the following:

- Monitoring for signs of suicidal thoughts
- Encouraging compliance in taking antidepressant medications
- Encouraging follow-up visits with her health-care provider
- Encouraging the patient to seek counseling
- Advising the patient to get rest and nap when the baby sleeps
- Making referrals to community agencies such as depression support groups
- Encouraging the patient to verbalize her feelings and reinforce her personal power and autonomy (Joy, 2014)

Care of the Woman With a Postpartum Psychiatric Disorder

Postpartum psychosis is the most severe form of postpartum psychiatric illness. Psychosis causes the patient to lose touch with reality and inaccurately perceive the environment. It occurs in 1 to 2 per 1,000 postpartum women. The women at highest risk for postpartum psychosis have a history of bipolar illness or a previous episode of postpartum psychosis. This disorder typically has an abrupt onset within 48 to 72 hours of birth. Most women manifest signs and symptoms by 2 weeks postpartum (Joy, 2014). Signs and symptoms of postpartum psychosis are:

- Restlessness
- Insomnia
- Irritability
- Incoherent conversations
- Rapidly shifting mood from depression to elation
- Delusional beliefs that may relate to the infant; for example, she may think the baby is better off dead
- Auditory hallucinations that may tell her to harm herself or the infant

Postpartum psychosis is a medical emergency and requires hospitalization. The woman needs to be admitted to an in-patient psychiatric facility to begin mood stabilizers, antipsychotic medications, and psychotherapy.

Nursing care for the woman experiencing postpartum psychosis includes the following:

- Immediately reporting any abnormal psychiatric symptoms to the health-care provider
- Reorienting the patient to her surroundings

- Providing for safety for the patient and her baby
- Arranging for admission to a psychiatric facility
- Providing emotional support for the patient and her family

SAFETY *STAT!*

If a woman is suspected of experiencing postpartum psychosis, she should never be left alone with her infant. She may harm the infant while in the acute stages of her illness.

CULTURAL CONSIDERATIONS

The Chinese cultural practice of a lying-in period is practiced by some Chinese women. During this time, they rest in bed in a warm, draft-free room for a month. The body is considered to be weak and susceptible to illness. The new mother is encouraged to avoid bathing and exercise. Traditional Chinese believe that the woman who does not practice the lying-in month will experience aches, pains, and arthritis in old age (Galanti, 2015).

Key Points

- In the first hour after birth, it is critical that the nurse carefully monitor the patient for signs of PPH by assessing uterine involution and the amount of lochia.
- Postpartum assessment can be organized with the mnemonic BUBBLE LE, which stands for **b**reasts, **u**terus, **b**ladder, **b**owels, **l**ochia, **e**pisiotomy/laceration, **l**egs, and **e**motions.
- The woman who experiences a Cesarean birth requires the usual postpartum care, along with postoperative care to manage pain and prevent postoperative complications such as atelectasis and thrombophlebitis.
- The postpartum adolescent patient will require positive reinforcement for her attempts at taking on the mother role, and teaching to prepare her for newborn care.
- Nurses need to provide sensitive and empathetic care to the postpartum patient who plans to relinquish her newborn for adoption.
- All discharged postpartum patients should be provided with guidelines for recognizing complications and knowing when to call the health-care provider.
- PPH is an emergency. The nurse should recognize early signs and notify the health-care provider for assistance.

- PPH is usually caused by one of the Four Ts: **t**one, **t**issue, **t**rauma, and **t**hrombin.
- A hematoma is a collection of blood outside a blood vessel. In the postpartum patient, it is usually caused by the trauma of birthing. It can cause significant pain.
- A postpartum infection can occur in the uterus, incisions, bladder, or breasts. Any signs or symptoms of an infection should be reported immediately.
- Preventing thrombophlebitis is important in the postpartum patient. It can be a serious complication that results in death from a PE. Pain, redness, and swelling of the leg must be reported immediately to the health-care provider.
- Postpartum depression can be debilitating. The patient and her family should be taught the signs and symptoms so that they can be identified early and reported to the health-care provider.
- Postpartum psychosis is an emergency situation. Safety for the mother and newborn is the focus of care until the patient can be hospitalized and treated.

REVIEW QUESTIONS

1. A patient delivered a 9-pound infant 1 hour ago. She had a forceps delivery and has just been transferred to postpartum care. She puts on her call light and complains of severe rectal pain and pressure. The patient is exhibiting signs of:
   1. PPH
   2. Postpartum hematoma
   3. Postpartum blues
   4. Postpartum cramping

2. A postpartum patient states that she had postpartum depression with her first baby 3 years ago. The best response by the nurse is:
   1. "It will probably not happen again."
   2. "Don't worry about that."
   3. "Have you mentioned this to your nurse midwife?"
   4. "Were you hospitalized last time?"

3. A postpartum focal assessment includes the following: *(select all that apply)*
   1. Neurological assessment
   2. Uterine assessment
   3. Episiotomy assessment
   4. Respiratory assessment
   5. Breast assessment
   6. Bowel assessment

4. Which patient is at the highest risk to develop a postpartum infection?
   1. The patient who had a 23-hour labor
   2. The patient who delivered a 10-pound infant
   3. The patient who delivered her fifth child
   4. The patient who plans to bottle feed

5. A patient has developed mastitis. Which statement indicates that further teaching is needed?
   1. "I need to completely finish the antibiotics."
   2. "I need extra rest and fluids while on the antibiotics."
   3. "I must limit the time I feed on the infected breast."
   4. "I need to wash my hands before I breastfeed."

6. When observing the legs during the postpartum assessment, the nurse is looking for:
   1. Bruising from pushing
   2. Calf tenderness
   3. Range of motion
   4. Signs of infection

7. A woman calls the postpartum unit 2 weeks after discharge. She reports that her lochia has suddenly become heavier and she is passing bright red clots. The nurse should:
   1. Advise her to rest and call back if the bleeding does not slow down.
   2. Reassure her that it is the normal progression of lochia.
   3. Suggest that she eat a diet high in iron since she is losing more blood.
   4. Advise her to call her health-care provider.

8. During the postpartum focal assessment, the nurse notes that the patient has a fever of 38.9°C and foul-smelling lochia. The nurse reports the findings to the health-care provider. The nurse expects the health-care provider to order: *(select all that apply)*
   1. Methylergonovine (Methergine 0.2 mg IM)
   2. Gentamicin (Garamycin) 1 to 2 mg/kg every 8 hours IV
   3. A culture of the lochia to be sent to the laboratory
   4. Strict isolation of the mother
   5. Pelvic ultrasound
   6. CBC

9. A patient who had a Cesarean birth is 3 days postpartum. She reports to the nurse that she gets a sudden urge to urinate and has to hurry to the bathroom and then is only able to urinate a small amount. The nurse should:
   1. Report the symptoms.
   2. Reassure the patient that it is normal.
   3. Insert a Foley's catheter.
   4. Place a bedside commode near her bed to make it easier for her.

10. A man calls the postpartum unit and says, "My wife had a baby 5 days ago. Today she started crying over nothing! I can't seem to do anything right today. Is this normal? I'm a little worried." The nurse should:
    1. Advise him to call the health-care provider immediately.
    2. Reassure him that it is normal but if she continues to be sad for several days to call the health-care provider.
    3. Tell him to stop worrying.
    4. Advise him to stop any behaviors that may be causing her to be upset.

CRITICAL THINKING QUESTIONS

1. What is the nurse looking for when assessing the fundus in a postpartum patient?
2. What is the cause of sluggish bowels in the postpartum patient and what are appropriate nursing interventions?
3. Why are pregnant women and postpartum women predisposed to develop venous thrombosis?

DavisPlus

For additional resources and information, visit **www.DavisPlus.com.** Post-Conference Questions and Activities, Answers, and References can be found on Davis*Plus*.

unit FIVE

The Newborn

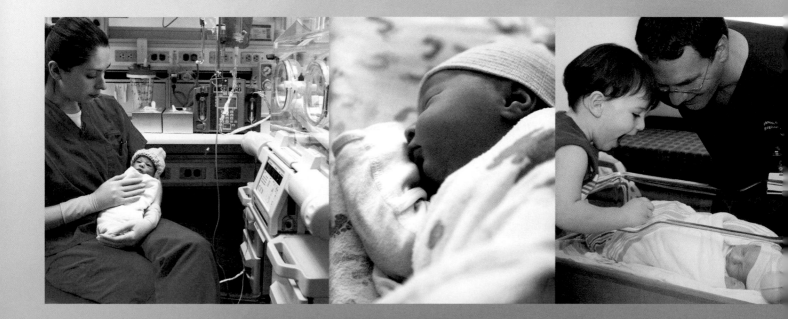

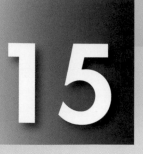

Physiological and Behavioral Adaptations of the Newborn

KEY TERMS

bilirubin
brown fat
catecholamines
conduction
convection
direct or conjugated bilirubin
evaporation
glycogen
hypothermia
indirect or unconjugated bilirubin
jaundice
probiotics
radiation
surfactant

DavisPlus For audio pronunciation guide, visit www.DavisPlus.com

CHAPTER CONCEPTS

Assessment
Oxygenation
Pregnancy
Sleep, Rest, and Activity
Thermo-regulation

LEARNING OUTCOMES

1. Define the key terms.
2. Identify ways in which heat loss occurs in infants.
3. Describe how infants can produce body heat.
4. List nursing interventions that support thermoregulation in the newborn.
5. Discuss the role of external and internal stimuli in the initiation of breathing in the newborn.
6. Identify the changes that occur as fetal circulation transitions into newborn circulation after birth.
7. Plan appropriate nursing interventions to assist with the transitions of the renal and gastrointestinal systems after birth.
8. Discuss the role of the liver in conjugating bilirubin.
9. Differentiate between unconjugated and conjugated bilirubin.
10. Define normal physiological jaundice.
11. Provide family-centered care by teaching parents about the behavioral changes and wake-sleep cycles of the newborn.

REAL-WORLD CASE STUDY

Paloma

■ Paloma, aged 18, delivered her new daughter 3 hours ago. The nurse walks into her postpartum room and observes that Paloma is sitting upright on her bed with her legs folded and her newborn baby girl lying on the bed in front of her. The blanket and cap are off the baby and she is dressed in a T-shirt and diaper only. Paloma is obviously happy about the baby and states to the nurse,

"I'm just checking out her fingers and toes again. She is so precious."

1. What concerns should the nurse have regarding these observations in Paloma's room?
2. What mechanisms of heat loss could the newborn be experiencing?
3. What nursing interventions are appropriate for this situation?

CONCEPTUAL CORNERSTONE

Thermoregulation

Thermoregulation is the ability for the human body to regulate body temperature at a constant value. Although all humans can be at risk for alterations in thermoregulation, infants have a significantly greater risk for **hypothermia**, which is a body temperature below normal. Babies are born with an under-developed temperature regulation capacity. Infants can produce heat but lack the ability to conserve heat because of a large surface area relative to body mass and limited subcutaneous fat to insulate. Premature and low birth weight (LBW) babies are at even higher risk for hypothermia, which can lead to cold stress. Hypothermia in the newborn is preventable by reducing risks. The nurse needs to be vigilant about monitoring the environment and the body temperature of the newborn, and provide appropriate interventions to maintain a stable body temperature for the newborn.

Immediately after birth, the newborn begins critical adaptations to extrauterine life. All organ systems are involved at some level but the most significant adaptations are in the respiratory and cardiovascular systems. Newborns also experience behavioral transitions after birth. The nurse can assist the parents to become more comfortable meeting the needs of their infant by educating them about the behavioral transitions. This chapter discusses the physiological adaptations made by the newborn and nursing interventions that support the newborn in this transitional phase. Behavioral adaptations of the newborn are also discussed, along with patient teaching guidelines to assist the parents with understanding newborn behavioral adaptation.

PHYSIOLOGICAL ADAPTATIONS

The transition to extrauterine life actually begins before birth. The fetus prepares for extrauterine life through the following:

- The fetal lungs develop and mature during the last trimester to support gas exchange at birth. **Surfactant,** a mixture of phospholipids and lipoproteins, is produced in the lung cells. The production of surfactant begins at

34 weeks' gestation. It is important for the newborn because it prevents the alveoli from sticking together when the newborn takes the first few breaths and makes it easier for gas exchange to occur in the lungs.
- **Brown fat** is a body fat that is used by infants to regulate body temperature. An infant does not shiver to raise his body temperature; he or she burns brown fat instead. The main function of brown fat is to protect the infant from hypothermia. It is deposited during the last few weeks of gestation. Brown fat is located in the scapular area, the thorax, and behind the kidneys (Fig. 15.1).
- Glucose is stored in the liver as **glycogen** to provide an energy source for the newborn at birth.
- During labor, the fetal adrenal glands are stimulated to produce **catecholamines,** which are hormones. The hormones produced by the fetal adrenal glands are dopamine, norepinephrine, and epinephrine. These hormones help the newborn by causing an increase in the level of surfactant in the fetal lungs; increasing blood flow to the heart, lungs, and brain; increasing energy; and stimulating white blood cell production in the immune system (Hillman, Kallapur, et al, 2012).

Immediately after birth is a time of significant physiological adaptation for the baby. Physiologically, the infant must adapt from being dependent on the placenta for oxygen and nutrients to independent functioning. Practically every body system undergoes transition at birth, with the most significant changes requiring the successful initiation of respiratory function, cardiovascular function, and thermoregulation.

SAFETY *STAT!*

Before the baby is delivered, it is extremely important for the nurse to identify infants who may need support for the initial transition to extrauterine life. Infants who may need assistance with transition include premature infants, infants with a non-reassuring fetal heart rate pattern in labor, infants with shoulder dystocia, those who went through assistive deliveries, and those with the presence of meconium. This will help prevent delay in an infant receiving supportive and resuscitative interventions and will help improve the outcome.

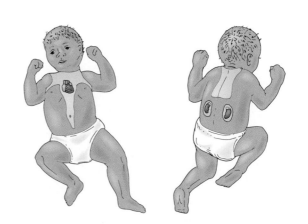

FIGURE 15.1 Sites of brown fat stores in the newborn.

Thermoregulation System

The temperature of a newborn is about 37.2°C at birth because of the warm environment of the uterus. The infant begins to lose heat immediately after birth through four mechanisms:

- **Evaporation** is the loss of heat as the amniotic fluid on the infant evaporates (Fig. 15.2A).
- **Conduction** is the transfer of heat from the infant's body to cooler surfaces, such as towels or the cold base of a warming unit (Fig. 15.2B).
- **Convection** is the transfer of the infant's body heat to the surrounding cool air (Fig. 15.2C).
- **Radiation** is the transfer of the infant's body heat to a cooler object that the infant is not in contact with, such as a window (Fig. 15.2D).

The newborn's thermoregulation system is immature and it is difficult for a newborn to conserve heat. It can take up to 4 hours for a newborn's temperature to stabilize. The newborn has a large skin surface area to body weight ratio, which increases heat loss. Infants do not have subcutaneous fat to provide insulation and the blood vessels are close to the surface, so they have to rely on brown fat to provide additional heat if needed. Preterm infants may have no brown fat to assist with temperature regulation. To produce heat, the infant begins to metabolize the brown fat, also known as *nonshivering thermogenesis.* The infant's body constricts blood vessels in the skin and the deeper vessels pick up heat from the metabolized brown fat to warm the body. The brown fat reserves can be quickly depleted if the newborn experiences prolonged cold stress. When this happens, brown fat breaks down into fatty acids, which can lead to metabolic acidosis in the newborn (Keehn and Lieben, 2014).

Newborns can also attempt to raise their body temperature by crying and by kicking, but will quickly become fatigued from this effort (Hillman, Kallapur, et al, 2012).

Careful attention needs to be paid to the thermal environment of the newborn until the infant is able to regulate body temperature. The prevention of cold stress is a priority. As the infant tries to increase body temperature, an increase in the metabolic rate occurs. The consequences of an increased metabolic rate in the cold newborn are:

- An increased need for oxygen
- A decrease in surfactant production
- An increase in the use of stored glycogen, which can lead to hypoglycemia
- Rapid metabolism of brown fat, leading to metabolic acidosis

Nursing interventions for assisting the newborn's thermoregulation transition include the following:

- Drying the infant immediately after birth and removing the wet towels
- Placing the infant skin-to-skin with the mother as soon as possible
- Covering the head with a hat as soon as possible
- Monitoring the newborn's temperature every 15 min for the first hour
- Avoiding uncovering or exposing the infant's entire body for procedures
- If unable to maintain skin-to-skin contact with the mother, placing the infant under a pre-heated radiant warmer for procedures
- Not bathing the newborn until the temperature has been stable for at least 2 hours
- Not placing the baby's crib near a draft or a window (Phillips, 2013)

HEALTH PROMOTION

Preventing Conductive Heat Loss

Conductive heat loss can be prevented by:

- Prewarming objects that come into contact with the infant, such as the mattress, towels, stethoscope, and blankets
- Placing a prewarmed blanket on the scale before weighing the infant

---

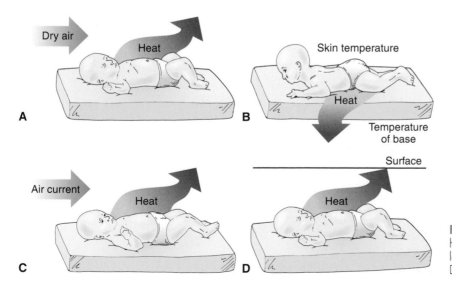

FIGURE 15.2 A, Evaporation mechanism of heat loss. B, Conduction mechanism of heat loss. C, Convection mechanism of heat loss. D, Radiation mechanism of heat loss.

SAFETY *STAT!*

Do not overheat surfaces or place the infant on a surface hotter than skin temperature. Heat blankets in a temperature-controlled blanket warmer only.

 ## CULTURAL CONSIDERATIONS

Traditional Latino health theories are related to cold and heat. Cold can sometimes cause illness by chilling the body and hot can cause illness by heating the body. Babies at birth do have trouble with body temperature regulation for a few days, but after that they can usually maintain body temperature without overwrapping. Parents need to be cautioned that overdressing or bundling the newborn excessively can make the baby uncomfortable and cause problems such as heat rash. In addition, overdressing a baby while sleeping has been linked to a higher risk of sudden infant death syndrome (Alcaniz, 2011).

Respiratory System

While in the uterus, the fetus receives its oxygen through the umbilical cord. The fetal circulation picks up oxygen from the placenta with the umbilical vein and transports the oxygenated blood to the fetal heart. Most blood bypasses the lungs because the placenta is supplying oxygen to the fetus instead of the lungs. In the uterus, the fetal lungs are full of fluid. When the infant is born, a sequence of events must happen in order for the infant to breathe, including internal and external stimuli. The internal stimuli are chemically focused and the external stimuli are related to mechanical, sensory, and thermal changes in the newborn's body.

First, the external stimuli begin as the fetus moves through the birth canal. Pressure on the chest causes the lung secretions and amniotic fluid inside the lungs to be squeezed out through the airway. Next, when the chest fully emerges from the birth canal, the chest re-expands or recoils, causing an intake of air to fill the lungs. The first few breaths are critical: the lungs are adjusting to pressure changes from intrauterine to outside the mother's body; there is increased blood flow to the lungs; and the first breaths are forcing the alveoli to open. Surfactant secretion increases to keep the alveoli open after the first few initial breaths (Hillman, Kallapur, et al, 2012).

After the first few breaths, breathing is easier for the infant. As the infant is dried vigorously, sensors in the skin are stimulated, which further encourages the respiratory center to begin the first sequences of breathing.

The internal stimuli are the chemical factors that influence the newborn to breathe. After the umbilical cord is cut, the newborn will experience a decrease in oxygen concentration, an increase in carbon dioxide, and a drop in the pH in the blood, triggering the medulla to stimulate the respiratory center in the brain to begin functioning (Fig. 15.3) (Posner, Dy, et al, 2013).

Nursing interventions for assisting the newborn with the respiratory transition after birth include the following:

- Counting the respirations per minute
- Suctioning the mouth and nose with the bulb syringe to clear mucus
- Monitoring the respiratory effort
- Observing the abdomen because newborn breathing involves the use of the diaphragm and abdominal muscles

SAFETY *STAT!*

Allowing the newborn short bursts of crying will increase the depth of respirations and aid in opening the alveoli at birth. However, prolonged crying is not safe for the newborn because it will tire the infant and force the infant's body to use up stored glycogen for energy.

NURSING CARE PLAN for Regulating the Newborn's Body Temperature

Nursing Diagnosis: The newborn has a risk for imbalanced body temperature related to a large surface area in relationship to mass and lack of subcutaneous fat for insulation.

Expected Outcome: The newborn's axillary body temperature will remain in the normal range of 36.5°C to 37.2°C.

Nursing Interventions:
- Monitor body temperature frequently to identify abnormalities and implement interventions.
- Keep the baby wrapped appropriately with a blanket if not skin-to-skin with the mother.
- Keep the head covered with a cap.
- Do not place the infant's crib near a draft or a window.
- Bathe the newborn when the temperature is stable. Do not uncover the entire body for the bath. Wash the newborn in sections and dry thoroughly.
- Teach the parents to keep the newborn covered appropriately.

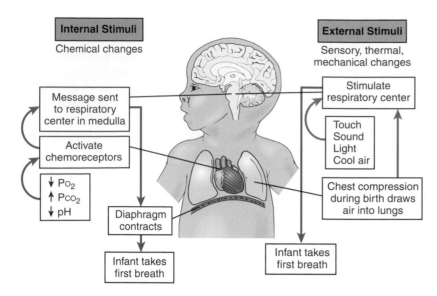

FIGURE 15.3 Chemical, sensory, thermal, and mechanical factors involved in the initiation of respirations. Pco_2, partial pressure of carbon dioxide; Po_2, partial pressure of oxygen.

Cardiovascular System

After the newborn starts breathing and the umbilical cord is cut, changes occur in blood flow, pressure, and volume within the heart. The fetal circulation is no longer effective and blood flows in a new route (Fig. 15.4). See Table 15.1 for circulation changes that occur during newborn transition.

A newborn's blood volume is 80 to 110 mL/kg and a newborn has more red blood cells than the average adult. The blood cells provided extra oxygenation for the stress of labor.

A newborn's hemoglobin averages 17 to 18 g/100 mL of blood and the hematocrit is between 45% and 50%.

After the stress of labor has passed and oxygenation through the lungs is established, the large number of red blood cells is not needed by the newborn. Within days, the extra red blood cells begin to break down. As they are broken down, **bilirubin,** the waste product of the breakdown of the red blood cells, is released and the serum indirect bilirubin level rises.

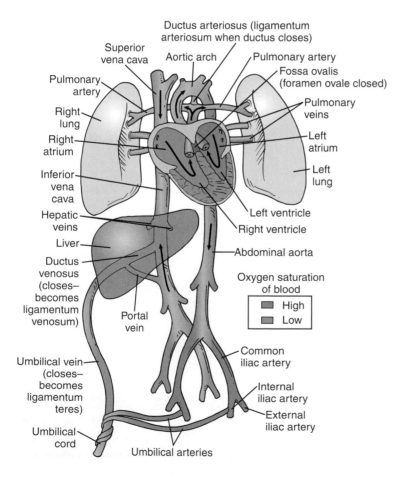

FIGURE 15.4 Neonatal circulation.

TABLE 15.1 CARDIOVASCULAR CHANGES AFTER BIRTH

Fetal Circulation	Postbirth Status
Pulmonary Circulation	
• Decreased blood flow through the lungs	• Increased blood flow through the lungs
Systemic Circulation	
• Higher pressure in the right ventricle	• Decreased pressure in the right ventricle
• Lower pressures in the left atrium, left ventricle, and aorta	• Increased pressure in the left atrium, left ventricle, and aorta
Ductus Arteriosus	
• Allows blood to bypass the fluid-filled lungs by shunting blood from the pulmonary artery to the aorta	• Closes almost immediately after birth or may remain open or partially open for up to 15 hours after birth to allow increased blood flow to the lungs to permit oxygenation
	• May remain open if the lungs fail to expand
	• Anatomical obliteration within 1–3 months
Ductus Venosus	
• Shunts a portion of the left umbilical vein blood flow to the inferior vena cava, allowing blood to bypass the liver	• When the cord is clamped and blood flow is stopped, it closes completely by day 3 and forms a ligament.
Foramen Ovale	
• An opening that allows blood to flow directly to the right atrium and bypass the lungs	• Functionally closes at birth when increased pressure in the left atrium and decreased pressure in the right atrium occurs
	• Constant circulation leads to permanent closure within a few months
Umbilical Arteries	
• Carry deoxygenated blood from the hypogastric arteries to the placenta	• Blood flow disrupted when the umbilical cord is cut
	• Closed within hours of birth and permanently gone by 2–3 months
Umbilical Vein	
• Carries blood from the placenta, ductus venosus, and liver to the inferior vena cava	• Closed when the umbilical cord is cut and eventually forms a ligament

Sources: Hillman NH, Kallapur SG, & Jobe AH. (2012). Physiology of transition from intrauterine to extrauterine life. *Clinical Perinatology* 39:769-783; Keehn NF & Lieben K. (2014). *Newborn assessment*. Retrieved from NetCE at http://www.NetCE.com

The normal term newborn also has an elevated white blood cell count, ranging from 15,000 to 30,000 cells/mm³. An elevated white blood cell count in a newborn does not reflect infection but does reflect how stressful the birth was for the infant.

Newborns have a diminished ability to clot blood because of the absence of vitamin K. Vitamin K is essential for the formation of factor II (ie, prothrombin), factor VII (ie, proconvertin), factor IX (ie, plasma thromboplastin component), and factor X (ie, Stuart-Prower factor) in the clotting sequence. Vitamin K is synthesized in the intestines. A newborn has a sterile intestine at birth and does not have enough intestinal flora to synthesize vitamin K until about 24 hours after birth.

Nursing interventions for assisting the newborn with the cardiovascular transition after birth include the following:

• Monitor the heart rate immediately after birth. If less than 100 bpm, stimulate the baby to breathe. If ineffective in

increasing the heart rate, use positive pressure ventilation with room air at a low pressure to increase oxygenation, which will increase the heart rate.

• Begin chest compressions if the heart rate is below 60 bpm.
  When beginning chest compressions, monitor the color of the trunk and mucous membranes, and the capillary refill time of the trunk. Keep in mind that the normal newborn may have decreased peripheral circulation and bluish hands and feet (Goodling and McClead, 2015).

Renal System

The kidneys of the newborn are immature at birth and do not concentrate urine well until the baby is about 6 weeks old. The urine of a newborn will be odorless and a light color or clear. The newborn should void within 24 hours of birth with a volume of about 15 mL. For the first 2 days of life, the total daily output should be about 30 to 60 mL. As the newborn ingests more breastmilk or formula, the volume should rise to 300 mL per day.

Nursing interventions for assisting the newborn with the renal transition after birth include the following:

- Monitoring the first void
- Weighing diapers if concerned about urinary output
- Encouraging frequent breastfeeding to increase fluid intake and therefore urine output

PATIENT TEACHING GUIDELINES

Parents do not have a way to measure urine output except by diaper count. They should be instructed to expect the number of wet diapers per day to equal the age of the baby for the first week. For example, a 2-day-old baby should have a minimum of two wet diapers. A 3-day-old baby should have a minimum of three wet diapers. By the end of the week, most breastfeeding mothers have a good milk supply and the wet diaper count should be six to eight per day.

Gastrointestinal System

The newborn's gastrointestinal tract is sterile at birth, but bacteria begin entering the mouth shortly after birth through vaginal secretions, hospital linens, and contact at the breast. These bacteria become **probiotics,** intestinal bacteria that aid in digestion and synthesize vitamin K.

The capacity of the newborn stomach is about 60 to 90 mL. The pancreas is immature in the newborn; the enzymes lipase and amylase, which help to digest fat and starch, are deficient for the first few months of life. In addition, the cardiac sphincter between the esophagus and stomach is weak, which allows the infant to regurgitate easily.

The meconium stool, which is composed of sticky, blackish green material made from mucus, vernix, lanugo, hormones, and carbohydrates that accumulated in the bowel during fetal development, should be expelled within 24 to 48 hours of birth (Norwitz, 2013).

Nursing interventions for assisting the newborn with the gastrointestinal transition after birth include the following:

- Monitoring for the meconium stool and reporting if not expelled within 24 hours
- Teaching parents not to overfeed the newborn
- Teaching parents about the immature cardiac sphincter and regurgitation

THERAPEUTIC COMMUNICATION

The nurse observes a mother bottle feeding her 1-day-old infant. The infant is showing no interest in the feeding and is taking his mouth off the bottle nipple. The nurse notices that the mother is trying to force-feed the infant to finish off the bottle of formula. Using therapeutic communication, the nurse discusses newborn feeding with the mother.

Nurse: "It looks like your little guy is done eating."

Mother: "But he hasn't finished. I want him to get enough to eat."

Nurse: "Actually, it looks like he has taken in about an ounce. That's about all his tiny stomach can hold today."

Mother: "Really? That's not much."

Nurse: "Yes, he can hold about an ounce or a tiny bit more. Every day his stomach gets a little bigger. He will give you cues when he is hungry or done eating. Sometimes overfeeding makes babies spit up even more. If he wakes up and acts hungry, offer him more."

Hepatic System

At birth, the liver stores glycogen and iron. It is immature and does not detoxify medications or break down bilirubin from red blood cells efficiently at birth. Extra red blood cells that were necessary to provide extra oxygenation during the stress of birth begin to break down within days of birth. The liver's job is to take this **indirect or unconjugated bilirubin** that causes the yellow discoloration of the skin (ie, **jaundice**) out of the system.

During the conjugation process, the liver changes the yellow pigment from the breakdown of the red blood cell into a water-soluble pigment that can be excreted by the body. The removal of unconjugated bilirubin begins when phagocytes remove old red blood cells from the circulation. As the red blood cells break down, heme, the oxygen-carrying component of hemoglobin, is broken down into iron, carbon monoxide, and biliverdin. The biliverdin is broken down further into bilirubin. The bilirubin attaches to albumin in the blood and travels to the liver. In the liver, an enzyme called glucuronyl transferase acts upon the bilirubin to change it into a water-soluble pigment called **direct or conjugated bilirubin,** which is excreted into the common duct and duodenum. Once the direct bilirubin is in the intestine, the normal intestinal flora reduces the direct or conjugated bilirubin into urobilinogen and stercobilinogen. These are excreted mainly in the stool, causing the yellowish brown color of the stool, but a small amount is excreted in the urine (Fig. 15.5). Because the newborn liver is immature and the number of unneeded red blood cells is large, the job of breaking down and removing the bilirubin is not accomplished efficiently, causing a large number of babies to develop a normal physiological jaundice by day 2 to 4 (Tharp, Farley, et al, 2013).

Nursing interventions for assisting the newborn with the hepatic transition after birth include the following:

- Monitoring for yellow sclera and skin and reporting findings
- Teaching the parents about normal physiological jaundice

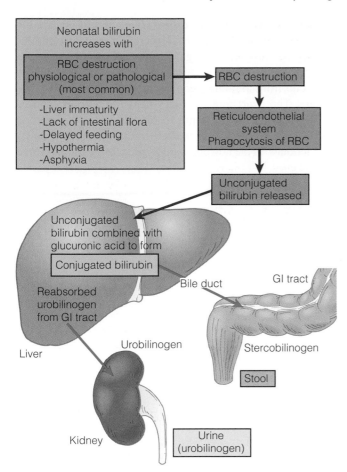

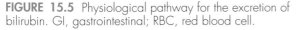

FIGURE 15.5 Physiological pathway for the excretion of bilirubin. GI, gastrointestinal; RBC, red blood cell.

LABS & DIAGNOSTICS

The bilirubin and bilirubin fractions laboratory test is also known as the *conjugated/direct bilirubin, unconjugated/indirect bilirubin test*. This test provides the health-care providers with the level of bilirubin in the newborn's body. An expected range for a newborn is less than 5.8 mg/dL total bilirubin. However, the total bilirubin level will rise and should peak by day 5 but should be below 11.7 mg/dL to be considered normal physiological jaundice. Elevated levels must be reported (Van Leeuwen and Bladh, 2015).

SAFETY *STAT!*

The appearance of jaundice before 24 hours of life indicates an abnormally rapid destruction of red blood cells and could indicate an ill newborn.

 LEARN TO C.U.S.

The nurse is assessing a 2-hour-old infant and notices a faint yellow tint to the skin. Knowing that normal physiological jaundice is not visible until days 2 to 4, the nurse is concerned and calls the pediatrician, using the C.U.S. method of communication.

Nurse: "Hello doctor, I am calling because I am **concerned** about baby Ramirez. I noticed that his skin is slightly yellow and I am **uncomfortable** waiting for you to make rounds later today to see the infant. I feel like we have a patient **safety** problem. He could be sick. Can I order a bilirubin test?"

Immune System

The newborn is born with passive antibodies (ie, immunoglobulin G) passed to him or her from the mother through the placenta. The newborn is protected by the mother from polio, measles, diphtheria, pertussis, chicken pox, rubella, and tetanus. This passive immunity from the mother protects the infant for 2 to 4 months (Waaijenborg, et al, 2013). A newborn cannot produce his own antibodies until about 2 months of age.

Nursing interventions for assisting the newborn with the immune system transition after birth include the following:

- Maintaining strict hand washing for everyone who cares for the newborn
- Protecting the newborn from infection
- Screening health-care personnel and visitors for illness
- Teaching the parents about hand hygiene for themselves, family members, and visitors
- Encouraging the parents to begin immunizations at 2 months of age

SAFETY *STAT!*

A newborn has no immunity against herpes simplex. Any health-care personnel with a herpes simplex outbreak (ie, cold sores) should not care for an infant until the lesions are crusted over. If the newborn contracts herpes simplex virus it can progress to a systemic form of the disease, which could be fatal.

BEHAVIORAL ADJUSTMENT TO EXTRAUTERINE LIFE

Even though babies are nonverbal, they are extraordinary communicators. They have the social skills of initiating interaction by crying, quieting when soothed, and mutual gazing. A newborn will demonstrate that he or she likes something by focusing his or her eyes and tracking an object or person moving around the room. Newborns also demonstrate behaviors that indicate their dislikes, such as turning away, crying, and yawning. As babies transition into extrauterine life, they also learn to self-soothe themselves by thumb or hand sucking.

Every baby is different, and parents will begin to learn the personality and behaviors of their baby from the start. Nurses can assist parents to understand the behaviors of their newborn

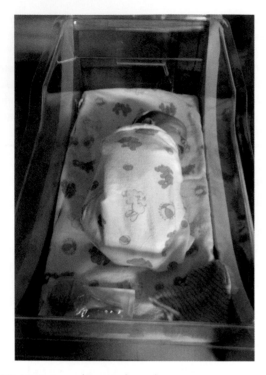

FIGURE 15.6 A newborn in deep sleep.

through education and by providing positive reinforcement to the parents as they care for and interact with their newborn.

Periods of Reactivity

All healthy newborns go through expected periods of alertness and sleepiness. The first period of reactivity occurs in the first 30 to 60 min after birth; during this time the newborn is usually alert, active, and cooperative. A vigorous suck reflex is usually present, which makes this an excellent time to introduce latch-on for breastfeeding.

After this brief period of alertness, the newborn will fall into a deep sleep that can last 2 to 4 hours or longer. This is called *the period of relative inactivity* (Fig. 15.6). The newborn will be in a deep sleep and is unresponsive to external stimuli. The heart rate and respiratory rate both decrease but stay within the normal limits. The mother may have trouble waking the baby for feedings.

The second period of reactivity begins when newborn wakes up from the long sleep and is again alert, active, and hungry. The heart rate will vary depending upon external stimuli, and periods of rapid respirations may be noted in response to stimuli. This is the time to encourage family interaction with the newborn and to educate the mother about hunger cues.

PATIENT TEACHING GUIDELINES

Sleep and Awake States

Parents can learn about their baby's mood by how he or she responds to touch, sights, and sounds. Newborn behavior typically falls within the following states:

- **Deep sleep:** The baby lays very still, with an occasional twitch. Usually there are no eye movements and breathing is regular. It is difficult to awaken the baby.
- **Light sleep:** This state is also known as *rapid eye movement sleep*. The eye movements may be visible beneath the eye lids and the baby may occasionally fuss or make sucking movements. This state typically occurs right before the baby wakes up.
- **Drowsy:** The baby's eyes may open. The baby is not fully asleep and may go back to sleep or wake up more.
- **Alert:** The baby's eyes will be open. Breathing is regular and the baby is attentive to what is going on around him. At this time the baby is most interested in eating.
- **Active alert:** In this state the baby is more active and may begin to chew on his hands or foot, and may try to get in position for feedings. The baby is sensitive to hunger, discomfort, and fatigue. He may require comforting in this state.
- **Crying:** Crying is the way that a baby conveys that something is bothering him or her. The baby may need to be fed or burped, need to have the diaper changed, be bored or overstimulated, or need close physical contact (Tharp, Farley, et al, 2013).

Key Points

- Thermoregulation can be difficult for the newborn because of inability to conserve heat, which is caused by a large surface area relative to body mass and limited subcutaneous fat for insulation.
- Hypothermia in the newborn is preventable by reducing risks. The nurse needs to monitor the environment and the body temperature of the newborn and provide appropriate interventions to maintain a stable body temperature for the newborn.
- Brown fat aids in body temperature regulation. It is found in term newborns in the scapular area, the thorax, and behind the kidneys. The infant metabolizes the brown fat to produce heat. This metabolism of brown fat is known as *nonshivering thermogenesis.*

- Glycogen is stored in the liver to provide an energy source for the newborn at birth.
- The infant begins to lose heat immediately after birth through four mechanisms: evaporation, conduction, convection, and radiation.
- The sequence of events that causes the newborn to begin breathing includes internal stimuli and external stimuli.
- After birth, the fetal circulation is not effective and changes occur that increase blood flow to the lungs and liver. The ductus arteriosus, ductus venosus, and foramen ovale close to redirect the blood flow through the newborn's body.
- The newborn's kidneys are immature and do not concentrate urine well for about 6 weeks. The urine will be

odorless and a light color or clear. The newborn should void within 24 hours of birth.

- Bacteria begin entering the gastrointestinal tract shortly after birth through vaginal secretions, hospital linens, and contact at the breast. The bacteria aid in digestion and the synthesis of vitamin K.
- The meconium stool, which is composed of sticky, blackish green material made from mucus, vernix, lanugo, hormones, and carbohydrates that accumulated in the bowel during fetal development, should be expelled within 24 to 48 hours of birth.
- The immature liver is unable to change bilirubin from the breakdown of red blood cells into a form that can be excreted by the body, causing a deposit of bilirubin in the skin (ie, jaundice) to occur.

- The newborn is born with passive antibodies passed to him or her from the mother through the placenta. A newborn cannot produce his own antibodies until about 2 months of age.
- The first period of reactivity occurs in the first 30 to 60 min after birth and this is an excellent time to introduce breastfeeding and encourage bonding.
- The second period of reactivity begins when newborn wakes up from the long sleep and is again alert, active, and hungry. This is the time to encourage family interaction with the newborn and to educate the mother about hunger cues.
- Newborns have periods of sleep and awake states. Nurses can educate and assist parents to understand the needs and behaviors of their newborn.

REVIEW QUESTIONS

1. A newborn is in the active alert state. Which of the following would the nurse expect to see?
   1. The newborn is crying vigorously.
   2. The newborn is attentive to what is going on around him.
   3. The newborn's eye movements are visible under the eye lids.
   4. The newborn is showing signs of hunger.

2. A term newborn has just been born. Which intervention should require the highest priority?
   1. Conducting the 5 min Apgar score
   2. Injecting vitamin K
   3. Removing wet blankets
   4. Applying the identification band

3. A newborn is in the first period of reactivity. Which of the following actions should the nurse take at this time?
   1. Place the infant under the radiant warmer.
   2. Encourage bonding and breastfeeding.
   3. Perform a head-to-toe assessment.
   4. Invite extended family in to meet the baby.

4. A newborn has just been delivered. Which of the following physiological changes is of highest priority?
   1. Passing meconium stool
   2. Closure of the ductus venosus
   3. Spontaneous respirations
   4. Thermoregulation

5. A nurse has been teaching a mother of a 2-day-old infant about the risk for infection in the newborn. Which statement indicates that the mother needs further teaching?
   1. "The baby received some immunity from me through the placenta."
   2. "I plan to drop by my 5-year-old niece's birthday party at the pizza restaurant with my baby tomorrow."
   3. "I will ask any family or friends that want to hold by baby to wash their hands first."
   4. "Anyone who's sick should not visit my baby."

6. A baby can lose heat by evaporation if which of the following situations occurs?
   1. The mother unwraps the baby to show a visitor.
   2. The nurse places the baby crib near the air conditioner vent.
   3. The baby is placed in a cold crib.
   4. The baby is wet from amniotic fluid.

7. How can the nurse assess the successful transition of the respiratory system in the newborn? *(select all that apply)*
   1. Count the number of respirations per minute.
   2. Dry the baby thoroughly.
   3. Observe the chest and abdomen.
   4. Observe the capillary refill time of the foot.
   5. Observe the color of the mucous membranes.

8. Which of the following changes occur in the cardiovascular system when the newborn transitions from the uterus to extrauterine life? *(select all that apply)*
   1. The right ventricle has increased pressure.
   2. There is increased blood flow through the lungs.
   3. Blood is shunted from the pulmonary artery to the aorta.
   4. The ductus arteriosus closes.
   5. Blood flow to the liver increases.

CRITICAL THINKING QUESTIONS

1. The nurse is preparing to bathe a newborn. How can the nurse promote the newborn's thermoregulation during this procedure?

2. Describe the process the heart and blood vessels undergo when converting from fetal to neonatal circulation.

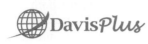 Davis*Plus*

For additional resources and information, visit **www.DavisPlus.com.** Post-Conference Questions and Activities, Answers, and References can be found on Davis*Plus*.

Assessment and Care of the Newborn

16

LEARNING OUTCOMES

1. Define the key terms.
2. Define *physical assessment.*
3. Identify normal newborn vital signs.
4. Demonstrate a head-to-toe assessment of the newborn.
5. Summarize abnormal findings from the head-to-toe assessment that must be reported.
6. Identify normal newborn skin variations.
7. Differentiate between cephalohematoma and caput succedaneum.
8. Explain the effects of maternal hormones on the newborn's physical characteristics.
9. Identify the normal newborn reflexes.
10. Discuss nursing care of the newborn.
11. Summarize the usual newborn screenings that are completed for health promotion.
12. Discuss Ballard's tool, which is used to determine gestational age.
13. Demonstrate the correct technique for an infant heelstick.
14. Demonstrate the correct technique for a newborn's bath.
15. Develop a discharge teaching plan on newborn care basics.
16. Plan family-centered care by including the family in discharge teaching.
17. Instruct the parents on newborn safety.

KEY TERMS

acne neonatorum
acrocyanosis
apnea
caput succedaneum
cephalohematoma
circumcision
dermal melanosis
erythema toxicum neonatorum
fontanel
gynecomastia
hemangioma
lanugo
melanocytic nevi
milia
nevus flammeus
nevus simplex
preterm
post-term
pseudomenstruation
retractions
vernix caseosa

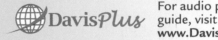 **DavisPlus** For audio pronunciation guide, visit **www.DavisPlus.com**

CHAPTER CONCEPTS

Assessment
Communication
Critical Thinking
Development
Safety

REAL-WORLD CASE STUDY

■ A student nurse is at the bedside of a postpartum patient and has just completed a physical assessment of a 3-hour-old male newborn. As the student reviews her notes, she is concerned about the following findings: axillary temperature of 36°C, respiratory rate of 42 breaths/min, heart rate of 150 bpm, crackles were heard bilaterally in the lower lung bases, the newborn's hands and feet are slightly blue, there are little "white heads" on the nose, and the infant actively moves the left arm but barely moves the right arm. When the student

continued on page 228

removed the diaper, she noted that the infant has a swollen scrotum and had passed a large, black, sticky stool.

1. Which of the assessment findings are normal for a 3-hour-old infant?
2. Are any of the student's assessment findings abnormal?
3. Are there any abnormal assessment findings that should be reported to the charge nurse immediately?
4. Are there any nursing interventions that the student nurse should implement after the assessment?

CONCEPTUAL CORNERSTONE

Assessment

Nursing assessment is a systematic method of collecting data to identify problems and then plan safe and effective care for the patient. There are three different types of assessments that the nurse may use while providing care in the hospital for the patients. The first type is the initial or baseline assessment that is done on admission to establish a baseline for reference and future comparison. The second type of assessment is problem-focused and is done to determine the status of a particular problem. The third type is emergency assessment, which is done to identify any life-threatening problems. Data-collecting techniques include observation, interviewing, and physical examination.

For this chapter, the concept of assessment or data collection will focus on the baseline physical examination of the newborn. The nurse will need an understanding of normal newborn physical characteristics and behaviors to be able to identify abnormal findings and potential problems to report to the health-care provider.

The nurse has an important role in the care of a newborn. The nurse is often the first health-care professional to physically examine and provide initial care for the newborn. Nurses also have the responsibility to teach parents basic newborn care so that they are prepared for discharge from the hospital. This chapter will provide information about physical assessment, nursing care of the newborn, and discharge teaching.

PHYSICAL ASSESSMENT OF THE NEWBORN

Immediately after a baby is born, a 1-min and 5-min Apgar score is given. This is a quick method of assessing the newborn to determine if any emergency interventions are needed. Within 2 hours of birth, an initial head-to-toe assessment should be done to determine if there are any problems that require medical or nursing interventions. This section of the chapter discusses the normal newborn vital signs, initial measurements, and an in-depth head-to-toe assessment.

Assessment and observation of the newborn begins at birth and should continue regularly through the first 24 hours of life to monitor successful transition to extrauterine life. Nurses need to be familiar with the normal features of the transitional period to detect problems with transition, report the problems, and develop a plan of care.

Before beginning the physical assessment, the nurse should ensure that the infant is in a warm and well-lit environment. Proper lighting is important for observing the skin color. The assessment consists of observation, auscultation, and palpation. If possible, conduct the observation portion of the assessment before touching the newborn.

At the onset of the assessment, before stimulating the newborn with touch, the nurse should observe the infant's:

• Position
• Sleep or wake cycle
• Skin color
• Respiratory pattern

Vital Signs

Vital signs indicate physiological functioning and include heart rate, respiratory rate, temperature, and blood pressure. The blood pressure is not routinely assessed in a newborn unless there are suspicions of a congenital cardiac anomaly. Hospital policies vary on timing for newborn vital signs but they are usually taken every 30 min for the first 2 hours after birth, then every hour for 3 hours, and then every 4 to 8 hours for 24 hours. See Table 16.1 for normal newborn vital signs.

Newborn Measurements

Each newborn should be weighed and measured for length, head circumference, and chest circumference. To prevent inaccuracies, the infant should be weighed on the same scale each day in the hospital. When weighing the infant, the diaper should be removed. The standard range for a term newborn weight is 2,500 to 4,000 g (Keehn and Liehen, 2014) (Fig. 16.1).

To obtain an accurate length, the newborn's leg must be fully extended and the nurse should record the distance from head to heel. It is easier to obtain an accurate measurement if one nurse holds the infant in place while another nurse measures from

TABLE 16.1 NORMAL NEWBORN VITAL SIGNS

Vital Sign	Normal Ranges
Temperature	36.5°C–37°C axillary
Heart Rate	Asleep: 100 bpm; Awake: 110–160 bpm; Crying: 180 bpm
Respiratory Rate	30–60 breaths per minute
Blood Pressure	Not routinely assessed; average for a 1–3-day-old infant is 66/40 mm Hg

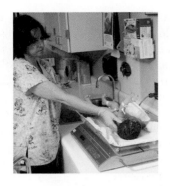

FIGURE 16.1 Weighing the infant.

head to heel. The standard range for a term newborn is 48 to 53 cm or 19 to 21 in. (Keehn and Liehen, 2014) (Fig. 16.2).

Chest circumference is measured by placing the tape measure around the infant's chest at the nipple line and noting the number at midway between inspiration and expiration. The standard range for a term newborn chest circumference is 30.5 to 33 cm or 12 to 13 in. (Fig. 16.3).

Head circumference is measured by placing the tape measure just above the ears and eyebrows. The expected range for the head circumference is 33 to 35.5 cm. or 13 to 14 in. (Fig. 16.4).

Skin Assessment

The skin assessment can give the nurse information about the infant's cardiac function, respiratory function, gestational age, and thermoregulation. The skin color should be assessed in good natural lighting if possible. There are always variations in skin tone, but an infant with good cardiac and respiratory function will have pink mucous membranes and nail beds. In darker-pigmented infants, the mucous membranes may be light pink

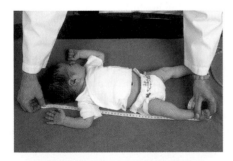

FIGURE 16.2 Measuring the infant's body length.

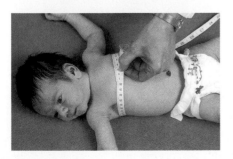

FIGURE 16.3 Measuring the chest circumference.

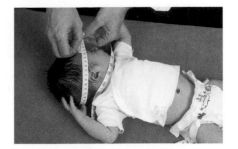

FIGURE 16.4 Measuring the head circumference.

with a slight yellow or red tinge (Keehn and Liehen, 2014). It is normal for newborns to have **acrocyanosis** for the first 24 to 48 hours after birth. Acrocyanosis is a bluish color of the hands and feet because of immature peripheral circulation. It is also common for newborns to have petechiae on the scalp, forehead, and cheeks. These are tiny pin-point bruises that occurred from pushing during delivery or from a rapid delivery.

A skin temperature range of 36°C to 36.5°C is acceptable for the term newborn. The term newborn should have good skin turgor to indicate adequate hydration. To assess for skin turgor, the nurse should gently pinch the skin on the thigh or chest. The skin should immediately recoil. If the skin remains "pinched," the newborn has poor turgor and may be dehydrated.

The palms of the hands and the soles of the feet should have creases. The creases in the sole develop from toe to heel. An absence of creases could indicate a motor defect. It is thought that sole creases develop in the uterus because of fetal movement of the lower extremities (Keehn and Liehen, 2014). A preterm infant will have minimal creases and a post-term infant will have increased creasing of the soles.

Lanugo is fine, downy hair that covers the forehead, ears, and body of the newborn (Fig. 16.5). Lanugo develops at 19 weeks' gestation and is very obvious at 27 to 28 weeks' gestation. After 28 weeks, the fetus begins to slowly lose the hair and any hair present at birth will fall off within the first weeks of life (Keehn and Liehen, 2014). A post-term newborn will have very little or no lanugo.

Vernix caseosa is a white protective coating on the skin of the newborn. It is usually more prominent in the folds of the legs, arms, and neck (Fig. 16.6). It protects the skin from the emersion in amniotic fluid and disappears as the fetus

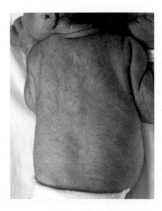

FIGURE 16.5 Lanugo.

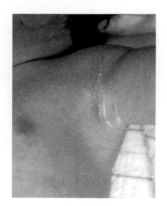

FIGURE 16.6 Vernix caseosa.

ages. A term newborn will usually have vernix in the folds of the armpit or groin area. A premature newborn will have vernix covering the entire body.

Birthmarks, Rashes, and Skin Lesions

Birthmarks are not uncommon and may cause some anxiety for the family. Most birthmarks are benign but some will require further investigation by the health-care provider. Some birthmarks fade away over time and others persist into adulthood.

A strawberry **hemangioma,** also known as a *nevus vascularis,* consists of newly formed capillaries in the dermal and subdermal layers of the skin. The strawberry hemangioma has sharp demarcation and is raised and dark red. It may be present at birth or may appear in the first few weeks of life. Usually no medical intervention is required unless the hemangioma is larger than 5 cm. The hemangioma gradually fades away over a few years; 50% of hemangiomas are gone by age 5, and 70% are gone by age 7 (Antaya, 2015).

DRUG FACTS

The Food and Drug Administration (FDA) has approved an oral pediatric formulation of propranolol hydrochloride (Hemangeol) for the treatment of large hemangiomas in infants (Antaya, 2015).

Nevus flammeus, also known as *port wine stain,* is usually present at birth and grows with the child. It is made up of dilated skin capillaries. The nevus flammeus is frequently located on the face and is red to purple in color. This birthmark is not raised and does not blanch if pressure is applied. This lesion will not fade on its own, and laser surgery is the treatment of choice if the parents desire to have it removed (Antaya, 2014).

Nevus simplex, also known as *stork bites, angel kisses,* or *salmon patches,* appear in 40% of all newborns. It may be found on the forehead or nape of the neck. It is pink in color and does blanch when pressure is applied (Fig. 16.7). It may be more prominent when the newborn cries. No treatment is required, and it frequently fades by 18 months of age (Ngan, 2015).

Congenital **melanocytic nevi,** also known as *moles,* are uncommon in the newborn but have a potential for malignancy. A nevus may be flat or raised. The congenital melanocytic

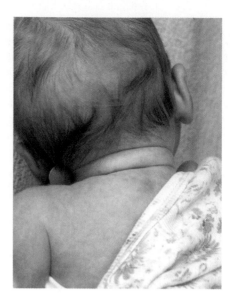

FIGURE 16.7 Nevus simplex, also known as *stork bites.*

nevus is usually evenly pigmented and brown or black in color. Hair may be present. A hairy nevus noted along the base of the spine could indicate a spina bifida congenital spine abnormality. The nurse should document and report any nevi noted. Melanocytic nevi can be removed surgically for cosmetic considerations or if the parents are concerned about the potential for malignancy later in life (MacCalmont, 2013).

Erythema toxicum neonatorum, also known as *newborn rash,* may appear as macules, papules, or vesicles. The rash appears on any part of the body except the palms and soles of the feet. It appears suddenly and also disappears quickly, rarely lasting more than 7 days. It does not cause any discomfort for the newborn and does not require any medical treatment.

Acne neonatorum are clogged hair follicles or pores in the skin. On the newborn they are found on the forehead, nose, and cheeks and may be white or black. The newborn acne will resolve without treatment and causes no scarring.

Milia are sebaceous glands occluded with keratin. They look like tiny white papules about 1 mm in size located on the nose, chin, cheeks, and forehead (Fig. 16.8). Milia usually disappear within 4 weeks and require no special care.

Dermal melanosis, also known as *Mongolian spots,* is a common finding in infants of darker skin, particularly infants

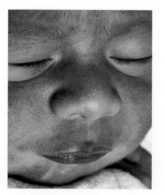

FIGURE 16.8 Milia.

of Asian, East Indian, or African descent (Keehn and Lieben, 2014). The spots are caused by melanocytes trapped deep in the skin, appear flat and bluish-gray or brown, and are located on the back or buttocks (Fig. 16.9). This lesion can be mistaken for a bruise. The presence of any should be documented in the infant's medical record. No medical interventions are required. Most Mongolian spots disappear by 2 years of age. Occasionally they may be observed through childhood, finally fading away by adolescence (James, Berger, et al, 2015).

The nurse should report the following abnormal skin assessment findings:

- Cyanosis, which could be caused by a cardiovascular or respiratory problem
- Thin skin with abundant lanugo, which could indicate prematurity
- Meconium staining, which may be caused by hypoxia in the uterus before birth
- Poor skin turgor, which may be caused by dehydration
- Pallor (ie, paleness), which could be caused by anemia or hypothermia
- Any nevus or mole

Head Assessment

At the beginning of the head assessment, the nurse should first observe the general appearance, including the shape, circumference, and suture lines. A newborn born vaginally will generally have a head with a flattened forehead that rises to a point at the posterior skull over the occiput. This shape reflects the molding that occurred to the skull as the suture lines came together when the head passed through the pelvis during birth. Overriding sutures are normal findings that result from molding and resolve spontaneously. The molding or "cone head" appearance resolves within 3 to 5 days after birth.

Another condition that may be noticed on the head is a **cephalohematoma,** which is a swelling on the head that does not cross the suture line. It is caused by birth trauma that causes a rupture of blood vessels between the skull and periosteum. It usually appears by day 2 of life and may worsen over a few days. The cephalohematoma will resolve over days or weeks as the blood is reabsorbed (Moses, 2015) (Fig. 16.10).

Caput succedaneum is a swelling of the scalp of the newborn. It is caused by pressure from the uterus or vaginal wall

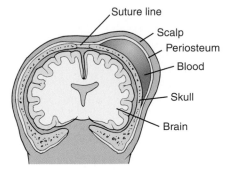

FIGURE 16.10 Cephalohematoma.

during delivery. The scalp will be soft and spongelike with possible bruising. Caput succedaneum is swelling of the scalp, so it will cross the suture lines. No treatment is needed; the swelling will decrease over a few days (Kaneshiro, 2013) (Fig. 16.11).

The newborn head circumference, referred to as the *occipital-frontal circumference,* is determined by measuring around the head from the frontal to occipital area by placing the tape measure above the ears. The nurse should measure the largest part of the head. As edema and molding from the birth subside, the head circumference may decrease as much as 2 cm over a week. The acceptable head measurement for a term newborn is 33 to 37 cm or 13 to 15 in.

A term newborn will have a diamond-shaped anterior **fontanel** located between the coronal and sagittal suture lines, approximately 4 to 5 cm in size. A fontanel is sometimes referred to as the "soft spot" on the baby's head. It is a fibrous membrane that lies between the bones of the cranium. The anterior fontanel closes by 18 months of age. The posterior fontanel is located midline on the back of the head between the sagittal and lamboid sutures, and is approximately 0.5 to 2 cm in size. The posterior fontanel should close by 2 months of age. Both fontanels should be flat. Missing or small fontanels could indicate a potential problem of fused cranial bones that could interfere with brain growth. When a newborn cries or vomits, the nurse may observe that the fontanel fluctuates, but it should never be tightly bulging. A tight, bulging fontanel may indicate an increase in intracranial pressure. Sunken fontanels are associated with dehydration and decreased intracranial pressure.

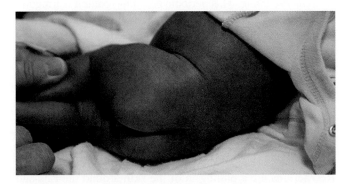

FIGURE 16.9 Dermal melanosis, also known as Mongolian spots.

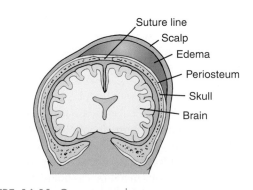

FIGURE 16.11 Caput succedaneum.

The nurse should document and report the following abnormal findings:

- Enlarged fontanels
- Abnormally small fontanels
- Bulging or sunken fontanels

Eye Assessment

The eyes and eyelids should be examined for symmetry in size and location on the face. The outer portion of the eye should be at the same height as the top of the ear. The sclera should be white or bluish-white. A yellow appearance indicates jaundice. Birth trauma may cause a subconjunctival hemorrhage. The pupillary reflex can be determined by shining a bright light into the eye and observing an instant constriction of the pupil. The newborn's visual field is approximately 8 to 12 in. with a visual acuity of 20/200.

The nurse should document and report the following findings:

- Yellow or red sclera
- Any exudate noted in the eyes
- Drooping eyelids

Ear Assessment

The nurse should note the ear size, shape, and location. A mature infant will have firmer ear cartilage than a premature infant. The nurse should note any abnormal folds, discharge, or irregularities of the pinna. The placement of the ear should be in a horizontal line from the inner canthus of the eye. If the ears are lower than that line, it is referred to as low-set and may indicate a chromosomal abnormality. Infants with normal hearing should have some response to loud sounds and voices. The nurse should document and report:

- Any abnormal anatomical findings
- The newborn's lack of response to loud noises

Nose Assessment

The nurse should observe a nose that is midline with symmetrical nares. A small amount of clear nasal discharge is expected in the newborn. Newborns are obligatory nose breathers, which means that the newborn breathes through the nose much easier than through the mouth. The nurse can check for air movement through the nose by placing a finger under the nose. Newborns who are experiencing respiratory difficulty will often flare the nostrils as an attempt to breathe in more air. The nurse should document and report:

- Obstructed nasal passages
- Any discharge from the nose that is not clear
- Any anatomical abnormalities
- Any nasal flaring

Mouth Assessment

The lips, mouth, tongue, and gums should be inspected. The nurse should note any asymmetrical movement of the mouth or tongue, which could indicate nerve injury from birth trauma. The lips and mucous membranes should be pink and a small amount of saliva should be present. If the infant has a large amount of mucus that bubbles, the nurse should suction it with the bulb syringe. If there continues to be a large amount of bubbly saliva, the health-care provider should be notified to evaluate the patency of the esophagus. A pen light can be used to visualize the palate. The nurse can also place a gloved finger in the mouth to palpate the palate for intactness and to elicit the sucking reflex from the infant.

The nurse may notice white papules, known as *Epstein's pearls,* on the roof of the mouth or gums. Sometimes they appear as little emerging teeth, but are really cysts. The cysts contain trapped mucous membrane cells. They are commonly found on the midline of the palate and formed when the palate fused during early fetal development. They are not painful and they disappear within a few weeks.

The nurse should document and report:

- Asymmetrical movement of the lips or tongue
- Mucous membranes that are not pink
- Excessive bubbly saliva
- Absent suck reflex
- A hole in the palate

Chest Assessment

The nurse should observe the infant's chest for shape and symmetry of movement. The newborn chest should be round and 1 to 2 cm smaller than the head circumference. The size, shape, nipple formation, and nipple placement should be noted. Frequently, in both genders, the breasts are enlarged because of the maternal hormones. This condition is called **gynecomastia** and resolves within days as the level of hormones the baby received in utero from the mother declines. Neonatal gynecomastia is sometimes accompanied by galactorrhea, also called "witch's milk." Galactorrhea is a milky-appearing discharge from the nipples that resolves spontaneously as the hormone level in the infant drops. The nurse should document and report:

- Any variation in chest size from the norm, either too large or too small
- Any abnormalities in the placement or size of the nipples
- Any purulent or bloody discharge from the nipples

Respiratory Assessment

A respiratory assessment includes observation of the newborn's breathing effort, chest movement, and auscultation of the lung fields. Newborns experience a breathing pattern known as *periodic breathing.* This periodic breathing pattern is irregular and the infant can pause breathing for 5 to 15 sec. When the infant is in a deep sleep, the breathing pattern is generally more even and regular, and as the infant becomes more awake, the breathing pattern may change to periodic breathing. The infant's work of breathing should be unlabored and the infant should appear to be breathing easily. The chest movement should be smooth. The nailbeds can be inspected for color; a bluish color would indicate decreased oxygenation of the blood.

Infants with respiratory distress may exhibit seesaw movements of the chest and abdomen, nasal flaring, and retractions. **Retractions** are a pulling in of the skin around the ribs and sternum when inhaling becomes hard work for the infant.

When auscultating the newborn's lung fields, it is recommended that the nurse use a pediatric or newborn stethoscope. The smaller sized 2.5-cm diameter diaphragm of the pediatric or newborn stethoscope makes it easier to hear the lungs without hearing other body sounds at the same time. The nurse will listen to a lung field and cross over to the opposite side to compare the two lung fields. The normal newborn will have wet sounds, such as crackles, for the first 24 hours after birth because of the long immersion in fluid during gestation.

The nurse should document and report:

- A respiratory rate of less than 30 or more than 60 breaths/min
- Cessation of breathing (ie, **apnea**) of more than 20 sec
- Any abnormal sound other than crackles in the first 24 hours
- Any increased work of breathing noted, especially seesaw chest movements and retraction of the skin around the ribs and sternum

Cardiovascular Assessment

Listening to the heart sounds of a newborn can be difficult because of the normally fast rate. Using a pediatric stethoscope and minimizing extraneous noise and distractions will help. When assessing the heart sounds, the nurse should first focus on identifying the following heart sounds: S_1 (ie, closure of the mitral and tricuspid valves) and S_2 (ie, closure of the aortic and pulmonic valves). Next, notice the regularity or irregularity of the rhythm. Finally, the nurse should systematically listen for heart tones by using the following sequence:

1. The aortic valve area by placing the stethoscope at the second intercostal space at the right of the sternum
2. The pulmonic valve area by placing the stethoscope at the second intercostal space to the left of the sternum
3. Erb's point, also known as the left lower sternal border (LLSB), is located at the third intercostal space and does not reflect a particular valve sound, but is a good location to evaluate the S_2 heart sound
4. The tricuspid valve area by placing the stethoscope at the fifth intercostal space at both the left and right side of the sternum
5. The mitral valve area by placing the stethoscope at the fourth intercostal space at the left of the midclavicular line

The newborn's peripheral pulses should be assessed for quality and equality by comparing them side to side. The pulse rate and rhythm should match the apical pulse.

The capillary refill time (CRT) can be evaluated by pressing firmly on the foot for approximately 5 sec, causing the foot to blanch, and then by counting the number of seconds for the skin to return to natural color. Normal CRT should be less than 3 sec. However, the test for CRT in the newborn is controversial because the refill time can be affected by decreased peripheral circulation, the temperature of the foot, and the environmental temperature (Keehn and Lieben, 2014). The nurse should document and report:

- A heart rate below 110 bpm or above 160 bpm at rest
- Any extra heart sounds other than the normal S_1 and S_2 heart sounds
- Any abnormal heart sounds, such as blowing, clicking, or mechanical sounds, which could indicate a murmur
- Any discrepancy between the peripheral pulses side to side and with the apical heart rate
- A CRT greater than 3 sec

Abdomen and Gastrointestinal Assessment

To assess the abdomen, the nurse will first observe the shape, contour, and movement. The abdomen should have a domed appearance owing to immature abdominal muscles. The umbilical stump should be white and gelatinous in appearance and have three vessels, two arteries, and a vein. The umbilical stump begins to dry within hours of birth. The nurse should note any bulging around the umbilicus, which could indicate failure of the umbilical ring closure, resulting in an umbilical hernia. The anus should be inspected for patency.

Auscultation of the abdominal bowel sounds should be completed before any touching of the abdomen, which could stimulate the bowel, producing peristalsis. There should be bowel sounds within 1 to 2 hours of birth. A stool assessment is an important part of the abdominal and gastrointestinal assessment. The first newborn stool is the meconium stool. It is made up of bile salts, bile acids, epithelial cells, lanugo, and debris shed from the intestinal mucosa during intrauterine life (Hekmatnia, 2013). Meconium is dark and sticky. The meconium stool should be passed within 24 hours of birth. By the 2nd or 3rd day, the stool is called *transitional* because it will have a green or yellowish seedy appearance. After a few days, the breastfed infant's stool will have the appearance of mustard, and the bottle-fed infant's stool will have a tan, yellow, or greenish appearance.

The nurse should document and report:

- Failure to pass a meconium stool within 24 hours
- A closed anus
- Absence of bowel sounds after 2 hours
- A flat abdomen

Genitourinary Assessment

During the initial head-to-toe assessment of the newborn, an examination of the genitalia should be included. The female genitalia should be inspected for placement of the labia and urinary meatus. In a healthy newborn, the labia will cover the clitoris. Maternal hormones may cause the labia to be swollen and darker than the surrounding tissue. Mucus and blood-tinged vaginal discharge is not uncommon and is called **pseudomenstruation.** The discharge may be present for a few days until the maternal hormone level in the newborn decreases.

The male infant's penis should be midline and straight, with the urethral opening midline at the tip of the penis. The length of the nonerect penis is 2 to 3 cm at birth. Until 3 to 4 years of age, the foreskin is usually tight, but it does not affect the stream of urine. The scrotum will appear large and loose, with a dark appearance because of maternal hormones. The nurse should lightly palpate for the presence of testes. Testes usually descend by the third trimester and are approximately 1 cm in size at birth.

Urinary output should be evaluated. The newborn should urinate within 24 hours of birth. Normal urine output is 1 to 2 mL/kg/hour.

The nurse should document and report:

• A lack of or decreased urinary output
• Any structural abnormality of the genitalia
• Undescended testicles

Neurological Assessment

The newborn's neurological system is immature at birth. The nurse may notice periodic jerking or twitching, which is considered normal. Tremors are not considered a normal finding in a newborn. The newborn's cry can provide information about the neurological status. A high-pitch cry can indicate an increase in intracranial pressure. When assessing the reflexes, the nurse needs to consider the gestational age, not the birth weight. Premature infants will have a reduced response to reflex evaluation. Table 16.2 provides information about newborn reflexes. The nurse should document and report the following warning signs:

• Tremors
• A high-pitched cry
• Abnormal pupil responses
• Hypertonic or hypotonic positions
• Absent newborn reflexes

Musculoskeletal Assessment

To begin the musculoskeletal assessment, the nurse should first observe the resting posture. The normal resting posture for a newborn is flexed with good muscle tone. The limbs should be inspected for symmetry, webbing, range of motion, length, and number of digits (Keehn and Lieben, 2014). Uterine position can sometimes cause the feet to be turned inward. The nurse can gently try to straighten the foot. If the foot can be straightened, it is usually caused by uterine position and will straight out over time. If the foot cannot be straightened because of resistance, the nurse should never force the foot and the findings should be reported.

The nurse can assess the hips for developmental dysplasia of the hip, also known as *congenital hip dislocation*. Two tests are recommended to determine hip instability in the newborn. Ortolani's maneuver is performed with the infant in a supine position. The examiner holds the infant's thigh with a thumb and places the index finger of the same hand over the greater trochanter area. The hip is gently lifted and abducted while pushing gently down on the knee. If the hip is not stable, a "clunk" sound will be heard or felt by the examiner. For Barlow's test, the examiner places a thumb on the infant's thigh and uses the palm of the same hand to press down the knee. While applying gentle pressure, the examiner feels for a dislocation with the middle finger of the same hand. If the hip is

TABLE 16.2 NEWBORN REFLEXES

Reflex	Description	Age the Reflex Disappears
Babinski Reflex (Babinski reflex)	When the sole of the foot is stroked, the newborn's big toe moves upward toward the top surface of the foot and the other toes fan out.	2 years of age
Plantar Grasp (Plantar grasp)	The newborn's toes curl downward in response to pressure applied to the sole of the foot at the base of the toes.	8 months of age

TABLE 16.2   NEWBORN REFLEXES—cont'd

Reflex	Description	Age the Reflex Disappears
Rooting Reflex 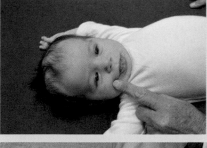 (Rooting reflex)	The newborn turns the mouth to the same side of the cheek that is stroked.	Becomes a voluntary reflex around 3 weeks of age
Gag Reflex	The newborn coughs in response to stimulation of the posterior oral cavity.	Continues into adulthood
Moro's (ie, Startle) Reflex 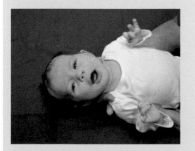 (Moro's [startle] reflex)	In response to a slight drop, sudden movement of the crib, or a loud noise, the newborn quickly makes a symmetrical abduction of the extremities and places the index fingers and thumbs into a "C" shape.	6 months of age
Palmar Grasp 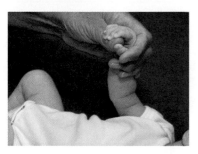 (Palmar grasp)	The newborn wraps the fingers around the examiner's finger when it is placed in the newborn's palm.	4–6 months of age

Continued

TABLE 16.2 NEWBORN REFLEXES—cont'd

Reflex	Description	Age the Reflex Disappears
Stepping Reflex (Stepping reflex)	The newborn simulates walking when held in an upright position and the sole of the foot touches a flat surface.	2 months of age
Tonic Neck Reflex (Tonic neck reflex)	In a supine position, if the newborn's head is turned to one side with the jaw over the shoulder, the arm and leg on the same side extend while the opposite arm and leg flex.	4–6 months of age
Extrusion Reflex (Extrusion reflex)	The newborn uses the tongue to push foreign objects out of the mouth.	3–4 months of age

Sources: Keehn NF & Lieben K. (2014). *Newborn assessment*. Retrieved from NetCE at http://www.NetCE.com; Moses S. (2015). *Newborn reflexes.* Retrieved from Family Practice Notebook at http://www.fpnotebook.com/NICU/Exam/NwbrnRflxs.htm

not stable, the examiner will feel the hip dislocate. Both tests are considered "positive" if a dislocation is observed.

The newborn's spinal cord and back should be observed for curvatures and asymmetry. Any nevi, dimples, or skin tags that appear on the midline of the back along the spine could indicate a spinal cord condition and are not considered a normal finding in the newborn.

The nurse should document and report:

- Absence of limbs or digits
- Structural abnormalities of any bones or muscles
- Lack of movement of a limb
- Asymmetrical thigh creases
- Unequal length of limbs
- Positive Ortolani's or Barlow's tests
- The presence of any nevi, skin tags, or dimples on the spinal cord

SAFETY *STAT!*

Warning signs observed during the physical assessment that must be reported immediately include:

- Axillary temperature of less than 36.1°C or greater than 37.2°C
- Cyanosis

- Heart rate less than 110 bpm or greater than 160 bpm (180 bpm if crying)
- Respiratory rate of less than 30 or greater than 60 breaths/min
- Hypotonic or hypertonic muscle tone
- Lack of movement of arms and legs
- Jaundice
- Periods of apnea longer than 20 sec (Keehn and Liehen, 2014)

Pain Assessment

Some hospitals require a newborn pain assessment to be done once a day and before, during, and after a painful procedure. A commonly used pain scale is the Neonatal Infant Pain Scale (NIPS) (Alcock, et al, 1993). This pain scale is considered to be appropriate for infants less than 1 year of age. For 1 min, the nurse observes facial expression, cry, breathing pattern, arms, legs, and state of arousal, with a numeric score assigned to each. A score of greater than 3 indicates that the neonate or infant is in pain.

▊ NURSING CARE OF THE NEWBORN

Most hospitals encourage rooming-in of the newborn with the mother. Fathers or a support person are often encouraged to stay with the new mother. Even though the infant spends most of the time in the mother's room, the nurse has the ultimate responsibility for the newborn's care. In addition to the initial assessment and ongoing assessments, the nurse has the responsibility to provide physical care and to complete the basic newborn screening to promote the health of the newborn. This section discusses the nurse's role of administering medications, determining the gestational age, completing the first bath, and coordinating newborn screenings before discharge.

Medications

The nursery nurse will review the infant's medical record to verify that the vitamin K and erythromycin ointment were given right after delivery. If not, the nurse will administer those two medications. Some health-care providers also order the first hepatitis B vaccine to be given to the newborn. The complete hepatitis B vaccine series is given as three injections over a 6-month period. Starting the hepatitis B vaccine series in the hospital reduces the risk of the newborn getting the disease from family members who may not know they are infected with the disease (CDC, 2015).

 DRUG FACTS

If the mother has hepatitis B, an additional medication is given within 12 hours of birth to protect the baby against catching hepatitis B. The medication is called *hepatitis B immune globulin (HBIG)*. This medication provides antibodies to help the newborn's immune system fight off the virus (CDC, 2015).

Estimation of Gestational Age

During pregnancy, the gestational age is determined based upon the mother's last menstrual period, fundal measurements, and ultrasonography. After birth, every newborn does not receive a gestational age assessment. Most hospitals have a policy regarding which infants should have gestational age assessments completed. A gestational age assessment should be completed on babies that are **preterm** (ie, born before 37 weeks' gestation), **post-term** (ie, born after 42 weeks' gestation), babies of diabetic mothers, and babies weighing less than 2,500 g or more than 4,000 g (Moses, 2015.) Classifying the newborn provides information that assists the health-care provider and the nurse to plan and provide appropriate care for the newborn.

NURSING CARE PLAN for Educating Parents About Their Newborn's Appearance

Nursing Assessment: New parents are surprised that their newborn does not look like the babies in television commercials. The newborn has a long head that is slightly misshaped, a hemangioma on the leg, and a red, raised rash on the trunk and legs.

Nursing Diagnosis: There is a risk for ineffective parenting as evidenced by the mother's remark of "His head looks so strange. Is he normal? It's bad enough that he has a rash, but he has that red birthmark on his leg!"

Expected Outcome: Parents will verbalize understanding that their newborn's appearance is normal, the head and rash will improve within days, and the hemangioma will fade over time.

Nursing Interventions:

- Allow the parents to verbalize their fears without condemnation from the nurse.
- Educate the parents about normal newborn characteristics.
- Explain the process of molding that occurs as the fetus moves through the birth canal.
- Explain that hemangiomas usually fade over a few years.
- Point out the positive physical characteristics of the newborn.

The most widely used clinical tool for assessing gestational age is the Ballard's tool. It was developed by Dr. Jeanne L. Ballard and assesses the newborn's gestational age by evaluating six areas of neuromuscular activity and six areas of physical maturity. The scores from the neuromuscular activity assessment and physical maturity assessment are combined to classify the newborn as preterm, term, or post-term. Ballard's tool is depicted in Figure 16.12.

Bath

The purpose of the initial bath is to remove blood and body fluids that could contaminate health-care workers. Amniotic fluid can contain viruses, such as HIV. Nurses must practice universal precautions and wear gloves until the initial baby bath is given. The risks of bathing the newborn are hypothermia, respiratory distress, and an increased oxygen need. Most babies cry at some point during the bath experience because of stimuli never experienced in the uterus, such as undressing, temperature changes, and the touch of the washcloth and towels (McManus Kuller, 2014).

The Association of Women's Health, Obstetric, and Neonatal Nurses (AWHONN) (2013) recommends that the newborn be bathed between 2 and 4 hours after birth if the newborn's temperature is at least 36.8°C. The World Health Organization (WHO) recommends waiting 6 hours after birth to avoid interfering with bonding and the initiation of breastfeeding.

Hospitals use a variety of methods to bathe the baby, including sponge bathing, small tub bathing, large tub or immersion bathing, and swaddling immersion bathing. The initial bath can be given at the mother's bedside or in the nursery. When preparing for the bath, the room should be warm and free of drafts. For all methods of bathing, a pH neutral cleanser is used and the skin is gently washed. Blood and body fluids are removed, but any vernix should not be scrubbed off.

Newborn Screening

Newborn screening is a state-based public health program that provides newborns with testing to determine if a medical condition is present that requires early interventions to maintain the health of the newborn. Newborn screening tests for a variety of genetic, metabolic, and endocrine disorders; infectious diseases; hearing loss; and congenital heart disease. The four most commonly diagnosed conditions in the United States are hearing loss, congenital hypothyroidism, cystic fibrosis, and sickle cell disease (ACOG, 2015).

The newborn is primarily tested by blood samples obtained from a heelstick at least 24 hours after the first feeding. These samples are placed on special filter paper and sent to the state laboratory. Noninvasive testing is used to test for hearing loss, and an oxygen saturation meter is used to test for congenital heart disease.

LABS & DIAGNOSTICS

The correct technique for obtaining blood specimens for newborn screening is to:

1. Warm the newborn's heel to increase circulation.
2. Cleanse the newborn's heel with alcohol and allow to dry.
3. Use a spring-activated lancet to puncture the skin no deeper than 2.4 mm on the outer aspect of the heel.
4. Collect the blood directly on the collection paper or pipet.
5. Apply gentle pressure to the heel with gauze and cover with an adhesive bandage.
6. Provide comfort to the newborn.

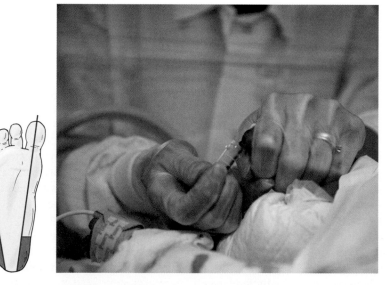

(Heelstick)

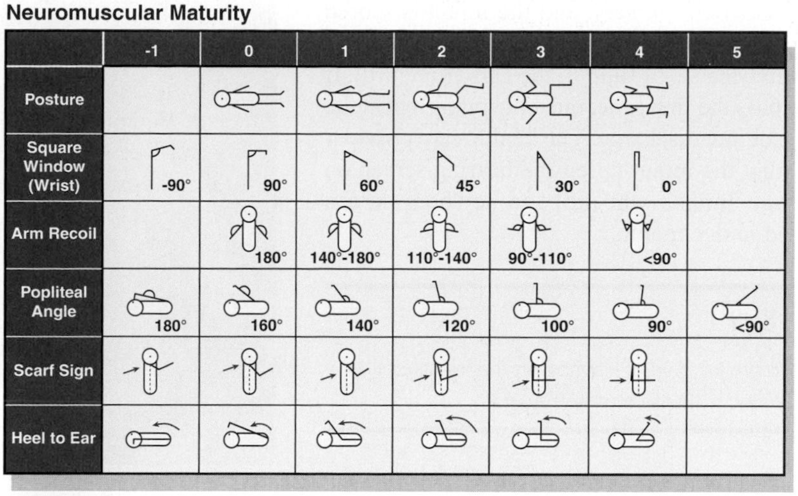

Neuromuscular Maturity

	-1	0	1	2	3	4	5
Posture							
Square Window (Wrist)	-90°	90°	60°	45°	30°	0°	
Arm Recoil		180°	140°-180°	110°-140°	90°-110°	<90°	
Popliteal Angle	180°	160°	140°	120°	100°	90°	<90°
Scarf Sign							
Heel to Ear							

Physical Maturity

Skin	Sticky Friable Transparent	Gelatinous Red Translucent	Smooth pink Visible veins	Superficial peeling or rash, few veins	Cracking Pale areas Rare veins	Parchment Deep cracking No vessels	Leathery Cracked Wrinkled	
Lanugo	None	Sparse	Abundant	Thinning	Bald areas	Mostly bald		
Plantar Surface	Heel-toe 40–50 mm: -1 <40 mm: -2	>50 mm No crease	Faint red marks	Anterior transverse crease only	Creases over anterior 2/3	Creases over entire sole		
Breast	Imperceptible	Barely perceptible	Flat areola No bud	Stippled areola 1–2 mm bud	Raised areola 3–4 mm bud	Full areola 5–10 mm bud		
Eye/ear	Lids fused loosely: -1 tightly: -2	Lids open Pinna flat Stays folded	Barely curved pinna; soft; slow recoil	Well-curved pinna; soft but ready recoil	Formed and firm Instant recoil	Thick cartilage Ear stiff		
Genitals (Male)	Scrotum flat, smooth	Scrotum empty Faint rugae	Testes in upper canal Rare rugae	Testes descending Few rugae	Testes down Good rugae	Testes pendulous Deep rugae		
Genitals (Female)	Clitoris prominent Labia flat	Prominent clitoris Small labia minora	Prominent clitoris Enlarging minora	Majora and minora equally prominent	Majora large Minora small	Majora covers clitoris and minora		

Maturity Rating

Score	Weeks
-10	20
-5	22
0	24
5	26
10	28
15	30
20	32
25	34
30	36
35	38
40	40
45	42
50	44

FIGURE 16.12 Ballard Gestational Age Assessment Tool

TEAM WORKS

Newborn screening programs are effective for early diagnosis because of the collaboration among nurses, hospitals, laboratories, pediatricians, and specialists. The team functions to screen all babies, identify screen-positive babies, diagnose conditions, communicate with families, and provide referral to treatment centers.

Newborn Congenital Heart Defect Screening

The American Academy of Pediatrics (2015) recommends that all babies be screened for a critical congenital heart defect (CCHD). In the United States, 18 of every 10,000 babies are born with a critical heart defect that requires medical intervention. The newborn may not exhibit signs of a heart defect immediately after birth; therefore this simple screening test can help in the early identification of newborns with a heart defect.

The screening is conducted on a 24-hour or older infant. Pulse oximeter probes are placed on the right hand and right foot to obtain a pulse oximeter reading of the oxygen saturation of the blood. If there is a difference of more than 5% between the hand and the foot, the test is considered positive. The health-care provider must be notified so that further testing can be ordered.

Newborn Hearing Screening

The National Institutes of Health (NIH) recommend hearing screens on all newborns, and this recommendation has been implemented by many hospitals. Most states in the United States have implemented mandatory newborn hearing screening programs. Hearing loss occurs in 2 to 4 infants per 1,000 (Delaney, 2014). Early identification of hearing problems with early treatment can prevent severe psychosocial, educational, and speech problems for a child. Screening is usually completed before discharge.

One method of evaluating hearing is the otoacoustic emission test (OAE), which measures a response produced the inner ear by placing a probe in the ear. The other test is the auditory brainstem response (ABR), which measures the hearing from the ear to the brainstem. Information is obtained by placing electrodes on the infant's head. Both tests are easy to perform in the newborn nursery, and the infant is scored as a pass or a fail. Occasionally a newborn does not pass the first hearing screen because of fluid in the ears from birth. If the infant did not pass the first time, most hospitals repeat the test one final time before discharge. The health-care provider must be notified that the infant failed the hearing screen on the second attempt. Infants who fail the newborn screen should be re-tested in one month.

SAFETY *STAT!*

Every time a newborn is taken to his mother, the identification band must be verified with the mother's band.

DISCHARGE TEACHING FOR NEWBORN CARE

The nurse has the responsibility to prepare parents for discharge by teaching and demonstrating basic newborn care. Establishing rapport with the parents will make them feel more comfortable to ask questions. The nurse should encourage parental participation in newborn care in the hospital. There is more than one correct way to provide basic newborn care, and the parents should be encouraged to modify the care to meet their needs or cultural preferences. Reassure the parents that a baby does not know or care if the parents are experts at baby care; the infant just needs basic love, food, warmth, and safety needs to be met. The nurse should focus on safety and basic care while reassuring parents that they will become more comfortable in their new role of providing newborn care.

The nurse should assess the parents' readiness to learn and their teaching needs. Ideally, teaching should occur in short segments. It is difficult for new parents to absorb all the information if the nurse waits until an hour before discharge to begin the teaching. Experienced nurses know that effective discharge teaching is started well before discharge and that printed material to take home for reference is also important. This section will focus on discharge teaching for the healthy term newborn.

Use of the Bulb Syringe

Parents should be instructed about how to use a bulb syringe. The bulb syringe can be used to remove excess mucus, breast milk, or formula if the infant chokes. The bulb in the syringe should be compressed to remove the air, with the tip placed along the cheek or gently into the nostril, and then the fingers should release the bulb to provide suction. The mucus or milk can be squeezed out onto a tissue. The tip of the bulb syringe can scratch the throat, so the parents should never stick the syringe straight back into the mouth and throat area (Fig. 16.13).

Car Seat Safety

From birth to 12 months, the baby should ride in a rear-facing seat that is compliant with current safety standards for car

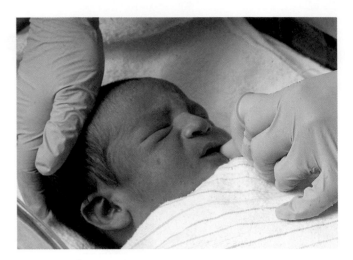

FIGURE 16.13 Bulb syringe used to remove mucus.

seats (NHTSA, 2015). The harness cradles and protects the child's neck and spinal cord in the event of a crash. The car seat should be installed according to the manufacturer's instructions. A car seat that is involved in any accident should be replaced.

Trimming the Baby's Nails

At birth, some babies have long nails. They can easily scratch and cut their own skin. Nurses in the hospital do not cut fingernails. Long-sleeved undershirts with cuffs are used to cover the nails and protect the skin. The parents can be instructed to trim the nails with baby nail scissors or baby clippers. The nail edges should be rounded to avoid sharp edges. It is sometimes easier to cut the nails when the baby is sleeping.

SAFETY *STAT!*

Instruct the parents that if they accidently draw blood or cut the finger when trimming nails, they should apply pressure with a sterile gauze pad. Never apply an adhesive bandage because babies put their fingers in their mouths and can dislodge the bandage and choke on it.

Diaper Rash

Diaper rash can be caused by persistent wet or soiled diapers or by use of some baby products such as commercial baby wipes, creams, and powders. If the baby develops diaper rash, the recommended treatment is to:

• Change diapers often.
• Clean the skin with warm water and avoid commercial premoistened cleaning cloths.
• Apply a barrier of zinc oxide to the skin.
• Keep the diaper area open to air as long as possible before applying a clean diaper (American Academy of Dermatology, 2015).

Umbilical Cord Care

The baby's umbilical cord will slowly change from whitish blue to black over a period of several days. The umbilical stump will fall off within 10 to 21 days. The American Academy of Pediatrics (2015) recommends that the parents:

• Keep the stump dry by folding the diaper below the stump so that it is exposed to air.
• Sponge bathe the baby until the cord falls off.
• Keep the cord clean. If the cord becomes soiled, clean with warm water and pat dry. Some health-care providers instruct the parents to clean the stump once daily with alcohol. The nurse will reinforce the instructions of the pediatrician or pediatric nurse practitioner.
• The stump should be allowed to fall off on its own. Parents should be instructed to avoid pulling on the cord to dislodge it. When the cord falls off, a small amount of bleeding may be noticed by the parent.
• Parents should report any signs of infection such as pus or redness around the umbilical stump.

 CULTURAL CONSIDERATIONS

In the Mexican culture, an attractive umbilicus, also known as the belly button, is important. A protruding belly button is considered unsightly. The mother may place a coin over the umbilicus and wrap a belly band over the coin and around the abdomen to hold the coin in place over the umbilicus. This tradition is not harmful. The nurse should respectfully encourage the mother to clean the coin with alcohol before placing it over the umbilicus (Galanti, 2015).

Circumcision

Circumcision is the surgical removal of the end of the foreskin of the penis. Circumcision can be a controversial topic. The parents may choose circumcision for the newborn because it is a personal preference or a cultural practice. The role of the nurse is to provide information, not personal opinion about whether or not the newborn should be circumcised. Newborn circumcision may be performed in the hospital nursery or at the pediatrician's office.

Before the procedure, an informed signed consent is obtained from the mother. A numbing cream may be applied to the penis 30 to 40 min before the procedure. Some physicians also inject an anesthetic prior to the procedure. In studies, sucrose solution in small amounts has been shown to be effective in reducing the pain response in infants undergoing painful procedures and may be given to the infant (Harrison, Beggs, et al, 2012). Ringlike clamps are tightened over the foreskin and the skin is removed with a scalpel. Another method of circumcision involves the use of a ring called a Plastibell that is left on and falls off on its own, along with the dead foreskin, after 10 to 12 days. The doctor will usually wrap the penis in petroleum gauze to prevent the penis from sticking to the diaper (Fig. 16.14).

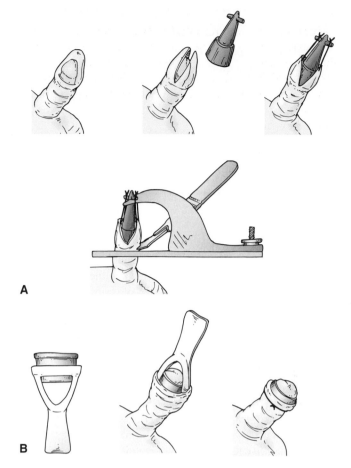

FIGURE 16.14 Removal of the foreskin during circumcision. A, Yellen's clamp procedure. B, Plastibell procedure.

A small amount of blood-tinged drainage may be noted on the diaper after the procedure, and a yellow crust may form on the circumcision site. The nurse should document when the newborn urinates for the first time after a circumcision.

The nurse should instruct the parents to do the following:

• For a few days, wrap the penis in a small amount of gauze with a dab of petroleum jelly to keep the sensitive penis from sticking to the diaper.
• Do not remove or try to wash off the yellow crust. It is not a sign of infection.
• Give a sponge bath until healing is complete and the "ring" falls off, if a Plastibell appliance was used.
• Keep the penis clean and dry.
• Call the doctor if:
  • There is discoloration of the penis.
  • There is discharge from the penis or surgical site that includes pus.
  • There is a spot of blood in the diaper larger than 2 in.
  • The baby does not urinate.
  • A fever greater than 37.8°C axillary occurs.
  • The parents are unable to calm and soothe the baby.

HEALTH PROMOTION

Preventing Flat Spots on the Newborn's Head
A baby sleeps flat on the back several hours a day, which can lead to flat areas on the back of the head. Parents can prevent flat spots on the newborn's head by arranging for "tummy time" each day. Placing the baby on his or her tummy on a blanket on a clean floor for several minutes each day will prevent flat spots. Tummy time also makes the neck and shoulder muscles stronger so that the baby can start to sit up and crawl.

Feeding Schedules

Feeding consumes most of the day with a newborn. It is difficult to get a newborn on a schedule; therefore the American Academy of Pediatrics recommends feeding the baby "on demand" for the first few weeks. When the baby shows signs of hunger such as crying, rooting, and chewing on hands, the mother should feed the baby. The general guideline is that a breastfed baby should be nursing every 2 to 2½ hours and a bottle-fed baby should be fed every 3 to 3½ hours during daytime and evening hours. Unless recommended by the pediatrician, the baby does not need to be awakened at night for a feeding. The baby can wake the mother if hungry.

Elimination

The breastfed newborn should be passing 4 to 5 seedy yellow bowel movements by day 5. A breastfed newborn may have a bowel movement at each feeding or every other feeding. Once the mother's breast milk supply is established, the infant should void clear or pale yellow urine 6 to 8 times daily. The bottle-fed infant should have at least one large tan or yellow bowel movement per day and 6 to 8 wet diapers (American Academy of Pediatrics, 2015).

Positioning and Holding

The caregiver should always support the infant's neck when holding or positioning the infant. The neck is weak and the infant has no control over the head. In the infant seat or car seat, the neck can be supported with a rolled blanket or towel placed around the outside of the head and neck.

There are two ways to safely hold an infant: the cradle hold and the football hold. In the cradle hold, the infant is supine across the adult's chest with the infant's head in the elbow area, which supports the head and neck, with the other arm supporting the back and lower body. The football hold allows the adult to hold the infant with one arm. The infant is placed along the inner aspect of the adult's forearm, with the hand and wrist supporting the head and neck. The rest of the infant's body is supported by the forearm and held snuggly against the adult's body.

Clothing

Any new clothing should be washed before dressing the newborn. To prevent a skin rash, parents should use detergents that are hypoallergenic and free of dyes.

Parents should be cautioned about overdressing the newborn. Typically, the healthy newborn only requires about one layer more of clothing than the parent. The newborn's head accounts for a significant amount of heat loss; therefore, a cap to prevent heat loss should be encouraged when the infant is taken outside or if the room is cool.

Swaddling

Swaddling is a method of wrapping the baby to provide security and warmth. Parents can swaddle the newborn using the following steps:

1. Place the blanket on a flat surface with one corner of the blanket pointing away. Fold that corner down a few inches.
2. Place the baby face up on the blanket with the neck at the edge of the folded-over corner.
3. Fold the left corner of the blanket over the baby and tuck it under the back. The newborn's hands can be left close to the face to allow hand-to-mouth behaviors, which are calming for the newborn.
4. Fold the bottom corner over the feet and chest. Allow the baby to be in a comfortable position, such as flexing his legs.
5. Bring the right corner around the baby's body, covering the bottom corner.

SAFETY *STAT!*

The infant's crib should be free of toys, pillows, and blankets. For safety, the American Academy of Pediatrics (2015) recommends that babies be dressed in layers or swaddled in a blanket for sleep, and that parents should avoid loose blankets in the crib. Infants should always be placed on the back for sleeping. Research has shown that the rate of sudden infant death syndrome (SIDS) in newborns has declined since parents have been educated to place infants on their backs to sleep. The baby's crib should be close to the mother at night, such as in her room, but for safety, the newborn should not sleep in the same bed as the parents.

Sponge Bathing

Sponge bathing should be done until the umbilical cord falls off and the circumcision site is healed. A newborn does not require a complete bath every day. However, the genital and buttock area should be cleaned daily to prevent irritation in the diaper area. The procedure for sponge bathing is:

- Gather all supplies before beginning the bath: a mild or hypoallergenic baby soap, wash cloths, towel, clean diaper, and clean clothes.
- A towel should be placed on a firm surface next to the sink or basin of water filled with lukewarm water. The parents should always test the water on their forearm.
- Undress the baby and cover with a towel. To avoid chilling the baby, only the parts of the body being washed should be exposed.

- Always keep one hand on the baby.
- Start with the eyes. Using a clean cloth and no soap, wipe gently from the bridge of the nose outward.
- Move next to the ears and the rest of the face. No soap is needed for the face.
- Uncover the chest and, using gentle soap, clean the neck, chest, arms, and hands. Pay attention to creases in the skin. Rinse carefully, keeping the umbilical stump dry. Pat the skin dry.
- Cover the chest and uncover the lower body. Wash, rinse, and pat dry the toes, feet, and legs.
- Turn the baby over and wash and rinse the back.
- The genitals and buttocks are washed last. For a girl, wash from front to back. If the boy is circumcised, do not wash the penis until it is healed.
- After drying the baby, the diaper should be replaced and the baby wrapped in a towel before washing the hair.
- To wash the hair, the baby can be held in the football hold, supporting the neck and head; use the other hand to wash and rinse the hair. Tilt the head slightly back to keep water and shampoo from running into the eyes.

Skin Care

Babies have delicate skin. The mother should be encouraged to avoid washing the baby with any products that have fragrance or unnecessary additives. Some commercial baby wipes can be irritating to the skin. If that is the case, plain water with cotton squares are sufficient for cleansing the diaper area. Talcum powder is not used for babies because of the risk of inhaling the talcum into the lungs.

Infant Follow-Up Care After Discharge

Most pediatricians schedule a 2-week follow-up appointment for the newborn. However, a newborn who is not feeding well and has lost 10% or more of the birth weight will probably be scheduled for an appointment 2 days after discharge for a weight check.

PATIENT TEACHING GUIDELINES

Before discharge, parents should be educated that any of the following signs of newborn illness requires a call to the pediatric or family practice office:
- Breathing more than 60 breaths/min
- Grunting sounds when breathing
- Blue color of the face, tongue, or lips
- Abdominal distention (ie, a hard belly) accompanied by vomiting or no bowel movement for more than 1 day
- Jitters or shakiness of the whole body
- Vomiting that is forceful and shoots out several inches
- Persistent choking during feedings
- Heat-to-toe yellow skin color
- An umbilical cord that is red and has pus around the base
- Diarrhea (ie, more than six watery stools per day)
- Poor feeding
- Excessive crying

Key Points

- An assessment is a systematic way of obtaining data to identify problems. The newborn should have a complete head-to-toe assessment within 2 hours of birth.
- Initial measurements of the newborn include head, chest, length, and weight.
- A complete head-to-toe assessment includes vital signs and assessment of the skin, head, eyes, ears, nose, mouth, chest, and abdomen, as well as the respiratory, cardiovascular, genitourinary, neurological, and musculoskeletal systems.
- Throughout the newborn assessment, the nurse should identify warning signs to report.
- There are a variety of normal newborn skin variations, including rashes, birthmarks, and lesions.
- There are many newborn reflexes that indicate healthy neurological functioning.

- A gestational age assessment may be indicated if the newborn appears preterm, post-term, small for gestational age, or large for gestational age.
- Nursing care for the newborn includes medications, the initial newborn bath, and coordination of newborn screening for health maintenance.
- The nurse is responsible for discharge teaching regarding newborn care, including umbilicus care, circumcision care, feeding schedules, and elimination.
- To promote safety, the parents need to be instructed about the use of the bulb syringe, sleeping positions, holding and positioning, trimming the nails, bathing, car seat safety, and skin care.

REVIEW QUESTIONS

1. The white protective coating on the skin of the newborn is called:
   1. Lanugo
   2. Milia
   3. Galactorrhea
   4. Vernix

2. A mother asks the nurse, "Why does my baby have blue hands?" The best response by the nurse is:
   1. "He is just cold."
   2. "He may have been born with a heart problem."
   3. "The circulation in the hands is not fully developed."
   4. "The hands are always blue in the newborn."

3. Normal newborn rash is also known as:
   1. Erythema toxicum neonatorum
   2. Nevus simplex
   3. Hemangioma
   4. Nevus flammeus

4. Swelling on the head caused by birth trauma that does not cross the newborn's cranial suture lines is termed:
   1. Molding
   2. Caput succedaneum
   3. Cephalohematoma
   4. Melanosis

5. The nurse notes that the newborn's respiratory rate is 42 breaths/min, the pulse is 140 bpm, and the CRT is less than 3 sec. The nurse should:
   1. Report the findings to the charge nurse.
   2. Document the findings as normal.
   3. Repeat the examination to verify abnormal findings.
   4. Return the newborn to the nursery for observation.

6. The nurse is most concerned about which of the following assessment findings?
   1. Gynecomastia
   2. Positive Ortolani's test
   3. Pseudomenstruation
   4. Dermal melanosis

7. A sponge bath should not be given to the newborn until: *(select all that apply)*
   1. The baby is able to sit up on his or her own.
   2. The umbilical cord falls off.
   3. Both parents can help with the bath.
   4. The circumcision is healed.
   5. The infant is 1 month old.

8. Which of the following assessment findings should be reported? *(select all that apply)*
   1. Undescended testicles
   2. Periodic mild twitching
   3. Yellowish skin color
   4. Stork bites on the forehead
   5. Bulging anterior fontanel
   6. Absent Moro's reflex
   7. Irregular breathing pattern

9. The purpose of starting the hepatitis B vaccine series is to:
   1. Prevent the infant from contracting hepatitis while in the hospital.
   2. Comply with state law regarding immunizations.
   3. Prevent the infant from contracting hepatitis B from family members.
   4. Prevent the infant from acquiring a sexually transmitted disease later in life.

10. A new mother asks the nurse if she should get her baby circumcised. The best response by the nurse is:
    1. "Of course, everyone does it."
    2. "What are your questions or concerns about it?"
    3. "I didn't circumcise my son."
    4. "It's up to you; you're the mom."

CRITICAL THINKING QUESTIONS

1. A new mother questions why her baby needs the newborn screening. She states, "He is perfect. He had 8 and 9 Apgar tests at birth, and he doesn't look sick." How should the nurse answer the patient about the newborn screening tests?

2. Why should an infant of a diabetic mother receive a gestational age assessment?

For additional resources and information, visit **www.DavisPlus.com.**
Post-Conference Questions and Activities, Answers, and References can be found on DavisPlus.

Newborn Nutrition

17

LEARNING OUTCOMES

1. Define the key terms.
2. Discuss infant nutritional needs.
3. Describe the process of human milk production.
4. Describe the stages of milk production.
5. List the advantages and disadvantages of breastfeeding.
6. Identify contraindications for breastfeeding.
7. Identify cues of infant readiness to nurse.
8. Teach a mother how to correctly latch-on a baby for breastfeeding.
9. Discuss common breastfeeding problems and how to manage those problems.
10. Identify warning signs of inadequate breastfeeding in the newborn.
11. List the advantages and disadvantages of bottle feeding.
12. Teach bottle feeding parents how to prepare formula.
13. Discuss bottle feeding and safety issues for parents.
14. Identify signs of bottle feeding problems.
15. Provide patient-centered care when assisting parents to implement their choice of feeding method for their newborn.

KEY TERMS

areola
engorgement
fore milk
galactosemia
hind milk
immunoglobulin
inverted nipples
lactoferrin
lactogenesis
prolactin

DavisPlus For audio pronunciation guide, visit www.DavisPlus.com

CHAPTER CONCEPTS

Development
Nursing
Nutrition
Promoting Health

REAL-WORLD CASE STUDY

Samantha

■ Samantha is 25 years old and pregnant with her first baby. She is planning to return to her job as a kindergarten teacher after a maternity leave of 4 months. At her 20-week prenatal appointment, the nurse introduces the subject of breastfeeding. Samantha is interested in breastfeeding, but no one in her family has ever breastfed before and she does not really know much about it. She is wondering if it will be hard to be a working breastfeeding mother.

continued on page 246

How can the nurse:

1. Explain to Samantha the advantages of breastfeeding?
2. Provide Samantha with resources for learning about breastfeeding?
3. Make suggestions for assisting Samantha with working and breastfeeding?

CONCEPTUAL CORNERSTONE

Nutrition

Nutrition is a fundamental concept for nursing practice because it is directly related to health. Good nutrition is important for a healthy lifestyle. The newborn who receives proper nutrition will grow appropriately and meet physical, mental, and emotional developmental milestones. Underfed or improperly fed infants run the risk of organ damage, dehydration, and failure to thrive, and do not meet developmental milestones. The infant is at risk for altered nutrition owing to immature organ development that requires certain nutrients for maturation, and the infant's total reliance on others for feeding. Nurses can have an effect on the nutritional needs of the newborn by educating parents about infant nutrition, encouraging breastfeeding, supporting correct bottle feeding, and monitoring the growth and development of the infant. Early support of healthy nutrition can set the foundation for a lifetime of healthy food choices.

Whether parents decide to breastfeed or bottle feed, learning the skills to feed their infant can produce some anxiety for them. Nurses need to be informed and educated about infant feeding practices. Parents look to nurses to provide education, guidance, and support when choosing a feeding method. Infant nutrition is important because it has an effect on the infant's growth and brain development. This chapter focuses on feeding the full-term infant of normal birth weight in the context of both breastfeeding and bottle feeding.

RECOMMENDED INFANT NUTRITION

The American Academy of Pediatrics (2012) recommends exclusive breastfeeding for the first 6 months of age, with the addition of solid foods along with breastfeeding for another 6 months. The World Health Organization (2015) recommends exclusive breastfeeding for 6 months, and then the addition of appropriate food along with breastfeeding for 2 years or more. Women who receive education and family support are more likely to continue breastfeeding to 6 months or longer postpartum (Brown, 2013). Nurses play a crucial role in facilitating success with lactation. The mother makes her decision about whether or not to breastfeed before delivery in

90% of cases. Therefore her choice of feeding should be discussed with her starting in the second trimester and throughout the pregnancy and postpartum (Wagner, 2012).

In 2014, the percentage of infants breastfed at birth in the United States was 79%. By 6 months of age, only 49.4% were still being breastfed, and at 12 months of age, only 26.7% were being breastfed (CDC, 2014).

Nutritional Needs of the Infant

The estimated calorie need for infants is based on their age, size, and sex. Estimated calories by the National Institute of Health (2013) are:

- 105 to 108 kcal/kg/day (Term infant)
- 110 to 120 kcal/kg/day (Preterm infant)

The estimated fluid requirements for a newborn are:

- 140 to 160 mL/kg/day (Term infant)
- 60 to 80 mL/kg/day (Preterm infant) (Ambalavanan, 2014)

Calorie needs per pound of body weight are higher during the first year of life than at any other time. For the first 4 to 6 months of life, breast or formula feeding can provide sufficient calories. The infant's health-care provider will measure weight and length and plot this information on a standardized growth grid to determine the adequacy of an infant's caloric intake.

The calories in an infant's diet are provided by protein, fat, and carbohydrates. Of the protein requirement, 50% is used for growth in the first 2 months of life, which declines to 11% by 2 to 3 years of age. Fat provides 40% to 50% of the calories supplied during infancy and is a source of essential fatty acids. Carbohydrates, primarily lactose, are the principal source of dietary energy. Water requirements for the first 6 months are met when adequate amounts of breast milk or infant formula are consumed.

The newborn infant frequently eats only small amounts the first few days; parents should be educated about the size of the infant's stomach to avoid overfeeding (Wickham, 2013).

Infant stomach capacity is the following:

- Day 1: 5 to 7 mL
- Day 3: 22 to 27 mL
- Day 10: 45 to 60 mL

THE BREASTFEEDING MOTHER AND INFANT

The *Healthy People 2020* breastfeeding objective includes an increase in exclusive breastfeeding to promote infant health and reduce mortality. The Academy of Breastfeeding Medicine (2013) recommends that all health-care professionals promote breastfeeding early in prenatal care and recognize that breastfeeding is superior to bottle feeding. The promotion of breastfeeding by health-care providers may help to increase support from families and employers, making it easier for the woman to continue breastfeeding. Parents need to be provided with complete and current information on the benefits of breastfeeding and breastfeeding techniques.

After delivery, postpartum unit policies on breastfeeding should support and encourage breastfeeding by placing the newborn in direct skin-to-skin contact with the mother after delivery and assisting her with latch-on during the first hour after birth. The mother and infant should not be separated on the postpartum unit and should be encouraged to sleep in close proximity to facilitate breastfeeding. Postpartum units should not sabotage breastfeeding by providing supplements such as water or formula unless medically indicated and ordered by the health-care provider. Women can be successful with breastfeeding when nurses and lactation specialists provide education and support as the new mother learns breastfeeding techniques.

THERAPEUTIC COMMUNICATION

Not all women are comfortable with the idea of breastfeeding their infants. They may have never seen or been around a breastfed baby. They may be embarrassed to breastfeed around people. It is very important that nurses enthusiastic about breastfeeding do not make a patient feel badly about her choice to bottle feed. The nurse should educate and support the patient's decision regarding feeding methods. When discussing breastfeeding choices, use open-ended questions and general leads. Some examples are:

"What are your thoughts about breastfeeding?" (Open-ended question)

"What do you know about breastfeeding?" (General lead)

"What are your concerns about breastfeeding?" (Open-ended question)

Lactogenesis

Milk production, or **lactogenesis,** includes all the processes needed to transform the mammary gland from its nonproducing state to one of milk production.

At puberty, estrogen stimulates breast tissue to enlarge through growth of mammary ducts into the mammary fat pad. The effects of estrogen and progesterone enable the formation of the structure of the adult female breast, but full alveolar development and maturation of the epithelium requires the hormones of pregnancy.

The basic unit of the mammary gland is the alveolus that connects to a ductule. Each ductule drains to a duct, which then empties into the lactiferous sinuses. Milk is stored in the lactiferous sinus. At the end of each ductule is a cluster of small, grapelike sacs called *alveoli.* A cluster of alveoli is called a *lobule;* a cluster of lobules is called a *lobe.* Each breast contains between 15 and 20 lobes, with one milk duct for every lobe. The 15 to 20 milk ducts merge, with eight or nine ending at the tip of the nipple to deliver milk to the baby (Gabriel, 2013) (Fig. 17.1).

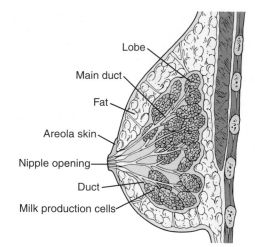

FIGURE 17.1 Cross section of a lactating breast.

After childbirth and the delivery of the placenta, estrogen and progesterone levels drop quickly. Nipple stimulation occurs from latching-on the infant to the breast, which stimulates the pituitary gland to trigger a rise in the hormone **prolactin.** Prolactin causes the alveoli to take proteins, sugars, and fat from the blood supply and make breast milk (Fig. 17.2).

The first substance produced by the breasts is colostrum. It is produced in very small amounts during the second and third trimesters. The pregnant woman may notice a small amount of a sticky substance on her bra or nightgown occasionally. Colostrum is the perfect first food for the newborn. It is easy to digest and highly concentrated with carbohydrates and fat. It also contains secretory **immunoglobulin** A (IgA), which is a new substance to the newborn. IgA is a protein that functions as an antibody to protect the baby from infections in the mucous membranes in the throat, lungs, and intestines.

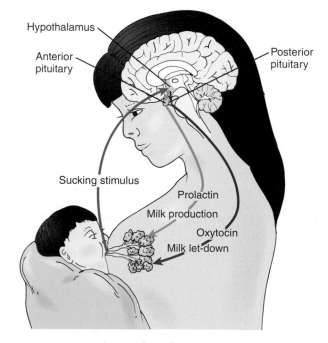

FIGURE 17.2 Mechanism for milk production.

Leukocytes are also present in colostrum, which protects the newborn from infections. Colostrum also has a laxative effect, which aids in the passage of the first meconium stool after birth (La Leche League, 2012).

Frequent breastfeeding at least 8 to 12 times a day stimulates the pituitary to increase levels of prolactin, which causes an increase in the volume of breast milk. Mature milk is produced around the 3rd and 4th postpartum day.

For the baby to receive the milk from the breast, the let-down reflex must occur. The baby sucking the nipple stimulates the pituitary gland to release prolactin to produce the milk and oxytocin, another hormone, to release the milk. Oxytocin causes the cells around the alveoli to squeeze the glands to push the milk into the ductules and into the ducts. The mother may notice the let-down reflex and a tingly or warm sensation in her breasts. She may notice the milk drip or spray during let-down. The let-down reflex can also be triggered by the mother hearing a baby cry or thinking about her baby. As the baby suckles, the combination of the let-down reflex, compression of the areola, and negative pressure created by suckling allows the milk to be delivered to the infant (Wagner, 2015).

Components of Breast Milk

The following list provides an overview of the components and nutrients in breast milk:

- **Proteins**: The balance of the proteins, approximately 60% whey and 40% casein, allows the infant to digest breast milk easily. Other specific proteins in breast milk are:
  - **Lactoferrin,** which has bactericidal and iron-binding properties
  - **Secretory IgA,** which protects the infant from viruses and bacteria
  - **Lysozyme,** an enzyme that promotes the growth of healthy intestinal flora and has anti-inflammatory functions
- **Bifidus factor** supports the growth of lactobacillus, which creates an acidic environment in the intestines.
- **Cholesterol and fats** are essential for brain development and the absorption of fat-soluble vitamins, and are a primary calorie source.
- **Vitamin** amount and types in breast milk are directly related to the mother's dietary intake.
- **Carbohydrates, especially lactose:** Lactose is the primary carbohydrate found in human milk, accounting for approximately 40% of the total calories provided by breast milk.
- **Antibodies** from the mother reduce the risk of neonatal infections (Wagner, 2015).

DRUG FACTS

Vitamin D

The American Academy of Pediatrics (2012) recommends vitamin D supplementation (400 IU/d) starting after delivery. There is widespread vitamin D deficiency in the United States, and breastfeeding mothers deficient in vitamin D are unable to pass vitamin D in the breast milk to the infant.

Stages of Human Milk

During the establishment of lactation, there are three stages of milk production: colostrum, transitional milk, and mature milk.

- Stage 1: Colostrum
  - Yellowish fluid that is present for 2 to 3 days
  - Contains high levels of protein, and lower levels of carbohydrates, fats, and calories than mature milk
  - High in immunoglobulins G and A, which protect the infant from infections
  - Has a laxative effect to promote passage of the meconium stool
- Stage 2: Transitional Milk
  - This stage is from day 3 to day 10.
  - Contains increasing levels of carbohydrates and fat with decreasing levels of protein
- Stage 3: Mature Milk
  - **Fore milk** is the milk produced and stored between feedings. It has higher water content than hind milk.
  - **Hind milk** is produced after several minutes of feeding and has a higher fat content and contributes to the feeling of fullness and satisfaction for the infant (Wagner, 2015).

CULTURAL CONSIDERATIONS

Nurses know that colostrum is rich in antibodies and is very healthy for the newborn. It is also known that milk production is enhanced by the nipple stimulation that comes with early breastfeeding. Some cultures, such as the Hispanic culture and the Vietnamese culture, do not encourage putting the newborn to the breast until the actual milk comes in. The best way to deal with this situation is to educate the new mother on the advantages of colostrum and early breastfeeding, and be understanding if she prefers to wait a few days to begin breastfeeding (Galanti, 2015).

Advantages of Breastfeeding

The advantages of breastfeeding for the mother and infant include the following:

- Breast milk provides the exact nutrients required for an infant's growth and development.
- Breast milk provides immunological protection. A mother will pass on some of her immunities to the baby.
- Breast milk is convenient and economical for the mother. She does not need to prepare bottles. It is always ready and available for the infant.
- Breastfeeding promotes close physical contact between a mother and child to enhance bonding and attachment.

Disadvantages of Breastfeeding

The disadvantages of breastfeeding for the mother and infant include the following:

- The mother must be available for feeding or provide pumped milk if she is absent.
- Feeding in public may cause embarrassment.

- Certain medications can interrupt breastfeeding.
- Early breastfeeding may be uncomfortable.
- Leaking of breast milk may occur and require nursing pads to be worn in the bra.

DRUG FACTS

Most drugs pass from the mother through the breast milk to the baby. If the mother requires medication while breastfeeding, the health-care provider should check for risks to the baby before prescribing the medication and fully inform the mother of the risk.

Contraindications for Breastfeeding

There are some contraindications for breastfeeding. The health-care provider and nurses should be aware of the following contraindications:

- An infant diagnosed with **galactosemia,** a rare genetic metabolic disorder that makes it difficult for the infant to metabolize milk sugar; breastfeeding an infant with galactosemia can damage the liver, kidneys, and brain
- The infant whose mother:
  - Has been infected with HIV
  - Is taking antiretroviral medications
  - Has untreated, active tuberculosis
  - Is infected with human T-cell lymphotropic virus type I or type II, which is the virus that causes some leukemias and lymphomas
  - Is using or is dependent upon an illicit drug
  - Is taking prescribed cancer chemotherapy agents, such as antimetabolites that interfere with DNA replication and cell division
  - Is undergoing radiation therapies; however, such nuclear medicine therapies require only a temporary interruption in breastfeeding (CDC, 2013)

LEARN TO C.U.S.

Kari, aged 28, gave birth 1 day ago at the local hospital. She did not have prenatal care and admits to alcohol and drug use. She plans to breastfeed and states, "I can't afford to buy formula; I have to breastfeed." The nurse is concerned about breastfeeding and substance abuse. The nurse uses the C.U.S. method of communication with the pediatrician.

Nurse:

C: "I am very **concerned** about Kari and her baby.

U: I am **uncomfortable** with assisting her with breastfeeding. I am not sure it's the right thing for her to do.

S: I feel that we have a **safety** issue because Kari admits to substance abuse and alcohol use."

Correct Breastfeeding Techniques

The breastfeeding mother can be supported in her plan to breast-feed by first providing a relaxed and supportive environment.

The nurse should be available to assist with positioning, education, and positive feedback during the process. Minimizing interruptions and visitors will facilitate the process. The father should be included in education and feeding sessions. Women with partners who support and encourage breastfeeding are more likely to choose this method of infant feeding.

Newborn Cues

The new mother needs to be taught signs that the newborn is interested in nursing. However, if the newborn does not demonstrate signs of hunger, she should still offer the breast every 2½ hours until breastfeeding has been established and she is more aware of her infant's cues. Newborns indicate hunger by rooting, making hand-to-mouth movements, and making mouth and tongue movements while in an awake/alert state (Womenshealth.gov, 2014).

PATIENT TEACHING GUIDELINES

As the new breastfeeding mother's milk flow increases, the contraction of the milk-filled alveoli may create a tingling, stinging, burning, or prickling sensation in her breasts. The milk may drip or even spray during letdown. Sometimes, just the sound of any baby crying will cause milk let-down. If this happens at an inconvenient time, she can try crossing her arms in front of her breasts and apply gentle pressure to stop the flow.

Positioning

The position of the infant is an important part of successful breastfeeding. First, the mother should wash her hands to avoid transferring bacteria to her breast. Next, she should be in a comfortable sitting position or side-lying in bed. Pillows should be placed around the mother to support the baby and prevent the mother from hunching her back. Pillows can be placed to support her arm. The infant should be placed in the mother's arm with his or her stomach flat against the mother's abdomen (Fig. 17.3).

Another position is the football hold, in which the infant is cradled in the mother's arm with the infant's head in her palm and the toward the mother's elbow. This position puts less stress on the abdomen if the mother is recuperating from a Cesarean birth.

Achieving Latch-On

The mother should position her hand around the breast, cupping it with her fingers close to the chest wall. Her hands are usually in a "C" position as she supports her breast: The thumb is on top and her fingers are underneath the breast. She should avoid covering the **areola,** the dark area around the nipple. This part of the breast goes into the infant's mouth. After positioning her hand, the mother should lightly brush her nipple across the lips of her infant to elicit the rooting reflex. The infant will instinctively open his or her mouth and extend the tongue. The mother should bring her baby to her breast and maneuver the nipple and areola into the infant's mouth. These actions will initiate the sucking reflex (Figs. 17.4 and 17.5).

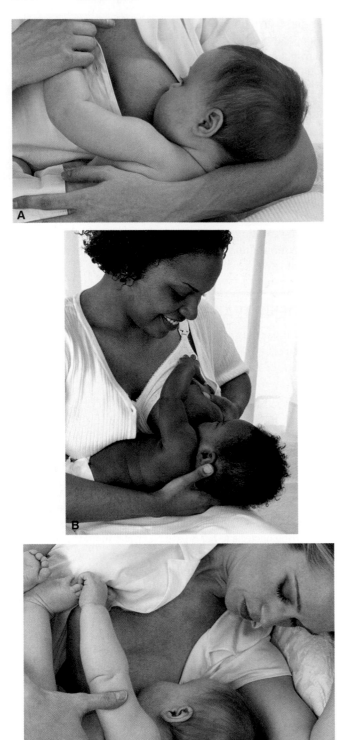

FIGURE 17.3 Common positions for breastfeeding. A, Cradle hold position. B, Football hold position. C, Side-lying position. (*Courtesy Medela Corporation, McHenry, Illinois.*)

The mother should put the infant on the breast every 2½ hours during the first 4 to 5 days after birth to assist with creation of the milk supply. Generally, it takes about 30 to 40 min of sucking for an infant to have a complete feeding. If the infant falls asleep on the breast, the mother should be encouraged to take him or her off the breast, change to the

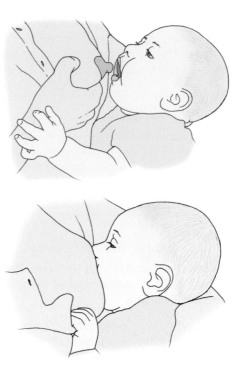

FIGURE 17.4 Correct latch-on position. When properly latched-on, the tip of the infant's nose, cheeks, and chin should all be touching the breast.

other breast, and resume the feeding session. The baby should be burped between breasts. The mother should alternate the breast at which the feeding begins. She should avoid supplemental formula or water because some babies will suck on a bottle even if full of breast milk.

The new mother should be reassured that even though feeding a newborn can take up much time initially, after breastfeeding is established, the infant becomes stronger and feedings proceed much faster. Instruct the breastfeeding woman that her baby will have several wet diapers and two to three dirty diapers per day. A breastfed infant's stools are looser than formula-fed infants.

HEALTH PROMOTION

Checkpoints for Correct Latch-On

- Observe the position of the mother. Is she comfortable, with pillows in appropriate locations? Reposition if needed.
- Observe the position of the baby. Is he or she lying "tummy to tummy" with the mother? If not, reposition.
- Observe the position of the baby on the areola. Usually the lips need to be 1 to 2 in. beyond the base of the nipple.
- Observe the infant's lower lip. It should not be folded in.
- Observe the motion of the masseter muscle and listen for sounds of swallowing. A clicking sound indicates improper positioning.

  Observe the comfort level of the mother. If she is experiencing any nipple pain, she should take the infant off the breast and latch-on again.

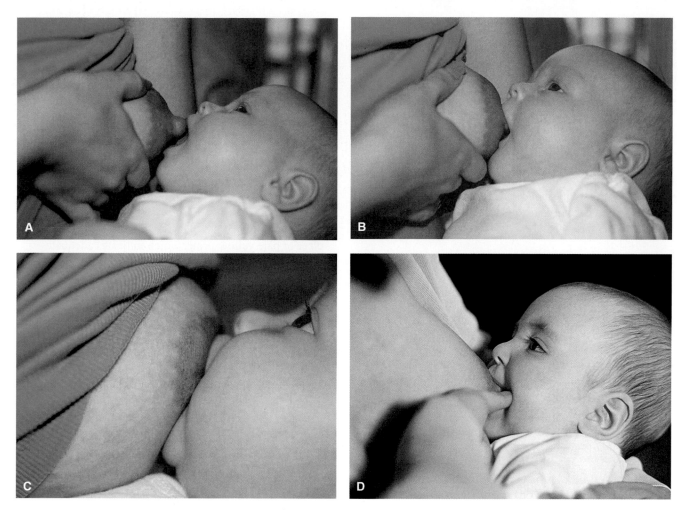

FIGURE 17.5 Infant latch-on. A, Nipple is aligned with the baby's nose. B and C, As the baby latches to the nipple, the baby's mouth is placed 1 to 2 in. beyond the base of the nipple. D, To remove the baby from the breast, the mother inserts her finger into the corner of the baby's mouth to break the seal.

Signs of Effective Breastfeeding

The infant is getting sufficient intake from breastfeeding if:

- The mother's breasts soften during and after a feeding.
- The mother can hear the infant swallowing during the feeding.
- The number of wet diapers increases to at least six to eight by the time the infant is 6 days old.
- The infant has two to three yellow stools by the 5th day after birth.

Breastfeeding Challenges

Breastfeeding can be a challenge in the first few days or weeks. The nurse can provide guidance to support the breastfeeding mother with common problems.

Sore Nipples

Sore nipples are a common occurrence but can be prevented or managed with the following interventions:

- Make sure the infant has correct latch-on every time the baby is placed on the breast.

- Try changing positions from sitting to side-lying or football hold to move the infant's mouth to a different position on the breast.
- Change nursing pads often to avoid trapping moisture on the nipple areas.
- Expose the nipple to air to promote healing.
- Avoid harsh soaps on the breast.
- Apply modified anhydrous lanolin after nursing to keep the skin soft.
- Gentle massaging of colostrum or breast milk into the nipple can soothe an irritated nipple.

Nipple Confusion

A latex nipple fits into the infant mouth differently than a breast nipple. An infant that is learning to breastfeed can have difficulty with learning how to place her or his jaws and tongue if a latex nipple is introduced too early. If the mother wants to avoid nipple confusion and be able to leave the baby with a bottle, she should first establish breastfeeding *for at least 2 to 3 weeks before introducing a bottle.*

Low Milk Supply

Most women make plenty of milk, but during the baby's growth spurts at 3 weeks, 6 weeks, and 3 months, the supply may be a little low to satisfy the baby.

- Breastfeed more often and allow the baby to decide when to end the feeding. Feeding the baby in this method is sometimes called "cluster feeding." The baby is allowed and encouraged to breastfed as often and as long as he or she wants. This method of feeding will increase milk supply for the growing baby.
- Offer both breasts at each feeding. Have the baby stay on the first breast as long as he or she is still suckling and swallowing. Offer the second breast when the baby slows down.

Engorgement

Engorgement can happen when the body is adjusting to the amount of milk to make. It can also occur the first time the baby sleeps through the night. The breasts may feel heavy and swollen, with a flat nipple.

- Breastfeed every 2½ hours when the baby is awake.
- Soften the breasts with a warm cloth or in the shower and express enough milk by hand to soften the breast to allow correct latch-on by the infant.
- Latch-on the infant correctly and the feeding will take care of the engorgement.

Flat or Inverted Nipples

Flat or **inverted nipples** may make it difficult to latch-on the baby. Flat nipples do not stand out from the areola and inverted nipples tend to retract or pull inward. Women with these types of nipples may require more assistance with breastfeeding.

- Breast pumping may be used to pull out the nipple.
- Before delivery, the lactation specialist may recommend that the pregnant woman wear a special device called a *breast shield* or a *supple cup* to encourage the nipple to protrude from the breast.

LABS & DIAGNOSTICS

Inverted or Flat Nipples

Women who are screened for flat or inverted nipples early in the pregnancy can benefit from consulting a lactation specialist regarding options for preparing the nipples for breastfeeding. Women with flat or inverted nipples can breastfeed, but it does cause some degree of difficulty. The La Leche League recommends early detection and using nipple shields, breast pumps, and techniques to encourage the nipple to protrude more from the breast to aid in latch-on.

TEAM WORKS

The first few weeks of breastfeeding can be difficult for new mothers. They frequently have many questions and may have problems such as sore nipples and engorgement. A team consisting of the postpartum nurse, lactation specialist, pediatrician, nurse practitioner, and perhaps another experienced breastfeeding mother can assist her to be successful in her desire to breastfeed.

Warning Signs of Breastfeeding Problems

Warning signs in the healthy term breastfed newborn include:

- Losing more than 7% of birth weight
- Not gaining back birth weight by 10 days of age
- Not having at least two to three bowel movements per day after day 2
- Not having four or five wet diapers per day by day 4 with clear or pale yellow urine, which indicates adequate hydration of the newborn

THE FORMULA-FEEDING PARENTS AND INFANT

The infant formula industry acknowledges the importance of human milk and recognizes breastfeeding as the preferred method for feeding babies. The formula industry is committed to producing infant formulas modeled on breast milk. Commercially prepared formulas meet the nutritional requirements based on the recommendations of the Committee on Nutrition of the American Academy of Pediatrics to provide the infant with the right combination of protein, fat, carbohydrates, vitamins, and minerals.

The American Academy of Pediatrics (2012) states that cow's milk is not suitable for infants under 1 year of age. It is not appropriate for infants because it contains a higher level of protein than the infant requires; the fat is difficult for the infant to digest; it is a poor source of iron; it contains only a small amount of vitamins C, E, and copper; and the sodium level is too high for an infant.

Bottle feeding can be a warm, loving experience for the parents and their infant. If the parents choose this method of feeding, they should be supported and educated without disapproval from the nursing staff.

Advantages of Formula

The advantages of bottle feeding for the parents and infant include the following:

- It may be the appropriate choice for a mother with a chronic illness who requires medications harmful to the infant.
- It provides adequate and acceptable nutrition for the infant.
- Anyone can feed the infant.
- It may be more comfortable for the mother to feed in public.
- The mother does not need to worry that her food or alcohol intake may affect the baby.
- It may be easier to leave the infant with a sitter or family member to give the parents a break.

NURSING CARE PLAN for the Patient with Ineffective Breastfeeding

Elaina has arrived at the hospital lactation clinic with concerns about breastfeeding. Even though she is feeding her infant every 4 hours, she reports that he often falls asleep on the breast and only nurses for 10 to 15 min. She is concerned that her 5-day-old son is not getting enough milk. She reports that he is having only two wet diapers a day and has not had a bowel movement since yesterday.

Nursing Diagnosis: There is ineffective breastfeeding related to the mother's lack of knowledge of breastfeeding techniques as evidenced by infant's inadequate number of wet and soiled diapers.

Expected Outcomes:
- The infant will have at least six wet diapers and two to three stools per day.
- The infant will breastfeed every 2½ hours with 30 to 40 min of sucking time.

Interventions:
- Provide verbal encouragement so that Elaina will not quit breastfeeding.
- Weigh the infant and compare the weight with the birth weight.
- Review infant cues of hunger with the mother.
- Review feeding requirements of offering the breast every 2½ hours and encouraging the infant to nurse for 30 to 40 min each feeding.
- Encourage her to wake the baby up if he falls asleep while nursing and have him latch-on again.
- Observe the mother latch-on the infant and give suggestions if needed.
- Review infant elimination patterns with the mother.
- Provide written instructions.
- Ask Elaina to maintain a feeding diary to monitor the infant's intake, as well as wet and soiled diapers.
- Follow up with a weight check and feeding diary review in 2 days.

Disadvantages of Formula

The disadvantages of bottle feeding include the following:

- Formula costs can be expensive for parents on a budget.
- Bottles, nipples, and formula must be purchased.
- Bottles and formula must be carried along with the infant.

Types of Formula

Most infant formulas have 20 calories in each ounce. It is important that parents are aware of correct bottle preparation. Prepared formula should be in a covered container in the refrigerator, and unused formula should be thrown out after 24 hours. Hypoallergenic formula should be given if an allergy to milk-based formula is suspected. Soy-based formula should be given to infants who cannot take dairy-based products for health, cultural, religious, or personal reasons, such as a vegan lifestyle.

Parents should be taught the following about formula:

- Ready-to-feed formula is available in a can or carton and should not be diluted.
- Liquid concentrated formula is formulated to be diluted with equal amounts of water.
- Powder formula should be dissolved in water.

SAFETY *STAT!*

If the parents are concerned about the safety of tap water, the water should be sterilized before making formula. Water can also be checked for lead, nitrates, and bacteria. The steps to sterilize the water are:
- Let the cold water run until it is a cold as it gets. It may take 2 min. This process reduces the amount of lead and other contaminants in the water.
- Bring the cold water to a boil and let it boil for 1-2 min.
- Let the water cool before preparing the bottles (Mayo Clinic, 2015).

SAFETY *STAT!*

Well water in rural agricultural areas can be contaminated with nitrates, which can be dangerous for babies under 6 months of age. The nitrates can cause a problem with the infant's blood oxygen level. Families relying on well water should be cautioned to have the water evaluated for safety before using it for formula preparation.

Bottle Feeding the Infant

When the nurse educates the parents about bottle feeding, the following information should be included:

- Before purchasing, check the expiration date on the formula container.
- After purchasing, sterilize the bottles and nipples. After initial sterilization, bottles do not need to be sterilized unless the family water supply is not safe. Washing bottle

and nipples with soap and water or in the dishwasher is sufficient to kill bacteria.

- Make sure to follow the package directions to dilute the formula or to mix the bottles correctly.
- If the water supply is not proven to be safe, the water for mixing the formula should be boiled first.
- Wash the formula container with soap and water before opening it.
- Some babies will drink a bottle straight from the refrigerator. Others prefer a bottle warmed in a bowl of warm water. Parents should always check the temperature of warmed formula to avoid burning the infant.
- Make sure the nipple is not too large to cause gagging or too small to cause frustration for the infant.
- Parents should wash their hands before every feeding.
- Before feeding the infant, find a comfortable place to sit and have a burp cloth nearby.
- Cradle the baby in one arm with the head slightly elevated and hold the bottle with the opposite arm.
- Angle the bottle so that the baby is not sucking in air.
- Keep the nipple filled with formula.
- Stop and take burping breaks.
- Try different nipple shapes to see what the baby prefers.
- Do not use a bottle that has been sitting out for more than 2 hours.
- Continue to feed until the newborn gives indications of being full, such as a decrease in sucking, spitting out the nipple, turning away, or pushing away the bottle.
- Never force a baby to finish a bottle.
- When the baby begins to cut teeth, do not let the baby fall asleep with a bottle in the mouth because this can lead to tooth decay from the milk sugar.

SAFETY *STAT!*

Warming a Bottle

Never warm a bottle of formula or breast milk in the microwave. Microwaves heat unevenly and a baby could be burned.

SAFETY *STAT!*

Propping a Bottle

Bottle-fed babies should never have the bottle propped for feedings. There are two major problems with this practice. First, the baby could choke and aspirate without adult observation. Second, the baby who falls asleep with a propped bottle has residual milk left in the mouth that pools around the teeth. The milk sugar can cause breakdown of the teeth and cause nursing-bottle syndrome.

Warning Signs of Bottle Feeding Problems

Parents should be warned about the following practices that are not healthy or safe for the infant:

- Infant cereal fed through a bottle
- Water or fruit juice given before 6 months of age
- Overdiluting the formula to reduce expense
- Formula mixed with private well water that has not been tested for safety
- Allowing a baby to sleep with a bottle in the crib

Key Points

- Parents need to be informed of the nutritional needs of the newborn.
- Newborns need to be breastfed or fed commercially prepared formula for the first year of life. Cow's milk is not appropriate nutrition until the child is 1 year old.
- Breast milk is convenient and economical for the mother. The milk is always ready and available for the infant.
- Teaching the mother correct latch-on technique will promote successful breastfeeding and help the mother to avoid sore nipples.
- Breastfeeding challenges such as engorgement and inverted nipples can be overcome by the mother with assistance from nurses.
- Bottle feeding may be the appropriate option for feeding if the mother is not comfortable with the idea of breastfeeding, has a chronic illness that requires medications, is HIV positive, or has an addiction problem with alcohol or drugs.
- Parents who bottle feed need education about formula preparation and bottle feeding techniques to be successful with bottle feeding.

REVIEW QUESTIONS

1. A new mother is concerned because her 2-day-old infant is only taking ½ ounce of formula at each feeding. The best response by the nurse is:
   1. "The baby is not getting enough to eat."
   2. "You need to feed the baby less often so he can eat more at the feeding."
   3. "His stomach is so small right now, that's about the right amount for a 2-day-old infant."
   4. "There must be a problem with the baby's digestive system."

2. A breastfeeding mother is complaining that she has sore nipples. The nurse should: *(select all that apply)*
   1. Observe her latch-on technique with the infant.
   2. Suggest that she only breastfeed for 5 min on each side.
   3. Suggest that she change breastfeeding positions.
   4. Suggest that she give the baby a bottle for a couple of feedings.
   5. Suggest that she switch to bottle feeding.

3. A new father states, "As soon as we take the baby home, I am going to be feeding him a little bit of cereal between feedings." The best response by the nurse is:
   1. "Babies don't need solid food until about 6 months of age."
   2. "Your baby should sleep through the night if you do that."
   3. "That's the wrong thing to do."
   4. "You'd better ask your pediatrician about that."

4. A new mother is excited and wants to begin breastfeeding as soon as possible. The nurse can facilitate the first breastfeeding experience by helping the mother to hold her baby:
   1. With her hand holding the cheeks.
   2. With the baby turned in toward her body, in straight head and body alignment.
   3. With the baby flat on his back and his head turned toward the breast.
   4. With his arms folded over his chest.

5. Teaching for bottle feeding parents should include: *(select all that apply)*
   1. Warm the bottle in the microwave.
   2. Formula is available in three forms: ready to eat, concentrated liquid, and powder.
   3. Never prop a bottle.
   4. Discard unused formula in a used bottle after 2 hours.
   5. Store prepared bottles in the refrigerator.

CRITICAL THINKING QUESTION

Are there any hospital policies that may have a detrimental effect on supporting and encouraging breastfeeding?

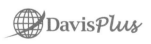 **DavisPlus**

For additional resources and information, visit **www.DavisPlus.com**. Post-Conference Questions and Activities, Answers, and References can be found on Davis*Plus*.

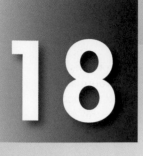

18

Newborn at Risk: Conditions Present at Birth

KEY TERMS

hematochezia
hyperinsulinemia
hypocalcemia
hypoglycemia
hypomagnesemia
hypoparathyroidism
hypoxia
intrauterine growth restriction (IGR)
large-for-gestational age (LGA)
necrosis
necrotizing enterocolitis
polycythemia
small-for-gestational age (SGA)
spina bifida

DavisPlus For audio pronunciation guide, visit www.DavisPlus.com

CHAPTER CONCEPTS

Addiction
Collaboration
Development
Ethics

LEARNING OUTCOMES

1. Define the key terms.
2. Identify factors present at birth that can help identify a high-risk newborn.
3. List risk factors that can lead to an SGA newborn.
4. Compare and contrast the SGA newborn and the premature newborn.
5. Discuss possible complications that can occur at birth for the LGA newborn.
6. Identify risk factors for a premature delivery.
7. Discuss potential complications of prematurity.
8. Describe the physical characteristics of a post-term newborn.
9. Explain the situation that causes the condition of polycythemia in the infant of a diabetic mother.
10. Explain possible complications for the infant of a diabetic mother.
11. Plan nursing care for a chemically exposed infant.
12. Discuss medical management and nursing interventions for the newborn exposed to HIV.
13. Use the nursing process to plan nursing care for the high-risk infant that includes teamwork and collaboration, patient-centered care, and evidence-based practice.

REAL-WORLD CASE STUDY

Jade

■ Jade, aged 17, is admitted to the hospital labor and delivery unit in early labor. She is accompanied by her boyfriend, Eddie. The contractions are 5 min apart and mild. This is Jade's first baby and her due date is 2 weeks away. As the nurse is taking a pregnancy history, Jade confides that she "smoked a little weed" during her pregnancy.

Eddie quickly tries to silence her by saying, "Don't tell anyone, they might take away our baby!"

1. What additional questions would the nurse want to ask Jade regarding her marijuana use?
2. How should the nurse respond to Eddie's comment?
3. What concerns should the nurse have about Jade's delivery?

CONCEPTUAL CORNERSTONE

Ethics

Ethics, as applied to nursing, is defined as a system of moral principles governing behaviors and relationships that is based on professional nursing beliefs and values. Simply put, *ethics* refers to standards of right and wrong that influence human behavior. Morals are similar to ethics; they are private personal standards of right and wrong in conduct and character that are based upon values and beliefs.

Nurses have a code of ethics that includes respect for human rights and the right to life, choice, dignity, and being treated with respect (Butts and Rich, 2015). Nurses are human, and when providing care to high-risk newborns and their families, the nurse may personally disagree with choices a parent has made. For example, a woman who uses illicit drugs during pregnancy and causes harm to the fetus may cause the nurse to experience strong feelings of anger. That patient with different morals and values deserves the same level of care as any other patient.

Another situation that may cause issues with ethical beliefs could be the parental decision to stop care for a critically ill preterm infant, or to continue care when there is little likelihood that the newborn will recover. When parents are faced with difficult decisions regarding care of their newborn, the nurse can assist them with thinking through their values and beliefs, but the nurse should not offer an opinion based upon the nurse's ethical beliefs.

This chapter provides an overview of the care of the high-risk newborn. Care of these newborns is a subspecialty of maternity nursing. Nurses who work in this highly specialized area need to gain in-depth knowledge of the care of high-risk newborns by attending advanced educational courses and spending time in a preceptorship with an experienced nurse.

IDENTIFICATION OF THE AT-RISK NEWBORN

During pregnancy, women should be screened for factors that could place the newborn at risk for problems. Factors such as premature labor, diabetes, hypertension, placenta abnormalities, HIV infection, and an unhealthy lifestyle can place a fetus at risk. On admission to labor and delivery, the nurse should review the pregnancy health of the woman and be alert for possible risk factors for newborn problems. Predicting a possible high-risk situation for a newborn allows the nurse to plan appropriate interventions and arrange for sufficient help at the time of birth. Advanced planning and swift action may prevent long-term complications for the high-risk newborn (Fig. 18.1).

CARE OF NEWBORNS WITH PROBLEMS RELATED TO GESTATIONAL AGE AND DEVELOPMENT

The length of a term pregnancy is 40 weeks (ie, 280 days) from the first day of the last menstrual period to the estimated date of delivery. In the past, the period from 3 weeks before the estimated due date to 2 weeks after the due date was considered "term." Research has shown that respiratory complications for the newborn vary upon the exact time that a baby is born in that 5-week range. To facilitate delivery of quality health care for the neonate, the American Congress of Obstetricians and Gynecologists (2013) has created terminology for identifying preterm, term, and post-term births:

- A preterm birth is less than 37 weeks, 6 days.
- An early term birth is from 37 weeks, 6 days through 38 weeks, 6 days.
- A full term birth is from 39 weeks through 40 weeks, 6 days.
- A late term birth is from 41 weeks through 41 weeks, 6 days.
- A post-term birth is 42 weeks and beyond.

This section will discuss problems related to gestational age and development.

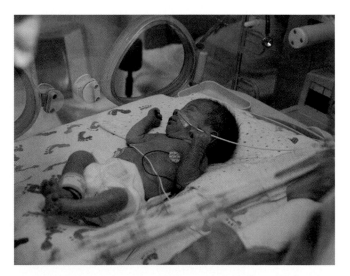

FIGURE 18.1 A high-risk newborn in the NICU.

The Small-for-Gestational-Age (SGA)/ Intrauterine Growth Restriction (IGR) Newborn

A **small-for-gestational age (SGA)** newborn is defined as an infant whose weight is less than the 10th percentile for his gestational age. The SGA newborn may have been affected by **intrauterine growth restriction (IGR),** which is decreased fetal growth caused by a decrease in placenta perfusion during gestation. There are many possible causes of SGA:

- Abnormalities of the placenta or vessels that restricted nutrients and oxygen to the developing fetus
- Maternal hypertension
- Uncontrolled, severe diabetes
- Poor maternal nutrition
- Drug use
- Heavy smoking
- Exposure to teratogenic substances
- Alcohol consumption
- Twins, triplets, or other multiples
- Small parents (Ross, 2013)

IGR is often diagnosed during pregnancy at routine visits when the health-care provider measures fundal height and also through ultrasound examinations. If poor placental perfusion is thought to be the cause, labor may be induced and the fetus delivered early.

Assessment findings would include:

- Weight, length, and head circumference all below the 10th percentile for gestational age
- Large head in relationship to the rest of the body
- Thin extremities and trunk
- Loose skin caused by absence of subcutaneous fat
- Thin umbilical cord

Term SGA infants do not have complications related to immature organs such as a premature baby does; however, they do have risks for:

- Perinatal asphyxia during labor if the SGA was caused by placental insufficiency; the fetus may not receive enough oxygen during the stress of labor.
- Meconium aspiration may occur during asphyxia. The infant may pass meconium into the amniotic fluid and then aspirate it into the lungs at birth, causing respiratory distress.
- **Hypoglycemia** (ie, low blood sugar) may occur because of a lack of stored glycogen. Neonatal hypoglycemia is defined as a plasma glucose level of less than 30 mg/dL in the first 24 hours of life and less than 45 mg/dL thereafter (Cranmer, 2014).
- Hypothermia may occur because of a lack of subcutaneous fat (Kendig and Nawab, 2015).

Nursing interventions for the SGA infant are:

- Performing a gestational age assessment
- Assessing for respiratory distress
- Assessing for tremors or jitteriness, which are early signs of hypoglycemia
- Instituting early feeding to prevent hypoglycemia
- Monitoring for hypothermia
- Monitoring vital signs and daily weight
- Teaching the parents about the need to keep the infant warm and to provide frequent feedings

---

HEALTH PROMOTION

Prognosis for a Small-for-Gestational-Age Newborn

- If asphyxia was avoided at birth, the neurological prognosis for the SGA infant is excellent.
- If the growth restriction was because of placental insufficiency, adequate nutrition after birth will allow the infant to "catch up."
- A SGA situation caused by maternal drug use and smoking may contribute to a smaller child and adult.

The Large-for-Gestational-Age (LGA) Newborn

The **large-for-gestational-age (LGA)** newborn is an infant whose weight is greater than the 90% for gestational age (Fig. 18.2). The predominant cause of LGA is maternal diabetes (Kendig and Nawab, 2015). Delivery complications during a vaginal delivery can occur because of the large size of the fetus. A Cesarean delivery should be considered to prevent injury to the large infant. The most common complications for an LGA newborn are:

- Shoulder dystocia
- Fracture of the clavicle or limbs
- Perinatal asphyxia
- Meconium aspiration
- Respiratory distress
- Hypoglycemia

Assessment findings would include:

- Large, obese baby
- Listless, apathetic baby

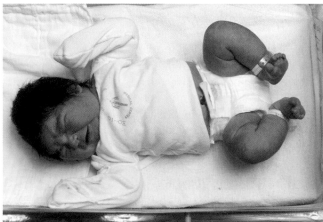

FIGURE 18.2 An LGA newborn.

Nursing interventions for the LGA newborn include:

- Performing a gestational age assessment
- Assessing respiratory status
- Assessing for signs of birth injuries and reporting them immediately
- Monitoring for tremors, which are an early sign of hypoglycemia
- Providing frequent feedings to decrease the risk of hypoglycemia

The Preterm Newborn

The length of gestation and birth weight are two important predictors of an infant's ability to survive outside the uterus. Preterm infants are born before 37 weeks' gestation and have an increased risk of complications and mortality. In the United States, 12% of infants are born prematurely (Furdon, 2014). Prematurity is classified as:

- Extremely premature: Born less than 28 weeks' gestation
- Very premature: Born less than 32 weeks' gestation
- Moderately premature: Born less than 34 weeks' gestation
- Late preterm: Born between 34 and 37 weeks' gestation (Kendig and Nawab, 2015).

Some neonatologists and neonatal intensive care nurseries also classify premature infants by weight:

- Low birth weight: Less than 2,500 g (ie, 5 lbs. 8 oz.)
- Very low birth weight (VLBW): Less than 1,500 g (ie, 3 lbs. 5 oz.)
- Extremely low birth weight (ELBW): Less than 1,000 g (ie, 2 lbs. 3 oz.) (Goldman-Luthy, 2015) (Fig. 18.3)

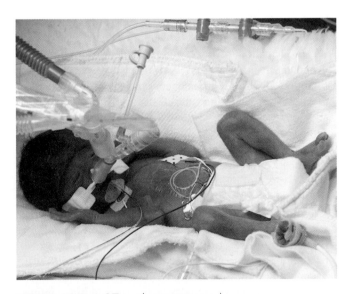

FIGURE 18.3 A 27-week-gestation newborn.

Etiology

There are many risk factors for a premature birth. Sometimes the cause of a premature birth is never really known. Known risk factors for a premature delivery include:

- Low socioeconomic status
- Cigarette smoking
- Prior premature births
- Multiple prior therapeutic or spontaneous abortions
- Little or no prenatal care
- Poor nutrition
- Untreated infections
- Pre-eclampsia
- Multiple gestation (Furdon, 2014)

Assessment

Confirmation of prematurity is based upon a gestational age assessment. The Ballard's scoring system is the main tool used to determine gestational age. The major anatomical parts used in determining gestational age are:

- Ear cartilage: For example, a preterm infant at 28 weeks has little ear cartridge.
- Sole creases: For example, a preterm infant at 33 weeks has only an anterior crease.
- Breast tissue: For example, a preterm infant at 28 weeks has no breast tissue.
- Genitalia: For example, extremely preterm infant males will have undescended testicles.

During physical assessment of the premature infant, the nurse will also notice that:

- The skin is thin and arteries and veins are visible.
- The skin is fragile and looks smooth and shiny.
- A moderately premature infant will have abundant lanugo.
- Fingernails and toenails may only be partially formed.
- The ears may fold over.
- Very preterm infants have less muscle tone.
- The premature baby does not lie in a fetal position until 35 weeks.

TEAM WORKS

When a premature delivery is expected, a team of professionals should be at the delivery to provide prompt stabilization, which is crucial to the long-term outcome for the newborn. In addition to the obstetrician and labor nurse, there should also be a neonatologist, newborn intensive care nurses, laboratory technician, and respiratory care practitioners in attendance.

Potential Complications

Being born too early predisposes the newborn to short- and long-term complications. The age and weight of the premature newborn influence the severity of the complications. In the first few weeks, the premature newborn can experience a variety of short-term complications.

- A premature baby may have problems with breathing because of an immature respiratory system and the absence of surfactant to keep the alveoli open. Medical management and nursing care for respiratory distress syndrome is discussed in Chapter 19, Newborn at Risk: Birth-Related Stressors.
- Thermoregulation is difficult for the premature infant because of the lack of subcutaneous fat and the infant may not have developed brown fat to assist with heat production during stress. Cold stress can occur easily in a premature newborn. Management and nursing care for cold stress is discussed in Chapter 19.
- Heart problems are common in premature babies. The most common problems are a patent ductus arteriosus (PDA) and hypotension. The PDA is supposed to close on its own to allow more blood flow to the lungs, but in a premature infant, it may stay open, causing heart failure (Fig. 18.4).
- Intraventricular hemorrhage in the brain of the very premature infant can occur because of the fragile underdeveloped blood vessels in the brain. The blood vessels rupture and bleed into the ventricles of the brain. There may be no symptoms or the nurse may observe:
  - Apnea
  - Decreased muscle tone
  - Decreased reflexes
  - Excessive sleep
  - Weak suck
  - Seizure and other abnormal movements.

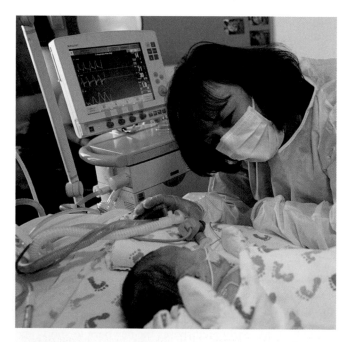

FIGURE 18.4 Most premature newborns are on a cardiorespiratory monitor. *(Courtesy St. Luke's Hospital, Bethlehem, Pennsylvania.)*

There is no way to stop the bleeding. The health-care team will keep the infant stable and treat any symptoms. The prognosis depends upon the amount of bleeding that occurs and if there is an accompanying swelling of the brain (Lee, 2015).

- Premature babies have immature gastrointestinal systems, which predisposes the newborn to **necrotizing enterocolitis.** This complication occurs in the second to third week of life for a premature, formula-fed infant. The exact cause is unknown, but it is associated with formula feeding and characterized by damage to the intestinal tract that may have occurred from abnormal intestinal flora, immaturity of the intestinal mucosa, intestinal ischemia caused by decreased placental blood flow, and possibly a genetic predisposition. The damage may affect only the mucosal lining, or there may be full-thickness **necrosis** (ie, death of the tissues) and perforation of the bowel. The signs and symptoms are:
  - Vomiting
  - Diarrhea
  - Delayed gastric emptying
  - Decreased bowel sounds
  - Lethargy
  - Increased abdominal girth
  - Visible intestinal loops
  - Palpable abdominal mass
  - **Hematochezia** (ie, bright red blood in the stool)

Medical management includes stopping formula feedings, insertion of a nasal gastric tube, feeding with breastmilk, and the administration of antibiotics. Surgical intervention may be required to remove perforated or necrotic intestinal tissue (Springer, 2014).

- Premature infants are at risk for anemia and jaundice. Anemia is caused by a lack of red blood cells. All infants experience a drop in red blood cells after birth, but it may be more profound for the premature infant if frequent blood draws are required for tests.
- Infection can occur easily in the premature newborn because of an immature immune system. Infection can quickly spread to the newborn's bloodstream, causing sepsis. Detection, management, and nursing care for neonatal sepsis are discussed in Chapter 19.
- Fluid and electrolyte imbalances can be a problem for the premature infant because of the immature circulatory and renal system. Close monitoring of IV fluid intake and electrolyte balances are important to prevent fluid overload and heart failure.
- The most common problem of the premature neonate is apnea. Apnea of prematurity is the cessation of breathing for more than 20 sec, or the cessation of breathing for less than 20 sec accompanied by bradycardia or oxygen saturation levels of less than 85%. Apnea of prematurity is related to immaturity and/or depression of the central respiratory drive to adequately stimulate the muscles of respiration (Nimavat, 2014). Medical management of apnea of prematurity includes tactile stimulation, administration of oxygen, the use of continuous positive airway

pressure (CPAP), and pharmacotherapy. As the infant matures, the apnea will resolve.

 DRUG FACTS

Caffeine is the preferred drug for treating apnea of prematurity. Caffeine stimulates the respiratory center and relaxes smooth bronchial muscles. It can be administered IV or by mouth and has a rapid onset. The usual dose is 5 mg/kg every 24 hours (Vallernand and Sanoski, 2013).

Possible long-term complications of prematurity include:

- Retinopathy of prematurity, a potentially blinding disease caused by abnormal development of the retinal blood vessels. The retina receives light and turns it into visual messages that are sent to the brain. Retinopathy occurs in extremely low birth weight infants. A premature birth results in the cessation of normal growth of the blood vessels of the retina. Long-term outcomes include visual impairment and blindness. The American Academy of Pediatrics recommends that all premature infants be tested for retinopathy. Early surgical laser treatment is the treatment of choice (Silva & Subramanian, 2015).
- Cerebral palsy, a disorder of muscle tone and movement, can be caused by infection or inadequate blood flow to the developing premature infant's brain. A study by Oskoui et al (2015) indicates that there may be a genetic component that influences whether prenatal or birth stressors will cause cerebral palsy. This may explain why newborns with similar prenatal or birth stressors may have no disabilities or different types of cerebral palsy.
- Premature babies are usually behind on meeting developmental milestones, may have learning disabilities, and are more like to have psychological problems such as attention-deficit hyperactivity disorder (Mayo Clinic, 2014).

The Post-Term Newborn

A post-term newborn is born after 42 weeks' gestation. The cause of postmaturity is unknown, but a previous post-term delivery increases the risk. Usually, fetal growth between 39 and 43 weeks' gestation results in a large infant. However, in some cases the placenta begins to involute and the villi begin to degenerate, causing placental insufficiency syndrome for the fetus (Kendig and Nawab, 2015). The fetus receives inadequate nutrition and oxygen from the placenta, resulting in an SGA infant who is undernourished. The fetus may have used stored glycogen for energy before birth. In addition, the amniotic fluid volume begins to decrease with postmaturity.

Assessment

A gestational age assessment should be done to confirm that the newborn is postmature. Physical assessment characteristics of a postmature newborn are:

- The infant will be more alert after birth
- Decreased subcutaneous fat
- Loose skin
- Dry and peeling skin
- Lack of vernix and lanugo
- Long fingernails and toenails
- Meconium staining on the umbilical cord

Potential Complications

Post-term infants have a higher rate of death and disease than term infants. Possible complications that can occur are:

- The incidence of stillbirth or neonatal death is increased in post-term infants (Norowitz, 2015).
- The larger body size can lead to prolonged labor and birth trauma.
- Hypoglycemia can occur owing to lack of stored glycogen.
- During labor, the post-term infant is more likely to have a bowel movement in the uterus because of stress. There is a chance the newborn may inhale the meconium, causing breathing problems. Meconium aspiration syndrome is discussed in Chapter 19.

CARE OF THE INFANT OF A DIABETIC MOTHER

Neonatal complications for the infant of a diabetic mother (IDM) are directly related to inadequate glucose control in pregnancy (Mimouni, Mimouni, et al, 2013). Fetal malformation can occur because of poor glucose control in the first trimester. High levels of glucose in late pregnancy can lead to macrosomia, hypoxia, polycythemia, and cardiomegaly. Infants born of diabetic mothers have an increased risk of complications; therefore the nurse should be watchful for complications and intervene as appropriate. The major complications and nursing interventions will be discussed in the following section.

Fetal Macrosomia

Macrosomia, or an LGA infant weighing more than 4,000 g at birth, occurs in 15% to 45% of diabetic pregnancies (Potter, 2013). High levels of maternal glucose during gestation lead to fetal hyperglycemia and **hyperinsulinemia** (ie, excess insulin), which causes increased growth in the fetus. The large infant is at risk for birth injuries caused by shoulder dystocia. Frequently, the macrosomic IDM is delivered via Cesarean birth because of the large size. At delivery, the macrosomic IDM appears ruddy, fat, puffy, and may have decreased muscle tone (Potter, 2013).

Nursing interventions for the macrosomic infant include:

- Notifying the pediatrician or nurse practitioner of birth weight and signs of macrosomia
- Performing a gestational age assessment
- Observing for signs of birth injuries
- Observing for signs of hypoglycemia

Hypoglycemia

IDMs often have a rapid fall in glucose within an hour of birth. Hypoglycemia can occur faster in an IDM than normal infants. This is linked to fetal hyperinsulinism that occurs during

NURSING CARE PLAN for the Post-Term Infant

Nursing Diagnosis: There is a risk for hypoglycemia related to lack of glycogen stores.
Expected Outcome: The newborn maintains a blood sugar between 30 to 40 mg/dL.
Interventions:
- Monitor for signs of low blood sugar, such as tremors.
- Check blood sugar at birth.
- Assist the mother to breastfeed as soon as possible.

Nursing Diagnosis: There is a risk for ineffective thermoregulation caused by an absence of subcutaneous fat because of weight loss in the uterus.
Expected Outcome: The newborn maintains an axillary body temperature of 36.5°C.
Interventions:
- Monitor body temperature every 30 min.
- Place the infant skin-to-skin with the mother.
- Avoid procedures that expose the infant.

Nursing Diagnosis: There is a risk for altered parenting related to the appearance of the newborn.
Expected Outcome: Bonding with the parents will occur.
Interventions:
- Unless the baby is unstable, keep him or her with the parents.
- Educate parents on the physical signs of postmaturity.
- Provide positive reinforcement for bonding behaviors.
- Point out positive aspects of the infant's physical condition.
- Encourage parents to ask questions.

---

gestation; maternal glucose comes across the placenta but insulin does not. The fetus produces high levels of insulin in response to the maternal glucose, and when the cord is cut and the glucose influx is over, the fetus has a high level of insulin in the blood, causing hypoglycemia (Mimouni, Mimouni, et al, 2013).

Prevention of hypoglycemia is a goal. Early feeding immediately after birth is suggested for the IDM. Identification, management, and nursing interventions for hypoglycemia are discussed in Chapter 19.

Congenital Malformations

High blood sugar concentration is toxic to cell growth in the first trimester and explains cardiac and central nervous system (CNS) abnormalities of the IDM (Mimouni, Mimouni, et al, 2013). Cardiomegaly with an enlarged left ventricle occurs in approximately 30% of IDMs; the risk of **spina bifida** (ie, a defect of the spinal cord) is 20 times higher for the IDM (Potter, 2013).

Nursing interventions include:

- Promptly identifying the congenital abnormality, if obvious, at birth
- Notifying the health-care provider of any physical abnormalities or abnormal vital signs

Fetal Hypoxia

Poorly controlled diabetes can lead to a **hypoxia,** a decreased supply of oxygen to the fetal tissues. Uncontrolled high levels of glucose can cause vascular disease in the mother, leading to decreased blood flow to the placenta. In addition, the fetus develops an increased need for oxygen consumption related to high levels of glucose coming from the mother. Chronic fetal hypoxia can lead to intrauterine death and respiratory depression at birth. While in the uterus, the fetus attempts to compensate for the decreased oxygen by producing extra red blood cells.

This condition of extra red blood cells is known as **polycythemia.** Polycythemia is diagnosed when the hematocrit is greater than 65% (Lessaris, 2014). The polycythemia makes the blood more viscous (ie, thicker or sticky), which can cause strokes or seizures in the fetus or newborn. Polycythemia contributes to an increased risk of hyperbilirubinemia after birth when the extra red blood cells break down and the immature liver cannot manage the breakdown of the bilirubin.

Signs of polycythemia are:

- A "ruddy" (ie, red) appearance of the skin
- Sluggish capillary refill time
- Respiratory distress
- Poor feeding
- Lethargy
- Seizures
- Apnea
- Cyanosis
- Hematuria

Medical management of polycythemia is controversial. The vital signs, hematocrit, and blood glucose will be monitored frequently. The hematocrit levels usually peak 6 to 12 hours after birth and then decline until the infant is 24 hours old. More than 60% of infants with a hematocrit level greater than 64% at 2 hours will have a high value 12 hours later (Lessaris, 2014).

Some physicians will perform a partial blood exchange transfusion with saline to decrease the hematocrit quickly in symptomatic infants. In asymptomatic infants, the common approach is to observe for the onset of any symptoms and let the newborn's body adjust the hematocrit. Some physicians will hydrate the newborn with IV fluids to decrease the hematocrit.

Nursing interventions for the polycythemic infant include:

- Notifying the health-care provider immediately of any signs and symptoms of polycythemia
- Infusing IV fluids, if ordered, and observing closely for signs of fluid overload

SAFETY *STAT!*

Newborns are at risk for fluid overload. Careful calculations of appropriate fluid amounts based upon the infant's weight should be confirmed by two licensed nurses.

Mineral/Electrolyte Metabolism

Hypocalcemia and **hypomagnesemia** can occur in the neonate if the mother had poorly controlled diabetes. In the newborn, hypocalcemia is defined as a calcium level less than 8 mg/dL; hypomagnesemia is defined as a magnesium level less than 1.7 mg/dL (Malhotra, 2014). The mother's poor glycemic control leads to maternal glycosuria (ie, glucose in the urine), which is accompanied by magnesium loss. Low maternal levels of magnesium lead to fetal deficiency. Magnesium and calcium metabolism are closely related. Magnesium controls calcium in the body. If the magnesium level is insufficient, calcium will be lost in the urine and not deposited in the bones and soft tissues. Severe hypomagnesemia causes a secondary hypocalcemia and **hypoparathyroidism,** because magnesium is needed for the appropriate secretin of the parathyroid hormone (PTH). Medical management includes screening for hypocalcemia and hypomagnesemia and administration of calcium and magnesium to obtain normal levels.

Signs and symptoms of mineral/electrolyte imbalances in the newborn are:

- Poor feeding
- Lethargy
- Tremors
- Seizures
- Cardiac arrhythmias
- Respiratory distress

Nursing interventions for the infant with an abnormal electrolyte balance includes:

- Recognizing abnormal signs and symptoms and reporting them immediately to the health-care provider

- Maintaining close observation of the newborn to detect deterioration
- Administering calcium and/or magnesium as ordered by the health-care provider
- Providing education and emotional support to the family

SAFETY *STAT!*

The symptoms of an electrolyte imbalance are very similar to hypoglycemia in the newborn. If symptoms persist with a normal blood sugar, the health-care provider should be notified immediately.

CARE OF CHEMICALLY EXPOSED INFANTS

Prenatal substance abuse is a significant problem in the United States. Almost all drugs cross the placenta and have an effect on the fetus. Drugs can affect the fetus in many ways. In early gestation, drugs can have a teratogenic effect, causing structural birth defects. After that initial period of development is complete, drugs have a subtler effect, such as alterations in neurotransmitters, their receptors, and brain organization (Behnke and Smith, 2013).

Caring for a newborn that was prenatally exposed to illicit and prescription drugs can be challenging for the nurse. The mother may admit her use of drugs during the pregnancy or may be fearful of losing custody of her newborn and not report her use. The health-care provider may order a drug toxicology screen on a newborn's urine or meconium sample to be prepared for appropriate care for the infant in withdrawal.

Neonatal abstinence syndrome (NAS) is a group of similar behavioral and physiological signs and symptoms in the neonate caused by withdrawal from various pharmacological agents. Withdrawal symptoms will vary depending upon the age of the neonate, the drug, the drug's half-life, and the mother's last use (MacMullen, Dulski, et al, 2014). See Table 18.1 for information on approximate withdrawal onset and symptoms of withdrawal from various drugs.

Newborn nurseries and neonatal intensive care units (NICUs) use neonatal abstinence scales as tools to evaluate newborn reflexes and behaviors that indicate the severity of withdrawal symptoms and help the nurses and physicians to plan for medical intervention.

Medical management of the newborn with NAS may include:

- Transferring any infant with signs of NAS to the NICU
- Providing supportive therapy with IV fluids to prevent dehydration from nausea and vomiting
- Providing pharmacological therapy to reduce symptoms and gradually wean the newborn from the substance; morphine is the most frequently used medication for

TABLE 18.1   DRUG WITHDRAWAL FOR THE NEONATE

Drug	Onset of Withdrawal Symptoms	Symptoms of Withdrawal
Opioids	24–72 hours	Hyperirritability Tremors High-pitched cry Nasal congestion Hyperthermia Tachycardia Poor feeding Regurgitation Diarrhea
Alcohol	3–12 hours	Jitteriness Irritability Hypertonia Hyperreflexia Seizures Poor suck Poor sleep Tremors Diaphoresis Hyperactivity
Cocaine	2–3 days	Irritability Hyperactivity Tremors High-pitched cry Some neonates have no symptoms of withdrawal
Marijuana	Depends upon mother's last use (symptoms may occur if the mother used marijuana heavily during pregnancy and during labor) Tremors Exaggerated startle reflex Disturbed sleep cycles	Hypoglycemia Tremors Impaired sleeping Jitteriness
Selective serotonin reuptake inhibitors (SSRIs)	Hours to days	Continuous crying Restlessness Sleep disturbances
Barbiturates	1–14 days	Irritability Tremors Excessive crying Restlessness Increased muscle tone Vomiting Diarrhea
Caffeine	At birth	Jitteriness Vomiting Tachypnea Bradycardia

Sources: Behnke M & Smith VC. (2013) Prenatal substance abuse: Short and long term effects on the exposed fetus. *Pediatrics* 131(3); Hamdan AH. (2014). *Neonatal abstinence syndrome.* Retrieved from Medscape at http://emedicine.medscape.com/article/978763; Hudak ML & Tan RC (2012). Neonatal drug withdrawal. *Pediatrics* 129(2); Jaques SC, Kingsbury A, Henshoke P, Chomachai C, Clews S, et al. (2014) *Cannabis, the pregnant woman and her child.* Retrieved from Medscape at http://emedicine.medscape.com/article/826443; MacMullen NJ, Dulski LA, and Blobaum P. (2014). Evidence-based interventions for neonatal abstinence syndrome. *Pediatric Nursing* 40(4) 165-172.

opioid-addicted newborns to reduce symptoms and to wean slowly (Hamdan, 2014)
- Administering phenobarbital, which is effective in controlling seizures

---

SAFETY *STAT!*

Avoid the use of naloxone at the time of delivery if the mother is suspected to be opioid dependent. Naloxone will cause abrupt withdrawal and seizures for the neonate.

Nursing interventions for a newborn with NAS are:

- Assessing daily for signs of withdrawal and reporting any signs and symptoms immediately
- Administering and monitoring pharmacological treatment
- Monitoring for skin breakdown and applying barrier ointments for prevention of diaper rash from diarrhea
- Bottle-feeding with high-calorie formula to promote weight gain
- Encouraging breastfeeding if not contraindicated
- Providing parenting education to the caretakers of the infant
- Communicating with and providing a referral to a social worker for postdischarge care and follow-up

Some drug exposures during gestation do not cause severe withdrawal symptoms for the newborn. However, it is likely that brain chemistry and function have been changed because of the exposure. Long-term effects related to prenatal drug exposure may be:

- Poor growth through childhood
- Hyperactivity and attention-deficit disorder
- Impaired cognition, leading to learning disabilities
- Poor language development
- Higher rates of criminal behavior and substance abuse (Behnke and Smith, 2013; Hudak and Tan, 2012)

PATIENT TEACHING GUIDELINES

Care for the Chemically Exposed Newborn
Home care for a newborn who has been exposed to drugs in the uterus can be challenging. Helpful tips for the parents or caregivers should include:
- Provide a calm quiet environment.
- Swaddling is usually very calming for the newborn.
- Avoid unnecessary handling.
- Use a light dimmer to keep lights low.
- Respond quickly to cries.
- Limit stimuli such as stroking, direct speech, and strong fragrances.
- Provide "space" by positioning the baby to face outward, away from the caregiver's body.

CARE OF THE NEWBORN EXPOSED TO HIV

HIV transmission from mother to child during pregnancy, labor and delivery, or breastfeeding is known as perinatal transmission. The Centers for Disease Control and Prevention (CDC) recommends routine HIV testing for all persons aged 13 to 64 years in health-care settings, including women during pregnancy. It has been proven that women who take antiretroviral medications in pregnancy can reduce the risk of transmission of HIV to the fetus to less than 1% (CDC, 2015).

The CDC recommends that infants born to mothers with unknown HIV status should receive rapid HIV testing as soon as possible either during labor or immediately after birth with immediate implementation of prophylactic medication.

Medical management of the HIV-exposed newborn is:

- Zidovudine (ZDV) 4 mg/kg twice a day through 6 weeks of age if the mother received antiretroviral medications during pregnancy
- If the mother did not receive prenatal antiretroviral medications, the newborn should receive:
  - ZDV 4 mg/kg twice a day through 6 weeks of age plus Nevirapine (NVP) – three doses in the first week of life, 12 mg PO per dose if birth weight is greater than 2 kg and 8 mg per dose if birth weight is 1.5 to 2 kg (AIDS Institute, 2014)
- Follow-up consultation with a pediatric infectious disease specialist
- Obtaining a complete blood count for a baseline

Nursing interventions for the HIV-exposed newborn includes:

- Strictly maintaining standard precautions to avoid exposure
- Making sure gloves are worn by anyone handling the newborn (including family members) until the first bath
- Notifying the health-care provider of any abnormalities noted during physical assessment
- Administering medications as ordered
- Educating parents about the importance of following the drug prophylaxis plan after discharge
- Advising the mother not to breastfeed

 CULTURAL CONSIDERATIONS

The prevalence of HIV infections in Asia and Europe varies considerably because of cultural practices and lack of national reporting centers in many countries. The sex-worker industry in places such as Thailand and the Caribbean islands is responsible for increased HIV transmission to young women. They transfer the virus to their infants during pregnancy (Rivera, 2015).

Key Points

- Early identification of risk factors for a high-risk newborn will facilitate rapid interventions at birth to help prevent complications for the newborn.
- An SGA newborn is defined as an infant whose weight is less than the 10th percentile for his or her gestational age. The SGA newborn will have mature organs but can have complications related to asphyxia and thermoregulation.
- The LGA baby weighs greater than 90% for gestational age. The predominant cause is maternal diabetes.
- For a preterm infant (ie, born before 37 weeks' gestation), the gestational age and weight are important factors in determining the infant's ability to survive outside the uterus.
- Confirmation of gestational age is based upon a gestational age assessment.
- Premature infants are at risk for problems related to almost every body system.

- The most common problem for the premature infant is apnea of prematurity.
- A post-term newborn is born after 42 weeks' gestation. Post-term infants have a higher rate of death and disease than term infants.
- The IDM has complications at birth directly related to glucose control during pregnancy.
- Complications for the IDM include hypoglycemia, polycythemia, and electrolyte imbalances.
- Fetal exposure to drugs in early pregnancy can cause fetal anomalies, and exposure throughout pregnancy can alter brain chemistry and cause long-term effects on the child.
- Some drugs cause severe withdrawal symptoms in the newborn that require medical and nursing interventions.
- Newborns who have been exposed to HIV during pregnancy should receive prophylactic medications to reduce the chance of acquiring HIV from the mother.

REVIEW QUESTIONS

1. The SGA newborn:
   1. Was born before 37 weeks' gestation
   2. Was born between 34 and 37 weeks' gestation
   3. Weighs less than the 10the percentile for gestational age
   4. Weighs less than the 25th percentile for gestational age

2. A physical characteristic of a preterm infant is:
   1. Dry skin
   2. Lanugo
   3. Long toenails
   4. Hypertonia

3. An IDM may develop polycythemia. A physical characteristic of polycythemia is:
   1. Abundant lanugo
   2. A ruddy appearance of the skin
   3. Temperature instability
   4. Constant crying

4. Possible complications of prematurity are: *(select all that apply)*
   1. Retinopathy
   2. Color blindness
   3. Apnea
   4. Cerebral palsy
   5. Learning disabilities

5. A symptom of necrotizing enterocolitis is:
   1. Constipation
   2. Hyperactivity
   3. Fever
   4. Bloody stool

6. A 10 lb, 6 oz infant of an insulin-dependent diabetic mother was just admitted to the nursery. The priority of care is:
   1. Administer the vitamin K injection.
   2. Check the blood sugar.
   3. Bathe the baby.
   4. Complete a head-to-toe assessment.

7. When observing a drug-exposed newborn, what symptom suggests that the newborn may be exhibiting withdrawal symptoms?
   1. Sleepiness
   2. Constipation
   3. Irritability
   4. Alertness

8. The nurse is completing an assessment on a macrosomic infant. The nurse is aware that the most common reason for macrosomia is:
   1. Maternal diabetes
   2. Maternal drug use
   3. Postmaturity
   4. Chemical exposure

Chapter 18

9. Risk factors for a preterm birth include: *(select all that apply)*
   1. Cigarette smoking
   2. Prior preterm births
   3. Small mother
   4. Eating spicy food
   5. Infections

10. A physical characteristic of a post-term newborn is:
    1. Abundant lanugo
    2. Dry skin
    3. Abundant vernix
    4. Absent toenails

CRITICAL THINKING QUESTIONS

1. Why is it important to maintain good glucose control throughout pregnancy?

2. Why would it be beneficial to place the infant of a diabetic mother at the breast immediately after delivery?

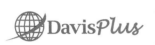

For additional resources and information, visit **www.DavisPlus.com**. Post-Conference Questions and Activities, Answers, and References can be found on Davis*Plus*.

Newborn at Risk: Birth-Related Stressors

KEY TERMS

anoxia
brachial plexus
dyspnea
echocardiography
hypercapnia
hyperinsulinism
hypoxic-ischemic encephalopathy
neonatal sepsis
respiratory distress syndrome (RDS)
tachypnea

DavisPlus For audio pronunciation guide, visit www.DavisPlus.com

CHAPTER CONCEPTS

Family
Metabolism
Oxygenation
Thermo-regulation

LEARNING OUTCOMES

1. Define the key terms.
2. Identify possible causes of birth asphyxia.
3. Discuss the risk factors for RDS.
4. Recognize signs of respiratory distress.
5. Plan nursing care for a newborn with transient tachypnea (TTN).
6. Identify physical signs of a newborn with meconium aspiration syndrome.
7. Discuss the underlying pathophysiology of persistent pulmonary hypertension of the newborn (PPHN).
8. Plan nursing interventions to manage cold stress in the newborn.
9. Recognize signs of hypoglycemia in the newborn.
10. Discuss nursing interventions for the newborn with hypoglycemia.
11. Plan nursing interventions for a newborn with a brachial plexus injury.
12. Discuss the nursing interventions for the jaundiced newborn undergoing phototherapy.
13. Summarize the risk factors, medical management, and nursing interventions for the newborn with sepsis.
14. Formulate a plan to provide family-centered care in the neonatal intensive care unit (NICU).

REAL-WORLD CASE STUDY

Baby Daniel

■ Baby Daniel was born at 42 weeks' gestation. Immediately after birth he demonstrated signs of respiratory distress. The physician and nurses were unable to stabilize him in the labor and delivery room, so he was quickly transferred to the NICU. Daniel was diagnosed with meconium aspiration syndrome and has a collapsed lung. His parents are very concerned and confused about what has happened to their son.

1. What are signs of respiratory distress?
2. How would you explain meconium aspiration syndrome to the parents?
3. How could you facilitate bonding for the parents?

CONCEPTUAL CORNERSTONE

Gas Exchange

To survive, all cells need a supply of oxygen and removal of waste. A lack of oxygen or a buildup of waste can cause the death of cells. Gas exchange is the process in which oxygen is transported to cells and carbon dioxide is transported from cells. The terms *hypoxia* (ie, insufficient oxygen reaching the cells) and *anoxia* (ie, no oxygen reaching the cells) relate to this concept. Ventilation, the process of inhaling oxygen into the lungs to the alveoli to exchange oxygen for carbon dioxide that is exhaled, can become a problem for the at-risk newborn.

There are many problems that can interfere with gas exchange. The newborn may have hypoxia because of delivery problems, such as placental insufficiency or cord compression. After delivery, a lack of surfactant, fluid in the lungs, or meconium plugging the bronchioles or alveoli can contribute to hypoxia. Regardless of the exact cause, the newborn will exhibit many of the same signs and symptoms. The basic nursing interventions to treat hypoxia are the same even if the nurse may not know the exact cause of the hypoxia. The nurse who is alert for subtle and early signs of hypoxia in the newborn can promptly implement care that can prevent a state of anoxia and possible long-term health consequences for the newborn.

Nurses play a vital role in the care of high-risk newborns. The labor and delivery, postpartum, and newborn nurses often identify problems in the newborn and initiate care until the baby can be transferred to the NICU. Nurses in the NICU provide family-centered care as they work alongside the physicians and neonatal nurse practitioners to provide medical and nursing care for the sick newborn.

CARE OF THE NEWBORN AT RISK BECAUSE OF BIRTH ASPHYXIA

Birth asphyxia is also known as *perinatal asphyxia, asphyxia neonatorum,* or ***hypoxic-ischemic encephalopathy*** and is described as acute brain injury caused by asphyxia when the baby did not get enough oxygen during the birth process (Zanelli, 2015). Birth asphyxia occurs in 4 out of 1,000 births in the United States (Monnaf, 2013). Possible causes of asphyxia during the birth process are:

• The mother does not get enough oxygen during labor.
• The mother's blood pressure is too high or too low during labor.
• The placenta separates from the uterus too quickly, resulting in loss of oxygen.
• The umbilical cord becomes wrapped too tightly around the neck or body.
• The fetus is anemic and does not have enough red blood cells to support the fetus during contractions.
• The newborn's airway becomes blocked.
• The delivery is too long or too difficult.

Whatever the cause, when the baby becomes asphyxiated and breathing slows or ceases, there is a lack of perfusion of blood to the brain and other organ systems. Hypoxia forces cells to undergo anaerobic respiration, which produces less energy. Lactic acid forms as a byproduct of cell respiration, the cells cannot function normally, and tissues become affected and damaged. The tissues affected first by the lack of oxygen in the cells are in the brain, muscles, and heart. The heart dysfunction causes hypotension, leading to damage in a variety of organs. As the brain begins to receive adequate blood perfusion again, it can begin to swell, which causes more neurological problems for the newborn.

Signs and symptoms of birth asphyxia are:

• Cyanosis
• Difficulty breathing
• Gasping respirations
• Bradycardia
• Hypotonic muscles
• Low Apgar score
• Meconium-stained amniotic fluid
• pH less than 7
• Apgar score of less than 3 for more than 5 min
• Seizures
• Multiorgan dysfunction in the immediate neonatal period (Monnaf, 2013; Zanelli, 2015)

At birth, immediate medical care is to perform cardiopulmonary resuscitation (CPR) if needed. The newborn with birth asphyxia may be transferred to the NICU if symptoms are severe or persist (Fig. 19.1). Additional medical management may include:

• Blood pressure management with medications
• Ventilation support and oxygen therapy if needed
• Careful fluid management
• Avoidance of hypoglycemia or hyperglycemia
• Avoidance of hyperthermia
• Treatment of seizures
• Hypothermia therapy (33°C to 33.5°C for 72 hours), followed by slow rewarming (Zanelli, 2015)

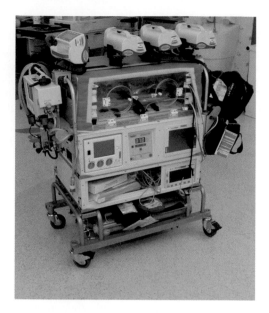

FIGURE 19.1 Neonatal transporter. *(Courtesy McLeod Regional Medical Center, Florence, South Carolina.)*

NICU nursing care for the baby with birth asphyxia may include:

• Administering ordered medications and fluids
• Monitoring ventilation and oxygenation of the baby
• Monitoring fluid balance
• Monitoring and reporting signs of hypoglycemia, hyperglycemia, and hyperthermia

Prognosis depends upon the severity of the asphyxia. Long-term complications may be:

• Cerebral palsy
• Epilepsy
• Blindness
• Delayed motor development
• Mental retardation
• Learning disabilities

CARE OF THE NEWBORN WITH RESPIRATORY DISTRESS

Respiratory distress is a common problem of the neonate. It can be caused by asphyxia at birth, a lack of surfactant with a premature birth, fluid in the lungs, meconium aspiration, pulmonary hypertension, cold stress, and other conditions that affect the ability of the newborn to breathe. Nurses need to be able to identify early signs of respiratory distress and initiate care to provide oxygenation and improve gas exchange to prevent more complications or death for the newborn.

Respiratory Distress Syndrome

Respiratory distress syndrome (RDS) is caused by a lack of surfactant and immaturity of the fetal lungs. It is a disease almost exclusively seen in premature infants, but it does occur in infants experiencing birth asphyxia, in infants of diabetic mothers, and in infants born by Cesarean section.

RDS is also known as *hyaline membrane syndrome* because of the formation of hyaline membranes that line the alveoli and impair ventilation. Surfactant decreases surface tension in the alveoli and assists the alveoli to stay open for ventilation. If surfactant is absent, the alveoli cannot open for oxygenation; therefore hypoxemia and **hypercapnia** (ie, elevated carbon dioxide) occur, leading to respiratory acidosis. Acidosis causes vasoconstriction and damages the epithelium of the lungs, causing an exudate that forms the hyaline membrane inside the alveoli and impairs oxygen exchange.

The signs of RDS will be evident either at birth or within 8 hours of life (Pramanik, 2015). The most common signs are:

• **Tachypnea** (ie, rapid breathing)
• **Dyspnea** (ie, labored or difficult breathing)
• Grunting with expirations
• Nasal flaring
• Intercostal retractions
• Cyanosis

Medical management includes:

• If a premature birth is likely, administration of antenatal corticosteroids will reduce the risk of RDS (Pramanik, 2015)
• Transfer to NICU
• Surfactant therapy
• Oxygen therapy (Fig. 19.2)
• Continuous positive airway pressure (CPAP) to keep the alveoli open at the end of respiration
• Mechanical ventilation support if needed
• Vapotherm: heated and humidified high-flow oxygen through a nasal cannula

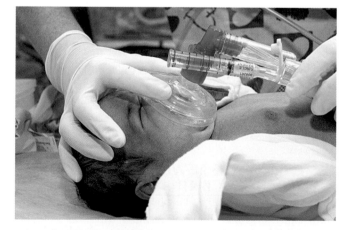

FIGURE 19.2 During respiratory distress, some newborns require oxygen administered through a mask. *(Courtesy St. Luke's Hospital, Bethlehem, Pennsylvania.)*

- Inhaled nitric oxide (NO) to decrease lung inflammation and promote lung growth (Pramanik, 2015; Keehn and Lieben, 2014)

Nursing interventions for a newborn in respiratory distress would include:

- Administering CPR if indicated
- Administering ordered medications and fluids
- Monitoring respiratory and oxygenation status
- Providing emotional support to the family

TEAM WORKS

A newborn with RDS will require a team approach to decrease the chance of long-term complications. The labor and delivery nurse, NICU nurse, obstetrician, neonatologist, laboratory technician, and respiratory care practitioner will all be involved in the care.

Transient Tachypnea of the Newborn (TTN)

TTN is a common self-limiting condition of infants in which **tachypnea,** increased oxygen needs, and mild respiratory distress occur. TTN occurs more often in infants sedated from maternal pain medications in labor, prolonged labor, macrosomia, and babies born via Cesarean section. It is thought to be caused by residual fluid in the lungs and usually resolves within 48 to 82 hours.

Medical management of TTN includes:

- Supportive care with IV fluids and gavage feedings until the respiratory rate has decreased enough to allow breast or bottle feedings
- Oxygen support to maintain oxygen saturation levels above 93%
- Chest x-ray
- Arterial blood gas (ABG) assessments (Subramanian, 2014)

Nursing interventions for a newborn with TTN include:

- Administering and monitoring ordered IV fluids
- Monitoring oxygenation by physical assessment, ABGs, and O_2 saturation levels
- Administering gavage feedings
- Minimizing stimulation
- Preventing hypothermia or hyperthermia
- Providing emotional support to the family
- After TTN has resolved, focusing on bonding and breast-feeding support

Meconium Aspiration Syndrome

During labor and delivery, a fetus may become stressed because of a decrease in oxygen caused by placental insufficiency, cord compression, or infection, causing the fetus to pass meconium into the amniotic fluid. Approximately 5% of the newborns who pass meconium before birth will inhale it into the lungs, causing lung injury and respiratory distress (Kendig and Nawab, 2015). The meconium can block bronchioles, causing difficulty with oxygenation, pneumonia, and pneumothorax (ie, collapsed lung).

The nurse should be observant for signs of possible meconium aspiration if the newborn has a greenish yellow staining of the skin, nail beds, or umbilical cord. Additional signs are:

- Tachypnea
- Retractions
- Nasal flaring
- Grunting
- Decreased oxygen saturation levels
- Decreased breath sounds

If meconium is evident at birth, thorough suctioning should occur with the first breath. If the newborn progresses into respiratory distress, endotracheal intubation and mechanical ventilation may be required. The infant will be transferred to the NICU and the medical and nursing care is the same as discussed for the newborn with respiratory distress.

Persistent Pulmonary Hypertension of the Newborn (PPHN)

When the fetus is delivered, the fetal circulation begins the transition to normal circulation, in which the blood flows from the right ventricle into the pulmonary arteries to the capillaries in the alveoli for gas exchange. Oxygen is picked up and carbon dioxide is released. In PPHN, the fetal circulation persists, or remains, as it was in the uterus: the ductus arteriosus and/or foramen ovale remain open, blood is shunted away from the lungs, the lungs have high pressure, and there is inadequate blood flow to the lungs for oxygenation of the newborn (Sallaam, 2014). This condition can be life-threatening. The most common causes of PPHN are:

- Perinatal asphyxia
- RDS
- Neonatal sepsis
- A congenital defect of the heart or lungs

Signs and symptoms of PPHN are similar to RDS except for the additions of cyanosis that does not improve with administration of oxygen, symptoms of shock (ie, low blood pressure and tachycardia), and the possibility of a heart murmur caused by the open ductus arteriosus and/or foramen ovale. Medical and nursing care will begin with transferring the infant to the NICU. Additional medical and nursing management includes:

- **Echocardiography** (ie, a test that looks at how blood flows through the heart vessels, valves, and chambers) to diagnose heart defects
- Chest x-ray to diagnose lung defects
- ABGs to monitor oxygenation
- Oxygen therapy
- Administration of dopamine to elevate blood pressure
- Administration of surfactant, if caused by lung disease
- Administration of vasodilators after the infant is stable to reduce lung hypertension
- Mechanical ventilation
- Continuous monitoring of vital signs and oxygenation
- Maintaining a normal body temperature

- Nutritional support
- Minimal handling of the newborn to reduce oxygen consumption
- Teaching and emotional support of the family (Sallaam, 2014)

The prognosis of PPHN depends upon the initial cause. It may resolve or the infant may have ongoing health problems. Because of the hypoxemia the infant experienced, survivors of PPHN have a higher risk of neurosensory hearing loss and neurodevelopmental problems later. These babies should be monitored closely for problems and receive early interventions.

SAFETY *STAT!*

PPHN has been linked to babies whose mothers use antidepressant medications, or selective serotonin reuptake inhibitors, during the late stages of pregnancy (Whiteman, 2015). Patients should be encouraged to discuss the risks and benefits of any medications taken during pregnancy.

CARE OF THE NEWBORN WITH COLD STRESS

Thermoregulation is extremely important for any infant, but even more so for the high-risk infant. The risk of cold stress is highest during the immediate transitional period after birth. Normal rectal temperature for term and preterm infants is 36.5°C to 37°C. Cold stress is likely if a newborn is born outside of the hospital environment. Infants at risk for cold stress are:

- Premature
- Small-for-gestational-age (SGA) infants
- Infants who require CPR
- Infants who have an infection or a congenital anomaly

When the infant's body temperature drops, the body attempts to adapt and raise the temperature by:

- Peripheral vasoconstriction conserves heat for the core of the body.
- Core blood volume increases, causing an increase in heart rate and blood pressure.
- An increase in metabolic rate can lead to increased oxygen needs and hypoglycemia.
- Brown fat is metabolized, causing a release of fatty acids and subsequent acidosis.

Prevention of cold stress should be the focus. At delivery, the infant should be dried thoroughly with a prewarmed blanket. A cap should be placed on the head and the infant placed for skin-to-skin contact with the mother. For any necessary procedures, the infant should be placed under a radiant warmer. Signs that an infant is experiencing cold stress are:

- Temperature below 36.3°C
- Weak cry
- Respirations that become slow and shallow
- Jitters from low blood sugar
- Refusal to eat
- Lethargic
- Respiratory distress

If the signs of cold stress are not noted, the infant can progress into cardiopulmonary arrest from hypoxia. Nursing interventions for cold stress will depend upon the severity of the problem. Interventions may include:

- Monitoring the temperature every 15 min
- Providing skin-to-skin contact with the mother
- Placing the infant under a radiant warmer
- Double-wrapping the newborn
- Placing the infant in an incubator and gradually rewarming
- Using special rewarming blankets
- Infusing warmed IV fluids
- If bottle fed, warming the formula
- Treating hypoglycemia according to the nursery protocol

LEARN TO C.U.S.

A newborn was just delivered in his parent's car 20 min ago on the way to the hospital. The parents and the newborn arrive in the emergency room with the baby wrapped in the father's shirt. The emergency room physician places the infant on a bed and begins a quick assessment of heart rate and respirations. The newborn is breathing but not crying and seems lethargic. The nurse notes that the newborn has been uncovered for several minutes. Using the C.U.S. method of communication, the nurse says, "Doctor, I am **concerned**. I am **uncomfortable** seeing this examination done on a regular bed. We have a **safety** issue. The infant may be cold stressed. We need to move him under a radiant warmer."

NEONATAL HYPOGLYCEMIA

Neonatal **hypoglycemia** is defined as a plasma glucose level of less than 30 mg/dL in the first 24 hours of life and less than 45 mg/dL thereafter. It is the most common metabolic problem in newborns (Cranmer, 2014). Both healthy and ill-appearing infants can be affected by hypoglycemia during the first few days of life. Risk factors for hypoglycemia are:

- Premature or postmature birth
- Infant of a diabetic mother (IDM)
- SGA
- Large-for-gestational-age (LGA)
- Stress at birth, for example, cold stress or asphyxia (Sinha, 2014)

Newborns need glucose for energy and most of the glucose is used for brain function. Long-term complications from frequent or prolonged hypoglycemia are neurological damage, such as mental retardation; developmental delays; personality disorders; decreased head size; lowered IQ; and seizures (Cranmer, 2014). If the newborn has risk factors for hypoglycemia, the blood sugar should be checked with a heelstick blood sample. The nurse should be aware that the newborn's blood glucose levels can drop if the newborn:

• Has no glycogen stored in the liver; for example, a premature newborn
• Has used up stored glucose for heat production or a birth stress, such as asphyxia
• Is an IDM and has **hyperinsulinism** (ie, increased levels of insulin)
• Cannot feed enough to keep the glucose level in an acceptable range (Lee, 2013)

The signs and symptoms of hypoglycemia in the newborn are:

• Jitteriness or tremors
• Lethargy or irritability
• Hypotonia
• Weak or high-pitched cry
• Apnea
• Hypothermia
• Poor feeding

Most hospital nurseries have protocols instituted by the physicians on the unit for nurses to follow in the event of hypoglycemia. This saves time and allows the nurse to begin prompt treatment of hypoglycemia.

Nursing interventions for hypoglycemia include:

• Obtaining a blood sample via heelstick as soon as possible after birth for high-risk infants; if results are normal, repeating 30 min, 1 hour, 2 hours, 4 hours, 8 hours, and 12 hours after birth (Potter, 2013)
• Obtaining a blood sample on any infant who exhibits signs and symptoms of hypoglycemia
• If the glucometer reading is between 20 and 40 mg/dL, and if the newborn is term and able to feed:
  • Making sure the infant is breastfed or bottle-fed
  • Rechecking the blood glucose 20 min after the feeding
• If:
  • The glucometer reading is less than 20 mg/dL *or*
  • The glucometer reading is 40 mg/dL and the newborn is unable to feed or is preterm *or*
  • The newborn is symptomatic *or*
  • The glucometer reading is 40 mg/dL after feeding:
    • Draw blood for a STAT blood glucose from the hospital laboratory.
    • Give an IV bolus of 2 mg/kg of D10W (10% dextrose in water).
    • Notify the health-care provider.
    • Recheck glucose after bolus; if below 40 mg/dL, begin a continuous infusion of D10W at 4 to 6 mg/kg/min (Sweet, Gray, et al, 2013).

SAFETY *STAT!*

Always check the blood sugar immediately after birth for any large or small birth weight newborn. Early detection and treatment of hypoglycemia will prevent complications for the newborn.

CARE OF THE NEWBORN WITH BIRTH INJURIES

Injuries to the newborn can occur as a result of traction and compression during the birthing process. These injuries are known as *birth trauma*. It occurs occasionally and unavoidably with an average of 6 to 8 per 1,000 live births (Laroia, 2015). Risk factors for birth trauma include:

• Fetal macrosomia
• Cephalopelvic disproportion
• Prolonged or very rapid delivery
• Use of forceps or vacuum extraction
• Abnormal presentation, such as breech
• Large fetal head

Common soft tissue injuries are cephalohematoma, caput succedaneum, and abrasion or lacerations from instrumental deliveries. These injuries resolve within days and cause no long-term problems for the infant. Brachial plexus injuries, cranial nerve injuries, and fractures are less common, but have the potential for more complications for the newborn. Those injuries are discussed in the following sections.

Brachial Plexus Injuries

A **brachial plexus** injury to the newborn occurs from an increase in the infant's neck-shoulder angle resulting in a traction force to the brachial plexus. The brachial plexus is a network of nerves that originate in the neck area and branch off to form the nerves that control movement and sensation in the shoulders, arms, and hands. Brachial plexus injuries occur in 0.5 to 5 infants per 1,000 live births and are associated with large birth weight, long labors, vaginal breech delivery, and shoulder dystocia (Snyder-Warwick, 2014).

Nurses are usually the first to suspect or detect a brachial plexus injury right after delivery or when completing the first physical assessment. Symptoms of a brachial plexus injury in the newborn are:

• Limited movement on one side of the body
• No Moro's reflex on the affected side
• Clawlike appearance of the newborn's hand on the affected side
• Abnormal muscle contractions on the affected side

Definitive diagnosis of a brachial plexus injury may include x-rays to determine if there is a fracture of the clavicle, shoulder, or arm; imaging studies; and nerve conduction studies. Medical management of a brachial plexus injury will depend on the severity of the injury. Approximately 93% of infants with brachial plexus paralysis demonstrate spontaneous improvement by 4 months of age (Snyder-Warwick, 2014). Medical management may include:

- Physical therapy such as range-of-motion activities, massage, and stretching to help the infant develop muscles on the affected side
- Surgical treatment, such as grafting a nerve from a less-used muscle to the affected area

Nursing care for the newborn with a brachial plexus injury includes:

- Reporting symptoms of a brachial plexus injury immediately
- Protecting the affected arm from dangling when held or moved
- Not lifting the infant under the axillae
- Teaching the parents how to support the affected arm with rolled blankets when the infant is in the car seat and crib
- Monitoring for signs of pain and reporting to the healthcare provider
- Positioning the infant with good body alignment to prevent complications from muscle contractures
- Providing emotional support to the family

TEAM WORKS

When a newborn has a brachial plexus injury, team work is an important part of promoting a good outcome and recovery. The nurse will be providing the initial care and educating and supporting the parents. The health-care provider will make the diagnosis along with consultation with neurologists and physical therapists. The parents will be part of the team as they will be learning exercises from the physical therapist that can be done at home with their baby. Later, if complete recovery does not occur, a surgeon will join the team.

Cranial Nerve Injury and Spinal Cord Injury

Cranial nerve and spinal cord nerve injuries result from hyperextension, traction, and overstretching with rotation during the delivery (Laroia, 2015). The damage may range from a temporary loss of sensation and motor function to a cord transection (ie, complete tear).

The physical findings for a cranial nerve injury are usually asymmetrical movements of the face, with eye and mouth drooping noted. Most infants recover within weeks to months.

Spinal cord injuries often result in a stillborn or rapid neonatal death because the damage usually occurs in the cervical and upper thoracic spine. An injury at that level of the spinal cord makes it difficult to establish respiratory function.

Fractures

A fractured clavicle is the most frequently fractured bone in the newborn during delivery (Laroia, 2015). It is associated with macrosomic infants and infants with large shoulders, which can make a vaginal delivery difficult. After the delivery, the nurse will notice that the newborn does not move the affected arm. In addition, a palpable bone irregularity may be noted during physical assessment. Diagnosis is made with an x-ray of the clavicle and affected arm.

Healing occurs in 7 to 10 days. To decrease pain, the arm is immobilized by pinning the undershirt sleeve to the shirt. The newborn should also be observed for a possible brachial plexus injury associated with a fractured clavicle.

◼ HYPERBILIRUBINEMIA

Hyperbilirubinemia is also known as jaundice. Jaundice is the most common condition that requires medical attention in newborns (Hansen, 2014). Physiological jaundice is a normal occurrence in newborns; unconjugated bilirubin is slowly conjugated (ie, paired with proteins in the liver) for excretion in the gastrointestinal tract and by the kidneys.

However, in some infants the serum bilirubin level rises excessively and requires treatment to accelerate the removal of bilirubin from the blood before complications can occur. This type of hyperbilirubinemia is known as pathological or nonphysiological jaundice. When the serum bilirubin is excessively elevated, the skin becomes saturated with bilirubin, causing the yellow coloration. After the skin is saturated, the bilirubin begins to deposit in the brain and can cause a neurotoxicity; this is known as *kernicterus*.

Risk factors for pathological jaundice include:

- Prematurity
- A blood type incompatibility
- Lack of effective breastfeeding
- Excessive bruising

Detection and diagnosis of pathological jaundice begins with a physical assessment. Jaundice can usually be detected visually when the level reaches 5 to 6 mg/dL (Hansen, 2014). Jaundice first appears on the face. The sclera may be tinted yellow also. As the bilirubin level rises, it spreads down the body. A transcutaneous bilirubinometer is a noninvasive instrument that can give an estimate of the total bilirubin before a serum bilirubin test is performed. Definitive diagnosis of hyperbilirubinemia is made through laboratory testing. See Table 19.1 for common laboratory tests that may be ordered to determine the severity of the hyperbilirubinemia and possible causes of the problem.

Medical management is based upon the gestational age, weight, and bilirubin level. Health-care providers have charts and tools based on gestational age and weight for determining at which bilirubin level to begin phototherapy. Breastfeeding, phototherapy, and exchange transfusions are the usual medical management.

Breastfeeding at least 8 to 12 times a day will help with decreasing bilirubin levels. A baby who is having at least six wet diapers and three stools per day will help to eliminate the bilirubin through the gastrointestinal tract and kidneys.

Generally, many health-care providers will institute phototherapy when the total serum bilirubin level is at or above

TABLE 19.1 LABORATORY TESTS FOR THE NEWBORN WITH JAUNDICE

Test	Purpose
Total or Direct Bilirubin Level	Measures the amount of bilirubin in the blood that is produced when the liver breaks down red blood cells
Direct and Indirect Coombs'	Detects antibodies against red blood cells seen in Rh and ABO blood incompatibilities
CBC	Detects anemia or infection, which would raise the bilirubin levels
Albumin	Detects the amount of albumin available to bind with bilirubin for excretion
Blood Culture	Detects infection that could raise bilirubin levels
Peripheral Smear	A follow-up test if the CBC is abnormal; used to closely evaluate the blood cells under a microscope
Reticulocyte Count	Useful if the infant is anemic; measures red blood cell production by the bone marrow

Source: Van Leeuwen AM and Bladh ML. *Davis's Comprehensive Handbook of Laboratory & Diagnostic Tests.* 6th ed. FA Davis: Philadelphia, 2015.

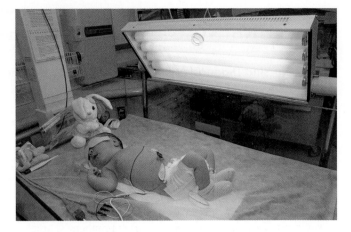

FIGURE 19.3 A newborn undergoing phototherapy. The eyes and genitals are covered for protection. *(Courtesy St. Luke's Hospital, Bethlehem, Pennsylvania.)*

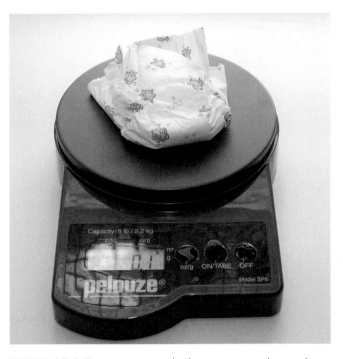

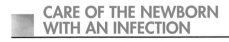

FIGURE 19.4 Diapers are weighed on a gram scale to calculate accurate urinary output.

15 mg/dL in infants 25 to 48 hours old, 18 mg/dL in infants 49 to 72 hours old, and 20 mg/dL in infants older than 72 hours (Sawyer, 2013). Phototherapy using a "blue light" converts bilirubin molecules into water-soluble compounds that can be excreted by the body (Sawyer, 2013). The infant can be exposed to the blue light through overhead lights, pads, or blankets (Fig. 19.3). The infant can be removed from the light for feedings, especially since feedings are an important part of the treatment plan.

A blood exchange transfusion in the neonatal intensive care nursery may be required if the bilirubin levels are rising so quickly that kernicterus may occur. Serious neurological damage may occur if the bilirubin levels do not drop with feedings and phototherapy.

Nursing interventions for the infant with jaundice requiring phototherapy may include:

- Encouraging breastfeeding 8 to 12 times a day
- Monitoring the number of stools
- Weighing diapers to obtain accurate urine output information (Fig. 19.4)

- Placing eye patches on the newborn's eyes to protect the retina from damage from the phototherapy light
- Undressing the newborn except for the genital area to expose the maximum amount of skin to the light
- Monitoring the newborn's behavior; irritability or lethargy could be signs that the bilirubin level is irritating the brain
- Monitoring the infant's body temperature for hypothermia from being undressed.

CARE OF THE NEWBORN WITH AN INFECTION

Newborns can be exposed to infection through vertical transmission from the mother, from organisms that enter the

NURSING CARE PLAN for the Infant with Jaundice

Nursing Diagnosis: There is a potential for hypothermia or hyperthermia.
Expected Outcome: Maintain a temperature between 35.5°C and 37°C.
Interventions:
- Check the body temperature and vital signs every 2 hours.
- Dress the baby appropriately when removing him or her from the phototherapy.

Nursing Diagnosis: There is deficient fluid volume related to phototherapy and poor feeding.
Expected Outcome: The infant will produce six wet diapers per day.
Interventions:
- Encourage breastfeeding 8 to 12 times per day.
- Document the number of wet diapers.
* Weigh diapers on a gram scale to get an accurate amount of urine output.

Nursing Diagnosis: There is a risk for injury from the effects of phototherapy.
Expected Outcome: The jaundice will resolve without injury to the patient.
Interventions:
- Place the newborn at the appropriate distance from the light source per hospital protocol.
- Cover the infant's eyes and genitals.
- Ensure that the eye patches do not cover the nose and mouth.
- Turn the infant every 2 hours.
- Note the activity level every 2 hours. Lethargy or irritability are early signs of kernicterus.

vagina during labor, from contaminated hospital personnel and equipment, and from family and visitors. Nurses need to be constantly on the watch for signs of infection. A newborn has an immature immune system that is unable to mount an attack against a severe infection before it becomes systemic. The newborn may only exhibit subtle signs of infection that an experienced nurse can observe and report immediately to begin appropriate care. This section discusses neonatal sepsis and infection from herpes virus.

Sepsis

Neonatal sepsis is a blood infection that presents within the first 7 days of life but may occur up to 90 days after birth. Sepsis is an invasive infection in which chemicals released into the blood to help fight the infection cause inflammation over the entire body. The most common causes of neonatal sepsis are group B streptococcus (GBS), *Escherichia coli*, and herpes (Anderson-Berry, 2014). Risk factors include:

- Preterm delivery
- Maternal infection with GBS
- Amniotic membranes ruptured for longer than 24 hours
- Chorioamnionitis (ie, infection of the amniotic membranes)
- Frequent vaginal examinations during labor in which the examiner inadvertently transports *E coli* from the rectal area into the vagina and cervix

Because of an immature immune system, the newborn may exhibit vague symptoms at the onset because any or many organs could be infected. Prompt recognition of signs of sepsis and initiation of treatment are vital to the survival of the neonate. Signs and symptoms of neonatal sepsis are:

- Poor temperature control (ie, hypothermia or hyperthermia)
- Irregular respirations
- Dyspnea
- Grunting and retractions
- Cold clammy skin
- Abnormal heartbeat
- Lethargy
- Poor feeding
- Diminished activity or hyperactivity
- Bulging fontanel
- Diarrhea
- Abdominal distention

The septic newborn may require transfer to a level III perinatal center. Medical management of sepsis could possibly include:

- Cardiopulmonary support
- IV fluids
- Placement of a central venous line for antibiotic administration
- IV antibiotics, such as aminoglycosides, penicillins, and vancomycin
- Antiviral medication, such as acyclovir, may be given if the infection may be from herpes

- IV total parenteral nutrition (TPN) during the acute phase to support the immune system and for growth and development (Ambalavanan, 2014; Anderson-Berry, 2014)

Nursing intervention for the newborn with sepsis includes:

- Monitoring vital signs and laboratory results, and reporting abnormalities promptly
- Promoting thermoregulation
- Administering IV fluids, antibiotics, and antiviral medications as ordered
- Monitoring fluid balance
- Administering TPN and observing for complications
- Supporting the family emotionally and providing opportunities for bonding

LABS & DIAGNOSTICS

A complete diagnostic evaluation of the infant with suspected sepsis includes:

- A complete blood cell count (CBC) with differential; this test is not always reliable because the immature immune system of the newborn may not be able to produce neutrophils to fight infection and therefore the newborn with sepsis could have normal neutrophils or even decreased neutrophils
- Chest x-ray if respiratory symptoms are present
- Lumbar puncture if neurological symptoms are present

SAFETY *STAT!*

Aminoglycosides and vancomycin have the potential to be ototoxic (ie, cause damage to the hearing) and nephrotoxic (ie, cause damage to the kidneys). Therefore the dose based on weight must be calculated carefully and the serum drug level should be evaluated after the third dose or 48 hours after the start of treatment to avoid overdosing and causing complications. Infants should receive an audiology screening before discharge (Anderson-Berry, 2014; Vallerand, Sanoski, et al, 2014).

Herpes

Newborns can become infected with the herpes virus during pregnancy, labor, or delivery. The herpes virus type 2 (ie, genital herpes) is the most common cause of herpes infection in the newborn, but type 1(ie, oral herpes) can also cause infection. If the mother has an active case of herpes type 2 at the time of delivery, the fetus can be exposed while passing through the birth canal. The newborn may only develop a skin infection that blisters, crusts over, and then heals. However, the herpes infection can become systemic like neonatal sepsis and be life-threatening to the newborn. The symptoms of a systemic neonatal herpes infection are identical to the signs and symptoms of neonatal sepsis. The medical management and nursing interventions are also the same, with the exception of antibiotics. Antibiotics are not effective against

a virus. The newborn would receive antiviral medications instead (Kaneshiro, 2014).

SAFETY *STAT!*

If a woman has a suspected case of genital herpes, she should have a scheduled Cesarean birth to reduce the risk of transmission of the herpes infection to her newborn.

CARE OF THE FAMILY OF AN AT-RISK NEWBORN

As most parents are planning for the birth of their baby, they are expecting a normal birth and a healthy newborn. Even a woman who experiences complications during her pregnancy holds on to the hope that her newborn will be born without problems and leave the hospital with her. Admission of their baby to the NICU places the parents and other family members into a stressful situation. When the unexpected complication of having a sick newborn happens, the parents will experience a range of emotions:

- Fear of the unknown and the environment of the NICU
- Anger that the birth experience was not what was planned
- Guilt, because the mother often blames herself
- Loss of bonding and attachment time because the parents and child are separated
- Loss of control because the staff does not always communicate openly with the parents
- Frustration because the other women on the postpartum unit have their babies in their rooms
- Anxiety caused by worry about the baby's health
- Helplessness because the baby needs high-level skilled care and the mother cannot provide care to her infant

Nurses must develop strategies to provide family-centered care and reduce the stress and anxiety that the parents are experiencing. Nursing interventions that support family-centered care in the NICU include:

- Providing opportunities for the parents to hold and bond with their newborn
- Developing a therapeutic relationship with the parents
- Providing positive reinforcement for the concerns the parents demonstrate
- Encouraging the parents to talk about the NICU experience
- Never behaving as if the parents are in the way or interrupting
- Answering all questions honestly
- Including the parents in an open dialogue with the entire NICU team
- Demonstrating care for the parents and the baby
- Referring to the baby by his or her first name
- Allowing the parents to provide care such as bathing and feedings (Fig. 19.5)

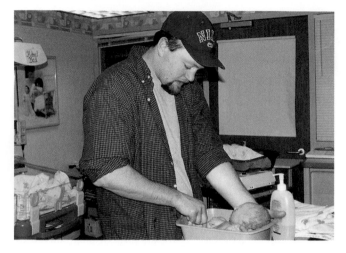

FIGURE 19.5 A new father bathes his infant.

• Starting to teach home care before discharge so that the parents will not be overwhelmed (Fig. 19.6)

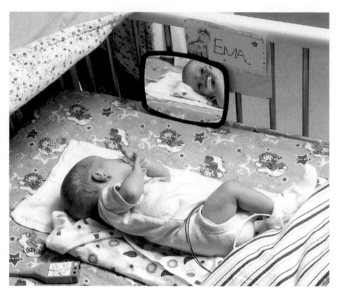

FIGURE 19.6 A 10-week-old infant born at 27 weeks' gestation, who will be going home soon.

THERAPEUTIC COMMUNICATION

It is very important to establish a therapeutic relationship with the parents of a sick newborn. Communication with the parents needs to be sincere and honest. False reassurance is not therapeutic for the parents. Some examples of therapeutic communication are:

"Tell me how you're feeling today..."

"What questions do you have?"

"You look worried, what's on your mind?"

"I have time; can I sit with you and talk about your baby and your concerns?"

CULTURAL CONSIDERATIONS

The babies in the NICU come from a variety of cultural and religious backgrounds. The parents may want to have their seriously ill newborn baptized in the NICU. They may want to place religious items in the incubator with the newborn or place a religious symbol under the mattress. The family might request to have a spiritual leader place hands on the baby and pray. Nurses should establish a therapeutic relationship with the parents and encourage them to engage in their spiritual beliefs because it will provide them comfort and reduce their stress while their baby is ill.

Key Points

■ Birth asphyxia occurs when the newborn's brain does not receive enough oxygen during the birth process.

■ Respiratory distress can be caused by lack of surfactant, immature lungs, fluid in the airways, meconium blocking the airways, and other conditions that make it difficult for the newborn to initiate or maintain respirations after birth.

■ The most common signs of respiratory distress are tachypnea, dyspnea, nasal flaring, and chest retractions.

■ Prompt recognition of the signs of respiratory distress is required so that interventions can be started before CPR is required.

■ Transient tachycardia is self-limiting and manifested by mild respiratory distress and tachypnea.

■ Meconium aspiration syndrome is caused by the fetus inhaling meconium during the birth process. The meconium can block small bronchioles, thus inhibiting gas exchange.

■ Cold stress can compound problems for an ill newborn. Careful management of the newborn's temperature is extremely important.

■ Neonatal hypoglycemia is the most common metabolic problem for newborns. Long-term complications from untreated or poorly treated hypoglycemia include developmental delays, seizures, and mental retardation.

■ Birth injuries most often occur with macrosomic infants delivered vaginally. The most common birth injuries are fractured clavicles and brachial plexus injuries.

■ Hyperbilirubinemia that is excessive can cause neurological problems for the newborn if not treated. Hyperbilirubinemia is treated with breastfeeding, phototherapy, and exchange transfusion.

■ Newborns can become infected in a variety of ways. The immature immune system often cannot produce obvious symptoms. The nurse needs to be alert for subtle signs of neonatal sepsis and report promptly to initiate care.

■ The nurse has an opportunity to provide family-centered care by including the parents in the care of the ill newborn.

REVIEW QUESTIONS

1. A nurse may suspect a brachial plexus injury if:
   1. The newborn has tremors.
   2. The newborn cries continually.
   3. The newborn does not demonstrate a Moro's reflex.
   4. The newborn has hypotonia.

2. Signs of hypoglycemia include: *(select all that apply)*
   1. Tremors
   2. Hunger
   3. Weak cry
   4. Lethargy
   5. Jaundice

3. The nurse checks the blood sugar of a 2-hour-old newborn and the glucometer reading is 32 mg/dL. The nurse should:
   1. Recognize that this is a normal reading and document it.
   2. Initiate breastfeeding.
   3. Call the laboratory for a STAT blood glucose level.
   4. Transfer the newborn to the NICU.

4. A nurse has been explaining TTN to the newborn's mother. Which of the following statements indicates that the mother understands the teaching?
   1. "My baby will probably go home on oxygen therapy."
   2. "I can breastfeed my baby while he is breathing so fast."
   3. "This breathing problem may have happened because I had a Cesarean birth."
   4. "My baby may be in the NICU for about 2 weeks."

5. Which of the following are risk factors for neonatal sepsis? *(select all that apply)*
   1. Preterm birth
   2. Cesarean birth
   3. Precipitous delivery
   4. Frequent vaginal exams
   5. Mother has GBS infection

6. A sign that a newborn may be at risk for meconium aspiration syndrome is:
   1. Acrocyanosis
   2. Yellow-green tint on umbilical cord
   3. Asymmetrical breathing
   4. Born before 38 weeks' gestation

7. Physical findings that would alert the nurse to immediately report a possible problem of PPHN would be: *(select all that apply)*
   1. Cyanosis after administering oxygen
   2. Blue hands and feet
   3. Bradycardia
   4. Heart murmur
   5. A cephalohematoma

8. Which infant is most likely to develop cold stress?
   1. The LGA infant
   2. The IDM
   3. An infant with a cardiac birth defect
   4. A premature infant

9. Which of the following physical signs could indicate a risk for hyperbilirubinemia?
   1. Acrocyanosis
   2. Cephalohematoma
   3. Newborn rash
   4. Tremors

10. The nurse is *not* providing family-centered care with the following intervention:
    1. Allowing the mother to bathe the baby
    2. Inviting the parents to participate in a care planning conference
    3. Bottle-feeding a breastfed baby because the mother is tired
    4. Allowing the family to place a crucifix inside the infant's crib

CRITICAL THINKING QUESTIONS

1. Discuss the signs that the nurse would notice if gas exchange is impaired in a newborn.

2. Why would it be important to uncover the eyes of an infant undergoing phototherapy for feedings?

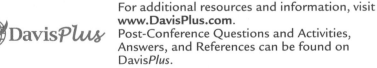

For additional resources and information, visit
www.DavisPlus.com.
Post-Conference Questions and Activities, Answers, and References can be found on Davis*Plus*.

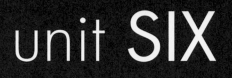

Growth and Development

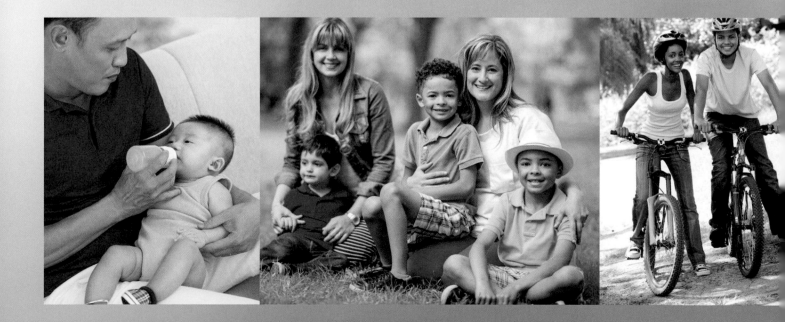

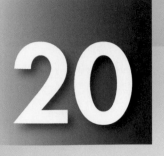

20

Introduction to Pediatric Nursing

KEY TERMS

empowerment
enabling
new morbidity

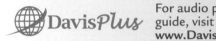

For audio pronunciation guide, visit www.DavisPlus.com

CHAPTER CONCEPTS

Family
Development
Safety

LEARNING OUTCOMES

1. Define the key terms.
2. Discuss contemporary issues facing children and their families in the 21st century, including social issues, and morbidity and mortality outcomes.
3. Analyze national pediatric health goals as identified from professional and government organizations.
4. Apply principles of family-centered care to families receiving care in a hospital or home setting.
5. Describe the anatomical, physiological, social, and emotional differences between adults and children, emphasizing the critical components that are pertinent to safe, emergent care of children across health-care settings.
6. Analyze care environments for safety concerns across childhood.
7. Describe issues of growth and development within the eight stages of childhood including newborn, young infant, older infant, toddler, preschooler, early school-aged child, later school-aged child, and adolescent.
8. State the importance of play across childhood and the theory that contributes to selecting play for specified situations such as promoting development, procedural distraction, and complimentary therapy for symptom control.

REAL-WORLD CASE STUDY

Leon

■ Leon, an 11-year-old child, has been admitted into the pediatric nursing unit for pain and a significant rash around his gastrostomy tube (GT) insertion site on the upper left quadrant of his abdomen. His GT insertion site requires a surgical revision because acidic gastric content is spilling out onto the skin of his abdomen, causing

REAL-WORLD CASE
STUDY *continued*

redness, irritation, and infection. Leon is developmentally delayed with a minimal vocabulary to express his needs. The hospitalist suggests his cognitive age to be approximately that of a 2 to 3-year-old. Because of the discomfort of his skin wound and his minimal communication skills, the staff expresses challenges caring for Leon's needs. Pain assessment, simple instructions, maintaining an intact IV site, and administering medications have all posed challenges for the staff.

1. Who best knows the most effective way to assess and communicate with Leon?
2. What is an innovative means to provide basic communication with this child?
3. What challenges can be anticipated for the family of Leon as he is treated for his skin infection and prepared for a surgical revision of his GT site?

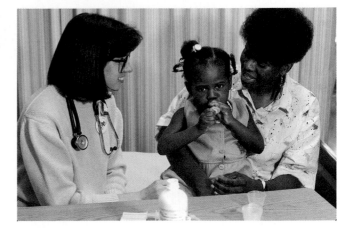

FIGURE 20.1 Pediatric nurses care for children of all ages.

will help a pediatric nurse be more successful in care. These skills include developmental approaches to assessment and pain assessment tools that are appropriate for various ages and stages of development. Pediatric nursing is considered a specialty area with specialty practice protocols.

CONCEPTUAL CORNERSTONE

Safety

Children need to be monitored for safety. Across childhood, safety remains one of the most important aspects of care of children. Safety includes providing anticipatory guidance to parents and caregivers as to what they can expect currently and in the future for their child's particular developmental stage. Pediatric nurses are key players in role-modeling safety for parents, caregivers, grandparents, siblings, and visitors.

Nurses caring for children of any age require a unique set of knowledge, skills, and behaviors. Pediatric nursing is considered a specialty practice requiring a body of knowledge acquired through study and experience. Pediatric nursing involves caring for children between birth and 18 years of age, as well as their families, in a variety of clinical settings focusing on normal growth and development; acute, chronic, and critical care issues; and end-of-life and palliative care (Fig. 20.1). Not all children experience a hospital stay during their childhood. Pediatric nurses must be prepared to interact with children and their families in settings that span both health promotion and health restoration from illnesses. Children with chronic conditions require professional health-care relationships so the family can manage complex care issues. These types of ongoing professional relationships encourage self-care, disease management, early assessment of complications, and overall wellness for the child and his/her family.

The assessment of pain is one of the most difficult challenges in pain management within the specialty of pediatric nursing. Using a set of pediatric-based pain assessment skills

CHALLENGES IN THE CARE OF CHILDREN IN CONTEMPORARY TIMES

Families today are faced with a variety of stressors that interfere with daily life. Homelessness rates have increased across the nation; violence in schools, neighborhoods, and communities has increased; and the number of families without funds for health-care access or full insurance coverage is increasing. The lack of consistent health-care provider visits contributes to lower immunization rates, less support for new parents, delayed interventions for children experiencing acute health issues, and delayed support for children with chronic illnesses.

There are many challenges that face pediatric health-care teams as well. Childhood obesity levels have sky-rocketed; unsafe neighborhoods prevent vigorous outdoor play; gang violence and social pressures influence decision making of older school-aged children and adolescents; child abuse can leave lasting emotional scars; and troubled economic times that reduce a family's choices all can influence a child's experience in normal growth and development. Pediatric nurses need to be comfortable in evaluating a family's concerns about parenting and child-rearing, and they need to be educated on how to guide family members to locate resources, health information, injury prevention ideas, and recreation within any given community.

Pediatric nurses are in a unique position to support families facing stressors. Providing anticipatory guidance that supports a safe and healthy lifestyle improves the health outcomes of children across the developmental stages. Refer to Box 20.1 for a list of challenges facing pediatric health-care team members related to the influence of poverty on children's health care.

Box 20.1 Pediatric Challenges: Influence of Poverty and the Uninsured

- Percentage of children without health insurance in 2013 ranged from 4.8% (CDC.gov, 2014) to 7.6%, but children living in poverty had a higher rate of 9.8% (U.S. Census Bureau, 2013)
- Breakdown of the percentage of children within each category who are within the poverty level:
  - African American: 38%
  - Latino: 30%
  - Native American: 29%
  - White: 10.1%
  - Asian: 9.8%
- 14.9% of American children, including 25% of African American children, report the experience of food insecurity in 2014
- 26.3% of American children (32.1% of children aged 0 to 3 years) are covered exclusively by public health insurance
- 25% of children 3 to 9 years of age living in poverty had untreated dental caries

Source: United States Census Bureau (2014) found at www.census.gov/content/dam/Census/library/publications/2014/demo/p60-250.pdf

ISSUES THAT INFLUENCE CHILDREN'S HEALTH-CARE OUTCOMES

National registries follow the causes of death and illness in children. The term *morbidity* is used to describe the prevalence of an illness, disease, or infection within a given population. Morbidity data show incidences, or new cases, of illness, including those associated with chronic disorders, injuries/accidents, infectious diseases, and those that lead to disabilities. The term *mortality* is used to describe the causes of death in each childhood development level or age bracket. Mortality data show the causes of death in all age groups so decisions and corresponding resources can be allocated to preventing deaths across childhood. Morbidity and mortality data collected aid in regional, state, and national policy making. These data therefore aid in subsequent resource allocation, including immunization recommendations, school attendance policies, and accident prevention strategies.

The term **new morbidity** refers to contemporary factors that influence the health and well-being of children in the 21st century. These factors include increasing use of childcare; latch-key children who are left alone after school while parents need to work; indiscriminate use of antibiotics that leads to resistant strains of bacteria; single parent households with limited resources; homelessness; drug use; and multiple social stressors.

SAFETY *STAT!*

Overview of Critical Pediatric Nursing Issues: Issues of New Morbidity

The term *new morbidity* is used to distinguish contemporary social issues that influence the general health and safety of children, as well as their sense of well-being. Examples of current concern include the following:

- Society violence and unsafe neighborhoods with limited forms of safe recreation across childhood
- Increased divorce rates and increased single parent households
- Increased drug and alcohol abuse by teens, parents, and extended family members
- Continued lack of thorough prenatal care and health promotion/disease prevention screening processes
- Increased numbers of medically underinsured or uninsured children and families in the nation with restricted access to health care
- Increased poverty levels, which lead to families being unable to fill prescriptions, follow through with ordered diagnostics, or complete needed health promotion/disease prevention health-care appointments
- Bullying in school settings
- Increased injury and accident rates across childhood
- Poor nutrition and increasing pandemic childhood obesity rates across childhood
- Exposure to peer pressure with drugs, alcohol, and early sexual activity
- Rates of sexually transmitted diseases
- Mental health issues including depression, anxiety, and low self-esteem
- Eating disorders
- Teen pregnancy rates
- School drop-out rates
- Child abuse and neglect

NURSING CARE ACROSS CHILDHOOD

Pediatric nurses have the joy and privilege of caring for children from prematurity through older adolescence. Because of the widespread ages of the pediatric population, children are grouped into developmental stages. There are eight stages of childhood that can be encountered:

1. Newborns: First 28 to 30 days of life
2. Early infancy: 30 days to 6 months of life
3. Older infancy: 6 months to 1 year of life
4. Toddler: 1 year of life to third birthday
5. Preschooler: Third birthday through 5th year
6. Early school-aged child: 6 years old up to the 10th birthday
7. Late school-aged child: 10 to 12 years old
8. Adolescent: 13 to 18 years old

Roles of the Pediatric Nurse

Care of children should not focus exclusively on the treatment of injuries or illness. The care of a pediatric patient may take place in a well-child setting, an acute care or critical care setting, a school setting, or in hospice, and therefore should focus on the goal of the child's health-care experience (Fig. 20.2). In well-child settings, care should focus on health promotion and disease prevention, including anticipatory guidance for all adults involved with the child's care. In acute care hospital environments, care should be focused not just on the illness or injury requiring hospitalization, but should include health education and the promotion of healthy lifestyles. For instance, if a child is admitted for a surgical procedure, the nurse should take the opportunity to assess the child's development, social skills, activity levels, disease prevention strategies (eg, dental care, healthy eating, and exercise), and self-care knowledge base. Because children make up approximately 25% of the nation's population, all nurses should be educated about the basics of pediatric care across childhood. These basics should include teaching families about providing a safe home environment, the prevention of childhood diseases, and health maintenance when a child is inflicted with an acute or chronic disease (Box 20.2).

Definition of Family

A family is considered a biological, legal, and/or emotional relation between two or more persons. There may be a variety of constellations including nuclear, alternative, adoptive, foster, and communal families (Figs. 20.3 and 20.4). See Box 20.3 for a summary of family structures. The most important factor in discussing the structure of a child's family is: *A family is who they say they are.*

Family-Centered Care

The philosophy of family-centered care recognizes the family as the constant in the child's life and that all members of the family are affected by the illness, injury, or hospitalization that the child is experiencing. Furthermore, the foundation of

> ## Box 20.2 The Roles of the Pediatric Nurse
>
> - Fostering family-centered care (ie, family unit–based care focusing on partnerships and collaboration)
> - Educating families in the prevention of common injuries and accidents across childhood
> - Providing health promotion through education, screening, and prevention measures
> - Teaching principles of anticipatory guidance and expected behaviors for developmental stages
> - Providing for care during acute illnesses or exacerbations of chronic conditions
> - Providing community-based nursing care focused on communities and client groups
> - Providing complex care coordination for children with multiple morbidities
> - Advocating for the child when families are unable to secure necessary care
> - Providing death and dying care, and symptom management at the end of life

family-centered care includes the need to provide support based on respect, encouragement, the enhancement of strengths, and the encouragement of competence. Health-care institutions across the nation are incorporating the principles of family-centered care into the care team's approach to strengthen the family unit, include all members, and enhance the communication and outcomes of the experience. The issues that the health-care team focuses on, other than the critical issues surrounding the child's illness or injury, are the self-identified needs of the family to encourage moving toward healing and a high level of functioning. Normalization, or the process of living one's life as normally as possible,

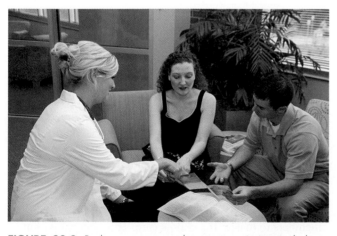

FIGURE 20.2 Pediatric nurses work in many settings, including schools and community organizations.

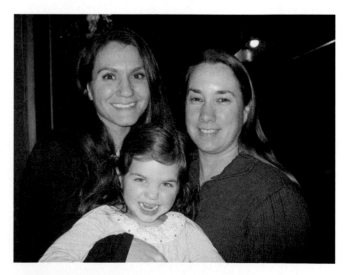

FIGURE 20.3 An alternative family.

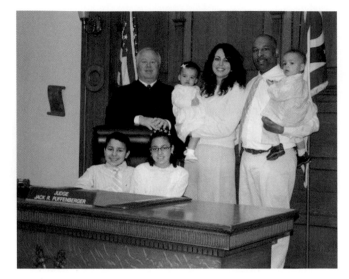

FIGURE 20.4 An adoptive family.

is promoted; personal identities are encouraged to grow beyond the child's illness state.

Family-centered care involves nurses providing a safe, child-friendly, and decorative environment, along with the support needed to assist the child and family as one unit. According to one hospital that successfully incorporated family-centered care into their pediatric unit, the provision of hope, love, and engaged care in which the family was supported and strengthened was the basis of a collaborative partnership between the family and health-care providers (Frost, Green, et al, 2010). See Box 20.4 for a list of family-centered care principles.

Box 20.3 Family Structures

- Nuclear or conjugal family: Husband, wife, and children living in the same household
- Reconstituted or step family: Both parents may contribute children from previous relationships or marriages to a new household
- Single-parent family: One parent responsible for running a household
- Same-sex family: Two members of the same sex are significant others and care for the household
- Extended family: Any constellation of family members lives together in one household
- Binuclear family: A child's time is divided between two households
- Foster family: A family that takes care of a child in either a long-term or temporary relationship
- Adoptive family: A family that permanently and legally accepts all responsibilities for a child from the biological parents
- Communal family: A group of people who may not be related live together and share responsibilities for household

Box 20.4 Family-Centered Care Principles

The philosophy of family-centered care includes the following principles:

- The family is recognized as the constant in the child's life.
- The family is recognized as being made up of who they say they are.
- The family is treated as one unit because the entire family is affected by the child's illness.
- Health-care providers are acknowledged as providers of collegial support.
- The two core concepts are enabling and empowerment.
- Natural care giving is supported.
- Decision-making roles within the family structure are supported.
- The unique strengths of the individuals and family unit are built upon.
- Living at home and within the child's greater community is promoted.
- Siblings and extended family members are included in care provisions.
- Diversity among structures is acknowledged and cultural diversity is promoted.
- Normalization is promoted and identities are encouraged beyond the illness state.
- A parent-professional partnership is promoted.
- The child is helped to cope with hospitalization.
- The child is helped to cope with separation anxiety that begins at 8 to 10 months and peaks at 16 to 30 months.
- Family goals, dreams, strategies, and activities are supported.
- Support systems, services, education, and information for all members are located and provided to the family.

Two important overarching goals of implementing family-centered care are to foster the development of empowerment and enabling:

- **Empowerment:** The interaction between the family and health-care providers is such that the family's sense of control over their lives continues while family members are supported so they can foster their own strengths, abilities, and actions through the care giving/helping role. This concept within the family-centered care principles addresses assisting a family to feel as though they are supported, listened to, and competent.
- **Enabling:** Professionals provide opportunities for family members to master the child's care. This concept within family-centered care principles describes the teaching, supporting, and enabling that allows a family to care for their child.

Family-centered care is provided regardless of the practice setting where the encounter takes place. Families need to be encouraged to be present with the child whenever it is safe and possible. If the child is hospitalized, the parents should have access to the child 24 hours a day and therefore should be encouraged to stay with the child throughout the required care. Examples of this include encouraging parents to accompany a child during a minor medical procedure or staying in a provided bed in an acute or critical care setting. This closeness supports parents to feel welcomed to participate in the child's care, and to provide emotional support to the child around the clock. With current economic times placing financial stress on families, parents are not always able to stay with their hospitalized child because they must complete work duties and provide for the families' needs. No judgment should ever be expressed about this as the functioning of the family may rest on the ability of a parent to provide.

Siblings are an important aspect of family-centered care. Siblings should be encouraged to interact with the hospitalized child while also being provided the opportunity to play and develop. Play rooms should include sibling time and participation. Child Life Specialists should be called upon to provide healthy and educative opportunities for siblings while present. If a child is being hospitalized for care of a chronic condition, information on sibling support groups should be provided and involvement encouraged.

Pediatric Care Settings

Children are cared for in a variety of clinical settings. Some settings are geared toward the well child and offer care for maintaining health and preventing illness, and other settings are for restoring health, such as clinics geared to children with special needs or chronic disorders. The following list includes examples of care environments:

- Acute care hospital units, which can be either general hospitals serving people across the lifespan, or hospitals geared for children; they either focus on general medical needs or a subspecialty such as surgery, rehabilitation, oncology, burn, and orthopedic units
- Critical care or intensive care units
- Specialty clinics for children with special needs, such as cystic fibrosis, endocrine disorders, or oncology
- Outpatient clinics, such as well-child immunization clinics
- Public health departments
- Home care for children
- Hospice care for children
- Private primary care providers (ie, private practice clinics)
- Nurse practitioner-run pediatric or family care clinics
- School nursing programs

Children are not just small adults and should be treated accordingly. Nursing must take into account children's uniqueness, strengths, and resiliency. The focus of care for children is not based on the child's chronological age, but rather the child's developmental level within a developmental stage.

Nursing Care for Children on Medical Surgical Units

In many health-care settings there will be no specific pediatric unit staffed with experienced pediatric nurses. In these cases, nonpediatric nurses will be required to provide care for children who are assigned to adult units. When this is the structure of care, specific competencies should be required for all health-care team members that provide care to the child and family. Developmentally appropriate care and communication skills are imperative for the successful care of hospitalized children and include medication dosage calculations; pediatric-specific skills; neonatal, infant, and child resuscitation techniques; play therapy; and family-centered care principles. New technologies, such as pediatric simulation education, can help with keeping pediatric skills up-to-date (Fig. 20.5). Practicing pediatric cardiopulmonary resuscitation (CPR) via mock codes is also helpful in keeping confident in emergency skills (Fig. 20.6). Keeping care focused on safety and injury prevention is important to prevent problems associated with nursing units not designed for the specific care of children.

 LEARN TO C.U.S

You are working in a large outpatient surgical center that specializes in adult day surgical procedures. In a staff meeting, you are told that the center will be starting to perform procedures on children. How might you express your concerns during the staff meeting?

C: "I am **concerned** about taking care of children who will be having surgical procedures here."

U: "I am **uncomfortable** with my pediatric skills and competencies. Without having pediatric-focused skills such as developmental theory, physical assessments on children, safe medication administration for children, and a review of infant and child CPR, I would be uncomfortable as an adult nurse having to care for children after surgery."

S: "I think we have a **safety** issue here."

QUALITY AND SAFETY IMPERATIVES

National accreditation organizations for hospitals and health-care environments specify quality and safety imperatives for caregivers to provide the safest environment possible for patients across the lifespan (The Joint Commission, 2015). The following are the identified imperatives for nurses working in pediatrics:

- Identify patients correctly before treatments, diagnostics, medications, or any form of medical/nursing care.
- Implement and test the quality and effectiveness of improvements in staff communications including:
  - **Read back verbal orders (RBV):** The nurse legibly writes the verbal orders received and reads them back in person or over the phone. (Most institutions now

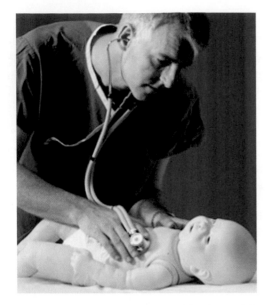

FIGURE 20.5 Pediatric simulation is helpful to keep skills current. *(PediaSIM pediatric simulation photo courtesy CAE Healthcare. © 2011 CAE Healthcare.)*

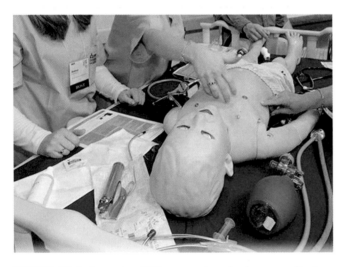

FIGURE 20.6 Practicing CPR via mock codes keeps pediatric nurses confident in their skills. *(PediaSIM pediatric simulation photo courtesy CAE Healthcare. © 2011 CAE Healthcare.)*

do not allow any form of verbal orders unless in an emergency.)
- **Do Not Use Abbreviations list (DNUA):** The nurse makes sure that no member of the health-care team, in any department, uses the DNUA that are identified as contributing to errors.
- **Hand-off reports:** With all patient hand-offs or reports given between nurses or care providers within any care environment (eg, between surgical nurses and postanesthesia care unit nurses and surgical floor nurses, or between pediatric intensive care nurses and medical floor nurses), nurses ensure the hand-off report is thorough, precise, comprehendible, and complete enough to provide the next phase of care safely without neglecting

any aspect of care. Omissions would include failing to state the child's previous intake and output (I&O) or the timing of the next antibiotic medication ordered.
- **Critical test results:** The nurse makes sure that when laboratory personnel call the pediatric nursing unit with a critically high or critically low laboratory value, the correct health-care provider is notified of the result in a timely fashion so an intervention can be provided.
- Use medicines safely by following the Rights of Medication Administration every time a medication is ordered, dispensed, and administered.
- Prevent infections by following national communicable disease prevention measures, including standard precautions and infection-specific precautions (eg, droplet, airborne, contact, and reverse isolation techniques).
  - Hand hygiene is the most important nursing responsibility in the reduction of transmission of disease.
- Check patient medications carefully, following institutional policy using at least three checks between obtaining the medication and administering the medication to the child.

National Patient Safety Goals

National patient safety goals are created annually to encourage institutions, health-care teams, professionals, and individuals to focus on areas found to be most important for the health and safety of people of this nation. Although these goals do not specifically focus on the child, all of them can be applied to situations where a child requires health care, including home, hospital, and ambulatory care. The Joint Commission updates its National Patient Safety Goals annually and nurses should visit The Joint Commission Web site (www.jointcommission.org) for the current goals so that they provide the safest and most meticulous care possible. The National Patient Safety Goals for 2016 for hospital-based nursing include the following three examples:

- Improve the accuracy of patient identification:
  By using at least two ways to properly identify patients, such as the patient's name and date of birth, the pediatric nurse makes sure the correct child receives the correct care. Do this to make sure that each patient gets the medicines, treatments, and transfusion products meant only for them.
- Communicate results of blood tests and other diagnostic exams right away to the appropriate provider:
  This is especially true when the results are of a critical nature (ie, outside of normal ranges).
- Insure safe administration of medications:
  Ensure that all medications are labeled correctly. Even medications in syringes, cups, and basins must be labeled and kept in their original packaging with clear labels of the correct dosing instructions.

Preventing Medical and Medication Errors in Pediatrics

Children are especially vulnerable to medication errors because they are dependent upon the caregiver's accuracy.

Whereas adults may question a medication they have never seen before or taken for their particular condition, children are not at the developmental level to do this. Children also experience physiological aspects that contribute to the effect of medical errors. These include delayed medication clearing times, rapid absorption because of increased metabolic rates, easy transmission across the blood brain barrier, greater percentage of body water, diminished ability to absorb water-soluble drugs, and delayed excretion, all of which can put a child at greater risk for overdose, toxic reactions to the drug, and even the possibility of death.

Pediatric caregivers need to recognize that medications are administered to children based on their unique body differences. Consideration is given to a child's height, weight, body surface, age, and medical condition, and doses are calculated for each child and medication to ensure safety. To prevent medication errors in pediatric care environments, the nurse needs to accurately measure the child's height and weight before the two most common calculations are performed: milligrams of medication per kilogram weight of the child, or body surface area (BSA) measured in square meters (m^2). Astute assessment of a child after administering a medication is warranted because many drugs have not had the same pharmacological research performed on them with children as compared with adults. Frequent evaluation is important to quickly identify untoward reactions, allergic reactions, or dangerous side effects of medications delivered to children. See Appendix E for guidelines about safe medication calculation.

Medical Errors

Medical errors, which are types of errors considered broader than medication errors, encompass distinct groupings. The following represent groups of medical errors that can occur in pediatric care.

- Medication errors
- Wrong site surgeries
- Lack of follow-up to ensure medical treatments were successful
- Misread diagnostics or lost specimens
- Hospital-acquired conditions (HACs)
- Hospital-acquired infections (HAIs), such as nosocomial infections
- Multidrug-resistant organisms developed when hospitalized
  - These can include vancomycin-resistant *Enterococcus* (VRE) and methicillin-resistant *Staphylococcus aureus* (MRSA)
- Central line–associated blood stream infections (CLABSIs)
- Catheter-associated urinary tract infections (CAUTIs)
- Hospital-acquired pressure ulcer (HAPU)
- Observed over expected (OE) mortality where patients suffer conditions within a health-care institution above and beyond what is expected
- Falls with injury taking place within a health-care institution
- Slaying sepsis, a condition in which a patient dies of septic shock from a HAI such as MRSA

Medication Errors

There are four basic types of medication errors. Children are vulnerable to each of the following four types.

- **Acts of omission:** These occur when the nurse does not administer a medication when the medication is due. Acts of omission can be dangerous, such as when a child requires a medication to fight infection and the nurse omits administering the antibiotic as prescribed. Hanging a secondary piggyback line of a medication and failing to open the clamp for administration is a specific example of an act of omission.
- **Acts of commission:** These occur when a nurse administers a medication that breeches one of the "7 rights for safe medication administration": right patient, right drug, right dose, right route, right time, right family education, and right assessments before and after medication administration. Acts of commission in pediatrics can be dangerous and need to be prevented. Additional rights for safe medication administration include right assessment and evaluation, right documentation, and, for those of consenting age, the right to refuse.
- **Scheduling misconceptions:** These occur when a nurse or family member responsible for the child's medication misinterprets the prescribed medication and neglects to administer the drug as ordered. An example of this is when a nurse receives an order for a once a day medication and does not clarify if the first dose is to be administered the day it is ordered, and subsequently administers the first dose of the medication the next day. This type of error can be dangerous if the child's condition warrants the administration of the first dose right away.
- **Scheduling noncompliance:** This occurs when a family member receives a prescription for a medication and does not fill the prescription as needed, or when the caregiver does not adhere to the scheduled dosing requirement of the medication. An example of this is when a child does not receive a daily dose of an inhalant to prevent asthma symptoms.

TEAM WORKS

Interventions for Preventing Medication Errors

Because of the numerous potential or actual errors that can occur in the field of pediatric nursing care, interventions have been developed to reduce the possibility of errors. The following represent examples of interventions developed to reduce medication errors with children.

- Computerized order entry and computerized medication administration records for nurses
- Ward-based pharmacists who provide a double-check of the physician's order and administration processes
- Improving communication between physicians and nurses, and nurses with nurses, when medications are first ordered, doses are reduced or increased, administration schedules are changed, or medications are discontinued

- Two nurses double-checking all medications administered to infants under 12 months
- No interactions with nurses who are preparing medications in the medication room
- Use of colored vests or sashes worn by the nurse who is calculating, preparing, or administering medications to warn others that he or she is concentrating and should not be disturbed

 DRUG FACTS

Certain medications should always be double-checked by two nurses. Institutional policy and procedures will guide the pediatric health-care team in how to best administer medications safely to a child; some may require that an RN be present as part of the safety check. Always know your health-care institution's policies about double-checking medications. The following represents a partial list of high-alert medications that should have two nurses double-check for safety:

- All cardiac medications
- All blood products
- All insulin medications, including oral hypoglycemic
- Total parenteral nutrition and lipids
- All medications associated with cancer therapy
- All anticoagulants
- All narcotics
- All electrolytes

Medication Reconciliation

Medication reconciliation is a term used for the process of accurate history taking on a child's home medication regimen. When a child is admitted for a complication associated with a chronic condition, the admitting nurse carefully interviews the primary caregivers on the medications being administered at home, including the doses, schedules, and the indication for the medication according to the family. This process allows the health-care team to use caution when ordering new medications to prevent medication interactions, double dosing, or mismanagement. Accurate documentation of the child's home medications should be performed so that all team members, specialists, pharmacists, and interdepartmental personnel are aware.

Maintaining Safe Environments and Preventing Injuries

Hospitals are inherently unsafe places with a chaotic environment full of unsafe equipment, dangerous chemicals, and a multitude of personnel and visitors. Children are not accustomed to the new environment, and with any stressors, they can quickly become disoriented. Young children require assistance with their environment, including:

- Bed positioning should be set at the lowest setting at all times unless the nurse is performing an intervention. Proper body mechanics should be supported by raising the bed. Do not ever walk away from a bed in the high position. Leave the upper bed rails up.

- Crib rails must be left up at all times. Even when reaching for an item such as a diaper, do not leave a young child in a crib with the rails down for even a moment. They may reach for you and suffer a significant head injury after a fall.
- Do not leave supplies, toys, or any items in a crib (Fig. 20.7).
- Children should be taught how to call for a nurse using the call button. Maintain the call button next to the child at all times.
- Suction should be set up at the bedside for emergent use. The suction machine and collection container/tubing should be checked every shift for proper function in all settings.
- Oxygen should be secured and ready for use in an emergency.
- Electrical equipment should be out of reach of all children and approved covers should be used on all electrical outlets to prevent electrocution.
- Young children should be assessed frequently for possible strangulation. IV tubing can easily wrap around an active young child's neck.
- Young children should have an alarm device either on their wrist or ankle that will alert the health-care team if a child is abducted.
- Medications should never be left at the bedside.
- Arts and crafts items, such as glue or scissors, should not be left at the bedside.
- Know your institution's safety color codes for various emergency responses. These codes may change based on each institution's preference.

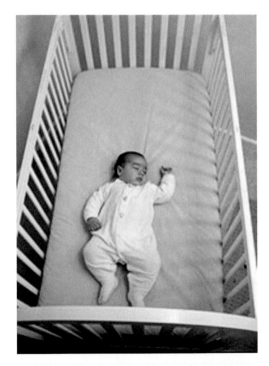

FIGURE 20.7 To provide safety, keep cribs empty of supplies, toys, and any items. (Photo courtesy the Safe to Sleep campaign, Eunice Kennedy Shriver National Institute of Child Health and Human Development, National Institutes of Health and Human Services [www.nichd.nih.gov/sids].)

Extra Safety Needs of the Preverbal Child

Keep an accurate name badge on a preverbal child at all times. If parents leave their young child for any period of time, the health-care team must have accurate patient identifiers on all children, especially preverbal children who cannot confirm their name, birthday, or any identifying information.

Walking on the Pediatric Unit Barefoot

All ambulatory children are required to wear slippers, shoes, or socks with a fall-prevention sole. Children cannot be allowed to walk the pediatric unit without the safety of some type of foot covering. Children being transported between units also require safe foot coverings to prevent injury. Children attending play sessions in the play room must wear appropriate safe clothes and shoes or socks. Slipping on newly cleaned floors, such as after cleaning up spills of juice or other liquids, can be very dangerous for an ill child. Children receiving narcotic pain control or other medications that alter perception or information processing should be reminded to wear shoes or slippers when they get up to use the bathroom. Supervision is required for young children or those susceptible for injury while ambulating.

Toddlers Allowed to Sleep in Adult-Size Hospital Bed

Health-care institutions may have a policy on whether or not they allow children younger than 3 years old to sleep in large adult-sized hospital beds. Precautions must be taken to prevent falls when young children sleep in adult-sized beds. When a parent leaves the room or even goes to the bathroom for just a few minutes, the young child must be kept safe while not supervised. Young children may try to get out of the bed to find their parent. Some hospitals require that all unsupervised children (even for just a minute) must be placed in a safe metal crib with the side rails up. Safety top cribs are used for children who are at the age of crawling up and over the crib side rails. Check institutional policies concerning young children (ie, infants or toddlers) being allowed to sleep in adult beds, and discourage adults from sleeping with their young child in a hospital bed.

Crib Safety

Cribs should not be used for storage of personal items or care items. Diapers, diaper wipes, thermometers, extra blankets, and toys should not be stored in a young child's crib. Young children have been known to stack items and climb on them to crawl over crib side rails. Make sure an appropriate bed is selected for a young child.

SAFETY STAT!

Children who are hospitalized and who can stand should be in what are called "high top" or "climber" cribs. These metal cribs have safety covers so a child cannot climb out and potentially suffer a serious head injury.

Medicine and Scissors Left at the Bedside

Under no circumstances should any metal objects, scissors, hemostats, hazardous medical equipment, or medications be left at the bedside. If a child does not take his/her medication immediately, the medication should be brought back to the medication room for proper and safe storage. Young children are at risk for finding medications and taking medications that are not prescribed for them.

Older Infants or Toddlers Left in a High Chair or Another Device

Infants and toddlers should never be left unsupervised in bouncy seats, high chairs, infant swings, toddler cars, wagons, or any such motility, play, or feeding device. Nurses who place children in these items need to ensure the child is under constant supervision. Children left alone in their rooms in one of these items may attempt to climb out and suffer an injury. Make sure parents are involved with the child's care and are providing supervision with the use of these items.

PEDIATRIC GROWTH AND DEVELOPMENT

The term *growth* is used to describe the physical changes that take place during childhood. The terms *growth* and *development* are often used together but they have very different meanings. While the term *growth* refers to an increase in the child's height and weight over time, it does not refer to the child's cognitive, emotional, and psychosocial *development*. Children typically grow in a predictable pattern and their development includes mastery of specific milestones; yet, families need to be taught that each child is unique and will grow and develop in their own unique pattern and way. Pediatric nurses teach families that the mastery of milestones is described in ranges so that parents are patient with each child's unique mastery plan. For instance, walking is described as a normal milestone that takes place between 10 and 16 months. When parents hear ranges, they tend to accept their child's unique pattern while still being aware of when to report deviations in expected patterned growth.

Anatomical and Physiological Differences Between Children and Adults

Children are not little adults and cannot be cared for as such. There are 13 important anatomical and physiological differences between children and adults that provide a framework for safety for pediatric health-care team members.
- Children's airways are anatomically small
- Young newborns are obligate nose breathers for first several weeks
- Children's heads are disproportionately large
- Infants have a large posterior head bone occiput, which makes airway occlusion more likely
- Children have poorly developed intercostal chest muscles; fatigue leads to respiratory failure
- Children have less tidal volume in their lungs
- Young children have a larger BSA, which results in a greater heat loss and greater insensible losses

- Infants and young children have less total circulating blood volume (ie, 80 to 90 mL/kg)
- Young children have high glucose needs and poor glycogen stores, which results in a higher metabolic rate
- Across childhood, kids have relatively healthy cardiovascular systems; primary hypertension and cardiovascular disease are rare
- Young children have immature temperature regulation; young infants can rapidly experience hypothermia if not dressed and wrapped appropriately
- Young children have immature immune systems and less overall organ maturation (especially kidney function and the concentration of urine)
- Young children pose challenges in assessment and treatment of the six human symptoms (ie, pain/discomfort, dyspnea, fatigue, sleep disturbances, nausea, and emotional distress); use vital signs and developmentally appropriate pediatric tools to measure symptoms such as pain

All of these anatomical and physiological differences affect the following aspects of the child's status, but by adolescence, differences lessen compared with adults:

- How the child, overall, is affected by trauma and/or injuries
- The presentation of the child's physical illnesses in relation to severity
- A child's rapid rate of decompensation under stress, injury, or trauma
- Blood pressure changes that demonstrate a late sign of shock
- Slower rate of metabolism of medications

Children's patterns of growth and development are of importance to the pediatric nurse in teaching families what to expect at the various developmental levels. Although children grow uniquely and at their own pace, there are consistent patterns that are demonstrated at each stage. Table 20.1 provides information about the growth, development, and perceptions experienced among the various pediatric populations.

Children's patterns of development follow three progressions:

- **Cephalocaudal:** Development is from head to toe. For example, infants have head control before they are able to crawl, stand, or walk (Fig. 20.8A).
- **Proximal-distal:** Development is from the trunk to the distal extremities. For example, the young infant can move his/her legs and arms but cannot pick up objects with a finger grasp (Fig. 20.8B).
- **General to specific:** Development is from mastering simple tasks to the advancement of more complex tasks. For example, the young child will typically master slow crawling behaviors and then fast crawling behaviors, and then, progressively, standing, running, and skipping.

Parents need to be reassured that many factors influence the rate and pattern of their child's growth. Factors that influence childhood growth and development include the following:

- Health status
- Family function
- Socioeconomic status
- Basic human needs
- Cultural influences and values
- Genetics and heredity
- Personality and temperament

Theoretical Frameworks in Childhood Development

Pediatric nurses rely on their knowledge of developmental theory to guide their interactions, expectations, and teaching. Theory provides a framework to make sense of childhood behaviors. Four significant theorists have provided frameworks to understand childhood behaviors and cognitive development. The concepts should be applied to all children regardless of age or care setting. These theoretical frameworks are:

1. **Erik Erikson, psychosocial development:** Erik Erikson's theory of psychosocial development is widely accepted as a universal means to understand the dichotomy of met and unmet tasks within each of the developmental stages.
2. **Jean Piaget, cognitive development:** Jean Piaget's theoretical framework is widely accepted as a means to understand and predict children's cognitive development.
3. **Sigmund Freud, psychosexual development:** Sigmund Freud proposed a theoretical framework about how children develop in the psychosexual realm.
4. **Lawrence Kohlberg, moral development:** Lawrence Kohlberg developed the theory of moral development in children.

Temperament

Temperament is defined as the combination of intellectual, emotional, ethical, and physical characteristics of a specific individual (Venes, 2005). Parents and care providers require an understanding of a child's unique and natural style of reacting to and interacting with others to craft a positive approach to each child (Oliver, 2002). There are many temperament traits, including activity level, the ability of the child to either approach or withdraw from a situation, mood, adaptability, intensity, distractibility, and the child's threshold of sensory stimulation (Oliver, 2002).

Temperament is displayed in various ways. Although children are unique, there are types of temperaments that can be identified and therefore prepared for. If a pediatric nurse knows a child fits into a type of temperament, then planning can be done for simple tasks such as bathing, medication administration, or undergoing a procedure or assessment (Oliver, 2002).

- **Easy children who demonstrate flexibility:** Tend to demonstrate behaviors that are predictable or regular; will generally approach new situations, people, and circumstances with a positive attitude. Easy children tend to be more flexible in new situations. They come across as calm and not easy to upset (Fig. 20.9).

(Text continued on page 300)

TABLE 20.1 GROWTH, DEVELOPMENT, AND PERCEPTIONS ACROSS CHILDHOOD

Age Group	Anatomical and Physiological Growth	Fine and Gross Motor Skills	Cognitive, Emotional, and Social Development	Spiritual Development	Perceptions of Family	Perceptions of Safety
Younger Infant (1 month up to 6 months)	Anatomical and physiological growth in infants is the most rapid compared to the other developmental stages: • Height increases 1 in. per month • Weight doubles at 5–6 months • Weight increases by 1.5 pounds per month • Teeth emerge: 6–8 in first year expected • Head circumference (HC) increases by 0.5 in./month • Young infants have variable sleeping habits but need 12–14 hours of sleep plus 2–3 naps	• Gross movement slowly replaced by fine movements • Holds chin up at 1 month and chest up at 2 months • Rolls back to side by 3 months • Holds head erect at 4 months • Sits supported at 4 months • Has voluntary grasp at 5 months • Rolls from front to back at 5–6 months	• Language consists of cooing; slowly develops mimicking sounds • Laughs at 2–4 months • Makes consonant sounds at 3–4 months • Regards a person's face at 1 month • Displays social smile and follows object 180 degrees at 2 months • Recognizes familiar faces at 3 months • Experiences stranger anxiety beginning at 6 months	• The young infant is too young to comprehend or demonstrate spiritual development	Perceptions of family begin to occur during the first year of life: • The young infant recognizes familiar caregivers by sensory interpretation of voice and smell.	Perceptions of safety are very limited in the infant: • No perceptions of safety exist. Young infant responds to statement of "no" by reflex withdrawal, whereas older infants may stop what they are doing momentarily when they hear "no" but may not connect their action with this.
Older Infant (6th month up to 12 months)	Anatomical and physiological changes continue at a rapid pace during the second half of infancy,	• Gross motor movements are replaced with finer motor movements	Cognitive/ emotional/social development is demonstrated as early language development	• The young infant is too young to comprehend or demonstrate spiritual development	Perceptions of family begin to occur during the first year of life: • By 8 months of age separation	Perceptions of safety during the second half of infancy become important as the infant learns to

Continued

TABLE 20.1 GROWTH, DEVELOPMENT, AND PERCEPTIONS ACROSS CHILDHOOD—cont'd

Age Group	Anatomical and Physiological Growth	Fine and Gross Motor Skills	Cognitive, Emotional, and Social Development	Spiritual Development	Perceptions of Family	Perceptions of Safety
	although they decrease in pace toward the end of the first year: • Height increases by 50% of birth height by 1 year • Weight increases 1 pound per month • Weight triples by 1 year of age • HC increases by 33% • Posterior fontanel closes by 2–3 months • Anterior fontanel closes by 12–18 months of age • Central incisors erupt at 5–7 months • Older infants need 9–11 hours of sleep plus two naps	• Sits unsupported (alone) at 8 months • Pulls up to a stand at 9 months • Crawls at 10 months • Drinks from a closed ("tippy") cup at 9 months • Feeds self at 9 months • Builds two-block tower at 12 months • Pincer grasp mastered by 12 months • Stands alone at 12 months, walks holding onto one hand at 11 months, walks alone at approximately 12 months	and meaning of emotions: • Pronounces syllables (eg, dada, mama) at 8 months • Says 2–10 words at 12 months • Experiences marked stranger anxiety at 8 months • Emotions are experienced, such as jealousy, at 12 months • Plays patty-cake and waves good-bye by 12 months		anxiety starts and the child demonstrates a strong preference for their parents • Family is seen as familiar and comforting to the infant • Stranger anxiety begins in later infancy at approximately 8–10 months of age • The older infant experiences a deep attachment to their caregivers and separation anxiety begins in this second half of infancy (8–10 months) and peaks at 16–30 months	roll, crawl, and walk: • Because older infants are becoming locomotive, they require vigilant supervision to prevent injuries, accidents, toxic exposures, and toxic ingestions; older infants move from rolling to crawling to walking very quickly and are then at risk for falls, injuries, ingestions, and accidents
Toddler (1–3 years)	Anatomical and physiological development in the toddler slow down compared with the fast growth during	Development of fine and gross motor skills of toddlers becomes more tuned as they explore their	Cognitive/ emotional/social development during the toddler stage changes as they become more	Toddlers are too young to develop a sense of spirituality but may explore preliminary ideas through choices of story-telling and	• Family is important to toddlers even if they express negativism and challenging behaviors • Toddlers enjoy family time and	Perceptions of safety continue to be a concern as toddlers will test their environments and parental limits; these aspects of

	the first year of life: • Cephalocaudal and proximal-distal growth begins to slow down • Child gains 3–5 pounds a year • Birth weight is quadrupled by 2 years • Abdomen protrudes, child may be slightly bowlegged • Walks with confidence and balance • Child is approximately 50% of adult height by 2 years • Major task is beginning to toilet train • Toddlers need 12 hours of sleep a night plus one nap	environment and continue to master locomotion: • Pulls to a stand and then stands alone • Stoops and recovers from the motion • Walks backward and runs by 18 months • Walks up steps by 2 years • Throws ball overhand and jumps up for ball by 3 years	aware and secure in their environments: • Child begins to tolerate some separation from parent • Child engages in parallel play, acknowledging other children but not playing with them • Child develops strong need for rituals • Toddlers use negativism in their quest for individualism • Toddlers are very egocentric • Temper tantrums are common as a method of expressing frustrations • Masturbation at this time is considered normal	readings offered by the parent	will engage in playful activities	development inherently lend themselves to an unsafe stage and toddlers need constant supervision: • Toddlers are very busy, fast, and prone to accidents and falls • Toddlers do not have a sense of safety and require constant supervision • Toddlers fall a great deal and have many expected bruises on forehead and shins • Toddlers with unusual bruises, such as linear bruising or bruising on the back or abdomen, should be investigated for abuse
Preschooler (3rd birthday through the 5th year)	Anatomical and physiological development in the preschool period focus on	Development of fine and gross motor skills during the preschool period	Cognitive/emotional/social development of the preschooler moves	Spiritual development in the preschool period can be demonstrated in responses to	Perceptions of family during the preschool period become very important to the	Perceptions of safety of the preschooler remain paramount; preschoolers enjoy testing limits and

Continued

TABLE 20.1 GROWTH, DEVELOPMENT, AND PERCEPTIONS ACROSS CHILDHOOD—cont'd

Age Group	Anatomical and Physiological Growth	Fine and Gross Motor Skills	Cognitive, Emotional, and Social Development	Spiritual Development	Perceptions of Family	Perceptions of Safety
	slower overall growth but changes in teeth eruption and toileting: • Average growth is 2.5–3 in. per year • Average weight gain is 5 pounds per year • All 20 deciduous teeth should be in by 3 years; tooth brushing should be well established • Most children are toilet trained by the end of the preschool period (with potential accidents) • Preschoolers will have more stable blood glucose levels but should be provided snacks throughout the day for energy • Preschoolers need 11–13 hours of sleep	demonstrates increased mobility and grace: • Preschoolers enjoy drawing and can draw circles and crosses by 3 years • Most can build a 9–10 block tower by 3 years • Most children can lace shoes by 4 years • Preschoolers can use safety scissors, copy triangles, draw a few letters and numbers, and print their name by 5 years • Preschoolers become more graceful in their motor abilities and enjoy mastering balance, skipping, hopping, and tricycle riding	to becoming more and more social; peer interactions increase and are governed by learning manners, patience, and early cooperation: • Preschoolers experience many fears during this period, more than any other • Fears include the dark, monsters, dogs, separation from family, being left alone, bedtime • Magical thinking is used to make sense of a complex world • Preschoolers need regular social experiences with peers to learn acceptable behaviors such as sharing and the beginnings of manners • Preschool programs are	emotions and early spiritual explorations: • Preschoolers learn and experience the sense, feeling, and meaning of love • Preschoolers enjoy participating in religious and cultural practices (i.e., Sunday school activities and learning)	child. The desire to be accepted and part of a family unit become important: • The preschooler's significant "other" is the child's family unit • The child understands he or she is separate from the parent (ie, autonomy) • The family's acceptance is important and clashes in expectations cause anxiety and fears	remain at risk for injuries: • Preschoolers are less accident prone than toddlers but they are still at risk for burns, falls, and aspirations • Preschoolers need to learn safety rules; parents should consistently reinforce and explain safety rules in simple terms (eg, cars, roads, tricycle use, kitchen hazards)

Continued

School-Aged Child (6–12 years)	Anatomical and physiological changes occur more slowly during this longest period of development; the school-age period spans just under 7 years from the child's 6th birthday until just before the child's 13th birthday: • Girls typically grow faster than boys during this time period • The average school-aged child grows 2 in. per year • Average weight gain is 4.5–6.5 pounds per year • The school-aged child's immune system grows stronger with greater immunity developing with exposures to common childhood infections and illnesses	available to foster socialization, creativity, and safety rules Development of fine and gross motor skills for school-aged children focuses on mastery of socially expected skills: • School-aged children master bicycling, rollerblading, skateboarding, and swimming • School-aged children demonstrate rapidly increasing balance and motor skills	Cognitive/emotional/social development of the school-aged child focuses on peer interactions and family dynamics: • School-aged children need social peer networks; best friends become paramount • Achievement is important and children need to be offered chances for industry, homework, chores, and activities they can complete and feel good about; praise for work is important • Preschool fears are replaced with fear of namecalling or social embarrassment and teasing • Team sports become important; group activities should be stressed and rules followed	Spiritual development emerges as important to many school-aged children: • School-aged children begin to ask questions about the meaning of life, presence of "God," and question aspects of thoughts and meanings that cannot be seen • School-aged children ask parents and adults about their beliefs and question the roots of their beliefs	Perceptions of family for the school-aged child begin to change in the later stage as the child becomes more involved with social interactions with peers: • Family function remains important but peer relationship importance grows • School-aged children need a parent or family member they can trust to be listened to and heard, and have questions answered honestly • Family time and meal time should be important; limit TV watching and encourage family interaction and caring behaviors	Perceptions of safety may become an issue for school-aged children as they continue to test their limits and desire autonomy. Parents and figures of authority must continue to insist on the use of safety gear and devices: • Helmet use and safety pads for skating must be communicated • Safety guidelines around biking/swimming are important • Reinforcement around talking with strangers must continue • Importance of seat belts must be communicated consistently

TABLE 20.1 GROWTH, DEVELOPMENT, AND PERCEPTIONS ACROSS CHILDHOOD—cont'd

Age Group	Anatomical and Physiological Growth	Fine and Gross Motor Skills	Cognitive, Emotional, and Social Development	Spiritual Development	Perceptions of Family	Perceptions of Safety
	• School-aged children need 9–10 hours of sleep per night; bedtimes should be firmly established • Child may experience enuresis (15% of 6 year olds) • During the period of preadolescence (ie, older school-aged), there is a rapid growth experience • Diet and nutrition is important during the period of rapid growth in later school-aged children; the food pyramid should be learned and applied; less picky eating occurs		• Play becomes more rough, competitive, and complex, requiring greater fine motor skills and growth of motor movements • Secret clubs, scouts, collections, and reading all acquire importance • Need for conformity exists and they enjoy pleasing adults around them, such as teachers			
Adolescent (13–18 years)	• Puberty begins for girls between ages 8 and 14; boys between 9 and 16 • Menses begin approximately 2.5 years after the onset of puberty	Development of fine and gross motor skills during adolescence reaches that of an adult: • Overall gross motor development reaches	Cognitive/emotional/social development continues as they move closer to independence and young adulthood: • The significant social structure	Spiritual development takes a different turn as the adolescent develops cognitively; they begin to question and test spiritual concepts and ideas: • Teens question their spirituality and are	Perceptions of family continue to remain important to the teen and they continue to be influenced by the structure, function, and	Perceptions of safety become of upmost importance during the adolescent stage when feelings of invincibility are present and

- Boys' voices deepen, nocturnal emissions occur
- Girls can grow between 2 and 9 in.; boys between 4 and 12 in.
- Girls gain between 15 and 55 pounds; boys between 15 and 65 pounds
- Good nutrition and regular meals are of paramount importance; missed meals because of activities and sports must be discouraged
- Acne begins as sebaceous glands become activated
- Overall body size and mass increase to adult size; hair growth patterns resemble adult patterns by the end of adolescence
- Tanner's stages of sexual development occur with breast enlargement and genitalia development (see Chapter 25 about adolescents for a full description)

that of full adulthood
- Fine motor development can continue to develop if the adolescent challenges themselves with mastery of such activities as musical ability

of the adolescent is the child's peer group
- They continue to refine who they are, where they are going, and life goals
- Group socialization and parties are important
- Teens continue to need firm limit setting and rules of behavior
- Teens need choices and a sense of control, offer this when appropriate (i.e., let them decide medication administration times, respiratory therapy schedules, and meal times)

influenced by family practices and spiritual values

dynamics of the family unit:
- Teens need a safe adult they can go to for questions and active listening, feelings of safety around their emotions, and support
- Teens look at family values as they make life decisions and seek emancipation from parents
- Families should be supportive, encouraging, but noninterfering, offering assistance with problem solving in peer group/dating and other relationships

boundaries are stretched:
- Adolescents may feel invincible and not prone to accidents and injuries
- Avoiding sports injuries becomes essential and competition increases
- Driving safety and rules must be established and held consistent
- Teens may demonstrate recklessness, drug, tobacco and alcohol experimentation, and engagement/experimentation in sexual activity

Sources: Muscari, 2005; Selekman and Jakubik, 2007.

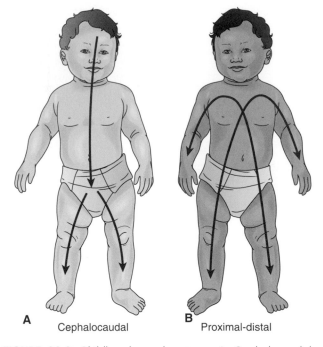

A Cephalocaudal **B** Proximal-distal

FIGURE 20.8 Childhood growth patterns. A, Cephalocaudal. B, Proximal-distal.

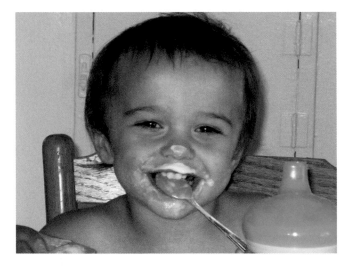

FIGURE 20.9 Temperaments differ in children and range from difficult and feisty to easy.

- **Active, feisty, or difficult children:** Tend to demonstrate more intense reactions to new situations and may fight against change or react with a sense of negative withdrawal. These children may be easily upset by commotion and demonstrate difficult feeding, sleeping, and social behaviors.
- **Slow-to-warm-up or cautious children:** Tend to demonstrate the need for more time to accept new situations, activities, and social interactions. They may display a moodier temperament with inactivity before acceptance. These children may appear to withdraw or have trouble with new people and situations.

No matter what the child's temperament is, during the implementation of pediatric nursing care, all children should be treated with the same level of respect, taking into account their developmental level and social needs. Children's adaptability, intensity of reaction, attention span, and approach may be quite unique for each child; it is the pediatric nurse's joy and challenge to provide each child's care according to the influence of his or her attitude and temperament.

PLAY ACROSS CHILDHOOD

The work of a child is play…

The universal language of children is play. Play is an essential component of the joy of childhood and presents opportunities for valuable lessons. Children learn to share, interact cooperatively, and socialize with peers. Play provides opportunities to test one's skills, knowledge, and abilities. Pediatric nurses are responsible for providing play situations to promote development, socialization, and stimulation, especially when a child is ill. See Table 20.2 for ideas of play for each developmental stage of childhood.

Play promotes a variety of cognitive and physical development, regardless of the child's age. Positive outcomes to play include:

- Physical-motor development and ability
- Intellectual learning
- Cognitive processes
- Social skills
- Lessening of symptoms
- Moral development
- Reduces anxiety
- Learning about procedures (medical)

PROFESSIONAL PEDIATRIC ORGANIZATIONS

Nurses working in the field of children's health care benefit from the opportunities of networking, education, professional development, and research dissemination. The Society of Pediatric Nurses (SPN), existing since 1990, gives a platform for support and development. State and regional meetings allow for geographical networking on issues shared between all subspecialties of the field. This society's Web site is a strong resource for conferences, regional meetings, policy updates, clinical information and guidelines, professional support, and other numerous Web links. A discussion board allows for communication between its members. The mission statement of the SPN is:

> *The mission of the Society of Pediatric Nurses is to promote excellence in nursing care of children and families through support of its members via clinical practice, education, research and advocacy. (Society of Pediatric Nurses, www.pednurses.org)*

There are many other pediatric-based national organizations with regional or local chapters that can provide support and information. See the list of online resources provided at the Davis*Plus* website.

TABLE 20.2   IDEAS FOR PLAY ACROSS CHILDHOOD

Age Group	Play Characteristics and Ideas
Newborn (birth to 30 days)	• Low stimulation; en face pleasurable interactions with caregivers; promote attachment • Allow uninterrupted sleep • Give soft touch with warm palms • Soothing soft music • If the newborn is premature and demonstrating signs of stress (eg, decreased oxygen saturation, increased heart rate, and increased respiratory rate), give rest periods
Younger Infant (1–6 months)	• Participates in solitary play • Black and white mobiles, music boxes, crib boxes, rattles, safe mouthing toys (eg, oral teething rings), mirrors, contrasting colors such as black and white
Older Infant (6–12 months)	• Participates in solitary play • Encourage activities that promote development of the crude pincer grasp at 8–10 months • Challenge older infant to pick up items • Give child items to bang together: pots and pans, plastic containers with lids • Hide and seek to encourage development of object permanence • Nesting cubes, stacking challenges (just 2–3 at a time)
Toddler (1–3 years)	• Participates in parallel play (next to but not with other toddlers or children) • Dress-up games • Practicing putting clothes on and off; buttons and zippers and Velcro fasteners • Toy phones, picture books, pail and shovel, safe water play (supervised at all times), stacking cubes
Preschooler (3–5 years)	• Participates in associative play; play with loose rules • Play kitchens, tool chests, medical and nursing kits, and work surfaces • Tricycles, wagons, trucks, cars • Large-piece puzzles • Arts and crafts with drawing, gluing, and creating
Young School-Aged Child (6–10 years)	• Participates in structured and cooperative play with other children of the same gender • Best friend activities • Collections • Books, games, puzzles
Older School-Aged Child (10–12 years)	• Participates in structured and cooperative, competitive games, with same gender • Team play, making up new games with distinct rules • Secret clubs • Board games, computer technology and games
Adolescent (13–18 years)	• Participates in social activities • Activities that represent adult behavior: studying the drivers' training books • Access to peers via computer social technology, phones, letter writing • Scrap books, journal writing • Challenging arts and crafts such as jewelry making • Social clubs, dances, movies

Key Points

- Nurses caring for children of any age require a unique set of knowledge, skills, and behaviors. Pediatric nursing is considered a specialty practice requiring a body of knowledge acquired through study and experience.
- Pediatric nursing involves caring for children between birth and 18 years of age, as well as their families.
- The care of a pediatric patient may take place in a well-child setting, an acute care or critical care setting, a school setting, or a hospice, and therefore should focus on the goal of the child's health-care experience.
- Contemporary issues facing children and their families in the 21st century include social issues, and morbidity and mortality outcomes.
- National pediatric health goals have been identified by professional and government organizations and include topics such as preventing infections, preventing errors, and promoting safety.
- Applying the principles of family-centered care to families receiving care in a hospital or home setting is essential. Two foundational principles are empowering and enabling.

- There are distinct anatomical, physiological, social, and emotional differences between adults and children that emphasize the critical components pertinent to the safe emergent care of children across health-care settings.
- Nurses must understand foundational growth and development phases within the eight stages of childhood, including newborn, young infant, older infant, toddler, preschooler, early school-aged child, later school-aged child, and adolescent. Each phase is unique and provides challenges, obstacles, and rewards.
- Play is very important across childhood. Nurses should work directly with members of the Child Life team to select play for specified situations such as promoting development, procedural distraction, and complimentary therapy for symptom control.
- Providing safety in all aspects of care is an important role for the pediatric nurse. Safety includes the prevention of medication errors including acts of omission, acts of commission, scheduling misconceptions, and issues with scheduling noncompliance.

REVIEW QUESTIONS

1. While talking with a group of young mothers at a support group, one mother tells the group that she is tired of always changing her 18-month-old's diapers and wants to start toilet training right away. The nurse would be correct in telling the group that:
   1. "Her readiness is dependent on the age of toilet training of the child's siblings."
   2. "You should discuss your child's readiness with your pediatrician."
   3. "If this is the most convenient time to being toilet training, you and your husband should begin."
   4. "When your child indicates readiness through her behaviors, then it is time to begin."

2. While teaching young parents about the importance of vaccines for their infant, the nurse explains that vaccines reduce childhood morbidity. The term *morbidity* is defined by the nurse as:
   1. The incidence of infectious diseases in the nation.
   2. The top three causes of death in each childhood level.
   3. The prevalence of an illness, disease, or infection within a population.
   4. The number of children with a particular infectious disease within a given institution.

3. While educating a family with a toddler, the nurse tells the parents, who are expressing concerns, that masturbation is:
   1. Abnormal for this age
   2. Normal for this age
   3. Harmful for the child's growth and development and considered promiscuous
   4. To be encouraged as a form of self-expression

4. While giving well-child teaching for a young father about his infant daughter, the nurse explains to the father that most infants can sit up unsupported by which age?
   1. 4 months
   2. 7 months
   3. 8 months
   4. 12 months

5. What findings on a 2-year-old child would be most indicative that the child has experienced physical abuse?
   1. A scalding burn on his anterior trunk with an irregular shape
   2. Bilateral shin bruises in various stages of healing
   3. A black eye where bruising extends from the outer eye to just under the eye
   4. Bruises on the back or abdomen

6. A mother informs the nurse that her 2-year-old daughter does not want to engage in play activities with her peers. The nurse explains that it is normal for the child to participate in which form of play:
   1. Cooperative
   2. Associative
   3. Parallel
   4. Solitary

7. The predominant challenge in providing pain management for hospitalized children is:
   1. Obtaining a physician's order for narcotics
   2. Administering opioids to young children orally
   3. Assessing children accurately in their pain level
   4. Educating family members concerning their children's pain experience

8. Children who display "slow-to-warm-up" temperament types will typically be okay with new situations and new activities—they just have difficulty warming up to new people.
   1. True
   2. False

9. Jean Piaget's theoretical framework is widely accepted as a means to understand and predict children's cognitive development.
   1. True
   2. False

10. A nurse should understand that no matter what a child's particular temperament is, all children should be treated with the same level of respect. When caring for children, nurses should take into account which the following? *(select all that apply)*
    1. The child's developmental level
    2. The child's social needs
    3. The child's adaptability
    4. The child's intensity of reaction to situations
    5. The child's attention span

CRITICAL THINKING QUESTIONS

1. Describe resources available to patients and their families in your clinical setting that promote normal growth and development, provide play opportunities, and foster sibling interaction with a hospitalized child.

2. List resources in your community that assist families with children who have identified special needs. How do families locate and tap into these resources? How are referrals made? Search local organizations that focus on the care of children with special needs. What services do they offer families?

For additional resources and information, visit **www.DavisPlus.com.** Post-Conference Questions and Activities, Answers, and References can be found on Davis*Plus*.

DavisPlus

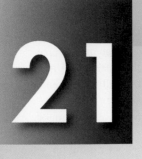

21

Health Promotion of the Infant: Birth to One Year

KEY TERMS

anthropometric measurements
chromosomes
congenital
failure to thrive (FTT)
genetics
hereditary
immunizations
myelination
separation anxiety
thermoregulation

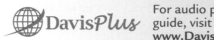 For audio pronunciation guide, visit www.DavisPlus.com

CHAPTER CONCEPTS

Bowel Elimination
Cognition
Comfort
Family
Development
Mobility
Nutrition
Promoting Health

LEARNING OUTCOMES

1. Define the key terms in this chapter.
2. Describe the unique needs of the newborn and infant as compared to older children in relation to safety, bonding, communication, and development.
3. Describe the differences between infants and older children and adults in relation to body systems, anatomy, and physiology.
4. Describe the patterns of rapid growth and development of the newborn, young infant, and older infant.
5. Compare the nutritional needs and eating patterns of the infant, including accurate kilocalorie and fluid maintenance calculations.
6. Discuss the elimination patterns of the newborn, young infant, and older infant.
7. Describe the need infants have for stimulation, play, and sleep to promote normal growth and development.
8. Differentiate the various schedules, infectious diseases, and care required for infants undergoing immunizations.
9. Differentiate various nutritional disorders that can be found during infancy, including organic and nonorganic FTT.
10. Describe respiratory distress in the infant, including assessment and interventions.
11. Describe the phenomenon of sudden infant death syndrome (SIDS) and the needs of the family immediately after the infant's death through the period of grief and loss.
12. Discuss the interventions that can assist a caregiver who is caring for an infant experiencing colic.
13. Describe key assessments and interventions for an infant demonstrating dehydration.
14. Understand the importance of discussing safety issues for infants with parents, including maintaining a clear airway and preventing severe injuries such as shaken baby syndrome.

REAL-WORLD CASE STUDY

Danielle

■ Danielle is a 9-month-old, first-born daughter whose mother had a healthy pregnancy; Danielle is now considered a well infant, experiencing expected growth and development. On a national growth chart, Danielle is at the 50th percentile for both height and weight. She is rolling over, crawling slowly, trying to pull herself up in a standing position, smiling a lot, and babbling frequently. Danielle's only medical concern is that her parents to do not "believe" in immunizations and although she has attended all of her well-child checkups to date, her parents have not agreed to any of the childhood immunizations that should have been administered thus far. Her parents say they are concerned with the side effects of childhood vaccines and plan on keeping her exempt from immunizing when she starts school. Danielle and her family live in a county where pertussis has been considered an epidemic, and the annual influenza has been commonly found across the lifespan. Danielle's parents are planning on raising her as a vegan; she is currently breastfed 4 times a day, and has had organic rice cereal, vegetables, fruits, and tofu introduced successfully to her diet.

1. How does a nurse interpret an infant whose anthropometric measurements are plotted in the 50th percentile?
2. How is pertussis contracted during infancy?

CONCEPTUAL CORNERSTONE

Family-Centered Care

Families with newborns and infants need support, education, and anticipatory guidance. The concept of family-centered care provides a foundation in which to interact with and support new families. Family-centered care encourages collaboration, engagement, and respect, and promotes the concept of enabling parents to care for their child through demonstration and education, especially if the child has special needs or a chronic illness. Infants are born very dependent, yet rapidly progress and change over the 12 months of this first developmental stage. Family-centered care provides a foundation for interacting with new families with young infants to reduce anxiety, promote safety, and provide guidance about what to expect of their infant.

The period of infancy is a remarkable experience for the child and those involved with his or her care. Infants are born very dependent and undergo a rapid and progressive change toward gaining independence over the 12 months of their first developmental stage. Infants not only grow exceptionally fast, but they achieve a large number of milestones all within the first year of life, including holding up the head, rolling over, crawling, standing, and beginning to walk.

Milestones are defined as general patterns of growth and development achievements during the stages experienced by the infant. Infants grow with an expected series of orderly steps, but the growth of an infant is not in a steady pace. Each infant grows and develops in his or her own timeline and within his or her own unique growth pattern. No two infants develop in exactly the same way. Each infant also has his or her own unique temperament and personality. Parents need to understand that each infant is unique; therefore nurses teach parents about ranges in the expected development of their infant. For instance, a pediatric nurse would explain to new parents that the expected timeframe for walking is 10 to 16 months, emphasizing that expectations for each child during the infancy period will be unique, and they should not try to compare each child's unique development.

One of the most important topics to cover with parents of an infant is the importance of keeping well-child checkups (Fig. 21.1). A healthy infant needs to have a series of **immunizations;** measurements, including head circumference (HC) checks, weight checks, and length checks; and developmental milestone checks, assessing for dysfunctions or delays in the infant's development. The earlier problems in growth and development are identified, the earlier referrals can be made for interventions to assist the child. Nurses must encourage parents to maintain all records of infant well-child checkups so that important information is available as needed.

With the rapid development during infancy comes many concerns about safety. Pediatric nurses must teach families about these concerns to prevent injuries. Anticipatory guidance, or education focusing on what to expect and planning a safe and healthy environment before an incident or injury happens, is paramount.

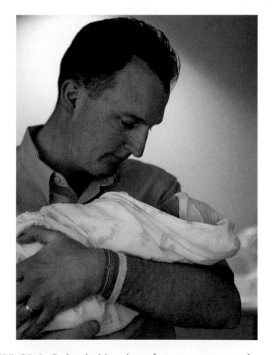

FIGURE 21.1 Father holding his infant in a moment of joy.

GROWTH AND DEVELOPMENT OF THE INFANT

Infancy begins with the newborn period. The newborn period spans the first month, or first 30 days, from birth. Following the newborn period, infancy is categorized as *early infancy,* which is the first 6 months, and *older infancy,* which is the second 6 months. After infancy, the child moves to the toddler period. See Box 21.1 for a description of all of the developmental stages.

Heredity and Genetic Influences

Genetics is the study of how our genes, chromosomes, and genotypes, or sequencing and combinations of genes, are expressed and responsible for health or disorders. During the early infancy period, the newborn is assessed for genetic abnormalities. Although rare, it is important that any genetic abnormality is identified early so appropriate medical care can be implemented. Each human cell contains 46 **chromosomes** in each nucleus, or 23 pairs. Each chromosome then contains thousands and thousands of genes. Genes are those elements that are responsible for **hereditary** characteristics (ie, the transmission of genetic characteristics from the parent to the offspring). Genes may or may not be expressed or passed on to the next generation. Mendel's law states that each parent contributes one gene for each hereditary property, one gene being dominant and the other being recessive. Dominant genes will determine the infant's characteristics, such as hair color, skin color, eye color, and height. In a dominant health disorder in an infant, only one defective gene, or a set of genes, is passed by one parent to the child. In recessive health disorders, both of the infant's parents must pass the defective gene to the infant. Some inherited, or genetic, disorders, known as ***congenital,*** are present at birth, and other genetic disorders will not manifest or become apparent until later in childhood or adulthood.

"Carriers" are children or adults who carry the defective gene but usually do not experience the symptoms of the disease or disorder. A carrier would have one defective gene and one healthy gene.

Box 21.1 The Nine Stages of Childhood

1. **Premature infants:** Born before 36 weeks' gestation
2. **Newborn infants:** Birth to 28 to 30 days
3. **Early infancy:** 1 to 6 months
4. **Older infancy:** 6 months to 1 year
5. **Toddler:** 1 to 3 years
6. **Preschooler:** 3 to 5 years
7. **Early school-aged:** 6 to 10 years
8. **Late school-aged:** 11 to 13 years
9. **Adolescent:** 13 to 18 years

In autosomal diseases and disorders, the autosomal chromosomes represent the first 22 pairs. In a dominant disorder, only one defective gene or set of genes is passed on to the child by one parent. A heterozygous carrier is one in whom there are two different alleles (ie, pairs) for the same trait (Dd). Parents need to understand that when one parent is a heterozygous carrier, there is a 25% chance of having a child with a disease or disorder, a 50% chance of having a child who is a carrier of the genetic trait, and a 25% chance of having a child who does not have the genetic disease or disorder. Examples of autosomal dominant disorders include osteogenesis imperfecta, night blindness, and neurofibromatosis.

In recessive autosomal diseases and disorders, both parents must pass the defective gene or set of genes to their child. Examples of an autosomal recessive disease are sickle cell anemia, phenylketonuria (PKU), and albinism. Genetic counseling is offered to parents who are known to carry a defective gene, or who have previously given birth to a child with a genetic disorder.

Some genetically linked disorders found in infants are genetic sex-linked. Sex-linked disorders are carried on the X chromosome and are passed only by women to their children. Examples of sex-linked disorders include hemophilia, glucose-6-phosphate dehydrogenase (G6PD), and color blindness.

A genetically related syndrome is a group of recognizable characteristics appearing together to present a clinical picture. Trisomy 21, also known as *Down's syndrome,* involves a genetic disorder in which three chromosomes can be found on the 21st pair. This means there is an extra chromosome, resulting in a total of 47. Infants with trisomy 21 genetic disorder present with distinct features. These features include a small head; a flat and broad nose; a small oral cavity, which leads to the appearance of a large and protruding tongue; short stature; hypotonia; and bilateral low-set ears. Many children with trisomy 21 are found to have mild to moderate cognitive delay, formally known as *mental retardation.*

The Newborn Period: Physical Growth and Development

The newborn period is birth to 30 days. During this period, the physiology of the newborn is different than any other developmental stage. The newborn has unique physical characteristics that are used to guide nurses in safe care. Newborns are susceptible to a variety of injuries and health problems, including hypoglycemia and hypothermia. The newborn period has the highest mortality rate (ie, death rate) than any other time period during childhood. Assessing the newborn requires knowledge in each of the body systems because the newborn has unique needs for the first hours, days, and weeks of life. A review of each body system aids the nurse in identifying areas of concern for the vulnerable newborn infant.

Transition to Extrauterine Life

Transition to extrauterine life refers to the first 24 hours of life. The newborn leaves the stable, warm, and nourishing environment of the womb and enters life. The newborn faces profound physiological changes, including the transition from fetal or placental circulation to newborn circulation patterns, closure of the fetal ducts, and development of an independent respiratory pattern. Complete metabolic support from the mother stops and the newborn adjusts to an independent supply of oxygen, nutrients, and thermal regulation.

Several factors can interrupt the normal transitional period from fetal life to newborn life. Incomplete removal of the amniotic fluid can lead to respiratory distress and tachypnea of the newborn. Fetal asphyxia, hypercapnia, and subsequent acidosis will contribute to a troubled adjustment to postfetal life. The most critical first step in the transitional period from fetal life to newborn life is the onset of breathing and the establishment of a successful breathing pattern. Some infants require mild tactile stimulation to induce a regular breathing pattern, but few require a resuscitative effort to assist the newborn to independent breathing. The simple act of drying off the newborn's skin may be enough stimulation to assist the infant. According to the American Academy of Pediatrics, gentle back, arm, or trunk rubbing and gentle flicking of the soles of the infant's feet are acceptable means to stimulate a newborn to breathe (American Academy of Pediatrics, 2000).

The assessment of Apgar scores is important in predicting a newborn's health status. Apgar scoring is performed at the birth site and is considered the most frequently used method to assess a newborn's adjustment to extrauterine life. Five areas are assessed at birth and then at 1 and 5 min after birth. These are the newborn's heart rate, respiratory effort, muscle tone, reflex irritability, and overall skin color. Each of these five signs is scored with a 0, 1, or 2. See Table 10.1 for a summary of the Apgar scoring system. The range of Apgar scores is 0 to 10. An infant is considered to be in severe distress if the score is between 0 and 3, in moderate distress if the score is between 4 and 6, and in no distress if the score is between 7 and 10. Apgar scoring is repeated every 5 min after birth if the scores represent distress, and are continued until the child is transferred to a higher level of care or is considered to be adjusting well. If a newborn requires cardiopulmonary resuscitation (CPR) after birth, the Apgar score should not determine this need because CPR should be started well before the 1 min check (Hockenberry and Wilson, 2007).

Cardiovascular System

The newborn is adjusting to external uterine life. The newborn's cardiovascular system must go through a series of events, including the closure of the three fetal shunts. The foramen ovale, the ductus arteriosus, and the ductus venosus must all close during the transitional period to successfully transition from fetal circulation to postnatal circulation. As the newborn takes his or her first breaths, the inspired oxygen dilates the pulmonary vessels and pulmonary blood flow increases, supporting ventilation and gas exchange. It is important for the nurse to assess the newborn's cardiac system.

Newborn cardiac assessments should include:

- Assessment for cyanosis, mottling, edema, discolored or blue nail beds, and clubbing as signs of cardiac abnormalities and poor perfusion
- Inspection for heaves and lifts of the chest
- Auscultation of heart sounds starting at the aortic area and moving to the pulmonic, Erb's point, tricuspid, and then mitral areas; assess the quality, rate, intensity, and rhythm of the heart; normal innocent heart murmurs may be found in up to 50% of infants
- Palpation of all central and peripheral pulses and comparison of femoral to brachial, looking for discrepancies in rate and rhythm
- Percussion of the heart; in infancy, the heart is large in relation to body size

Thermoregulation

The newborn has an important need for the preservation of the core body temperature. **Thermoregulation,** which is the process of maintaining a core body temperature, is a challenge for the newborn and is considered absolutely crucial for survival. Factors that influence thermal regulation include the thin layer of subcutaneous fat, the large body surface area for weight, the lack of ability to shiver, and the newborn's gestational age. At birth, the newborn has a layer of brown fat, which is mitochondria-rich and is used to generate heat. Prematurity reduces the amount of brown fat available.

PATIENT TEACHING GUIDELINES

It is important for the nurse to teach the new parents that swaddling or wrapping the newborn in clean dry blankets is essential to maintain body temperature. Newborns should consistently wear a soft hat and be dressed in appropriate layers of clothing. One tip is to dress the infant in one layer more than the adults are wearing in the same environment, plus a blanket.

Thermoregulation is important to prevent fluctuations in blood glucose. While trying to regulate their body temperature, newborns can experience hypoglycemia.

Newborn temperature assessments should include:

- Frequent assessments of rectal or axillary temperatures with a calibrated thermometer
- A notation of temperatures above 37.5°C or below 36.0°C; these temperatures should be reported and an intervention initiated.
- Wrapping a newborn in extra blankets or removing a layer of blankets may be enough to support thermoregulation. Continue to check the newborn's temperature until stable.

Respiratory System

The infant has a proportionally large head for the body size with a short neck, small mandible, and large tongue. This makes young infants more susceptible for airway compromise and they may require a sniffing position for comfort during periods of respiratory distress.

The infant has a compliant rib cage with poorly developed intercostal muscles with few type 1 fatigue-resistant fibers. This causes the infant to progress from respiratory distress to respiratory failure to respiratory arrest without intervention. If retractions are noted, they must be reported immediately so an intervention can be initiated.

The infant has cartilaginous tracheal rings and the cricoid ring is the narrowest part of the airway. This is in opposition to the adult, in which the larynx is the narrowest part of the airway.

Young infants are obligate nose breathers and have narrow nasal passages that are easily obstructed by mucus. Infants will need to be suctioned in the presence of increasing nasal mucus. Teaching parents how to use a bulb suction device is appropriate. Even a small amount of resistance to airflow from edema or mucus will cause increased work of breathing (WOB).

Newborn respiratory assessments should include:

- Inspection of the lip color, nail color, and pulse oximetry; blood gases and hemoglobin (Hgb) may be ordered as part of the assessment of the respiratory system if the newborn demonstrates respiratory distress
- Inspection for retractions, nasal flaring, use of accessory muscles, tachypnea, head bobbing, and shoulder rolling, which all can indicate respiratory distress
- Auscultation for adventitious or abnormal breath sounds such as rales, rhonchi, wheezing, or stridor
- Inspection for irregular respiratory rates and patterns

Gastrointestinal System

The newborn will demonstrate an immature gut from an absence of normal flora and reduced gastric enzymes, which puts the newborn at risk for infection in the gastrointestinal systems. Breastfeeding is a natural way of introducing normal flora.

Newborns are at risk for fluid and electrolyte imbalances. At no time should a newborn be given free water unless specifically ordered. If a small amount of water is ordered, it should always be sterile water. Formula should be mixed with sterile water during the first few months of infancy to prevent the introduction of unwanted microbes that lead to diarrhea. Overall fluid requirements for the newborn and young infant up to 6 months are, on average, 125 to 150 mL/kg/day. Solid foods should not be introduced to a newborn or young infant until 6 months of life. See Table 21.1 for details of the stool patterns of infants.

Newborn gastrointestinal assessments should include:

- Inspection for visible peristalsis
- Auscultation of bowel sounds in all four abdominal quadrants
- Palpation for masses
- Frequency, quantity, and consistency of stool

Genitourinary System

The newborn's bladder capacity is about 15 to 20 mL. The urine is very light yellow because the newborn's kidneys

TABLE 21.1 STOOL PATTERNS OF INFANTS IN THE FIRST YEAR OF LIFE

First stool: Meconium	• Usually passed in first few days of life • Consistency is thick and sticky • Color is black/green and composed of amniotic fluid, mucosal cells, ingested blood, and secretions from intestinal lining
Transitional Stool	• As the meconium is passed, the stool transitions in color and consistency • The transition occurs at about 3 days of life • Consistency is less thick and sticky • Color is green/brown to yellow/brown
Breast Milk Stool	• Color is orange-yellow • Consistency is soft and even • Appears after the fourth day of life • Breastfed newborns will have several stools a day
Formula Stool	• Color and odor of formula stools is dependent on the formula fed • Consistency is soft

do not concentrate urine effectively. This leaves the newborn at risk for fluid loss and dehydration. Newborns do not cope well with electrolyte fluctuations because their kidneys are immature and unable to concentrate or excrete electrolytes well.

The newborn girl's urethra is very short, which leaves her at risk for the development of urinary tract infections (UTIs). It is important to show parents how to clean the infant girl's genitalia so that they can demonstrate a thorough cleansing and removal of all stool.

Newborn assessments of the genitourinary system include:

- Inspection of the outer genitalia for hygiene and rashes
- Inspection of the quality and color of urine
- Olfaction for malodorous urine

Musculoskeletal System

At birth, the newborn's skeletal system has more collagen present than it does ossified bone. Rapidly, the bones mature and become less pliable. The musculoskeletal system is intact and growth occurs via hypertrophy, not hyperplasia or new cellular growth. Because of the risk of injury, careful handling of the newborn is essential. Parents need to be taught how to carefully position, dress and undress, and carry their infant with head support.

Newborn assessments of the musculoskeletal system include the following:

• Inspection for skeletal deformities
• Inspection of bilateral muscle movements
• Palpation of extremities for masses and deformities

Endocrine System

The newborn's endocrine system is influenced by the mother's hormones. It is not uncommon to see a newborn's nipples secrete a small amount of milky substance called "witch's milk," or a newborn girl's vagina produce a small amount of blood-colored secretion called "pseudomenstruation." The newborn's blood glucose levels fluctuate widely as the pancreas adjusts to secreting insulin. Other hormones are produced, but the endocrine glands are considered immature. The pituitary gland can only secrete limited amounts of antidiuretic hormone (ie, vasopressin), leaving the newborn at risk for dehydration caused by diuresis.

SAFETY *STAT!*

The newborn's blood glucose levels fluctuate widely as the pancreas adjusts to secreting insulin. Stressed or sick newborns require their blood glucose levels to be monitored. They are prone to hypoglycemia.

Assessment of the newborn endocrine system includes inspection for symptoms of fluctuating blood sugars.

Integumentary System

The newborn's skin is thin, but all structures within the newborn's skin are present and functional. Because of the thin nature, any topical medications or ointments will be readily absorbed. Care should be taken to clean the newborn's skin gently but thoroughly to prevent tissue injury, rashes, or tears; two layers, the dermis and epidermis, are loosely bound. The newborn is at risk for skin breakdown and should be assessed regularly.

Assessments of the newborn's integumentary system include:

• Inspection for rashes, clogged sebaceous glands (ie, milia), and bruises
• Palpation of skin for lesions and masses

Neurological System

Maturation of the neurological system takes time because the newborn has immature nerves. **Myelination,** the process of a myelin sheath growing around nerve fibers, continues during *cephalocaudal–proximal-distal development,* and the young infant slowly masters movements. The first movements are primitive reflexes that, over time, become purposeful movements. The most important aspect of the newborn's neurological system is the autonomic system; this is what stimulates the initiation and maintenance of a respiratory pattern after birth.

Assessments of the newborn's neurological system include:

• Inspection of primitive reflexes
• Inspection for equality and symmetry of movements

Sensory Organs

At birth, the sensory organs are all present. Olfactory, tactile, taste, and hearing abilities (ie, upon removal of amniotic fluid) are all intact. Vision is not mature for quite some time. Expect the newborn and young infant to have about only 20/200 visual acuity, needing objects to be within 6 to 8 in. of the face to be seen. Parents are encouraged to hold their infant close, also known as *en face* position (Fig. 21.2). The eyes are structurally incomplete with immature ciliary muscles. This means the newborn will have trouble accommodating and fixating on an object. The newborn's sense of smell is intact and he or she will react strongly to unpleasant odors. Newborns are able to distinguish their mother's breast milk from others and will cry for their mother's milk if her breasts begin to leak (Hockenberry and Wilson, 2007).

Nutrition

Infant nutrition changes rapidly throughout the first year of life.

• The newborn starts with breastfeeding or formula feeding exclusively until the infant is 6 months old. Feedings number about 8 to 12 per day in the newborn period and then slowly become larger and less frequent as the infant grows.
• Food is then introduced in a sequence one at a time to allow for the assessment of food sensitivities or allergies. Iron-fortified infant cereals are introduced first, only after the infant both shows an interest in the food and accomplishes the developmental milestone of being able to swallow a small bolus of food placed on the tongue.
• Green vegetables are introduced after cereals are well established, followed by the yellow and orange vegetables.
• Pureed fruits are introduced one at a time, after eating vegetables is well established.

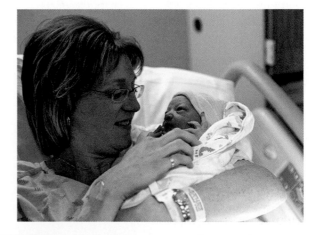

FIGURE 21.2 Mother holding young infant in en face position of bonding.

- Lean meats and egg yolks can be given starting at about 10 months.
- Egg whites are introduced after 10 months.
- No cow's milk should be given to an infant until after 12 months because it can cause inflammation and microbleeds in the intestines. Cow's milk also contributes to milk anemia when young children consume more than 32 ounces a day, thus replacing other iron-rich foods. When cow's milk is introduced, the young child should be given whole milk for the first 2 years to provide the fat needed for brain growth. After 2 years, the child should be offered whichever milk the family drinks, preferably skim milk.

BREASTFEEDING. The American Academy of Pediatrics recommends breastfeeding for all infants for at least the first year of life. The World Health Organization (WHO) recommends human milk as the exclusive food for full-term infants for no less than the first 6 months. The goal of *Healthy People 2020* is to have over an 80% rate of breastfeeding initiation. See Table 21.2 for a list of benefits of breastfeeding. Many mothers need breastfeeding instructions and support. This can include initial teaching by the nurse and follow-up teaching for lactation education. Breastfeeding education should take place regardless of previous births because each infant's feeding patterns and behaviors are unique.

When the infant requires even a short hospitalization, there may be a disruption of breastfeeding. During hospitalizations, the mother should be supported with a breast pump and storage of the milk. Follow institutional policy for breast milk storage. Typically, extra pumped breast milk can be stored in a freezer compartment with its own door for up to 3 months, in a refrigerator compartment for 3 days, and on the counter at room temperature for up to 3 hours. For evidence-based research about breastfeeding and cognitive development, see Box 21.2.

Overall recommendations should include 8 to 12 breastfeeding sessions per day on demand. The goal is to prevent maternal fatigue and anxiety, which can negatively affect milk production. When the newborn or young infant is producing six to eight wet diapers a day, breastfeeding is considered adequate. Breast milk supplies 100% of the healthy young infant's nutrition; therefore no supplemental water, glucose water, or formula should be given unless medically indicated.

USING FORMULA. While nurses consistently promote breastfeeding and provide education and support, there are situations in which the infant's status requires formula feeding, or it is the decision of the mother to use formulas. Examples of conditions in which infants require formula include enteric tube feedings, anatomical abnormalities, gastrointestinal diseases, or severe FTT. Conditions in which it is the mother who may not be able to perform breastfeeding include birth injuries, breast disease or infection, and lack of production of breast milk. If formula is going to be used as the infant's primary nutrition, or is going to be used to supplement breast milk, iron-fortified formula is often suggested because maternal iron stores are depleted in the infant by 6 months of age.

TABLE 21.2 BENEFITS OF BREASTFEEDING

Benefits for the Infant	Benefits for the Mother
1. Breast milk allows for faster gastric emptying, reducing the likelihood of reflux.	1. Breastfeeding provides the mother more rapid postpartum weight loss.
2. Breast milk provides host defense immunity factors, immunoglobulin A (IgA), growth factors, cytokines, lactoferrin, lysozymes, and nucleotides. All of these substances provide protection from infections.	2. Breastfeeding allows faster uterine involution after birth, reducing the chance of excessive bleeding.
3. Breastfeeding reduces the incidence of OM, gastrointestinal diseases, respiratory diseases, and atopic conditions (eg, asthma, eczema, and dermatitis).	3. Breastfeeding can contribute to the spacing of subsequent pregnancies, although this phenomenon is quite unreliable and should not be promoted as a form of birth control.
4. Breast milk contributes to the protection of the neonate from necrotizing enterocolitis.	4. Breast milk is sterile and provides economic advantages in comparison with formula.
5. Breastfeeding improves long-term cognitive and motor abilities.	

Box 21.2 Research Summary of Breastfeeding and Cognitive Development

Research findings suggest that one or more constituents of breast milk facilitate cognitive development in infants, particularly premature infants. According to a 2009 study on the effect of the human mother's breast milk on the infant's brain size, white matter development, and intelligent quotients (IQ), breast milk has been found to be more beneficial than previously expected. White brain matter growth is positively associated with breastfeeding in infants. The findings support the public health implications for the encouragement and support of breastfeeding to promote higher cognitive levels.

(Isaacs, Fischl, et al, 2009)

There are several categories of infant formula, all of which provide nutrition and fluids to the newborn or infant. Some infant formula is prescribed by the primary provider to replenish specific vitamins, electrolytes, and levels of kilocalories or protein. Newborns with congenital anomalies or those with feeding disorders are provided with premade and premeasured formula.

During the newborn and young infant period, all formulas are mixed with sterile water and the baby bottle is warmed in a water bath. Even with the use of a water bath, the nurse needs to teach the family to consistently test the heat level of the formula.

SAFETY *STAT!*

Under no circumstances should the nurse ever use a microwave to warm formula. Microwaves are inconsistent in their power. Microwaving formula leaves "hot spots" within the liquid and can cause a severe burn. This education should also be provided to the infant's caretakers.

The type of formula used is based on a number of factors, including the quantity of calories, water, and nutrients needed. Begin with the quantity of calories needed. The calculation is performed by multiplying the infant's weight in kilograms by the scale of calories required per age. See Table 21.3 for a list of calorie needs. There are a variety of commercial formulas available. Pediatricians or primary caregivers can provide information about the selection of an appropriate formula. Families are encouraged to follow the manufacturer's specific instructions for preparing formulas. Deviations from the exact recommended mixture can lead to the infant failing to gain weight if it is too dilute, or dehydration and metabolic acidosis if it is too strong.

CULTURAL INFLUENCES ON INFANT NUTRITION. The family's cultural background can have a profound effect on the nutrition of the infant. Perspectives on breastfeeding, length of breastfeeding, introduction of foods, and selection of foods during infancy are highly influenced by the family's cultural background. For instance, introducing rice, beans, various types of meats not traditional to the American diet, and types of milk including goats milk may vary according to the cultural norms of the family.

Sleeping Patterns and Requirements

Young infants require about 22 to 23 hours of sleep a day for first few weeks of life. Rest is imperative for health and growth/development. Older infants require about 16 hours of sleep a day, including two naps. Typically, an older infant will nap for 1 to 2 hours in the morning, and nap again in the later afternoon.

PATIENT TEACHING GUIDELINES

Encouraging parents to not let their older infant nap too late in the day improves night sleep behaviors. Although waking a napping infant is difficult for many caregivers, longer afternoon naps will cause the infant to stay up too late or have difficulty with a bedtime routine.

Infants will begin to sleep through the night at 4 to 6 months, but children vary greatly in this. Parents need to understand that each of their children will be unique in their sleeping patterns and flexibility is warranted. Frustrations can occur when parents expect siblings to have similar sleeping patterns. Tips for successful infant sleeping include:

- Expect **separation anxiety,** a situation in which the child expresses anxiety when parents leave or the child is taken from the parents, to start at 8 to 10 months. Separation anxiety intensifies at about 12 months; therefore going to bed becomes more difficult. Use routines and be firm and consistent. Provide a safe bed where the infant cannot easily crawl or climb out of the crib.
- Place the infant on the back to sleep; this greatly reduces the incidence of SIDS. See further information from the American Association of SIDS Prevention Physicians' Web site.
- Do not place pillows or stuffed animals in crib because they may cause suffocation.
- Do not place infants to sleep on waterbeds; this may cause overheating and provides a suffocation risk.
- Although some families choose to, do not sleep with an infant because injuries can occur. The infant should have a safe and separate sleeping area.
- Do not use electric blankets in an infant's crib because this can cause overheating.
- Do not leave on a TV or radio because this might influence quality of sleep.
- Provide a consistent sleeping situation by establishing a routine before bedtime with a positive interaction.
- Help the infant to feel safe and secure at bedtime by using a night light.

Infant Development

Infant development includes psychosocial needs and bonding, as well as physical, cognitive, and communication development.

TABLE 21.3 KILOCALORIE REQUIREMENTS

Developmental Age	Kcal Requirements
0–30 days	100–110 kcal/kg/day
1–4 months	90–100 kcal/kg/day
5 months to 5 years	70–90 kcal/kg/day
Older than 5 years	1,500 kcal for first 20 kg of weight, plus 25 kcal for each additional kg/day

Physical Growth and Development

The physical development of the infant from the newborn period through the first year is astounding. The infant will grow to triple his or her birth weight and double the birth length in the first 12 months. The infant's weight increases by about 1.5 lb or 0.68 kg per month for the first 6 months of life, then increases by about 0.75 lb or 0.34 kg per month the second 6 months. The infant's length grows at an average of 1 in. (2.54 cm) per month in the first 6 months, with an average length of 29 in. (73.66 cm) by 12 months of age. Measurements of children's growth are also called **anthropometric measurements** and can include weight, height, and HC. National standard growth charts are used to follow the natural physical development of the infant and are kept as records for referral if problems are identified. Figures 21.3 and 21.4 provide examples of growth charts.

Several factors influence the infant's physical development. These factors include hereditary influences such as the size and weight of the parents, plus the nutritional status, the level of overall health, cultural factors, and growth patterns known as *spurts* and *lags*. An infant who is born prematurely will take several months to gain weight and height, eventually matching the average size of other infants the same age. Growth measurements are followed and plotted from birth to 3 years, and then new charts are used to follow growth from 3 to 18 years. The plotted measurements are interpreted as percentiles. An infant's measurements, plotted on a growth chart, that fall within the 5th to 95th percentile are considered acceptable.

The infant's HC is measured at each well-child visit and plotted on standardized growth charts. The nurse uses clean, disposable paper measuring tape and places the tape at the level of the largest part of the head, usually right above the brow line. The infant's HC, also known as the *occipital frontal circumference (OFC)*, increases by 0.5 in. or 1.25 cm per month for the first 6 months and increases a total of 33% by the end of the first year. The average value for the HC is 17 in. (43.18 cm) by age 6 months, and 18 in. (45.72 cm) by age 12 months. The infant's posterior fontanel closes at 2 to 3 months of age. The infant's anterior fontanel, the larger of the two, closes later at 12 to 18 months of age. Fontaneles come in a variety of shapes and sizes and are therefore unique for each infant. The purpose of the fontanel is to allow the infant's cranium to expand or contract as needed during the birth process.

The nurse will also measure the infant's chest circumference. The chest circumference is typically 2 cm (.78 in) less than the infant's HC. The nurse places the paper measuring tape at the level of the nipples.

The infant will produce six to eight teeth during the first year, with central incisors erupting first at about 5 to 7 months. See Figure 21.5 for a description of development of the infant's dentition. Parents should begin daily dental health by cleaning the infant's teeth with a damp cloth as soon as they erupt. Infants are at risk for dental caries if they have a bottle or are breastfed while they sleep. This should be discouraged and infants should be weaned from a bottle by 12 months of age to continue to promote dental health.

Normal vital sign ranges in infancy are demonstrated as a heart rate range of 120 to 180 bpm in the newborn period, slowing to 100 to 120 bpm by the first year. The respiratory rate is 40 breaths/min, fluctuating greatly in the first few weeks of life; the axillary temperature ranges from 36.5°C to 37.5°C; the blood pressure of 70 to 85 mm Hg systolic over 41 to 49 mm Hg diastolic in the newborn period rises to an average of 90/60 mm Hg by 12 months.

An infant's metabolic rate is almost twice that of an adult. Infants require more calories, nutrients, and water for their body size in comparison to an adult. The gross and fine motor milestones of an infant are noted in Boxes 21.3 and 21.4.

SAFETY *STAT!*

New parents need to receive explicit guidelines about maintaining safety for their newborn. Topics to cover include, but are not limited to:

- Head support while handling the newborn
- Maintaining an appropriate body temperature to avoid heat loss, including covering the newborn's head at all times
- Laying the newborn on his or her back to sleep to reduce the incidence of SIDS
- Never drinking hot liquids near or above an infant, especially when holding the infant
- Using a bulb syringe to clear secretions in the nose and mouth; preventing choking
- Safety while changing clothes to prevent overextending joints and causing injuries
- Using only an approved newborn-ready car seat and installing the seat safely (ie, rear-facing, in the center of the back seat)
- Preventing falls, burns, suffocation, sunburns, animal bites or scratches, or other home injuries
- Never shaking the baby; prevents shaken baby syndrome

Challenging a young infant during play is a wonderful means to promote fine motor development. The pincer grasp, which is mastered by 7½ to 8½ months, can be encouraged by providing a food treat such as Cheerios, and giving positive reinforcement for success in picking up the food treat and placing it in the mouth. This is now a dangerous time because the infant has mastered locomotion and will get around the floor, picking up any small item and placing it in the mouth. Infants require constant supervision when they move around the home.

Cognitive Development

The infant is experiencing the sensorimotor cognitive developmental period according to Piaget. During this period, the infant is beginning to discriminate between persons, comprehend word meaning, and learn object permanence (ie, the infant realizes an object exists when it is no longer in view).

The infant is experiencing the oral stage according to Freud. Here the infant finds enjoyment, pleasure, and satisfaction

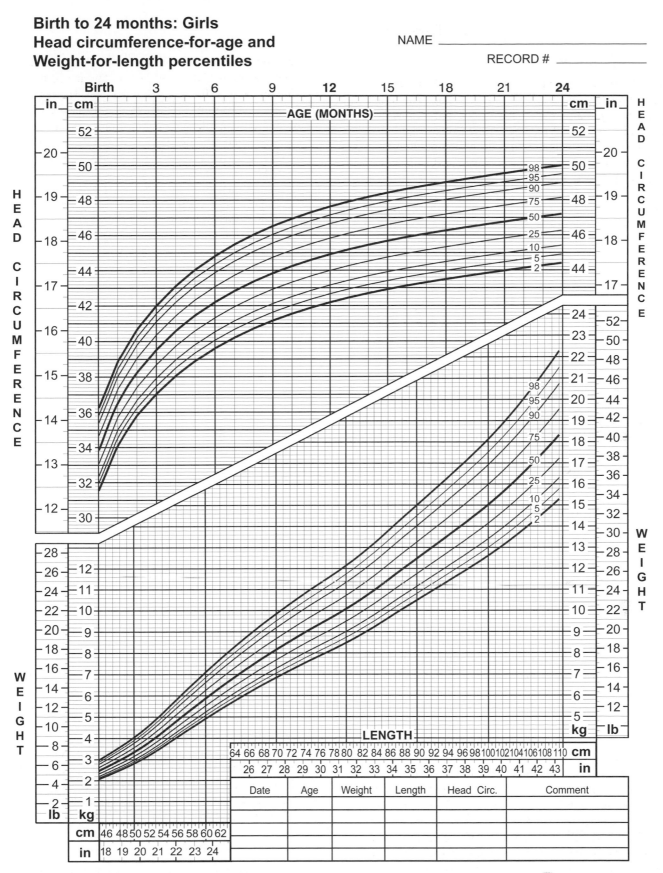

Birth to 24 months: Girls
Head circumference-for-age and
Weight-for-length percentiles

NAME _____

RECORD # _____

Published by the Centers for Disease Control and Prevention, November 1, 2009
SOURCE: WHO Child Growth Standards (http://www.who.int/childgrowth/en)

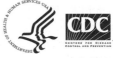

FIGURE 21.3 WHO growth chart for girls from birth to 24 months old. *(From Centers for Disease Control and Prevention. Published by the Centers for Disease Control and Prevention, November 1, 2009. Source: WHO Child Growth Standards, www.who.int/childgrowth/en. Retrieved from www.cdc.gov/growthcharts/who_charts.htm#The%20WHO%20Growth%20Charts.)*

Birth to 24 months: Boys
Head circumference-for-age and
Weight-for-length percentiles

NAME _____

RECORD # _____

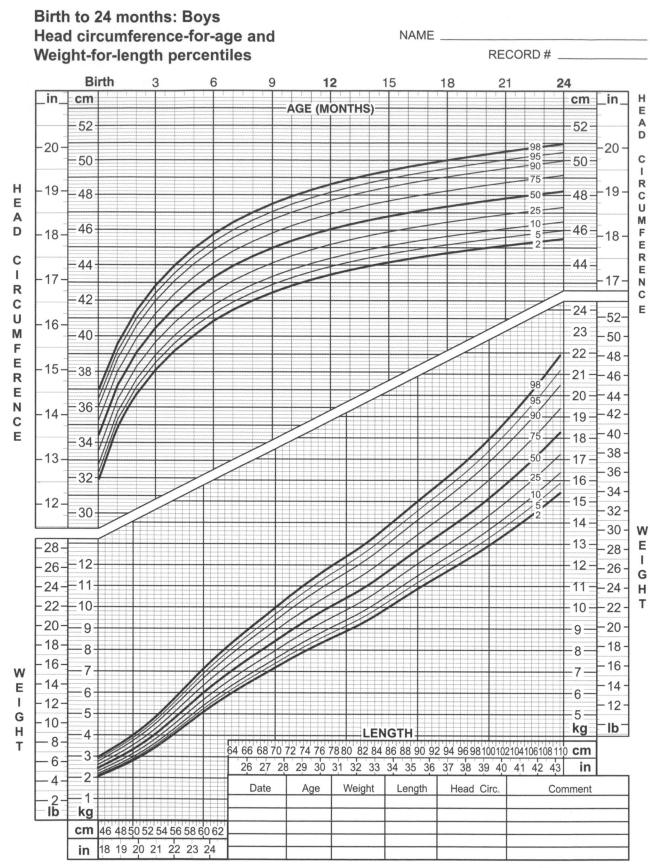

Published by the Centers for Disease Control and Prevention, November 1, 2009
SOURCE: WHO Child Growth Standards (http://www.who.int/childgrowth/en)

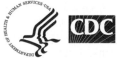

FIGURE 21.4 WHO growth chart for boys from birth to 24 months old. *(From Centers for Disease Control and Prevention. Published by the Centers for Disease Control and Prevention, November 1, 2009. Source: WHO Child Growth Standards, www.who.int/childgrowth/en. Retrieved from www.cdc.gov/growthcharts/who_charts.htm#The%20WHO%20Growth%20Charts.)*

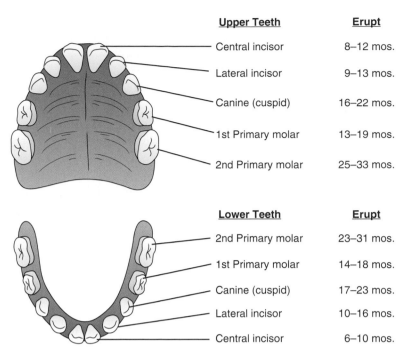

Upper Teeth	Erupt
Central incisor	8–12 mos.
Lateral incisor	9–13 mos.
Canine (cuspid)	16–22 mos.
1st Primary molar	13–19 mos.
2nd Primary molar	25–33 mos.

Lower Teeth	Erupt
2nd Primary molar	23–31 mos.
1st Primary molar	14–18 mos.
Canine (cuspid)	17–23 mos.
Lateral incisor	10–16 mos.
Central incisor	6–10 mos.

FIGURE 21.5 Dentition in children (ie, tooth eruption pattern).

Box 21.3 Gross Motor Milestones of the Infant

1. Holds head up by 3 months while lying prone
2. Rolls over by 5 to 6 months, starting from prone to supine
3. Holds head steady when sitting by 6 months
4. Sits leaning forward by 7 months
5. Sits unsupported by 8 months
6. Gets to a sitting position alone by 9 months
7. Pulls up to a stand by 9 months
8. "Cruises" by standing and holding on to surfaces such as a coffee table by 10 months
9. Stands alone by 12 months
10. Begins to walk independently between 9 and 12 months

Box 21.4 Fine Motor Milestones of the Infant

1. Identifies hands by 3 months
2. Brings hands together by 3 months
3. Grasps rattle voluntarily by 4 months
4. Transfers objects from hand to hand by 6 months
5. Uses finger and thumb to grasp items by 9 months; called prehension
6. Bangs two lightweight items together by 9 months
7. Drinks from a cup at 9 months (needs tippy cup or covered cup to accomplish this task)
8. Begins to nest two items by 12 months
9. Builds two-block tower at 12 months

sucking, and meets the world orally, bringing most items he or she encounters to the mouth for exploration and stimulation. Parents should be taught examples of safe toys for oral play for their infant. See Figure 21.6 for infant toy ideas. Table 21.4 provides information on the key developmental theorists.

Communication Development

The development of communication throughout infancy is a marvelous achievement. Parents enjoy the rapid changes that take place in this first year of life. The infant will begin to regard a person's face at about 1 month and he or she will display a social smile and follow objects 180 degrees at 2 months. As a parent or caregiver plays with the infant, he or she will express delight by cooing at 1 to 2 months and laughing at 2 to 4 months. The infant will make consonant

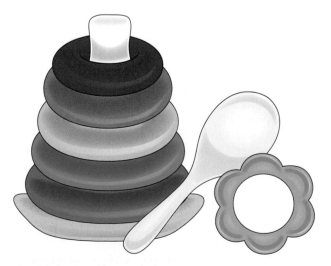

FIGURE 21.6 Appropriate and safe toys for the infant include items such as rattles, teething rings, noisemakers, stuffed animals without buttons, crib mirrors, and crib busy boxes.

TABLE 21.4 DEVELOPMENTAL THEORISTS

Developmental Theorist	Theory

Psychosocial Development: Erikson	• The crisis of infancy is the development of "trust versus mistrust."
	• The infant must develop a sense of trust as a foundation for future psychosocial tasks across childhood.
	• Having a sense of predictability assists the infant with mastering a sense of trust in the caregiver's behaviors and in the environment. This can be done by providing warmth, nutrition, elimination needs, and play/stimulation upon demand in a predictable manner.
	• Social interactions are very significant for the infant. Progression of socialization occurs monthly:
	  • Socially smiles at 2 months
	  • Recognizes familiar faces at 3 months
	  • Smiles at a mirror at 5 months
	  • Fears strangers at about 6 months

Psychosexual Development: Freud	• The predominate psychosexual development is demonstrated in the oral stage found between birth through 18 months of age. • The infant displays the desire to suck, bite, chew, taste, and swallow, learning the environment through the mouth.

Cognitive Development: Piaget	• The infancy period is described as the sensorimotor stage, where the infant gains knowledge of the environment through the senses.
	  • Birth to 1 month: The infant demonstrates survival sucking reflexes.
	  • 1–4 months: The infant explores own body as the center of interest.
	  • 4–8 months: The infant now focuses on the environment and gives great attention to objects within reach.
	  • 8–12 months: The infant actively searches for hidden objects and readily explores the environment for stimulating objects and play items. Object permanence is now intact and the infant sees himself or herself as separate from others.

sounds at 3 to 4 months of age. The infant will recognize familiar faces at 3 months of age. As the infant continues to interact with his or her caregivers, the infant will make imitative sounds at 6 months, demonstrating the importance of frequent interactions in language development. Finally, at the end of this first developmental stage, the infant will be able to say one to two words at 12 months. These first words will carry meaning to the infant. The first words may be "Ma-Ma," "Da-Da," "No," "Ba-Ba," or some word that the primary caregiver has emphasized and the infant associates with something he or she wants.

Interacting with the primary caregivers is an easy and effective way to show language learning. When others attempt to interact with the older infant, stranger anxiety starts and may prohibit the interactions between nurse and child. Stranger anxiety will begin at 6 to 8 months and last for several months. This is an expected behavior and parents should be reassured that it is normal.

Psychosocial Needs and Bonding

Bonding is a process of developing a meaningful relationship between the infant and the caregiver. Bonding provides a sense of security that is needed for the infant to feel safe. Bonding should be encouraged right after birth by having the mother hold the infant close to her, talking to the infant in a quiet, nurturing, and calm tone. The infant quickly learns to connect those close feelings with the parent and develop a sense of connection. The infant's sensory organs are intact and assist the infant in recognizing the parent and developing their bond. Even ill infants should have the opportunity to bond with their parents and all steps to promote close time together should be provided, as medically indicated.

ANTICIPATORY GUIDANCE FOR PARENTS OF THE INFANT

With the rapid development during infancy come many concerns about safety. Pediatric nurses must teach families about these concerns to prevent injuries. Anticipatory guidance, or education focusing on knowing what to expect and planning a safe and healthy environment before an incident or injury happens, becomes paramount. See Box 21.5 for information about how to guide and educate the parents of an infant.

Box 21.5 Anticipatory Guidance for Parents of an Infant

- Promotion of overall health and well-being:
  - Well-child checkup appointment schedule
  - Immunization schedule
  - Guidelines for nutrition in the first year of life; introduction of new foods after 6 months
  - Safe sleeping areas and patterns; no sleeping with infant; place infant on the back to sleep to help prevent SIDS
  - Promotion of infant/child CPR classes
  - Prevent sun exposure and only use sunscreen with SPF 15 or higher after 6 months of age
  - Avoid television for children under 2 years old
- Promotion of a safe home environment:
  - Prevention of exposure to pollution, mercury, water contaminants, chemicals used for hobbies, bleach-containing cleaning solutions, and mold
  - Assessment of the presence of lead to prevent poisoning
  - Avoid the use of pesticides in and around the home/garden
  - Maintain working smoke alarms and check batteries
- Promotion of healthy growth and development:
  - Provide for the need for sucking
  - Encourage sensorimotor learning and play
  - Encourage and foster language development
  - Promote daily dental hygiene
  - Foster bonding and a trusting relationship/ environment

During the infancy period, taking purposeful steps to promote health is imperative. Parents and the pediatric health-care team work collaboratively to provide health promotion to form a foundation of health for all of the infant's childhood years. Adequate nutrition, an appropriate sleeping pattern, balance between play and napping, proper hygiene, and bonding are all important to promote health in the infant. Families need education and support concerning health promotion so the infant can experience a healthy beginning and deviations in health are identified early. Categories of health promotion in the infant stage include well-child checkups and immunizations, dentition, pacifier safety, immunizations, car seat safety, infant device safety, and toy safety. Toy safety is of particular concern because infants are at such high risk for aspiration, choking, and injury from toys that are developmentally inappropriate.

Dentition

Teaching parents how to care for an infant's emerging teeth is very important. The health of children's teeth impacts many aspects of his or her health. Understanding the growth of teeth and how to care for them provides a foundation for good dental care throughout childhood.

Teething

The infant will have about six to eight teeth erupt during the first year of life. This causes discomfort for the infant as the baby teeth, or deciduous teeth, break through the gum line. Parents should be taught to expect this discomfort and to talk to their caregiver about ideas for comforting the infant. Infant teething rings, including those that can be frozen, should be used under supervision.

SAFETY *STAT!*

Use only commercial teething rings and teething products to promote safety. Allowing the infant to chew on such items as frozen bagels may cause choking.

As soon as the first tooth erupts through the gum line, nurses need to teach parents to clean the new tooth and gum line. Cleaning the infant's teeth with a wet washcloth is sufficient. Toothpaste should not be used because the fluoride level may be high and cause poisoning. Providing this daily routine sets up the infant for appropriate tooth care later in childhood.

Using Bottles

The infant should be weaned from the bottle completely before his or her first birthday. Juice should never be given through a bottle. Infants who are put to bed with a bottle of juice or milk may develop early tooth decay because of small amounts of the liquid bathing the infant's teeth during sleep. A bottle of water may be given to the older infant at bedtime but should be removed from the infant's bed.

Using Pacifiers

Specific guidelines should be followed if a pacifier is introduced to an infant. Only pacifiers that are made of one piece of plastic should be offered to prevent a teething infant from chewing the pacifier into parts and creating a choking risk (Fig. 21.7). It is always a necessity to obtain caregiver permission before introducing a pacifier to an infant because some parents do not want pacifiers introduced to their infant.

Safety Measures in the Home

Pediatric nurses can be very influential to the promotion of a safe home environment. Providing anticipatory guidance concerning what to expect as an infant rapidly grows and

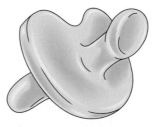

FIGURE 21.7 Example of a safer one-piece pacifier.

becomes mobile can save lives. The next section describes several aspects of home safety.

The Use of Infant Devices in the Home

Parents have choices on a variety of infant feeding, sleeping, resting, mobility, and play devices. These include high chairs, bouncy seats, walkers, swings, strollers, and play stations. It is imperative that infants not be left alone in these devices because lack of supervision can lead to accidents and injuries. Health promotion education includes explaining that safe, intact, and approved devices where the infant is placed in a safe environment with constant supervision is part of a healthy start. Older infants left in high chairs can rock themselves over; pets can have access to unsupervised infants in these devices; and walkers can plunge down stairs if left unsupervised or without gates to prevent a fall, causing severe injuries. If parents have questions about a certain device, they should be instructed to contact the manufacturer for specific safety checks and recommendations for use. Parents must be reminded that they should never leave a child unattended on a changing table or in a swing, highchair, bouncy seat, or wagon. The American Association of Pediatricians' Web site has links to guidelines for the use or nonuse of specific types of devices.

Toy Safety

Parents should provide safe toys for the teething infant. Infants should not be given toys that have unsafe buttons or any small item that can be gummed or chewed off, placing the infant at an aspiration and choking risk. The infant experiences the world through sensory experiences and benefits highly from solitary play, visual and auditory stimulation, and touch.

Crib Selection

Parents need to be instructed in safe crib selection. Older cribs may not be safe if there is peeling paint or larger gaps between the crib slats. Space between crib rail slats should not be wider than $3\frac{5}{8}$ in. because the young child might place the head between the bars and suffocate. The crib should be free from toys, stuffed animals, or any other suffocation risk.

Car Seat Safety

Health promotion includes providing infants with safe car restraints. Infants should be in the back seat, center, facing backward. In pickup trucks where there is no backseat, the infant should be placed in the middle, facing backward. Infants should always be placed in certified car seats appropriate for their age and size. Children with special needs, or those with orthopedic devices such as spica casts, will need specialized car seats.

SCREENING AND HEALTH PROMOTION FOR THE INFANT

Infants require several well-child checkups during this first year of life to ensure problems with growth and development are identified early and interventions are initiated. Providing regularly scheduled appointments to allow measurements, nutritional checks, education, and anticipatory guidance will promote healthy growth and development, as well as safety. First-time parents need a lot of guidance and support during this year of rapid change.

Well-Child Checkups and Immunizations

One of the most important topics to cover with the parents of an infant is the importance of keeping well-child checkups. A healthy infant needs to have a series of immunizations; measurements, including HC checks, weight checks, and length checks; and developmental milestone checks that assess for dysfunctions or delays in the infant's development (Table 21.5). The earlier problems in growth and development are identified, the earlier referrals can be made for interventions to assist the child. Nurses must encourage parents to maintain all records of infant well-child checkups so that important information is available as needed.

The development and use of immunizations globally has eradicated previously devastating diseases such as smallpox and polio in the nation. Immunizations are given to infants to produce antibodies (ie, active immunity) against various diseases that can be acquired in the community. The purpose of immunizations is to prevent the acquisition and spread of infectious diseases and prevent complications from the diseases, some with quite profound consequences. Schedules are published for health-care professionals and are published regularly. Recommendations for specific immunizations and schedules for the vaccine shots are made by the Centers for Disease Control and Prevention (CDC) for all infants. See the CDC Web site for more information including consultation and printed materials on the vaccines required for all healthy infants. Although immunizations are administered at set intervals for healthy infants, schedules may vary because of office visit timing, the wellness state of the infant, missed doses, and a limited vaccine supply.

There are four types of immunizations offered during childhood. The first type is the live attenuated type, such as the measles, mumps, and rubella vaccine (MMR) and the oral polio vaccine (OPV). The second type of immunization is the inactivated type, such as the *Haemophilus influenza* type B (Hib) and the hepatitis B (hep B) vaccines. The third type is the inactivated toxoid, such as tetanus and diphtheria, and the fourth type is the immunoglobulins (IVIG), such as the respiratory syncytial virus (RSV).

Immunizations may take weeks to months for a full effect, but then offer lasting protection against specific infectious diseases. Make sure that families receive written information about each disease and immunization, possible side effects, and schedules. Document the discussion of concerns, questions, refusals, or delays. Informed consent must be secured before administration.

Some parents/caregivers refuse immunizations for their infants. This must be immediately reported to the physician or primary caregiver for further evaluation as to the reasons cited. See the latest CDC immunization guidelines (CDC, 2014) for information on:

- Schedules and off-schedules when doses are missed
- Guidelines for administration

TABLE 21.5   SCHEDULE FOR WELL-INFANT CHECKUPS AND IMMUNIZATIONS

Patient Age	Well-Infant Checkup	Immunizations
Birth/Neonate	*Neonate:* Infant may need weight, HC, and hepatitis B (hep B) vaccine if not administered after birth; may need hearing screening if not conducted within the first few days of life	*Birth:* hep B
1 Month	Immunizations if not administered at the 1 month visit, and weight, HC check	*n/a*
2 Months	Immunizations and weight, HC check	hep B, rotavirus, diphtheria and tetanus toxoids and pertussis (DTaP), *H influenza* type b (Hib), pneumonococcal vaccine (PCV), and inactivated poliovirus
4 Months	Immunizations, growth and development	rotavirus, DTaP, Hib, PCV, and inactivated poliovirus
6 Months	Immunizations, growth and development, interactions with caregiver, achievement of expected milestones	hep B, rotavirus, DTaP, Hib, PCV, and inactivated poliovirus
12 Months	Immunizations, growth and development, possible laboratory analysis for anemia if concerns exist, interactions with caregiver, achievement of motor and language milestones	DTaP, Hib, PCV, varicella, MMR

- Guidelines for premedications
- Care for the child after immunizations

SAFETY PROVIDED TO THE INFANT WHILE HOSPITALIZED

When infants are hospitalized, a safe environment must be provided (Table 21.6). There are many medical equipment devices and situations that place an infant at risk. Nurses provide a clean, safe, and well-protected environment for the infant to recover and rest (Table 21.7). Infants are vulnerable to a host of scenarios that can be threatening to their safety.

- **Identification:** All infants must have a hospital-provided identification wrist band or ankle band. The band information should include the infant's full name, date of birth, medical record number, and any other identifying information required by the particular institution. A second band should be added if the infant has demonstrated an allergic reaction to any medication or food. Many institutions also require that each parent or primary caregiver also wear a band for safe identification. Learn your hospital or institution child abduction policy and procedure.
- **Prevention of infection:** Hospital environments place the infant at risk for acquiring a nosocomial, or hospital-acquired, infection. Meticulous hand washing prior to all

patient contact and the use of aseptic technique during any medical procedures is imperative. Young infants are considered immuno-immature and are at a higher risk for acquiring infections. Newborns are administered eye medication before discharge to prevent infectious diseases after birth.

- **Safe handling and neck support:** Nurses are role models for parents to learn proper neck support during handling of the infant. Care must be taken when dressing the infant to ensure that the limbs and neck are protected from injury. When an infant is ill, the nurse follows precautions to position the infant into proper body position to provide alignment and support for limbs and the neck.
- **Body temperature control:** Young infants are at particular risk for hypothermia. Nurses must take precaution to ensure the infant's temperature is stabilized during medical procedures and interventions. Infant blanket warmers can be used to warm blankets but the nurse should always check for level of heat. Under no circumstances should a nurse prepare a hot pack and place it against an infant's skin for temperature stability because burns can occur.
- **Crib selections:** There are several styles of cribs available for infants during hospitalization, including high top cribs for standing infants to prevent climbing over rails and falls.
- **Infants sleeping in a large hospital bed:** Hospital policies exist to ensure that infants do not sleep in a large bed with

TABLE 21.6 CHECKLIST FOR MAINTAINING SAFETY IN THE PEDIATRIC TREATMENT ROOM

Introduction to Treatment Rooms	• Many pediatric units have a treatment room where minor procedures are conducted that do not require a surgical team. Saving the crib as the child's safety zone and using the treatment room aids in developing a trusting environment. • Treatment rooms can be stocked with toys and visual distractions to use during procedures. • Whenever possible, members of Child Life should be included in any procedures performed on children in a treatment room.
Equipment Used in Treatment Rooms	• The health-care team should be well prepared for an untoward reaction of a child to a procedure. Having clean resuscitative equipment in close proximity to the child is life-saving. Even during simple procedures such as an IV insertion, an infant with a respiratory infection can become distressed, cry, and demonstrate respiratory compromise. Being prepared is essential.
Safety Checklist for Treatment Rooms	1. Crash cart 2. Treatment table manual resuscitator bags and masks 3. Source of suction with clean tubing, collection bucket, and new suction tip still in packaging 4. Source of oxygen with tubing and various delivery devices, including nasal cannula, simple mask, partial rebreather, and nonrebreather masks 5. Cardiac monitoring equipment with adequate supply of chest leads (small and regular size) 6. Blankets for restraining wrap procedures 7. Vital sign equipment 8. Blood drawing devices, storage bags, and labels 9. Stool/seat for parents 10. Distraction equipment, safe toys 11. Proper source of light 12. Call light equipment to rapidly get help/assistance 13. Code button 14. Time-out reminder poster

TABLE 21.7 SAFETY CHECKLIST FOR HOSPITAL NURSES CARING FOR INFANTS

Patient Identification	• Infants must always have a secure hospital wrist or ankle band that identifies their full name, medical record number, and birth date. At no time should the nurse remove the identification band and place the band on any surface, around crib rails, or on IV poles or bedside equipment. • The infant's identification must be checked before all medications are administered or any procedures are performed. • Parents are often required to have an identification band on with the infant's identification information.
Crib Safety	• Older infants will try very hard to climb out of their crib to either find their parents or to be with the parents in the room. It is important that the side rails are up to their maximum height at all times. Infants close to 12 months of age should have a high-top crib where they are boxed into the crib for safety. • Every time the crib rails are lowered, the nurse should anticipate the infant trying to immediately climb out of the crib or roll to the edges.

TABLE 21.7 SAFETY CHECKLIST FOR HOSPITAL NURSES CARING FOR INFANTS—cont'd

	• At all times the nurse should have a firm hand on the infant and all equipment within easy reach. • Every year infants fall out of hospital cribs onto hard floors and suffer injuries. Prevention is key and the nurse should anticipate a distressed infant trying to climb, roll, or push out of the hospital crib. • Older infants may try to pull themselves to a standing position, climb on top of toys, stuffed animals, or equipment, and attempt to climb out of the crib if these items are left in the bed. The only items that should be in the crib at any time are blankets and a personal item such as a "blankie" or favorite stuffed toy that the child brings from home. Be aware of older infants trying to get out of their crib any way they can.
Airway Safety	• Every hospital crib or isolette should have airway resuscitation equipment within reach. This includes a manual resuscitator bag and three sizes of masks. • Each bed should have a newborn size mask, a pediatric mask, and an adult mask. This equipment should be stored in a clean clear plastic bag out of reach of the infant and should be checked on a regular basis. • A source of oxygen should always be available for respiratory emergencies, and a complete suction setup should be available at all times for emergency aspirations or emergencies.
Parental Involvement	• Parents or a significant caregiver, such as a grandparent, should be highly encouraged to stay with the child during the entire hospitalization. • Young children without parents present require high-top cribs because they will climb out of bed to search for family members. • Hospitalized children have better clinical outcomes if they are comforted by the presence of their family.
Monitoring Systems	• If medically indicated, hospitalized children will be monitored for heart rate, respiratory rate, and oxygen saturation. • As the child's vital signs demonstrate stress, the monitor system alarms the nursing staff of the clinical change. • Other monitoring systems can be used to alert the nursing staff if the child is taken off the unit; this prevents infant/child abduction.
Use of Car Seats in Cribs	• Some nurses ask the family to bring in the child's car seat and place the seat safely within the crib. This sitting up position helps some children who are in respiratory distress. • Check with the institution's guidelines about this practice because not all hospital policies allow for the use of the car seat.
Hot Water Bottles, Hot Pads	• The only heating devices that should be used for children are those that are commercially made and approved by the hospital. • Heating pads should not be prepared on the unit and microwaved. These homemade devices have a history of leading to burns and should never be prepared and used on children. • Hot water bottles, if approved for use by the institution, should only be used by following the manufacturer's instructions. Children are at tremendous risk for burns, and diligence is required for the use of any warming or heating device.
Microwaving Formula and Infant Foods	• Infant formula and breast milk should never be placed in the microwave for heating. Only warm water baths should be used to slowly heat any form of infant nutrition. Microwaving leads to unpredictable "hot spots" that can cause burns.
Safety Around Tubes and Preventing Strangulation	• Active older infants and young children in cribs are at risk for strangulation by medical tubing and cords. These children must be monitored frequently to prevent strangulation. IV tubing and oxygen tubing, as well as nasogastric tubes (NGTs) and Foley's catheters, all provide an opportunity for injury or strangulation.

an adult. Even if the infant shares a "family bed" at home, in the hospital infants must sleep in an appropriate size crib with side rails up at all times.

- **Falls:** Infants are at risk for falls in the hospital setting. Nurses must keep crib rails up when not with the child or with their hands on the child for safe holding. Infants who roll over or lunge at the caregiver when the rails are down can suffer head injuries if they fall down to the linoleum hospital floor. Parents must be reminded to have all infant supplies readily available at easy reach so that they do not turn their back on the infant who can then suffer a fall.

SAFETY *STAT!*

Most hospitals and health-care settings that care for infants require that two nurses double-check medications. This double-check includes the safe dose range for each medication and a double-check of the final concentration prior to administering.

 ## DISEASE AND INJURY PREVENTION FOR THE INFANT

Infants have anatomical and physiological differences compared with older children and adults. Because of these differences, pediatric health-care team members must assess an infant for conditions especially found during this vulnerable age. This section provides information about diseases and injuries that are associated with this age group.

Otitis Media

Otitis media (OM), which is an inner ear infection, is a common diagnosis in infancy and early childhood. OM is the inflammation of the inner ear caused by pathogens such as *Streptococcus pneumoniae, H influenza,* or a variety of viruses. In the neonate, *Staphylococcus aureus* may be the culprit. Occurring most often between 3 months of age and 3 years, it is children who are bottle fed, especially while they are in the supine position when being fed, who are most prone to infection. Prevention of OM includes instruction to the family about the importance of breastfeeding to provide immunity and only bottle feeding while the infant is held in an upright angle.

Aspiration

Because infants are focused intently on mouthing anything within their reach and because they are teething, they are at high risk for aspiration. Carpets and wood floors must be keep free from any debris; the infant, when crawling, will pick up and place anything he or she finds into the mouth. The infant is also at high risk for suffocation. Plastic bags, shopping bags, dry cleaning bags, and garbage bags all place the infant at risk because the bag can be easily pulled over the head.

Drowning

Infants are at very high risk for drowning in even just an inch or two of water.

- Infants should never be left unsupervised during a bath. The use of bath rings that prop up the infant in a sitting position do not provide water safety. Infants can easily tip and fall forward or backward and drown.
- Crawling infants can fit through pet doors and fall into swimming pools.

Parents must be instructed to constantly hold their young infant while in the bath and stay within easy reach when the infant is sitting up in a tub.

Poisoning

Older infants who spend their time exploring their environments are at great risk for poisoning. Medicines, cleaners, cosmetics, and any other potentially harmful substances must be stored in their original containers behind locked cabinets. Several varieties of cabinet locks are available. Parents should be instructed to post the national poison control hotline phone number by the telephone.

Burns

To prevent burns during the infancy period, the following four procedures should be followed:

1. Caregivers should be instructed to never microwave formula, baby food, or breast milk. Only warm water baths should be used to heat food or drinks.
2. Caregivers should never hold an infant in one arm and drink a hot beverage in their other arm. This balancing act can lead to severe hot liquid burns.
3. Never use hot packs on infants because their skin is particularly susceptible to burns. Under no circumstances should hot packs be microwaved and placed on the infant's skin.
4. Home water heaters should not be turned up to over 48.8°C (120°F). Above this, the infant can suffer a severe burn from bath water.

DISORDERS OF THE INFANT

Specific ailments can affect the child during the infancy developmental stage. The pediatric nurse must become familiar with common ailments and the signs and symptoms of unexpected illnesses to find evidence of disease and report these findings to primary care providers. Disorders of young infants cross all body systems and may present symptoms from as early as the newborn period. The following sections present information about health problems of the newborn and infant. Subsequent chapters discuss other body system–specific illnesses that can also occur during infancy.

Sudden Infant Death Syndrome (SIDS)

The National Institute of Child Health and Human Services defines SIDS as a sudden, unexpected death of a previously healthy infant under the age of 1 year that remains unexplained after a thorough case investigation, including autopsy, examination of the death scene, and review of the clinical history. The incidence of SIDS is 7,000 annually, or one out of every 1,000 live births in the United States, occurring mostly in males, during night hours, while the infant is positioned prone. There is a higher incidence of SIDS in infants of African American and Native American descent. The peak age is between 2 to 4 months of age. Socioeconomic risk factors include low income status, low educational level of the mother, a history of drug abuse or high alcohol consumption in the house, and maternal anemia.

One theory is that the infant's respiratory center in the brain is immature and cannot sustain a strong respiratory pattern. Factors associated with SIDS include smoking in the home, putting the infant to sleep in a prone position, and having a sibling who died of SIDS. Infants who have had acute life threatening events (ALTE) are considered to be a greater risk. Nurses should assess at-risk infants for inspiratory pauses, impaired arousal, and decreased O_2 or increased CO_2. Most infants (ie, 80%) present with bloody mucus in the mouth or nares, cyanosis of the nail beds and lips, and an autopsy report of inflammation in the upper respiratory tract, petechiae on the lung pleura, thymus and pericardia, and pulmonary edema. Central nervous system abnormalities, such as delayed myelination or scarring in the tissues surrounding the respiratory control center within the brainstem, have also been detected.

Parents need to be taught that infants should be placed on their back to sleep, making sure there are no fluffy pillows or heavy blankets in the bed that could cover the infant, and that the infant should not become overheated while sleeping. The parents should check that there are no gaps or spaces between the crib mattress and the crib rails, and that the crib mattress is firm and nonmoldable.

Additional resources for SIDS are provided in Box 21.6.

Dehydration

Infants are particularly at risk for severe dehydration because of their large body surface area, immature kidney function, and susceptibility to gastrointestinal infections, especially viruses. Significant amounts of water and electrolytes can be lost in a very short period of time. Dehydration can become complicated when the ill infant not only has frequent stools, but then decreases oral intake. The goal for dehydration treatment is to replace fluids and electrolytes rapidly while monitoring for ongoing fluid losses. Signs of mild dehydration (ie, 5% body weight loss or less) are harder to assess because the infant's vital signs will remain close to normal. Clinical signs and symptoms of moderate dehydration (ie, 10% body weight loss or less) in the infant include elevated heart rate, deeper respirations, and decreased urinary output (UOP). Severe dehydration (ie, 15% body weight loss or greater) includes the previous signs plus delayed capillary refill time, absent tears, dry mucous membranes, and sunken fontaneles. Nurses must assess for lowering in BP measurements, which is a late sign of dehydration.

Colic

Colic, also known as *paroxysmal abdominal pain,* can occur in as many as 30% of infants. Rarely is there an organic cause associated with colic symptoms. Infants present with what appears as severe abdominal pain or cramping that is accompanied with persistent, loud crying. Colic can present as crying longer than 3 hours a day for more than 3 days per week. Colic has an abrupt start and an abrupt resolution. Most children are under 3 months of age when colic starts and almost all infants stop with colicky symptoms by 6 months of age. Despite the obvious symptoms of abdominal pain, infants with colic eat, gain weight, and thrive. Parents, often frazzled and exhausted by their persistently crying infant, will need reassurance that colic will indeed stop. Fruit juices should not be administered to infants because juice carbohydrate malabsorption may contribute to some cases (Duro, Rising, et al, 2002). Parents should also be encouraged to take a break from their crying infant and compose themselves during the long crying episodes. Some cultural groups have found that herbal teas may decrease the irritability and crying associated with colic.

Failure to Thrive

Failure to thrive (FTT) is a term used when a child is not gaining weight, growing in height, or thriving in a healthy state. FTT exists when a child's measured weight and height (ie, physical growth) is considered significantly less than normal. FTT can be identified by consistent plot points on a national growth chart that fall below the fifth percentile. Some references will say FTT is found when the consistent points fall below the third percentile. Growth retardation may be accompanied by delayed developmental and emotional functioning.

FTT is associated with families living in poverty. There are two main types of FTT: organic and nonorganic. Organic FTT is when there is an identifiable underlying medical condition, whereas in nonorganic FTT there is not an identifiable underlying medical condition, and the condition is therefore associated with psychosocial factors. This disorder is typically found in children younger than 5 years old (most often infants) with difficult parent/child relationships.

Box 21.6 Resources for Information About Sudden Infant Death Syndrome

- American Sudden Infant Death Syndrome Institute, 1-800-232-SIDS
- National Sudden Infant Death Syndrome Foundation, 1-800-638-7437

You may also visit these organizations' Web sites for additional information.

NURSING CARE PLAN for the Child with Failure to Thrive (FTT)

The creation of a nursing care plan for a child with FTT can include the following nursing diagnoses and corresponding nursing goals:

Nursing Diagnoses:
- There is delayed growth and development related to inadequate calorie intake as evidenced by low percentile weight plot on the national standardized growth chart.
- There is altered maternal-infant interaction related to lack of understanding of the infant's needs as evidenced by poor weight gain.

Expected Outcomes:
- The infant will demonstrate a growth plot point on a national standardized growth chart at the 50th percentile.
- The mother will verbalize the nutritional needs of her infant to the pediatric health-care team staff, including the appropriate daily caloric needs of the infant.

Assessments for FTT include the nurse identifying the knowledge base of the parents concerning infant nutrition and the feeding needs of their infant. Because the problem may stem from the parents'/caregivers' failure to offer and provide adequate calories for growth, the nurse must assess for a history of poor eating habits or difficulty with feedings. The nurse must also assess for sleep disturbances, vomiting, recurrent infections, and dermatitis. Further assessments should include a loss of subcutaneous fat, and a reduced muscle mass and tone. Developmental milestones should be assessed because the infant with FTT may be delayed in motor, cognitive, and language skills. Mothers should be assessed for depression; this has been found to be associated with FTT.

Treatments for FTT include providing a feeding environment free of stress, allowing 30 min for mealtimes, and providing encouragement and support while eating. The nurse must offer the young infant high-calorie supplements and formulas that provide more than 20 kilocalories per ounce. Preventing associated complications such as vitamin deficiencies, dehydration, electrolyte imbalances, and anemia are important. The nurse must secure a multidisciplinary approach for the care of the infant with FTT, including assistance from a nutritionist for screening, education, and support.

Key Points

- The infant time period is from birth through the first year, ending right before the child's first birthday.
- The newborn and infant experience rapid physical growth, development, and the achievement of many new motor milestones.
- The first year of life has an increased caloric and fluid requirement that far exceeds the other childhood developmental stages.
- The infant experiences the world through sensory experiences and benefits highly from solitary play, visual and auditory stimulation, and touch.
- Older infants develop objective permanence, which allows them to search for a hidden toy or play object.

- Older infants rapidly acquire locomotion, place everything in the mouth, and become very interested in the environment. These behaviors cause tremendous risks, require constant supervision, and require the provision of a safe environment throughout the home.
- Parents and caregivers should allow the infant to develop a sense of what Erikson's developmental theory describes as trust versus mistrust by providing the child immediate attention to their needs (eg, warmth, play, rest, diaper hygiene, and oral gratification through sucking and nutrition).

REVIEW QUESTIONS

1. At what point in an infant's development would you expect the birth weight to triple?
   1. At 6 months
   2. At 12 months
   3. At 9 months
   4. At 18 months

2. While the nurse is assessing the neurological development and milestones of a 3-month-old infant, which of the following would the nurse expect to find?
   1. Parachute reflex
   2. Moro's reflex
   3. While prone, lifting head and neck off surface
   4. While supine, rolling from back to front

3. While assessing an infant with moderate dehydration demonstrating a 10% body weight loss, which of the following would the nurse expect to find?
   1. Decreased pulse
   2. Bulging fontanels
   3. Lethargy
   4. Decreased urine output

4. While reinforcing a teaching session between the nutritionist and a mother of a 5-month-old infant who has stopped breastfeeding, you explain that the maternal iron stores are present in the infant's body until what time frame?
   1. 3 months of age
   2. 1 month of age
   3. 6 months of age
   4. 12 months of age

5. The most important aspect of care of an infant, according to Erik Erikson, is to develop a sense of what?
   1. Belonging
   2. Family
   3. Trust
   4. Warmth

6. When administering medications to an infant in the hospital, the best way to ensure medication administration accuracy and safety is to:
   1. Double-check all medications and calculations with a second nurse
   2. Make sure the parents are present to identify their infant
   3. Have a representative from the pharmacy present to double-check medication calculations
   4. Document with a black ink pen immediately after the medication administration

7. All of the following represent ways to communicate with infants except:
   1. Emphasizing vowels and consonants
   2. Close contact with primary caregiver
   3. Promotion of security through immediate need gratification
   4. Providing simple conversations that encourage autonomy

8. While providing anticipatory guidance to the parents of a 4-month-old during a routine scheduled well-child visit, the nurse would explain which psychosocial stage is the infant expected to accomplish during the first year of life?
   1. Sensorimotor
   2. Trust versus mistrust
   3. Autonomy versus shame and doubt
   4. Oral fixation

9. Which of the following foods should the nurse teach the parents to introduce to their infant's diet first?
   1. Pureed fruits
   2. Runny oatmeal
   3. Strained green peas
   4. Iron-fortified cereal

10. Which of the following immunizations would be given to a 4-month-old infant? *(select all that apply)*
    1. MMR vaccine
    2. Varicella vaccine
    3. Rotavirus vaccine
    4. Hib vaccine
    5. Polio vaccine (IVP)
    6. PCV
    7. DTaP

CRITICAL THINKING QUESTIONS

1. Where can parents go online to receive reputable information on congenital anomalies, inborn errors of metabolism, and other syndromes found in infancy?

2. How would a nurse assess a family home for safety concerns? What would a checklist look like to guide a nurse in the assessment of a safe environment within a home?

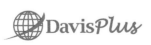

For additional resources and information, visit
www.DavisPlus.com.
Post-Conference Questions and Activities, Answers, and References can be found on DavisPlus.

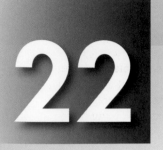

22

Health Promotion of the Toddler

KEY TERMS

autonomy
food lags and jags
iron-deficiency anemia
negativism
parallel play
separation anxiety
stranger anxiety
temperament

DavisPlus For audio pronunciation guide, visit www.DavisPlus.com

CHAPTER CONCEPTS

Bowel Elimination
Cognition
Comfort
Development
Elimination
Infection
Mobility
Nutrition
Promoting Health
Safety
Self
Sleep, Rest, and Activity

LEARNING OUTCOMES

1. Define the key terms.
2. Describe the unique needs of the toddler as compared with older children in relation to safety, bonding, communication, and development.
3. Describe the differences between toddlers and older children and adults in relation to body systems, anatomy, and physiology.
4. Compare the nutritional needs and eating patterns of the toddler including accurate kilocalorie needs and socialization at the dinner table.
5. Describe the need toddlers have for stimulation, play, and sleep to promote normal growth and development.
6. Differentiate the cognitive development during the toddler period including causality, spatial relationships, object permanence, and learning through toys.
7. Differentiate the psychosocial development of the toddler in relation to social engagement, temperament, stranger anxiety, separation anxiety, moral development, and spirituality.
8. Analyze the importance of discipline for the toddler and how anticipatory guidance can be used while families are caring for a toddler's social development, motor milestones, active lifestyle, injury prevention, and safety needs.
9. Describe child abuse during the toddler developmental period including assessment and interventions.
10. Describe the phenomenon of autism, which is often first noticed in the toddler developmental period.
11. Discuss the interventions that can assist a caregiver who is caring for a toddler experiencing iron-deficiency anemia.
12. List the assessments and interventions that assist a child experiencing common childhood infectious diseases.
13. Understand the importance of discussing safety issues for toddlers with parents including maintaining a safe environment for an active and explorative child.

REAL-WORLD CASE STUDY

Rachael

■ Rachael, a nursing assistant who is helping to care for a toddler girl hospitalized for cellulitis of the face requiring IV antibiotics, reports to the health-care team that the parents are planning on leaving for the day to attend to their other children and check in with work. The family told Rachael that the child can be left in the twin hospital bed for the day because they felt she would be content in watching movies and napping until their return. The nursing assistant explained to the parents the policy that toddlers who are left alone must be placed in a high-top "climber" crib designed to prevent children from crawling over the crib rails. The parents are quite upset and want to have permission to bypass the policy to make their toddler girl happy while they are away. The toddler has an IV in her left arm with the placement of a gauze wrap around the site to prevent her from seeing the site and pulling at it.

1. How should the nurse approach the family to discuss safety concerns? What are the safety concerns of leaving the toddler in a twin hospital bed unsupervised by parents?
2. What injuries could this toddler suffer because of the request to be left in the bed?
3. Who can the health-care team call to request assistance in this situation?

CONCEPTUAL CORNERSTONE

Safety

Safety is a large concern for the toddlers who want to explore their environment and do so independently. They quickly move from fast crawling to more efficient locomotion, mastering walking and then running. Whenever given the chance, toddlers may run away from parents and adults to explore a new environment or to see a new sight. Toddlers require constant supervision to be kept safe from such things as bodies of water (eg, lakes, pools, and rivers, as well as buckets or trashcans with water), playground structures, and traffic. They inherently do not understand and process rules for safety and may rebel against limitations. Toddlers enjoy climbing and quickly learn that by pulling a chair or stool over to a counter, they can climb up and reach items they desire. They are very curious and will open cabinets, storage closets, or any compartment. Tantrums, especially when told "no," is normal behavior but should be handled with care. Parents of toddlers have much to learn about safety and control. Pediatric nurses are in the perfect position to offer parents anticipatory guidance about how rapidly toddlers develop, how curious they are, and how inherently unsafe their actions may be.

The period of toddlerhood follows the rapid changing and exponential growth period of the infant. Toddlerhood, the period of time between the first birthday up to the child's third birthday, represents a slower period of growth in height and weight compared with infancy, but a fast period of growth in communication and other developmental milestones. The toddler understands his or her mastery over mobility and cruises through the environment at a faster and faster pace. Not all 1-year-old toddlers have learned to walk. With the average age of mastering walking being 9 to 16 months, the toddler may begin this developmental period with walking being the first major accomplishment. Very quickly the toddler develops a sense of exploration and is determined to get up, walk, and steady himself or herself, and will explore every inch of the environment.

SAFETY *STAT!*

Exploration and curiosity put a toddler at risk for injuries, accidents, and poisoning. It is very important that the nurse stress to the parents the importance of providing both a safe home environment and constant supervision for their toddler.

As compared with the infancy developmental stage, the toddler period is marked by a period of slow growth. Toddlers grow in a steplike pattern rather than a linear pattern. This steplike pattern is caused by sudden spurts of growth in height and weight, with lags that can be several months long.

The toddler period brings new challenges for parents. The toddler is very curious, very active, and will attempt to explore every inch of the home, leading to potential injuries and poisonings. The child may approach many interactions with negativity, choosing to use the word "no" as a source of growing independence and **autonomy** (ie, being self-governing). This can cause the parent or caregiver distress, so it is important that they understand this as a normal and healthy process for the child to express himself or herself. Toddlers are very impulsive and cannot be trusted for a second around a body of water such as a pond, pool, or bath tub. Raising a toddler can be very exhausting and the parent or caregiver needs reassurance and support.

SAFETY *STAT!*

Tantrums are common during the toddler period and the parents should not give in to the toddler's demand. The best way to handle a tantrum is to ignore the behavior while keeping the toddler safe.

GROWTH AND DEVELOPMENT OF THE TODDLER

The toddler developmental period is different from the infant in that the growth in height and weight slows down, the need for kilocalories is less, and the toddler is becoming very mobile. Safety becomes the primary concern for the toddler as the growing sense of autonomy, the desire to learn and explore, and the lack of safety judgment places the toddler at risk. Parents need to balance safety with encouragement to satisfy curiosity and manipulate objects (Ball, Bindler, et al, 2014).

Physical Growth and Development

The physical development of the toddler is quite different from the previous period of infancy. The toddler, through growth spurts, will grow an average of about 3 in. (7.62 cm) per year. On average, the parents of a toddler can be told that their child's height at 24 months typically represents half the expected height of the child at adulthood. For instance, if the child's height is 36 in., the parents can expect their toddler to be 72 in. as an adult, or 6 feet tall. The average 2-year-old is approximately 33 in. The annual weight gain of a toddler is 4 to 6 pounds (1.8 to 2.72 kg) per year. The parents should expect their 2½ year old to have an average weight of 27 pounds (12.24 kg) because their birth weight quadruples by this age.

Head circumferences (HCs) continue to be measured until at least 24 months of age. From the first birthday to the second, the toddler's HC equals the chest circumference. During the second year of life the HC will increase on average 1 inch per year, and the HC slows to 0.5 in. per year between the second and third birthday.

The toddler presents with a distinct stance. Their abdomens protrude because of their underdeveloped abdominal muscles (ie, lordosis; Fig. 22.1). The bowleggedness (ie, tibial torsion) of the walking older infant continues through early toddlerhood as the weight of their trunk produces a burden on the growing legs. These two distinct toddler characteristics are typically gone by the preschooler period.

The toddler typically walks by no later than 15 months. Some primary caregivers will want to see the toddler if they are not walking by 16 months. The toddler will walk up stairs, one at a time, holding an adult's hand, by 18 months. The toddler will walk up and down stairs, one step at a time, placing both feet on each step, at the average age of 24 months. Toddlers will jump with both feet at 30 months, and ride a tricycle by their third birthday.

The toddler will demonstrate far greater sophistication in their play as compared with the older infant. The toddler likes to scribble spontaneously at 15 months, and will attempt to build a tower with two to three blocks at 18 months. Toddlers are very exploratory (Fig. 22.2). Although quite uncoordinated, the toddler demonstrates rapidly greater mastery of his or her hands. In early toddlerhood the child will be clumsy, full of energy, and demonstrate an overwhelming desire to move around constantly. Although the growing toddler may seem like a supernova of unfocused movement, the physical skills development has a predictable sequence from cruising (ie, holding on to furniture) to walking to running to climbing to jumping, all within the course of several months.

During the toddler developmental stage, the child becomes a picky eater and slows down in his or her consumption. Fewer calories are required during the toddler period because this time is marked by slower growth. It is very important that the parents understand that the toddler's milk consumption should be monitored. No more than 24 to 32 ounces of milk should be consumed daily because this will greatly reduce the toddler's consumption of other sources of protein and vitamins. Calorie requirements for the toddler average 70-90 kcal/kg/day and protein requirements average 1.2 g/kg/day. During the beginning of the second year of life, the toddler should be eating the foods that the rest of the family is consuming, taking into account smaller portions for their decreased appetite and their need for their food to be chopped up to small bite-sized pieces to prevent choking. Emphasizing three complete meals and three snacks per day provides the toddler with their needed calories without having drops in blood glucose. Toddlers do not have the physiological ability to regulate their blood sugar well, so to prevent fluctuating blood glucose levels, a nutritious no-sugar snack should always be available.

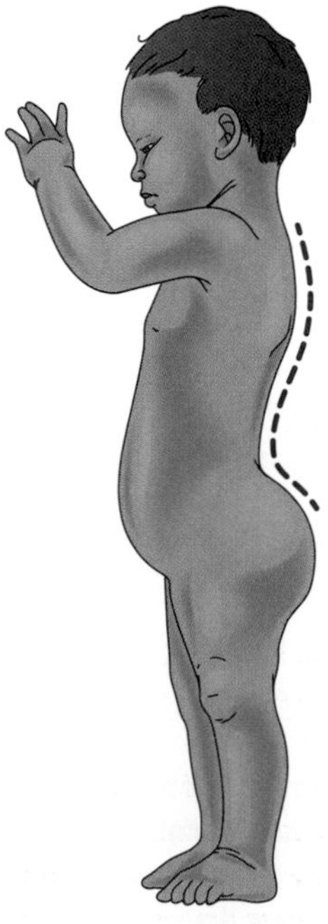

FIGURE 22.1 Toddler with exaggerated lumbar lordosis.

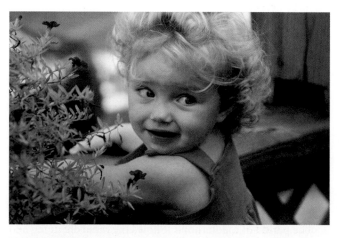

FIGURE 22.2 Toddler in a state of exploration.

SAFETY *STAT!*

Toddlers are at risk for **iron-deficiency anemia** (ie, fewer circulating red blood cells [RBCs] caused by a deficiency of dietary iron) associated with poor nutritional intake. Too much consumed milk fills the toddler up and he or she will not desire to eat the variety of foods needed during this time period.

Some parents worry about getting enough well-balanced nutrition into their toddler's diet. Adding chopped or pureed carrots and zucchini to spaghetti sauce, adding chopped fresh fruit to yogurt, making fresh fruit smoothies, or cooking apples with cinnamon and sugar are some ideas to increase intake of fruits and vegetables.

SAFETY *STAT!*

A rapid nutritional status assessment of a toddler includes three items: the child's hair is evenly dispersed across her head, the skin is not overly dry, and the child has neither the appearance of being underweight nor overweight (Rudd and Kocisko, 2014).

Toddlers should be given a spoon to try to eat on their own. Often they will hold the spoon in one hand, picking up their food in the other hand and putting the food in their mouths with their fingers. Giving the toddler a chance to eat their food with a spoon gives them a growing sense of autonomy, which is what they need to master. Patents need to allow for self-feeding opportunities (Ball, Bindler, et al, 2014). Finger foods are safe, provided they are not hard, posing a choking risk. A toddler should not be given hot dogs, raw carrots or celery, or peanuts because these foods carry the risk of aspiration and choking.

Fine motor milestones of the toddler should be encouraged by offering them challenging toys. Placing objects within appropriately shaped slots is a great way to encourage eye-hand coordination while introducing the toddler to shapes, colors, and mental challenges.

The normal vital sign ranges in the toddler period include a heart rate between 80 and 110 bpm, a respiratory rate between 23 and 25 breaths/min, systolic blood pressure between 90 and 105 mm Hg, diastolic blood pressure between 55 and 70 mm Hg, and an expected temperature of 37.2°C.

Nutrition

The toddler period marks an age of challenge in nutrition. Because they are at a slow rate of growth, their appetite decreases, they become erratic, and their kilocalorie needs change dramatically from infancy. Toddlers may display definite dislikes in certain foods and adamantly refuse to eat them; these are known as *food lags and jags.* "Food jags" occur when the child will be willing to eat only a few foods for several days (eg, peanut butter and jelly sandwiches, cold milk, and fruits). "Food lags" can be described as a very apparent lack of interest in eating and the missing of meals, much to the parents' distress and concern. These are normal behaviors and should be included in family teaching.

Toddlers at 1 year of life have an average weight of 10 kg (22.04 lb), and the 2- to 3-year-old's average weight increases to only 12 to 14 kg (26.45 to 30.86 lb). Over the period of time from the first to the third birthday, the toddler may only gain 4 kg, or 8.8 pounds. This is dramatically different from the infant who triples their birth weight. Estimated body weight for the toddler can be calculated by Weight (kg) = (Age in years + 4) multiplied by 2. The average kilocalorie need for a toddler ranges between 70 kcal/kg/day and 90 kcal/kg/day.

Assessment of nutritional status can be effectively done by conducting an oral intake history over a 3- to 5-day period using a food diary given to the parents or primary caregiver. When complete, a registered dietitian should assess the diary and make recommendations. The child should be observed for gross changes in body composition including edema, inadequate or excess adipose tissue, dehydration, and increased or decreased muscle mass. The child's height, weight, and body mass index should be assessed and plotted on growth charts (ie, World Health Organization [WHO] charts for children 0 to 2 years of age and Centers for Disease Control and Prevention [CDC] charts for children 2 years of age and older; see the WHO and CDC Web sites). Further evaluation and referrals should be made if the child's growth demonstrates being under the 5th percentile or above the 95th percentile.

LABS & DIAGNOSTICS

If there is an indication of malnutrition in the toddler, laboratory tests should be drawn, including a complete blood cell count (CBC) with differentiation, comprehensive electrolyte panel, and albumin.

SOCIALIZATION AT THE TABLE. Toddlers should be included at the family dining table. Although their attention span is short, they will benefit from the structure and socialization that occurs at the family meal. A young toddler should be placed in a high chair and an older toddler may be comfortable in a booster seat. The child should be allowed to participate in the conversation even if their language skills are limited. The child should be praised for participation and then be allowed to leave the table even if the other family members are not done eating. Toddlers have no concept of manners and they should not be expected to demonstrate them.

Sleeping Patterns and Requirements

The toddler requires, on average, 14 hours of sleep per day. During early toddler months, the child will move from two naps a day to one nap in the afternoon. Parents should be encouraged to not put their toddler down for a nap too late in the afternoon as this disrupts the bedtime routine. Putting the toddler down to sleep may carry the challenge of **separation anxiety.** The toddler fears being alone and may cause a parent distress; he or she will fight being put to bed, fearing the separation.

As months progress during the toddler period, the child may develop a particular desire for a bedtime routine. They may want the same book read to them a couple of times before bed each night for weeks on end, or they may want a sequence of events to take place just the same each night. For instance, using the toilet followed by a story, followed by three kisses, another story, a picture book, and then more kisses, in the same order every night. Parents should be encouraged to follow this routine whenever possible to create a sense of bedtime security.

Security items may become very important to the toddler. Typical security items may be a particular loved stuffed animal, a small soft blanket, or a particular toy. Sometimes the toddler has a surprising security item such as a necktie, a clothing item of the mother's, or some unexpected household item. It is very important that the pediatric nurse respect what is important to the child and protect it from loss or damage.

CULTURAL ASPECTS OF THE FAMILY BED. Many cultures around the world participate in the belief and practice of bed sharing. During the first year of life, parents should not sleep with their infants because of the risk of suffocation and injury. During the toddler period, in which the child expresses both the fear of the dark as well as separation anxiety, the family may practice the family bed. For young toddlers, the same concerns for injury remain and this should be discussed with the family so risks and benefits can be determined.

Cognitive Development

According to Piaget, the toddler period marks the sensorimotor cognitive development period. The toddler is experiencing two stages. First the child must experience trial and error experimentation to develop appropriate understanding of the environment. This is also the time of relentless exploration. The toddler is independently mobile and, while awake, needs constant play and stimulation. The second stage of this developmental period is marked by more complex mental combinations that allow the child to devise new means for task accomplishment.

Mastering the Environment

The toddler needs to master his or her environment. The toddler is actively exploring and experimenting throughout the environment to achieve what were previously unattainable goals. The toddler moves from crawling to standing to walking to running, all within a short period of time. This gives the toddler a real sense of autonomy and a deep desire to understand what is around him or her. It is very common to see a toddler explore the environment, pick up a toy or item, look at it, shake it vigorously to see if it makes noise, listen to it, smell it, lick it to see if there is a taste, and then throw it to see what happens. It is very important that the caregiver allows for this environmental exploration and experimentation because the toddler needs this for new learning and mastery of new skills.

Understanding Causality

Causality becomes important to the cognitive development of the toddler. As children explore their environment, they become aware that there is a causal relationship between two events. Turning on a light switch makes the room bright. Although the toddler learns that *x* causes *y*, he or she cannot then apply this to new situations. Parents will find that toddlers will explore the same cause and effect relationship over and over in new situations even if it was experienced in a previous situation. For example, sitting in a highchair at home, the toddler learns that if he or she drops her spoon, someone will reach over and pick it up over and over until the parent gets frustrated. When the child is at a grandparent's home or in a restaurant, he or she will do the same behavior over again to see what happens in this new environment.

Exploring Spatial Relationships

Spatial relationships are also being explored by the toddler, who is developing an awareness of shapes and sizes. A very good toy or activity for a toddler to practice these relationships is through the use of nesting cups, where the larger container must be placed below the smaller one as the tower is built. A toy that has several holes with specifically shaped blocks that require the toddler to identify which shape fits into which opening is also an effective way to practice spatial relationships. As their fine motor skills develop, mastery and speed over these types of activities improve rapidly.

Understanding Object Permanence

Toddlers enjoy the game of hide-and-go-seek, peek-a-boo, and challenges to object permanence. They enjoy searching for a favorite object that has been placed in a drawer, closet, or cupboard. By the end of the toddler period, the child will understand that if they drag a chair over to a counter or surface, the height will allow further access. This poses great dangers, so baby gates should be used throughout the toddler period to prevent injuries, burns, and access to toxic or harmful substances. Just telling a toddler "no, do not touch that," does not work to secure a safe environment.

SAFETY *STAT!*

It is imperative that parents secure toxic substances, medications, cleaning supplies, and dangerous objects such as scissors in locked cabinets or on high enough surfaces that toddlers cannot get them.

Learning Through Toys, Crafts, and Games

Toys, simple crafts, and games should be provided to challenge the toddler in both motor development and cognitive/psychosocial development. An appropriate selection of these activities will help the toddler to develop a sense of autonomy by letting the toddler perform developmentally appropriate tasks such as "cleanup," self-feeding, and beginning to self-dress. Undressing skills come long before dressing skills. Toddlers also enjoy imitating adults (Fig. 22.3).

Games and toys for toddlers can be divided into six areas (Table 22.1). All of these promote healthy development and improve motor skills.

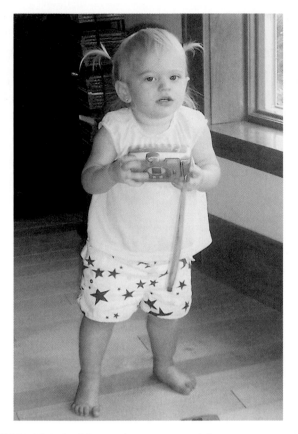

FIGURE 22.3 Toddler at play imitating adults.

Communication Development

Language development occurs rapidly in the toddler period (Table 22.2). The toddler begins the second year with only one to two words, ending the toddler period at the third birthday with between 300 to 500 words. The toddler will use two to three word sentences, learn to use pronouns, and will state their first and last name by 2½ years of age.

Multilingual families are rich in providing cultural experiences but may provide further challenges in language development. Households where two languages are spoken have been known to cause small delays in toddler language development. Homes with three or more spoken languages can cause further delays. The toddler may demonstrate an understanding of what is said around him or her, but responses may be delayed.

A direct link between a young child's language development and positive parenting has been found by Glascoe and Leew (2010). Researchers found that language development gaps occur in homes where the child is experiencing negative or problematic parenting. Talking, reading, and playing with young children are related to the development of language skills during the toddler period.

Psychosocial Growth and Development

According to Erikson's theory of psychosocial development, the crisis the toddler is experiencing is "autonomy versus shame and doubt." A parent can be highly influential in the mastery of autonomy, defined as functional independence, by providing not only opportunities for the toddler to demonstrate independence, but also by providing emotional support and encouragement to learn. The toddler may display frustration because this stage is marked by the need to learn to wait a little longer for need gratification and learn that his or her behaviors have a reliable and predictable effect on others.

The toddler period is marked by distinct psychosocial challenges. The toddler experiences a deep fear of the dark and should be provided a night light for sleep. The child might protest loudly at bedtime. If there is an expression of fear concerning the dark, the parent should not disagree or challenge the fears, but provide support. If the toddler has mastered the previous developmental stage of trust versus mistrust, then he or she is ready to give up dependence and start to assert autonomy and control. This may be distressing for a parent of a toddler because the child will say "no" frequently, demonstrate tantrums, and show an ever-increasing sense of individualism. Separation anxiety remains intact during the early toddler period, even though growing independence

TABLE 22.1 TOYS FOR TODDLERS

Activity	Examples	Rationale
Push/pull toys	Child grocery carts, large trucks/cars, popcorn popper with handle	Combines skills of pushing up/pulling
Rocking and rolling	Large plastic balls/soft mats	Provides motor control
Throwing and catching	Soft "Nerf" style foam balls	Promotes eye/hand/arm coordination
Climb and balance	Toddler outdoor structures	Encourages confidence and body balance
Running and jumping	Games with music	Promotes large motor coordination
Swimming/splashing	Safety flotation devices/noodles	Promotes large motor coordination and promotes confidence, but needs constant parent supervision

TABLE 22.2 LANGUAGE DEVELOPMENT OF THE TODDLER

Milestones in Expression	Age	Notes
First word:	11 months	Often "Ma-ma", "Da-da", "No", "Bye-bye"
Second word:	12 months	Needs audience, encouragement, and response
Jargon:	14 months	Truly enjoys interacting and soliciting a response, will talk in nonsensical language, making up sounds and words
Four–eight words:	16 months	Accumulation of words becomes exponential
Two-word sentences:	20 months	Examples include "Daddy bye-bye," "Mo milk"
Three-word sentences:	30 months	Toddler puts nouns and verbs together
Use of pronouns:	36 months of age	Understands "me," "my," and "you"

is important. The toddler may interpret separation as desertion. Toddlers also do not understand the depth of importance of items to others (part of egotistical thought) and will test this importance by manipulating other's possessions. This includes jewelry, eye glasses, car keys, and sentimental home belongings. A typical toddler will identify the importance of an item to an adult, pick it up, look right at the adult, and throw the item, waiting for the response to his or her triumph. The adult must keep calm, verbalize behavioral limits, and be consistent. All valuables must be out of sight and reach, and kept safe from toddlers. Again, the toddler period is marked with caregiver challenges and frustrations, so a safe environment free of potential catastrophes is essential. According to Sigmund Freud's theory of psychosexual development, the toddler is now experiencing the "anal" stage. This particular stage can last until the child is in the preschool period, up to four years of age. The buttocks and the anus are the sexual centers. The task requiring mastery is the cognitive awareness of the need for expulsion or retention of feces and urine as the toddler learns toilet skills. As the child gains neuromuscular control of the anus, more control is gained over toilet behaviors. When control is firmly established, the toddler feels mastery of "letting go or holding on."

Socialization

Toddlers understand they are members of a family. The family structure is very important to their development. Understanding roles and responsibilities during this time period helps them to understand family dynamics, interactions, and responsibilities. The toddler should be included in all family activities but will need constant supervision. Adapting the family activity to include a toddler may be stressful; the toddler participates in **negativism** (ie, a tendency of being negative in attitude), tantrums, and egocentric behavior. These behaviors should be discussed by the family and the importance of showing patience for the toddler's demands should be acknowledged. This is a difficult period for many because the toddler is unable to share without guidance and is only able to see the world through his or her own eyes.

Toddlers are slow to warm up to strangers and this poses specific challenges for health-care providers trying to assess and intervene for an ill child. Physical assessments are difficult because the young child will not cooperate nor can they be reasoned with.

TIPS ON ENGAGING TODDLERS. Pediatric nurses can use certain means to successfully engage a fearful or uncooperative toddler. Using hand or finger puppets to distract a young child during procedures, reading a simple and familiar book, and providing the child with a "magic wand" full of glitter suspended in oil or water can be helpful if the nurse needs cooperation.

TEAM WORKS

If a procedure is required to be performed in the treatment room, the child's safety should be secured first, such as a mummy wrap for an IV start, but whenever possible, the child should be provided a distracting age-appropriate toy. Solicit the assistance of a member of the Child Life team to come and assist during any procedure. They are masterful in engaging toddlers and distracting them during procedures.

STRANGER ANXIETY. **Stranger anxiety** is a very real experience for young children. Starting at about 9 months, the older infant protests when he or she is given over to someone else to be held and fears the new person in her presence. Stranger anxiety continues throughout the toddler period, lessening toward the end of the second year. The parent's response to the new person will greatly influence the child's responses to a new caregiver, child care provider, or overall new person to the family. For some young children, any new and unfamiliar situation or person can set the child off with an emotional response of anxiety; for other children, the reaction can be milder. Tips to lessen the child's stranger anxiety response are to establish a positive rapport with the parent first, then approach the child in a calm, quiet, and positive manner, encouraging engagement with smiles and soft words. The child should be offered a form of play from the nurse to engage the frightened child. Whenever possible, the nursing staff should plan care by the same providers to offer consistency and familiarity.

SEPARATION ANXIETY. When a toddler must be left alone in a hospital environment, having the parent leave a personal item may assist the toddler's fear of separation. The toddler is not yet able to understand the function of time, so it is not helpful to try to make a toddler understand that their parent will be back. The three stages of separation anxiety can be seen throughout the toddler period: protest, despair, and detachment. These stages of separation anxiety peak at 18 months and are readily apparent during hospitalizations. The duration of separation anxiety varies depending on the child but typically begins in late infancy and lasts until the child is older than three years of age.

- **Protest:** This is the first stage of separation anxiety from the primary caregiver. In this phase the toddler protests the separation with loud crying and may demonstrate physical aggression toward others. The toddler fights to cling on to the parents before they leave, then becomes agitated as he or she struggles to search for the parents. The toddler in this phase may be inconsolable and may need to be placed safely in a high-top crib to prevent him or her from climbing out. No items should be left in the bed other than his or her security item(s) because he or she may stack them to climb out of the crib.
- **Despair:** This is the second stage of separation anxiety. Here the young child becomes quiet, may lie on his or her side facing away from the door or others, and demonstrates behaviors of depression. The child may be disinterested in eating or refuse to eat. The toddler may refuse to participate in play activities or show great passivity in playing with favorite toys. This phase may last hours to days.
- **Detachment:** The third stage of separation anxiety is detachment, sometimes also referred to as *denial*. Here, the toddler demonstrates a slow reentry into interactions with others and play. Although the child is still detached, he or she may demonstrate an artificial adjustment to the separation from the parent. This phase is not always seen in the hospital, because lengths of stay are decreasing.

When pediatric nurses are aware of these three phases of separation anxiety, they can provide support and comfort to the child. Encourage the parents to never sneak out of the hospital while the toddler is sleeping or distracted. The toddler, although protesting will occur, should be told in a simple straightforward manner that the parent must leave and will come back. A personal item of the parent's can be left with the child as part of the comfort.

TEAM WORKS

The child may be highly resistant to interactions with the nurse in the protest phase, but later, as the child recognizes the nurse as the one who will provide for basic needs and play opportunity, improvements in behavior may occur.

INTRODUCTION TO CHILDCARE. Families often return to work before or during the toddler period. With the increasing need for both parents to work to make ends meet, safe and reliable child care becomes very important to secure. Since 1992, women with infants to care for have become the fastest-growing members of the contemporary workforce (Leifer, 2007). In some urban environments, it is difficult to secure child care for infants and toddlers because of competition and lack of selection. Some child care is provided in private homes, some licensed by the state and others not. Other alternatives include formal child care institutions of various sizes and child care facilities offered by city, region, or state offices. For instance, Head Start, a program offered by state funds, provides structured child care within settings for families with young children at no cost or low cost. Along with child care, the centers provide continuing education for providers and education seminars for parents on safety, nutrition, and local health provider referrals. Head Start programs provide screening of all of the children for nutrition, dental health, blood pressure, and height and weight measurements.

Making the decision about what type of child care a child will have may take considerable planning. Selecting from a nanny, a home child care environment, and a formal child care institution should include an assessment of the child's needs, family's needs, and the **temperament** (ie, the mental, physical, and emotional traits) of the child. A nanny provides consistency and one-on-one care, but a licensed care facility provides toddler socialization, structure, parent interaction, and a more stable arrangement versus an individual provider.

Parents can be offered assistance and support in the selection of a local child care facility. Web sites, such as the National Association for the Education of Young Children, offer ideas for selecting sites, curriculum styles, and site assessments. Offering parents a checklist to determine the right fit for their needs and the child's temperament can help with the anxiety parents can feel about providing safety for their young child while they work. See Table 22.3 for an example of such a checklist.

Moral Development

Kohlberg's theory describes the toddler period as the preconventional stage in which punishment, obedience, and obtaining rewards are the central focus of the child's moral development. How and when a parent disciplines the toddler highly affects the young child's moral development. With egocentrism and the inability to see others' points of view, the toddler develops a negative view of morals because privileges are withheld and punishments are applied. It is extremely important that the parent or caregiver provide the young child a developmentally appropriate explanation as to why he or she is being punished. Examples include telling the child immediately, as he or she is being placed in a time-out, a simple explanation that running into the street is dangerous because cars might hit him or her, or that touching the tools in the garage is dangerous because he or she may get hurt.

TABLE 22.3 CHECKLIST FOR SELECTING SAFE CHILDCARE

Items to Investigate	Diversity in Settings
Types of providers	• Family home care in private homes • Child care centers (eg, nursery schools, preschools) • In-home caregivers (eg, nanny, babysitter) • Shares, where several families get together to share one provider • Play group exchanges • Babysitting co-ops, where parents rotate caring for their children and others • Child care facilities that specialize in children with special needs/technology dependence
Licensing and accreditation	• All child care providers of licensed facilities take a 15-hour course called *Early Childhood Education* (ECE) that includes cardiopulmonary resuscitation (CPR) and basic first aid
Teacher preparation	• Some facilities have providers with early childhood education degrees
Child-to-staff ratio	• State regulated; often 4:1 for infants, 6:1 for toddlers (check state regulations)
Curriculum	• Structured or free play • Use of standardized toddler curriculum
Napping stations	• Cots versus lying on floor; quiet, clean; flexible for children to rise on their own time
Schedules	• Flexible hours or rigid for all participants
Costs	• Daily, weekly, or monthly fee, early drop off or late pickup fees • Forms of payment, fees for late payments
Site visit checklist	• Visit first without child and then second visit with child • Facility philosophy, mission, goals, length of time in business, staff turnover • Written emergency response plan and posted emergency numbers • Published guidelines for child with food allergies • First impressions of safety; first impression of child • Children with joy, engaged in play, interacting with providers • Quality, quantity, and safety of toys present • Type of discipline used, consistency and appropriateness, alignment with family values and practices • Well lit, clean, organized, attractive • Toilet-training facilities, hand washing station and practices, support for training, praise/rewards • Kitchen facilities clean, selection of food served, teachers eating with children

Temperament

Parents will describe to the nurse how "different" each of their children's temperaments are. Each child is different and unique. Temperament refers to the combination of mental, physical, and emotional traits of a person, marking the toddler's predisposition for interactions with others and the environment. The toddler's temperament will influence how he or she views the environment by providing a unique personal attitude or nature toward feelings, reactions, and social makeup.

Some toddlers are prone to frequent tantrums. Preventing and managing tantrums take skill on the part of the parent. Not giving in to the toddler's demands is very important because the child learns quickly that the tantrum works in gaining what

is wanted, and therefore reinforces the negative behavior. Whenever possible, the parent needs to ignore the behavior while keeping the child safe. Tantrums can be so severe that the child holds his or her breath or falls to the floor, hitting the head.

An appropriate and successful way to approach a toddler is to offer two choices. The choices should be visual (eg, this toy or that) or the choices should be offered in a comprehensible manner. For instance, if the pediatric nurse needs to administer an oral antibiotic, the toddler should be offered not whether or not to take the medication, but whether they want to have it mixed with chocolate syrup or cherry syrup, making sure the toddler understands that the medication will be taken.

DISCIPLINE. Discipline is very important in the toddler stage. The young child demonstrates frustrations, and then acts out of anger via tantrums. This is normal and universal behavior for a toddler and can be found regardless of culture, ethnicity, or socioeconomic level. No discipline beyond the use of the word "no" should ever be shown during the infancy period, so the concept of discipline is new to the toddler. When a toddler demonstrates unwanted or unsafe behaviors such as writing with crayons on the wall, jumping on the bed, or running out the front door of the family home, the discipline mechanism of choice is time-outs. Time-outs should begin early in the toddler period with a very short removal of the child from his or her activity and play, and then not interacting with the child. As the toddler gets older, the time-out period should also extend. According to Muscari (2001), the length of the time-out should be 1 min for each year of life, increasing as the child grows. It is acceptable if the family chooses to use a time clock such as a cooking timer with a bell to alert the child when the time-out is over. It is better for the child if this is used regularly during the time-out.

Consistency is an essential component of positive discipline. All caregivers should be in agreement about providing the toddler with a consistent discipline program. Discipline should be initiated immediately after the misbehavior, planned in advance, oriented to the behavior itself and not to the child, and should be conducted in private and in a nonshame–inducing fashion (Muscari, 2001). The toddler needs to associate the unwanted behavior with the subsequent discipline to learn what is and what is not acceptable.

Caregivers should never try to reason, threaten, promise, hit, or give in to a toddler having a tantrum. Overcriticizing and restricting may cause increased feelings of shame and doubt. Patience is required with toddlers' persistent use of the word "no" and their growing assertiveness. Box 22.1 lists ideas for discipline during the challenging toddler period.

Play

The toddler has moved from individual play to **parallel play** (Fig. 22.4). The toddler will desire to play near, or actually alongside, another toddler, but will not yet want to share toys or craft supplies. Often the parent or caregiver will see toddlers play back to back, almost touching, but not interacting with their play activities. Sharing is a learned process that requires parental intervention and positive reinforcement. Toys are quickly played with and often discarded for the next new experience. The toddler is happiest with a variety of large, colorful toys all within reach. Their energy levels allow them to be quite active, progressing from toy to toy, or activity to activity, quite rapidly.

Appropriate types of toddler play are those that promote learning, challenges, and stimulation of all of their senses. Toys should be large, colorful, and safe by being free of detachable parts. Young toddlers will still explore certain items orally, leaving them at risk for choking and aspiration. Large dolls with clothes that come off and on easily with Velcro and snaps, play phones, busy boards, and cloth books are excellent choices for the toddler. They are able to build

---

Box 22.1 Ideas for Discipline During the Toddler Years

- Immediate positive reinforcement for good or wanted behavior
- Ignoring unwanted behavior and tantrums
- Distracting the young child from participating in unsafe or unwanted behaviors
- Keeping routines simple and consistent, such as at meal times and bedtimes
- Setting reasonable limits; giving simple rationales as to why the behavior is unsafe or unwanted
- Trying to provide two selection choices when possible
- Identifying if the toddler is being intentionally destructive or is exploring the environment with unintentional vigor; decide then if discipline is warranted or if the child needs instructions
- Always following through on discipline, not just stating threats of time-outs or toy removal
- Becoming aligned with spouse and/or other caregivers

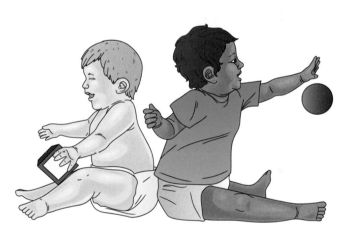

FIGURE 22.4 Parallel play.

towers of three to four blocks, and truly enjoy building, knocking over, and building again. Towers that require the toddler to stack larger blocks on the bottom provide added challenges.

Toilet Training

Toilet training is a universal task of early childhood. The toddler period is the most common time that a child masters this task because the child tends to be both physiologically and psychologically ready (Box 22.2). Assessment of readiness can be found when the toddler demonstrates certain behaviors, including being able to stay dry for 2-hour periods of time, the ability to sit and squat, and having regular bowel movements. Emotional readiness is demonstrated by the child's desire to willfully please the parents, as well as being able to verbalize the desire to void or produce a bowel movement. Because the young child has full

Box 22.2 Psychological Readiness for Toilet Training

- Toileting training begins with emotional readiness
- Toddler acts to please others
- Toddler will imitate others who he or she can see using the toilet
- Feeling of wetness or messiness leads to personal motivation
- Toddler will remove clothes, walk to the potty, and sit on it on his or her own
- Begin potty sitting at 18 months, without expectations
- Toddlers should achieve day dryness by age 18 months and night dryness by second to third year
- If toddler is not trained by 5 years of age, seek further evaluation
- Toddler may fear being sucked into toilet
- Toddler may fear the sound of a loud flush
- Toddler will demonstrate great curiosity with excrement
- Toddler girl will not wipe front to back and must be taught to prevent urinary tract infections (UTIs)
- Stressors such as illnesses and hospitalizations cause regression; toilet training may need to be retaught

kidney function and anal sphincter control by 2 years of age, toilet training should not be expected to start until after this time. Typically, the child demonstrates fecal control before bladder control. The young child must master the act of toileting and have the willingness to let go of waste on command.

Wanting to Watch a Family Member

Toddlers often learn about their environment from watching others interact and perform duties. Toilet training is no different. It is not uncommon to see a toddler drag his or her little chair into the bathroom to watch how a parent or sibling goes to the bathroom. Watching others pull up or down clothing, sit comfortably on the toilet, defecate and urinate, and use bathroom tissue is intriguing to the toddler while they are learning toilet training. This watching may be acceptable to some families and not acceptable to others.

Assistive Devices for Toilet Training

The toddler should have a specific age-appropriate toilet when toilet training. Small plastic or wooden child toilets are available and are an excellent choice to assist the child. The child's toilet should be placed where the toddler has access to it. It may take the child several attempts to learn to sit on the device. At first the toddler may choose to sit on the potty fully clothed. Later, after a successful attempt, the toddler may want to drag the potty chair around the house and keep

it nearby. Praise should be offered at each attempt. The potty should be emptied immediately, because the toddler will want to manually explore their "prize" after a successful defecation. Toddlers need supervision with both the child potty chair and the full-size toilet; they may place toys or objects in the toilet or use the water for play.

A wonderful book to purchase or check out from the local library is titled *Everyone Poops* by Taro Gomi (Kane/Miller Book Publisher, 2001). This delightful developmentally appropriate children's book demonstrates the daily regimen of defecation and shows members of the animal world and people participating in toileting. The book can be seen as humorous but is also quite educational for the young child learning the ropes.

Positive Reinforcement

The most important aspects of toileting training are providing the young child with enough time to master the act, being patient with accidents, and providing lots of positive reinforcement. Some families reward the young child with a small treat after each attempt, as well as smiling, clapping, and stating, "Good job! We are proud of you!" This is a very important step in a child's autonomy, or independent function, and the parent, caregiver, or nurse's response to the child's attempts and successes are very important to the child. Even while hospitalized, toilet training should continue. The nurse needs to explain to the family that regressive behaviors are common and toddlers may lose or regress in their toilet training skills while hospitalized.

ANTICIPATORY GUIDANCE FOR PARENTS OF THE TODDLER

Preventing injuries during the toddler period is of ultimate importance; the toddler wants to exert autonomy. Every room of the home, the garage, and the front and back yards need to be assessed for potentially dangerous items or situations. A trashcan with only a few inches of standing water poses a drowning risk because the toddler may step on something, fall head first into the receptacle, not be able to push himself or herself up, and drown. Every year, thousands of toddlers experience severe injuries, drowning, and accidents as their natural tendency to explore without understanding consequences leads them to dangerous situations. Anticipatory guidance aids the pediatric nurse in teaching parents and caregivers of toddlers to identify harmful situations and avoid tragic consequences. Some families use harnesses to promote safety (Fig. 22.5).

Dentition

The toddler's tooth eruption pattern includes the presentation of 10 to 14 deciduous, or baby teeth, for a total of 20 teeth by the third birthday. The first and second molars and canines erupt. Processed sugar, which is known as a *cariogenic substance,* should be minimized and the toddler's teeth should be brushed twice a day. To promote success and decrease negativity during toothbrushing, the toddler should be given a large

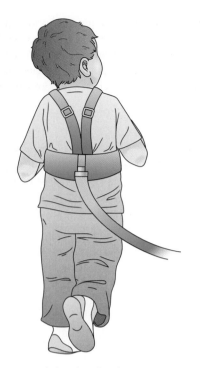

FIGURE 22.5 A single-leash safety harness.

soft-bristled toothbrush to hold and play with while the parent proceeds with actually brushing the child's teeth with another toothbrush. Only a very small amount of nonfluoride toothpaste should be used during this period because the toddler will swallow the fluoride foam, which can be toxic. Regular toothbrushing at this age sets the child up for tooth hygiene throughout childhood. Flossing a toddler's teeth poses challenges but should be attempted on a regular basis until accepted by the child. The toddler should be seen by a dentist by the third birthday. Parents should be encouraged to investigate if their community water supply is fluoridated. If not, a discussion with the pediatrician should take place concerning the addition of fluoride supplements into the child's daily nutrition.

Tooth decay can occur during late infancy and toddlerhood (Fig. 22.6). At no time should a young child be put to bed with a bottle of juice or milk. Toddlers do not need refined sugar, and sweets should be eliminated or reduced.

Visual and Auditory Acuity

The toddler's sensory organs continue to mature. Visual acuity continues to progress from 20/200 during the infancy period

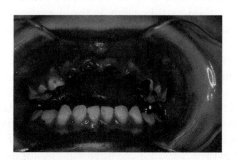

FIGURE 22.6 Tooth decay in a toddler.

to 20/40 to 20/60 in the toddler period. A toddler's hearing acuity is completely intact. Although a hearing screening test should have been completed in infancy, and is not conducted again until the child is seen for the prekindergarten well-child check, the pediatric nurse should question the family about any hearing concerns, especially if there has been a history of inner ear infections. With a pattern of inner ear infections, the toddler may have a conductive hearing loss, which warrants further screening and possible interventions. Because the period of toddlerhood marks a tremendous growth in vocabulary, it is important that the toddler is not delayed in speech development caused by a hearing impairment.

Home Safety

As difficult as it may be, the toddler needs constant supervision. Although the toddler is very demanding, it is imperative that the family provide a safe home. Toddlers are at great risk for the ingestion of toxic substances; they continue to mouth many items in their environment, and they will try to explore unsafe areas of the home to make new discoveries. Toddlers cannot be trusted because they are very active every minute they are awake and they have increasingly accelerated locomotion, running away when then can. Safety gates are important to prevent toddlers from exploring unsafe rooms such as the kitchen, garage, and bathroom without supervision, or attempting to master stairs before they are developmentally ready.

Kitchen Safety

The kitchen poses extreme risks for the fast-moving and exploring toddler. It is essential that kitchen cabinets and drawers have child-proof locks placed on them. These devices are relatively inexpensive and can be purchased at most drug or hardware stores. Handles from cooking pots must be directed away from the front of the stove, and only the back burners should be used. Stove and oven buttons should be removed or a device placed on them to prevent a toddler from turning the oven or stove on. Drinks that are not hot should be within reach of a toddler so they are not climbing in an attempt to reach drinks that may be hot. Providing one unlocked cabinet with safe plastic tubs and pots and pans allows toddlers to have their own play center where they can interact with the parent and make loud noises while banging the pots together, but still be maintained in a safe environment.

Gates and Barriers

Child safety gates and barriers should be purchased and established before the infant begins to rapidly crawl, and long before the toddler walks. Safety gates should protect the child from the kitchen area, the bathroom, any pets who are not yet well established with the presence of the child, and on top of any stairs, even just one step. Several models are available that have either swinging doors or levers that allow the parent quick access to the next room. Under no circumstances should the toddler have free rein of the house or ever be left without supervision in the kitchen, bathroom, or near the front door.

Swimming Pools

Pools create another level of safety risk. Toddlers are very explorative and fast in their movements. Two locked gates should separate the young child from the family swimming pool. Toddlers have drowned when they crawl through a pet door out into the back yard and into the pool. A drowning can be silent because the child is too young to know to fight to rise to the surface. A complete safety check must be performed on a regular basis. Pool covers should not be seen as a mechanism for safety because toddlers will walk out on them, fall through, become trapped below the surface, and drown.

Only federally approved swim safety devices or swim suits should be used. Upon purchasing, the parent should look for a label that describes safety approval. At no time should a toddler be left to float in a flotation device; the parent should have their hand on the child and floatation device at all times (Fig. 22.7).

Until more clear-cut scientific evidence exists on the effects of infant and toddler aquatic programs, the American Academy of Pediatrics (AAP) Committee on Sports Medicine and Fitness recommends the following (AAP, 2000; AAP, 2010):

- Children are generally not developmentally ready for formal swimming lessons until after their fourth birthday.
- Aquatic programs for infants and toddlers should not be promoted as a way to decrease the risk of drowning, as even advanced swimmers can drown.
- Parents should not feel secure that their child is safe in water or safe from drowning after participation in such programs.
- Whenever infants and toddlers are in or around water, an adult should be within an arm's length, providing "touch supervision."
- All aquatic programs should include information on strategies for prevention of drowning, and the role of adults in supervising and monitoring the safety of children in and around water.

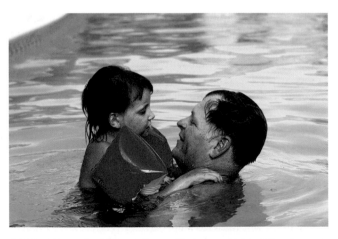

FIGURE 22.7 Toddler using a safety swim device. *(From National Institutes of Health. Retrieved from http://visualsonline. cancer.gov/details.cfm?imagineid=2097)*

- Hypothermia, water intoxication, and communicable diseases can be prevented by following existing medical guidelines and do not preclude infants and toddlers from participating in otherwise appropriate aquatic experience programs.

Preventing Accidental Poisoning

Young children are at risk for ingesting toxic substances, especially during infancy and toddlerhood. Crawling infants, active toddlers, and curious preschoolers are at extreme risk for coming in contact with toxic substances and tasting them as part of their exploration. Common toxic exposures leading to poisoning include:

- Acetaminophen or salicylate toxicity or overdose
- Iron or lead
- Carbon monoxide
- Alcohol
- Anticholinergics
- Antihistamines
- Toxic plants
- Muscle relaxants
- Opioids, narcotics, benzodiazepines, and barbiturates
- Cardiac medications such as calcium channel blockers and digoxin
- Tricyclic antidepressants
- Paint thinners
- Certain cosmetics
- Car antifreeze

Suspected overdose or poisoning managements include a four-step process:

1. **Ensure adequate ABCDs:** Step one is to ensure the young child has adequate ABCDs (ie, airway, breathing, circulation, and disability/minineurological examination).
2. **Empty the child's mouth:** Step two is to terminate exposure by emptying the young child's mouth. Under no circumstances should vomiting be induced until informed to do so by the poison control center. The poison should be washed from the eyes per instruction and the child's clothes should be removed and skin washed as instructed.
3. **Identify the poison:** Step three is to identify the poison. The child, family, caregiver, and any witnesses should be questioned about the type of substance, amount consumed, and time of consumption. All parties should look for environmental clues such as empty containers, nearby spills, and odor on breath, and all evidence, such as containers, vomitus, and urine, should be saved. The child must be taken to the closest emergency room for immediate care (911 should be called for transport).
4. **Prevent poison absorption:** The final step in the process is to prevent poison absorption. The child should be positioned in a side-lying fashion and the drug antidote, or activated charcoal PO or by nasogastric tube (NGT), should be administered as directed by the poison control center (even the emergency room personnel will call for assistance

from this national organization). The child may require whole bowel irrigation with polyethylene glycol electrolyte solution, a cathartic such as magnesium citrate or sulfate, or the performance of a gastric lavage may be warranted. The nurse should monitor for symptoms of shock and a full body systems assessment should be done. The family will be in great emotional turmoil and will need support and clear communication during the resuscitative process.

DRUG FACTS

The poison control center should be called immediately for guidance in treatments by calling 1-800-222-1222. The family should attempt to locate the poisonous substance and be able to state the time since ingestion, if possible.

Car Seat Safety

During the toddler period, the young child will transition from a backward-facing infant car seat to a toddler transitional car seat. There are many products available. If the family is going to use a previously owned toddler car seat, they should be instructed to research the product's continued safety by contacting the manufacturer. Once the young toddler is more than 20 pounds and older than 1 year, he or she can be placed forward-facing in the center seat in a transitional car seat. See the National Highway Traffic Safety Administration Web site for further guidelines.

An air bag can save an adult's life. However, air bags and young children are a dangerous mix. The following information is provided as guidelines to help keep young children safe:

- The safest place for *all* infants and children younger than 13 years to ride is in the back seat.
- *Never* put an infant or toddler in the front seat of a car, truck, SUV, or van with an air bag.
- Infants must always ride in rear-facing car safety seats in the back seat until they are at least 20 pounds AND at least 1 year of age. Infants ride rear-facing until they reach the maximum weight and height allowed by the manufacturer for use of the car safety seat.
- All children should be properly secured in car safety seats, belt-positioning booster seats, or the shoulder/lap belts correct for their size.
- Seat belts must be worn correctly at all times by all passengers who have outgrown booster seats; fit shoulder/lap belts properly to provide the best protection.
- Side air bags improve safety for adults in side-impact crashes, but children who are not properly restrained and are seated near a side air bag may be at risk for serious injury. Vehicle owner's manuals should provide information about side air bags.

SCREENING AND HEALTH PROMOTION FOR THE TODDLER

During the toddler period, the recommendation is for the child to be seen three times: at 15 months, 18 months, and 24 months. At the first two visits, immunizations are administered. At the 24-month visit, the child will have his or her blood drawn for hemoglobin and lead levels. Wellness promotion is stressed at these well-child visits and the results of the screening exams are explained to the parents or caregiver (Table 22.4).

SAFETY PROVIDED TO THE TODDLER WHILE HOSPITALIZED

Hospital environments are inherently unsafe for young toddlers who have mastered locomotion. The toddler's incessant desire to move, explore, investigate, and manipulate objects leaves him or her at great risk for injuries while in a hospital setting, whether the setting is an exclusive children's hospital or a traditional hospital serving those across the lifespan. Toddlers require constant supervision when out of their high-top cribs, and frequent assessments even when in the metal cribs. Nurses need to check on toddlers on a frequent basis and, if medically indicated, the toddler's hospital room door should remain open at all times.

The toddler child may become aggressive while hospitalized because of loss of autonomy, confinement, separation from family members, separation from familiar home environment and toys, and from the constant flux of new strangers interacting with them. The nurse must be prepared for a toddler to aggressively fight against any procedure. Asking for assistance in a gentle restraining position is imperative during

TABLE 22.4 RECOMMENDATIONS FOR WELL-TODDLER CHECKUPS

Assessments:	15 months	18 months	24 months

History
  Family
    routines
  Sleep habits
  Nutrition
  Home
    safety
  Toilet
    training
  Tantrums/
    negativity
	X	X	X

Physical exam
  Growth
    patterns
  Fine and
    gross motor
    skills
  Skin
    integrity
	X	X	X

Screenings
  Hearing
  Lead
	X	X	X

Hemoglobin			X
Immunizations*	X	X	
Nutrition	X	X	X

Anticipatory
  guidance
  education
	X	X	X

*Immunizations: At 15 months the toddler should have hepatitis B (hep B); *Haemophilus influenza* type B conjugate (Hib); diphtheria, pertussis, and tetanus (DTaP); measles, mumps, and rubella (MMR); and varicella zoster virus (VZV) for chicken pox.

At 18 months the toddler should have hep B, DTaP, and VZV.

even minor procedures. Vital sign measurements may be very difficult to assess in a toddler. If possible, the nurse should take vital signs when the toddler is sleeping or resting in the parent's arms.

Medicating Toddlers

Toddlers can be profoundly difficult to administer medications to. During medication administration, the nurse can expect resistance, negativity, and aggression from the toddler. Assume a young child will be uncooperative and secure assistance for positioning or use of gentle, appropriate restraining holds. Try to offer a toddler two choices concerning oral medical administration such as offering to mix the medication with two different syrup flavors to mask the medication taste. Allow the older toddler to take the medicine cup or syringe and administer the medication under strict supervision if appropriate. A young toddler may take the cup or oral medication syringe and throw it. Never call medications "candy" to any age child. Do not leave medications at the bedside, in unlocked drawers in the patients' room, or on a food tray. Mix the toddler's oral medications in the smallest amount of fluid as possible to have a greater chance of the entire dose being consumed. Do not mix medications in a cup of juice or any other larger volume because the young child will most likely not consume the entire quantity. Discourage stalling behaviors; be calm and firm.

Solicit the parent's or caregiver's assistance whenever possible. Assume the child will go home on the oral medication; including caregivers' assistance helps to empower them to administer the medication at home. Compliment the child for taking the medication and give positive reinforcement with the presentation of a sticker or small token.

Safe Sleeping Practices and Policies

Parents who have their toddler hospitalized may want to share a big bed with their child rather than place the child into a covered crib. This poses safety risks. Toddlers who wake up when their parent is not present will quickly climb out of bed to seek the family member. Even a quick trip to the restroom or shower gives the unattended toddler the opportunity to go searching. Young toddlers may fall out of the large bed, get caught in the upper side rails, or suffer an injury by climbing. Most hospitals do not allow toddlers to sleep with their parents outside of the crib and will publish rules on this behavior. The nurse may be held responsible for an injury caused by allowing the toddler to sleep in a big bed. This behavior must be monitored for and institutional rules should be explained to prevent the toddler from becoming injured.

Ideas for Play

Hospitalized toddlers pose special challenges for the pediatric nurse. Toddlers are not at ease in the hospital setting and require a development of trust. Having consistent caregivers assists with the development of trust. The toddler, depending on type of illness, will want to participate in play activities offered by Child Life specialists. Soliciting the help of members of the Child Life team can prove to be invaluable. If the child's illness allows him or her to leave the room (ie, no infectious diseases or immunocompromised immune system) then the toddler should be given opportunities to participate in age-appropriate activities in the play room. If the child is confined to the room, toys and simple crafts should be provided under supervision. At no time should scissors be left at the bedside. Toddlers have been known to cut their urinary catheter tubing, central line catheters, and IV tubing with scissors.

Appropriate toddler toys for the hospitalized child include finger paints, clay, plastic dinosaurs, dolls, busy boards, puzzles with very large pieces, and large blocks. Toys that make noise, such as music boxes and airplanes with runway sounds, are enjoyable.

or caregivers of toddlers in preventing injuries that could be life-threatening or cause serious harm.

■ INJURY PREVENTION FOR THE TODDLER

Parents must understand the need to provide adequate and constant supervision for children in the toddler developmental stage. Table 22.5 provides specific guidelines for parents

■ DISORDERS OF THE TODDLER

Certain disorders are more commonly found in the toddler period than during the rest of the childhood. Pediatric nurses should become familiar with the basics of these disorders so

TABLE 22.5   INJURY PREVENTION TIPS DURING TODDLERHOOD

Injury	Injury Prevention Guidelines
Suffocation	Do not leave any plastic wrapping, dry cleaning bags, plastic grocery bags, or crib mattress plastic covers within reach of the toddler. Explain to the child and older siblings how dangerous it is to place plastic bags over the head. Do not allow young children to play around or in appliances such as the washing machine, dryer, or refrigerator. Do not allow older siblings to place a pillow over the toddler's head during play.
Choking and Asphyxiation	Always cut the toddler's food into small bite-size pieces. Toddlers should not be given foods with the highest choking risk, such as hot dogs, carrots, whole grapes, ice cubes, or hard candies. Do not allow older siblings to feed a young toddler until they are old enough to understand the child's need to chew thoroughly before the next bite. Asphyxiation occurs when the child who is choking cannot exchange air and dies. Toddlers should not be allowed to walk around or run while eating or with food in their mouths. It is good practice to insist from an early start that the young child sits throughout all snacks and meals.
Drowning	Toddlers are at high risk for drowning in even a small pool of water. Do not leave toddlers unsupervised in the bath tub. Never leave buckets or trashcans of standing water near the house. Provide the required double-locked gating system around pools. Never allow a toddler to swim alone; always be touching the child or within arm's reach. Only use federally approved swim safety devices and swim safety suits.
Electrocution	Always place safety covers on all electrical outlets in every room in the house. Do not let toddlers play with electrical equipment or with electrical cords. They are too young to understand the danger of electrical appliances being around water. Do not store curling irons, hair dryers, or electric shavers anywhere near bathroom sinks or tubs. Do not leave electrical appliances plugged in around the kitchen where a toddler can drag a chair over and reach.
Animal Bites	Even well-behaved pets can turn aggressive toward a playful toddler. Toddlers do not understand how to be gentle when playing with animals. Do not allow a toddler to approach a restrained dog or pet an unfamiliar dog because many are not comfortable with children and will bite. Cats will readily scratch an aggressive toddler. Cat scratches are especially dangerous because of the potential to transmit bacteria (*Bartonella henselae*) that often requires antibiotic therapy
Traffic Safety and Playing Outdoors	Toddlers will readily chase a ball out into traffic. It is important to stress to the toddler that he or she must look before crossing, but the caregiver should not trust a toddler around a street. Developmentally, they cannot process caution and safety around traffic. Toddlers require constant supervision when playing outdoors. Some families choose to use chest harnesses when taking their toddler to busy areas. Harnesses can be basic, where the parent holds a "leash" style handle, or there is also a "belt to belt" style. Harnesses allow exploration while avoiding dangers by containing the child. Some associate harnesses with animal control practices and are against their use, while others say harnesses are less restraining than strollers.

Continued

TABLE 22.5   INJURY PREVENTION TIPS DURING TODDLERHOOD—cont'd

Injury	Injury Prevention Guidelines
Falls and Climbing	Toddlers will readily drag a chair over to reach a taller surface. Prevent injuries in the kitchen, especially around the stove, by using baby gates to prevent access to dangerous home areas.
Motor Vehicle Accidents	Always use federally approved and size-appropriate car seats when transporting children. Place the child in the center of the back seat. Children younger than 12 years or under 100 pounds should not be in the front seat with an air bag because severe injuries, including decapitation of small children, have occurred. See the AAP for further information on air bag safety.
Burns	Burn injuries can occur during toddlerhood in both the kitchen and the bathroom. Water heaters should be turned below 48.9°C (120°F). Toddlers should wear a high SPF sunscreen on all exposed skin while in the sun, even for short periods of time, and it should be reapplied after sweating or swimming. Toddlers should be required to wear hats while outdoors.
Bodily Damage	Toddlers should never have access to sharp items such as needles or scissors that are not child safety scissors. Children should not run around the home holding items near their face; impalements occur with such items as pens, pencils, toothbrushes, and kitchen utensils. Never remove an impaled object until the child has been transported to an emergency room because excessive bleeding and further tissue damage can occur.

they can be of assistance in early identification and intervention. Four of the most common disorders are child abuse, iron-deficiency anemia, autism, and common infectious diseases. In addition to the information included in the sections that follow, all of these disorders are addressed in a more in-depth discussion in subsequent chapters.

Child Abuse

Child abuse is most commonly seen in the infancy and toddler period. Child abuse is also called *child maltreatment* and is considered a nonaccidental injury or trauma that leads to sexual violation, emotional trauma, physical harm, or death. Child abuse is considered an intentional act of abuse (eg, physical abuse, such as traumatic injuries, or emotional abuse, such as consistent belittling) or neglect (eg, such as not providing for the child's medical, nutrition, clothing, and supervision needs). Categories of child abuse include physical abuse, physical neglect, emotional abuse, emotional neglect, verbal abuse, and sexual abuse. Infants, toddlers, and preschoolers are the most common victims of physical abuse, whereas school-age children and adolescents encounter emotional abuse and sexual abuse more often.

Contributing Factors

Contributing factors are categorized in three areas: child factors, parental/abuser factors, and environmental factors.

Although not all of the factors will be present in each case of abuse, they should be considered as influencing factors.

- **Child Factors:** These factors include the child being a special needs child, technology dependent, having a difficult or demanding temperament, having learning disabilities, being premature with or without a congenital anomaly, or those with a chronic illness.
- **Parental/Abuser Factors:** These factors include adults who are having substance abuse or addictions, unemployed, experiencing frequent moves, socially isolated, at the age of adolescence, experiencing multiple stressors, lacking parenting skills, having anger control issues and/or a low tolerance for frustration, having low self-esteem or low confidence, and who have experienced abuse in his or her own life.
- **Environmental Factors:** These factors include the family living in low-income, unsafe neighborhoods; being of low economic status themselves; living in areas of low employment rates; living in crowded conditions; and having a lack of educated adults present. Keep in mind that child abuse can occur in any socioeconomic level.

Prevention Strategies

Prevention strategies include parenting classes for young parents or high-risk parents, promotion of role modeling from other family members, encouragement of respite care for stressed caregivers, education to prevent shaken baby syndrome, and support groups for parents who are socially isolated.

Assessment and Reporting

Assessment includes the type, location, and severity of the injury, with meticulous documentation and reporting, and the assessment of incompatibility between the history told of the injury and the presentation of the injury. Failure to thrive may be evidence of physical and emotional neglect. The pediatric nurse must follow state and institutional policies carefully concerning the assessment of an abused child. Some institutions will want the nurse to initially assess the child alone and then include the parents/caregivers. Photographs may be required in the reporting of child abuse. There are a number of categories of mandatory reports (see state laws). Lack of reporting can lead to heavy fines and imprisonment. See Chapter 28 for an in-depth presentation of child abuse.

Iron-Deficiency Anemia

Anemia is the overall reduction of the number of RBCs or of the hemoglobin that RBCs carry. Iron-deficiency anemia is the most common childhood form of anemia. Anemia is not typically classified as a disease process, but a manifestation of an underlying condition. When circulating hemoglobin is significantly reduced, clinical symptoms present because of hypoxia. Risk factors include poor nutritional intake of iron. A common phenomenon is the overconsumption of milk. Young children whose daily diets include more than 24 to 32 ounces of milk become full and therefore are at risk to consume too little of iron-rich foods, thus leading to iron-deficiency anemia. Mild cases can be managed via diet. Moderate cases need iron supplements, and severe cases require blood transfusion of packed RBCs.

Autism

Autism generally presents before the child reaches 36 months of age. It can be severely disabling. The key indicators are impaired nonverbal and verbal communication, as well as impaired or absent reciprocal social interactions. Parents report considerable delays in communication patterns and social play compared with other children of the same age and development. The child may display stereotypical body movements and preoccupation with body parts.

Autistic children often fall into the functionally retarded range of the intelligence scale. Autism is more common in males than in females and may be associated with other neurological disorders. The cause is unknown at this time. Pediatric nurses should assess the young child for impaired social interactions, impaired communications, repetitive patterns of behavior, and lack of interest in activities expected at the child's age and level of development. The child with suspected autism may demonstrate abnormal electroencephalograms (EEGs) and may display a seizure disorder.

Treatment for younger children with autism focuses on speech and language; the child may require special education. Families should be referred to support groups for caregivers and parents of autistic children. Physical contact should be minimized while the child is in a health-care setting or hospital as it may cause anxiety and distress for the autistic child. Research has demonstrated that there is no connection between autism and childhood immunizations (AAP, 2010).

Common Infectious Diseases

Toddlers are at a particularly high risk for the acquisition and transmission of common communicable infectious diseases (Fig. 22.8). Because toddlers do not have the developmental cognitive processing to understand germ theory, nor do they demonstrate independent personal hygiene such as effective hand washing, they are at a higher risk for infections than older children. Toddlers who are still in diapers are at risk for become infected or transmitting fecal parasites such as pinworms. Other infectious diseases include the common cold (ie, the most common illness of childhood), influenza, varicella zoster (ie, chicken pox), dermatological infections such as fungus, or infestations such as pediculosis (ie, lice). Pediatric nurses must always use universal precautions when touching potentially contaminated body secretions, applying standard precautions such as droplet, airborne, and contact precautions for particular illnesses (see Appendix C for infection control precaution guidelines). Pediatric nurses routinely assess young children for infectious diseases, apply appropriate precautions, treat as ordered, and educate family members on the disease process, transmission, incubation period, symptoms, and treatments.

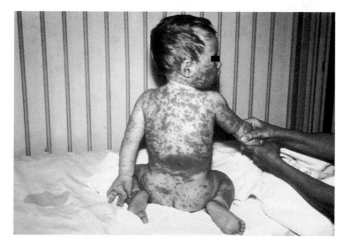

FIGURE 22.8 Toddler with rash associated with roseola. *(From the Centers for Disease Control and Prevention, Department of Health and Human Services. Retrieved from http://phil.cdc. gov/phil/details.asp, ID#3318.)*

NURSING CARE PLAN for the Toddler with an Infectious Disease

Because most children are immunized, the vast majority of children in the United States do not experience the complexities of a serious infectious disease. When a pediatric health-care team encounters a child with an infectious disease, the following nursing care plan can assist with the creation of safe care.

Nursing Assessments:
- Assess the child's history of exposure and report to the team. Some childhood infectious diseases such as pertussis are reportable to the local public health department.
- Assess the child's skin for rashes and lesions that indicate explicit childhood communicable diseases (eg, see Fig. 22.8 for an image of a toddler with a roseola rash).
- Assess the child's respiratory system for the development of pulmonary involvement such as cough and coryza (ie, runny nose).
- Assess the child's intensity of associated symptoms such as pruritus, mouth sores, fatigue, myalgia, upper respiratory congestion, irritability, and overall discomfort.

Nursing Diagnoses:
- Risk for infection: Secondary infections can occur when the child scratches rashes and lesions.
- Risk for pain: Discomfort can occur when a child has a rash associated with a childhood infectious disease.
- Risk for fatigue: Many communicable diseases cause extreme fatigue and irritability.

Expected Outcomes:
- The toddler will not transmit the infectious disease to other peers or family members while in the acute infectious state.
- The toddler will conduct simple infection control measures such as hand washing and sneezing into a tissue.
- The toddler will have a reduction of symptoms (eg, pruritus, fatigue, irritability, sleep disorder) during the acute phase of the infection.

Key Points

- The toddler period is marked by slower growth, fewer calorie needs, food lags and jags, picky eating, tantrums, and negativity. Families need specific anticipatory guidance during this challenging developmental stage.
- Toddlers need to be introduced to consistent discipline. Time-outs should be used and should last as many minutes as the child is old in years. Time-outs should be conducted in a private place.
- Because the developmental period is marked by increasing locomotion and exploration, the toddler requires constant supervision to provide protection against injury, harm, and dangers. The developmental milestone the toddler is struggling to accomplish is Erikson's psychosocial stage of autonomy versus shame and doubt. Toddlers need opportunities to exert their independence and separation from their primary caregiver.

- A major task for the toddler is toilet training. This task requires instruction, experimentation, support, and patience.
- Toddlers are participating in parallel play. They are not able to share naturally and need to be taught how to share. Toddlers are egocentric and cannot process the views or needs of another.
- Toddlers experience both separation anxiety and stranger anxiety. Measures should be taken to reduce the effect of these experiences.
- Toddlers are at risk for aspiration and choking. Foods should be cut into bite-size pieces and only low-risk foods should be served.
- Child abuse is most commonly found in children between the ages of infancy and 3 years. Nurses need to be aware of this risk and assess for all types of child abuse (Hockenberry and Wilson, 2012)

REVIEW QUESTIONS

1. Which of the following activities within the hospital environment is the child in the toddler developmental stage most likely to be fearful of?
   1. Going into the treatment room for a minor procedure
   2. Having to leave the play room for a nap
   3. Seeing the parents pack up their belongings to leave for work for the day
   4. Watching a roommate being placed on a gurney to go to surgery

2. According to Erikson, the milestone that the toddler must achieve can best be supported by which of the following activities:
   1. Activities that support family and sibling interaction and bonding
   2. Creative thinking and play activities that promote exploration
   3. Art activities that promote the sense of completion of a task
   4. Activities that provide the child a sense of individuality and control

3. A frustrating behavior displayed by a toddler that a parent should acknowledge as a normal response to the cognitive development of a toddler is:
   1. The toddler's persistence to eat only what they want
   2. The toddler's lack of sharing with others
   3. The toddler's egotistical thought process
   4. The toddler's need for the consistent presence of their security item

4. The number of words mastered by a toddler by the third birthday is:
   1. 50
   2. 1,000
   3. 300
   4. 750

5. Bedtime fears are a very real experience for the toddler. Which of the following creates the greatest fears?
   1. The unreasonable thought that their security item will become lost
   2. The fear of monsters under the bed
   3. The loss of time with older siblings who get to stay up later
   4. The fear of separation from parents at bedtime

6. A parent comes into the clinic with a toddler for a well-child appointment. The topic of food preferences and refusal has been brought up as a concern that the child is not eating enough and is refusing to consume what the rest of the family eats for dinner. The nurse's best response is:
   1. "This is unacceptable and the child should be kept in the high chair until dinner is consumed."
   2. "This is normal because the toddler is experiencing strong food preferences."
   3. "This is worrisome because the toddler experiences exponential growth and requires more calories at this time."
   4. "This is normal and food lags should be expected during this time of slowed growth."

7. Stranger anxiety is a common experience for the toddler. The nurse should practice which of the following to assist in the minimization of stranger anxiety in the hospital?
   1. Do not touch the toddler unless absolutely necessary.
   2. Establish a positive rapport with the parents before approaching the child.
   3. Ask the older sibling to hold the child during measurement of vital signs.
   4. Assign as many different nurses as possible to the child's care to get them accustomed to new people.

8. Car seat safety for the toddler includes the following:
   1. Maintain the car seat facing backwards and in the center back seat until the age of 2.
   2. Maintain the car seat facing forward and in a reclining position.
   3. Use only booster seats because the toddler is tall enough to see out the car windows.
   4. Transition to a convertible seat and place it facing forward.

9. The prevention and identification of child abuse is important during the toddler years because:
   1. The demands of the care of a toddler cause parents to become frustrated.
   2. Tantrums can cause a parent to lose control.
   3. This is the most common age of child abuse in the nation.
   4. Child abuse is much more common in the infancy developmental period.

10. Iron-deficiency anemia is a common toddler nutritional problem. While teaching a parent about the greatest influence to the development of this disorder, the nurse explains that:
    1. Iron-deficiency anemia is related to the stopping of breast milk.
    2. Iron-deficiency anemia is correlated with teething and the development of pica.
    3. Food lags and preferences cause the child to stop eating enough iron-rich foods.
    4. Too much milk in the diet prevents the toddler from consuming enough iron-rich foods.

CRITICAL THINKING QUESTIONS

1. What is the process of reporting child abuse in your state? What paperwork is required? Who are mandatory child abuse reporters? What are the consequences of the nurse not reporting evidence of abuse?
2. When teaching families to prepare themselves for the demands of raising a toddler, what support mechanisms can be offered to caregivers experiencing frustration and fatigue, and questioning their modes of discipline?

3. What anticipatory guidance suggestions can a pediatric nurse provide to parents of toddlers who experience the conditions of common communicable diseases, injuries and accidents, and food dislikes?
4. How would a nurse assess a home for safety concerns for a family with a toddler? What would a checklist look like to guide the pediatric nurse in the assessment of a safe home environment?

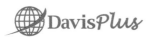 DavisPlus

For additional resources and information, visit **www.DavisPlus.com.**
Post-Conference Questions and Activities, Answers, and References can be found on DavisPlus.

23

Health Promotion of the Preschooler

LEARNING OUTCOMES

1. Define the key terms.
2. Describe the unique needs of the preschool-aged child in relation to children in other developmental stages and age groups.
3. Describe the differences between the preschool child and older children and adults in relation to body systems, anatomy, and physiology.
4. Differentiate the physical growth and development of the preschool period in comparison to other developmental stages.
5. Describe magical thinking in the preschool period and its effect on the child's view of his or her world.
6. Compare the nutritional needs and eating patterns of the preschooler to previous behaviors of the infant and toddler.
7. Identify the need to promote hand washing and hygiene practices in the preschool period.
8. Contrast the play needs and socialization practices of the preschooler to other developmental stages.
9. Teach the family of a preschooler anticipatory guidance practices to reduce injury and accidents.
10. Define the phenomenon of enuresis and encopresis in the preschool period and state appropriate resources for the parents of a child with these disorders.
11. Outline a plan of care that focuses on the safety needs of the preschool child, including prevention of illnesses, accidents, and injuries in both home and school settings.

REAL-WORLD CASE STUDY

Vanessa

■ Three-year-old Vanessa has been hospitalized for cellulitis associated with a spider bite that requires IV antibiotics and wound care. She is typically very communicative, expressive, and playful. Her parents share the responsibilities of her care, and one parent is

continued on page 348

KEY TERMS

animism
artificialism
encopresis
enuresis
imminent justice
intuitive thinking
magical thinking
nightmares
night terrors
preconceptual thinking
selective attention
symbolic functioning

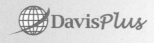 For audio pronunciation guide, visit **www.DavisPlus.com**

CHAPTER CONCEPTS

Comfort
Development
Family
Infection
Mobility
Nutrition
Promoting Health
Sensory Perception
Sleep, Rest, and Activity

REAL-WORLD CASE STUDY *continued*

always present at her bedside. Vanessa is experiencing pain associated with her wound and her peripheral IV site. She demonstrates discomfort by grimacing, moving her legs around in bed frequently, and refusing to get out of bed to sit in a chair or ambulate to the playroom for organized crafts. Her nurse, using an objective pain assessment tool (FLACC: Face, Legs, Activity, Cry, and Consolability of the patient), believes she is experiencing a 4 to 6 out of 10. When asked, Vanessa says she caused this spider to bite her and now caused her hospitalization because she has been "naughty." As a preschool child, her responses to her condition and her hospitalization are very expected because she is demonstrating magical thinking and preconceptual and preoperational thinking.

1. Is it appropriate to reorient this child and tell her that her hospitalization is not because she "is naughty?"
2. How can Vanessa be encouraged to get out of bed?
3. What is another pain tool that the nurse can use with Vanessa?

CONCEPTUAL CORNERSTONE

Growth and Development

As compared with the previous toddler period, the preschool developmental period is marked by slower overall growth in height and weight, but greater fine motor achievements. Preschool children learn to draw, craft, and develop skills that require greater eye-hand coordination. In relation to preschool growth and development, the concept of safety is very important during this period. Preschoolers are more independent than toddlers, yet they require frequent reminders about safety issues such as protective gear, street safety, car seat safety, and home safety. Growth and development for the preschooler is focused on physical, cognitive, and emotional achievements as they master more complex and creative play, and magical thinking.

The preschool developmental period spans from the child's third birthday through his or her fifth year. During this period, many children attend preschool, where they must learn to share and take direction from adults other than their parents. As a preschool child matures, he or she displays temperament and ease not previously shown during the toddler years, progress that is vital for when he or she begins school. By the fifth birthday, most preschoolers are quiet and contemplative and would rather participate in cooperative play than in parallel play.

GROWTH AND DEVELOPMENT OF THE PRESCHOOLER

The preschool period, unlike the infant and toddler periods, is a time during which the child is slowing down in growth and entering a period of creative play, fine motor achievements, and greater socialization with peers. Physical growth remains slow and steady, but finer movements and motor control become more prominent. Preschoolers learn to ride a tricycle, jump, skip, draw, paint, write basic letters, and participate in magical thinking.

Physical Growth and Development

The preschool child is marked by a slowing of physical growth. The preschooler gains only 5 pounds (2.26 kg) per year in weight and grows 2.5 to 3 in. (6.35 to 7.62 cm) per year in height. The toddler's classic stance changes as well. The slightly taller, leaner preschooler stands with an erect posture rather than with a protruding tummy. Other physical changes include the following:

- By the start of the preschool age, all 20 primary, or deciduous, teeth have erupted. Toward the end of the preschooler period, the child will begin to shed the primary teeth.
- Blood sugar begins to stabilize toward the end of this period, and less snacking will be needed.
- Expected vital signs include a heart rate range of 90 to 115 bpm, respiratory rate between 16 and 22 breaths/min, and a blood pressure range of 85 to 90 mm Hg over 55 to 60 mm Hg.
- Immunity continues to mature and the administration of immunizations continues. Diseases experienced during this time include lice, varicella (ie, chickenpox), influenza, cutaneous staphylococcus such as impetigo, and streptococcus infections such as strep throat.
- Visual acuity matures; most preschoolers will have visual acuity of 20/40 by their third birthday and 20/30 by their fourth birthday.
- Visual disturbances often present during the early preschool period. Both nearsightedness (ie, myopia) and double vision (ie, amblyopia) can present during this time.
- Hearing acuity is 100% intact with no expected deficits.

SAFETY *STAT!*

The continuation of childhood immunizations during the preschool period is important. During the preschool period, the child is exposed to more and more children, increasing the possibility of exposure to infectious diseases. The four immunizations that must be administered to the preschool child are varicella, MMR (ie, measles, mumps, and rubella), DTaP (ie, diphtheria, tetanus toxoids, and pertussis) and IVP (ie, inactivated poliovirus).

PATIENT TEACHING GUIDELINES

Immunizations

There is a growing concern for pediatric health-care providers that parents are refusing immunizations for their children. It is important to teach parents that there are three major concerns if young children are not immunized:

- The possibility of serious complications from childhood infectious diseases (eg, pneumonia, meningitis, or encephalitis)
- The mandate that states require immunizations for children to attend public school
- The spread of childhood infectious diseases to others within the family's community, especially to young infants who have a greater chance of serious complications

Gross Motor Development

As the preschool child ages, he or she will be able to accomplish new, independent tasks. The preschool child benefits from mastery of new tasks and will want to showcase accomplishments to parents, caregivers, and nurses (Fig. 23.1).

- Provide praise when a preschooler attempts a new accomplishment, whether or not he or she actually masters or fails at it. For example, if a preschooler attempts to tie his or her shoes, provide praise, whether successful or not.
- Do not reprimand a preschooler who fails at a task. When a preschool child hears frequent reprimands he or she will be less inclined to attempt a new motor skill.

The Health Promotion feature details the gross motor tasks that a preschooler will attempt at different ages.

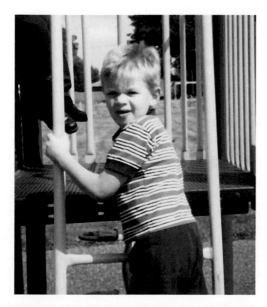

FIGURE 23.1 A preschooler at play.

HEALTH PROMOTION

Gross Motor Skill Development in Preschoolers
3-Year-Old
- Builds towers of six to nine blocks
- Catches a ball
- Climbs on higher structures
- Hops in place
- Jumps horizontally
- Marches
- Paints in circular motions with whole hands
- Rides tricycle
- Runs
- Smears or dabs paint
- Stands on one foot briefly

4-Year-Old
- Alternates feet going up a flight of stairs
- Gallops
- Goes up and down steps easily
- Jumps
- Pumps on a swing
- Runs on tip toes
- Skips on one foot
- Throws ball over head
- Walks heel to toe

5-Year-Old
- Displays good balance
- Dresses without help
- Hops and skips well
- Pulls wagons
- Rides scooters
- Skates
- Plays on playground equipment

Between the beginning of the third year and the end of the fifth year:
- Buttons and unbuttons
- Draws copies of shapes on paper
- Draws detailed stick figures
- Learns to write
- Pours from a pitcher
- Progresses from holding scissors to being able to cut a line with scissors
- Progresses from putting on shoes to lacing shoes to tying shoelaces
- Uses eating utensils
- Washes face and hands

Nutrition

During the preschool period, the child consumes about half of the calories of an adult, approximately 1,200 to 1,600 calories a day.

- Food preferences may still affect how a preschooler eats; he or she may continue to demonstrate picky eating behaviors well into the preschool period.

- The most important aspect of eating behavior during this period is to teach the parents to ensure that the preschooler is consuming a well-balanced diet, is taking in adequate calories, has limited salt and fat, and is exposed frequently to new foods.
- Preschoolers benefit from two cups of nonfat or low-fat milk per day.
- Total dietary intake of fat should not exceed 35% of total daily calories; 25% should be the goal for most children.
- Parents and caregivers should offer fruits and vegetables at every meal, encourage lean meats, introduce fish, and offer only low-sugar cereals.
- Nutritious snacks that are appealing to preschool children include peanut butter on graham crackers (assess for peanut or other food allergies), celery sticks with cream cheese, and carrot sticks dipped in ranch dressing.

SAFETY *STAT!*

Be aware of the increasing numbers of young children with food allergies. Preschool children attending child care or preschool classes, and their teachers, must be made aware of food allergies to prevent potential serious reactions including anaphylaxis.

FAMILY MEALS. The experience of the family meal is very important to the well-being of the preschooler. Parents and caregivers should use meals as an opportunity for the family to become close and demonstrate respect for one another:

- Children should not be allowed to eat in front of the television but should be set up at the family table at their own place in their own chair and engaged in conversation during the evening meal.
- The preschooler can add to the family conversation by offering a summary of what he or she experienced and learned in preschooler class that day.

OBESITY. Childhood obesity rates are increasing as more and more children are being exposed to high-fat diets, including fast food consumption, in combination with decreasing levels of activity. To combat this, the preschool child should be encouraged to eat a variety of nutritious foods and taught the importance of physical activity and rigorous play.

MYPLATE. The older preschool child might enjoy learning about the need for good nutrition and increased activity by being introduced to the MyPlate for Preschoolers. MyPlate, which provides guidelines for eating well, being active, and being healthy, can be found online.

- This family-appropriate Web site introduces children and their parents to healthy food choices while helping them to understand the calculation of calories and minutes of exercise needed for a healthy lifestyle by providing educational opportunities to learn sample meal patterns, meal ideas, and snack ideas.

- The site also assists with teaching young children to follow food safety rules, such as washing their hands before preparing foods or eating, refrigerating foods promptly, not cross-contaminating uncooked foods with cooked foods, and using a food thermometer.
- The site provides specific food preparation ideas, kitchen safety, and play ideas to enhance the child's experience in food preparation while teaching guidelines for safety.

Sleeping Patterns and Requirements

The preschooler needs, on average, 12 hours of uninterrupted sleep per night, though he or she may wake up and need reassurance from any fears during the night. Providing a bedtime routine and a night light might assist with the reduction of fears in the middle of the night.

- Parents need to be educated that their preschooler may demonstrate sleep disturbances, especially if the child is newly engaged in preschool, where there is a high level of activity and a new level of intense stimulation.
- Activities that help a child slow down before bedtime and the application of a bedtime routine can help the young child understand that bedtime is near and that no delay is acceptable. Young children should not be allowed to watch television before their bedtime as it has been shown to disturb the child's sleep routine.

NIGHTMARES AND NIGHT TERRORS. Both nightmares and night terrors are common during the preschool period:

- **Nightmares** are described as scary dreams that may awaken the child, producing crying and requiring reassurance and comfort.
- **Night terrors** cause the child to awaken from a deep sleep after the child demonstrates great fear, thrashing of arms and legs, yelling, and possibly running or walking out of her or his room or even out of the house. Parents need to be taught that night terrors are not uncommon during this time period and very little needs to be done for the child other than reassurance and safety during the episode.

NAPPING. As the child progresses from toddlerhood to the early preschool developmental stage, he or she will probably no longer take an afternoon nap. This varies greatly among children.

- Most preschool settings provide the early preschool child with an opportunity to nap or take a rest during the day. Some schools provide individual cots, and others require the families to bring in a pad.
- The child will slowly need less rest during the day but will need to maintain sufficient sleep during the night. A young preschooler who naps will still need 12 hours of sleep per night. The older preschooler may just need quiet time to lay down and look at a book or play with a stuffed animal instead of a nap.

Cognitive Development

Piaget's stages of the preschooler's cognitive development are described as *preoperational*. Although Piaget's theory does not have a specific theoretical period that covers the years of 3 through 5, his preoperational theory component covers the ages of 2 through 7 years. The preoperational stage is described as the transition that the young child goes through in which he or she leaves complete egotistical thinking and develops social awareness and the ability to consider other points of view. Although preschoolers are not able to think about more than one thought at a time, they begin to think about the various parts of their thought's whole meaning (Hockenberry and Wilson, 2013).

Preschoolers experience three phases of cognitive development:

1. **Preconceptual thinking:** This can be described as the young child's judgment of environment by visual experiences. There are three components: artificialism, animism, and imminent justice (Box 23.1).
2. **Intuitive thinking:** This type of thinking begins around 4 years of age and is defined as the preschooler's ability to classify information while becoming more aware of cause-and-effect relationships. Cause-and-effect relationships demonstrate the child's awareness of the prediction of responses, which requires a deeper level of understanding of the child's previous experiences.
3. **Symbolic functioning:** This relates to the experience of play and is demonstrated by a child who creates an image in his or her mind to mean something other than it is, such as using a pillow for a horsey, a cardboard box for a car, and a blanket for a cape.

Magical Thinking

The preschool period is marked by the experience of **magical thinking.** Preschoolers have rich fantasy lives and deep imaginations; because of this, they have trouble telling fantasy from reality and use the process of magical thinking to fill in the blanks when they do not understand their complex environments.

- When utilizing magical thinking, the preschooler will invent stories to explain the circumstances of confusing situations. For example, the preschooler will use magical thinking to reason why a sibling has cancer and is hospitalized. He or she may state that the sibling is being punished for denting their father's car or for poor behavior.
- Preschoolers may blame their behavior on imaginary friends or come to conclusions about complicated social situations by believing that their made-up reality replaces and explains their actual reality.

PATIENT TEACHING GUIDELINES

Preschoolers may struggle with the concept of death. They may see death as something temporary. It is important to not use euphemisms like, "went to sleep" or was "put to sleep" because they, as magical thinkers, will expect the person or animal to wake up. Give clear and honest answers and explanations. Feelings about death may come out in a preschool child's play activity.

Concept of Time

The preschooler begins to understand the concepts of *today, tomorrow,* and *later,* though also struggling to understand the concepts of past, present, and future. One goal is to have the preschooler comprehend the days of the week, the months, and the basics of the four seasons before his or her fifth birthday. By doing this, the child learns that he or she can anticipate future events and look forward to particular situations. Birthday celebrations are a classic example of this.

Selective Attention

Parents of preschoolers may question if their child has a hearing impairment when the child demonstrates periods in which he or she does not respond to their voices. This is known as **selective attention.** As the child is playing or is concentrating on a craft, puzzle, or fabric book, he or she may not respond to requests or even to his or her name, as the activity being worked on has captured the full attention. This is normal but can be frustrating to parents (Fig. 23.2).

Language Development

During the preschool period, the child makes great strides in communication:

- **2 years:** The toddler can be expected to say 50 words.
- **3 years:** The child is verbally communicating with up to 900 words.
- **4 years:** The preschooler is answering simple questions with simple answers.
- **5 years:** The child rhymes, uses complex and compound sentences, talks in future tense, and states his or her full name and address.

Box 23.1 Components of Preconceptual Thinking

There are three components of preconceptual thinking:

1. **Artificialism:** The preschooler believes that everything is made by humans.
2. **Animism:** The preschooler believes that inanimate objects are alive.
3. **Imminent justice:** A belief that everything has a determined universal code of law and order.

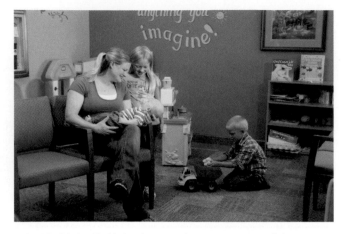

FIGURE 23.2 Child displaying selective attention while engaged in self-play.

What the preschooler likes to talk about also changes during this period:

- **3 years:** The early preschooler likes to tell simple stories and enjoys describing what he or she sees, hears, and experiences. Not all stories told will be completely truthful, as the child is in the magical thinking stage.
- **4 years:** The child may talk incessantly while exaggerating and boasting. At this age, the child likes rhymes, silly words, and playing with speech, and may also enjoy endlessly questioning parents.
- **5 years:** The child, who is very interested in his or her environment, tells long tales about daily experiences. He or she may also test parents by using profanity and forbidden words.

HEALTH PROMOTION

Expected Language Development of the Preschooler
3-Year-Old

- Asks many questions
- Displays a poor use of pronouns
- May repeat a sentence of up to six syllables
- Speaks a total of 300 to 900 words
- Talks incessantly, even when others are not listening or paying attention
- Uses three- to four-word sentences

4-Year-Old

- Asks questions at a peak of frequency
- Counts out loud
- May use forbidden words or mild profanity if in the presence of older children or siblings
- Names colors
- Speaks a total of 1,500 words
- States names of animals, people, and places
- Tells exaggerated stories
- Uses four- to five-word sentences
- Uses prepositional phrases, such as "in front of" or "in back of"

5-Year-Old

- Can state names of coins
- Enjoys telling long stories
- Learns time-oriented concepts, such as days of the week, months, seasons
- Names most colors
- Speaks a total of 2,100 words
- Uses five-word sentences

Preschool is a period of language growth. With that growth comes the potential of problems. Preschool children need encouragement to speak and explain their thoughts, as well as communicate their questions and their needs. Speech problems should be identified as early as possible.

Numbers, Colors, and Letters

The preschool child is exposed to a new world of symbolic meanings:

- Numbers are learned after practicing their meaning, sometimes in the incorrect order. Preschoolers delight in learning their numbers and should be able to identify 0 to 10 before their fifth birthday.
- Identifying colors becomes a game, and learning to mix colors while painting is exciting.
- Preschoolers learn to copy simple shapes, stick figures, and numbers, and should be encouraged to practice this new skill repeatedly. Upon seeing their child begin to practice drawing, some parents and caregivers may push to have their child use one hand rather than the other (right versus left, left versus right), which can discourage the child from practicing the skill. Instead, parents and caregivers should encourage their child in this activity, making it a positive experience. By the time the child is 4, however, the child's preference for hand use is well established.

Psychological and Developmental Growth and Development

During the preschool developmental period, Erikson describes the child's psychological and psychosocial development as needing to master *initiative versus feelings of guilt*. Here, the child must master the process of initiating activities that are independent and self-directed, receiving support and praise for their attempts at mastery.

- If the child is not given an opportunity to initiate these activities, he or she may be reluctant to try new processes.
- As the child takes on new experiences, even if he or she does not have all of the physical abilities to be successful, parents and caregivers need to support the child in the attempts so that the child does not develop guilt over any failures to master the task.
- This period can be a difficult balancing act for parents, as they have to guide and support the child while also setting limits and restricting the child from partaking in unsafe situations.

Frequent experiences of blame or negativity during skill exploration can cause the child to experience guilt and decreased feelings of worth. Support is needed while the child is trying out new experiences and wanting to do more things independently.

Socialization

The preschool child is now participating in greater social interactions. Unlike the toddler, who is egocentric and participating in parallel play, the preschooler is interacting with both adults and peers in greater depth during play and school. The development of socialization will depend on the opportunities offered the child.

Moral and Spiritual Development

According to Kohlberg's theory on moral development, during the preschool period, moral development and an orientation to what is considered "good" and "bad" through the eyes of the child is replaced with a basic understanding of what is considered socially acceptable. Preschoolers inherently want to please the adults in their lives and will do things to create a positive reaction from parents, teachers, and other adults. Children at this age should be given opportunities to help in small ways and should receive praise for their attempts to please others.

- In general, the preschooler wants to conform to rules, and will like to more and more as he or she ages.
- As the preschooler matures through this period, the child becomes easygoing with a positive attitude, is less resistant to change, and is more secure. The child has also developed a greater sense of personal identity (Fig. 23.3).
- The preschool period is a good time to discuss cultural diversity and to teach the child respect for differences in religious beliefs and cultural practices.

Children benefit from interacting in a diverse community. The preschool period is an excellent time to provide guidance to a child as their socialization expands and they interact with diverse cultural groups and families.

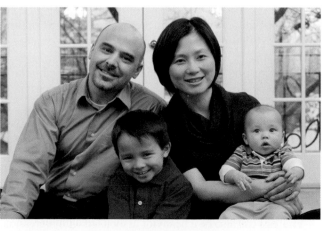

FIGURE 23.3 Cultural diversity in families.

CULTURAL CONSIDERATIONS

Teaching Diversity and Multiculturalism

Promoting tolerance, respect, and engagement in multiethnic activities produces well-rounded children with open minds and greater social abilities. The preschool period is considered a prime time to teach multicultural perspectives and multiethnic lifestyles because this is when the child begins to develop ideas of the world. Adults should:

- Set a good example for the preschool child by showing respect for all people
- Not expect gender to dictate choices of toys, such as girls not wanting to play with trucks or boys not wanting to play with dolls
- Point out similarities between people, as well as teaching differences
- Reinforce that people come in all shapes, sizes, looks, colors, and abilities

Ideas for preschool activities that promote cultural awareness and diversity include:

- Teaching how to count in different languages
- Holding parties that celebrate different cultures and ethnicities
- Providing food play sets of ethnically diverse meals
- Providing books that include pictures of children in wheelchairs, missing limbs, or using crutches
- Reading stories to preschoolers that share the experience of cultural diversity and respecting different views
- Providing dolls with various shades of skin color
- Encouraging conversations about diversity by providing a board of pictures of children with diverse skin color, body shapes, and sizes, and pictures of various constellations of family structure

Overall, do not make cultural diversity or multiculturalism a separate subject than everyday preschool activities. Rather, incorporate diversity in all aspects of the child's reading, play, and social activities.

As the preschooler progresses through the fifth year, he or she is becoming more self-assured and well-adjusted. The child is struggling to gain inner control while wanting to please those around them.

A successful way to teach parents about this age group is to explain that their preschooler needs to know clear and consistent rules and the consequences for breaking those rules.

Spiritual development surfaces during the preschool years as the young child explores his or her thoughts on the family's faith and religious practices. Preschoolers:

- Have a very concrete conception of a god and see God as a physical being they can draw, talk to, and think about
- May enjoy simple rituals during worship, such as prayers and spiritual stories
- May benefit from being able to see and touch religious representations such as statues, crosses, picture books, and crafts

Temperament

As the preschool child's life incorporates more social activities outside of the house, the child's temperament highly influences his or her ability to adapt to new social situations.

The preschooler's temperament influences his or her ability to adjust to group situations and adapt to distractions, moods, intensity of reaction, and amount of persistence. In order for the child to be successful at school, his or her temperament must adjust to the new preschool classroom structure and circumstance. Parents can be of assistance by selecting a preschool environment that will support their child's temperament. For example, a classroom that does not restrict movement will better serve a child with an active temperament and extra energy.

Discipline

The preschooler needs to be allowed to develop a sense of initiative while learning self-control and rules. The child should have a consistent discipline experience and be guided by parental desire for appropriate and safe behavior. Teaching self-control takes time and patience, but the rewards include the child being able to behave nicely while playing with other children or interacting with other adults.

- The pediatric nurse should assess the family's discipline strategies and maintain consistency while the child is hospitalized.
- According to Kohlberg's theory of moral development, the preschooler's conscience is emerging; the child is learning self-control and consequences. The preschooler learns what is right and wrong by listening, watching, and imitating others.
- As the preschooler grows, he or she learns how to avoid punishment or how to win rewards.

PATIENT TEACHING GUIDELINES

Appropriate Disciplining in the Preschool Period

The preschool child benefits from consistent discipline for unwanted or unacceptable behaviors. Guidelines for disciplining a child within the preschool period include the following:

- Time-outs should last 1 min for each year of age, meaning that a 3-year-old's time-out should last 3 min.
- Children in time-out should be placed in a quiet and restricted area where the child can regain control and think about his or her behavior.
- Adults who apply discipline should be fair, firm, and consistent.

Tips to avoid situations that require discipline include the following:

- Parents and other authority figures should do their best to prevent children from putting themselves in situations that are unsafe.
- Explanations should be very clear when it comes to expectations of the child.

- Parents and other role models should consistently demonstrate the behaviors that are desirable.

Family Relationships

As stated earlier, preschool children develop the desire to please their parents, grandparents, and other significant people in their lives.

- They want to conform to the patterns, rules, and expectations of the family structure and fit in as an important part of the family dynamics.
- The young child is acutely aware of the roles and functions of each member of the family and develops an understanding of sex-role functions.
- A challenge for a child in the early preschool years is to feel comfortable with separating from his or her parents for increasingly longer periods of time. The adjustment may start when the child enters a structured preschool educational environment.

When the preschool child turns 4 years old, some undesirable behaviors may surface within family dynamics:

- Sibling rivalry may present with either older or younger siblings. The child may become disruptive by invading an older sibling's privacy or touching the sibling's personal possessions.
- If a 4-year-old perceives that parents or family members are asking too much, he or she may act rebellious, aggressive, and provoke frustrations.
- As the child progresses into the fifth year, he or she becomes more in-tune with family expectations and desires to help by doing simple chores or errands around the house. The child may also seek out the company of family members more.
- It is important that the young preschool child is supervised in her or his care of younger siblings. For instance, a 3-year-old should not feed an infant sibling without constant supervision because a choking episode can occur.

Enuresis

Enuresis is inappropriate voiding after the child is successfully toilet trained, and it can be quite upsetting for the child and parent.

- Preschool children may experience enuresis, or bedwetting, especially if the child is experiencing nightmares or any type of anxiety.
- True enuresis is when the child experiences a minimum of two episodes of inappropriate voiding over at least a 3-month timeframe.
- Nocturnal bedwetting occurs at night, and diurnal enuresis occurs during the day.
- Boys experience enuresis more often than girls.
- For some children, enuresis can cause extreme frustration and distress, and may cause disruptions in the child's social life.

Enuresis can also be a behavior associated with regression, such as when a child is hospitalized, experiencing a stressful period, or when a new sibling is born, all of which are emotional situations. Parents need to demonstrate patience with their child and attempt to assess what led to the development of the enuresis.

Play

The preschool child actively engages in associative play, which does not have a common goal like cooperative or organized play. In this type of play, preschoolers:

- Interact and engage in a common activity with loose organization and rules
- Are willing to exchange materials, although with hesitation, until each child is finished with the materials they are playing with
- May attempt to control or limit participation

Parents and caregivers should encourage associative play, but they must also remember that the preschooler needs quiet play that is creative, manipulative, constructive, and educational in nature, as this type of play aids in the development of fine motor movements. Simple sewing projects in which the child uses thick yarn to lace through a design on cardboard, easy construction sets, and coloring projects provide for this type of quiet play.

Ideas for toy selection during the preschool period include toys that allow children to mimic adult activities and pretend-play adult work roles, such as:

- Play kitchens
- Tool chests
- Medical and nursing kits

According to Hockenberry and Wilson (2007), preschoolers should be offered no more than one simple project per year of age. For instance, a 3-year-old will be able to concentrate and have patience for decorating three eggs for a spring basket when they are 3 years old.

Preschoolers can benefit from learning via play. If facing a medical procedure or surgery, a preschooler can participate in medical play to learn about the upcoming experience and demystify the equipment and procedure. Medical play also helps a preschooler act out their fears and emotions, providing an avenue for release of their feelings.

TEAM WORKS

The Importance of Medical Play for Preschool-Aged Children

Preschool children have great fears associated with body mutilation and require age and developmental-stage appropriate explanations using language that fosters understanding. The entire health-care team needs to commit to not discuss in complex medical terminology anything associated with pathology, disease states, or medical interventions that will frighten the preschool child.

- Change of shift report, if given at the bedside while hospitalized, should be directed toward all members of family who are present, including the child. Use words that are positive and support the preschool patient's understanding of what is being said.
- To reduce the common experience of fear during the preschool period, play should be incorporated into all areas of the preschool child's interaction with the health-care team. If in a clinic environment, toys and books should be offered that provide appropriate distraction and comfort. Developmentally appropriate books that provide education about the condition, disease, and treatments or care should be provided, such as children's books on cancer, sickle cell disease, chickenpox, or diabetes. In the hospital, play should be designed so that the child can participate regardless of her or his disease, medical condition, developmental level, or symptoms.
- The entire health-care team needs to respect the child's play and should try to conduct physical examinations and interventions outside of play time.
- Whenever possible, the child's hospital bed should be considered the safe zone for rest, play, and eating. The pediatric health-care team should use the treatment room to perform painful procedures or examinations that produce discomfort.
- All members of the pediatric team should incorporate within their professional role a playful tone when interacting with a preschool child. A playful tone fosters security and demonstrates respect to the child. Baby words or a babyish demeanor should not be used; rather, the health-care team should use a developmentally appropriate and playful conversational tone.
- A Child Life Specialist's assistance should be secured to provide play ideas and play supplies for preschool children. These specialists are uniquely educated about developmental stages and are gifted in providing play opportunities, if needed, to reduce a preschooler's fear surrounding hospitalizations, diagnostic examinations, treatments and interventions, and separation from family.

IMAGINARY FRIENDS. A preschool child may develop imaginary friends. These friends may be harmless and somewhat comforting for the child, but parents should be aware of the relationships and monitor their effect on the child's safety.

- Imaginary friends can be very important if the child experiences periods of actual loneliness. The use of imaginary friends can come and go, but may surface with consistency during life-changing circumstances, such as the loss of a grandparent, a geographical move, a divorce, or when a best friend moves away.
- The child may blame the imaginary friend for certain behaviors, such as a lost item, a broken vase, or during discipline for an unwanted or unacceptable behavior.

Parents can become involved with the imaginary friend by:

- Calling him or her by name
- Including him or her in a game by setting up a marker for the imaginary friend during a board game

If the child begins to blame the imaginary friend for poor behavior, the parent should intervene and reinforce, in simple and straightforward terms, that the child is responsible for his or her behaviors and will experience the consequence of the unwanted behaviors. For instance, if the child blames the imaginary friend for sneaking restricted food, the parents need to teach the child that, although the imaginary friend was "there," the child will still experience the discipline for the misbehavior.

GAMES AND ARTS AND CRAFTS. One of the joys of the preschool age is that children very much enjoy artistic and creative play. Box 23.2 lists ideas for engaging the preschooler in cooperative activities or solo ideas.

Box 23.2 Preschool-Aged Play Activities

All of the following preschool play activities can be easily implemented into a hospital setting.

- Make leaf banners by gluing festive leaves onto pieces of fabric.
- Teach basic and simple math equations by patterning small objects and counting various colors, sizes, and shapes, and placing small objects into organized piles.
- Create "fingerprint trees or animals" that represent the current season, such as a turkey or snow-covered trees.
- Make a family photo album by gluing pictures to colorful paper and adding little shapes around them, such as frames with the person's name.
- Create a map of the hospital showing where the kitchen, nursing station, play room, and elevators are in relation to the child's room.
- Build a pinecone bird feeder by placing peanut butter into the cone, rolling in bird seed, and then attaching a yarn hanger.
- Create jewelry pieces by stringing large beads or flavored cereal loops onto string.
- Make tie-dye baby wipes by painting water-soluble colorful paints onto moist wipes and then drying them.
- Assemble a sensory table where the child can explore their five senses by squishing, sifting, sorting, digging, and pouring. Accept the mess and let the child explore freely.
- Create a paper plate wind spinner by painting one side of the plate or making glitter glue patterns. Cut the plate in a spiral and hang with tape. A paper plate face mask can also be created.
- Play dress up with adult-sized clothing to recreate adult occupations (eg, fireman, police officer, nurse, physician, store keeper, gardener, auto mechanic).

CHEATING TO WIN. During the preschool period, children hate to lose at games or any simple competitive activity. Parents need to understand that this a normal part of the preschooler's development and is universal for this age group.

Because most of the simple board games or card games for this developmental period are won by chance, not strategy, children should be taught manners and truth-telling while engaging in a game.

MINIMIZING TECHNOLOGY. According to the American Academy of Pediatrics (2013), preschoolers should not have more than 1 or 2 hours a day of any type of screen time. It is imperative that parents and caregivers place a limit on how much time they allow their preschoolers to spend watching TV and playing on the computer. Five consequences have been linked to potentially occur with longer screen times:

- Watching a screen more than 2 hours daily has been linked to childhood obesity.
- When exposed to screen time before bedtime, children have been known to have trouble falling asleep.
- Children in elementary school who have TVs in their rooms tend to have poorer performances on school-related work and also lower test scores.
- Children who watch excessive TV are more likely to participate in bullying behaviors, have attention problems at preschool, and show more signs of anxiety and depression as compared with children who have restricted screen time.
- Young children need to be encouraged to have creative and imagination-rich playtime. The more screen time a child participates in, the less imaginative playtime the child has (Mayo Clinic, 2015).

SAFE TOY SELECTION. Toy selection should begin with the parent, caregiver, or nurse assessing the child's motor and cognitive abilities. Because all children are unique and have preferences, including the child in toy, game, or craft selection is ideal. When choosing toys, keep these points in mind:

- Preferable toys include those that are large, brightly colored, and challenging but able to be mastered.
- Preschoolers enjoy giving the products of their play to important people as gifts. Games, toys, and crafts that require focused attention and produce an item that can be gifted are ideal.
- Because preschoolers have difficulty following rules, it is important to choose games that have simple rules.
- Most preschoolers place items in their mouths, so mouthing behaviors should be assessed during play to ensure that the child is not placing anything dangerous into his or her mouth.

PROTECTIVE EQUIPMENT. The preschool child is beginning to attempt greater independence and is graduating from one type of play equipment to the next, such as moving from tricycles to bicycles with training wheels, and from scooters to large skateboards. This is the time in the child's life to insist on the use of protective gear.

- Make sure that the child is using appropriate protective gear for the sports he or she participates in, such as shin guards for soccer, helmets for bike riding, and elbow pads, knee pads, and helmets for skateboarding.
- By setting rules for protective equipment early, the child learns their importance and remains safer in play.

Body Image

When speaking with a preschooler who is learning about his or her body, use correct anatomical language and teach the child that parts of the body are private, but in general, the body is normal and differences are acceptable. Parents need to promote an awareness of the positive aspects of both sexes, teaching the differences in simple explanations with a positive tone.

- Because the preschool period is marked with fears, the expression of fear of bodily harm or mutilation is real and should be expected.
- In sex education, the preschool child may ask many questions, including where babies come from and why. Using simple straightforward explanations will diminish the use of magical thinking to fill in the blanks or substitute the truth.

One game that can assist the child in developing a positive body image while learning simple anatomy is to have the parent trace the child's body while the child is lying on a large piece of paper. This gives the parent and the child an opportunity to use the paper as an educational tool. The parent names the body parts and the child draws in the details, and then the child names the part with the new vocabulary word and colors it to his or her liking.

SEXUAL DEVELOPMENT. According to Freud's theory of psychosocial development, the preschooler experiences the phallic phase. In this phase, the child is exploring his or her sexual identity by exploring the genitalia and masturbating, which is perfectly normal, healthy behavior. When parents and caregivers encounter this behavior, they must not pass judgment or show disdain. They must also be aware of their role during this period:

- When the child shows an interest in masturbation, parents and caregivers must set limits and teach privacy.
- Parents need to be aware that the Oedipus complex may develop in preschool boys, in which they fight for the attention of their mothers. Parents also need to be aware that the preschooler, regardless of sex, may cause conflict during the Oedipal phase as he or she competes against the same sex, exhibits jealousy and rivalry, and tries to win the love of the opposite-sex parent.

This phase typically resolves with a strong identity with the same-sex parent.

The preschool period is also a time when children want to play doctor to examine the opposite sex. Although they do not understand the function of the genitalia, they want to know the differences between the sexes. Sexual curiosity is normal and can be expected during this period.

Preschool

Preschool provides for group care before the primary school experience. Not all children between 3 and 5 years old are enrolled in a preschool experience as some families choose to provide a less structured day-to-day experience. Preschool is not a part of general education mandated for minors. Preschools can be public or private. Some preschools come with expenses that limit participation for many families.

The benefits of and preparation for the preschool experience include the following:

- Preschool provides the child with social engagement, fine and gross motor development, play opportunities, and skill development in preparation for kindergarten.
- Children attending preschool have the opportunity to adjust to social-cultural differences and engage in a relationship with a teacher who provides a new means to guide them differently than their parents.
- According to Hockenberry and Wilson (2013), children from a limited peer-group experience, such as an only child, and children from impoverished homes particularly benefit from the preschool experience because it provides extensive stimulation and social interaction.
- Readiness for preschool is based on the child's emotional maturity, attention span, successful toilet training, and sense of autonomy. All of these factors will influence the child's ability to happily engage in a structured environment in which he or she is encouraged to participate in a well-planned set of activities, napping periods, shared meal time, and outdoor play.
- Having parents read to their young children, encourage learning, and provide a positive perspective on the preschool period will assist the child in coping with the newness of the preschool experience.
- The first day of preschool may pose a particular challenge for both the child and the parent. The parent should behave with confidence, positivity, and support. The preschool child carefully watches the parent's response to the new environment, and will rely on the parent's support and encouragement to enter and engage. If the parent is confident, excited and ready, the child will see this and respond to the encouragement.

ANTICIPATORY GUIDANCE FOR PARENTS WITH A PRESCHOOLER

All throughout childhood the pediatric nurse supports the parents' education by providing anticipatory guidance for each of the developmental stages. Anticipatory guidance for the family of a preschooler continues to focus on health and safety. Preschoolers, although more cautious than toddlers, can still end up in unsafe situations concerning traffic, swimming, and other potentially hazardous predicaments.

Many preschoolers are at risk for injuries because of their inappropriate belief that they have higher skill levels than they actually do.

Anticipatory guidance for health and safety tips for the parents of a preschool child should include the following:

- Talking with the health-care professional to check on the child's development and expectations for behavior and motor skill development
- Participating in recommended health screenings, including blood pressure measurement and screenings for:
  - Vision
  - Hearing
  - Obesity
  - Hemoglobin
  - Hematocrit
  - Lead
  - Tuberculosis, if at risk
  - Cholesterol, if at risk caused by obesity or other disease states
- Making a vaccination schedule
- Assessing the home for lead-based paint, peeling paint surfaces, or any chewable surfaces painted with lead-based paint
- Proper storing of household cleaning products, pesticides, and automobile solutions such as antifreeze and windshield wiping solutions
- Supervising young preschoolers (ie, 3 year olds) in the bathtub to prevent near or actual drowning accidents; they should not be allowed to play with the water faucet
- Using safety gates at the top and bottom of stairs to prevent falls and serious injuries
- Maintaining safety around pets and teaching manners and gentle handling of family animals
- Providing at least 12 hours of uninterrupted sleep per night
- Reminding the family and child about safe eating habits and the prevention of choking by always sitting down to eat
- Providing injury prevention in relation to climbing and falls, swimming, playground structures, and tricycle and bicycle safety
- Evaluating the need for firearms in the house; if present, storing them safely by keeping them unloaded, with trigger guards in place, in a locked metal storage facility that is inaccessible to children of all ages

Medical Concerns

The child in the preschool developmental period needs to participate in at least one well-child assessment by a pediatric health professional. This is often done as a requirement for entry into formalized child care or a preschool classroom. Early identification of health problems in this period can assist the child in the prevention of later poor health consequences. Providing well-balanced nutrition and promoting early care of the child's emerging permanent teeth are important for the growing child's overall health and well-being.

Medication Safety

Preschool children are in need of developmentally appropriate (simple) education and at risk for medication errors for several reasons:

- They are in a developmental period in which the indication, scheduling, and side effects of their medications should be explained very simply: "To take your pain away," or "to treat your sore throat."
- They are magical thinkers and may believe that they are required to take medications, regardless of the route, as a punishment for a previous wrong-doing.
- They are unable to swallow pills effectively and may require that the pills be mixed or crushed, or that elixirs be created, which can be incorrectly calculated. In addition, they often refuse medications or fight off taking medications, putting them at risk for not finishing a prescription.

Parents must be involved from the very start in the process of administering medications. Tips to provide parents when administering medications to their preschool child include the following:

- Praise the child for adhering to medication scheduling and dosing.
- Never tell the child that medications are candy.
- Do not allow the child to negotiate when to take medications. Minimize stalling behaviors.
- Allow the child to take the medication cup or oral syringe and place the medication into his or her mouth.

Dentition

Dental hygiene practices are important during the early childhood years. Preschoolers experience the shedding of their primary teeth and the eruption of their permanent deciduous teeth. Also, the enamel on a child's primary teeth is much thinner than that found on permanent teeth, so the preschooler must brush regularly to prevent caries, which can occur rapidly because the distance from the tooth's pulp to the tooth's surface is thinner on primary teeth. Parents and caregivers should encourage the child to brush his or her own teeth while providing supervision to make sure that the child uses the appropriate amount of toothpaste and is thorough in his or her care.

- Pediatric nurses need to reinforce to parents that while the primary (deciduous) teeth will be shed, the health of these first teeth is very important to the well-being of the child. If the primary teeth develop caries, the decay and infection can affect the health of the permanent teeth located above.
- Severe tooth decay in primary teeth can lead to decay in permanent teeth that are budding.

THUMB SUCKING. Thumb sucking must be stopped if the child has continued to do this into the preschool period. This habit may provide the young child with a sense of security, but it can be disruptive to the child's tooth alignment. It can be difficult to stop when the child is experiencing fears, especially around going to sleep, so some parents choose to use over-the-counter products to apply to the child's thumb or nails to provide an undesirable taste.

Health-Care Terminology

Because preschoolers are afraid of bodily harm, they may become fearful when around health-care professionals using medical terminology. Follow these tips:

- Make sure preschool children are not present when parents are discussing specifics about their child's illness or injuries, as the child will become quite fearful of the unknown and subsequently show intense fear with the concern of their body being harmed. Have the parent step out of the child's room and discuss his or her clinical status away from the preschooler.
- When the time comes to inform the preschooler of his or her medical condition or health state, the pediatric nurse should contact the services of Child Life. Child Life provides professionals who specialize in child development, medical play, typical play, and distractions and strategies for healthy coping. See the Team Works box for a summary of Child Life services.

TEAM WORKS

Child Life Services

Child Life Specialists are experts in child development. They promote effective coping through developmentally appropriate education, preparation, play, self-expression activities, and family advocacy. In collaboration with members of the health-care team and parents, Child Life provides:

- Encouragement for the understanding of laboratory tests and other diagnostic tests
- Ease of fears around anxiety with hospitalization, separation, and the unknown
- Fostering of an environment of emotional support, especially with chronic illness
- Advocacy of the philosophy of family-centered care
- Engagement of children and family members in special events, such as holiday celebrations
- Prehospitalization tours of the medical units, operating rooms, and clinics
- Support for siblings of pediatric patients who are affected by the child's illness or trauma
- Provision of health literacy through information and resources, as well as engagement of parents whose children have similar health problems
- Collaboration with members of a multidisciplinary care team to provide a comprehensive plan of care and treatment
- Coordination of donations, program funding, gifts, and grants

---

Medical Play

Preschoolers have a measurable reduction of stress and anxiety while hospitalized if they are offered the opportunity to participate in medical play. It allows them to work through anxieties and fears associated with the unknowns of the health-care setting.

- Beginning 3 or 4 days before the procedure, Child Life professionals can provide the child with mock situations. Medical kits, plastic syringes, cotton balls, adhesive bandages (eg, Band-Aids), tape, gauze, and anatomically correct dolls can be used to simulate a previous experience or an expected experience.
- Parents can help by encouraging and then allowing their child to express himself or herself during medical play.
- Aggression, anger, and sadness may be expressed during this play. These are normal responses and should be supported.
- Both parents and health-care professionals should listen and watch to see if an explanation or correct guidance is needed, such as when playing out a presurgical experience.
- A doll or stuffed animal acts as the patient and the child can imitate experiences or fears of the upcoming unknown. A child who re-enacts stressful medical experiences may experience a catharsis. See Figure 23.4 for a picture of a child at medical play.

Misconceptions are common in the preschool period and medical play can be used specifically to help with misunderstanding.

- After a child is allowed to act out his or her feelings on the medical play equipment, it is appropriate for a health-care professional to then assist the child with

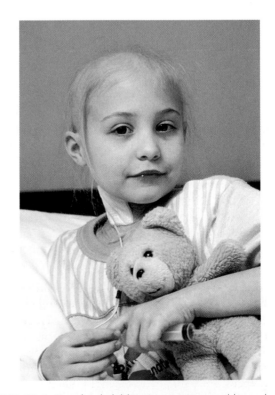

FIGURE 23.4 Preschool child using a syringe and bear during medical play. (*From the National Cancer Institute. Photographer, Bill Branson.*)

misunderstood words or misconceived situations, or to correct the magical thinking processing of an incorrect situation. For instance, if the child is to have a central venous catheter placed in his or her chest the next morning, the child can be allowed to play with the equipment and medical doll, and then be guided through the expected process by a member of Child Life to prevent any misunderstandings or provide simple answers to the child's questions about the procedure and after-care.

• Special attention should be paid when a preschool child demonstrates fears of the unknown, body mutilation, pain, needles, loss of body function, bleeding, and when a child communicates a belief that the hospitalization or procedure is a punishment for misbehavior. See Box 23.3 for ideas for medical play.

Regression of a preschooler's previously acquired developmental milestones and skills is also a reaction to the stress and anxiety felt during hospitalization.

• Parents who identify post-hospital regression should not reprimand the child but assure him or her of how the child acted bravely during a scary experience (Gannon and O'Malley, 2008).
• The regression shown by a child after hospitalization may last a while and may be acted out in the preschool environment to teachers. Both the child's parents and teacher should remind the child that they are safe.

SCREENING AND HEALTH PROMOTION FOR THE PRESCHOOLER

Health screenings are an important aspect of early identification of health issues in children. The preschool period is an excellent time to begin to assess for health concerns. Most states mandate

---

Box 23.3 Ideas for a Preschooler's Medical Play

Medical play provides the preschool child a form of expression. When faced with feelings of anxiety about pending medical procedures and scary aspects of the unknown hospital environment, medical play can give the child the opportunity to work through emotions. Medical play includes:

• Playing with doctor's and nurse's kits, either made up with real equipment or commercially prepared for a preschool-aged child
• Using medical materials to make collages
• Reading books about health-care experiences
• Painting with water colors or tempera paints using syringes
• Using an anatomically correct doll to talk through the expected surgical or medical procedure

---

or promote visual screening for preschool children. Children at this age are particularly vulnerable to myopia (ie, nearsightedness) and amblyopia (ie, double vision). Further screenings should include evidence of neglect, child abuse, nutrition, obesity, and language development. Head Start programs offer further screening in height, weight, and blood pressure for children in their programs. Preschool children need immunizations to continue their childhood immunization schedule.

SAFETY *STAT!*

Immunization Booster Shots
Preschool children need four immunization booster shots: (1) DTaP; (2) IPV; (3) MMR; and (4) varicella. Parents need to know about the importance of these immunizations to prevent both the spread of infectious diseases and serious complications of diseases such as pneumonia, encephalitis, and meningitis. In addition, for the safety of the child and others, immunizations are required for public school attendance.

SAFETY PROVIDED TO THE PRESCHOOLER WHILE HOSPITALIZED

The hospital environment is a very unsafe place for a child. Concerns about electrical equipment, security and abduction prevention, falls from examination tables and large adult-size beds, as well as IV pumps and other medical equipment are legitimate and require that a pediatric nurse remain aware of potentially unsafe situations and circumstances.

• Preschool children are curious and explorative. Precautions must be in place to prevent injuries, accidents, and medical and medication errors within the complex and often hectic hospital environment.
• Many institutions require that young children wear a security alarm device on the ankle or wrist for rapid notification of a child leaving the nursing unit.
• Devices, such as electrical outlet covers, and safety measures to prevent free-flowing IV fluids are used to reduce the probability for injuries.

If a preschool child is left alone while hospitalized, measures must be taken to reduce the chance that the child will wander off in search of family members.

• If there are no hospital personnel that can safely monitor a young preschool child, the child may need to be placed in a high-top crib.
• 4- and 5-year-olds will need someone at the bedside or to be placed in a bed close to the nursing station for observation.

The safest way to maintain an environment free of injuries, accidents, or wandering is to have a family member remain with the child.

• Pediatric nurses should request that an extended family member such as an uncle or aunt, grandmother or grandfather, older sibling, or family friend come and

stay with the child if parents or caregivers cannot remain at the bedside.
- Under no circumstance should the preschool child be allowed to stay in a nursing unit play room without constant supervision by an appropriate member of the family, health-care team, or hospital volunteer.

INJURY PREVENTION FOR THE PRESCHOOLER

Preschool children are curious and active. Pediatric health-care team members must provide anticipatory guidance to parents and caregivers on how to prevent injuries or accidents during this developmental period. Prevention of injuries and accidents should be in the following six areas: drowning, poisoning, fires/burns, falls, sports injuries, and motor vehicle–related injuries. Preschool children should not play in the garage, kitchen, or yard without supervision. Preschool children must be taught safety in both their home environments and at school.

SAFETY *STAT!*

Preschool children must use an approved front-facing car seat in a back seat without air bags. Many preschool children can be in a booster seat with snug-fitting straps over the shoulder and against the top of the legs. Children should not ride in a car with a seat belt only unless they are at least 57 in. tall (4 feet 9 inches, 144.78 cm).

DISORDERS OF THE PRESCHOOLER

During the preschool period, particular disorders are of concern. This next section will address two concerns found during this developmental period: common infectious diseases and the experience of encopresis, or soiling after completing potty training.

Infectious Disease

Preschool children are particularly vulnerable to common infectious diseases. These diseases include a variety of viral, bacterial, and parasitic infections. Parents, preschool teachers, and health-care professionals need to know the basics of prevention and early recognition of the most common childhood infectious diseases to prevent the spread of disease to others and to minimize the risk of complications. Promoting healthy behaviors early in childhood can reduce illnesses.

HEALTH PROMOTION

Teaching Preschool Children to Avoid Germs

Young preschool children do not comprehend germ theory and require instruction, supervision, and support in learning how to reduce the chance of acquiring or spreading infections:
- Have children wash their hands immediately upon returning home from preschool. Research has shown that the common cold can be reduced by 50% in households with preschool children who are instructed to wash their hands upon coming home from school.
- Have children wash their hands right before sitting down to eat. Preschoolers often use eating utensils as well as their fingers when consuming snacks and meals.
- Instruct children not to share dishes, cups, and eating utensils with others to reduce the chance of spreading germs. Discourage feeding younger siblings bites of their food with their own eating utensils.
- Encourage children to wash their hands after they play outside to reduce the amount of soil, dirt, animal dander, and germs from playmates entering the house.
- Teach children to cough into their elbows to reduce the spread of germs.
- Teach children to use tissues when sneezing and blowing their nose. Often young children wipe their noses on their sleeves or blow their nose into their hands and wipe mucus on their clothing.
- If a child is exposed to a cold or other infectious disease during play, wipe off all toy surfaces with a commercial cleaner such as antiseptic household cleaning wipe.
- Clean thermometers after each use, even when used repetitively by the same child.

Varicella Zoster

Varicella zoster, or chickenpox, is caused by a virus spread by both close contact and airborne exposure via coughing and sneezing.

- The disease causes fever and an intensely itchy rash with lesions. The lesions resemble blisters with characteristic weeping that heal by developing yellow crusts.
- The child will experience a fever just before the eruption of the rash.
- Varicella is highly contagious and is prevented by childhood administration of two vaccines.
- Children hospitalized with the chickenpox require isolation, preferably in a negative pressure room to avoid transmission.

Croup

Croup, also called *laryngotracheobronchitis*, is marked by a very harsh and repetitive cough that has been compared with the sound of a barking seal.

The vocal cords, larynx, and trachea become inflamed with the parainfluenza virus, which can cause a cough that is frightening to the young child and parents.

- Because children younger than age 5 have small airways, the symptoms are worse in these children.
- Croup is usually not serious and can be treated at home with moist air and oral fluids.

Fifth Disease

Fifth disease, or erythema infectiosum, is a viral infection caused by the parvovirus B-19.

- The virus causes a mild rash with a characteristic "slapped cheek" appearance on the face and a lacy red rash on the child's limbs and trunk that resolves in approximately 7 to 10 days.
- Only occasionally does the rash cause the child to itch.
- The infection produces a low-grade fever.
- Before the rash appears, the child's infection is contagious via respiratory secretions while the child appears to just present with a common cold.

Impetigo

Impetigo is a bacterial infection caused by either group A streptococcus or staphylococcus.

- The bacteria that cause this mild illness produce contagious lesions.
- Small, round bacterial infections are common on the face and have a characteristic yellowish crust. Young children should not be allowed to touch these lesions, as the bacteria can spread or the lesions can get secondary infections.
- Impetigo lesions do not produce scars.

Head Lice

Head lice are parasites that can be found on the head and body, including the pubic area. There are three types of lice:

1. Pediculus humanus capitis: head louse
2. Pediculus humanus corporis: body louse
3. Pthirus pubis: pubic louse
    - Lice infestations are spread between children in close contact, especially when hats, sweaters, play clothes, bed clothes, sports gear such as helmets, and combs and brushes are shared.
    - Lice move between people only via a surface; they do not fly or jump.
    - Lice infestations cause intense itching from the feeding and crawling behaviors of the adult lice. Females lay their eggs at the base of the hair shaft, and the eggs, also called nits, hatch in 7 to 9 days.
    - The adult louse is the size of a sesame seed and lives approximately 30 days.
    - Over-the-counter pediculicides are effective in the treatment of a lice infestation.
    - Children should not return to school until they are free of nits.

Pertussis

Pertussis, also known as *whooping cough,* is a highly contagious bacterial respiratory infection caused by *Bordetella pertussis.*

- The hallmark symptom is an uncontrollable and violent cough, sometimes followed by vomiting.

- The whooping sound associated with this disease occurs when the child takes one or several breaths before or between coughing episodes.
- Transmission occurs from person to person via coughing or sneezing while in close contact.
- Children develop symptoms between 7 and 10 days after exposure.
- The pertussis immunization is very effective in protecting the preschool-aged group.

Ringworm

Ringworm infections are caused by a fungus called a *dermatophyte*—not a worm at all.

- Ringworm infections in children most commonly appear on the scalp, called *tinea capitis,* or on the moist areas of the skin.
- The child who presents with ringworm will demonstrate a red scaling or fissure on the skin typically appearing 4 to 14 days after exposure. They may also demonstrate hair loss if infestations occur on the scalp.
- Early treatment with antifungals can prevent complications of abscesses or cellulitis.
- Hand washing is the most effective means to prevent transmission.

Hand washing should be taught in a consistent manner and modeled by adults. Young children benefit from lifelong health habits and therefore should be taught hand washing from a very early age with positive reinforcement.

PATIENT TEACHING GUIDELINES

Hand Washing for Preschoolers

- Provide an accessible stack of paper towels that the child can reach with ease.
- Teach the child to make the water warm, not hot, when turning it on.
- After applying a small amount of liquid soap from preferably a hands-free dispenser, instruct the child to sing a pleasant song, such as "Happy Birthday," for the duration of lathering her or his hands up to the wrists.
- Demonstrate the need to pay special attention to the surfaces between the fingers and under the nails.
- Rinse the hands by holding the hands downward.
- Take a small supply of paper towels and dry the hands thoroughly, and then dispose towels directly into a hands-free waste basket after turning off the faucet with the wet paper towel.
- Instruct the child to wash hands after outside play, before meals, after toileting, and after waking up from a nap. Consistency in reminders of hand washing creates a pattern of positive behaviors carried on throughout childhood.

Rotavirus

Rotavirus is the most common cause of severe diarrhea among young children.

- Under electron microscopic examination, the virus demonstrates a wheel-like appearance.
- The primary mode of transmission is from the fecal-oral route, though the virus can survive on surfaces, contaminating them.
- Transmission of the virus follows a winter seasonal pattern, is self-limiting, and only lasts for a few days for those children with a healthy immune system.
- Prevention via the rotavirus vaccine is effective in the prevention of the associated gastroenteritis.

Respiratory Syncytial Virus (RSV)

Respiratory syncytial virus (RSV) is a contagious respiratory virus that infects the lungs, causing a form of bronchiolitis. It is a mild infection in older children, but a potentially severe infection in infants. Preschoolers do not have as high a risk for complications as infants do, but can be very symptomatic.

- Almost all children will demonstrate antibodies that show they have had an infection before their second birthday.
- Infection is most common in the late fall and winter months. People are generally contagious for 3 to 8 days, and those with weakened immune systems can remain infectious and shed the virus for several weeks.
- Hand washing and disinfecting hard surfaces are required to minimize the transmission of the virus.

Strep Throat

Strep throat is caused by the bacteria group A streptococcus.

- The classic infection causes severe sore throat and pain on swallowing (ie, dysphagia).
- Parents should seek medical attention for fevers greater than 38°C, pus located on the back of the throat, sore throat symptoms lasting for more than a week, or known contact with someone with strep throat.
- A throat swab confirms the infection.
- Antibiotics treat this infection and children should not return to preschool until cleared by a primary caregiver because it is highly contagious via saliva.

SAFETY *STAT!*

Strep throat is associated with pain. Children as young as 3 can use a Wong-Baker FACES pain scale to rate their pain. The caregiver provides the child with a tool that depicts a series of face pictures from a smiling face to a crying face; the child picks the picture that most represents their pain level. The FLACC pain tool can also be used between the ages of 7 months through the preschool period. Here the caregiver determines the pain level by matching the five areas (expressions on Face, positioning and movement of Legs, Activity level, Cry, and Consolability) to the child's clinical presentation.

Encopresis

Encopresis is a medical diagnosis given to a child, 4 years or older, who had previously achieved potty training and is now soiling his or her clothing during the day. This baffling, unexpected, and highly embarrassing fecal soiling is highly frustrating for both the child and the parents. The disorder affects 1.5% of children between 4 and 12 years of age and is more common than expected by pediatric nurses.

Stool retention in the colon begins the process of encopresis. With the enlargement of the colon, the intestinal walls and nerves located within them stretch and cause a diminishing of the nerve sensation. Eventually the child will lose the ability to contract and push the stool out. The child with encopresis does not have the sensation or urge to defecate, and the stool is passed without his or her feeling it until after defecation has occurred. As the intestinal wall continues to stretch, large, hard stools are retained and liquid stool is released by seeping out around the fecal mass. Typically, the soiling occurs in the late afternoon, after school.

Other symptoms include severe constipation with abdominal pain, lack of appetite, avoidance of bowel movements, and the passage of such large stools that they frequently clog the toilet. Some children are prone to this condition, as they are born with colonic inertia, or a tendency toward constipation. Parents often express exasperation that their child does not feel the soiling nor, with daily repeated exposure, becomes aware of the odor coming from his or her pants. However, the problem should be seen as a medical problem that requires intervention and less as an emotional, behavioral, or developmental issue.

Encopresis a chronic problem, but it is treatable:

- The child must take responsibility to sit on the toilet several times a day in an attempt to pass at least a half-cup sized stool. Some parents accomplish this by setting a timer in the bathroom and requiring the child to sit for at least 10 min.
- The child's diet must include high fiber and lots of water, and the family must work together to diminish the emotional aspect of this condition during the long treatment.
- The overall treatment goal is for the child to have a daily normal bowel movement; reduce stool retention, thus healing the stretched lower intestine; have the child gain control of defecation; and resolve any bad feelings, such as guilt and frustration, and family conflicts because of the symptoms of encopresis.

NURSING CARE PLAN for the Child with Encopresis

Encopresis is an elimination disorder that presents with challenges for both health-care professionals and families. Preschool children who are experiencing this disorder can benefit from the outcomes of a nursing process, including nursing diagnoses, goals, and interventions.

Nursing Diagnoses:
- Constipation is experienced, related to inconsistent patterns of elimination and stool retention.
- Bowel incontinence related to watery stool seeping around hardened stool is observed.
- Anxiety and emotional distress related to the discomfort of incontinence are experienced.
- There is pain related to discomfort during the elimination of hard and retained stool.

Expected Outcomes:
- The child will have normal bowel function as evidenced by passing soft stools on a daily basis without constipation or seeping liquid stool.
- The child will not experience anxiety, social isolation, or embarrassment.

Interventions:
- The child's current impaction of hardened stool will be evacuated with enemas, stool softeners, and suppositories per medical order.
- The child will be provided sufficient high-fiber foods and oral fluids to assist with daily elimination.
- The child will be given support and positive reinforcement for actively engaging in a plan of treatment including nutrition, fluids, and at least twice daily trying to pass a stool, for at least 5 to 10 min, after meal times.

Key Points

- The preschooler time period is from 3 years old through the fifth year, ending right before the child's sixth birthday.
- The preschooler experiences rapid language development, often through imitation.
- The young preschooler remains egocentric and slowly grows to being able to identify another's point of view or feelings.
- Preschoolers have very active imaginations and enjoy play that allows them to act out adult roles.
- The experience of magical thinking denotes how the preschooler has a minimal distinction between what is reality and what is fantasy, believing he or she can cause actual events.
- The preschool child fears body mutilation, death, and blood, and may show signs of regression in response to these fears.
- Parents and caregivers should allow the preschooler to develop a sense of what Erikson's developmental theory describes as initiative by allowing the child the opportunity to show what they can do, try out new skills, and develop new roles.

REVIEW QUESTIONS

1. The pediatric nurse should explain to the parents of a preschooler that they can expect their 3-year-old child to be able to accomplish which of the following skills?
   1. Tie tennis shoe's laces
   2. Boogie board small waves
   3. Ride a tricycle
   4. Use a jump rope

2. A 4-year-old child has been admitted to the in-patient pediatric unit for a course of antibiotics to fight cellulitis. Which of the following bed assignments would be most appropriate for this preschooler?
   1. In a bed in a single room away from the other children
   2. In a high-top crib
   3. In a multibed room with three other children
   4. In an isolation room to prevent the spread of the infection

3. Which behavior demonstrated by a preschooler would confirm the child is in an appropriate developmental level?
   1. She takes her oral antibiotic without hesitation.
   2. She cries loudly when her mother leaves the hospital room.
   3. She is distressed about a scar from a previous abdominal surgery.
   4. She is requesting a ballerina bandage after having her blood drawn.

4. Which of the following conditions can occur when a preschooler frequently scratches chickenpox vesicle lesions?
   1. Secondary bacterial infections
   2. Cellulitis in opposing arm
   3. Scabies infection
   4. Neurological sequela

5. Which of the following infections experienced by a 5-year-old child in a preschool center must be reported to all parents?
   1. Facial cellulitis
   2. Strep throat
   3. Pediculosis
   4. Urinary tract infection

6. A preschooler is requesting to have the same lunch for school every day. An appropriate response to the parent would be:
   1. "That is unacceptable and variety is required for sound nutrition."
   2. "That is OK; your young child will change his mind soon enough."
   3. "Try taking leftovers from last night's dinner."
   4. "Try to have the preschooler pack his own lunch the night before."

7. Which of the following would the pediatric nurse see as the reason for a preschooler describing her teddy bear as being in the hospital because she was "naughty"?
   1. Separation anxiety
   2. Magical thinking
   3. Intuitive thought processing
   4. Egocentrism

8. What heart rate would a pediatric nurse expect to find in a preschooler who is 4 years old?
   1. 90 to 115 bpm
   2. 120 to 125 bpm
   3. 80 to 100 bpm
   4. 60 to 90 bpm

CRITICAL THINKING QUESTIONS

1. What behaviors are considered "classic" for a preschooler to display while demonstrating regression during hospitalization?
2. In an ideal world, what health screenings would be worthwhile to conduct in a preschool classroom located in a high-risk neighborhood with families of a lower socioeconomic status?
3. Although laws vary from state to state, universally, in what car seat style and position within an automobile should a preschool child be placed for safety?

For additional resources and information, visit **www.DavisPlus.com**.
Post-Conference Questions and Activities, Answers, and References can be found on DavisPlus.

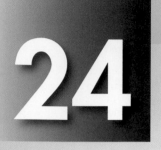

24

Health Promotion of the School-Aged Child

KEY TERMS

concrete operations
deciduous teeth
precocious puberty
prepubescence
puberty
sexual latency

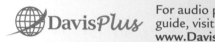 For audio pronunciation guide, visit **www.DavisPlus.com**

CHAPTER CONCEPTS

Communication
Development
Nutrition
Safety
Sleep, Rest, and Activity

LEARNING OUTCOMES

1. Define the key terms.
2. Describe the unique needs of the school-aged child as compared with older children in relation to safety, socialization, and communication.
3. Evaluate the slower growth period that represents the school-age time period.
4. Compare the nutritional needs and eating patterns of the school-aged child, including accurate kilocalorie and fluid maintenance calculations.
5. Contrast the play and sleep patterns of the school-aged child in relation to the other developmental stages.
6. Discuss the issues surrounding safety for the school-aged child, including the need for education about safety devices for organized sports, bike riding, skateboarding, and roller skating.
7. Describe the teaching needs of the entire family of a school-aged child in relation to prevention of child abduction, sexual assault, and other forms of societal violence.
8. Define the effects of bullying on a school-aged child's emotional health and well-being.
9. Critically evaluate the concerns associated with the current epidemic of childhood obesity.
10. Describe the concerns of the increasing incidence of asthma across childhood.
11. Discuss the care of a child with a pediculosis (ie, lice) infestation and how this may affect the child's perception of their body image.

REAL-WORLD CASE STUDY

Christina

■ Christina, a 10-year-old school-aged child, comes to the pediatric clinic for a well-child visit. Her height is 50 in. and her weight is 108.25 pounds. Before plotting her measurements on a national standardized growth chart, the pediatric nurse first converts her measurements to cm and kg. Findings indicate that her height is in the 25th percentile but her weight is in the 95th percentile. Her body mass index (BMI) (ie, weight in kg divided by height in meters squared) shows her size to be in the classification of obesity. The nurse notes that both of her siblings appear overweight and her mother is obese. The child's measurements are reported to the Registered Nurse Team Leader, who reports the situation to the pediatrician. A dietician is called for a referral for the family and meets with the mother to openly discuss the findings, as well as the medical risks and social problems associated with childhood obesity. Three week-long daily diet histories are analyzed by the dietician and it is noted that the child consumes fast food and foods high in corn syrup, and consumes very few fresh fruits and vegetables. Dietary changes are made and the entire family participates in a 6-month-long mild to moderate physical activity program. At the checkup 1 year later, the child's height remains in the 25th percentile but her weight is plotted in the 50th percentile. The pediatric team considers this family's commitment to healthier eating and increased activity to be a success.

1. How did the health-care team calculate her BMI?
2. Where are the ranges of BMI for children published for quick reference?
3. Do pediatric health-care team members share the results of the child's BMI with the parents?
4. How can the nurse assist with referring the family to community services that can provide nutritional support and low-cost, healthy foods?

CONCEPTUAL CORNERSTONE

Health, Wellness, and Illness

Because the school-age period is the longest of the five developmental stages, spanning 7 years, it is important for the pediatric nurse to be aware of the child's and family's health education, nutrition, activity and exercise, well-child checkups, and immunization needs during this important developmental period.

Part of educating patients and families about health, wellness, and illness is to understand the developmental and cognitive abilities of this stage. The school-aged child is in the developmental period of industry versus inferiority. It is very important to the school-aged child to have a sense of accomplishment. Pediatric nurses can provide opportunities for school-aged children to learn about their health and wellness

promotion by having them gain a sense of accomplishment via educational projects and activities. Furthermore, a school-aged child's ethnic and cultural background strongly influences his or her outlook on life; responses to illness, injuries, and hospitalizations; and participation in health and wellness programs. Setting the stage for health and wellness early in the school-age stage will influence the development of healthy habits during adolescence.

The time period of the school-aged child's developmental stage spans from the sixth birthday through the 12th year of life; the school-age period ends at the child's 13th birthday. This developmental stage, also referred to as "the middle years," is marked by tremendous emotional, language, and cognitive development, but slower physical growth than what has been experienced in the younger stages, and much slower growth than what will be experienced during the adolescent time period.

The developmental stage of the school-age period is considered to surround the experience and mastery of industry. Erikson's psychosocial developmental theory describes children of this stage as needing to master industry, or achievements, and confidence, versus the opposite, which is a sense of inferiority (Fig. 24.1). According to Erikson, the school-aged child needs many opportunities to demonstrate his or her academic, social, and cognitive achievements to perceive of himself or herself as successfully industrious.

GROWTH AND DEVELOPMENT OF THE SCHOOL-AGED CHILD

Overall growth and development of the school-aged child is represented by a slower, steadier pattern. The long span of the school-age period, which extends from the child's sixth birthday through the 12th year of life, denotes tremendous change in cognitive, psychological, and social aspects, but shows only slow and steady changes in physical development.

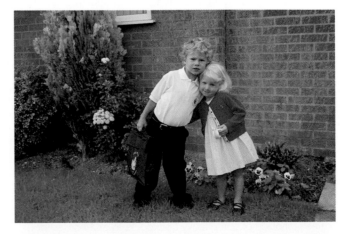

FIGURE 24.1 The school-aged child develops a sense of industry that provides the child with purpose and confidence in being successful.

Until the school-aged child hits the rapid growth spurt of preadolescence, the child's physical growth and development remains steady, paced, and slow.

Physical Growth and Development

Physical development of the school-aged child begins with the first accomplishment of shedding the **deciduous teeth** (ie, baby teeth, central incisors typically first) and then ends with the experience of puberty. Growth via height and weight slows down during this period and is considered steady and paced. During middle childhood, the average weight gain for boys and girls is 4 to 6.6 pounds (1.81 to 2.99 kg) per year, and the average height increase is 2 in. (5.08 cm) per year, with a total of doubling their weight during this time period and a total height increase of 1 to 2 feet (30.48 to 60.96 cm). Proportionally, school-aged children become more graceful in their movements and play and steadier on their feet. Activities such as bike riding, skateboarding, rollerblading, skiing, and climbing become more comfortable and much easier. As the middle years progress, the child becomes taller and thinner in appearance. Muscle tissue replaces fat and the child's body weight begins to represent a larger percentage of muscle tissue and less adipose tissue over these years. School-aged children experience a decrease in their head circumference growth, and an increase in their leg length growth. The skull itself experiences very little growth over these years, and the growth of the brain also changes relatively very slowly.

SAFETY *STAT!*

Muscles are still growing and are not as functionally mature as they will be in adolescence. Children of these middle years need to avoid injuries from overuse or overconfidence.

Body systems become more mature and functional. Blood glucose levels are maintained well and are balanced, requiring less snacking and less prompt feeding times. The total caloric requirement decreases but is dependent on the level of rigorous activity experienced at this time. School-aged children who participate in a great deal of sporting activities will need corresponding higher levels of daily calories. Bladder capacity is variable between both the middle school-ages and the genders, girls having a larger bladder capacity than school-aged boys. The immune system can now function quite efficiency and can launch both an appropriate antibody response and a localized inflammatory response to the presence of injury or infection. Bone and muscle tissue continue to mature throughout this period; until fully mature during adolescence, care must be taken to prevent injury.

SAFETY *STAT!*

School-aged children require solid, well-fitting shoes without heels, should not carry heavy backpacks to and from school, and should be offered well-adjusted school desks because they spend many hours per day sitting in them.

The greatest variation noted during the school-age period is at the end, when the children are reaching their 13th birthdays. Variation in height, weight, motor ability, coordination, and emotional maturation is noticeable and many children are quite sensitive to these variations. Nurses can be influential during this late school time period by being honest and supportive of these differences, assuring the older middle school-aged child that he or she is just about to enter a time of tremendous growth during adolescence.

Prepubescence is a term used to describe the time period of body and emotional changes reflected in a child right before puberty. This time period starts toward the end of the school-age developmental period and is marked by the development of clear secondary sex characteristics over an average of 2 years, ending with the ability to reproduce. These sex characteristics include body hair, breast development, testicular and penile growth, and body odor. This is also the time of rapid growth of bones and muscles. Pediatric nurses need to take the opportunity to offer education to the child and family because these times are marked with variability, perceived embarrassment, and possible negative self-image. **Puberty** normally begins in girls between the ages of 8 and 12, and in boys between the ages of 9 and 14.

Precocious puberty is the process of puberty that begins before the age of 8 for girls and before the age of 9 for boys. It can be specifically defined as breast development in girls before the age of 7 in Caucasians and before the age of 6 in African Americans. The cause of precocious puberty often cannot be found. Rarely, conditions such as hormone disorders, tumors, infections, injuries, or brain abnormalities cause precocious puberty to develop. Symptoms of precocious puberty include the following:

- For girls: Breast growth and first period (ie, menstruation)
- For boys: Enlarged testicles and penis, facial hair starting on the upper lip, and a deepening of the voice
- For both girls and boys: Pubic hair, underarm hair, early rapid growth, adult body odor, and acne

The best way to understand the process of puberty or precocious puberty is to understand how the process begins in the child's body:

1. **The brain begins the process**: The hypothalamus makes gonadotropin-releasing hormone (Gn-RH).
2. **The pituitary gland releases more hormones**: Gn-RH causes the pituitary gland to release luteinizing hormone (LH) and follicle-stimulating hormone (FSH).
3. **Sex hormones are produced**: LH and FSH cause the ovaries to produce estrogen and the testicles to produce testosterone. Both of these hormones are now responsible for the growth and development of sexual characteristics. Estrogen and testosterone are also now produced in the adrenal glands.
4. **Physical changes occur**: The physical changes brought forth by the presence of estrogen and

testosterone now cause the physical changes associated with puberty.

SAFETY *STAT!*

Particular factors place a school-aged child at risk for the development of precocious puberty:

1. Being a girl; girls are statistically more likely to develop this condition
2. Being of African American decent
3. Being significantly overweight or obese
4. Having medical conditions that place the child at risk, which include congenital adrenal hyperplasia, hypothyroidism, or McCune-Albright's syndrome
5. Being exposed to sex hormones such as estrogen or testosterone creams, ointments, adult medications, or dietary supplements

If warranted, the treatment for this condition includes the administration of medications to delay further development. Treatment includes Gn-RH analog therapy, which includes a monthly injection of a medication such as leuprolide. These medications stop further sexual development. The child continues to receive the medication until the normal time of puberty, at which time the medication is stopped and the process of puberty continues.

Nutrition

The period of development of the school-aged child is marked by slower growth in both height and weight. This time period demonstrates the need for the school-aged child to eat responsibly with portion control. Obesity is a major health problem in the nation and the school-aged child, if not supported to make healthy decisions, may face this challenge. The school-aged child is spending more time away from the family with longer school days and more social events. Food choices become more independent as the child eats more with others, attends more social events such as parties, and participates in more screen time. Nutrition education should begin in the early school-age period and the child should be encouraged to share their growing knowledge of healthy eating with the family. Promoting intake of fresh fruits and vegetables daily is one of the most important lessons the child must learn.

Until the child experiences the preadolescent growth spurt, school-aged children, on average, need fewer calories per kg of weight/body size than children in the faster-growing infant, toddler, and preschool developmental periods (Ball, Bindler, et al, 2014). School-aged children, on average, need only 1,500 calories for the first 20 kg of weight, plus 25 calories for each additional kg over 20.

Promoting well-balanced meals is a major responsibility of a pediatric nurse working with school-aged children. It is imperative to offer meals that include a variety of healthy, low-fat choices and to discourage anything more than very minimal consumption of fast foods and candy.

SAFETY *STAT!*

School-aged children like sweets and are drawn to high-calorie, low-nutrition foods. Food should never be used as a reward for good behavior, whether in the home or in the hospital.

PATIENT TEACHING GUIDELINES

Healthy snacks need to be reinforced at home, and family rules about after school snacking need to be set. Children should not come home from school, turn on the television or sit down to the computer, and start indiscriminately snacking.

Sleeping Patterns and Requirements

The overall sleep needs of the school-aged child are very important to success in school (Fig. 24.2). Children in these middle years may display avoidance of going to sleep, stalling behaviors, difficulty in falling asleep, or difficulty staying asleep as they contemplate concerns and worries. School-aged children may seek comfort during the night in the form of a hug or a drink of water. Knowing that they are not alone may help them get back to sleep.

The sleep needs of a school-aged child remain in the 10- to 12-hour range per night. Although they may not sleep in as long as an adolescent, when given the opportunity, they may enjoy staying in bed longer on the weekends. A lack of sleep causes a tremendous decrease in the child's energy at school and may cause poor academic performance. Sleep needs to be prioritized and the school-aged child needs a routine and a reasonable bedtime each night. A child's bedroom should not have a TV, computer, video games, or music playing while the child is attempting to go to sleep. A child may need time to unwind before sleep and some children during the school-age period may still enjoy being read to before sleep.

PATIENT TEACHING GUIDELINES

One important topic to discuss with families is the need to set limits on the use of technology right before the school-aged child goes to sleep. Technology use at bedtime may cause the child to have difficulty getting to bed and going to sleep. It is important to not only limit the use, but to set limits on when the technology, or screen time, should be shut off to allow the child to participate in a relaxing bedtime routine.

Cognitive Development

Cognitive development of the school-aged child is marked by an increase in the ability to think more abstractly, more concretely, and with more rational judgments (Rudd and Kocisko, 2014). The school-aged child is exposed to a great deal of academic work that highly influences thinking and cognitive development. Box 24.1 provides examples of tasks during this period that influence the cognitive development of the school-aged child.

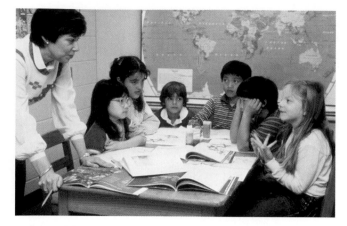

FIGURE 24.2 School-aged children working together in the classroom.

Box 24.1 Tasks Related to Cognitive Development in the School-Aged Child

- Learning to read: From learning to read to reading to learn, from single words to understanding the meaning of what he or she is reading, and from stumbling slowly to fluency and correct pronunciation
- Fully developing a sense of time, space, cause and effect, nesting (eg, building blocks, puzzle pieces), reversibility, conservation (ie, permanence of mass and volume), and numbers, including the distance between numbers and their meanings
- Understanding the relationship of parts to the whole (eg, fractions) and being able to focus on projects in which objects are divided into parts, put back together again, and taken apart in a new way, all representing one whole
- Learning to classify objects in more than one way
- Becoming interested in collections, board games with rules and rationales, and card games with progressively more difficult challenges (from "Go Fish" to hearts)
- Learning to spell and learning where to find resources to assist in progressively more complex spelling words
- Moving from very concrete and logical ways of thinking and interpreting their complex world to more abstract and meaningful views
- Moving from a very egocentric care-free world to one with problems, concerns, and worries

The school-aged child's teacher may be the first important adult in the child's life other than the child's parents. This relationship builds on the child's reflection of who they are, how they interact with others, and how others perceive them. A strong teacher will influence the child's cognitive development, social skills, manners, and self-esteem. It is imperative that the child be allowed creativity in the classroom to test out his or her various skills and improve the child's sense of industry versus inferiority. School is often referred to as the child's "job" in life during this developmental period. Homework becomes very important and the middle school child's sense of identity may be highly influenced by his or her quality of work and the grades earned on academic projects.

Psychological and Developmental Growth and Development

According to Erikson, the school-aged child must have accomplished mastery of the first three psychosocial developmental stages of trust, initiative, and autonomy to now master the stage of industry. Industry can be defined as the child's sense of worth. The child must feel as though there is safety and trust in their environment, must feel like they are encouraged to initiate tasks without guilt associated with failure, and must have a sense of complete autonomy in who they are. After the mastery of these quite foundational aspects of developmental growth, the school-aged child looks forward to demonstrating the completion of tasks. A school-aged child's sense of worth can come inherently from within himself or herself or may be influenced by his or her social environment or relationships with others, either within the family or outside of it. School-aged children need opportunities to assist with classroom structure and function (perhaps through successful experiences in assigned classroom roles and responsibilities) and to interact positively with adults and those with authority.

Pediatric nurses can help a child with a growing sense of industry by offering the child a task to perform while hospitalized. Organizing papers for new charts, drawing pictures of new ways to design a playroom, coming up with new games for younger children, or drawing maps between rooms and the fire alarms/escapes are examples of ideas to promote a sense of accomplishment and success. Pediatric nurses need to understand that the child's concept of successes and failures are very important to the child. If a child is experiencing a chronic illness, encouragement to master a task at the level of their ability will be important and should be planned for. For example, children with juvenile rheumatoid arthritis may experience a sense of accomplishment and industry if they are encouraged to successfully complete their activities of daily living (ADLs) on their own or are able to take their medications by themselves, and these successes are followed by acknowledgement and praise. Pediatric nurses should look for situations and opportunities that allow a school-aged child to feel as though he or she has contributed to and accomplished important responsibilities and tasks.

Sigmund Freud's theory on the psychosexual stages describes the time of the school-aged child as a period of **sexual latency:** a time when sexual desires are lessened. Sexual drives are considered dormant or hidden (ie, latent) while the school-aged child focuses his or her attention on school work, hobbies, friends, and expanding socialization and independence. In the early psychosexual stages of infancy, when the mouth (ie, oral) is the central focus, and during toddlerhood, when the anus is the central focus, the child orients themselves to these pleasures. During the latency period of the school-aged child, these previous experiences are no longer the focus and the focus on the genitalia that occurs in adolescence has not yet started.

Piaget's theory of development describes the school-age time period as categorized by *concrete operations.* This stage begins around age 7 or 8 and continues to about 11 to 12 years of age. Children in this stage of development are gaining a better understanding of their world through logical thinking of concrete events. They do continue to struggle with abstract or hypothetical concepts. Piaget believed that school-aged children begin to use inductive reasoning and logic to determine a particular outcome of a certain event. One important development in this stage is the child's understanding of the concept of reversibility. An example of this is a school-aged child learning to understand the reverse order of relationships of certain mental categories. For example: his or her pet is a turtle, the turtle is a reptile, and the reptile is an animal. This mental process also allows the child to understand that the reverse order of the relationship progression in this example is also true.

Socialization

By far the most important social developments of the school-aged child are the relationships they develop with their peers. School-aged children spend less time dependent on their parents and families for social activities, and branch out to establish relationships with school-aged peers. With these new relationships come certain developmental social rules: (1) the child must progress from free play to playing that may be elaborately structured with rules and be able to interrelate with peers according to the rules; (2) the child must progress from informal social structures during play to the demands of formal teamwork, such as baseball, basketball, and soccer; and (3) the child must learn to participate in social structures within the classroom, including group projects or group oral or written reports. See Box 24.2 for parental education information related to socialization during the school-age period.

A school-aged child learns that self-discipline is very important. The need for this discipline is most important in homework. Homework is a necessity and the need for self-discipline increases each year as the child progresses through ever more demanding courses. If the school-aged child has been successful in the resolutions of early psychosocial periods and is trusting, autonomous, and full of initiative (Erikson's theoretical stages), then he or she will learn easily to be industrious and demonstrate the required behaviors to succeed. A mistrusting child may doubt the future and feel defeated, whereas a shame- and guilt-filled child may have strong feelings of inferiority.

The three areas of a school-aged child's social circle in which he or she learns how to behave and respond to others are the family, the friends, and the school environment. The influence of these three areas affects how a child feels about

---

Box 24.2 Parental Education: Socialization: Is Your Child a Leader or a Follower?

- **Leaders:** If your child is a leader, he or she exhibits confidence in social situations. Leaders are not afraid to take risks in front of their peers and friends and may volunteer to answer questions, take leadership in a group project, or be a team leader in a sports activity. A school-aged child leader will be first to volunteer and first to get involved with activities. The child should be praised for this independence but encouraged to learn how to include and involve others who do not demonstrate leadership and would rather "follow the pack."
- **Followers:** If your child is a follower, he or she likes to watch how others make decisions and perform. Followers watch and mimic the behaviors of other school-aged children and wait to see what others are going to do in an activity. If a child follows the behaviors of someone who is demonstrating bullying behaviors or is disruptive in class, then the teacher or adult will need to encourage the child to get involved with kids who are a better influence. Followers need to learn specific skills about standing up for themselves and not letting others control them.

---

himself or herself and how the child will interact with others later in life.

- **Family:** The child wants very much to be accepted in the family structure. This is a need marked by spending more time away from the home and family life but needing to feel very much a part of the activities and togetherness of the family.
- **Friends:** As the school-aged child grows, he or she will spend less time with the family as a whole and with individual family members. The peer group becomes very important and influential. The school-aged child desires "best friends" as well as membership in social groups. Same-sex friends are the most important and being "important" to a friend is considered paramount. Sharing secrets and special memberships in clubs and a growing sense of trusting peers becomes very important. The school environment and friendships made there highly influence how a school-aged child perceives himself or herself. Bullying and negative social peer interactions can be devastating, with long-term consequences on self-image and self-worth.
- **School:** School teaches a school-aged child what is expected as far as discipline, in-class expectations, desired behaviors and demands, homework performance,

and rules of order. Much of a school-aged child's life is spent at school interacting with lines of authority, teachers, and peers. Standards of conduct, what is right and wrong, what is acceptable and what is not, and what consequences can happen for undesirable behaviors are all learned during the school-aged child's academic experience.

Moral Development

According to Kohlberg's theory of moral development, the young school-aged child sees rules and behavioral standards as coming from the expectations of those around them. Rules are not established from within but, rather, are created, established, and enforced by others. Conversely, as the young school-aged child grows and develops, their perception of rules and order begin to come from within as they interpret actions as either wrong or right. For the school-aged child, feelings of guilt may present if they have conducted themselves or made decisions that are considered wrong. School-aged children need standards because this is how they learn to know what is expected of them and whether or not their choices and decisions will be acceptable or perceived as wrong-doings. Experiencing punishment, such as a loss of privileges (eg, recess, play time, screen time, desserts) will highly influence the actions of the school-aged child. Rewards will provide a sense of desire and guide their judgment. According to Hockenberry and Wilson (2013), young school-aged children may interpret accidents, injuries, and misfortunes as being an outcome of punishment for their bad behavior, acts, or deeds.

Older school-aged children begin to judge a behavior, act, or outcome by the intention of the act, not by just the consequence. Rules are perceived as more authoritarian and older school-aged children are very keen on learning what exactly the rules are, how they are enforced and by whom, and what the consequences are of breaking the rules. They reflect on their perception of their intention, contemplating their own reasons, and begin to reflect on the consequences of the act on others' feelings and perceptions.

Children experiencing moral development in the school-age period are considered by Kohlberg as being in Stage Two, the emergence of moral reciprocity. The early stage of learning right and wrong, what makes adults happy, and the basic consequences of one's actions is now further developed. In Stage Two, the orientation focuses on the instrumental, pragmatic value of an action. One mental thought prevalent at this time is in the form of reciprocity: "If you scratch my back, I will scratch yours." The Golden Rule becomes very real with both "do unto others as you would want done to you" mixed with "if someone hits me, I am going to hit back." According to Kohlberg's theory, the school-aged child is processing situations with the rules, but choosing to apply rules only when it is in the child's immediate interest. Deals, agreements, and equal exchanges are prevalent. The school-aged child's concrete thinking and individualistic sense of self benefit from guidance to learn that, beyond one's own interest, one should pursue what is just, right, and expected for others.

PATIENT TEACHING GUIDELINES

The school-aged child needs adults' and parents' influence and guidance to move from this rule framework to one in which the child has empathy and makes decisions based on what is truly right, not just on what is considered moral reciprocity.

Spirituality

During this longest period of development, the school-aged child desires to explore his or her thoughts and beliefs around spiritual topics. The concrete thinking of school-aged children influences how they perceive their God and demonstrates how they progress toward adolescence. The young school-aged child may perceive God according to how he or she is taught by families or religious teachers, while the older school-aged child will begin to develop independent thoughts about his or her system of beliefs. The young school-aged child does best when presented with spiritual information that is concrete, systematic, and logical, while the older school-aged child will begin to view descriptions and definitions of spiritual terms and thoughts in a more abstract way. Many children in this developmental period enjoy learning about religious and spiritual aspects of their lives and are comforted by prayer and their faith.

Temperament

Temperament, also called *reactivity,* is a set of traits that influences behaviors. For the school-aged child, temperament is very much related to previous behavioral patterns or reactions to past situations. As children grow, they interact with their environment, allowing for experiences to help guide them in their reactions. Some school-aged children have what is considered a very easy temperament. These children fit in easily to new social situations, are flexible to schedule changes, do not react with passion when they encounter difficult situations, and generally have a temperament that is easy for peers and adults to relate to. For a child who is slow to warm up to new people and situations, encountering new social situations pose somewhat of a perceived threat and they exhibit a certain level of discomfort. This discomfort may be exhibited as shyness or mild aggression. These children need both warning and time to adjust to new circumstances, and need to be encouraged to engage but allowed to do so at their own speed.

PATIENT TEACHING GUIDELINES

A school-aged child with a difficult temperament has strong emotional reactions to new situations, new experiences, and new social events. These children benefit tremendously from rehearsals or practice situations in which they can try out the new situation and become accustomed to the new perceived demand. Raising a difficult temperament child, or teaching or providing nursing care to a difficult temperament child, requires special skills. These include patience, authoritarianism, consistency, support, firmness, prediction, and great understanding.

The temperaments of both parents and children will influence how a family interacts. If a highly organized and orderly parent has children whose temperaments express spontaneity, disorganization, impulsivity, and easy distractibility, the parent may find family time a challenge. How siblings relate to each other also is influenced by temperament.

Family Dynamics

The school-aged child enjoys participating in family activities. They enjoy pleasurable recreational time with their family, regardless of the family's constellation or size, and regardless of the age distance between or among siblings. School-aged children appreciate family interactions and enjoy planning vacations and time at the beach or park, and often request that all members participate in an activity. This valuable family time brings members together and solidifies the family structure. Each pair of family members has a unique relationship. A child will relate differently to each parent as well as to each sibling. Because the school-aged child can be quite sensitive to these different relations, family time is paramount. As much as possible, a family should try to spend time alone in recreation a few times every week. Participating in family meetings helps with both the planning of recreation and the feelings to togetherness (Box 24.3).

Box 24.3 Parental Education: Promoting Family Time: How to Create and Implement a Family Meeting

- The meeting should occur at a regular and pleasant time for all family members.
- The parent(s) should serve as the leader(s) of the discussion and make sure all ground rules are followed, such as allowing all members to have a chance to speak and share ideas and thoughts.
- The meetings should have the goal of emphasizing what members view as family needs, plans, and accomplishments, discussing positive efforts by each member.
- At no time should any family member experience criticism, interruption, or be held back by ridicule when sharing ideas and thoughts.
- All children should understand that the parents have the final say or word when difficult decisions are being made and that children are considered valuable "consultants" to the family decisions.
- Records should be kept that document goals, ideas, rewards, positive behaviors, and any new agreements.
- The family meeting should end with everyone sharing his or her perspective about how the meeting went and what could be done to strengthen or improve future meetings.

The school-aged child becomes fully aware of the social roles and responsibilities of each family member. The young school-aged child discovers what parents do for a living and takes pride in discussing these roles and responsibilities at school with peers. For older school-aged children, there is a realization of the meaning behind these roles. They learn to understand the experiences behind their parents' working roles and learn to adapt to variable schedules, demands, work time needed at home, and how finances influence family decisions.

School-aged children thoroughly enjoy coordinating family games. Ideas for fun family rituals and pleasures include the following:

- Family video night
- Sharing the Sunday newspaper over a special breakfast
- Cooking a large family dinner together
- Playing board games
- Collaborating on larger family chores or household projects
- Decorating the house for each seasonal holiday
- Making homemade birthday gifts from craft supplies, old jewelry, and candles
- Building a fire and roasting marshmallows or making s'mores
- Looking through family photo albums or older albums that show relatives
- Watching earlier family videos
- Participating in spiritual pursuits to bring families together: worship, prayer, or services
- Taking a spontaneous car ride and picnic

Play

Play continues to be an important part of a school-aged child's daily life. Young school-aged children enjoy competitive games in which same-sex teams compete. Through this early team play, children learn to cooperative and negotiate, and they learn how important rules are. Through team play, the school-aged child develops a sense of belonging, cooperation, and compromise. Although a young school-aged child may cheat to win, they learn quickly that cooperation has greater gains in the social network. Team sports become important and school-aged children often become involved with afterschool sports clubs and teams such as soccer, basketball, swim team, or baseball. Through these activities, the school-aged child learns to participate in group activities and to answer to an authoritative figure, the coach, rather than to a parent or teacher. Groups offer a testing ground for the child's interpersonal interactions, the development of a self-concept, and sex-role behaviors.

The school-aged child often develops his or her first true friendship. The concept of "best friend" becomes important. Special clubs, secrets, note passing, and unique code words are often shared in this best friend relationship. It is important for a parent to assess the impact of this often intense relationship to make sure the child continues to be social and engaged with others.

Play during the school-age period enhances the development of a sense of morality as the child conforms to social norms, customs, and expected behaviors. Cheating may continue throughout the school-age period, even when the child knows perfectly well what the rules are. Play remains important throughout the six years of the school-age developmental period, but it may shift from a group focus to more intimate recreation because video games and hand-held devices have become so popular.

ANTICIPATORY GUIDANCE FOR PARENTS OF A SCHOOL-AGED CHILD

Parents should be taught about safety, nutrition, obesity prevention, good dental practices, and the need for daily rigorous activity. Other anticipatory guidance counseling should include:

1. Promotion of school attendance and the value of consistently being on time and well-prepared for each school day
2. Promotion of successful homework behaviors through designated time, proper lighting, and a good desk/table and comfortable chair
3. Prevention of back injuries caused by heavy book bags and school backpacks
4. Rules for afterschool activities and checking in with parents about their location
5. Developmentally appropriate information on keeping safe after school to avoid physical harm, bullying, sexual assault, and other forms of societal violence
6. Limits on "screen time" such as video games, TV, and hand-held electronic devices
7. Safety through the use of helmets and pads to prevent sport injuries; properly fitting shoes
8. Rejection of offers for smoking, drugs, alcohol, and other illegal and harmful substances
9. Abstinence of any form of sexual activity
10. Prevention of dental caries and significant tooth abscesses through consistent brushing

DISORDERS OF THE SCHOOL-AGED CHILD

During the years of the school-age developmental period, a child can be exposed to a number of common infectious diseases, viral illnesses, and bacterial infections. Children are increasingly more social and spend more time away from their family and homes. Socialization within the school-age stage can be challenging for some children and a child may experience difficult interactions. The following section highlights a few common health and emotional experiences. Common disorders and challenges of the school-aged child include lice, asthma, obesity, and bullying.

Lice

Pediculosis (ie, lice) infestations are considered very common. There is no association with the socioeconomic level of the family, nor is there with race, culture, or ethnicity. Lice

infestations cross all geographical areas and affect genders equally. Lice prefer clean hair rather than oily hair; the female uses a type of biological cement to secure her eggs (also called *nits*) to the base of the hair shaft. Pediatric nurses must know how to identify the symptoms experienced by a child with a lice infestation, and be able to identify both the adult lice and the presence of nits and/or empty egg sacs. The pediatric nurse may be in the position of treating a child with lice and therefore should be knowledgeable about pediculicides (ie, chemical treatments for lice) and the procedure of meticulously removing all of the nits and egg sacs.

First and foremost, it is imperative that a child suffering from an intensely itchy lice infestation is not made to feel bad about the presence of lice. Teachers, peers, nurses, and family members should be educated about the emotional factors associated with lice infestations. The child may feel very bad, dirty, and sad about their condition and many children are made to feel worse by the teasing that can accompany treatment. Because lice are easily spread through a classroom or hospital ward, it is imperative that anyone involved become aware of the children's feelings associated with the infestation. Children need to understand that a lice infestation is a common childhood experience and it is fully treatable.

Lice are spread via combs, brushes, linens, coats, hooded jackets, play clothes, and hats. Lice can infest couches, beds, or car upholstery and therefore quite readily pose a communicable risk to others. Classrooms should not have coat racks where multiple clothes are hung on top of each other, and children need to be reminded not to share hats or hooded jackets. Lice do not fly or jump; rather, they need direct contact with another head of hair or clothing. The adult female louse prefers to lay her eggs at the very base of the hair shaft and uses a form of biological cement secreted by a gland next to her rectum to secure each egg sac, or nit (Fig. 24.3). Only via direct contact does the adult louse leave the primary host and infect a new host.

The adult female louse can lay hundreds of eggs during her short lifetime. The adult louse lives for 30 days and must eat almost daily. The nits hatch every 10 to 14 days, stay in their larvae stage for a short period of time, and then enter the adult louse phase of reproduction. Lice are considered parasites because they feed on human blood. As a child scratches their scalp intensely, blood scabs can form, which attract the feeding louse.

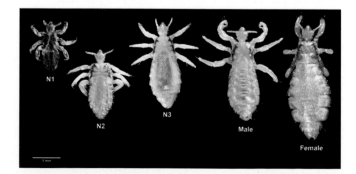

FIGURE 24.3 Head lice.

Symptoms of a lice infestation are marked by intense itching from three sources: (1) the crawling behaviors of the adult louse, (2) the feeding behaviors, and (3) the presence of waste products. When an adult witnesses a child with an intense head itch, lice should be suspected.

The treatment for lice is threefold. First, the hair must be treated with a pediculicide available over the counter. Then, each nit egg sac must be removed meticulously one by one with great care and patience, using fingernails or a fine-toothed lice comb. Thirdly, the child's environment must be treated. Combs and brushes must be replaced or washed with hot water. Linens and clothes must be washed in hot water. Car upholstery must be treated and carpets must be thoroughly vacuumed.

Nursing care of the child with lice begins with demonstrating no aversion to the child's situation. The pediatric nurse assesses the presence of the adult lice and nits. The nurse then assesses how long the child has been infected by determining the distance between the scalp and the nits. Adult female lice lay their eggs next to the scalp so the newly hatched larvae can begin to eat immediately. The further away the nit is from the scalp, the longer the child has been infected. Next, the nurse provides the child with emotional support and determines the best course of action for treatment. A school nurse may be able to send a child home with a lice removal/treatment kit, or the nurse may need to contact the parents to teach them the needed course of treatment.

TEAM WORKS

Neither the nurse nor any member of the health-care team should ever pass judgment or show any signs of disgust if a child is found to have lice because this can emotionally harm the child.

Asthma

Asthma is a disease process of the lungs that includes three conditions: (1) inflammation that causes a reduced total lumen surface area, (2) the production of mucus, and (3) the smooth muscle construction of the bronchioles. All of these lead to the symptoms of a tight chest, coughing, wheezing, and mucus production.

The diagnosis of asthma is becoming more prevalent in the United States. Annual new cases (ie, incidences) of asthma across childhood reached 8.3% in 2015 (CDC, 2015).

School-aged children have unique complications as they commonly do not want their peers to know about their asthma diagnosis. This poses challenges for the family and the school nurse when it comes to supplying asthma rescue medications at school. The school-aged child might be symptomatic and may not be willing to report their condition to an adult for fear of being ridiculed by his or her peers for needing medications (Fig. 24.4). Some states have passed legislation permitting school-aged children to carry their own rescue inhalants and other states are considering legislation. Nurses need to be supportive of the child with asthma but need to

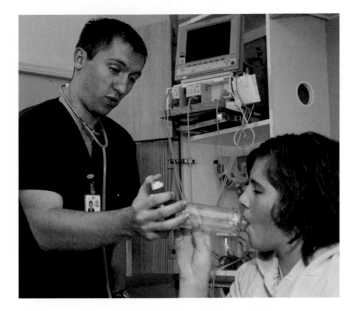

FIGURE 24.4 A respiratory therapist helps a child use a metered dose inhaler.

educate the child about the importance of taking rescue medications when symptomatic. See Chapter 32, Child With a Respiratory Condition, for further information about the pathology and treatments of asthma.

Obesity

Childhood obesity is defined as a child's weight being plotted at or above the 95th percentile on a national growth chart. Childhood obesity is now on the level of an epidemic in the United States.

Although geographically influenced, the overall rate of childhood obesity has reached a range of 10% to 32% in the United States. Influencing factors for obesity can be summarized into three categories: (1) lack of physical activity and too much "screen time"; (2) greater amounts of calories consumed than expended, especially in high-calorie foods, fast foods, and high-fat foods; and (3) genetic/familial factors. Childhood obesity has sociological (ie, peer responses), financial (ie, increased health-care costs), and health consequences (ie, poorer health outcomes).

 ## CULTURAL CONSIDERATIONS
Cultural and Ethnic Perspectives About Obesity

There are cultural and ethnic groups that do not place emphasis on a healthy weight for children. The American tradition is to place value on a child being trim, fit, and healthy. The concept of "health" is not the same in all parts of the world. Some cultural groups view larger children with heavier body weights as being a "picture of health" and place value on the child's heavier size as denoting family wealth and being more attractive. For instance, Burma has had a long history of valuing childhood overweight and obesity as a sign of the family's success. In some areas of rural China, a child with extra weight is seen as representing family financial success.

For other cultural groups, feeding children, even to the excessive, is a form of nurturing and is valued as a form of loving parenthood. Being overweight and obese in childhood is a known health risk factor, and in the traditional Western medical model, prevention, education, and interventions are used to prevent the health consequences of childhood obesity.

The severity of childhood obesity is identified by plotting the results of the calculation of the child's BMI. This calculation is performed by dividing the child's weight in kg by height in meters squared. BMI charts are readily available to use for referencing. See the National Institute of Health Web site for various growth charts categorized by gender and age, and information about BMI for children's ages. When a child is brought in for well-child checkups or for any pediatric clinic visit, the child's height and weight should also be plotted on a national growth chart. Families should be shown the result of the child's BMI and growth chart. Obesity is considered if the child's measurements demonstrate being at or above the 95th percentile for two consecutive plots. Pediatric nurses should initiate a professional nutritionist referral for the child and the child's family for immediate interventions concerning diet, food selections, and ideas to promote activity.

TEAM WORKS

Team Management of Childhood Obesity

- Obesity is now considered a national epidemic, with incidence data showing between 17% and 32% of children classified as overweight or obese. A team approach is required to assist families in committing to a plan of decreased total caloric intake along with increased activity. The entire family should be a part of the healthy eating and exercising plan.
- Pediatric nurses need the confidence to talk to families who have been identified as having obese children. Courage is required to bring up this sensitive issue, but by intervening, a team approach has been shown to promote success in changing unhealthy living patterns.
- Nurses, nurse practitioners, and pediatricians need to make referrals to health-care professionals who are specialists in the area of childhood obesity. Making a referral to a dietician or nutritionist who will create a plan of success is imperative for long-term weight management in children. Pediatric nurses can make referrals to food banks that provide free or low-cost nutritious foods in the community.
- At no time should the team working with a family with an obese child use the word *diet* or discuss *dieting*. Healthy food selection, healthy food preparation, healthy eating, and increased physical activity are phrases that should be used by all team members.
- When an overweight or obese child comes into the clinic or hospital, accurate measurements should be made each time the child is seen and the results should be shared with the interdisciplinary team.

- If a child is identified by a team member as being morbidly obese, Child Protective Services (CPS) may need to be contacted and a child abuse report filed in order for the family to receive the support, education, and services they need.
- The pediatric health-care team members must feel confident in talking openly to parents about the risks and long-term consequences of obesity (eg, bullying, hypertension, musculoskeletal disorders, heart disease). Conversations should be open, frank, supportive, and goal-oriented to the child's health.

Children can be taught about good eating and exercising habits by visiting an interactive Web site at the United States Department of Agriculture's home page at MyPlate. The site includes interactive learning activities on nutrition appropriate across the school-age developmental period.

The emotional factors associated with childhood obesity cannot be ignored. Bullying, discrimination, and social isolation can all occur for a child with obesity. Pediatric nurses need to be involved with community-wide initiatives to reduce the availability and consumption of fast foods, encourage daily rigorous activity, identify and intervene when children are identified as overweight, and provide a health-promotion program that includes the entire family.

Bullying

School-aged children are at risk for experiencing or witnessing the phenomena of bullying at some time during this developmental period. Bullying is a very real and devastating experience that can have long-term consequences on a child's social life, self-esteem, mental health, and overall life. Nurses must screen for bullying and report findings to parents who may not have been told about the experience. According to California Healthy Kids (2006), only 20% of seventh graders report feeling very safe at school and 29% report at least one incident of significant harassment at school. The pediatric nurse might be the first to be told about severe bullying. The child must be referred for immediate help from parents, teachers, and school administrators. The nurse should disclose the severe bullying to the pediatric team as the child might benefit from a referral to a child psychologist.

SAFETY *STAT!*

Extreme bullying has been associated with depression, anxiety, and suicide.

HEALTH PROMOTION

Identifying and Preventing Bullying of the School-Aged Child

Bullying is defined as:
- Punching, shoving, and other acts that hurt people physically
- Spreading negative rumors about people
- Keeping certain people out of a group
- Teasing people in a mean way

NURSING CARE PLAN for the Obese School-aged Child

A nursing care plan for a child with obesity can include the following nursing diagnoses and each of their associated goals:

Nursing Diagnosis: The child's body image is disturbed.
Expected Outcome: The child will demonstrate a healthy body image and describe contentment in elements of appearance to staff.

Nursing Diagnosis: The child demonstrates ineffective coping.
Expected Outcome: The child will show a reduced amount of eating of unhealthy snacks and nutrient-poor foods, especially when feeling stressed or responding to external stressors.

Nursing Diagnosis: The child's self-concept is disturbed.
Expected Outcome: The child will not state any degrading comments about his or her body during care.

Nursing Diagnosis: The child is experiencing ineffective health management.
Expected Outcome: The child will demonstrate increasing levels of activity every week and will state increasing levels of energy.
Expected Outcome: The child and family will demonstrate healthier eating habits as a family unit.

- Getting certain people to "gang up" on others
  Cyberbullying is defined as:
- Sending mean text, e-mail, or instant messages
- Posting nasty pictures or messages about others in blogs or on Web sites
- Using someone else's user name to spread rumors or lies about someone
  Those who experience bullying may:
- Be more likely to be depressed, lonely, and anxious
- Suffer with low self-esteem
- Feel sick
- Have suicidal thoughts
- Witnesses may feel helpless and guilty
  Signs that a child has been bullied:
- The child comes home with torn, damaged, or missing pieces of clothing, books, or other belongings.
- The child has unexplained bruises, cuts, or scratches.
- The child seems afraid of going to school, walking to and from school, riding the school bus, or taking part in organized activities with peers.
- The child appears sad, moody, teary, or depressed when he or she comes home.
- The child frequently appears anxious and/or suffers from low self-esteem.
  Intervention strategies to prevent or stop bullying include:
- Assessing the extent of the problem
- Establishing a coordinating team
- Establishing a code of conduct in the classroom and on the playground
- Establishing and consistently enforcing consequences
- Providing supervision before and after school as much as possible

- Building students' sense of community
- Distinguishing between "ratting" and "reporting"
- Training all school personnel how to assess bullying and about antibullying interventions
- Conducting school-wide antibullying activities using role-modeling and play-acting with positive resolutions
  Teaching children how to handle bullying experiences include
- Maintaining a poker face: Keep an emotionless and expressionless face while being teased and/or bullied. Some children do not know how to respond to being teased and bullied and show the embarrassment and anger on their faces. This is what bullies and teasers want. They want to see it bother the child. Children need to be taught to inform teachers, administrators, and parents if they are being bullied or if they see bullying.
- Teaching children that it is every student's right to inform staff of what is going on and it is every student's right to attend school without being bullied or teased.

INJURY PREVENTION FOR THE SCHOOL-AGED CHILD

School-aged children are at risk for a variety of injuries. Because of their interest in trying new sports and activities, it is imperative to provide information about injury prevention (Fig. 24.5). Preventing injury and promoting safety for the school-aged child includes varied safety information about sports and other physical activities, using protective gear, and

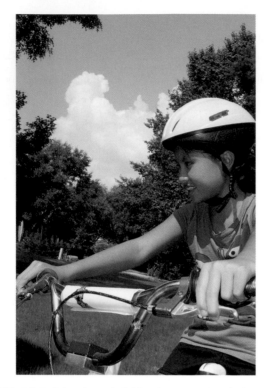

FIGURE 24.5 School-aged child with a protective helmet.

safety measures related to automobiles, water, strangers, firearms, and fireworks:

- **Sports Safety:** Parents should not allow a child to participate in a sports activity if they are not physically and developmentally ready to do so. School-aged children should try out for sports and have experienced coaches determine if the child is ready to participate. If a child experiences a head injury and has a loss of consciousness, he or she must be seen by a primary health-care provider. Emergency transport may be required.
- **The Use of Protective Gear:** School-aged children must be made to consistently wear protective equipment and padding for contact sports or activities such as scootering, snowboarding, or bicycling.
- **Skateboarding Safety:** Children should be taught the importance of not riding in the street and should be brought to skateboard parks and taught the rules.
- **Rollerblading and Roller Skating Safety:** This sport is prone to injuries. Children should be taught how to slow down and stop, how to protect themselves from falling injuries, and should be told never to go down sloping paths.
- **Avoiding Trampolines:** Trampolines are notorious for causing injuries and should be avoided. If necessary, only trampolines with secure-fitting safety nets should be allowed.
- **Automobile Safety:** School-aged children should always be made to wear their seatbelts. Young school-aged children may benefit from using a booster seat if

they are petite. Check state laws concerning each age group and required car safety devices. Some states continue to require booster seats for children between 4 and 8 years old and up to 80 pounds. Shoulder belts should always be used and, typically, children who weigh less than 120 pounds and who are under 5 feet tall should not be in a seat with an emergency air bag. All children aged 12 years and under should be required to sit in the back seat.

- **Water Safety:** School-aged children may act much more independently in water than younger children. They must be reminded about water safety and should not swim alone or unsupervised. Goofing off, rough play, dunking, and unsafe diving must be controlled to prevent water injuries or drownings.
- **Stranger Safety:** Many school-aged children are latch-key children who walk home from school and let themselves into the home. Parents should enforce rules concerning not talking to strangers or communicating to others that they are home alone. School-aged children must be taught about strangers trying to get their attention by such means as asking for directions or help, and children need to learn how to get away from potentially dangerous situations.
- **Firearm Safety:** Guns must be stored in a locked compartment and left unloaded with ammunition in a separate, locked area of the house. School-aged children are particularly vulnerable to firearm injuries and death, so in homes where firearms are present, precautions should include frequent family discussions on safety and no-touch rules.
- **Fireworks Safety:** Every year many children are harmed by the misuse of fireworks, including the loss of hands, limbs, and sight. School-aged children need constant supervision around the use of fireworks, should never be allowed to light the fireworks themselves, and need to be taught safety concerning distance and injury prevention.

SCREENING AND HEALTH PROMOTION FOR THE SCHOOL-AGED CHILD

School-aged children require systematic health screenings to ensure positive growth and development in all areas of their life. Healthy children learn better. Children who cannot hear well cannot concentrate on classroom presentations and discussions. A child who cannot see the blackboard or screen will not be able to comprehend a classroom lesson (Fig. 24.6). School nurses are typically involved with actual screenings or they help coordinate screening services. School nurses should educate teachers about the types of screenings being conducted so that they are aware of their role in identifying children who display problems in the classroom that influence the child's learning. The Labs & Diagnostics feature provides information about essential health screenings for school-aged children.

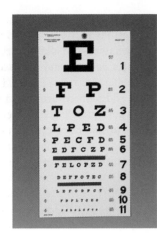

FIGURE 24.6 Visual screening chart used for school-aged children; Snellen's standard chart.

LABS & DIAGNOSTICS

Essential Health Screenings for the School-Aged Child

Specific protocols should be followed and may vary per school, district, or state.

- **Immunizations:** Immunizations in school-aged children include tetanus, diphtheria, pertussis, measles, mumps, rubella, human papillomavirus, meningococcal, and influenza.
- **Hearing Screening:** School-aged children should be screened annually, or at least four times between kindergarten and eighth grade. The American Speech and Hearing Association recommends that an audiologist train screeners. Screening is usually a single tone presented at varying levels of pitch. Rescreening can take place immediately if the child fails the first time. Other than failing a hearing screening test, children with a bad odor or discharge/drainage from their ears should have their hearing checked as soon as possible. Furthermore, if a child is easily distracted, frustrated in group learning, has difficulty finding the source of a sound, or needs repeated verbal instructions, hearing screening should be immediately recommended.
- **Visual Screening:** School-aged children should be screened annually, or at least four times between kindergarten and eighth grade. Most children are visual learners so it is imperative that early screening is conducted to promote academic success. According to Prevent Blindness America (2015), one out of four school-aged children and one out of 20 preschoolers are affected by vision problems. If left untreated, children can experience learning problems and school adjustment problems. About 80% of all school-age learning is visual. If a child's vision is found to be 20/40 or less, a second screening should take place. Snellen's chart is still considered to be the most reliable and most widely used instrument for visual screening.
- **Scoliosis:** School-aged children should be screened at least once before sixth grade. This screening checks for the physical condition of abnormal curvature of the spine, as well as its severity, if found, and is then followed up with an x-ray. Because the screening often includes forward bending to assess for a rib hump; obvious curves; and uneven shoulders, waist, or hips; a like-gender screener should be used. Privacy is essential as clothing may need to be partially removed or lifted during screening.
- **Child Abuse Screening:** School-aged children should be assessed for physical abuse, emotional abuse, and abuse associated with neglect. Children should be assessed for violence in their life, and risks for sexual abuse, sexual assault, sexual exploitation. School-aged children should also be assessed for safe afterschool supervision and problems with delinquency.
- **Lice Screening:** School-aged children should be screened monthly. Some school districts will allow and encourage parent volunteers to be trained for lice screening.
- **Dental Screening:** Schools are encouraged to coordinate a volunteer team of dental specialists to screen at least once in the early school-age period. Poor dental health may affect a child's academic performance, especially if the child is in chronic pain from dental disease or severe caries.
- **Blood Pressure Screening:** School-aged children should be screened at least every 2 years. Elevated blood pressure in children is overall not commonly found, but when identified early and treated, is then correlated with the prevention of heart disease, stroke, and kidney in later life. It is imperative that a correct-size cuff is used because children in the school-age developmental period can vary greatly in body size and shape. Only trained health professionals should assess blood pressures. The width of the rubber bladder should cover 75% of the child's upper arm.
- **BMI Screening:** Annual screening is needed in light of the national epidemic of childhood obesity. Volunteer screeners should be trained by professionals. A national standardized chart should be used to interpret the results. Screening children with potential or actual weight problems can contribute to positive health outcomes. Sensitivity and positivity should be used when discussing results with the child and family.
- **Well-Child Visits:** Well-child visits need to be encouraged by school staff on an annual basis. The completion of all vaccines and assessments for high-risk areas are covered.

Parents are notified of upcoming screenings and have a right to refuse to have their child screened. Confidentiality must be maintained no matter how old the child is or how severe the findings are. Confidentiality agreements must be signed for any organization or individual outside of the school system who performs health screenings on children. States vary in their mandates concerning contacting parents about the findings of the health screening. Many states encourage the nurse to participate in the "rule of threes" as the number of attempts to contact a parent or guardian concerning the need for a referral if the health screening produces results that require follow-up. It is imperative that the school nurse documents the findings as well as the contact or attempts to contact the family. Sending written communication home with the child is not recommended and may not be allowed by certain states.

SAFETY PROVIDED TO THE SCHOOL-AGED CHILD WHILE HOSPITALIZED

One of the most important areas of nursing care of the hospitalized school-aged child is to observe for maladaptive responses. Hospitalizations are almost always stressful, and although children in this middle developmental period do not suffer the same intensity of separation anxiety as children in the younger developmental stages do, being apart from family is stressful, fear-invoking, and can lead to regression, aggression, and feelings of isolation. Even if a school-aged child acts stoic when parents have to leave the hospital, the nurse should provide company, social interactions, play therapy, and distraction. Observe for behaviors of isolation because of school absenteeism, lack of peer contact, and increased dependence on caregivers.

Providing comfort and pain control is an important role for the pediatric nurse caring for a school-aged child who is hospitalized. Children at this developmental level can use subjective pain tools and should be encouraged to describe their pain, state the location, and respond to a numeric pain scale tool.

Key Points

- The school-age stage of growth, also considered the period of middle childhood, spans the longest developmental period and occurs from the child's sixth birthday up to the 13th birthday.
- This period is noted for slower physical growth but expansive social, developmental, communicative, and cognitive growth.
- According to Erikson's theory, the school-aged child must accomplish the task of industry or feelings of inferiority develop. The feelings of industry are associated with achievements at school. The experience of school is highly influential on the child's self-esteem and the development of friendships is paramount.
- Younger children experience the shedding of deciduous or primary (ie, baby) teeth, and the eruption of the permanent or secondary teeth.

- Older school-aged children experience the changes associated with entering puberty and see the development of adult sex characteristics including pubic hair, body odor, breast development, menarche, and changes in testicle and penis size.
- School-aged children are prone to injuries and must be guided to wear protective equipment and padding while participating in sports.
- Parents need anticipatory guidance concerning keeping the school-aged child safe and healthy. Prevention of tooth decay, injuries, and obesity is all important, as is the care of a school-aged child with a chronic disorder such as asthma.
- Immunizations needed during later school-age period include tetanus, diphtheria, pertussis, measles, mumps, rubella, human papillomavirus, meningococcal, and influenza.

REVIEW QUESTIONS

1. Evan, an 11-year-old child, has been hospitalized for a fractured femur caused by an all-terrain vehicle (ATV) accident while his family was on vacation in the snow. The injury requires 2 weeks of traction, and the nurse notes that boredom is setting in and making Evan restless. By understanding developmental theory, the nurse selects which of the following forms of play or distraction for this child?
   1. A multi-chapter adventure book on pirates in the seven seas
   2. A board game requiring multiple players
   3. A deck of cards to play solitaire whenever he chooses
   4. A video game for two on the large screen in the playroom

2. Parents of 7-year-old Heather bring her into the clinic for advice on her third pediculosis infestation in the last 6 months. Her mother describes her intense interest in performing arts and shares that she has been in two musicals in the last year. After listening, the nurse offers the family the following advice:
   1. Take a break from the theatre performances as it may be taking away from her homework.
   2. Encourage more dress up at home and less participation in children's theatre.
   3. Describe the importance of not sharing costumes with others and keeping personal items in a plastic bin away from other performing children.
   4. Be alert to other childhood parasite infections because lice is one of many the child might be exposed to in these developmental years.

3. Asthma is considered a chronic inflammatory process that involves three distinct characteristics. The pediatric nurse describes to the family of a newly diagnosed school-aged child that asthma's characteristics are:
   1. Mucus production, inflammation, and wheezing
   2. Wheezing, coughing, and mucus production
   3. Bronchoconstriction, coughing, and wheezing
   4. Bronchoconstriction, mucus production, and inflammation

4. Obesity has reached epidemic proportions. Influencing factors associated with most cases of childhood obesity include:
   1. Genetics, a sedentary lifestyle, and a high-fat diet
   2. Genetics, a high-calorie food intake, and minimal exercise
   3. A high-calorie food intake, a sedentary lifestyle, and genetics
   4. Depression, social isolation, and a high-calorie diet

5. Erik Erikson's theory of psychosocial development describes the opposing feelings of accomplishment or industry versus a school-aged child's feelings of inferiority. According to Erikson, the greatest influence to a school-aged child's success during this stage of development is:
   1. Successful mastery of the first three stages of psychosocial development
   2. Acknowledgment of the child's strengths and weaknesses
   3. Participation in school activities so that the child can demonstrate "industry" or accomplishment
   4. Support from parents on taking on new sports challenges

6. The loss of primary (ic, dcciduous) tccth and the eruption of permanent (ie, secondary) teeth take place during the early school-age years. The pediatric nurse explains to the family that, although shedding of the teeth can be quite variable, they can expect their child will lose which teeth first:
   1. First molars
   2. Central incisors
   3. First bicuspids
   4. Lateral incisors

7. While providing care at a summer camp for children, the nurse is approached by a counselor who asks about the process of puberty. The nurse explains that while puberty is considered the time when a child's sexual development is complete and the child is now able to reproduce, prepubescence is considered:
   1. The time period of initial sexual organ development
   2. The time period of intense emotional fluctuation
   3. The time period just before sexual maturity

8. Precocious puberty is the process of puberty that begins before the age of 8 for girls and before the age of 9 for boys.
   1. True
   2. False

9. According to Kohlberg's theory of moral development, the young school-aged child sees rules and behavioral standards as coming from the expectations of those around them. Rules are not established from within but, rather, are created, established, and enforced by others.
   1. True
   2. False

10. Precocious puberty can be specifically defined as breast development in girls before the age of 6 in Caucasians and before the age of 5 in African Americans.
   1. True
   2. False

CRITICAL THINKING QUESTIONS

1. What influencing factors exist in densely populated urban areas that lead school-aged children to be at risk for violence, isolation or supervision problems, and delinquency?

2. When does a pediatric school nurse need to become involved if a child is experiencing severe bullying?

3. How might a pediatric nurse approach the subject of childhood obesity with a family of a morbidly obese child?

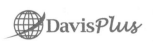 For additional resources and information, visit **www.DavisPlus.com.** Post-Conference Questions and Activities, Answers, and References can be found on Davis*Plus.*

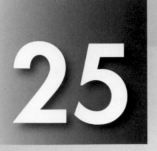

25

Health Promotion of the Adolescent

KEY TERMS

acne vulgaris
alcohol abuse
anorexia nervosa
bulimia
cyberbullying
human papillomavirus (HPV)
obesity
overweight

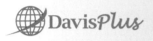 **DavisPlus**
For audio pronunciation guide, visit
www.DavisPlus.com

CHAPTER CONCEPTS

Communication
Development
Nutrition
Sexuality

LEARNING OUTCOMES

1. Define the key terms.
2. Describe the unique needs of the adolescent in relation to children in other developmental stages and age groups.
3. Describe the differences between the adolescent and adult in relation to body systems, anatomy, and physiology.
4. Differentiate the physical growth and development of the adolescent period in comparison with the earlier developmental stages.
5. Describe abstract thinking in the adolescent period and its effect on the teen's view of his or her world.
6. Compare the nutritional needs and eating patterns of the adolescent to the behaviors of the earlier developmental stages.
7. Identify the need to promote hygiene, self-care, disease prevention, and health promotion behaviors in the adolescent developmental period.
8. Contrast the recreation, play needs, and socialization practices of the adolescent to the earlier developmental stages.
9. Teach the adolescent and the family of an adolescent anticipatory guidance practices to reduce injury and accidents.
10. Define the phenomenon of sexuality, sexual practices, and sexually transmitted disease prevention in the adolescent period.
11. Describe the pathology of acne and discuss prevention and intervention practices to assist an adolescent with acne.
12. Analyze the relationship between suicide and depression as it relates to the developmental stage of adolescence. Integrate aspects of safety in relation to rapid assessments and interventions for adolescent depression to prevent suicide ideation, gestures, and attempts.

REAL-WORLD CASE STUDY

Katie

■ Katie, a 15-year-old teenage girl, has been admitted to your unit for a 2-week inpatient stay. She has a history of cystic fibrosis that has required many prolonged hospitalizations. Her height is in the 55th percentile and her weight is in the 5th percentile. Her mother, a single parent of four girls, struggles to balance her youngest daughter's chronic illness with working full-time, managing a home, and caring for her three other daughters. For this hospitalization, Katie requires respiratory treatment every 2 hours, chest vibrating physiotherapy every 4 hours, and triple antibiotics for both pneumonia and a questionable central line infection. Katie expresses a great deal of anger and despair about her hospitalization and often tries to refuse her respiratory treatments.

1. What developmental milestones should Katie be mastering during her teenage years?
2. How can the nurses offer Katie a sense of control over her situation while she is hospitalized for 2 weeks?
3. What distractions can the Child Life Specialist provide for Katie as she spends most of her hours alone?

CONCEPTUAL CORNERSTONE

Health, Wellness, and Illness

The concept of health, wellness, and illness is the most important concept to discuss when providing care to the adolescent population. Teenagers experience tremendous physical, emotional, and cognitive growth between the years of 13 and 18. Their personal decisions toward their health are highly influential to their overall wellness. Teenagers face many social pressures concerning experimentation with drugs, alcohol, and sexuality, and their decisions about these pressures influence their health. Pediatric nurses provide straightforward information to teens about health promotion and injury, disease, and infection prevention, as well as specific information about pregnancy and sexually transmitted infection (STI) prevention. Anticipatory guidance is given to teens and their family concerning adolescent milestones and expectations of behaviors, with an emphasis on the promotion of nutrition, effective sleep patterns, dental health, and safety.

Adolescence is considered to be the time period between the child's 13th and 18th years. Some child developmental specialists consider adolescence to extend beyond the 18th birthday, referring to this developmental period as "puberty to the 22nd birthday."

The developmental period of adolescents has mixed perspectives. It is a time of rapid growth and growing emotional maturity. Yet, the media portrays more of the problems associated with the adolescent time period than the positive aspects. For instance, the media often discusses the contemporary problems with high school drop-out rates, gang involvement, sexual activity, and depression rates. In reality, most adolescents succeed in school, have strong attachments to their families, involve themselves in their communities, and emerge without serious problems such as pregnancy, substance abuse, depression, or involvement with violence. When interacting with teens, families, and the community, the pediatric nurse can provide an important role in shifting away from the negative perspectives and illuminating the positive aspects of working together to teach, nurture, support, protect, and guide the teen through his or her journey. The pediatric nurse may find himself or herself in a unique relationship with teens in which trust and support create a closeness so that healthy advice, role modeling, and profound emotional support can take place. Helping a family direct an adolescent to healthy pursuits can be a rewarding experience for the pediatric nurse.

Creating an open communication pattern is one of the most important aspects of working with adolescents. The need to effectively communicate with teens is imperative to establish trust and an open dialogue. Teens do not simply "open up" to adults and a bond needs to form between the nurse and the adolescent for effective communication to take place. Because adolescents display a range of maturity, emotions, communication styles, and lifestyles, the nurse needs to be open, kind, flexible, and nonjudgmental, and be willing to work on the relationship. The rewards of gaining trust and closeness with a teen are worth the work because the nurse can be highly influential in health promotion and disease prevention behaviors in the teen's life. The pediatric nurse is in a unique position to offer a trustworthy and supportive relationship to coach and motivate the adolescent toward healthy choices and behaviors.

Just like adults, the adolescent population is becoming increasingly diverse relative to cultural and ethnic perspectives and lifestyles. It is important to assess the adolescent and his or her family for cultural influences to health-care decision making, literacy level, spirituality, and lifestyle.

GROWTH AND DEVELOPMENT OF THE ADOLESCENT

Physical changes are very apparent as the child progresses from the school-age period through the adolescent period. Most apparent are the physical changes in height, weight, body hair, and sexual development (eg, breast growth and the start of menses for girls; voice deepening, body hair, and nocturnal emissions for boys). What also must be acknowledged are the profound changes that happen in the adolescent's brain and social structure. The teen's developing brain experiences new cognitive skills, abstract thinking, and an enhanced ability to reason. The teen's frontal lobe neurons become fully myelinated and provide more critical thinking and reasoning. By 18, vital signs match those of adults. Socially, the teen transitions to new relationships with peers and adults, with tremendous emphasis on "fitting in." The rapid emotional and physical growth experienced by the adolescent must be recognized as influential to the care provided by the health-care team.

TEAM WORKS

Normal Vital Signs for Adolescents
Temperature: 36.6°C to 37.2°C
  Heart rate: 60 to 100 bpm (85 bpm average)
  Blood pressure: 100/61 to 121/70 mm Hg
  Respiratory rate: 12 to 20 breaths per minute

Hormones are known to affect an adolescent's physical changes, such as body mass increase; sebaceous gland activation; and hair growth in the axillary, breast areola, genital, and anal areas; there are also hormonal influences to a teen's emotional state. Stress hormones, sex hormones, and growth hormones are all being produced and they influence brain development. The time period of adolescence and puberty is multidimensional and includes intense sexual feelings, physical changes, increasing analytical capacity, and emotional maturity. Dramatic changes are occurring in every aspect of the teen's life. Teens are having an increased experience of independence and active participation in a more complex existence. The growth and sexual hormones being secreted have an effect on the teen's emotional life and therefore enhance and complicate the teen's interactions with the social environment.

Physical Growth and Development

Adolescence marks a period of rapid physical growth. The rapid skeletal growth, usually beginning at about 10 to 12 years for girls and 12 to 14 years for boys, finishes at about the teen's 17th year. The average gain in weight for girls during the teen years is 15 to 55 pounds (6.8 to 24.94 kg) and for boys it is 15 to 65 pounds (6.8 to 29.48 kg). The average gain in height for girls in the teen years is 1 to 3 in. per year, slowing at the onset of menarche and stopping at 16 years of age. For boys, the average gain in height in the teen years is 2 to 4 in. per year, with a significant growth spurt at 13; growth slows down and ends in the late teens.

Typical adolescent growth patterns can be expected unless there is preexisting or comorbid pathology present. Down's syndrome (ie, trisomy 21), Turner's syndrome, exposure to teratogens such as phenytoin (Dilantin) or alcohol, a history of extreme prematurity or TORCH infections (ie, toxoplasmosis, other infections, rubella, cytomegalovirus infection, and herpes simplex infections) all may cause a deviation in normal and expected adolescent linear growth.

Nutrition

The brief period of the teen growth spurt creates a greater need for calories. Often referred to as the "hollow leg syndrome," teens experiencing a growth spurt seem to be constantly hungry and are frequently eating. The calorie requirements are between 60 to 85 kcal/kg/day or 1,500 to 3,000 kcal/day for 11- to 14-year-olds, and between 2,100 to 3,900 kcal/day for 15- to 18-year-olds. More calories are needed if the teen participates in frequent sports activities.

Adolescents require an increase in oral calcium intake for their rapid skeletal growth. Foods rich in calcium are found in the Patient Teaching Guidelines feature. The prevention of dental caries should be reinforced. Teens should be following thorough dental hygiene by brushing their teeth at least twice a day and flossing once a day. Visiting a dentist should continue at least annually. The final molars erupt during the end of the adolescent period and may require an evaluation to ensure room to grow. Many teens and young adults need their wisdom teeth extracted.

PATIENT TEACHING GUIDELINES

Foods Rich in Calcium
Adolescents between 12 and 18 years need 1,300 mg/day of calcium. Magnesium (410 mg/day) is also important because it helps the body absorb and retain calcium. Vitamin D (600 units/day) is another critical nutrient that helps to regulate the use and storage of calcium. Calcium is essential for the adolescent's growth spurt. Vitamin K (75 to 120 mcg/day) also helps the teen regulate calcium and form strong long bones.

  Foods rich in calcium include:

- Yogurt
- Calcium-fortified orange juice
- Sardines
- Spinach
- Milk
- Soy milk
- Cottage cheese
- Cheddar cheese
- Salmon
- Tofu
- Almonds
- Beans
- Broccoli
- Kale
- Turnips
- Fortified cereals
- Enriched breads

The period of adolescence is associated with the potential of consuming high-fat, high-sodium, and low nutritional value "fast foods." With increasing independence and individual food/nutritional decision making, teens may gravitate toward easy meals on the go with friends. Rich in fat and calories and poor in nutrients, fast food is detrimental to the teen's health and may contribute to anemia. During the adolescent growth spurt, teens need education about proper diet to match their nutritional needs. Teenage girls with heavy menses may be at higher risk for iron deficiency. The teenage years are marked with an increased need for protein, calcium, zinc, and iron. Overall caloric needs are based on activity level. It is imperative that teens eat a nutritional breakfast, and snacks should be based on nutrition, not accessibility. National concerns about obesity across childhood continue and adolescents are at risk. Being overweight, obese, and underweight are nutritional problems that should be assessed for and intervened upon by the nurse.

Obesity and Overweight

Obesity and being **overweight** remain serious concerns across childhood. Teenagers are currently demonstrating higher incidences of obesity (ie, body mass index [BMI]

NURSING CARE PLAN for the Adolescent Patient's Nutritional Needs

During this period of rapid growth, the body has increased nutritional needs, requiring more calories, calcium, protein, vitamins, and minerals. Eating habits for teens affect their current health, and for female teens, the health of her future children is affected. Adequate calcium is imperative (ie, 1,300 mg/day of elemental calcium).

Nursing Diagnosis: The teen's nutrition is less than what the body requires.
Nursing Goal: The adolescent patient will consume adequate protein, calories, calcium, protein, vitamins, and minerals sufficient for bone growth, disease prevention, and tissue health.
Interventions
  • Teach the teen and his or her family appropriate nutrition needs, healthy dietary habits, and adequate health food intake.
  • Teach the teen where to find resources on how to prepare healthy food choices.
  • Encourage the teen to limit fat and empty calories, to not participate in unhealthy eating habits such as fad diets, and to reduce sedentary activities such as computer games.

---

greater than 30 kg/m²) and being overweight (ie, having a BMI greater than expected for height and weight) than previous generations. Nationwide, 14% of adolescents are overweight, which makes them at high risk for the development of type 2 diabetes, social discrimination, low self-esteem, and depression. Physical activity levels begin to decline during adolescence, less fruits and vegetables are eaten, and higher levels of "screen time" are engaged in; these are risk factors for obesity and being overweight.

Sleeping Patterns and Requirements

The average teen needs at least 8.5 to 9 hours of uninterrupted sleep per night. Many teens report that they do not get this requirement because of homework; TV watching patterns; the use of computers, cell phones, and texting; work schedules; and early school start times. Adolescents must understand the importance of quality and length of sleep to perform well in their academic lives. Sleep deprivation has a profound effect on the teen's ability to concentrate and perform well in school. Lack of sleep has been associated with emotional troubles, car accidents, poor grades, and illness.

Scientists have discovered that, compared with adults, the adolescent has a different sleep pattern based on a different circadian rhythm, or internal biological clock. Teens produce the brain hormone melatonin later at night than adults and therefore may complain of difficulty falling asleep.

Tips to help a teen improve quality of sleep include:

• Setting a regular bedtime schedule and planning ahead for chores and homework to be done
• Avoiding any stimulants such as coffee, tea, and caffeinated beverages or soda, especially after 4 p.m.
• Avoiding smoking; nicotine is a stimulant
• Keeping the lights out or low in the bedroom; computer screens are considered bright lights
• Waking up with a bright light as a signal to rise and get going
• Refraining from napping on a regular basis, especially no more than 30 min

• Not waiting to cram before a test by staying up late or all night
• Exercising regularly but not right before bedtime; exercise should be finished at least 3 hours before sleep
• Unwinding the mind before bed, including not playing violent video games and not watching scary movies or TV shows

Cognitive Development of the Adolescent

Physical changes in the adolescent can be considered less dramatic than the cognitive changes taking place in the teen's brain. How adolescents think, understand, and reason changes dramatically during the years from 13 to 18. They now analyze situations logically in terms of the situation's cause and effect, yet they do not always display mature decision making. Cognitively, they are able to entertain hypothetical situations, use metaphors, and participate in future-oriented and higher-level thinking.

Gender differences have been shown to exist in cognitive development. Adolescent girls demonstrate more confidence in their social skills and reading abilities, and adolescent boys demonstrate more confidence in math skills and athleticism. No matter what the gender, adolescents can make poor decisions and engage in risky behaviors. There is a relationship between immature adolescents and the increased likelihood of participating in risky behaviors, such as violence and the use of alcohol. Age and gender are less indicative of participating in risky behaviors than cognitive maturity and judgment. Adolescents are also more likely to fear social consequences to risky behavior, such as being shunned by peers, then they are to fear the potential consequences of their parent's discipline. As teens become more cognitively mature, their decisions about risky behavior and consequences become more mature.

CULTURAL CONSIDERATIONS
Adolescent Risk-Taking Behaviors
   A teen's cultural background may influence his or her perceptions about participating in high-risk behaviors.

The nurse should assess the child's perceptions related to the following categories:

Alcohol Use
- 81% of high school students report that they have tried alcohol.
- 32% of high school students report that they tried their first alcoholic drink before the age of 13.
- 50% of high school students report they have consumed more than one alcoholic drink in the last 30 days.
- 30% of high school students report they have consumed as many as five alcoholic drinks at one time during the last 30 days.
- Girls are as likely to drink as boys, but boys report more heavy episodic drinking experiences.
- 33% of high school students report they have ridden in a car of another teen who has been drinking within the past month.

Tobacco Use
- Smoking has been on the rise for girls, although more boys smoke more than girls.
- 70% of high school students report they have tried cigarettes.
- 25% of high school students report they smoked cigarettes before the age of 13.
- 25% of high school students report they smoke at least one cigarette per day.

Marijuana Use
- 47% of high school students report they have tried marijuana.
- 11% of high school students report they tried marijuana before the age of 13.

Other Drug Use
- 9% of high school students report they have used some form of cocaine.
- 14% of high school students report they have used some form of inhalants to get "high."
- 4% of high school students report they have used steroids.
- 9% of high school students report they have used methamphetamines.

Sexual Behaviors
- 50% of high school students report having had sexual intercourse.
- 8% of high school students report having had sexual intercourse before the age of 13.
- 19% of high school students report having had more than four sexual partners.
- 25% of high school students report using alcohol or drugs during their last sexual intercourse.
- 20% of high school sexually active girls report using birth control pills.
- 58% of high school students report using a condom during their last sexual intercourse.
- 6% of high school students report they have either been pregnant or have been responsible for someone getting pregnant.

Motor Vehicle Accidents
- 38% of high school students report that if they have ridden on a motorcycle, they did not use or rarely used a helmet.
- When learning to drive, teens may take life-threatening risks while driving, such as texting, placing others at risk.

Other High-Risk Behaviors
- 17% of high school students report they have carried a weapon (eg, club, knife, or gun).
- 44% of male high school students report they have been in a fight in the last 12 months.
- 9% of high school students say they have been forced to have sexual intercourse when they did not want to.
- Homicide rates are four times higher for high school students who are African American.

Theoretical Reasons for Participation in High-Risk Behaviors:
- Done for pleasure, fun, excitement, and the perception of being novel
- Feelings of intense danger
- Involve the need for peer approval, acceptance, and status
- Romanticizing and modeling adult behaviors
- Temptation to experiment with what is portrayed in the media
- Fear of intense teasing by peers if a virgin

The Pediatric Nurse's Influence
- Be a role model of health and decision making.
- Open a trustworthy channel of communication and listen.
- Provide honest information about the consequences of high-risk behavior.
- Do not pass judgment when a high-risk behavior has occurred.
- Praise and compliment the teen for well-thought-out decisions.
- Help the teen weigh the risks of the danger with the perceived benefits.
- Give ideas for and promote healthy behaviors, actions, and interests.
- Understand that any conversation brought up with an adult on these topics is a very positive sign.
- Know the signs of "normal adolescent experimentation" and troubled high-risk youth.
- Identify when a teen is participating in multiple high-risk behaviors.

(AACAP, 2011; American Psychological Association, 2002; CDC, 2000)

SAFETY *STAT!*

There is increasing concern about teen drivers being distracted by their cell phones. Texting while driving can be dangerous and deadly. According to the Centers for Disease Control and Prevention, car crashes are a leading cause of death for adolescents and about 7 teens die per day in America from texting and driving. Up to 3,000 deaths occur per year from adolescents driving and texting.

Because adolescence spans several years, theorists consider there to be three phases of adolescent cognitive development: early, middle, and late adolescence. Each of these phases has specific developmental markers.

- Early Adolescence, 12 to 13 Years
  - Beginning the use of formal logical operations in academic work

- Early formation of verbalizing one's own thoughts, opinions, and views
- Early questioning of authority figures and social standards
- Middle Adolescence, 14 to 15 Years
  - Posing intense questions concerning society standards and expectations
  - Using analysis with more depth and sophistication
  - Beginning to develop one's own code of ethics and what one considers right and wrong
  - Beginning to think about the long-term aspects of life
  - Thinking about making one's own life plans
- Late Adolescence, 16 to 18 Years
  - Thinking about greater global issues
  - Focusing less on one's self but continuing to argue views that oppose their own
  - A greater focus on future plans for education and career decisions

As teens develop higher levels of cognitive processing, it is very common for them to become argumentative. According to the American Psychological Association (2002), it is perfectly normal for adolescents to:

- **Argue purely for the sake of arguing with adults:** Teens need opportunities to experiment with their new skills of reasoning, even when creating frustration in the adults around them.
- **Be self-centered in life and conversations:** Teens must learn to take other people's perspectives and opinions into account instead of being "me-centered."
- **Rapidly jump to conclusions:** Even with the new skill of logical thinking, teens can jump to conclusions and defend their perspectives verbally. They need to be listened to, not corrected during debates.
- **Constantly find fault in positions that adults take (eg, parents, teachers, and others of authority):** Teens experiment with their new critical thinking, focusing on the exceptions, contradictions, and discrepancies they find in what adults say. Teens are known to be most critical to those adults they find particularly safe.
- **Consider everything a "big deal" and display overly exaggerated responses (ie, being "overly dramatic"):** Teens use social drama as a means to communicate, not necessarily as an indicator of worrisome actions.

Adolescents will display a range of higher level thinking. They still need adult supervision and guidance to help them make positive, healthy, and safe choices. Adolescents may seek adult input to their adultlike decisions regarding things such as finances, college choices, and career considerations. When these conversations come up, the adult should give the teen their full attention, support, and honest guidance so that trust continues and the lines of communication stay open.

The frontal lobe of the brain is the area for processing consequences and utilizing higher cognitive functioning. Completion of the myelinization of the neurons of the front lobe does not occur until the child is older than 16 years. The process of myelinization is a slow progression. Late frontal lobe neuron myelinization has been shown to interfere with thinking about safety and consequences of actions for young adolescents.

Sexual Development

Puberty and sexual maturity are associated with a slower process of development than physical growth. Sexual maturity, defined as achieving fertility, begins at around the age of 10 for girls and 11 for boys. Girls start with breast budding and progress to an increase in pelvic girth and the start of menstruation. For boys, the onset of puberty involves enlargement of their testes at around age 11 and progresses to the first ejaculation, which occurs, on average, between 12 and 14 years of age. During mid-adolescence, the teen progresses to secondary sexual characteristics such as increasing body hair and changes in voice. A male teen's voice changes occur at the same time as penis growth. Nocturnal emissions of seminal fluid (ie, wet dreams) seem to occur at the same time as the peak growth spurt of the boy's height. Race has been shown to be an influencing factor in the onset and progression of sexual maturity.

Many health-care professionals use Tanner's scale to assess and describe the external physical growth and developmental changes that take place during adolescence. This is a five-point scale that demonstrates the genitalia and pubic hair changes across childhood in boys (Fig. 25.1) and girls (Fig. 25.2).

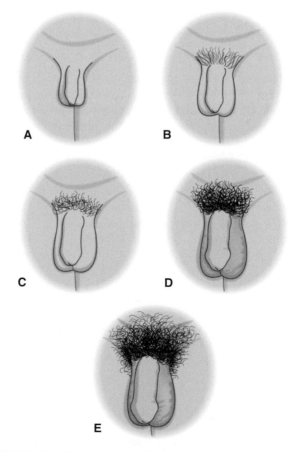

FIGURE 25.1 Tanner's stages for male genital and pubic hair development: A, Preadolescent; B, C, D, Adolescent; E, Adult.

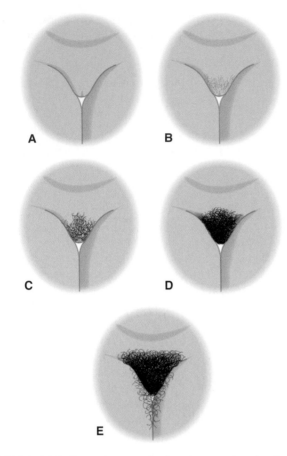

FIGURE 25.2 Tanner's stages for female genital and pubic hair development: A, Preadolescent; B, C, D, Adolescent; E, Adult.

Female breast development also takes place during adolescence (Fig. 25.3). When a teen demonstrates late physical and sexual maturity, the health-care team must be alert to the need for an investigation of metabolic health. Research has shown a relationship among depression, substance abuse, eating disorders, and disruptive behaviors for girls who mature physically and sexually early, and for boys who mature physically and sexually late. Research has also shown that boys who mature early are more likely to participate in early high-risk behaviors such as smoking, delinquency, and sexual activity. There is also a higher incidence of bullying for boys who mature late.

Adolescence is the period of time when some teens experiment with sex. Teens need to have honest education about protecting against pregnancy and STIs. Pediatric nurses might find that the teen is more comfortable talking with a nurse than talking to a family member about sex. Offering straight-forward information on sexuality, sexual activity, risks, and protection is an important nursing role.

 CULTURAL CONSIDERATIONS

Race and Ethnicity in Relation to Sexual Maturity

Research has shown that there is diversity in the onset of puberty and the progression of sexual maturity in various ethnic and racial groups. On average, African American girls begin menstruating 6 months earlier than Caucasian girls. Scientists are continuing to investigate the relationship between rural versus urban environments, genetics, dietary differences, and exposure to hormones in milk and meat as influences to earlier sexual maturation. Recent findings have shown that the onset of puberty is occurring 1 year earlier for Caucasian girls and 2 years earlier for African American girls than previous decades. One study showed that 27.2% of African Americans and 6.7% of Caucasians demonstrate some clinical signs of early puberty by the age of 7.

Regardless of cultural or ethnic influences, teens report that when they are prepared by adults for the changes in puberty, they feel more comfortable than those who were not prepared. With the range of puberty starting for boys between 9 and 14 (Healthychildren.org, 2015), starting the conversation about puberty in the later school age developmental period is important (Kaplowitz and Oberfield, 1999; Lerner and Galambos, 1998; Dounchis, Hayden, et al, 2001).

Psychological and Developmental Growth and Development

Overall, adolescents struggle with rapid growth, cognitive and emotional maturity, and spiritual exploration, all within the context of developing their self-identity and self-esteem. Adolescents become very involved with their peer group and peer pressure is highly influential to their positive and risky behaviors. Teens become progressively more interested in

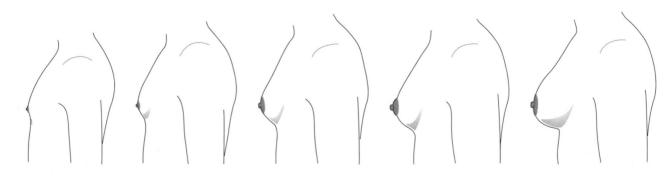

FIGURE 25.3 Breast development.

the opposite sex and many explore sexuality as a form of self-expression. Adolescents need positive role models and honest communication about adult-related activities. Familial expectations influence the teens' personal identity, work habits, and health perspectives. Pediatric nurses should offer guidance to families to keep channels of communication open and explain the emotional variability experienced by the adolescent.

Emotional maturity for teens includes their developing sense of identity. According to Erik Erikson's theory of psychosocial development, the teen is in the phase of development called *identity versus role confusion.* Here the teen is examining and redefining self, family, peer group, and community. While they are experimenting with different roles, if they are successful in this stage of development, they will develop confidence in their self-identity and optimism about their future. If they are not successful in this developmental stage, Erikson's theory suggests that they will be unable to have a meaningful definition of self and will therefore develop role confusion. The teen must determine their self-concept and their self-esteem. Self-concept includes their perception of their beliefs about who they are in relation to intelligence, physical appearance, personality, and attributes. Self-esteem includes how they view themselves, and is influenced through comments by others. Self-esteem has been found to have a direct relationship with negative outcomes such as eating disorders, depression, substance abuse, and delinquency behaviors (APA, 2002).

Freud considers adolescence as a phase of development called the "genital stage." The teen focuses on their genitals as an erogenous zone and will engage in masturbation and possible sexual relationships. Freud's theory of psychosexual development discusses the conflict the teen may have between society's expectations of restraint and his or her need for sexual satisfaction. This is a time for education concerning self-care and protection from pregnancy and STIs. It is not uncommon for the teen to experience homosexual thoughts and curiosity. Some teens may participate in bisexual relationships. The Oedipal complex, according to Freud, is a child's attraction to the parent of the opposite sex. This is common during early adolescent years.

Piaget's theory of cognitive development describes adolescence as a time of greater complex thinking, formal logical operations, and abstract thinking, all referred to as "formal operations." According to Piaget, the adolescent is able to logically manipulate abstract, observable, and nonobservable concepts with greater depth. This transition from earlier concrete thinking to formal logical operations occurs over time, with each teen developing at their own time and rate.

Emotional Development

Emotional growth and development during the adolescent period is highly variable. Regardless of where individual adolescents are in their development, their emotional status is influential to their well-being. The pediatric nurse must have an awareness of what to expect in relation to emotional variability when interacting with teens. Eight common emotional experiences that can occur anytime during adolescent emotional development are the following:

1. A period of high influence of the peer group on self-esteem, self-image, and self-worth
2. A period of feelings of invincibility
3. Emotional vacillation between the emotions experienced by children and young adults
4. Craving independence yet needing family time, parental influence, and support
5. Balancing conformity with the peer group and feelings of embarrassment when seen as unique or different than others
6. Feeling "grown-up" when participating in adult-type activities such as driving and voting
7. Feeling restless and complaining about being "bored" if not socializing, playing sports, or using technology
8. Feeling tremendous concern about appearance, and trying to balance "fitting in" with finding uniqueness and self-expression in relation to their looks

It is important to listen carefully when a teen is expressing concerns about his or her physical appearance. If the teen is complaining about eye glasses, acne, weight, or overall features, it is imperative that the nurse listen and offer support, never dismissing the conversation by saying, "You look fine" or "Don't worry, that is normal." To keep communication open, the nurse should be an attentive listener and offer support rather than close the opportunity for the teen to trust and open up about serious concerns.

Spiritual Development

U.S. adolescents demonstrate a high level of affiliation with a religious group. Between 84% and 87% of teens have reported being part of a religious group and the numbers have been rising. Religious and spiritual development in teens tends to be associated with providing the teen with security, reduced anxiety, meaningful processes to understand existential questions, and connection to a community (King and Roeser, 2009). According to Hockenberry and Wilson (2013), adolescents who have a greater level of spirituality and religiosity tend to demonstrate less of the high-risk behaviors associated with this developmental stage.

Kohlberg's theory about moral development describes adolescence as a time period when teens seriously question existing moral values and how these values have relevance to themselves, other individuals, and society. According to Kohlberg, this stage is called the *postconventional level of morality* and is marked by the development of a child's individual conscience and set of moral values. As the adolescent gains higher levels of maturity and autonomy, he or she begins to replace a set of morals and values presented by parents and family with his or her own. Concepts of duty, obligation, right versus wrong, and making amends for mistakes or misdeeds begin to emerge and become influential to decision making and actions. Some adolescents use the values and beliefs of their families as a stable foundation upon which to base their own beliefs and values.

Play

Adolescents need a "social community" as their main form of play and recreation (Fig. 25.4). The Internet, social media, cell phone, and portable computers have become the main sources of their "social communities," as well as sports, church groups, and, if the teen is old enough, work. Many researchers have determined that the average time spent by a teen in some form of media is 6 to 8 hours a day. Many teens participate in multiple forms of media or "screens" at the same time such as instant messaging, Facebook, and the Internet simultaneously. When interacting with teens, the pediatric nurse needs to promote positive media experiences while minimizing negatives such as violent video games and movies that portray unhealthy sexuality or any form of pornography. Appropriate choices of music are also a concern as many contemporary artists use profanity and violent references in lyrics. Rules must exist in the pediatric health-care setting concerning what teens are allowed to view or use for recreation and distraction. A Child Life Specialist should be consulted for healthy choices in recreation while hospitalized.

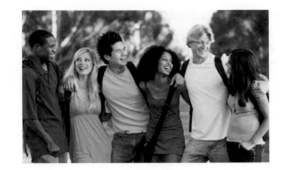

FIGURE 25.4 Teenagers socializing.

CONCEPTUAL CORNERSTONE

Growth and Development: Age-Appropriate Activities for Teens

- Organized and spontaneous sports activities with use of safety gear
- Caring for a pet, either one's own or volunteering to care for another's
- Volunteering for a lower-grade school, tutoring, or serving an institution such as a humane society or injured animal center
- Reading for pleasure
- Age-appropriate social media such as Facebook, chat rooms, instant messaging, or Internet use
- Movies at home with friends and popcorn
- Board games at an adolescent's developmental level (Monopoly, Clue, Beat the Parents, Backgammon)
- Video games that are nonviolent, nonsexual, and age-appropriate
- Social events (eg, movies, school dances, parent-supervised parties)
- Development of a secret code or secret languages
- Window shopping or visiting a mall
- Physical recreation such as surfing, hiking, running, kite flying, or hip-hop dancing
- Scrapbooking
- Journaling with writing and art work; making a flower press journal
- Making a "feeling" or "self-history" collage
- Beading and jewelry making

LEGAL ISSUES IN ADOLESCENT HEALTH CARE

State laws govern whether or not an adolescent can consent to treatment without parental knowledge. The three widespread requirements for a minor to be exempt from parental consent include emergencies, being an emancipated minor, and being a "mature minor":

1. **Emergencies:** A minor can be treated without parental consent if the child experiences an emergency need. This is based on the primary care provider's (eg, the nurse practitioner's or physician's) good judgment and when a delay to seek parental consent would jeopardize the health or life of the minor.
2. **Emancipated Minor:** Children who live away from their parents or legal guardians, are fiscally independent, are no longer subject to parental control, are in the military, or are married may seek and secure a legal status of emancipated minor. States vary in their definitions and requirements for emancipation.
3. **Mature Minor Rule:** Some states have laws that recognize that a minor may be of sufficient maturity to comprehend their illness, disease, or injury, and the need for health care, and therefore are allowed to provide consent for treatment.

ANTICIPATORY GUIDANCE FOR PARENTS OF THE ADOLESCENT

The period of adolescence requires knowledge about how to prevent injuries, disease, and illness. The major cause of morbidity and mortality during adolescence is not illness, but rather injuries and self-harming high-risk behaviors. However, the pediatric nurse needs to be prepared to discuss a range of topics concerning teen disease prevention and health promotion with parents and their teens. Health education can take place in a range of locations, including well-child clinic visits, hospital environments, schools, churches, and health fairs. Families need information and education about what to expect during the teenage years, how to prevent injuries and harm, and how to identify early signs of common problems.

Because teens need privacy and confidentiality, interviews and education may be appropriate during an individual session with the teen. Topics for discussion when providing anticipatory guidance for teens and their families include the following:

- **Dental health:** Teens need to be reminded that oral hygiene and regular dental checkups are a part of their overall health and well-being. Preventing gum disease and dental caries is an important part of their health promotion.
- **Hearing:** Many teens enjoy music as part of their daily routine. Teaching families to be aware of the danger of developing cochlear damage from sustained loud music is an important aspect of anticipatory guidance.
- **Posture:** Because of the inverse relationship between rapid skeletal growth and slower muscular growth, many adolescents demonstrate poor posture or slumping while seated. Identifying scoliosis from typical poor posture is important.
- **Preventing motor vehicle accidents:** The teenage years are associated with feelings of invincibility and the belief that harmful things, such as motor vehicle accidents, "won't happen to me." Requiring the teen to wear seat belts saves lives, is required in every state, and should be mandated by parents. Riding with underage drivers or allowing more riders in a car than there are seat belts is a concern that should be discussed.
- **Tanning and sun exposure:** Many adolescents feel the need to participate in tanning to improve their appearance. Sun exposure is associated with skin damage and the early development of skin cancer. Teens need to hear that sun tanning causes premature aging of the skin. Guidance must be offered to use a sunscreen of no less than 15 SPF (ie, sun protection factor) and UVA/UVB (ie, ultraviolet) protection sunglasses.
- **Social isolation:** Family members need to be able to identify when a teen is demonstrating social isolation. Because adolescence is characterized by social interactions, peer group association, and intimate friendships, the early identification of the lack of these relationships is important. Providing opportunities for teens to interact in groups such as clubs, sports, and youth groups is imperative for healthy social and emotional development.

SAFETY *STAT!*

When using headphones or ear buds to listen to music, the teen must have guidance about the level of sound that can be damaging. Music should not be turned up loud when the teen is using ear buds.

PATIENT TEACHING GUIDELINES

Tips for Talking with Teens

Families may need education about how to best talk to their teen.

The following tips provide suggestions for improving communication with teens:

- Listen nonjudgmentally and show a greater interest in their topic than in stating or discussing your own.
- Pose open-ended questions that inquire into the teen's interests and lifestyle.
- Do not ask "why" questions; rather, avoid making the teen defensive and get at what the teen is thinking rather than a quickly offered reason.
- Do not "attack" and put the teen on the defensive or make them feel accused of something.
- Try to match the teen's emotional state while talking, such as enthusiasm or sadness.
- Be emotionally authentic; do not communicate anger, hurt, or disappointment when you are not experiencing these emotions; similarly, do not communicate happiness and approval when you do not feel that way. Teens can read parents' emotions well, so express your true emotions.
- Talk about the news; discuss social or ethical dilemmas and interesting global issues of importance.
- Role-model decision making during conversations, such as explaining how you got to your position or how you arrived at a decision.
- Keep it short and simple by keeping the conversation to a reasonable length.
- Be yourself; do not try to act or talk like the teen or one of their friends.
- Seize the moment; be ready to identify a relaxing, good moment for conversation or a discussion; be around enough to grab a good moment to connect.
- Show genuine deep respect for what your teen has to say and what he or she wants to discuss with you.

SCREENING AND HEALTH PROMOTION FOR THE ADOLESCENT

Health screenings for teens help to prevent experimentation and risk-taking problems associated with the time period. Teens experience pressure to try new actions that can lead to health-related problems. Screening adolescents should take place during health checks and at school. With budget cuts, many teens are not offered comprehensive health screening sessions. During the developmental stage of adolescence, between the ages of 12 and 18, teens should be screened for:

1. Child abuse and neglect
2. Substance abuse
3. Risk for unprotected sex, and if so, for STIs; if sexually active, follow up for physical examination or treatment
4. Risk for unprotected sex and pregnancy; if sexually active and unprotected, follow up for physical examinations and referral
5. Signs and symptoms of depression, suicide risk, and other mental health issues

6. Alcohol, drug, and tobacco use
7. Learning problems, delinquency, and the need for special counseling
8. Blood pressure
9. Cholesterol if the teen's parents have a serum cholesterol level greater than 240 mg/dL
10. Multiple risk factors associated with cardiovascular disease or diabetes
11. Nutritional risks, such as anemia and eating disorders including **anorexia nervosa** (ie, an eating disorder marked by weight loss and disturbance of body image) and **bulimia** (ie, an eating disorder marked by episodes of binge eating followed by emotional distress and self-induced vomiting and diarrhea), and behaviors suspected of eating disorders, such as fixation on weight

HEALTH PROMOTION

Immunizations

The pediatric nurse should obtain a copy of the teen's immunization record. The teen should receive a single dose of the tetanus toxoid, reduced diphtheria toxoid, and acellular pertussis vaccine (Tdap), provided they have received the complete set of childhood immunizations. The one-time dose of tetravalent meningococcal polysaccharide vaccine (MPSV4) should also be administered to prevent meningitis and general body sepsis. This is now a mandate to begin many colleges. If a second dose of measles, mumps, and rubella (MMR) was not administered earlier, the second dose should be given by the end of the 12th year. Vaccination for the **human papillomavirus (HPV)**, which is a common sexually transmitted disease, is also recommended and will need to be followed with two more doses at 2 months and 6 months after the initial dose. Hepatitis B vaccine should be administered if not previously received, and Hepatitis A vaccine should be administered in a two-dose series. The annual influenza vaccine should also be administered.

INJURY PREVENTION FOR ADOLESCENTS

Because accidents remain the leading cause of teenage death via motor vehicle accidents, sports injuries, and firearms, families need to have continued teaching about injury prevention for their teens. Drug, alcohol, and sex education information should be readily available and the pediatric nurse must feel confident to bring up these subjects during hospitalization or routine visits to the pediatric clinic. Health promotion activities should include breast self-exams and Pap smears (if indicated) for teen girls and testicular self-exams for boys. More information about these health promotion activities for teens is available on the American Cancer Society Web site.

SAFETY *STAT!*

Teenagers need role models of safety when they are learning to drive. Parents should be reminded that everyone in the car must wear seat belts at all times. Parents, especially, can be influential role models for safety by consistently wearing a seat belt.

Teens must understand the importance of wearing safety equipment. When playing sports, it is imperative that appropriate helmets, protective padding, mouth guards, and safe shoes be worn. Seat belts must be worn whenever driving or being a passenger in a car. Drugs and alcohol should not be consumed by teens because this poses a tremendous safety risk.

Many teens desire body tattooing or body piercing. Although professional tattooing is illegal to perform on teens without adult consent, some teens seek self-tattooing or tattooing by peers. Understanding the consequences of the permanence of tattoos must be reinforced and should be taught in schools and wellness visits. Acquiring a tattoo from a nonprofessional using unclean practices and instruments poses risks of injury through the transmission of infectious diseases.

SAFETY PROVIDED TO THE ADOLESCENT WHILE HOSPITALIZED

If a teenager is hospitalized, they may be viewed as mature and independent. This perception poses risks for injuries, accidents, and high-risk behaviors. Hospitalized adolescents need supervision and need to understand the safety rules of the hospital unit. Policies exist to guide health-care professionals about how to best care for a hospitalized teen. These policies should include guidelines about peer visits, wandering through the halls or off the unit, going outside, and not leaving the grounds of the hospital. Teens may need rules explained about smoking and other high-risk behaviors. In rare cases, the health-care team may confront a teenager with behavioral issues that cannot be resolved by engaging the assistance of the family, and then a behavioral contract may need to be created and enforced. Work with Child Life and the social services team to create and implement a behavior contract if needed.

Hand washing and preventing the spread of infectious diseases must be reinforced with teen patients. Rules concerning use of teen lounges, the unit kitchen, and other common areas may need to be reinforced if the teen is hospitalized for an infectious disease.

CHALLENGES IN ADOLESCENCE

Challenges in adolescence include acne, dating violence, violence, depression, suicide, and self-harm. Experimentation with drugs, **alcohol abuse,** and sex are also challenges that need to be addressed with teens. Nurses need to take the opportunity to teach teens about social opportunities, how to say no to drugs, reducing risk and harm, saying no to sex, and preventing alcohol abuse.

Acne

Teens typically have some acne. It is so prevalent during this developmental period that it is often considered a common experience and a normal part of puberty. Acne can cause distress in teenagers who are conscious of their appearance and who are worried about how they look to others (Fig. 25.5).

There are four types of skin presentations of acne: (1) blackheads, called *open comedones,* (2) whiteheads that are pustules, also called *closed comedones,* (3) pimples, and (4) cysts. Acne is common during adolescence because the hormonal changes that occur contribute to the development of the skin presentation. The form of acne most common in teens is called **acne vulgaris** (*vulgaris* means "common type") and can present on the face, hairline, neck, chest, shoulders, and upper back.

Hair follicles contain pores called *sebaceous glands.* These glands, also known as *oil glands,* produce a substance called *sebum* whose function is to lubricate the hair and skin. Hormones secreted during adolescence stimulate the sebaceous glands to become overactive. This overproduction clogs pores and holds dead skin cells, and bacteria get trapped and begin to multiply, causing redness and swelling, which appears as acne. The most common bacteria associated with acne is *Propionibacterium acnes.* Closed, clogged pores become whiteheads; open, clogged pores become dark in color and are called *blackheads.* If the wall of the pore opens up, the sebum, dead cells, and bacteria make their way under the skin and cause a pimple. Very large infected clogged pores become painful nodules, which are cysts or boils.

Although some people find that eating certain foods like chocolate causes more acne, in general, foods consumed do not contribute to the production of acne. The most helpful action one can take to help prevent acne is to wash the face twice a day with a mild soap. Scrubbing the face with a washcloth does not help. Rather, gently cleansing the face is best. Washing one's face after having contact with oil, such as at a job at a fast food restaurant, and not using face products that contain oil may help. Many products exist that contain benzoyl peroxide and salicylic acid, which may help to prevent acne and reduce its presence. A teen should never try to pop or pick at acne as this can cause secondary infections and scarring.

Violence

For some teens, the threat of violence or actual violence is a daily occurrence. Violence in a teen's life can come from child abuse, domestic abuse, bullying, cyberbullying, gang violence, or street violence in unsafe living conditions. Being a victim of violence is associated with feelings of insecurity and anxiety. Even though their physical appearance mimics the size of adults, teens need to be protected from violence to thrive and develop into successful young adults. Teens facing violence need to be referred to counseling and offered support. Teens experiencing violence in their lives need interventions similar to younger children. When interacting with teens, it is appropriate to ask if they feel threatened by violence in their lives. If a teen discloses that someone is threatening him or her or is causing emotional or physical harm, further investigation and referral are imperative to provide the child safety and security. Teens must be encouraged to seek help from a trusted administrator, teacher, or adult when they are experiencing bullying or violence.

HEALTH PROMOTION

Cyberbullying

Cyberbullying is defined as emotional bullying using technological advances of social media to intimidate, harass, threaten, target, or embarrass another. Current data have shown that 43% of children between the ages of 10 and 15 have been cyberbullied in some form (Rainey, 2012). Social media is the new platform in which bullies can target and torment their victims.

Identifying if a child is being cyberbullied may be difficult. Children and teens may hide this form of bullying from parents, guardians, or teachers. Looking for signs such as withdrawing from family and friends; feeling uneasy or resistant to go to school; appearing jumpy or nervous when on the computer; or being angry, frustrated, or hurt after using the computer may help to provide clues if cyberbullying is taking place.

Posing as a child on social media sites, or setting up a Web site, social media post, or e-mail address to taunt and torment a child are forms of cyberbullying. Several cases of suicide have occurred from having been teased or ridiculed by others.

Prevention is the best solution for cyberbullying. Parents should know all of the child's login and password information. Time limits and computer access in open family areas help to prevent overuse of social media and to identify early

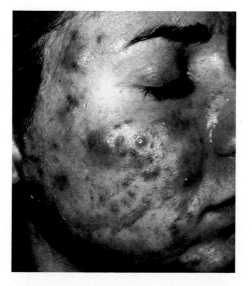

FIGURE 25.5 Acne generally begins in the teen years.

if cyberbullying is developing. Monitoring interactions on a regular basis also provides information on social media use. Parents must balance being overbearing with providing education and safety.

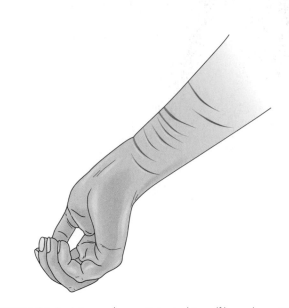

FIGURE 25.6 A teen who participated in self-harm by cutting.

Depression and Suicide

Adolescence is a period of adjustment and mood changes. Teachers, parents, and health-care providers must distinguish between normal teen emotional states and the development of clinical depression. Sadness is not considered clinical depression. See Chapter 31 for a discussion of adolescent depression.

Self-Harm

The period of adolescence may be associated with emotional pain, suffering, and depression. A teen may feel overwhelmed with a relationship breakup, a tumultuous relationship with a parent, losing someone very close to the teen, or trying to deal with day-to-day interactions. For some, these experiences cause a teen to participate in self-harm. Self-injury is one form of self-harm and can come in the form of cutting skin and tissue with utensils such as knives, razors, or sharp objects (Fig. 25.6). The cuts can be repetitive superficial cuts, or they can be deep gashes that cause significant blood loss and require surgical intervention. While most people will ask how someone can participate in this painful form of self-harm, some adolescents feel this form of self-harm causes them to focus on another form of pain other than their emotional pain. Adolescents have reported that the sensation of self-harm through cutting makes them release anger, but they then ask "Why do I cut?" and "How is this going to help me in the long run?"

Self-harm is serious. Adolescents who feel the need to cut must talk to a mental health professional about their problems. If the teen is not comfortable with this at first, they should be immediately encouraged to call a self-injury hotline.

Key Points

- Adolescence, the time period between the 12th birthday though the 18th year of life, is a time of tremendous physical and mental/emotional growth. The adolescent completes puberty and experiences gains in height and weight. Adolescents grow cognitively and begin to process more and more complex and abstract thoughts.

- Teens need information on appropriate self-care including good nutrition, healthy sleeping patterns, dental health, posture, and health social interactions. Nurses are in a good position to offer the family anticipatory guidance on what to expect during the teen years.

- Teens face challenges concerning peer pressures, society expectations, sexual maturity, and their future.

- Erikson's theory of psychosocial development describes this time period as "identity versus role diffusion"; this childhood stage focuses on the peer group, self-concept, self-esteem, and new roles. If the teen does not develop a sense of who he or she is in the family, peer group, and society, he or she may experience the inability to solve conflicts.

- Common fears associated with adolescence include relationships with the opposite sex and whether or not the teen can assume roles associated with being an adult.

- Teens still need their family and can appreciate limit setting and support without interference with their lives.

- Freud's theory of psychosexual development presents adolescence as the genital stage. Here teens focus on their sexual maturity, sexual feelings, need for masturbation, and interest in sexual relationships.

■ Piaget describes this as the formal operations time period, where the adolescent is developing abstract thinking and reasoning.

■ Kohlberg's theory of moral development discusses the postconventional level of morality; the teen is influenced by society and family, yet defines his or her own set of moral values.

■ Because of their tremendous physical, emotional, and cognitive growth, and the demands that accompany this growth, teens face challenges with mental health

issues, peer pressures, potential for injuries, and substance abuse.

■ Pediatric nurses must develop skills that make them comfortable with talking to teens and offering them nonjudgmental support.

■ Challenges in adolescence include acne, dating violence, violence, depression, suicide, and self-harm. Experimentation with drugs, alcohol abuse, and sex are also challenges that need to be addressed with teens. Nurses need to take the opportunity to teach teens about social opportunities, how to say no to drugs, reducing risk and harm, saying no to sex, and preventing alcohol abuse.

REVIEW QUESTIONS

1. After a female child experiences the first menses, there is an increase in linear growth.
   1. True
   2. False

2. When educating a teenage girl on her expected weight gain during adolescence, the nurse would be correct in stating the average weight gain between 12 and 18 years of age is:
   1. 15 to 55 pounds (6.8 to 24.9 kg)
   2. 20 to 40 pounds (9.07 to 18.14 kg)
   3. 5 pounds (2.27) a year
   4. None. With diversity in ethnic groups, there is no national average.

3. A girl will demonstrate sexual maturity by (1) increasing pubic hair, (2) breast bud growth, (3) menses, and (4) height. Place these clinical presentations in the order of occurrence.
   1. 4, 1, 3, 2
   2. 2, 1, 3, 4
   3. 1, 2, 4, 3
   4. 2, 4, 1, 3

4. Cyberbullying prevention includes the assessment of which of the following symptoms? *(select all that apply)*
   1. Appearing nervous when checking social media, texts, e-mail, or instant messages
   2. Closing the computer browser or e-mail windows in the presence of an adult
   3. Need for more time alone or privacy in one's room
   4. Appearing sad or depressed
   5. Demonstrating withdrawal from social interactions with friends and family
   6. Sudden and unexplained stopping of computer use

5. In many states, the adolescent is allowed to give consent for physical examinations and treatments of which of the following?
   1. Emergency treatment of a fractured arm
   2. Required prefootball physical clearance
   3. Treatment for staph infection on skin
   4. Medical treatment for a confirmed STI

6. The term *menarche* is used to describe which of the following?
   1. The time period of sexual development
   2. The teen's first menstrual period
   3. The time period between each menstrual period
   4. Tanner's fifth stage of sexual maturity

7. Hospitalized adolescents' concerns focus on all of the following *except:*
   1. Restricted independence and loss of choices
   2. Separation from peers
   3. Need for parental approval
   4. Illness as a punishment

8. When a young female nurse is caring for a hospitalized teen, it is appropriate to act as a peer to solicit compliance and adherence.
   1. True
   2. False

9. A minor may seek and secure a legal status of emancipated minor. States vary in their definitions and requirements for emancipation. The following are components of emancipation: *(select all that apply)*
   1. Teen cares for or lives with grandparents
   2. Teen lives away from their parents or legal guardians
   3. Teen is fiscally independent
   4. Teen is no longer subject to parental control
   5. Teen is in the military
   6. Teen is married

10. Acne is caused by the consumption of greasy foods, poor daily hygiene, and genetics.
    1. True
    2. False

CRITICAL THINKING QUESTIONS

1. Several social problems plague the developmental stage of the adolescent, including gang violence, school shootings, alcohol-related accidents, drug use, suicides, and date rape. How do the various sources of social media emphasize these problems? How do various avenues of general media portray the adolescent in relation to these problems? What is society doing to assist teens in the development of safety practices, the prevention of violence, and social maturity? What programs exist in your community to help teens? Are these programs being evaluated for their effectiveness? How? What are the outcomes of these prevention programs?

2. In health-care professional literature, the adolescent developmental period may be portrayed as a negative stage in life, and considered a period of emotional storm, stress, and social survival. What can be refuted in these negative perspectives? How can adolescence be considered a positive growth period that profoundly affects the rest of the child's adult life?

3. Setting boundaries may be difficult for many parents and adults working with teens. How can boundaries be negotiated? How can a pediatric nurse implement boundaries and rules within a health-care setting? Do adolescent behavioral contracts work in a hospital setting? Who creates them, implements them, and evaluates these contracts?

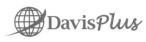

For additional resources and information, visit **www.DavisPlus.com.** Post-Conference Questions and Activities, Answers, and References can be found on Davis*Plus*.

unit SEVEN

Pediatric Concerns and Considerations

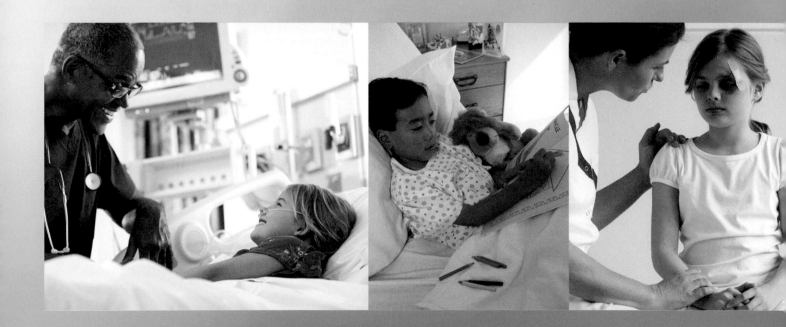

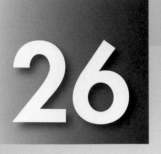

26

The Hospitalized Child

KEY TERMS

family-centered care
medical play
regression
restraints
therapeutic hugging

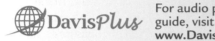 For audio pronunciation guide, visit www.DavisPlus.com

CHAPTER CONCEPTS

Comfort
Mobility
Nursing
Safety

LEARNING OUTCOMES

1. Define the key terms.
2. Describe the unique needs of a pediatric patient across childhood while hospitalized for a variety of acute and chronic conditions.
3. Discuss the safety concerns for young children while hospitalized in fast-paced, chaotic health-care environments.
4. Differentiate between adult hospital units and policies, and pediatric units and policies in relation to schedules, play environments, meals, equipment, and sleep needs.
5. Describe how bed selections, room selections, and staffing patterns differ between adult care environments and pediatric care environments.
6. State the three phases to hospitalization and separation for young children (ie, protest, despair, and detachment) and describe the behaviors expected in each phase.
7. Describe the basic guidelines for working with hospitalized children.
8. Analyze pain assessments and interventions for pediatric clients and describe both pharmaceutical and nonpharmaceutical nursing interventions to help relieve pain in children.
9. Describe the variations in frequently encountered nursing care procedures for pediatric patients across childhood.
10. State measures to administer medications safely to children who are hospitalized.
11. Describe the various methods for collecting specimens from children who are hospitalized.

REAL-WORLD CASE STUDY

Katrina

■ Katrina, a 27-month-old toddler, was admitted to a large city hospital pediatric unit for failure to thrive (FTT). Her mother, a 17-year-old adolescent, was with the child on admission 2 days ago but has not visited the child since a few hours after admission. She brought the child to the public health clinic for a well-child checkup and the pediatrician found the child to be under the 5th percentile in expected weight. The child was a direct admission to the hospital unit for an evaluation of her FTT. The toddler, still in the state of separation anxiety and "protest" with persistent crying, has not been visited by any other family member since the mother left 2 days ago. The charge nurse has made a referral to social services to assess the family dynamics and identify how the mother can be helped to be with her child more.

Upon assessment, it was determined by the social worker that the mother is unemployed and living with five others between the ages of 18 and 22 in a two-bedroom home. Her boyfriend, who is not the father of the child, lives in the house as well and is employed as a part-time construction worker. The mother is tearful on the phone with the social worker stating that she does not have transportation or bus money and is experiencing financial strain in providing for her toddler. The hospitalization is expected to be at least a week because the toddler is being evaluated for the etiology of her FTT, poor eating habits, delayed speech, and listless behaviors.

After several phone calls by the Department of Social Services, the mother comes in with the boyfriend for a visit. The mother is very affectionate and playful with the child and the boyfriend demonstrates a close relationship with the toddler. The family is encouraged to stay with the toddler throughout the hospitalization and a bed is brought in for the mother to sleep in. The mother is given toiletry items, a taxi voucher for discharge, and much support to stay with the child. With follow-up appointments in place with the public health department, the child is discharged after minimal weight gain for 5 days in a row.

1. What are the stressors the mother is experiencing during the child's hospitalization?
2. What are the three stages of "hospitalization" a young child can demonstrate?
3. What team members should be involved with this hospitalized toddler?

CONCEPTUAL CORNERSTONE

Discomfort

Being hospitalized produces a variety of unfamiliar, stressful, and uncomfortable experiences for children with acute illnesses and injuries. Hospitalized children are exposed to frightening surroundings, different timeframes, and unfamiliar people. Regression, protest, and despair are common reactions to being in the hospital and experiencing separation from parents. Discomfort is a very real experience for children across the developmental stages. Pain is caused by many sources of stimuli within a child's hospital experience. Pediatric nurses are leaders in pain assessment, management, and treatment, and must anticipate painful experiences while a child is hospitalized.

A hospitalization, for children of all ages, can be a very traumatic event. Not only does the illness, disease process, or surgical procedure cause anxiety and fear, but the strange environment with different rules, strangers, and unfamiliar timeframes and schedules can be frightening to a child. Hospitalization can be a negative experience for some children because separation from their primary caregiver, home environment, and familiar toys can cause stress.

Infants and young children cannot understand why they are hospitalized. The primary goal of infancy is the development of trust. Hospitalization reduces the building of trust because the child experiences inconsistent caregivers, fluctuating schedules, and a varying routine. Toddlers, while striving for a sense of autonomy, are faced with limitations, restrictions, and altered rituals and routines. Preschool children, in their magical thinking, may believe they caused the separation and hospitalization because of a behavior or action, and thus experience exaggerated fright. School-aged children better understand what is being told to them if explanations are straightforward and developmentally appropriate. School-aged children, while striving for productivity and independence, feel like they have less power in the hospital and become frustrated. It is up to the pediatric nurse to apply developmental theory to explain to children and their families why the hospitalization is taking place and what they can expect throughout the experience. See Appendix L for a summary of caring for the hospitalized child.

Applying the principles of the philosophy of **family-centered care** will help reduce the negative consequences of hospitalization for the child and family. Family-centered care provides guidelines to provide consistency, collaboration, and empowerment. Key elements of family-centered care include recognizing that the child's family is the constant in the child's life and no matter what is experienced in the hospital, the child will go back home to family. Therefore families need to be supported to learn all aspects of the child's care and should be empowered to care for their child. A partnership based on respect, support, education, and encouragement needs to be established with respect to the family's level of function, connectedness, spirituality, cultural diversity, economic level, and education. Parents should be invited and included in care conferences during which the child's condition will be discussed and treatment plans will be outlined. See Chapter 20, Introduction to Pediatric Nursing, for an in-depth discussion of the principles of family-centered care. Families should also be given access to read the hospital's version of the Bill of Rights for Hospitalized Children. This Bill of Rights varies per institution but most are based on that of the now defunct Association for the Care of Children's Health (ACCH).

PATIENT TEACHING GUIDELINES

Bill of Rights for the Child in a Pediatric Health-Care Setting

1. Right to evidence-based, quality health care based on national standards
2. Right to dignity, respect, and emotional support
3. Right to confidentiality and privacy
4. Right to the application of family-centered care
5. Right to religious and spiritual expression
6. Right to clear communication and use of interpreter services
7. Right to developmentally appropriate play and creative expression
8. Right to participate in informed decisions
9. Right to prompt pain assessment and symptom treatment and management
10. Right to access to the health-care institution's mission statement
11. Right to know the health-care institution's fees and charges
12. Right to access to interdisciplinary teams and social workers
13. Right to a second opinion on treatment plans or options

HOSPITAL SETTINGS FOR CHILDREN VERSUS FOR ADULTS

Not all hospitals offer the specialty of pediatric medical and nursing care. Some hospitals do not have a separate pediatric unit but rather have designated beds within an adult environment. Other hospitals have pediatric units constructed and devoted to help children feel comfortable while away from their homes. Some hospitals are completely devoted to the care of children only and these often are health-care institutions that are triage centers with specialty care teams such as pediatric oncology, gastroenterology, burn care, neurology/rehabilitation, and pediatric trauma. No matter what environment the child is hospitalized in, special child-friendly and child-focused care is required to achieve the best clinical outcomes.

Hospital Unit Overview and Orientation

When possible, the child and family should be oriented to the designated pediatric unit before hospitalization. A Child Life Specialist can provide tours and **medical play,** which is structured play that provides the opportunity for a child to learn about his or her diagnosis, procedures, surgery, and diagnostic or medical equipment. A Child Life Specialist can also navigate policies concerning visiting hours and sleeping arrangements to make the child more comfortable. During an acute hospitalization or an unexpected surgery, this preorientation may not be achievable. If a young child can see the hospital unit, the vital sign measurement equipment, and even an empty room in the unit where he or she will be staying, stress and anxiety may be reduced.

Designated pediatric units typically have a playroom for both the hospitalized child and the siblings. This is an area where no physical examinations, medication administration, or any medical assessments or discussions should take place. The child should be allowed, whenever feasible, to have a time of complete enjoyment in the playroom during his or her hospitalization. Adapting to mobility by bringing the child in a wheelchair or even on a gurney will help the child feel that he or she has an opportunity for recreation and enjoyment. Engaging Child Life Specialists in providing specific play opportunities for children with special needs is important and should be encouraged. For instance, a child with cancer who is immunosuppressed should be allow to have "neutropenic" playtime in the playroom where surfaces and toys are cleaned and the chance of acquiring an infectious disease from another child is minimized. Children enjoy getting out of their hospital beds and rooms and participating in developmentally appropriate play.

Admission Procedures

Hospitalized children require specialized admission assessments that differ from those of adults. Ask the parents the following basic questions in preparation for a child's hospitalization:

- Demographics, including the local home phone number and cell phone numbers to contact the family
- Chief complaint, associated symptoms, and past medical history
- Known allergies, including to food, medication, and environmental substances
- Medication reconciliation: List all medications and supplements the child is currently or has recently been on
- Developmental milestones
- Toilet training and patterns
- Immunization history and any need for updates
- Pain response, previous pain experiences, how the child expresses pain, and what soothes the child
- Eating patterns and typical diet
- Spiritual needs, religious practices, and cultural influences to the child's care
- Special comfort item such as a blanket or stuffed animal

Emotional Responses to Hospitalization

When a child is hospitalized, his or her relationship with parents and family becomes disrupted. In general, the child has barriers and challenges with many aspects of daily routines and interactions with parents. The child experiences an unpredictable routine and is forced to interact with many strangers under frightening circumstances. The hospital experience promotes a feeling of distrust. Children can feel as though they have a lack of control over their situation and the environment around them, and therefore perceive the hospital experience as a threat. Infants and toddlers between the ages of 6 and 36 months experience separation anxiety, which can lead to a particular reaction to the hospitalization called *stages of separation anxiety* or *reaction to hospitalization*.

The three stages of this reaction to separation are protest, despair, and detachment/denial (Robertson, 1958 found in Yawkey and Pellegrini, 1984).

PATIENT TEACHING GUIDELINES

Parents may need to be given difficult news about their child during the course of a hospitalization. Using the principles of family-centered care, parents should be given news about their child's condition at the bedside, where they can understand what is happening to their child. If the child's developmental level will make them vulnerable for fear, anxiety, or confusion, such as preschool children who engage in magical thinking, the team and parents may decide to step out of the room to discuss the news.

Protest

During the first stage, the young child protests loudly. This is displayed by crying, screaming, agitation, or demonstrations of anger. The child is often inconsolable and watches intently for the parent(s) to return. This period of time is difficult for the nurses and other health-care providers because the child does not readily respond to gestures of play or cuddling, or to offerings of comfort. This first stage of protest can last hours to 1 or 2 days.

Despair

In the second stage of separation, the young child withdraws and becomes inactive and uncommunicative. The child appears very sad and hopeless. Often, the child is lying on his or her side, turned away from the door or from others, lying quietly in despair. When the parents return during this second phase, the child may act ambivalent or sad. This is challenging for the parents because they desire to comfort the child.

Detachment/Denial

In the third phase, it appears that the child is adapting to the absence of their parents. The child starts to engage in interactions with others, may play in the bed, or may participate in activities offered in the playroom. The child appears to be adjusting but is actually still experiencing sadness and anxiety. When the parents return during this stage, the child may ignore his or her parents as a form of punishing them for leaving. Parents may be surprised, feel hurt, and feel guilt from this response to the reunion. Educating parents about how normal the child's reactions are may reduce their alarm and dismay.

Separation anxiety is further complicated by the child potentially having sleep deprivation because of the strange environment, noises, monitoring equipment, nighttime procedures, and the absence of the parents offering bedtime routines. Children with disrupted sleep may have more acute reactions because of their deep fatigue.

The goal for the nursing staff is to build trust with the child who is experiencing this negative response to separation and hospitalization. Continuing to offer the child support, positive and playful interactions, and consistency through routines helps to build this trust. Even at a young age, the child needs to hear from the nurses that the parents are coming back. Parents who must leave their child in the hospital should be encouraged to request extended family members to stay with the child if the parents need to go to work or be absent from the bedside. Leaving a personal item of the parents with the child also may make the child feel safe. This can be an article of clothing, a picture of the family, or a familiar item from the house. Parents need to know that the negative responses to hospitalization are transient. When separation is minimized, young children are able to demonstrate a strong capacity to withstand other stresses associated with illness, procedures, and hospitalization in general (Hockenberry and Wilson, 2007).

Stranger anxiety is also experienced when a young child is hospitalized. Stranger anxiety starts at approximately 8 months and continues through late toddlerhood and sometimes through the early preschool period. The most acute period of stranger anxiety occurs between 8 and 18 months. Children display anxiety with the close presence of a stranger, which is exacerbated by their lack of ability to verbalize their protests. Young children do not readily take to a stranger's touch or holding. Consistency in caregivers is one way to reduce stranger anxiety. Children also respond better to the caregiver establishing a rapport with the parents first, then slowly approaching the child with a soft, quiet voice. Whenever possible, the health-care team should perform assessments while the infant or toddler is in the parent's arms or lap.

Regression is also a common reaction from a young child being hospitalized and feeling loss of control. Regressive behavior is defined as a child displaying behaviors and achievements associated with a younger developmental stage. Children use regressive behaviors to help cope with stressful events. Behaviors can include regressing to incontinence with bedwetting and wanting to wear a diaper, desire for sucking on a bottle or pacifier, thumb sucking, frequent temper tantrums, food refusal, and the use of "baby talk." The child should be encouraged to behave as according to their age and developmental level, but should never be punished for the regression. Parents need to be taught that this is a normal response and the child will behave again at his or her level once the stress of hospitalization is over and feelings of loss of control subside.

Childhood Considerations for Hospitalization

Children are not little adults. They have physical, emotional, and play needs that are different than those of adults. The pediatric health-care team should conduct an assessment on the unique needs of each hospitalized child and provide an individualized plan of care. Children need undisturbed time for sleep, to have parents and familiar objects with them, and a bed selection that works with their medical diagnosis as well as their age and developmental level. The following section presents many ideas for individualized considerations while a child is hospitalized.

Time Demands and Potential Sleep Deprivation

A hospitalization can be detrimental on the rest and sleep patterns of children. Because hospitals run 24 hours a day, it is important to keep the child's rest and sleep needs in mind. Posting a sign stating that the child is napping is appropriate to allow uninterrupted sleep time during the day. Children should be encouraged to go to sleep as close to their normal bedtimes as possible because sleep is often disrupted for nighttime vital sign measurement, weight, and phlebotomy (Fig. 26.1).

HEALTH PROMOTION

Positive Sleeping Habits for a Hospitalized Child: Tips for Sleep Success

- Consistent lights out and bedtime while hospitalized
- Minimal nighttime disruptions for vital signs or assessments
- Bedtime rituals maintained while hospitalized (eg, bath, bedtime reading)
- Personal comfort items kept at bedside and offered to child at bedtime
- Lighting minimized to maintain safety (eg, bathroom light on only)
- Noise reduced to allow child to fall asleep and stay asleep
- Assignment of a bed to allow a roommate of a similar age and bedtime
- Fears assessed and addressed, such as strangers, monsters, and the dark
- Companionship of a parent or an extended family member supported so that someone familiar to the child is with the child overnight to provide support
- Medications administered before bedtime and as infrequently as possible at night, as well as grouped together for minimal sleep disruptions
- Aromatherapy such as a small lavender pillow
- Essential oils such as lavender drops to the spine area, or chamomile, marjoram, or valerian drops to smell (always mix topical essential oils with a base carrier oil such as apricot kernel oil to prevent stinging or burning the child's skin)
- Music therapy such as soothing jazz, light Disney tunes, or classical music before bedtime
- Massage therapy before bed, such as a soft foot rub or back rub with lotion
- Water intake minimized at bedtime to prevent the need to use the bathroom during the night (follow orders for IV therapy and required PO intake)
- Warmth provided before bedtime, such as a soft blanket from the blanket warmer

Bed Selection

Careful consideration is required when selecting pediatric bed assignments. Medical diagnoses and childhood infections influence how children are placed within the unit. Children with like diagnoses should be cohorted (ie, placed together)

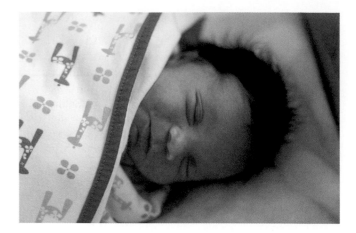

FIGURE 26.1 Hospitalized infant sleeping.

for support. For example, children with select infectious diseases, such as respiratory syncytial virus (RSV), can be cohorted according to institutional policy. Children of like ages may be positively influenced by enjoying similar activities and each other's company. Protect privacy at all times, regardless of the child's age.

Young infants require either an open crib or an incubator. Older infants should be placed in cribs. Toddlers and older infants who can stand and climb must be in cribs with high tops so that injuries can be avoided (Fig. 26.2). Check with each institution about the age that an older toddler or young preschool child can be given a full-size hospital bed to minimize falls.

SAFETY *STAT!*

Parents should not be allowed to sleep with their infants while hospitalized and infants must never be left on the parent's bed, even for a brief bathroom visit, because of the chance of a fall. Parents of young children should be given their own safe sleeping bed or convertible sleeping chair. Parents cannot be allowed to sleep or nap with the infant in the parent's hospital-provided sleeping arrangement. Remind parents to notify the nurse when they are going to shower or leave their infant or young child alone.

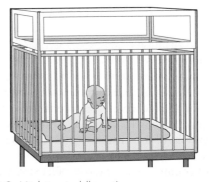

FIGURE 26.2 High-top toddler crib.

Visiting Hours

In the field of pediatrics, visiting hours are adapted to meet the needs of the family. Often, parents are encouraged and sometimes requested to stay with their young child around the clock. Parents should be provided essentials, such as access to unit kitchen areas, Internet service if available, meal guidelines or local restaurant menus for takeout or delivery, and privacy as required. It is common that hospitals provide either sleeping arrangements next to their child, or a boarding room for longer stays with more complicated or chronically ill children. Encourage the family's involvement and support the family's cultural, spiritual, and religious practices whenever possible during the stressful event of a hospitalization.

Parents at the Bedside

The positive impact of the presence of a child's parents at the bedside during hospitalization cannot be overestimated. Children fare better and have more positive clinical outcomes if their parents are present, engaged in the child's care, and offer the child comfort. Every effort should be made to assist the parents in maintaining a presence as much as possible each day. The immediate family should be offered no restrictions on visiting hours and should be offered sleeping arrangements next to the child's crib or bed. Nurses need to realize that parents may need to be away from the bedside to maintain employment or care for other siblings at home.

Cultural Factors

A hospital stay involves a disruption in a family's life. Cultural values and lifestyles influence how a family deals with the hospitalization of a child. There are many reasons why a family may not be able to allow an adult to stay at the bedside during the hospitalization. It may be easy for some caregivers to pass judgment on a family who has no or limited visiting behaviors, but it is very important to assess the situation and use the principles of family-centered care to empower and support each family member knowing that the family is the child's constant and the hospitalization is a stressor on the family structure and function. The factors that influence a family's reaction, adaptation, processing, and ability to stay present during a hospitalization include the child's age, whether the disease process is acute or chronic, the parents' employment status, the availability of extended family members, the family's trust in the hospital system to provide safety, the presence of a Child Life Specialist, and cultural and ethnic norms and practices.

THE CHILD'S AGE. Many first-time parents of newborns or young infants may be very reluctant to leave their child in the hospital without constant supervision. Mothers who are breastfeeding should be encouraged to stay to provide fresh breast milk or pump at home and bring in breast milk, either fresh or frozen. Parents of young infants often feel emotional distress if they have to leave their infant to attend to other siblings or work responsibilities.

Parents of children of all ages often feel torn when outside work or family responsibilities pull them from the hospitalized child's bedside. The parents must hear from the nurse that the child will be kept safe, supervised, and cared for in their absence.

NATURE OF THE DISEASE PROCESS. When faced with an unexpected hospitalization of an unknown timeframe, families of a child with an acute injury or disease process feel thrown off track. Because there is no time to plan a work absence, distress and frustration may occur when the unexpected event creates havoc in the family's life. The pediatric nurse must provide a clear understanding of what to expect such as estimated length of recovery or length of course of antibiotics. Parents must be supported in their need to be absent to take care of responsibilities that they may not have the power to change during the hospitalization.

An exacerbation of a chronic disorder such as sickle cell anemia or cystic fibrosis may influence the visitation of family members. Some families who are familiar with the hospital routine may not visit as much when the child has more frequent admissions.

PARENTAL EMPLOYMENT. Single parents may not be able to miss work if they are the sole providers of the finances of the family. There are times when a parent must juggle other children's needs, transportation, and employment, all during the hospitalization. The hospitalized child needs to know, at their developmental level, what the circumstances are and exactly when the parent will visit. Encouraging the child to keep a picture of the family, write letters to each family member, and draw pictures of the family, home, and pets may help the child feel connected in their absence.

AVAILABILITY OF EXTENDED FAMILY MEMBERS. Some fortunate families have grandparents, uncles or aunts, church members, neighbors, or good friends who can come and stay with the hospitalized child to provide distraction and comfort. Families who have recently relocated or who have a limited social network may not have family or community contacts who can visit the hospitalized child. Engaging hospital volunteers to play with the child, read the child books, or help them with homework may provide some distraction and comfort. Not all children's temperaments accept the presence of strangers.

TRUST IN THE HOSPITAL'S SAFETY SYSTEM. Parents with a perception that their child will be kept safe while hospitalized may feel more secure in leaving to take care of other family matters or work-related issues. Families who perceive that their child will be unsupervised or feel that their child's safety will be compromised will be less comfortable about leaving. It is acceptable to describe to the family how much supervision can be provided, but it is imperative to communicate that emergencies do happen on the floor and there may be times when the health-care staff is attending to an emergently ill child and cannot keep an eye on their child. Infants and toddlers must be secured in a high-top crib, or if able to stand and jump, they must be in a crib with a cover to prevent accidental falls from climbing out.

PRESENCE OF A CHILD LIFE SPECIALIST. Members of the Child Life department can work with the family to set up a system of communication, play, distraction, and comfort while a child is alone in the hospital. Although they provide visits and not around-the-clock supervision, Child Life can work with the child to help him or her feel more comfortable, secure, and engaged in play and activities that lessen feelings of homesickness or of missing the parents.

CULTURAL AND ETHNIC NORMS AND PRACTICES. There are some cultural norms that prevent a family from leaving a child in a hospital alone. Cultures whose norms are to be a collective group at all times will ensure the presence of a family member, extended family member, or family friend at all times.

Social customs related to the care of a sick, hospitalized child may involve a cultural diet, prayer sessions, and cultural religious practices, among other things. Families may want to provide their child cultural or ethnic food. Call the dietary department to work closely as a team to provide culturally acceptable foods. Cultural and ethnic practices include the following:

- **Filipino Families:** Family ties are considered of upmost importance. The family sees the extended family as the center of the child's community. Great effort will be made to make sure the hospitalized child is with a family member at all times. Children are fussed over and are provided physical affection and much attention. It is common to see a large number of visitors on a daily basis.
- **Mexican Families:** Elders have a prestigious status and may be the decision makers. Families stay together and rarely leave a child alone, if ever. Privacy is important and quiet time with lots of affection with the child is highly valued. Hispanics are emotionally expressive and expect to provide pampering to a hospitalized child, and receive pampering when hospitalized.
- **Vietnamese Families:** A hospitalization is seen as a disruption of harmony. Vietnamese families are close and will want to stay with their children. Touching and cuddling may be minimized during the hospitalization but the child will be provided with companionship and support.
- **African American Families:** Elders are seen as prestigious in the family structure and many African American families will have an elder stay with the hospitalized child if the parents need to work. Religion and spirituality are very important to many and prayer groups may be brought in to provide healing prayers. The establishment of trust is very important.

Whether a family is present or not, the child's well-being is the focus of the hospitalization and the pediatric nurse must support the entire family unit as they all adapt to the stress of a hospitalization and a disruption of family life and work schedules.

Sibling Reactions to Hospitalization

Siblings may experience negative consequences of a brother or sister being hospitalized. Fear, worry, anxiety, and loneliness may all surface at any time or throughout the hospitalization. When parents are absent and preoccupied with an ill child, the sibling may become angry and act out with jealousy and resentment. If the sibling is cared for by someone outside of the home, is being treated differently, or has unanswered questions about the hospitalized child's situation and status, reactions can be intensified (Hockenberry and Wilson, 2007). When possible, the older siblings should be included in the bedside rounds so they have a chance to comprehend what is happening to their hospitalized sibling and have a better understanding of the need for the hospitalization.

Meals for Pediatric Units

Hospitals will provide a child with specific diets that are medically indicated and developmentally appropriate. Choking hazards should be considered when making selections. Infant formulas and baby food are provided. Toddler snacks should be safe and should be provided by the dietician's office. Food from home is frequently allowed and should be discussed with the members of the health-care team to match the recommended consistency and tolerance desired.

Safety With Alarm Systems

Hospitals are required to provide an alarm system for young children to notify security in the unlikely event of an infant abduction. A policy will exist to inform the nursing staff how to handle such an event. Typically, the hospital provides an electronic banding system (wrist or ankles) that will notify the nursing station and the security office if the child is taken off the unit or moved far enough away to be considered a danger. Pediatric nurses should respond immediately to the sound of the alarm and follow procedures precisely to prevent abduction.

SAFETY *STAT!*

Under no circumstances should parents or children be allowed to remove their security alarm devices. If a device needs to be removed briefly for a procedure such as an IV placement, the nurse is responsible to replace the device immediately afterward to maintain safety.

Sensory Impairment

Hospitalized children who have a sensory impairment require special care and consideration. Hearing, visual, and tactile impairments place a hospitalized child at greater risk for stress, anxiety, and injuries. Policies must be in place to guide care of a child with a sensory impairment so that communication can be maximized and frustrations minimized. Children with significant hearing impairments should be offered all available technology to improve their understanding of the environment and care. The child's hearing aids should be used at all times, hospital sign language interpreters should be used, and television programs and technology for the hearing impaired should be used. If a child has learned lip-reading, guidelines should be followed for direct attention before speaking and a clear, slow, even rate of speech without exaggeration should be used. For visually impaired children, safety should be maintained and clear verbal communication should be emphasized to reduce anxiety.

PLAY THERAPY AND CHILD LIFE SPECIALISTS

The importance of play while hospitalized cannot be emphasized enough. Children of all ages need opportunities for play and expressive activities. The nurse should work with a Child Life Specialist to ensure a match between the child's medical condition and the form of play. Fatigue, infectious processes, chronic illnesses, disabilities, sensory impairments, and levels of cognitive and motor ability are just a few of the possible influences in the hospitalized child's ability to participate in play. No matter what the medical diagnosis, age of the child, or developmental level, some form of play should be offered on a daily basis. Play is known to provide six functions:

1. **Creativity:** Play promotes fantasy, imagination, exploration of talents, and the development of interests.
2. **Sensorimotor Development:** Play improves fine and gross motor skills by encouraging the child to explore his or her environments through visual, tactile, auditory, and kinetic stimulation.
3. **Intellectual Development:** Play provides learning through experimentation, exploration, manipulation, and comprehension.
4. **Socialization and Moral Development:** Play teaches the child about social rules and order, how to share, how to negotiate and interrelate with others, and about socially approved behaviors and moral standards.
5. **Self-Awareness:** Play provides an exploration of one's self identity and tests/expands the child's abilities.
6. **Distractibility from Stress, Anxiety, and Tension:** Play while hospitalized provides a source of positive distraction from the frightening environment of the hospital. Play allows the child to express his or her feelings, emotions, and anxiety while facilitating communication. Offering a child the opportunity for mastery over an unfamiliar environment, play allows for decision making and a sense of control, and lessens the child's stress.

Types of Play

Play is an essential component of healing for children from infancy through adolescence. Nurses need to ensure that every patient is provided the pleasure that play provides and that every patient has his or her hospital anxiety and fears reduced by play. Play can be offered no matter what the child's age, cultural background, or cognitive capacity. The information that follows describes the types of play for each developmental stage.

• **Infants:** Infants participate in solitary play in which the focus is on sensorimotor experiences and pleasure. Mirrors, mobiles, musical toys, and toys with a variety of textures, sounds, and motor challenges are used in the hospital. Because of mouthing in the older infant, toys must be washed thoroughly between infants. Toys brought from home should be inspected for parts that pose aspiration and choking risks.

• **Toddlers:** Toddlers participate in parallel play in which children play next to each other but are participating in their own play experience. The focus for the toddler is generally whole body, multisensory, and imitative of adult roles (eg, firefighter, police officer, ballerina, nurse, rock star, mother, or teacher). Providing opportunities for fantasy toys such as train sets, block towers, and dress-up clothes allows for toddlers to imitate their world experiences.

• **Preschoolers:** Preschoolers participate in associative play in which children play together with loosely regulated or poorly defined rules. Informal games allow preschoolers to learn social norms, sharing, and cooperation. Puzzles, games, and simple arts and crafts provide interactions and imagination.

• **School-Aged Children:** School-aged children participate in cooperative play via formal games, contests, competitions, and social groupings. Provide opportunities for a school-aged child to play games with family members, hospital staff, and visitors.

• **Adolescents:** Adolescents continue with cooperative play focusing on strong social interactions and abstract problem-solving. Teens need a means to keep in contact with their peers and should be provided opportunities to use technology to help them feel connected.

Functions of Medical Play

Medical play, also known as therapeutic play, is a form of play with a purpose of accomplishing therapeutic goals. The use of medical kits that a young child can manipulate and experiment with safely allows for expressions of emotions and fears, and mastery of the unknown. Giving a doll a shot with a toy syringe allows for the expression of fear and anger. Using anatomically correct dolls provides a learning opportunity for a child to increase understanding of a medical procedure or surgical outcome. Child Life Specialists can assist the nurse to teach a child what is going to happen to him or her during hospitalization, surgery, or diagnostics. As with all toys, the use of medical toys requires supervision, cleaning procedures, and safe storage.

PROVIDING A SAFE ENVIRONMENT

Hospitals can be inherently unsafe environments. Children who are hospitalized require measures to ensure safety. Follow hospital policy to instigate safety measures such as identification/name bands, security devices, and bed selection to keep young unattended children close to the nursing station. Teach the parents how to provide safety by instructing them about how to use the call bell, what symptoms or clinical signs they should watch out for, how and when to call for help, and how to use side rails on cribs. Patients and family members need to be reminded to have all electrical equipment that is brought in checked for safety by facility employees. With the parents, discuss supervised ambulation policies and never walking barefoot. Parents should not sleep with their infants or young toddlers in big beds. Any supplies kept in a pediatric hospital room should be out of reach or locked up. Children should not be allowed to touch monitoring or infusion equipment.

PAIN MANAGEMENT

Families are very fearful of their child experiencing symptoms, with pain being the most feared symptom. Children experience the same human response symptoms as adults but may perceive the experience differently. Most children by 5 years of age can answer specific questions about the location and severity of their symptoms. Pain in a young child is a frightening experience that provokes a variety of responses from anger to despair. There are many myths associated with the treatment of pain. Some health-care providers maintain a belief that, because of the immaturity of an infant's neurological system, they do not experience pain. See Box 26.1 for a list of myths, or untruths, that are still associated with the assessment, management, and treatment of pain in children.

SAFETY *STAT!*

It is very important that changes in a child's clinical status, especially changes in vital signs and overall appearance, be reported immediately. For instance, these changes include an increased level of pain, tachycardia, a change in color, a change in mental status, and a change in breathing pattern. The change in clinical status should be reported up the chain of command to the charge nurse and the hospitalist so that further assessments and interventions can be implemented. If there is a significant change in clinical status, report findings to the charge nurse and stay with the child while the team is notified.

Consequences of Untreated Pain in Pediatric Patients

Pediatric nurses are responsible for having comprehensive knowledge about the experience of pain in children. If left untreated, pain in children of all ages affects their ability to form trust with members of the health-care team.

Untreated pain has detrimental effects in many body systems. The physiological demands of adapting to injuries that cause pain place a child in a vulnerable position. Nurses must be aware of the detrimental effects and prioritize identifying and treating pain.

The immediate responses of untreated pain include the following:

• Decreased oxygen saturations
• Increased heart rate
• Increased blood pressure
• Heart rate variability
• Decreased peripheral skin blood flow

Box 26.1 Myths About Pain in Infants and Children

• *Infants do not feel pain.*
  • False! Infants have a definitive presentation of pain, just like older children and adults.
• *Young children cannot describe their pain.*
  • False! Children with language skills can talk about their pain.
• *Young children cannot localize their pain.*
  • False! Children can accurately place their hand over the place where it hurts.
• *Infants and children do not need pain medication.*
  • False! Children need pain medications, just like adults.
• *Children become easily addicted to pain medication.*
  • False! Children who take narcotics when in pain and not excessively do not become addicted.
• *Assessment of a child's pain is difficult.*
  • False! Use age-appropriate objective and subjective pain tools to accurately measure pain (see the Pain Assessment section and Table 26.2).
• *Children always tell the truth about their pain.*
  • False! Children may lie about their level of pain to avoid injections or oral medication.
• *Children's vital signs do not demonstrate pain.*
  • False! Pulse rate, respiratory rate, and blood pressure may increase, and oxygen saturation may decrease.
• *Children should never be given narcotics.*
  • False! Narcotics such as morphine are important treatments for severe pain during childhood.
• *Newborns do not experience pain.*
  • False! Even fetuses in the womb react to painful stimuli.
• *Children experience more severe side effects from narcotics than adults.*
  • False! Children experience side effects similar to those of adults.
• *If a child is playing, he or she is not in pain.*
  • False! Children play even when in severe pain.

• Increased caloric consumption; potential for periods of hypoglycemia
• Stress response leading to prolonged hyperglycemia
• Mistrust in the environment and with the health-care team

The long-term consequences of untreated pain in children include the following:

• Poor motor performance
• Poor adaptive behavior, learning disorders, and cognitive defects
• Temperament changes and psychosocial problems

Box 26.2 provides ideas for pain control by planning ahead for a painful procedure or experience.

NURSING CARE PLAN for the Hospitalized Child in Acute Pain

Assessments:
- Verbal children should be questioned about the word they want to use to describe their pain (eg, owie, booboo, sore, pain spot).
- Families should be questioned about any cultural or spiritual practices or beliefs that may influence how their child's pain is assessed and treated.
- Parents should be included in the assessment of their child's pain.
- An appropriate pain assessment tool should be identified and used consistently for the assessment of the child's pain severity.
- The location of pain should be determined by assessing the verbal description or nonverbal placement of the child's hand over the painful site.
- The location, onset, duration, quality, and intensity of the pain should all be assessed, if possible.
- Physiological measures of pain should be evaluated, such as the child's heart rate, blood pressure, respiratory rate, and oxygen saturation.
- Regardless of the value reported on the pain scale, the child's pain description should be believed and interventions should be provided. Work with the family to determine what has been used for pain relief in the past and use that as a foundation for providing the child with pain relief. Pain is a unique experience for each individual.

Nursing Diagnoses:
- The child is experiencing acute pain.
- There is a potential for injury.

Goals: Goals should have five components, including:
- Patient-oriented (The child…)
- Future-oriented (The child will…)
- Measureable (The child will state a pain scale value of less than two…)
- Time-oriented (The child will state a pain scale value of less than two by noon today…)
- Realistic for the child. Do not create a goal that cannot be accomplished realistically. When it comes to acute pain, the child's goal may be a large reduction of pain, but the child may still experience discomfort on both physical and psychological levels.

Interventions: Interventions for the reduction of acute pain should be multidimensional and must include pharmacological interventions, nonpharmacological interventions, distraction, family comforting, and support. Interventions can include:
- Narcotics and/or nonnarcotic analgesics should be administered. Determine if the medications are best delivered around the clock or PRN. Whenever possible, use the oral or IV medication administration routes to avoid the distress and discomfort of injections. Solicit the assistance of a pain nurse specialist if available. Assess the child's pain level before the administration of pain medications and 1 hour after, and carefully document the response the child has to the pharmacological pain intervention.
- Nonpharmacological interventions should be implemented, including:
  - Repositioning
  - Distraction and play therapy, if appropriate
  - Parental holding, cuddling, and touching, if appropriate; if the child is a teenager, just having the parent be present and close by may be a great comfort
  - Decreasing the environmental stimuli, such as noise, smells, and lights, and providing a sense of calm support for the child
  - Providing massage, warm or cold packs as indicated, and warm blankets and other tactile stimulation that is comforting to the child

Evaluation of Outcome: It is imperative that each intervention be assessed for effectiveness to see if the value of the pain scale or physiological measurement has been reduced. No more than 1 hour should go by without an evaluation of the effectiveness of the intervention. Note if the child is beginning to show a normal and an expected resumption of activities, play, and interactions. Assess the child's sleep and activity patterns and note if the child's physiological measurements are returning to the expected levels. Report if the pain interventions are not effective and document all aspects of the nursing process.

Box 26.2 Pain Control Methods for the Hospitalized Child

Plan ahead and intervene before pain starts:

- Offer a sucrose-dipped nipple or prescribed quantity of sucrose to infants before procedures
- Use nonpharmacological pain management techniques as well as pharmacological pain control measures before a painful procedure, including:
  - Distraction
  - Relaxation
  - Deep breathing
  - Guided imagery
  - Heat or cold to site
  - Positions of comfort
  - Favorite blanket, stuffed animal, toy, or personal possession (ask child or parent for ideas)
  - Warm blankets wrapped around child
  - Being held or rocked in a rocking chair
  - Lowered noise environment
  - Reduced lighting
- Use topical cream anesthetics, such as lidocaine and prilocaine (EMLA), before starting IVs or giving injections (but not on young infants).
- Use a variety of words to describe pain: Take into account the child's developmental level (eg, ouch, ouchie, booboo, owie, hurtie) and the words the family uses. Ask the parents what words they use and write them on a card and keep at the bedside; document for the interdisciplinary team.
- Use a team approach for pain control; involve Child Life Specialists.
- Understand the side effects of narcotics administration including gastrointestinal (GI) distress, constipation, and sedation. Educate parents about what to expect.

- Child Life departments and play therapists should be involved with all painful procedures.
- An accurate weight is the key to safety in calculating pain medication doses.
- Always medicate a child for pain before the pain experience becomes intense.

TEAM WORKS

Principles of Pain Management

- Children continue to be undermedicated for pain; the pediatric health-care team must include individualized pain assessment and management for each hospitalized child.
- Pain should be assessed on a frequent basis. Check level of pain with an appropriate pain scale at least with every set of vital signs, and more frequently if the child is experiencing pain.
- Remember that culture has an influence on the pain experience and may affect a child's expression of pain, verbalization of the experience, and/or the meaning given to the pain experience.
- Children have painful experiences in the hospital on a regular basis.

Key points to keep in mind when caring for a child who is experiencing pain and discomfort include the following:

- Evaluate pain and discomfort regularly and frequently.
- Try to prevent pain, not treat it after it occurs.
- Believe the child's reports of pain.
- Use pain scales that are developmentally appropriate; use behavioral indexes.
- Use the QUESTT protocol (Baker and Wong, 1987):
  - **Q**uestion the child about his or her pain.
  - **U**se appropriate pain tools.
  - **E**valuate the pain experience: Identify physiological and behavioral changes.
  - **S**ecure the parents' and caregivers' involvement.
  - **T**ake all influencing factors into account.
  - **T**ake action; report; re-evaluate after each pain reducing intervention.

Pain Assessment

Thorough pain assessment is the first step in managing acute and chronic pain. Children who are hospitalized can be expected to have various experiences that cause pain and discomfort. Providing assessments that are frequent (ie, no less than with every set of vital signs), thorough, developmentally appropriate, and that use standard, well-accepted, and respected pain tools are key. Assessments should be performed immediately when there are indications of pain, and pain should be assessed again no more than 1 hour after a pain intervention is initiated. Pain assessments, interventions, and re-evaluations must be carefully documented.

The assessment of pain should be threefold: (1) physiological indicators of pain, such as changes in vital signs; (2) behavioral aspects of pain, such as withdrawal and physical signs of depression; and (3) the results of pain tool assessments. Table 26.1 provides potential assessment findings for each developmental stage and the appropriate tools to be used.

Pediatric pain assessment tools have been developed and widely tested for validity and reliability. The gold standard of pain management is to use a pain tool that is appropriate for the child's developmental stage. Infants and toddlers need to have *objective* pain tools with which the nurse uses sets of behaviors to determine the child's level of pain. Preschoolers, school-aged children, and adolescents should be an active part of pain assessment. Therefore *subjective* pain tools are used to rate their pain and communicate the result to the nurse. Behavioral cues and vital signs should also be used by the nurse to help determine the level of pain a patient is experiencing. It is imperative that the nurse believe the child's pain rating. Common pain tools that have been determined to be effective in the assessment of pain in children are found in Table 26.2.

TABLE 26.1   ASSESSMENT OF PEDIATRIC RESPONSES TO PAIN

Developmental Age	Patient Response to Pain	Pain Scale Assessment Tool
Neonates	Rigidity; thrashing; generalized body response	CRIES pain scale
Infants	Local reflex withdrawal; high-pitched loud crying with eyes closed; pushes stimulus away after it is applied; localized body response	CRIES pain scale or FLACC scale
Toddlers	Loud crying; screaming; verbal expressions of one word; uncooperative; pushes stimulus away before it is applied; thrashing	CRIES pain scale or FLACC scale
Preschoolers	Loud crying; screaming; may put hand on site or misrepresent actual location of pain; may describe pain but not intensity	CRIES pain scale, FLACC scale, OUCHER pain scale, or the Wong-Baker FACES pain rating scale
School-Aged Children	Often see stalling behaviors; clenched teeth; body stiffens; closed eyes	• FLACC scale or the Wong-Baker FACES pain rating scale for younger school-aged children (ages 6–10) • Wong-Baker FACES pain rating scale, the numerical version, for older school-aged children (ages 11–13)
Adolescents	May talk about pain openly; less protesting; uses expressive words to describe pain experience	Wong-Baker FACES pain rating scale, the numerical version, or adolescent-specific tools such as the Adolescent Pediatric Pain Tool

Pharmaceutical Interventions for Pain

Therapeutic nursing management of pain may require both nonpharmaceutical measures and pharmaceutical agents. For the sake of the child's safety, the pediatric nurse must understand the indication, action, dosage, administration, side effects, and interactions of pain medications. Extra precautions are needed with the administration of IV narcotic medications. Mild pain can be treated with nonopioids and nonsteroidal anti-inflammatory drugs. Moderate to severe pain needs opioids (ie, narcotics) for complete pain control. General procedures for using pharmaceutical interventions for pain include:

• Consulting a current drug guide for correct safe dose ranges for both opioids and nonopioid medications; follow institutional policy
• Having the child's most current weight to accurately determine dose for pain medications; most medications are dosed as milligrams per kilogram of weight
• Following safety procedures for narcotics; children who are narcotic naive (ie, those who have not had narcotics previously) require frequent assessment for sedation and respiratory suppression; hospital protocols often dictate the documentation of hourly respiratory rates when a child is on narcotic pain control for the first time
• Double-checking infant and young children's pain medication doses with a second nurse to reduce medical errors
• Involving the parents in the assessment and management of pain; teaching parents how to safety administer pain medications to their child

• Understanding that pain is a unique experience and expressions of pain will vary; using many assessment techniques when deciding pain severity and choosing dosages of pain medications
• Documenting carefully both nonpharmaceutical and pharmaceutical interventions given for pain, and documenting all assessments of pain, including re-evaluation of pain after interventions are administered

Table 26.3 provides the drugs, dosages, and frequency of dosing of medications used in pediatric pain control.

DRUG FACTS
Topical Local Anesthetics

• Should be used during invasive procedures such as IM injections and IV starts; EMLA and NUMBY STUFF are two examples
• May be used on infants
• Must secure a physician's order
• Apply according to manufacturer's directions and allow ample time to work
• Place the cream on several areas where the needlestick may take place in case it takes more than one stick to be successful (eg, insertion of an IV)
• Cover cream with a clear dressing
• Remove the cream with a clean dressing before any needlestick

(Text continued on page 414)

TABLE 26.2　PAIN ASSESSMENT TOOLS

Pain Assessment Tool	Developmental Age of the Patient	Scale Description	How to Use It
Wong-Baker FACES Pain Rating Scale	Used for children as young as 3 years old	• Six cartoon faces ranging from smiling (0) to a tearful face (10) • 0–5 numbers can replace the 0–10 numbers if desired • The face selected by the child represents a numerical value • This scale provides three scales: Expressions, words, and numerical values	• Tell the child that the faces represent, from left to right, a person with no pain all the way to a person with the worst pain imaginable. Point to each face and describe the words with each face. Ask child to select the face that represents his or her own pain.
CRIES Pain Scale	Best used with infants who are 32–60 weeks' gestational age	• 0 = No Pain, 10 = Worst Pain • Based on assessment of five presentations with a scoring of 0 to 2: 　• Crying 　• Requires oxygenation 　• Increased vital signs, such as heart rate (HR) and BP 　• Expressions, especially grimacing 　• Sleeplessness: Waking at frequent intervals or being constantly awake	• Used for infants who are preverbal • Used for neonatal postoperative pain • Assess for crying, requirement of oxygen, increased HR and BP, facial expressions, and sleepless state • A score of 4 or higher indicates need for pain management

Wong-Baker FACES® Pain Rating Scale

0	2	4	6	8	10
No Hurt	Hurts Little Bit	Hurts Little More	Hurts Even More	Hurts Whole Lot	Hurts Worst

©1983 Wong-Baker FACES Foundation. www.WongBakerFACES.org
Used with permission. Originally published in *Whaley & Wong's Nursing Care of Infants and Children.* ©Elsevier Inc.

FLACC Scale
(Face, Legs, Activity, Cry, Consolability)

Can be used for children between 2 months and 7 years

Based on the assessment of child's:
- Facial expressions, such as grimacing, frowning
- Legs: Relaxed to tense, restless, or kicking
- Activity: Quiet to arched, rigid, or jerking
- Crying: None to crying steadily, sobbing
- Consolability: Content to difficult to console

Scale is scored between 0 and 2 in each of the five categories for a total score between 0 and 10

FLACC Pain Scale

Categories	0	Scoring 1	2
Face	No particular expression or smile; disinterested	Occasional grimace or frown; withdrawn	Frequent to constant frown, clenched jaw, quivering chin
Legs	Normal position or relaxed	Uneasy, restless, tense	Kicking, or legs drawn up
Activity	Lying quietly, normal position, moves easily	Squirming, shifting back and forth, tense	Arched, rigid, or jerking
Cry	No cry (awake or asleep)	Moans or whimpers, occasional complaint	Crying steadily, screams or sobs, frequent complaints
Consolability	Content, relaxed	Reassured by occasional touching, hugging, or talking to; distractible	Difficult to console or comfort

Each of the 5 categories—(F) Face; (L) Legs; (A) Activity; (C) Cry; (C) Conso ability—is scored from 0 to 2, which results in a total score between 0 and 10.

From: FLACC Pain Scale, from The FLACC: A behavioral scale for scoring postoperative pain in young children, by S. Merkel et al, 1997, Pediatr Nurse 23(3), pp. 293–297. Copyright 1997 by Jannetti Co., University of Michigan Medical Center. Reprinted with permission.

Numerical Pain Scale, 0–5 or 1–10

No pain	Mild pain	Moderate pain	Severe pain	Worst pain
0 1	2 3	4 5 6	7 8	9 10

Use only when a child is old enough and developmentally ready enough to conceptualize numerical values and distance between digits

Children as young as 5 years may be able to conceptualize these numbers and their values

Explain to child and family that one side of the scale (0) represents the absence of pain and the other side of the scale (10) represents the child's perception of the worst pain he or she could imagine

Continued

TABLE **26.2** PAIN ASSESSMENT TOOLS—cont'd

Pain Assessment Tool	Developmental Age of the Patient	Scale Description	How to Use It
OUCHER Pain Scale 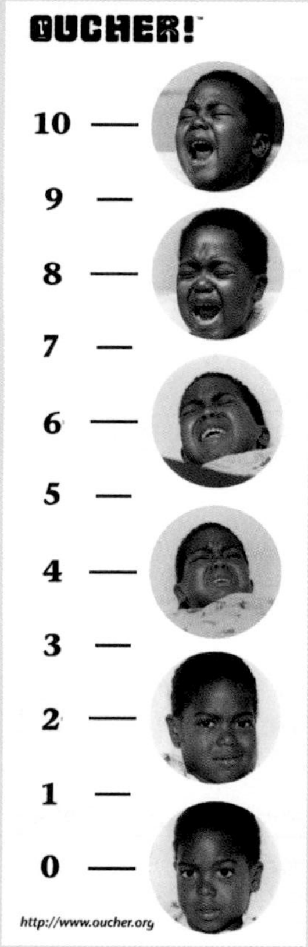	Can be used for children as young as 3 years old	Series of photographs used to evaluate pain, scored on 0–10 scale • Pictures include Caucasian, African American, Hispanic, Asian, and first world children • Children's faces range from laughing to crying • Each photograph is translated into a numerical value	Ask the child to choose the photograph of the child on the tool that best matches his or her pain experience

OUCHER!

10 —

9 —

8 —

7 —

6 —

5 —

4 —

3 —

2 —

1 —

0 —

http://www.oucher.org

Visual Analog Scale (VAS)	Older school children (eg, ages 10–13) and adolescents	A straight line or a numbered line used to describe no pain to the worst pain the child can imagine	Ask the child to draw a perpendicular line across a line exactly 100 mm in length, with the left side representing zero and the right side of the line representing 100, or worst pain the child can imagine
Adolescent Pediatric Pain Tool (APPT)	Adolescents	A multifaceted pain assessment tool available online for download that covers numerical values and a variety of categories of descriptive words (eg, burning, stinging, aching, throbbing) and temporal measurements (eg, constant, infrequent); there is also a drawing outline of the body where the child can note exactly where the pain is located	Teens have options to use color markers or shades of pencil markings to denote the severity of their pain experience on the body outline; for the descriptive words and temporal words or phrases, they circle the items that match their pain experience

TABLE 26.3 DOSAGES OF SPECIFIC DRUGS USED IN PEDIATRIC PAIN CONTROL (ALWAYS FOLLOW INSTITUTIONAL POLICES AND ACCEPTED FORMULARIES)

Drug	Dosage	Frequency of Dosing
Acetaminophen	10–20 mg/kg PO	Every 4–6 hr (do not exceed five doses in 24 hr)
Ibuprofen	5–10 mg/kg	Every 4–6 hr
Morphine	0.05–0.2 mg/kg, IV	Every 2–4 hr
Codeine	0.5–1 mg/kg PO	Every 4–6 hr
Oxycodone	20–30 mg PO	Every 3–4 hr
Hydrocodone	30 mg PO	Every 3–4 hr
Tylenol with Codeine	Follow institutional policy	Follow institutional policy
Meperidine	1–2 mg/kg, intramuscular (IM)	Every 4–6 hr
Methadone	0.1–0.2 mg/kg PO	As ordered

CULTURAL CONSIDERATIONS

Pain Management

Members of various cultures may express concerns about the administration of narcotics to their children. Some cultures do not support the use of any narcotics that may change the child's mental status or clarity of thinking. Parents need to be offered education on the importance of managing pain; especially acute pain from surgical procedures. Parents need to be reassured that addiction to narcotics during childhood is very rare and medications are only used to treat a level of pain confirmed through professional assessments. Culture has been known to influence pain experience, including the expression of pain, verbalization of the pain experience, and the meaning given to the pain experience.

SAFETY *STAT!*

An accurate weight is the key to safety in calculating and administering pain medications. Hospitalized children on pain medications, regardless of which route they are being administered (PO, IM, or IV) should be weighed daily.

Conscious Sedation

Children undergoing painful procedures should be placed in a treatment room or should be monitored in a pediatric intensive care unit (PICU). Many procedures require sedation at a level that requires close monitoring during and after the procedure. Conscious sedation medications such as propofol may be used during a procedure that leaves a child vulnerable, such as lumbar puncture, bone marrow aspiration, and peripherally inserted central venous catheter (PICC) line placement. Constant airway monitoring and management is imperative.

PEDIATRIC CONSIDERATIONS IN NURSING CARE: HOSPITAL PROCEDURES WITH CHILDREN IN MIND

Children should be prepared for procedures while they are hospitalized. The child's developmental level should be taken into account. The nurse should first assess what the child and family understand about the upcoming procedure and then a teaching session should be planned that is presented in a very supportive, calm, and appropriate level. Time should be allowed for the child and family to process the information and ask any questions that arise. Medical terms should be explained and visual aids should be used. Simple, straightforward, and concrete explanations should be offered and, when possible, literature with explanations and drawings or pictures should be offered. Many books are available to explain procedures to children in various age groups.

Preschool children are especially at risk for misunderstanding. Their fears of body mutilation and their use of magical thinking should be taken into consideration. To minimize separation anxiety, the parent should be encouraged to stay with the child whenever feasible and to be there when the child wakes up from sedation or anesthesia.

Informed Consent

A parent or guardian of a minor child must sign a consent form for the hospital admission, any procedures or surgeries, all blood product transfusions, and for diagnostic procedures such as magnetic resonance imaging or a computed tomography (CAT) scan. The nurse's responsibility is to make sure there are no further questions about the procedures and to act as a witness to the parent's or guardian's signature. The physician or advanced practitioner performing the procedure, or the anesthesiologist administering the child's sedation, are required to explain the procedure, risks, benefits, and alternatives to the family. Explanations should be done with the use of an interpreter if the family's primary language is not English. Explanations should be described to the depth of the parent's or guardian's understanding, and the parent or guardian should then state that he or she has no further questions. Special consent is needed from the parent or guardian for taking photographs of the child. Other reasons for a parent's signature can include special circumstances, such as the parent making the decision to leave the hospital or health-care institution against medical advice (AMA), postmortem examinations, or the release of the child's medical history or records to another health-care provider or institution. Lastly, when a child is being asked to participate in a clinical trial or research study, informed consent must be obtained by the child's parents or guardian.

Assent is the term used when a child participates in the consenting procedure. Typically, the age group for assent begins at the child's seventh birthday. Although the literature describes numerous perspectives on the process of assent, the American Academy of Pediatrics (AAP) has stated that a child should participate in the decision-making process to the extent that it is appropriate to the child's development.

Activities for Recovery After Medical Procedures

To help a child cope with recovery following medical procedures, there are many playful ways to engage the child. Ideas to engage a child and assist with the procedural experience include the following:

- **Early ambulation:** Prepare a game or age-appropriate craft activity in the playroom and have the child ambulate to the room to participate.
- **Increasing fluid intake:** Offer popsicles, decorate a cup, provide a silly straw, have the child keep track of his or her own intake and output (I&O) on a colorful chart, provide stickers as an incentive, or have a tea party for family.
- **Deep breathing and/or the use of an incentive spirometer (ICS):** Blow cotton balls across the table, have the child make and use a colorful construction paper pinwheel, blow bubbles, pretend to be a fire-blowing dragon, or use a pediatric ICS decorated as an animal.
- **Dressing changes:** If indicated, use premedicated dressings and then allow the child to wash his or her hands, remove his or her own dressing, and decorate the new dressing with colorful stickers. Provide a special prize or activity afterward.
- **Removal of monitoring devices:** Allow the child to participate in postprocedural activities, such as the removal of cardiac leads.

Preparing for Surgery

When not in an emergency situation, the nurse prepares the child for surgery. Emotional, cognitive, and physical preparation are all required. The child should have the procedure explained by both the nurse and a member of the Child Life team. The child's emotional well-being should be taken into account, with every effort made to comfort the child. You can assist in reducing anxiety over the unknown by talking in a quiet, soft voice with direct eye contact to establish trust and calm. The child should be kept with the

parent at all times up to the last minute before sedation. Physically, the child should have all jewelry removed, her or his hair tied back, skin surfaces washed, fingernail polish removed, and any loose teeth reported to anesthesia. Make sure the child is wearing readable identification before transport to the procedure. The child should be transported on a gurney or in a wheelchair, or should be carried by the parent and accompanied by a health-care team member (Fig. 26.3).

TEAM WORKS

For the safety of a child going from the pediatric unit to the surgical suite, implement a preoperative checklist. Using a checklist improves communication between teams.

- Assess vital signs (ie, temperature, blood pressure, pulse, respiration rate, oxygen saturation, and pain scale).
- Assess the last food and drink consumed or the last breast-feeding session. Document the exact time and content of the last oral intake.
- Assess the last stool and urination. Document the time and quantity.
- Using symptom assessment tools, assess for symptoms, including nausea, general discomfort, fatigue, emotional distress, dyspnea, and sleep deprivation.
- Assess for the presence of a signed and dated consent form for the procedure and assess for the need for a consent form for a blood product transfusion.
- Assess the child's mouth for the presence of loose teeth and report to the surgical team if found; loose teeth can become dislodged during intubation for surgery.
- Assess for the presence of any metal in or on the child's body, including implants, implanted central line ports, hardware, screws, and braces.
- Assess for the need for preoperative medications, such as presurgical antibiotics.
- Report any concerns to the surgical team that arise before surgery.

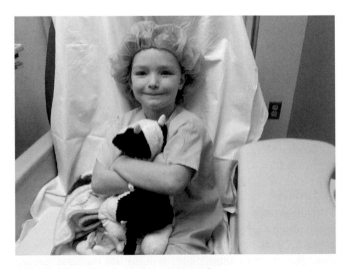

FIGURE 26.3 Young child preparing for surgery.

Postoperative Care

Begin assessment of a postoperative child as soon as the patient arrives on the unit. Have the family stay near the child, touching the child if appropriate, so that the child feels supported. Carefully transfer the child from the surgery gurney onto the hospital bed or crib, trying not to jar or move the child too roughly, which could cause discomfort or fear. Lock the gurney and bed to prevent injury and use a transfer sheet to provide the child with support when transferring.

Implement postoperative care:

- Assess the child's airway, breathing, and circulation.
- Assess the neurological status, including the mental status and level of alertness.
- Assess vital signs and oxygen saturation.
- Assess for pain using the most appropriate pain assessment tool for the child's developmental level.
- Assess for the need for oxygen.
- Assess IV lines, pumps, and catheters.
- Assess wound or surgical incision areas, and document the presence of drainage.
- Assess safety, including ensuring crib rails are up, side rails are up (the upper rails), and rails are padded as needed.
- Position the child for comfort.
- Assess the need for elimination.
- Provide emotional support for parents/caregivers.

Positioning for Procedures

Some medical procedures require a particular patient position to ensure procedural success. For instance, with a lumbar puncture, the child is side-lying in fetal position to maximize the spinal column for needle insertion. For pulmonary toileting, such as chest physiotherapy percussion, the child will be placed in a variety of positions during the procedure to maximize sputum drainage. Check the institutional policy and procedure manuals to identify the position required for each medical procedure. Positioning can vary according to the preference of the physician or nurse practitioner performing the procedure.

Restraints

The purpose of **restraints** is twofold: The child's safety is ensured by preventing movement during a procedure that could lead to harm, and the restraint provides safety by protecting a procedural site, wound, or medical device

from being touched, manipulated, or removed by the child. The use of restraints for any situation other than for gently holding a child safely and restricting movement during a short procedure requires a physician's order. The family should be informed about the use of a medical restraint and a discussion about the need for the restraint should be offered.

- Always provide the least restrictive form of a restraint and encourage the family to provide company to the child during the use of the restraint. During the use of a restraint, follow the institutional policy for assessing the child frequently and assess the skin perfusion and circulation frequently.
- Follow institutional policy meticulously about the use of restraints and the essential assessments of a child in a restraint. The Joint Commission on Accreditation of Healthcare Organizations (JCAHO) mandates the use of standards for acute care hospitals. These standards provide the health-care team with guidelines about the use of, orders for, alternatives to, application of, assessment of, and documentation of restraints. A medical order must be received within 1 hour of applying a restraint to a child. The medical order must include the indication for use, both the initiation and release times, the date, the type of restraint, and a signature. If needed, a registered nurse (RN) can receive a verbal order or telephone order for the initial use of a restraint.
- Whenever possible, use **therapeutic hugging** instead of physical restraint during a procedure. Therapeutic hugging includes a chest-to-chest straddle hold in a sitting position by a parent, or a back-to-chest sitting position in which the child's legs are held down securely during the procedure.
- Types of restraints include:
  - No-no's, or extremity restraints (ie, elbow restraints), to protect an IV line or to prevent a child from bending his elbow to get access to a nasogastric tube (NGT) or a medical device that could be removed by the child
  - Mummy (ie, swaddle) restraint, which is used for short-term positioning and extremity control during a minor procedure
  - Leg and arm restraints, which immobilize extremities for healing or during procedures

Phlebotomy

When a child requires a blood test via venipuncture during hospitalization, special pediatric considerations are needed. When possible, the use of a superficial numbing cream such as EMLA (lidocaine/prilocaine) helps to reduce the child's pain. Heelsticks are common during infancy for blood collection (see Labs & Diagnostics section in Chapter 16). Double-checking the accuracy in two patient identifiers should take place to prevent an error in handling and processing the specimens. If possible, any painful procedures such as phlebotomy should not be performed in the child's bed because this is considered the child's "safety zone." Use a treatment room for any shots, laboratory draws, or painful dressing changes.

SAFETY *STAT!*

Newborns and very small young infants who require multiple blood draws may need to have their blood loss calculated as output. Keeping accurate records on blood loss per day may be required.

IV Therapy and Central Lines

A hospitalized child may require IV hydration or IV medications (Fig. 26.4). It is imperative that safety considerations are implemented to prevent an accident leading to significant injury. When a child is hospitalized with an IV, make sure to take the following prevention steps:

- Prevent an accidental bolus of fluids or drugs by using only IV pumps with safety devices that clamp tubing whenever removed from the pump mechanics.
- Prevent medication infiltrations into tissues surrounding the vein that can cause significant tissue damage by assessing the site hourly.
- Prevent strangulation in a young child inadvertently wrapping tubing around his or her neck while in the crib.
- Prevent tissue injury by assessing and reporting a child who is crying inconsolably or is fussy with no other reason, as this may indicate an infiltration, phlebitis, or site infection.

FEEDING CONSIDERATIONS FOR SICK AND HOSPITALIZED CHILDREN

Children who have experienced anesthesia, certain procedures with side effects, many infectious processes, and chemotherapy do not have an expected appetite. Providing visually appealing and tasty foods may prove challenging. Having the family bring foods from home that are familiar and culturally oriented may assist with the child's food intake. Allow the child and family to select foods from the food service, encouraging them to choose foods that are colorful and mild in flavor. Giving the child ample time to complete his or her meal may increase oral intake. Hot, spicy, strongly aromatic, and greasy foods may deter the child from eating. Smaller portions with appetizing snacks or fruit smoothies between meals may help. Work with dietary services to calculate the required daily kilocalories based on the child's age and weight, and choose foods that are age-appropriate and appealing to each child.

Diets

During the hospital stay, children typically progress through an advancement of their diet after a surgical procedure. Children start with NPO status, meaning the withholding of all oral foods and fluids right after surgery. They then progress to the introduction of clear fluids (eg, broth, apple juice, frozen pops), then to full liquids (eg, milk shakes, yogurt smoothies), and then to soft foods (eg, apple sauce, mashed potatoes). If the child is successful in this progression, he or she will move to a regular diet appropriate and safe for his or her age and developmental stage. Before providing food

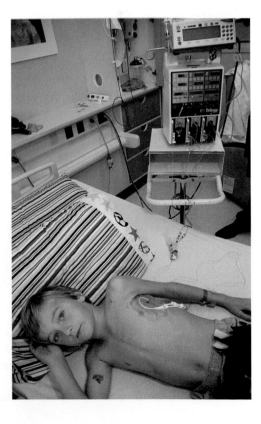

PICC line enters body here

PICC

FIGURE 26.4 Child with a central line. *(Photo by the National Cancer Institute.)*

or fluids after surgery, assess the child carefully for active bowel sounds in all four quadrants to make sure the child tolerates the food and does not vomit. Passing flatus also demonstrates the child's bowels are active and moving, which makes introducing clear fluids safer.

SAFETY *STAT!*

Pediatric nurses must adhere to diets that are ordered. The following list represents various diets ordered after surgery and while hospitalized, and ideas for items on each.

- Clear liquid diet: broth, JELL-O, ice pops, clear juices, ice chips
- Full liquid diet: cream soups, milk products, ice cream, liquid yogurt drinks without pulp
- Soft diet: mashed potatoes and other veggies, soft meats, pureed fruits, yogurt
- Regular diet: any foods considered safe for the child's developmental stage (eg, infants should have baby foods after they are introduced at home; toddlers should have foods that are considered to have low choking risk)
- Always call the dietary office and speak to a nutritionist if there are questions about appropriate foods for a child's diet

---

Calorie Counts

Because children often stop eating when they are sick, it is important to be aware of the kilocalorie needs of a child based on weight and age. The following guidelines are helpful in determining the amount of calories needed on a daily basis. If a child has a GI disorder or a diagnosis of FTT, alternative calorie requirements may be warranted (Table 26.4).

Fluid Maintenance Calculations

Determination of a child's minimal fluid maintenance can be performed by using the following calculation:

- If the child weighs between 0 and 10 kg, the fluid requirement is 100 mL/kg.

TABLE **26.4** DAILY KILOCALORIE REQUIREMENTS FOR INFANTS AND CHILDREN

Age of Infant or Child	Daily Kilocalorie Requirements
0–30 days	100–110 kcal/kg/day
1–4 months	90 to 100 kcal/kg/day
5 months–5 years	70–90 kcal/kg/day
Greater than 5 years	1,500 kcal for first 20 kg plus 25 kcal for each additional kg/day

---

- If the child weighs between 11 and 20 kg, the fluid requirement is 1,000 mL plus 50 mL for each kg between 11 and 20 kg.
- If the child weighs between 21 and 70 kg, the fluid requirement is 1,500 mL plus 20 mL for every kg between 21 and 70 kg.

Example:
If a child weighs 46 pounds:

Divide the pounds by 2.2 (ie, 46 / 2.2 = 20.9 kg)
1,000 mL + (10.9 x 50 = 545 mL)
Minimal fluid maintenance for a child weighing 46 pounds (20.9 kg) = 1,545 mL per 24 hours

Gastrointestinal Feeds

Children whose medical condition requires feedings and medication administration through an NGT or a GI tube need specialized care to ensure safety from aspiration and protection from skin breakdown. During hospitalization, after the placement of a feeding tube, the nurse should teach the family how to assess, clean, flush, and administer medications and feedings through the tube. If a child has had an NGT or a GI tube at home, then the hospitalization period provides an opportunity to assess how the family is doing, reevaluate their skills, and provide more teaching. Medications are either administered in a liquid form, or are crushed and mixed with water or formula and administered into the tube. Always assess for patency before administering medications or starting a continuous or bolus feeding in either an NGT or a GI tube.

Calculation of Intake and Output

Children who are medically frail, are at risk for fluid or electrolyte imbalance, or are receiving medical treatments that affect a child's fluid status, such as long periods of NPO, are placed on strict I&O measurements. If it is unclear how many mL are in a certain size cup, an ice pop, or a food container, call the dietary office for assistance. The health-care team typically assesses the child's 24-hour total I&O balance and then makes decisions. The term *positive fluid balance* is used to denote that the child has had more intake than output and may be at risk for fluid overload. The term *negative fluid balance* is used to describe a child who has lost more fluids than he or she has taken in. This occurs with a severe case of diarrhea, vomiting, or diuresis. Report discrepancies of fluid balance to the health-care team so that action can take place to correct a hospitalized child's fluid and electrolyte needs.

ADMINISTERING MEDICATIONS TO HOSPITALIZED CHILDREN

Hospitalized children often require a course of a variety of medications, including oral, topical, IV, injections, ear, eyes, nose, and suppositories. Safety is paramount because children require very specific doses that are often based on their most current weight (ie, milligrams per kilogram calculation or by their body surface area [BSA]). Follow institutional policy about double-checking the "10 rights" of accurate medication administration:

1. Right patient
2. Right drug
3. Right dose
4. Right route
5. Right time
6. Right method of administration for the child's developmental stage
7. Right preadministration assessment
8. Right family education
9. Right postadministration assessment
10. Right documentation

Medicating children requires a focus on safety. Many aspects of safety related to medicating children include storage, dosing, and accuracy. Safe storage, which includes locking medications in cabinets or drawers, is a very important measure to take when caring for children. Most pediatric medications are dosed according to milligrams per kilogram and therefore require accuracy in the child's measurements. Check a current pharmacology book for the safe dose range, safety considerations, and preparation guidelines for all pediatric medications. If a dose is found to be outside of the safe dose range, the nurse must check with the person who prescribed the medication, and also with pharmacy for guidelines as indicated.

SAFETY *STAT!*

All medications must be stored away from a child's reach and should never be left at the bedside or in a child's hospital room for later administration. If a delay in administration is required, bring the drug back to the safety of the nurse's medication room for storage and make sure the medication is labeled with the child's name, medical record number, date, time, and dose.

Oral Medications

Most pediatric oral medications come in a flavored liquid or a chewable tablet. If the medication is not palatable, mix it in a small amount of flavored or chocolate syrup. Accurately draw up the medication in an oral syringe and hold the syringe at eye level to assess accuracy in dosing. Older infants and toddlers may prove challenging for medication administration. Solicit the assistance of a parent and give choices to the child when able, but do not allow stalling behaviors. However, do not force a crying infant or young child to take a medication because this may lead to aspiration.

SAFETY *STAT!*

Never leave medications at the bedside of a hospitalized child to be given later. Take the medication from the room and store it, fully labeled, in the locked medication room.

Sublingual Medications

Some medications are ordered to be given sublingually (SL). Here the child places the medication under the tongue or against the buccal mucosa, where it rapidly dissolves and absorbs.

Subcutaneous and Intradermal Medications

Subcutaneous and intradermal (ID) routes are used frequently in pediatrics for some vaccines, insulin, hormone replacement, allergy desensitization, tuberculosis skin testing, and biotherapies, such as granulocyte colony-stimulating factor (GCSF). Using the smallest gauge needles (ie, 26 to 30), the nurse injects the child with the smallest volume (typically 0.5 mL or less). Using either a 45-degree angle for children with little subcutaneous tissue or a 90-degree angle for children with adequate tissue, insert the needle carefully with the bevel up. Common sites for both subcutaneous and ID injections in pediatrics are the same as in adults: the upper outer arm, central thigh, or abdomen (Fig. 26.5). Rotate sites to prevent inflammation or soreness.

Intramuscular Medications

IM medications are given to a hospitalized child most commonly for the administration of antibiotics or pain medication. Three aspects of the medication are taken into consideration:

1. The amount of medication to be administered will determine the size of the syringe.
2. The viscosity of the medication to be administered will determine the gauge of the needle.
3. The depth of the tissue to be penetrated will determine the needle length.

Most institutional guidelines will state that the maximum amount to be administered into one IM site is 1 mL for infants and young children up to 5 years of age, 1.5 mL for older children (ie, 6 to 10 years of age), and 2 mL for older school-aged children or adolescents (ie, 11 to 18 years of age). The volume will ultimately depend on the amount of muscle present. Some medication volumes require two injections. When possible, solicit the assistance of another nurse and give the shots simultaneously to reduce fear.

Common sites include the vastus lateralis, ventrogluteal, and, less commonly, the deltoid muscles. If two shots are required because of volume, then the needle is inserted at a 90-degree angle with a quick, dartlike motion. Aspirate for blood and discontinue the injection at the site where blood is found. Massaging the site is not necessary. Change the needle and select an alternative site. Medications should be injected slowly to reduce discomfort. If ordered, both the air-bubble technique and the Z-track technique may be warranted in pediatrics to prevent tracking the injected solution through the subcutaneous tissues. Two caregivers may be required to hold the child during the procedure. EMLA cream may be ordered to provide topical analgesia. Place a colorful bandage over the site and praise the child for his or her cooperation.

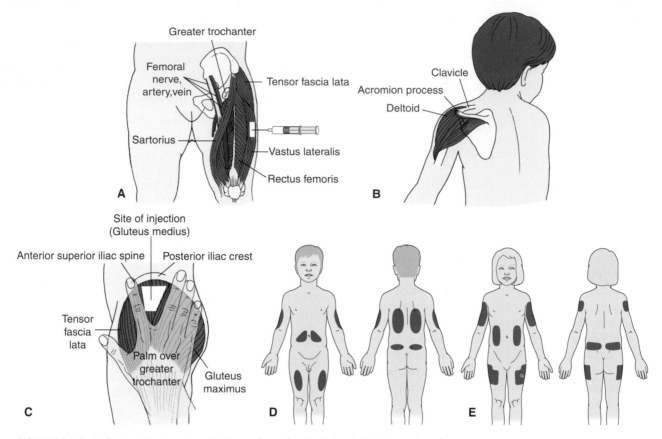

FIGURE 26.5 Pediatric injection sites: A, Vastus lateralis; B, Deltoid; C, Ventrogluteal; D, Subcutaneous; and E, ID.

IV Medications

Medications are often administered to children through IV routes while in the hospital.

Special care is needed to take care of these sites because it is difficult to insert an IV into many children. This is especially true for infants. Figure 26.6 illustrates venous access sites for infants.

Ear Medications

Otic medications are used in children to treat infections or inflammations of the outer ear and ear canal. Medications are instilled using a specialized dropper to administer a specific number of drops as prescribed. Ear drops should be instilled while the child is side-lying. After administration, a small cotton ball can be placed to prevent the medication from

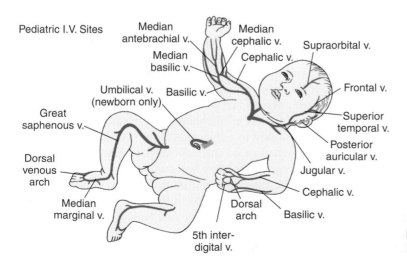

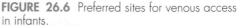

FIGURE 26.6 Preferred sites for venous access in infants.

running out. If possible, refrigerated otic medicine solution should be allowed to reach room temperature to prevent an uncomfortable sensation.

Eye Medications

Eye medications are administered to children in the same fashion as they are administered to adults. If the medication is in a drop form, the child should be placed in a supine position and the drops should be administered directly into the eye. If the medication is an ointment, the child should be either sitting with his or her head back, or in a supine position. The ointment is placed in a thin line from the inner canthus to the outer canthus on the bottom inner lid.

Topical Medications

Children younger than 6 months readily absorb topical medications directly through their skin. Therefore it is imperative that an order is received before any topical medications are applied to young infants. Topical medications should be administered in a thin layer and infants and toddlers should be held or gently restrained so they do not immediately lick or rub the medications off their skin. Only administer the medications in the timeframe ordered and carefully instruct parents to follow orders carefully. Only the skin affected should have the topical medication applied and care should be taken not to stain clothes.

Rectal Medications

Medications administered in the rectum cause most children to be quite fearful. This route is used most commonly when a child is unable to tolerate oral medications. Suppositories should never be inserted in a child with a bleeding disorder or with a low platelet count. The suppository should be lubricated with a water-soluble lubrication and inserted gently with a gloved finger.

▇ SPECIMEN COLLECTION

Specimens are frequently collected on a variety of body fluids to assist the health-care team with an appropriate medical diagnosis or evaluate progress of healing. Always wear gloves when handling body specimens. All specimens should be placed in the appropriate container (if there is a question, call the laboratory for guidance) and labeled with the collector's initials and the date and time of collection.

Urine Collection

The assessment of a child's urine is a very common diagnostic procedure performed in hospitals and clinics. The pediatric nurse will be responsible to collect either a clean sample of urine or a sterile sample of urine.

Clean-Catch Method: An Undiapered Child

For a clean-catch urine specimen, the child's genitalia should be cleansed with commercial saline wipes or gently with soap and water using a clean washcloth. Ideally, the specimen should be collected midstream and in a sterile collection cup that is labeled with the nurse's initials, date, time, and

the patient's medical record number. It should be immediately sent to the laboratory for processing.

Clean-Catch Method: A Diapered Child

When the patient is diapered, cotton balls can be placed in the diaper to collect urine. Wearing gloves, the nurse retrieves the saturated cotton balls and wrings them out in a sterile specimen cup. Processing the specimen is the same as a clean-catch urine specimen for a nondiapered child. The use of a urinary collection bag is also common (Fig. 26.7).

Sterile Catheterization

When contamination is probable, or if the ordering primary caregiver requests a specimen for culture and sensitivity, an in-and-out procedure using a sterile catheter may need to be performed to retrieve a urine specimen. Some institutions provide a sterile urinary catheterization kit, while others require the nurse to collect individual equipment. The size of the catheter must be correct for the child's physical size. The child's genitalia are cleansed with a povidone-iodine (Betadine) solution and the sterile catheter is inserted for urine collection. Young children may be very frightened of this procedure and may physically protest. Two or three nurses may be required to perform the procedure. A young girl's urinary meatus is very small and a flashlight may be required to locate the meatus opening.

Twenty-Four-Hour Urine Collections

The pediatric nurse may receive an order to collect a child's urine for a 24-hour period of time. This is done for laboratory evaluation of the secretion of a material over time, such as creatinine clearance. The storage container must be received from the laboratory and the specimen should be timed clearly from when the first urination was collected and stored. The container is kept in a specimen refrigerator where no breast milk or foods are stored. Check with the hospital environmental services department for storage guidelines.

Stool Specimens

Stool specimens are collected in the hospital environment to evaluate the presence of blood, parasites, or ovum. Small

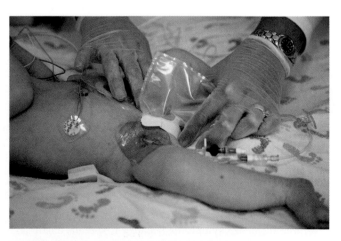

FIGURE 26.7 Pediatric urine collection bag.

amounts are required and should be sent to the laboratory immediately after collection. Placing a urine collection hat in the toilet or scraping stool off a diaper is acceptable.

Sputum Specimens

During cold and flu season, there is an increased incidence of hospitalization for children with respiratory infections. Collecting sputum is difficult in young children because they typically cannot follow instructions to produce sputum and spit in a cup. Children often cough and swallow their sputum. Respiratory therapists are skilled in sputum collection and should be utilized for assistance, especially with young children.

Respiratory Syncytial Virus (RSV) Specimens

RSV is a common respiratory infection during the fall and winter seasons. For infants and children with chronic conditions, an RSV infection can be very serious and require hospitalization (see Chapter 32, Child With a Respiratory Condition, for further information). When RSV is suspected, the nurse performs a nasal wash specimen to send to the laboratory for a rapid enzyme-linked immunosorbent assay (ELISA) evaluation to detect the presence of RSV antibodies. Care should be taken to prevent self-infection, so the nurse should wear a mask, goggles, gloves, and gown for RSV specimen collection. A small amount of sterile saline is injected via a sterile 3-mL syringe without a needle, aspirated right back, capped, and sent off to the lab. Because of the uncomfortable sensation of this collection procedure, a second nurse or nursing aide should assist to hold down the child's arms in a firm comfort hold. RSV is very communicable and care should be taken to prevent the spread of infection.

Methicillin-Resistant *Staphylococcus Aureus* (MRSA) Specimens

Because of the rampant spread of the resistant strain of methicillin-resistant *S aureus* (MRSA), testing is common in hospital environments. To identify risk and stop the spread, institutions are requesting that patients be tested by a nasal swab upon admission to critical care environments, and sometimes to the pediatric units. Ask the laboratory for the correct swab because there are differences between swabs for viral and bacterial specimens. The procedure can be frightening to young children, so use a comforting swaddle or a therapeutic hold. Explain to the school-aged child and adolescent there is a small level of discomfort that resolves immediately.

Influenza Specimen Collection

The influenza epidemic has affected the entire world. When a child presents with flulike symptoms, the nurse will obtain a nasal specimen for a rapid antibody test. The child's nares will be swabbed with a sterile collection device and immediately sent to the laboratory for evaluation. Wash your hands carefully before and after the procedure. Follow the institutional policy meticulously to determine if a child's symptoms resemble influenza symptoms because it spreads easily and the child must be placed in respiratory and contact isolation.

GUIDELINES FOR PARENTS IN ADMINISTERING MEDICATIONS AT HOME

Families need direct guidelines for the administration of medications at home. Whether a child is to have a PRN mediation based on the presentation of a symptom or if the child is to have an around-the-clock (ATC) medication regimen, it is the nurse's responsibility to assess the family's potential for compliance, ability to administer the medication accurately, and understanding of specifics of administration ***before discharge.***

Storage

All medications should be kept out of reach of the children who reside in the home. Medications should always remain in their original containers. Pediatric medications come in child-safe containers and should be kept completely closed at all times to prevent accidental ingestion and potential injury through poisoning.

Calculation

Before discharge, or under the direct instruction and supervision of the pharmacist, the family needs to be taught how to read the label and calculate the correct amount to be administered. The medication should be dispensed with simple directions about how to draw up the correct amount of the solution or identify the correct number of pills. The prescription should provide exactly the correct amount of medication for the full prescription, unless it is commercially made, such as eye drops, ear drops, or topical medications. Spoons with markers, syringes with larger fonts, and small medication cups with clear markings can all help the family's accuracy.

Preparation

If the medication prescribed requires any form of preparation, the nurse should demonstrate how to do the preparation before discharge. Medications such as powders, granules, or those that come in packets will require preparation immediately before administration.

Administration

The administration of a discharge medication can come in many forms. It is essential that the family understands how to administer the medication. Topical medications should be applied sparingly, and eye and ear drops must be applied correctly to be effective. NGT medication administration requires teaching and demonstrations, and injections such as insulin require specialized teaching to ensure the child receives the correct amount through the right administration procedure. Teaching checklists should be used to document the teaching being conducted. Teaching should be done over time with ample demonstration, return demonstration, and time for comprehension.

Assessment of Symptoms

When a home prescription requires that a parent or adult caregiver assess the child's symptom to determine whether or not a medication should be administered and how much, it is important that the nurse discuss a symptom scale appropriate for the child's development. Request an approved copy of a developmentally appropriate pain scale tool from the hospital to use at home.

Disposal

After the completion of the home medication regimen, the family should dispose of the remaining medication per the pharmacist's instructions. Medications should not be flushed down the toilet nor should a prescription medication be saved for future use unless specifically directed by the dispensing pharmacist.

Compliance

Adherence to the posthospital medication regimen is an important factor for the pediatric nurse to assess. If there is any reason that the nurse suspects the family will be unwilling or unable to obtain the prescribed medication because of financial, transportation, or social reasons, or if the nurse suspects the family will be unwilling or unable to administer the medication to the child, the nursing supervisor, charge nurse, and physician should be notified. In extreme cases, the child will be kept in the hospital to make sure a prescribed drug is administered and the prescription completed. In persistent cases of noncompliance with medical treatments, Child Protective Services may need to be notified.

SAFETY *STAT!*

Completing the Prescription

Because of the international concerns around the development of resistant microbes, it is imperative that the nurse remind the family that the entire dose of an antibiotic must be completed.

DISCHARGE PROCEDURES

With the shorter length of hospital stays and the greater dependence on home care and parents providing care, discharge procedures have recently evolved. It is more important than ever for a nurse to provide teaching and discharge instructions about all care required after the hospitalizations. Parents may need to learn specific skills, dressing changes, and medication administration, and will need to learn about follow-up visits. When a child is being discharged from a hospital, the following are imperative for the health-care team to provide to the parents:

- A follow-up appointment to assess the child's health after hospitalization; often, this is done with the child's community-based pediatrician, who has been following the child's growth and development
- Any needed referrals to specialists or specialized services, such as occupational therapy, physical therapy, developmental screening, or psychosocial care
- Any prescriptions that need to be filled for medications that are being initiated or that are being continued from the hospital stay
- A thorough assessment of the child's hospital room so that no personal items are lost or left behind

SAFETY *STAT!*

Discharge procedures are crucial times for the pediatric health-care team to stress important follow-up plans, including further appointments, diagnostic examinations, and follow-up laboratory draws. Use interpreter services as needed to confirm understanding of discharge plans and follow-up appointments.

Key Points

- During hospitalization, pediatric patients across childhood have unique needs for a variety of acute and chronic conditions. These include paying special attention to reactions to being separated from home, siblings, toys, pets, parents, and familiar environments.
- Young children experience anxiety described as both separation anxiety and stranger anxiety. The three phases of separation during a hospitalization experience can be described as protest, despair, and detachment/denial.
- There are many safety concerns for young children while hospitalized in fast-paced, chaotic health-care environments. These safety concerns include falls from beds and cribs, aspiration, choking, strangulation, and medical/medication errors. Nurses are in a unique position in being at the bedside to monitor for safety concerns.

- Pediatric and adult hospital units differ in their policies for schedules, play environments, meals, equipment, bed assignment, and sleep needs. Children are not considered to be "small adults" and therefore should not be treated as such. Hospitalized children should be supported based on the child's developmental stage and should be provided opportunities for growth, development, play, and social interactions.
- Careful consideration is required when selecting pediatric bed assignments. Medical diagnoses and childhood infections influence how children are placed within the unit. Children with like diagnoses should be cohorted (ie, placed together) for support.
- Several activities for recovery after medical procedures exist to assist the child. These activities include early ambulation to a fun activity, increased oral fluid intake through play such as a tea party, deep breathing using

toys and pinwheels, and having the child assist with post-procedure skills such as bandage application or removal of cardiac monitoring leads.

■ Pain is a unique experience for each child. Pediatric-specific assessments and interventions for pain are required. Pediatric pain tools developed for each stage of pediatric development have been validated by research and are considered very specific and effective. Hospitalized pediatric clients should be offered both pharmaceutical and nonpharmaceutical nursing interventions to help relieve pain.

■ Pediatric-specific calculations must be applied to children in the hospital. This includes calculating accurate medication doses, accurate calorie requirements, accurate fluid maintenance, and accurate I&O, especially with diapered infants.

■ Specific measures should be taken to administer medications safely, accurately, and effectively to children who are hospitalized. Double-checking weight-based pediatric medications and preventing choking should all be considered while caring for hospitalized children.

■ There are a variety of specimen-specific guidelines required to collect blood, urine, sputum, and other body fluids from children. Unique collection requirements of children include the inability to produce sputum on demand, emotional responses to having specimens collected, and urine and stool samples from infants and toddlers who are diapered.

REVIEW QUESTIONS

1. What is the best way to measure the height of a hospitalized 16-month-old toddler?
   1. Plastic tape measure
   2. Horizontal measuring board
   3. Asking the parents about the results of the last height measurement
   4. Having the child stand on the unit scale and using the measuring arm

2. How does the nurse determine how many calories a child needs on a daily basis?
   1. By asking the dietician to calculate the child's caloric needs
   2. By asking the parents their average daily meal preparations
   3. By calculating the child's BSA and multiplying the result by two
   4. By using a child's age to estimate their daily calorie need per kilogram of weight

3. Two forms of pediatric pain assessment tools are used to collect information about a child's pain experience. These two forms are:
   1. Numerical and visual
   2. Subjective and objective
   3. Physical and emotional
   4. Objective and parent's descriptions

4. Which one of the following pain assessment tools is used for a newborn?
   1. Wong-Baker FACES pain rating scale
   2. FLACC scale
   3. CRIES pain scale
   4. VAS

5. By what age can most children answer specific questions about the location and severity of their presenting symptoms?
   1. Preschool-aged child, starting at 5 years
   2. School-aged child, starting at 7 years
   3. Older school-aged child, starting at 9 years
   4. Older toddler, starting at age 22 months

6. Oral morphine sulfate has just been administered to a 6-year-old in severe pain after a surgical appendectomy. According to the child's age and developmental level, which pain tool would the nurse use to assess this child's level of pain relief?
   1. 1 to 10 descriptive numerical pain scale
   2. Poker Chip Pain Assessment Tool
   3. Wong-Baker FACES pain rating scale
   4. VAS

7. Regression is a common response of a young child to the stressors of hospitalization. Regression can be defined as the:
   1. Desire to act as an infant
   2. Display of earlier developmental behaviors
   3. Anger toward healthy siblings when the family visits
   4. Absence of trust toward the health-care team

8. Children experience negative consequences to hospitalization, including fear, anxiety, and pain/discomfort. Parents also experience consequences. Potential responses families may have toward the experience of a hospitalized child include: *(select all that apply)*
   1. Fear
   2. Guilt
   3. Family cohesiveness
   4. Frustration
   5. Loss of control
   6. Normalcy
   7. Financial concerns

9. Lack of control is one of the most influential aspects of a young child's hospitalization. When a child perceives a decrease in or lack of control of his or her environment, the child experiences:
   1. A perception of a threat
   2. An overload of stimulation
   3. A reaction of anger and despair
   4. An acceleration of developmental growth

10. The nurse is preparing a young school-aged child to go to surgery. As the nurse is completing the preoperative checklist, special attention should be given to which of the following?
    1. The presence of braces
    2. An allergy band
    3. Loose teeth
    4. Assent to the procedure

CRITICAL THINKING QUESTIONS

1. How do children in each of the six developmental stages (ie, newborn, infant, toddler, preschool-aged, school-aged, and adolescent) differ in their response to being hospitalized for an acute or chronic disorder? How do children in each of the developmental stages differ in relation to feelings of separation from family, the need for distraction and play, and the need for continued cognitive, social, and emotional development?

2. What pain assessment tools work best for children in each of the six developmental stages? What nonpharmaceutical interventions can be implemented as adjunct pain control measures for children in each of the developmental stages?

3. What forms of communication between pediatric nurses and other members of the health-care team work best for reducing errors in the hospitalized setting? For instance, what are ways in which communication can be improved while moving or transferring pediatric patients between departments? What elements of a hand-off (more formally known as a *hand-off report*) between health-care professionals promote safety and continuity of care?

For additional resources and information, visit **www.DavisPlus.com**. Post-Conference Questions and Activities, Answers, and References can be found on Davis*Plus*.

27

Acutely Ill Children and Their Needs

KEY TERMS

apparent life-threatening event (ALTE)
Broselow's tape
central cyanosis
clinical status
code blue
epiglottitis
higher level of care
peripheral cyanosis
rapid response team (RRT)
safety precautions
SBAR
shock

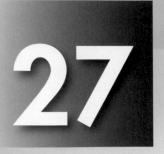 **DavisPlus** For audio pronunciation guide, visit **www.DavisPlus.com**

CHAPTER CONCEPTS

Comfort
Communication
Family
Safety
Trauma

LEARNING OUTCOMES

1. Define the key terms.
2. Discuss safety concerns when an acutely ill child is hospitalized and include every-shift safety checks for emergency equipment and safety precautions all pediatric nurses should perform.
3. Apply the principles of professional interdisciplinary communication through the use of the SBAR system.
4. State typical color-coding systems used within a hospital to call for rapid assistance from a variety of teams (ie, code red, code blue, code pink, code grey, code yellow).
5. Review the most current American Heart Association guidelines for cardiopulmonary resuscitation (CPR).
6. Discuss a comprehensive assessment of an acutely ill child who is hospitalized.
7. Define the system of emergency response with the color-coded, length-based resuscitation tape.
8. Analyze the use of and outcomes of an RRT.
9. Create a care plan that encompasses the needs of the family when a child is acutely ill and has a sudden change in clinical status that requires a higher level of care.
10. Describe the emergency response measures needed to assist a child in shock.

REAL-WORLD CASE STUDY

Maria

■ A licensed vocational nurse/registered nurse (LVN/RN) team is taking care of a young child, Maria, who was being seen in the pediatric clinic of a busy Public Health Department for difficulty breathing, rapid respiratory rate, congestion, and "feeling sluggish." The parents of the 2-year-old expressed concern that the 3-year-old at home caught a viral infection from preschool and brought it home to the younger sibling. The child presents with a respiratory rate of 48 to 56 breaths per minute, a heart rate of 146 bpm, blood pressure of 92/48 mm Hg, and an oxygen saturation of 89%. The child has very dry mucous membranes, no void thus far today, and presents with sleepiness, curling up in the father's lap. After the LVN takes the vital signs (VSs) and reports the condition of the child to the RN, the RN comes immediately to assess the child. Concerned, the RN calls for the doctor, who decides to place the child on oxygen in the clinic and to continuously monitor the child on an oxygen saturation probe. The child's saturation does not rise with 2 liters of oxygen administered via blow-by, and she is moaning and pushing away the oxygen delivery system. The team decides to call the local emergency room (ER) and request that the parents drive the child immediately to the ER for further evaluation.

1. What findings did this child present with that concerned the pediatric health-care team in the clinic?
2. Which primary finding led the team to insist on an immediate transfer to the local ER?
3. Why did the child not respond to the oxygen?
4. Why was the child so dehydrated? How does one look for clinical signs of dehydration? What level of dehydration was she in?

CONCEPTUAL CORNERSTONE

Safety

There are always safety concerns when a child is experiencing an acute illness or injury requiring hospitalization. Safety checks must be consistent and frequent. *Safety precautions* is the term used to describe multiple safety measures implemented by the pediatric health-care team to keep a child safe. Checking that emergency equipment functions, is present, and is the right size for the child is a responsibility for each nurse at the beginning of the shift. Being able to identify a change in clinical status for the worse, and being able and confident to call for help rapidly will save lives. Safe practice means using a RRT or a code blue team, and then clearly communicating the child's status and recent assessments. Using a communication tool such as SBAR will allow a nurse experiencing a stressful event to think clearly and communicate safely. Hospitals are inherently unsafe and the provision of safe care is a major responsibility for all members of the health-care team.

Working in the acute care environment requires that nurses have not only a certain level of confidence in responding to emergencies, but also a set of skills that can be performed quickly and smoothly to ensure a rapid response to a sudden change in **clinical status** (ie, the clinical well-being) of the acutely ill child. This chapter will present several strategies and skills to assist the nurse who is a part of a health-care team caring for a child whose level of acuity, or level of sickness, requires a team effort to provide safety and avoid harm.

Children, in general, are healthy and strong. When a child becomes very ill from an infectious disease, severe injury, or an exacerbation of a chronic illness, his or her internal resources to maintain homeostasis may falter. Acutely ill children may be able to compensate for quite a period of time before they suddenly demonstrate a severe decompensation. For example, a child with severe dehydration may not demonstrate hypotension until suddenly the blood pressure can no longer adjust to the loss of intravascular fluids. A child in severe respiratory distress may abruptly not be able to compensate and may go into respiratory failure and then respiratory arrest quite suddenly. Children need to be watched carefully when their clinical status is "guarded" because they may suddenly need to be moved to a **higher level of care,** such as the pediatric intensive care unit (PICU), to be provided an increased level of interventions and one-on-one nursing care.

PROVIDING SAFETY AT THE BEDSIDE

It is imperative that a nurse who first walks into a hospitalized child's room conducts an assessment of the safety of the layout of the room, the presence of emergency equipment that is the correct size for the child, and the functioning of the emergency equipment. The following checklist should be used to assess room safety for an acutely ill child who may need an emergency response:

- The presence of the bed in low position, with the side rails up and the call light within the child's reach
- The presence of a manual resuscitator bag (ie, Ambu) and a set of masks within a clean plastic bag away from the child's reach; practice attaching a mask to the manual resuscitator bag to feel the universal fit
- The correct size mask for the child for whom you are caring
- The presence of a suction setup with tubing and a clean canister; turn on the suction to make sure the equipment works effectively
- The presence of at least one suction device: tonsil tip, olive tip, bulb syringe, or deep sterile suctioning kit (Fig. 27.1)
- The presence of a source of oxygen, including a green color-coded "Christmas tree" connector that will allow the rapid placement of oxygen tubing onto the oxygen wall device
- The presence of an oxygen delivery system, such as a nasal cannula, a simple face mask, or a nonrebreather mask, depending on the severity of the child's illness
- The presence of a working **code blue** (ie, cardiopulmonary arrest) call system, such as a code button or a code string/pull
- The bedside phone with numbers for emergency response: code blue, code red, and the **rapid response team (RRT),** which responds to an emergency at the bedside
- Within the child's bathroom, the presence of a working emergency call button or string/pull

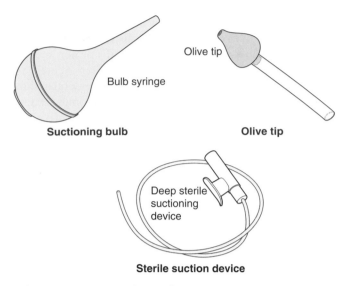

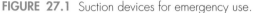

FIGURE 27.1 Suction devices for emergency use.

There are a variety of color-coded response systems that are used in large clinic and hospital settings. It is imperative that a nurse checks with his or her institution to learn the specific color codes for a particular health-care institution. Table 27.1 provides an example of color codes commonly used by direct caregivers to alert specific individuals, groups, security, or administration of an emergency and to communicate that help is required.

SAFETY *STAT!*

The four pieces of emergency equipment that must be at all bedsides are:
- Suction machine setup with tubing
- Source of oxygen
- A variety of manual resuscitator bags and different sizes of masks
- A code button to call code blue

SBAR Communication Techniques

Because communication has been determined to be the source of many errors in health-care environments, a tool was developed to create a prompt, organized, and effective means to communicate critical information between health-care team members. This tool, called **SBAR**, is especially effective in communications between the nursing staff and the medical staff. The technique provides a consistent framework to communicate about a patient's condition. It is easy to remember, can be used in person or over the phone, and is a concrete mechanism considered useful for communicating critical information that requires immediate attention. In high-urgency communications, the SBAR tool enables patient safety through concise communication that focuses on requesting assistance and recommendations. *SBAR* stands for *S*ituation, *B*ackground, *A*ssessment, and *R*ecommendation.

TABLE **27.1** COLOR-CODED RESPONSE SYSTEM

Code	Response
Code Red	Fire or smoke is present on the unit. Identify the exact location and begin patient removal from harm, as well as containment procedures.
Code Pink	A newborn, infant, or young child is missing or has been abducted. This process initiates a lockdown procedure or security watch of all elevators, stairs, and hospital exit doors.
Code Blue	CPR is needed, and a full team is required, including a pharmacist, laboratory personnel, a nursing supervisor, and a pediatric advanced life support (PALS)–certified response team.
Code Yellow	A disaster has occurred; prepare for a large number of incoming patients.
Code Gray	An adult is missing from his or her room or unit.
Code Dr. Strong Arm	There is a need for security to come immediately to the unit or location.
Code Rapid Response	There is a need for an emergency response team, but the child has not fully coded (eg, grand mal seizure; a fall accompanied by a head injury/loss of consciousness; tet spell for a child with congenital heart disease).

TEAM WORKS

SBAR Communication Tool
  Situation
- Identify yourself, your occupation/position, and the location where you are calling from.
- Identify the patient by name, date of birth, age, sex, and reason for hospitalization.
- Describe briefly the reason for the phone call; if urgent, say so.
  Background
- Give the patient's presenting complaint, such as being short of breath, in pain, or bleeding.

- Briefly describe the patient's pertinent past medical history relating to the immediate situation, such as the patient had surgery this morning, or is hospitalized for a cardiac procedure.
- Give a brief summary of the background of your concern, such as rapid development of chest pain or evidence of surgical wound infection.

   Assessment

- Provide important assessment information such as recent VSs, pain scale (see Chapter 26, The Hospitalized Child), a change in the status, or a change in the level of consciousness.
- State again if any VSs are outside of parameters, such as in tachypnea, bradycardia, or high temperature.
- Describe your impression of the severity of patient's situation.

   Recommendation

- Provide a brief suggestion of what action you think should be taken.
- Provide an explicit list of what you think you need.
- Wait to hear a response and write it down; read back any orders that are given.
- Ask if a provider will be coming to assess the child or what next steps are needed to provide safety and follow-through.

RESPONDING TO EMERGENCIES

Pediatric nurses must be prepared to quickly respond to an emergency when an acutely ill child's condition takes a turn for the worse and requires an RRT. Children are emotionally, anatomically, and physiologically different than adults. Their ability to compensate for a change in blood pressure, vascular volume, and respiratory status is limited and they often demonstrate a rapid demise. It is imperative that a pediatric nurse regularly practice emergency response procedures within the clinical setting and be prepared to rapidly be a part of a team that responds when a child's condition becomes worse.

Many acute care institutions offer regular practice mock code blue scenarios to allow a health-care team to practice a rapid response to an emergency. Practicing how to call for an RRT, call a code blue response, initiate a crash cart, and perform CPR are essential skills needed to help save a child's life during an emergency situation. Many conditions warrant a skilled emergency response for acutely ill children (Table 27.2).

Cardiopulmonary Resuscitation

Because of principles of growth and development, each developmental level and age group requires a set of rapid CPR response skills. Table 27.3 outlines the required steps for CPR for the neonate, infant, young child, and adolescent. It is imperative that a nurse remains certified in CPR. Changes in the sequence and content of CPR courses and guidelines are often made based on the most recent research on clinical outcomes and best practices. Check the American

TABLE 27.2 SKILLED EMERGENCY RESPONSE FOR ACUTELY ILL CHILDREN

Type of Condition	Emergency Response
Cardiovascular	• Cyanotic newborn • Infant in shock • Complicated postoperative care with bleeding • Cardiac arrhythmias • Septic shock
Metabolic	• Diabetic ketoacidosis • Severe hypoglycemia • Malignant hyperthermia
Neurological	• Change in consciousness • Child abuse/shaken baby syndrome • Increased intracranial pressure
Gastrointestinal	• Peritonitis • Appendix rupture • Gastrointestinal bleeding
Immunological	• Anaphylaxis • Acute blood product transfusion reaction
Toxicological	• Poisoning • Ingestion of an unknown substance
Respiratory	• Severe respiratory distress, significant increased work of breathing • Foreign body aspiration • Acute epiglottitis • Status asthmaticus • Dislodged tracheostomy tube
Burns	• Smoke inhalation • Chemical, thermal, or electrical burns

Heart Association's Web site on a regular basis to review any changes made on CPR guidelines. Implement only the most current guidelines for the best possible outcome and a coordinated team effort. It is the responsibility of the nurse to stay competent, confident, and ready to respond within a team to an acute pediatric emergency.

The majority of pediatric cardiopulmonary arrests originate from a problem in the respiratory system after a clinically significant respiratory event. Both infants' and small children's airway diameters are significantly smaller, anatomically, than adults' airways. Therefore even a small amount

TABLE 27.3 GUIDELINES FOR PEDIATRIC CARDIOPULMONARY RESUSCITATION

Age Group	Assessment	Circulation	Airway	Breathing
Newborns Birth–1 month	1. Airway clear of meconium? 2. Breathing? Effectively? 3. Muscle tone? 4. Color? 5. Heart rate? (Often Apgar scores will provide information concerning the need to intervene: respiratory effort, heart rate, reflex irritability, muscle tone, and overall color)	Universal compression to ventilation ratio for newborns is 3:1 • Start compressions if HR is less than 60 bpm within 30 sec • Compress at rate of 120 bpm with depth of ½ in.	• Open airway, attempt resuscitative breaths • Readjust airway if unsuccessful	• Provide resuscitative breathing at rate of 20–30 breaths per minute • If endotracheal tube or laryngeal mask airway is in place, then the rate should be 8–10 breaths per minute
Infants 1 month–1 year	• Determine unresponsiveness • Call for help	• Perform high-quality chest compressions at a rate of at least 100 bpm • Compress the chest at the level just below an imaginary line between the nipples • Compress the chest 1½ in.	• Open airway and maintain using the jaw-thrust or manual maneuvers, attempt resuscitative breaths Readjust airway if unsuccessful	• Perform bag-mask ventilations using 100% oxygen • Continue at a rate of at least 20 breaths per minute • Infant resuscitation (ie, 1 month to 1 year): Universal compressions to ventilation ratio is 30:2 for one rescuer and 15:2 for two rescuers
Children 1–8 years (Universal compression to ventilation ratio is 30:2 with one rescuer and 15:2 with two rescuers)	• Determine unresponsiveness • Call for help	• Compress the chest at the level just above the posterior sternal margin • Compress the chest 2 in.	• Open airway and maintain using the jaw-thrust or manual maneuvers, attempt resuscitative breaths • Readjust airway if unsuccessful	• Perform bag-mask ventilations using 100% oxygen • Continue at a rate of at least 20 breaths per minute

TABLE 27.3 GUIDELINES FOR PEDIATRIC CARDIOPULMONARY RESUSCITATION—cont'd

Age Group	Assessment	Circulation	Airway	Breathing
Older Children and Adolescents 8 years–adult	• Determine unresponsiveness • Call for help	• Compress the chest at the level just above the posterior sternal margin • Compress the chest 2 in.	• Open airway and maintain using the jaw-thrust or manual maneuvers, attempt resuscitative breaths • Readjust airway if unsuccessful	• Perform bag-mask ventilations using 100% oxygen • Continue at a rate of at least 20 breaths per minute

Source: 2010 American Heart Association guidelines for CPR and ECC – Part 4: CPR overview, Table 1: Summary of key BLS components for adults, children & infants. 2010, p S677. Reprinted with permission. 2010 American Heart Association guidelines for CPR and ECC – Part 4: CPR overview, Circulation. 2010;122 [suppl 3]: S676-S684.

of thick mucus, inflammation, or a foreign body obstruction can produce symptoms of respiratory distress. Pediatric nurses must be prepared to support a young child's airway by rapid suction, airway support, oxygenation, and possible resuscitation.

Choking Emergency

In children aged younger than 1 year, aspiration, obstruction, and choking are the leading causes of death. A young child's narrow airway lumen contributes to significant choking episodes. The airway remains small for size until the child is 5 years old. Anticipatory guidance for new parents should include explaining that an older sibling should not be allowed to feed an infant without constant supervision and that the mobile infant's environment should be frequently surveyed for choking and aspiration risks. A tracheostomy may need to be inserted if the child has upper airway obstruction. See Figure 27.2 for a depiction of tracheostomy equipment. Knowing how to clear a child's airway is a very important skill for a pediatric nurse (Table 27.4).

For children of all ages, expect continued airway symptoms after removal of the obstruction because of residual edema, inflammation, and irritation.

Child in Shock

Shock is a serious consequence of an acutely ill or critically ill child. **Shock** is the clinical outcome of poor perfusion, severe hypovolemia, low systemic vascular resistance (ie, severe hypotension), or systemic venous congestion. Shock requires immediate identification and a combination of aggressive treatments or the condition is fatal. There are four types of shock: hypovolemic, cardiogenic, distributive, and obstructive. Children who are hospitalized for trauma, severe infections, severe dehydration, or with cardiac complications are at risk for the development of shock. The highest priority in the early treatment of shock is to restore oxygenation to the tissues and the brain. In general, this is done by providing an oxygen source, improving volume and distributing the volume, reducing the increased oxygen demand, and correcting metabolic instability. Any change in perfusion, blood pressure, or level of consciousness must be reported rapidly and action taken. See Box 27.1 for a list of types of shock found in children.

SAFETY *STAT!*

Three common symptoms of early shock are hypovolemia, hypotension, and a change in mental status.

General Management of Shock

Shock is a very serious medical diagnosis that is associated with poor clinical outcome and death. Shock can only be reversed when it is identified early and there is a team effort

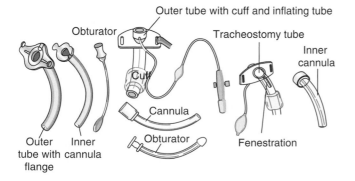

FIGURE 27.2 Tracheostomy equipment.

TABLE 27.4   GUIDELINES FOR AIRWAY CLEARANCE

Patient Population	Airway Clearance Guidelines
Newborn Airway Clearance (birth–1 month)	• Do not perform blind finger sweep; rapidly suction secretions or mucus • Place newborn on flat surface • Perform five chest thrusts with two fingers • Monitor respiratory status continuously after removal of object • Provide low-flow oxygen as required after event • Position newborn supine in sniffing position for maximal ventilation
Infant Airway Clearance (1 month–1 year)	• Do not perform blind finger sweep: remove foreign object via finger sweep only if visible • Place infant over leg, head down, and start in prone position, support the head and neck with one hand • Perform five back blows followed by five chest thrusts with the other hand • Monitor respiratory status continuously after removal of object • Provide low-flow oxygen as required after event • Position child side-lying and in sniffing position for maximal ventilation • Make sure child is seen by emergency personnel and transfer to appropriate level of care
Child Airway Clearance (1–8 years)	• Do not perform blind finger sweep; remove foreign object via finger sweep only if object is visible • If over 1 year of age, perform Heimlich's maneuver (ie, abdominal thrusts) • Continue until successful or child loses consciousness; then begin CPR • Monitor respiratory status continuously after removal of the object • Call for emergency backup and assessment; may require transport (ie, RRT or 911) • Position child for adequate ventilation • Provide low-dose oxygen as required after the event
Older Child/Adolescent Airway Clearance (8 years–adult)	• Do not perform blind finger sweep; remove foreign object via finger sweep only if object is visible • Perform Heimlich's maneuver (ie, abdominal thrusts) • Continue until successful or if patient loses consciousness, then begin CPR • Monitor respiratory status continuously after removal of object • Position child for adequate ventilation • Provide low-dose oxygen as required after event • Call for medical personnel to assess older child or adolescent after episode for possible transfer (ie, RRT or 911)

to stabilize the child's cardiopulmonary system. When there is evidence of the development of shock, call for help immediately! The following guidelines can help stabilize the child:

• Position the child in such a way as to increase cardiac output, such as supine Trendelenburg's position.
• Provide a rapid, high-flow source of oxygen and prepare for intubation and mechanical ventilation.

• Protect the child's vascular access because this is the lifeline to administer vasoactive medications; child might require a central line placement (Fig. 27.3 and 27.4).
• Secure either a rapid transfer to an intensive care environment or place the crash cart near the child.
• Make sure the team has an accurate height and weight of the child, or secure the use of a color-coded resuscitative tape, such as Broselow's system.

Box 27.1 Types of Shock Found in Children

Hypovolemic Shock

Hypovolemic shock occurs when a child presents in severe dehydration and then experiences severe vascular volume depletion. The child will require rapid administration of IVF with a reassessment of their fluid status via VSs after each fluid bolus to determine if more is required. Urine output is severely compromised during hypovolemic shock and IV potassium should not be administered until the child's urine output has been re-established.

Cardiogenic Shock

When the child demonstrates signs of pulmonary or systemic venous congestion such as increased work of breathing, distended neck veins, grunting, and signs of decreased perfusion, cardiogenic shock must be suspected. The focus of treatment is on the restoration of cardiac output. The child must be transferred to a critical care environment because mechanical ventilation is often required to support the child and vasoactive drugs may be needed to maintain adequate blood pressure and circulation.

Distributive Shock

Children who demonstrate a severe low blood pressure may be experiencing distributive shock. This condition is caused by a very low systemic vascular resistance, vasodilation, and the buildup of lactic acid. Monitor the child for change in level of consciousness. The most common causes of distributive shock are an overwhelming invasion of organism, leading to sepsis, or a complete loss of vascular tone from conditions such as spinal cord injury or anaphylaxis.

Obstructive Shock

Obstructive shock is identified via a diagnostic examination result demonstrating increased central venous pressure. The cardiac output is reduced and a decrease of blood flow from the heart is suspected. The goal of therapy is to initiate vasoactive drugs in an intensive care environment.

- Collect specimens for laboratory analysis.
- Provide a rapid source of vascular volume expansion through isotonic crystalloid IV fluids (ie, normal saline [NS]) via boluses that may be repeated several times.
- Administer required medications such as vasoactive drugs and antibiotics.
- Closely monitor the child for responses to the above interventions.

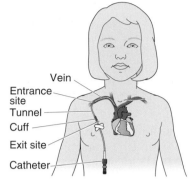

FIGURE 27.3 Tunneled catheter.

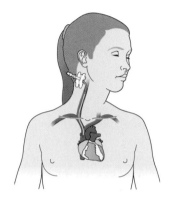

FIGURE 27.4 Jugular line.

LABS & DIAGNOSTICS

The pediatric health-care team may request specific laboratory analysis of a child's blood if the child is demonstrating signs and symptoms of shock. These analyses include venous blood gases, arterial blood gases (ABG), blood cultures, lactate, calcium, complete blood cell count (CBC), and glucose.

DRUG FACTS

For a child in shock, the most important medications to anticipate for administration are:
- Antibiotics STAT!
- Vasopressors (ie, vasoactive drugs that support blood pressure) such as dopamine, norepinephrine, or epinephrine
- Glucose for severe hyperglycemia
- Hydrocortisone

Cardiovascular Conditions

Pediatric patients with no previous cardiac pathology history are considered to be quite stable in the cardiovascular system. It is rare that a previously healthy child experiences a significant cardiac event that requires emergency response. Young infants, on the other hand, can experience circumstances where the airway, ventilation, and gas exchange are affected and they demonstrate serious symptoms requiring emergency care. An episode of acute cyanosis, tet spells, or acute life-threatening events are three examples of clinical situations where children need rapid emergency care provided by inter-disciplinary teams.

Cyanotic Infant

Cyanosis is defined as an episode in which a patient becomes suddenly purplish or blue in the skin and mucous membranes. The discoloration is related to a sudden decrease in oxygenation. The child may present with a central cyanosis or peripheral cyanosis. If the child has accompanying respiratory distress, then the health-care team should consider a respiratory etiology to the cyanosis. If the patient is tachycardic but otherwise quiet and without respiratory involvement, the team should consider a cardiovascular etiology.

- *Central Cyanosis:* Discoloration of trunk caused by reduced hemoglobin; associated with reduced oxygen saturation measurements
- *Peripheral Cyanosis:* Decreased cardiac output with an accompanying decrease in the peripheral blood flow; peripheral cyanosis (in the extremities) may not demonstrate a reduced oxygen saturation measurement

Assessments for cyanosis include signs and symptoms, allergies, medication reactions, past medical history, last oral intake, symptoms of illness, and fevers.

SAFETY *STAT!*

If a nurse encounters an infant with cyanosis, interventions required include:

- Assessing for breathing and circulation
- Opening the airway and assessing for the need for CPR
- Stimulating the child
- Giving 100% oxygen via mask
- Suctioning airway as needed to remove an obstruction
- Monitoring the child: placing on oxygen saturation and cardiac monitor
- Obtaining ABG

Tet Spells

A congenital (ie, existing since birth) heart condition called tetralogy of Fallot is an emergency cardiac anomaly that warrants open heart surgery for a repair of four conditions: overriding aorta, hypertrophy of the right ventricle, ventricular septal defect, and pulmonary stenosis. This severe condition causes acute and sudden central cyanotic spells referred to as *tet spells*. This is an emergency and requires the immediate application of oxygen. An RRT should be called to assist with this life-threatening emergency. See Chapter 33, Child With a Cardiac Condition, for a complete presentation of congenital heart defects and associated conditions.

Apparent Life-Threatening Event (ALTE)

An **apparent life-threatening event (ALTE),** also called an *acute life-threatening event,* is not a formal medical diagnosis, but a sudden, acute, and unexpected change in a young's infant's breathing pattern, which leads to a color change, apnea, limpness, and often choking or gagging. Often frightening to a caregiver who witnesses the ALTE, the child appears in acute distress and it may appear as if the infant has died. The episode requires immediate interventions from advanced pediatric health-care providers and the child should be hospitalized and monitored carefully during the diagnostic period. The child may require stimulation to bring him or her out of the episode, or may require resuscitation efforts.

SAFETY *STAT!*

Rapid assessments and interventions for a witnessed ALTE include positioning the airway open, simulating the child, assessing for obstructions, assessing for bradycardia or other abnormal heart rhythms, assessing for an airway obstruction, administering 100% oxygen, suctioning the airway if mucus is obstructing, and beginning CPR (ie, compressions, airway support, and breathing) as needed.

ALTE is not associated with sudden infant death syndrome (SIDS), but infants who demonstrate repeated episodes of ALTE should be monitored for an increased risk of SIDS. The incidence rate of ALTE is thought to be 0.05% to 1%. Prior episodes of ALTE occur in 5% of SIDS cases. SIDS is fatal, whereas ALTE is considered benign to near-fatal. Risk factors associated with SIDS are maternal smoking, a prone sleeping position, and a lack of breastfeeding. Risk factors associated with ALTE are different and include a history of cyanosis, difficulties with feeding, and episodes of repeated apnea.

Typically the child's health-care provider will bring the infant into the emergency department, describing the incident of ALTE as the "chief complaint." A thorough investigation into the cause of the ALTE needs to be conducted to rule out sepsis, gastroesophageal reflux, central nervous system (CNS) disorders, airway obstruction, metabolic disorders, or poisoning. ALTE is often associated with obstructive apnea.

The following should be conducted for all infants who demonstrate ALTE:

- Thorough medical history and detailed description of the event
- History of pregnancy, birth, and perinatal period
- Chance of ingestion of a substance, fall, and intentional or unintentional injury
- Physical examination of height, weight, VSs, signs of trauma, developmental assessment, and airway
- Unless the ALTE was determined to be a laryngospasm after gastroesophageal reflux, then further diagnostics should be performed, including:
  - Blood counts, cultures, and chemistries
  - Urinalysis
  - Metabolic screening

- Reflux screening
- Brain neuroimaging
- Skeletal survey
- Echocardiogram
- Chest x-ray

Management of an infant who presents with ALTE should include hospitalization with monitoring. Any serious underlying medical conditions must be ruled out, especially those concerning the child's airway. The family should be taught CPR before hospital discharge. Home-monitoring equipment may be ordered but often is used on a case-by-case basis.

Child in Acute Respiratory Distress

Children in acute respiratory distress need immediate attention and intervention. Young children are dependent on abdominal and diaphragmatic breathing and require rapid interventions to maintain an effective airway, air exchange, and breathing pattern. Early signs of respiratory distress include the following:

- Nasal flaring (Fig. 27.5)
- Head bobbing
- Anxiety
- Lethargy
- Decreased rate of responsiveness
- Retractions (ie, subcostal, intercostals, suprasternal, and sternum)
- Wheezing and stridor
- Use of accessory muscles
- Increased use of energy and effort needed to breathe

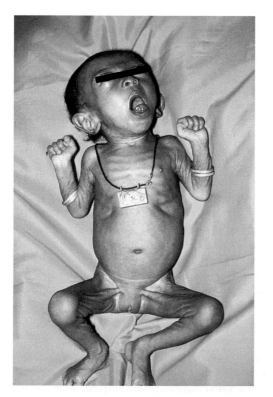

FIGURE 27.5 Infant demonstrating flaring of nares during respiratory distress.

- Feeding problems and refusal to eat (ie, fatigue and decreased ability to suck/swallow)
- Tachypnea and/or hyperpnea
- Hypoxia and hypercarbia

Late signs of respiratory distress include:

- Poor perfusion
- Bradycardia
- Decreased air movement and diminished breath sounds
- Expiratory grunting
- Apnea (ie, cessation in spontaneous breathing for greater than 20 sec)

Airway issues are the number one cause of emergency responses in children. Airway obstructions, inflammation, or occlusion will lead the child to have respiratory distress and need ventilator support. Pediatric nurses must think about airway issues first when a child demonstrates a change in clinical status. Common causes of decreased ventilation and respiratory distress can be found in Table 27.5.

SAFETY *STAT!*

Epiglottitis is a life-threatening infectious process that has the potential to cause complete obstruction in a child's airway. Patients who present with epiglottitis may need to have a tracheostomy if STAT antibiotics are not effective in reducing the infection and inflammation. The child may need rapid surgery if he or she does not respond to emergency interventions and antibiotics.

SAFETY *STAT!*

When a child is diagnosed with a severe respiratory illness and is experiencing respiratory distress, the team should place the child's condition on "guarded" or "critical" status. This designation will provide extra monitoring by health-care team members so a change in clinical status can be identified and rapid airway support provided.

TABLE 27.5 COMMON CAUSES OF DECREASED VENTILATION AND RESPIRATORY DISTRESS

Lower Airway	Upper Airway
- Respiratory syncytial virus (RSV) bronchiolitis - Asthma - Pneumonia - Foreign body in airway - Bronchospasm - Copious mucus	- Tracheal stenosis - Foreign body in airway - Croup - Epiglottitis - Tongue swelling (ie, allergic responses)

A smooth response to an acutely ill child needing emergency help is the responsibility of a team. Designated healthcare personnel must be available 24 hours a day to respond to emergencies. A team approach is needed to provide rapid comprehensive care to a child in a critical state. The following outlines the overall response needed for an acutely ill child needing critical care support:

- Ensure Compressions, Airway, and Breathing (CAB) through high-quality and effective CPR.
- Call for backup help immediately; do not hesitate to get help, and do not take a "wait and see" attitude!
- Do not leave the hospitalized acutely ill child alone or unsupervised under any circumstances if there is a decline in the child's condition.
- Bring the crash cart to the child's room and position it close to the child; it is much better to have it and not need it than to delay a resuscitative effort to retrieve it.
- Monitor the pulse oximetry continuously if you suspect a change in condition.
- Provide supplemental oxygen therapy.
- Position the child for maximal air exchange, such as the sniffing position.
- Monitor the child's blood pressure because hypotension is often a late sign of an eminent emergency.
- Apply a cardiorespiratory monitor; place on lead II for ease of interpretation. Place lead using "white on right, smoke above fire," meaning to place the white lead on the second intercostal space, midclavicular line; the black lead on the left second intercostal space, midclavicular line; and the red (sometimes green) lead on the left fifth intercostal space, midclavicular line.
- Establish an effective and patent IV access.
- Be prepared to rapidly draw pertinent laboratory tests (eg, chemistry, hemogram, ABG).
- Communicate child's history/present clinical status/ medical diagnosis to responding interdisciplinary RRT or code blue team.
- Provide support to the family.
- Call the nursing supervisor for leadership and coordination of all unit activities during the emergency.

Children who have severe allergies may need to have an EpiPen (epinephrine injector) prescribed. An allergen that causes severe respiratory distress may need to be treated with epinephrine in an outpatient setting and then the child may be transferred to an acute setting for further evaluation and treatment. Parents must know how to identify when the EpiPen is needed, how to check for the expiration date, how to administer the medication, and how to call for help after administration. Further guidelines include:

- The pen should remain in the original manufacturer's packaging so that the administration instructions can be referred to quickly.
- At least two pens should be maintained so that there is one at home and one stored per protocol at the child's school.

- The pen's expiration date should be checked on a regular basis and the pen replaced before it expires.
- The parents and any other caregivers for the child should periodically practice administering the medication to maintain competence and confidence.

HIGHER LEVEL OF EQUIPMENT PROVIDED IN HOSPITAL ENVIRONMENTS

Children who experience a significant change in clinical status that warrants a move to a higher level of care will also need specialized emergency equipment. Becoming familiar with emergency equipment can save lives. Even if the pediatric nurse is not directly responsible for using the equipment, a basic level of understanding should be secured. Having knowledge on where the equipment is stored, what it is used for, how to determine what equipment will be used when, and how to determine the right size of equipment for a child's particular height and weight can be extremely helpful for the response team.

Various clinical settings will have emergency equipment available. At the very least, a crash cart and a defibrillator should be made available. The following section outlines the purpose and content of several pieces of emergency equipment.

Crash Carts

Emergency response carts (ie, crash carts) are available throughout the acute care hospital environment. It is imperative that the pediatric nurse knows where to locate these carts and be familiar with how the equipment is organized. Some crash carts are organized by the child's weight in kilograms; others are organized in systems such as airway support/ intubation drawer, medication drawer, or IV access and fluids drawer. In general, the following list represents what a pediatric nurse can expect to find:

- Emergency response drugs for various emergency conditions and situations
- Oxygen equipment, including a variety of masks and various sizes of manual resuscitator bags and masks
- Airway supplies, including a variety of sizes of equipment for intubation
- IV therapy/fluids such as NS, lactated Ringer's (LR) solution, and IV start supplies; both peripheral IV catheters and interosseous needles must be present in the cart (Fig. 27.6)
- Laboratory specimen collection equipment and containers such as ABG, hemogram, electrolytes, and chemistry
- Back board to rapidly provide a hard surface for efficient chest compressions
- Broselow's tape in case the child's weight is unknown
- Suction equipment for rapid airway clearance
- Cardiac monitoring equipment and cardioversion equipment (Fig. 27.7)
- Oxygen tanks

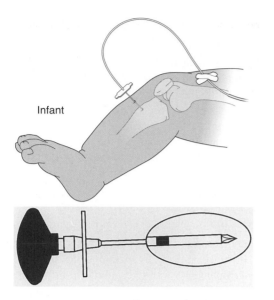

Infant

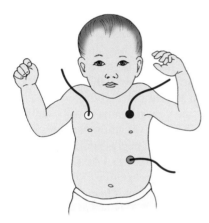

FIGURE 27.6 Intraosseous needle inserted in bone.

FIGURE 27.7 Child with a cardiac monitor on.

DRUG FACTS

An interosseous needle is used if traditional peripheral or central IV access is not possible or is unsuccessful during the care of a critically ill child. The needle is placed into the marrow of one of the child's long bones, such as the anterior superior area of the tibia. This use of the interosseous needle and the site of the flat area of a long bone has been found to be as effective a system of medication administration and distribution as IV injections.

Crash carts must be checked every 24 hours. One person, such as the charge nurse, will be responsible to check on the function and status of crash cart contents. Checking for expiration dates of the emergency medications is a very important aspect of maintaining emergency response equipment. All crash cart checks must be documented for state or regional inspectors.

Color-Coded, Length-Based Resuscitation Tape

Color-coded, length-based resuscitation tape, for example Broselow's pediatric emergency tape (Broselow-Luten system), is a tool used to determine the correct equipment and dosage of medication needed for children of various sizes during an emergency response (Fig. 27.8). The tape is recommended for use on any child under the age of 12 years. Because pediatric medications are most often calculated by milligrams per kilogram, rapid decision making can be made more easily and correctly if the child's exact weight is known. Under emergency situations in which the child cannot be weighed, the color-coded resuscitation tape is used to determine the best estimate of the child's weight based on the child's length. The tape is retrieved rapidly from the crash cart and placed next to the critically ill pediatric or trauma patient. Where the child's heel falls on the tape determines the color-coded "zone" where medication doses and equipment size are presented. Each zone has a color code. The team reads the information given on the zone and then the prepared medications, IV fluid boluses, and emergency equipment (eg, endotracheal tubes, suction catheters, and urinary catheters) are selected based on the child's respective zone. The response team does not need to rely on memory to determine the appropriate size of equipment or medication dosing during an emergency. Research has shown that pediatric health-care teams who estimate the child's weight without the use of the **Broselow's tape** are as much as 15% off (Frush, 2011).

For the color-coded length-based pediatric emergency tape to be effective, it must be used correctly. The child is placed supine on a flat surface with the color-coded side of the tape visible. The team places the red end of the tape even with the top surface of the child's head and smoothes the tape out along the child's side. The zone appropriate for the child is determined by where the child's heels fall, not the child's toes. Think "Red to Head."

SAFETY *STAT!*

The child should never be measured for the color-coded length-based emergency resuscitation tape while sitting up or having the head of the bed up. Pull the foot up in a 90-degree flexed position before measuring "Red to Head."

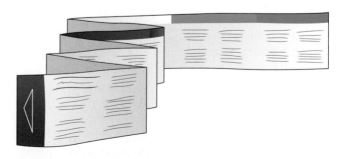
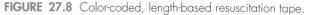

FIGURE 27.8 Color-coded, length-based resuscitation tape.

Other than using a color-coded, length-based, pediatric emergency resuscitation tape, the acute care facility may also have crash carts that are organized according to the color-coded system. Here, instead of organizing the crash cart by body system, the color-coded crash cart will have all of the equipment needed for the child in each color zone. For instance, the orange zone cart is for children whose measured height will average a weight that falls between 24 and 28 kg.

Rapid Fluid Resuscitation

Children whose condition rapidly deteriorates often require resuscitative vascular volume expansion. This is done by the rapid instillation of IV fluids (IVF). A common order is to provide NS (0.9%) IVF boluses at 20 mL per kg. The rate at which the boluses are delivered is up to the emergency response medical team. A common order would be to administer between 1 and 3 boluses, the first over 20 min with VSs rechecked after, and then subsequent IVF boluses over 30 to 60 min each. Follow orders carefully for safe clinical practice.

DRUG FACTS

A child requires a rapid bolus to correct dehydration. The child presented with a viral illness that caused a significant sore throat. His symptoms lead him to have poor oral fluid intake over several days. He has presented to the clinic with a weight of 18 kg and requires rapid volume expansion for hypotension with 0.9% NS (ie, an isotonic crystalloid fluid). To calculate his IV fluid bolus, the nurse would:

- Multiply his weight of 18 kg by 20 mL (IV boluses are 20 mL per kg per bolus)
- The total would be 360 mL of fluid
- The fluid IV bolus is 0.9% NS
- The rate of infusion is standard; infuse each bolus ordered over 1 hour unless otherwise directed

The nurse will then take a set of VSs to see if the child's clinical status has improved.

SERVICES PROVIDED TO FAMILIES IN HOSPITAL ENVIRONMENTS

Families who must hospitalize a child will need education, comfort, and support. When a child experiences a condition that warrants hospitalization, the pediatric nurse provides specific services to make sure that the child is cared for. If the child's condition worsens, then the nurse makes sure services are provided that protect the child from serious harm.

Pediatric nurses must be able to identify when a child's condition is deteriorating. Then, the pediatric nurse coordinates calling for rapid assistance from a multidisciplinary team. In providing assistance during emergencies, the nurse works within a pediatric health-care team to assist a child whose conditions require rapid, safe, and supportive emergency care.

Providing Assistance During Emergencies

Pediatric nurses can assume various roles during an emergency response in an acute care environment. Roles include airway management, compressions, taking serial VS measurements, running laboratory specimens, passing equipment from the crash cart to the response team, and providing emotional support to the family. Various hospitals have protocols to determine the role of the response team. Follow institutional policy and offer assistance within your scope of practice.

Caring for Families Present During Emergencies

It has been determined that families who witness at least part of an emergency resuscitative response to a critically ill or trauma victim have a shorter period of grief if the child dies. Determining if the family should be present during a code is a multifactorial decision based on hospital practice or hospital policy.

Follow these principles in providing care to families:

- Check the institutional policy for guidelines on family presence during resuscitation efforts.
- Understand that research has shown that most families would like to be present for at least part of the attempted resuscitative process (Boyd, 2000; Dolye, Post, et al, 1987; Hanson and Strawser, 1992).
- Families may be very reluctant to ask to remain present, so offer the opportunity. Family members may experience less anxiety, grief, and depression and have healthier grieving behaviors if they had the opportunity to be present during the resuscitative effort.
- If able, discuss the option of being present for resuscitation efforts before the child experiences a code blue.
- Notify the nursing supervisor of the family's wishes and provide physical room for them to be present.
- Assess the family's reaction and be sensitive to their need to leave during the resuscitation process.
- Provide emotional support after the resuscitation event and answer any questions the family may have.
- Make sure a referral is made to the social worker for the immediate assistance of professional support and clergy follow-up.

CULTURAL CONSIDERATIONS

Identifying the Decision Maker Within the Family Constellation

When an acutely ill child experiences a change in clinical status, a transfer to a higher level of care, such as an intensive care unit (ICU), may be warranted. During this stressful time, it is very likely that decisions will have to be made. For instance, if a child with a severe chronic neurological condition is hospitalized for an acute exacerbation of his or her condition and experiences a sudden decline, the health-care team will want to discuss treatment options with the family and secure consent. The team will need to identify who the legal decision maker is for the child, and who the primary decision maker is in the family. These may be two different family members, or they may be the same person.

Because of cultural and ethnic diversity, the primary decision maker for health-care treatment plans may not be the child's legal guardian. Although the legal parents or guardians will sign the treatment forms and consents, it is possible that the cultural makeup of the larger family constellation includes an elder who ultimately makes decisions for the family. Some families may have patriarchal decision-making lines; others may have matriarchal. Including the decision maker in the family conference is an important gesture of respect for the cultural or ethnic makeup of the family. Empowering the family to be included in treatment discussions ultimately creates more trusting and respectful collaborative interactions. Members of the health-care team must respect the family decision line while securing written consent from the legal guardian of the child.

According to Citko and Bourne (2002), questions should be posed:

1. Does the surrogate health-care decision maker have a close, caring relationship with the patient?
2. Is this person aware of the family's and the patient's (ie, child's) values and beliefs?
3. Is this person willing and able to make the needed medical treatment decisions?
4. Is there a consensus among the individuals as to the proper decision or decision maker?

The health-care team should document how medical decisions were made if someone other than the primary legal guardian or parent is involved with the child's health-care treatment decisions. Because children under 18 years of age do not have a Power of Attorney for Health Care or a Durable Power of Attorney for Heath Care, or an Advanced Directive of any sort, it is imperative that the health-care team support the family during difficult decision making and document the entire process that has occurred.

RAPID RESPONSE TEAMS

In acute-care settings there are situations where a child's condition worsens rapidly and the health-care team on the pediatric unit needs to have assistance immediately. RRTs were developed to offer family and staff an option to request and receive support from health-care professionals above and beyond those present on the floor. With the chaotic and hectic hospital environment, nurses need to have support in responding to emergencies when the child has not fully "coded," that is, has not experienced a full cardiopulmonary arrest. The activation of an RRT can be done by anyone who sees a child's condition change in such a level of severity that assistance is required right away, but the child is still breathing. Most institutions post the number to call for an RRT at each child's bedside.

TEAM WORKS

Essential members of a code blue team or RRT include the following:

- Pediatric hospitalist in house; he or she will be the leader of the code response
- RN assigned to the patient's care; he or she will have the most updated information about the child, including the admitting diagnosis, current medications, most current weight, and clinical picture of the child
- PALS-certified nurse to provide support during the resuscitative efforts
- Critical care nurse with expert knowledge on the calculating, drawing up, and administration of antiarrhythmic medications
- Respiratory therapist who will take leadership in the management of the child's airway
- Pharmacist who can assist with the management and replenishing of the emergency medications
- Member of central supply who can provide backup supplies for the crash cart
- Runner (ie, laboratory personnel member) for the specimens to be taken to the laboratory or to run the bedside laboratory evaluation equipment
- Nursing supervisor who can provide staffing support and support for the family

Historical Perspectives

In 1986, the First National Project on Quality Improvement in Health Care set out to explore how certain quality improvement methods within the health-care industry would affect clinical outcomes. Since then, in 2004, the nonprofit organization called the Institute for Healthcare Improvement started the "100,000 Lives Campaign" to implement certain quality initiatives and to save 100,000 lives. By 2008, the campaign increased the goal to 5 million lives. One key part of these lifesaving projects was to develop a plan to establish and evaluate the effectiveness of RRTs. The aim of the project was to identify patients across the lifespan before their conditions worsened and an intensive care transfer was needed.

Definitions

An RRT is a group of designated hospital personnel that carries an electronic device that alerts them to the need to respond quickly to a patient location. The following are essential components to the development of the team:

1. Establishment of an RRT membership and rotation schedule
2. Establishment of an RRT "criteria for activation" (ie, circumstances in which a parent or nurse or other team member would activate the team). This can be a list of diagnoses, clinical situations, or circumstances that lead to the need for a rapid response of a highly professional team.
3. Establishment of a range of RRT interventions

4. RRT education checklist
5. RRT event record

According to the American Association for Respiratory Care (www.AARC.org), an RRT will quickly respond to failing patients, in and out of the PICU and ICU, before their condition worsens, all which helps to ensure optimal clinical outcomes. RRTs have been reported to significantly lower mortality (ie, death) and cardiopulmonary arrests outside of ICUs (Sharek, et al, 2007).

Clinical situations in which an RRT should be called include the following:

- Airway compromise
- Grand mal seizures
- Change in neurological status/level of consciousness
- Dehiscence of a wound (ie, the separation of edges with or without the protrusion of intestines, called *evisceration*)
- Significant fall, resulting in an actual or potential injury
- Any unexpected or rapid change in clinical status in which the nurse or family becomes concerned for the child's welfare
- Head injuries
- Hemorrhage

How to Call a Rapid Response Team

Every hospital or health-care institution may have a slightly different procedure to call for the assembly of an RRT. The phone number to call should be posted in each child's room with an explanation of the purpose of the team. It should also be posted at the nursing station, the treatment room, the elevators, and the playroom. Typically, a placed call is transferred to an operator who then places the emergency notification out to the various team members. Many institutions promote the calling of an RRT by family members who are present during a change in the clinical status of their child. Research has shown that this system is not abused by families and that the RRT is used appropriately.

SAFETY *STAT!*

Calling for the Rapid Response Team

Many pediatric units and hospitals are now providing the family with a means to call the RRT without waiting to notify the nurse of the child's changing condition. Research has shown that this has not increased unwarranted calls and is considered an effective means to help save lives by early initiation of emergency response teams. Guidelines should include:

- Providing the family with education and reminders that they may call the RRT for rapid assistance for their child
- Teaching the family symptoms and/or clinical signs to be aware of that would warrant calling the RRT
- Providing the number to call RRT in large dark print located near the child's hospital room phone
- Letting the family know that if they are uncomfortable calling the RRT, they may call for help from the nursing station and help will be rapidly summoned

HELPFUL EMERGENCY RESPONSE MNEMONICS

Mnemonics (ie, memory devices) are tools to help rapidly remember and organize thinking about the steps to an assessment, response, or skill. The most commonly associated medical mnemonic is the steps of basic CPR: CAB (compressions–airway–breathing). Many mnemonics exist to support health-care professionals, but it is important to identify those that have been validated and supported by professional nursing and medical associations such as the American Heart Association, the Emergency Nursing Association, or nurse educators who have done research on the validity of the mnemonic. Many mnemonics exist to support acute care pediatric nurses who need to perform rapid assessments or interventions for children whose conditions are clinically unstable. Table 27.6 provides a list of example mnemonics considered useful.

SAFETY *STAT!*

The three medications the pediatric health-care team may require when a child is demonstrating acute respiratory distress (such as allergic responses to immunizations or antibiotics) are:

- Epinephrine 1:1,000
- Antihistamine, such as Benadryl
- Anti-inflammatory, such as Solu-Medrol

ASSESSING AN ACUTELY ILL CHILD

One method of assessing the stability of an acutely ill child is by using a systems approach. Table 27.7 provides comprehensive assessment information to determine the need to call for assistance from the pediatric hospitalist, RRT, or code blue team for the child. Any abnormal finding must be reported, acted on, and documented carefully.

DELEGATION AND REQUEST FOR A HIGHER LEVEL OF CARE

Pediatric nurses must always practice within their scope of practice. A licensed practical nurse (LPN), also called an LVN, must use the chain of command to immediately report any change in a patient's clinical status to the next appropriate person. If an RN is present and is a part of the health-care team, such as in a hospital or an acute/critical care environment, then the LPN/LVN would immediately solicit the involvement of the RN. If the setting does not include an RN, such as in some long-term care environments, then the LPN/LVN must follow the institutional policy on rapidly reporting a clinical concern. In some environments, such as a blood bank, the LPN/LVN may be required to call 911 for immediate assistance. It is imperative that the nurse know his or her scope of practice and reporting chain of command (Box 27.2).

When a hospitalized child experiences a change in clinical status that warrants a higher level of care, quick and efficient

TABLE 27.6   MEDICAL AND NURSING MNEMONICS FOR CARE OF THE ACUTELY ILL CHILD

Mnemonic	Definition
CAB	*The beginning steps of CPR* C = **C**ompressions A = **A**irway B = Resuscitative **B**reathing (bag-valve-mask of appropriate size)
ABC COPIME	*Means to organize a basic code blue response (Linnard-Palmer, 2012)* A = **A**irway assessment, open B = **B**reathing C = **C**ompressions after an assessment of presence of heart rate C = Grab the **C**rash **C**art, open drawers, and attach the equipment to the child. Place on three lead electrocardiogram (EKG) for monitoring or attach cardioversion pad (age appropriate), attach blood pressure cuff, and prepare suction device and tubing O = Place the child on an appropriate **O**xygen delivery device and flow rate for condition; if artificial breathing is required, attach high flow source of oxygen to the manual resuscitator rescue bag P = **P**lace the child on a back board, typically located on the back of the crash cart, to provide support for compressions I = Start **I**V access, rapidly draw laboratory tests, and have runner take to laboratory; begin fluid resuscitation with NS boluses (ie, 20 mL/kg rapid infusion) M = **M**ove all equipment, other patients, and any physical obstructions to make room for the resuscitative team E = **E**xplain to the members of the response team the medical history of the child, what happened, how long the child was requiring resuscitation, and what has been done

Source for CAB: 2010 American Heart Association Guidelines for CPR and ECC – Part 4: CPR overview, Circulation. 2010;122[suppl 3]:S676-S684.

TABLE 27.7   RAPID ASSESSMENT OF BODY SYSTEMS

Body System	Signs
General Appearance	• Work of breathing • Overall skin color • Level of consciousness • Poor feeding behaviors • Inconsolable crying in nonverbal children
Skin	• Presence of a rash • Mottling of skin • Cyanosis: central, peripheral, and/or circumoral • Presence of petechiae • Purpura spots on skin • Poor perfusion; delayed capillary refill time
Head, Ears, Eyes, Nose, and Throat (HEENT)	• Sunken eyes • Signs of traumatic head injury • Retinal hemorrhages • Epistaxis • Inability to swallow, drooling, dyspnea (epiglottitis?)
Cardiovascular (CV) System	• Presence of abnormal heart sounds; murmurs • Tachycardia • Apnea (ie, periods of no breathing lasting 20 sec or longer) • Hypotension (often a late sign)

Continued

TABLE **27.7 RAPID ASSESSMENT OF BODY SYSTEMS—cont'd**

Body System	Signs
Respiratory System: Adventitious Breath Sounds	• Hypoventilation • Wheezing • Rales • Retractions: subclavicular, substernal, intracostal, and/or subcostal • Paradoxical breathing/see-saw breathing • CNS disease or injury demonstrating respiratory distress without adventitious breath sounds, or pulmonary disease or pathology
Gastrointestinal System	• Abdominal pain • Vomiting • Projectile vomiting • Diarrhea • Abdominal masses • Signs of obstruction or peritonitis
CNS	• Irritability • Lethargy • Altered level of consciousness, especially a reduction in alertness • Seizures • Paralysis • Weakness • Coma

Box 27.2 Case Study: Reporting Chain of Command

A 4-year-old male child was admitted to the pediatric unit of a small community hospital after being stabilized for a fracture of his left femur within the emergency department (ED). A cast was placed on the child's left lower extremity and extended from the child's hips to the ankle (ie, spica cast). The child was transferred from the ED to the nursing unit on a gurney and placed into a double room bed. VSs were within an expected range and the child's pain score using the FLACC pain assessment tool and the Wong-Baker pain assessment tool both demonstrated a value of 1/10. The LVN performed VSs and an assessment of the child's foot and toes below the site of the fracture. Using a CCSMT (ie, color, circulation, sensation, movement, and touch) tool, the nurse found the neurovascular status of the child's affected foot was within normal limits (WNL). The child was comforted and given colorful developmentally appropriate books for distraction.

Two hours after being admitted to the unit, the child's father pressed the call button at the child's beside and requested an urgent response. The LVN found the child to be writhing in bed, diaphoretic, and demonstrating a pain assessment finding of 6 to 7/10. The child's left foot was pale, cool to the touch, and slightly swollen to the point that assessing the peripheral pulse was difficult. The pulse was weak. The LPN/LVN nurse immediately notified the RN who was in charge of the pediatric unit. He came in and assessed the child's CCSMT, confirming that there was a critical change in neurovascular status from expected findings. The RN called the ED physician who placed the cast on the child's left femur and after using the SBAR communication tool, was told to quickly call the orthopedic technician on call to come to the floor STAT to window the cast and provide relief from pressure. The ED doctor also told the RN to call the pediatric hospitalist in-house and have her come and assess the child's condition immediately. The health-care team was in action within 5 min and the child required the cast to be removed to restore adequate circulation and have full visual assessment of the site. The child was taken back to the ED and a new cast was placed. All members of the team debriefed quickly and found the chain of command effective. The RN expressed appreciation to the LPN/LVN for the rapid notification of the child's condition and made it clear that the processes and teamwork were effective.

processes must take place to move the child and his or her belongings. The pediatric nurse is responsible for assisting the health-care team to move a child from the acute care pediatric unit to the PICU. Communicating with the family is imperative so that their stress and fears about the move are reduced.

For instance, an asthmatic child who is experiencing greater wheezing, reduced ventilation, and a reduced level of consciousness will need to be transferred STAT to an intensive care environment to receive constant monitoring and more involved respiratory support.

THERAPEUTIC COMMUNICATION

The family needs to receive an explanation about the situation and the rapid move that will help them understand that the move is for safety, monitoring, and interventions that will allow the child's airway to be supported. The family needs to be talked to in a calm matter-of-fact manner with direct eye contact. One person should be assigned to support the family and calmly describe the steps of the move.

Transferring to a Higher Level of Care

The child should not be left alone during the preparation for the transfer. Ideally, one staff member should be assigned to the child until the transfer is complete, especially if CPR or other emergency support will be required. The move consists of the following steps:

1. The pediatric nurse should prepare all of the child's medical records, nursing chart, medication administration records, and identification card. (If all materials are electronic, make sure the process of transferring access to the PICU is complete.)
2. The nurse should call the receiving unit and give an oral report directly to the nurse who will be taking charge of the child. The following information should be included in the call for an effective hand-off:
   - Child's full name, date of birth, weight and height, date of admission, and admitting medical diagnosis
   - Short history of the hospital stay up to this time, including the severity of the child's condition and/or symptoms from admission to the present
   - Reason for the transfer, including any medical interventions that were attempted to stabilize the child's condition
   - Any pertinent results of laboratory, diagnostic, or radiological studies (ie, ABG, chemistry panels, and hematological panels such as a CBC)
   - Emotional condition of the family, which family members are present, and the depth of their knowledge about the need for immediate transfer

---

NURSING CARE PLAN for the Family of a Hospitalized, Acutely Ill Child

The family of a hospitalized, acutely ill child will need nursing care that supports the family's understanding of the events taking place. Teaching the family about the child's medical diagnosis, diagnostic examinations, medications, and expected length of stay are all critical components of providing supportive care.

Potential Nursing Diagnoses:
- Anxiety related to child's acute health state
- Fear related to unknown medical diagnoses
- Knowledge deficit related to medical treatments
- Family coping compromised because of acute events
- Caregiver role strain related to hospitalization and need to care for other family members
- Communication impaired because of language differences
- Fatigue related to disrupted sleep and inability to rest while child is hospitalized

Expected Outcomes:
- Family members will demonstrate less anxiety and more coping behaviors while the child is hospitalized by showing self-care practices such as adequate sleep, adequate nutrition, and participation in stress-reducing behaviors such as reading and watching movies and/or resting with the child during the hospitalization.
- Family members will demonstrate less fear by asking clarifying questions concerning the child's acute condition and receiving clear answers concerning the child's medical diagnosis throughout the child's hospitalization.
- Parents will demonstrate an understanding of the child's medical condition by being able to ask pertinent questions and describe basic information concerning the medical diagnosis, including diagnostics and treatment plan during the hospitalization.
- Family members directly involved with the child's care will demonstrate decreasing caregiver burden by sharing responsibilities for home chores and other child care duties, by providing respite (ie, time away for self-care) for the parents, and by providing support to one another during the hospitalization.

Key Points

- The pediatric nurse caring for an acutely ill child in a hospital needs to be able to determine a change in clinical status and quickly call for appropriate help.
- Having size-appropriate emergency equipment available in each child's room will provide safe care if a child's condition changes. Suction, oxygen, resuscitation masks of various sizes, and a working code blue button should be in every hospital room. A nurse should check for the presence, function, and size of equipment at the beginning of each shift.
- Using a body systems approach, the nurse identifies conditions that may warrant reporting to the next higher level of the care practitioner and possible transfer to an intensive care environment.
- Using tools such as SBAR for effective communication and mnemonics for rapid recall of emergency response steps allows a pediatric nurse to make significant contributions to the acutely ill child's clinical outcomes.
- Supporting the efforts of an RRT contributes to a child's clinical stabilization. Parents need to learn how to call for the RRT and should be encouraged to use this

system if their child's condition changes and they become concerned.
- The nurse must make sure to be familiar with the location and use of the pediatric color-coded, length-based resuscitation tape that provides information based on the estimated weight regarding equipment, fluids, and medications to be used during emergencies.
- Basic bedside emergency equipment should include suction, oxygen, a manual resuscitator bag, mask and valve, code button, telephone to call the RRT, and instructions for calling various codes for help (eg, code pink, code gray, code yellow).
- The nurse must be aware that certain conditions, such as severe reactive airway disease and epiglottitis, pose dangerous risks for a child's ability to ventilate. Therefore the child's condition must be considered "guarded," prompting extra attention, monitoring, clinical care, and concern.
- Shock is a serious condition for children that requires immediate identification, interventions, and transfer to an intensive care environment. Vasopressins, antibiotics, fluid boluses, and constant monitoring are required.

REVIEW QUESTIONS

1. SBAR is a system that a nurse can follow to prepare for and implement an effective phone call to a primary care provider. The components of SBAR include all of the following *except:*
   1. Situation of the child and the background of the concern
   2. Assessment of the child's current status
   3. Parents' presence in the child's room
   4. Recommendation of the pediatric nurse

2. Which of the following is considered incorrect when performing chest compressions on children?
   1. For an infant, the chest must be compressed ½ to 1 in. with a compression rate of at least 120 bpm
   2. For a neonate, the chest must be compressed ½ in. with a compression rate of at least 100 bpm
   3. For a toddler, the chest must be compressed ½ to 1 in. with a compression rate of at least 100 bpm
   4. For a 10-year-old child, the chest must be compressed 1 in. with a compression rate of at least 100 bpm

3. The following items are essential equipment that should be present at every hospitalized child's bedside area. *(select all that apply)*
   1. Suction device and tubing
   2. Blood sugar glucose monitoring device
   3. Manual resuscitator bag and correct size mask
   4. Access to code blue button and/or phone
   5. Source of oxygen with connector and tubing

4. The purpose of RRTs in the acute care pediatric setting is to provide a timely response to a child whose condition is worsening. Components of an RRT include the following: *(select all that apply)*
   1. Team membership
   2. Rotation schedule
   3. Criteria for activation
   4. Response team
   5. Response team event record

5. When working on a pediatric hospital unit, the nurse teaches the family about the RRT. When describing who is allowed to activate the RRT, the nurse would be correct in stating:
   1. Only the medical team who is asking for further team assistance
   2. The immediate family
   3. The nursing team who finds the child in distress
   4. Anyone who identifies the need to request help for the child

6. An LVN must use the chain of command to immediately report any change in a patient's clinical status to the next appropriate person. In the hospital setting, who should the LVN report a patient's clinical status changes to?
   1. The hospitalist on duty
   2. The nursing supervisor
   3. The ED attending doctor
   4. The RN working on the unit

7. The LVN and RN nursing team of a busy medical clinic is asked to participate in a "mock code blue." What are the components of this practice session? *(select all that apply)*
   1. Practicing how to call for an RRT
   2. Calling a code blue response
   3. Initiating the use of a crash cart
   4. Performing CPR

8. Pediatric nurses can assume various roles during an emergency response in an acute care environment. Roles include: *(select all that apply)*
   1. Airway management
   2. Compressions
   3. Taking serial vital sign measurements
   4. Running laboratory specimens
   5. Passing equipment from the crash cart to the response team
   6. Providing emotional support to the family

9. The primary intervention the pediatric nurse should perform when a child becomes cyanotic is to: *(select all that apply)*
   1. Provide a source of oxygen
   2. Suction
   3. Stimulate the child
   4. Call the parents to the bedside
   5. Call for pharmacy backup

10. An ALTE is not a formal medical diagnosis but a sudden, acute, and unexpected change in a young's infant's breathing pattern that leads to a color change, apnea, limpness, and often, choking or gagging.
    1. True
    2. False

CRITICAL THINKING QUESTIONS

1. How prepared are pediatric nurses to respond to a hospitalized child's sudden negative change of clinical status? How do pediatric nurses describe their level of comfort, education, and preparation to handle emergencies within the hospital?

2. Use an online literature database to discover how long, on average, a nurse retains CPR skills after the completion of a mandatory class. What can be done to help alleviate this rapid loss of effective resuscitation skills?

Which skills need frequent practice? Do mock codes help in increasing reported comfort and confidence in responding to emergencies?

3. Should parents be allowed to stay in a room when a child is requiring emergency resuscitation? Would the visual memory of the team's resuscitation efforts, including the use of emergency equipment, crash carts, and CPR measures assist or harm in the recovery of the family after the resuscitation attempts?

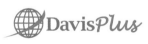

For additional resources and information, visit **www.DavisPlus.com**. Post-Conference Questions and Activities, Answers, and References can be found on Davis*Plus*.

28

The Abused Child

KEY TERMS

abuse
battered
Child Protective Services (CPS)
intentional injury
mandatory reporters of child abuse and neglect
Munchausen's syndrome by proxy (MSBP)
neglect
sexual abuse
unintentional abuse or injury

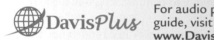 **DavisPlus** For audio pronunciation guide, visit www.DavisPlus.com

CHAPTER CONCEPTS

Development
Family
Safety
Stress
Trauma
Violence

LEARNING OUTCOMES

1. Define the key terms.
2. Describe global perspectives, historical perspectives, and legal aspects of child abuse, including the development of laws aimed at protecting abused children and preventing abuse in society.
3. Discuss the various types of abuse and their incidences and prevalence rates, and give examples of abuse scenarios in each of the developmental stages of childhood.
4. Analyze high-risk children and social/environmental influences to the development of child abuse.
5. Describe the child, parent, and environmental influences to child abuse situations.
6. Create a child abuse nursing care plan for a school-aged child including physical, emotional, and social implications.
7. Analyze the cultural influences to abuse identification and discuss the importance for members of the health-care team to investigate the differences between some cultural practices and evidence of child abuse.
8. State the essential nursing care of the abused child and family, including identifying signs and symptoms, supporting medical assessments, and documenting appropriately.
9. Describe how to maintain safety for a child who has been abused, including essential communication, team membership, and legal steps needed for protection.

REAL-WORLD CASE STUDY

Katrina

■ Katrina, an 18-year-old single parent, brings her child into the emergency room (ER) accompanied by her 19-year-old boyfriend because her 10-month-old infant is "sleeping too much, eating poorly, and is too thin." The ER pediatric nurse assesses the infant and notes the infant to have poor hygiene, a dirty diaper with dried stool, lower than expected weight (10th percentile on a national growth chart), lethargy, and large wide eyes. The infant does not

**REAL-WORLD CASE
STUDY** *continued*

demonstrate stranger anxiety and she does not smile when the nurse attempts to play with her and presents her with a brightly colored toy. Upon further assessment, the mother states that she is very stressed, has no support from her parents in the care of the child, has dropped out of high school, and has no child care for the infant during the day. The mother states she is home with the infant in her parents' home and "never has time away from the infant." The boyfriend is not engaged in the child and remains focused on his cell phone, texting during the entire time the nurse is interacting with the mother and child.

Upon further assessment, the child demonstrates a yellowish bruise on her low flank and a new bluish bruise on her upper right arm. The ER medical team orders a chest X-ray that shows the child has three rib fractures with evidence of healing. The team suspects child abuse and Child Protective Services (CPS) is notified. Within 60 min, a hospital social worker, a sheriff, and a member of the county CPS arrive to the ER and place the child on a 72-hour police hold. The child is transferred to the pediatric in-patient unit and is now awaiting a computed tomography (CT) scan of the body and a magnetic resonance imaging (MRI) of the head. Abuse is suspected and the mother is not allowed to visit her child without supervision.

The entire health-care team focuses on the well-being and healing of the child. The social worker identifies local support services for the mother, including a parenting class and a local mothers' support group. A family conference is held in the conference room on the floor of the pediatric unit and the following are present during the meeting: the mother, her parents, social worker, two CPS professionals, attending physician, charge nurse, nutritionist, Child Life Specialist, and ER physician. After the case conference, during which a plan of action was made for the mother, the CPS agency allowed the mother to reunite with the infant at discharge but will follow the family closely by agency visits and home visits. Mandatory parenting classes are required and the mother receives both group counseling and individual counseling. The child is discharged after she demonstrates progressive weight gain.

1. What specific conditions did the child present with that warrant a workup for abuse?
2. Why would the health-care team request the child have an MRI of the head?

CONCEPTUAL CORNERSTONE

Family

Families who are experiencing violence and abuse need help. Providing the child with a safe environment is the most important and immediate aspect of care. The entire family is affected by child abuse so safety for any family member involved in the abuse of the child must be provided. When a child presents with evidence or suspicion of child abuse of any form, the family will need help with parenting, anticipatory guidance, role modeling, counseling, and support services. The child who has experienced abuse will need to be provided comfort and a trusting relationship must be formed. Child abuse is a problem for the entire family, not just the child presenting with evidence of abuse or injuries who causes the pediatric health-care team to have suspicion.

Child **abuse,** also called *child maltreatment or **intentional injury**,* is a complex social problem. Pediatric nurses can be frontline care providers who identify the subtle or apparent evidence of child abuse. Understanding the influencing factors in the development of child abuse, learning the various types and clinical presentations of each, and understanding the required steps to reporting child abuse are all essential components in protecting the child from further harm. Pediatric nurses are **mandatory reporters of child abuse and neglect** and therefore it is essential to review all aspects of the complexity of child maltreatment. A mandatory reporter, because of his or her position, is legally responsible to report actual or suspected child abuse to authorities. All health-care providers are considered mandatory reporters. Other mandatory reporters include commercial film developers, child care custodians, and law enforcement agents from all branches of the law, such as law officers and correctional personnel.

- **Health-Care Providers:** All persons involved with the care of the child will be held responsible in assessing and reporting any actual or suspected symptoms or signs of child abuse. These include nurses, physicians, social workers, or anyone involved with the care of the child.
- **Child Care Custodians:** Although the definition of who is considered a child care custodian may differ from state to state, those who provide care and supervision for children, whether it is public or private, are considered mandatory child abuse reporters. Child care providers, clergy, coaches, and teachers are all included under this category of mandatory reporters.
- **Law Officers (All Branches) and Correctional Personnel:** Anyone who holds a legal position of authority in any branch of law is considered a mandatory reporter. This includes sheriffs, police, highway patrol, and other staff employed by those divisions. Persons who work for CPS are also mandated to follow up on all actual or suspected child abuse.
- **Commercial Film Developers:** Those who develop film are also held responsible to report pictures taken of children in sexually or physically abused circumstances. Because documentation of sexual abuse of children is not uncommon, commercial film developers are responsible, if it is identified, to report to law officers any photographs developed of children in sexually compromising positions or situations.

SAFETY *STAT!*

As a licensed health-care professional, nurses are required to report both suspected and actual abuse or neglect. It is not the responsibility of the nurse to determine who caused the abuse. It is mandatory that a report be filed with the local **Child Protective Services (CPS)**. This agency provides assessment, interventions, and treatment referrals for families who have a child who has been identified as experiencing maltreatment. The form should be faxed to the local Child Abuse Protection Agency within 24 hours of encountering the child. Lack of reporting, or delayed reporting, can result in severe legal consequences. All pertinent evidence should be collected, including verbatim quotes, pictures, radiographs, or any diagnostics that are associated with the child's clinical presentation or injury.

SAFETY *STAT!*

There are circumstances in pediatric health care where local law officers should be called in to the setting to provide immediate assistance. If the nurse suspects that the child, or other family members, are currently at risk for further abuse, law enforcements officers should be notified STAT.

Child maltreatment includes several types of abuse and **neglect** (ie, failure to provide for basic needs) concerning children younger than 18 years old by a parent, a person in a custodial role (eg, clergy, coach, or teacher), or a caregiver. The very few cases that are exposed in the media are just a small representation of abuse that happens in our society (Centers for Disease Control and Prevention [CDC], 2015).

CHILD ABUSE GLOBAL PERSPECTIVES

Internationally, child abuse has been recorded in science, art, and literature in most parts of the world. Reports of neglect, mutilation, infanticide, abandonment, casting out the weak child to fend for himself or herself, **sexual abuse,** and many forms of violence toward children have been documented dating back to ancient civilizations (Bensel, Rheinberger, et al, 1997). Unfortunately, child abuse did not come into the social limelight until 1962, when Kempe's seminal work was published: *The Battered Child Syndrome* (Kempe, 1962). Child abuse remains a global problem, with neglect being the most commonly found form of child maltreatment around the world.

Child abuse crosses all cultures, ages, economic levels, races, and religions, but is most prevalent in families living in poverty and those families composed of adolescent parents with young children. Nurses should never make assumptions about certain groups being at higher risk for child abuse but rather should be aware that social, economic, and personal stressors can contribute to the incidence of child abuse.

CULTURAL CONSIDERATIONS

Culture, too, has a very predominant role in the generally accepted principles of child-rearing and child care. Forms of child discipline accepted in one culture may be acts that are reportable and prosecutable in another. In societies of great cultural diversity, health-care professionals may be challenged to determine what practices are abusive or neglectful, and which might be considered culturally acceptable. The International Society for the Prevention of Child Abuse and Neglect compared definitions of child abuse in 58 countries and found common perspectives about what is considered abuse. Sexual abuse, physical abuse, emotional ill-treatment, neglect, or commercial exploitation resulting in potential or actual harm to the survival, dignity, or health of a child, all within the context of a relationship of power, trust, or responsibility, is considered child abuse (World Health Organization [WHO], 1999). The most important aspect is that the nurse, or any mandated reporter, follows state laws concerning reporting evidence of abuse, even if it is suspected and not perfectly clear. The consequences of not reporting are often harsh and should be avoided to protect the well-being of the child and family unit.

SAFETY *STAT!*

Protecting the child from further or continued abuse is of immediate importance. No matter what clinical setting the abuse is found in, the health-care team must protect the child from further abuse and report the suspicions or signs of abuse to the authorities.

CHILD ABUSE AND PREVENTION

Federal legislation was created in 1974 to provide definitions and guidance. The Child Abuse Prevention and Treatment Act (CAPTA), amended in 2003, offers evaluation, technical assistance, data collection, and supporting research, as well as minimal definitions of child neglect and child abuse.

Acts of commission in child abuse are situations in which the responsible person, often the parent, intentionally harms the child via physical, emotional, or sexual abuse. Acts of omission in child abuse are situations in which a parent or caregiver, to their best of abilities and often inadvertently, cannot provide adequate nutrition, shelter, warmth, appropriate seasonal clothing (eg, winter coats), safety, and education for his or her child. Both are considered major categories of child abuse and situations identified in both categories must be reported. The idea of responding to both acts of commission and acts of omission is to provide safety for the child, or provide what is necessary for the child to thrive and grow in a safe environment.

PATIENT TEACHING GUIDELINES

Parents who have unrealistic expectations of their children have been shown to be more at risk for abusing a child. Parents need to understand what appropriate expectations are for each of the developmental stages of childhood.

Parental expectations of their child's behavior are also associated with the incidence of child abuse. For instance, a parent who expects a very young child to behave outside the child's age or development, or a parent who expects a young child to perform chores above and beyond the child's physical, emotional, and cognitive development, may contribute to abusive situations and is considered a risk for being abusive (World Report on Violence and Health, 2002). A challenge for the health-care team is to determine if the abuse was intentional or unintentional. **Unintentional abuse or injury** occurs when a parent or caregiver lacks education on child rearing or basic needs, or neglects a child's basic needs because of lack of resources. See Table 28.1 regarding the etiology of abuse.

SAFETY *STAT!*

Providing anticipatory guidance to parents about realistic behavior for young children can help a parent understand appropriate expectations for each developmental stage. Nurses are in a good position to teach families about matching expectations with a child's ability to reduce the frustration the parent may feel if the child does not complete a chore or a task.

TABLE 28.1   ETIOLOGY OF ABUSE

Type of Factor	Factors
Parental	• The parent(s) experienced severe punishment when they were children • The parent(s) have poor impulse control • The parent(s) accept free expression of violence within the home • The family is experiencing social isolation, lack of parenting mentors, and little or no respite care • The parent(s) have poor social-emotional support systems • The parent(s) are participating in substance abuse • The parent(s) have low self-esteem • The parent(s) have a history of cruelty to animals • The parent(s) delay seeking medical treatment for the child and lack follow through • The parent(s) use multiple health-care providers, yet have a decreasing number of visits or increased no-shows
Child	• The child is under 4 years of age • The child has a difficult and/or demanding temperament • The child is perceived as a misfit within the family structure • The child has had numerous illnesses or has a chronic illness/disorder requiring extra demands • The child has a documented disability • The child has developmental delays • Typically, only one child is being abused; other siblings within the family are not usually abused • The child was a product of an unplanned or unexpected pregnancy • There was a difficult or problematic pregnancy and/or delivery • The child has a hyperkinetic disorder • There was an early failure to bond between the child and parent • The child was born prematurely • The child has a resemblance to someone the parent does not like
Environmental	• The environment the family functions in has chronic stress • Member(s) of the family are going through or have recently been through a divorce • The family has experienced frequent relocation to different geographical locations • The family is living in poverty and often times is living in an urban or rural area of impoverished homes • The family has experienced the consequences of unemployment • The family is living in inadequate or poor housing • The family is living in an unsafe neighborhood • The family is living in a community in which on-going violence is experienced; thus child abuse may be accepted

TYPES OF ABUSE

Child abuse comes in many types and forms. Types of child abuse include physical abuse, emotional abuse or neglect, physical neglect, and sexual abuse. Skills are needed to be able to identify all the different types of abuse, and teamwork is required to take evidence such as photographs or body secretions rapidly and thoroughly. Teamwork is needed to identify the variety of clinical manifestations of abuse (Box 28.1).

Box 28.1 Clinical Manifestations or Symptoms of Abuse

Pediatric nurses and health-care team members must be able to identify potential areas of abuse, including incompatibility of injuries noted and the given history of the injury or finding:

- Lack of or delayed normal growth and development
- Language delay
- Irritability, resists affection and cuddling, may be unresponsive to nurturing
- Vacant eyes and/or gaze aversion, also known as "radar gaze"
- Expressionless face, infrequent smile, may demonstrate anxiousness
- Weight is below the fifth percentile or a diagnosis of failure to thrive (FTT)
- Shaken baby syndrome (ie, subdural hematomas, fractures, bruises, and retinal hemorrhages)
- Falls and associated injuries in young children
- Bruises in various stages of healing and of various shapes (showing the object used for infliction)
- Slapping or grab marks, bruises demonstrating being tied up (ie, linear bruises on ankles and wrists)
- Gag marks
- Bilateral black eyes including upper eye lids
- External head, facial, and oral injuries
- Boggy scalp injuries from subgaleal hematomas (caused by lifting the scalp off the skull)
- Thermal injuries such as dry contact burns that are second degree
- Forced immersion burns such as sock, glove, dunking, or donut burns (ie, clear line of demarcation without accompanied splash burn marks)
- Traumatic hair loss (ie, alopecia)
- Unexplained fractures that may be in different stages of healing
- Spiral fractures
- Unexplained dislocations
- Sexual abuse: bruising, discharge, pain, and sexually transmitted diseases (STDs)
- Physical neglect, such as very poor hygiene

Physical Abuse

Physical abuse is defined as acts of true commission caused by either a parent or caregiver that result in actual physical harm or are considered to have the potential to cause physical harm. Examples of physical abuse include shaken baby syndrome; a **battered** child showing evidence of repeated injury to the skin, nervous system, or skeletal system; and visceral trauma from blunt force, especially with clinical evidence of repeated injury. Children who present with evidence of slapping, hitting, burning, or any other form of physical harm have most likely been experiencing the abuse for an extended period of time (American Academy of Pediatrics [AAP], 2010). Figure 28.1 provides examples of instruments that have been used for physical punishment and the marks left behind. Figure 28.2 illustrates the areas of a child's body where accidental injuries would be unusual.

SAFETY *STAT!*

New parents must be reminded to never shake their infant. One single episode of shaking can have lifelong devastating effects on a child's neurological system.

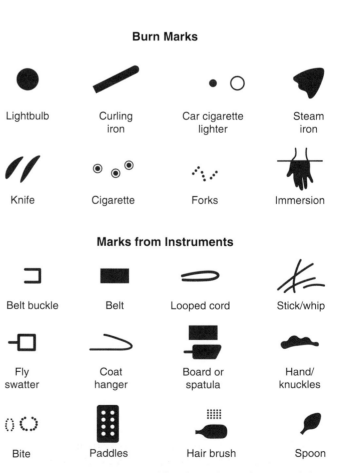

FIGURE 28.1 Instruments used for physical punishment and the marks they leave.

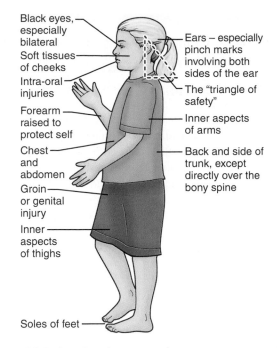

Black eyes, especially bilateral

Soft tissues of cheeks

Intra-oral injuries

Forearm raised to protect self

Chest and abdomen

Groin or genital injury

Inner aspects of thighs

Soles of feet

Ears – especially pinch marks involving both sides of the ear

The "triangle of safety"

Inner aspects of arms

Back and side of trunk, except directly over the bony spine

FIGURE 28.2 Accidental injuries in these areas are unusual.

Emotional Abuse or Neglect

Emotional abuse or neglect is defined as the failure of the parent or caregiver to provide an appropriate supportive environment. The child suffers because of an adverse effect on his or her emotional health and child development needs; examples include denigration, ridicule, intimidation, threats, hostility, discrimination, rejection, and restricting a child's movement (WHO, 1999). A child who, on a regular basis, is threatened, humiliated, ignored, repetitively blamed, called names, made fun of, or is found to be at fault is also considered emotionally or psychologically abused (AAP, 2010).

Physical Neglect

Physical neglect is when a parent or caregiver fails to provide for the appropriate development of the child by failing to provide nutrition, shelter, medical care, and safe living conditions. Physical neglect is differentiated by true circumstances of poverty in that there are reasonable resources available to the family, parent, or caregiver.

TEAM WORKS

Hunger from deprivation of food, a lack of physical development, medical noncompliance, and very poor hygiene are universal symptoms of physical neglect.

Sexual Abuse

Sexual abuse is when a parent, caregiver, stranger, or known family friend, relative, or neighbor uses a child for his or her own sexual gratification. A child who engages in a sexual situation with an adult or an older child, whether or not it is

a direct physical act, is considered sexually abused. Sexual abuse can occur when a child is forced to look at an adult masturbating, adult genitalia, or pornography, or is forced to be a part of the production of pornographic materials. Some sexually abused children are not forced to have sex but are persuaded, tricked, coerced, or bribed to do so. See Box 28.2 for factors associated with the sexual abuse of children.

Children who are victims of sexual abuse display classic symptoms of infection, abdominal pain, genital injury, constipation, urinary tract infections, sexually explicit behaviors, an increased interest in sexuality, and emotional disturbances. Health-care providers need a high index of suspicion and familiarity with the behavioral, physical, and verbal indicators of this type of abuse.

MUNCHAUSEN'S SYNDROME BY PROXY

When a parent intentionally creates an illness, fabricates the symptoms of an illness, or describes certain clinical presentations such as seizures, vomiting, or bloody diarrhea to be admitted into a hospital or health-care setting, the condition of **Munchausen's syndrome by proxy (MSBP)** must be suspected. This is a rare but real mental health disorder demonstrated typically by a mother who has some health-care knowledge and who displays behaviors of overinvolvement with her child. The perpetrator of this condition wants the child to experience multiple invasive tests and treatments, which allows the parent to receive a great deal of attention from the members of the health-care team. The symptoms described by the parent are not witnessed by members of the health-care team (eg, a grand mal seizure or prolonged episodes of nausea and vomiting) and the symptoms are not present when the parent is not around the child. Box 28.3 provides indicators of MSBP. The parent is typically viewed as very attentive and caring, until a pattern of bizarre attention-seeking behaviors is identified. The pediatric nurse must

---

Box 28.2 Factors Associated With Sexual Child Abuse

- Anyone can be an abuser: father, mother, sibling, or member of the extended family
- The person who is sexually abusing a child is typically male and known to the family
- Sexual abuse offenders come from all socioeconomic levels, cultures, and races
- Pedophiles often choose to work in environments in which children are present
- Father-daughter or step father-daughter abuse situations tend to be prolonged
- Eldest daughter is typically the victim
- Males are less likely to admit and report sexual abuse because of social stigmas

Box 28.3 Indicators of Munchausen's Syndrome By Proxy

1. Child is under 6 years of age
2. Perpetrator is usually the mother, who has some health-care knowledge
3. Father is not present in the health-care interaction, is uninvolved, or is absent from the home/family
4. Possible positive family history of parent with MSBP or another sibling who has experienced this type of abuse
5. Claimed history of the child by the mother is not supported by evidence found by health-care professionals
6. Child has both a history of multiple hospitalizations and experiences with multiple blood tests, x-rays, and other invasive procedures
7. The child does not display the symptoms during hospitalization and the child's condition improves when the mother is not present
8. The child's clinical signs and symptoms cannot be explained or substantiated by a known disease etiology

(American Psychiatric Association, 2013; National Institutes of Health, 2015)

Box 28.4 Case Study: Munchausen's Syndrome By Proxy

A 35-year-old mother brings her child to the ER of a large urban hospital claiming her infant daughter just had a period of a "blue spell" followed by a long grand mal seizure and then a period of not breathing. The mother rushes the pale and limp infant into the ER and the child is immediately brought in for a full diagnostic work-up. The mother claims a history of reflux, bloody stools found in the diaper, and a history of fevers. The mother is praised for her diligence of identifying the child's condition and the child is eventually transferred from the ER and admitted to the pediatric intensive care unit (PICU) for further observation and diagnostic procedures. After a long hospitalization, visits from multiple pediatric specialists, and many complex diagnostic procedures such as upper and lower gastrointestinal (GI) series, blood tests and electroencephalogram (EEG), no evidence is found to support the mother's claims.

identify this type of child abuse immediately before the child is subjected to multiple, sometimes painful, unnecessary diagnostic procedures. Box 28.4 presents a case study on a child identified as a victim of MSBP.

SAFETY *STAT!*

MSBP is rare. If a member of the health-care team suspects abnormal behavior by a parent displaying signs of this disorder, an immediate referral should be made to a social worker, and pertinent members of the pediatric health-care team who are caring for the child should be notified of the concerns. If the parent believes he or she may be a suspect, he or she is a flight risk and may leave the health-care facility against medical advice. Family members identified as flight risks should be reported to security and their assistance secured.

ABUSE STATISTICS

The incidence of reporting child abuse is considered a complex issue because the prevalence of abuse is predicted to be more widespread than what is identified and reported. According to the CDC, what is identified is only a small part of a widespread problem (2014). According to the CDC's 2012 statistics, 1,640 children died in the United States from neglect or abuse; 686,000 children under the age of 18 were found to be victims of child abuse by CPS; and the overall national rates of child abuse are predicted to be as high as 9.2 per 1,000 children. The breakdown of the types of child abuse is reported to be:

- 52% neglect
- 24% physical abuse
- 12% sexual abuse
- 16% other, which includes abandonment, congenital drug addiction, and threats to harm

The percentage total is greater than 100% because some children suffer multiple types of abuse.

FATAL ABUSE

It is difficult to collect data on the incidence of child abuse leading to the child's death. Based on an investigation of death registries and mortality data, WHO in 2015 estimated that 417,000 children die as a result of abuse. WHO found that infants and very young children are at greatest risk for death associated with abuse, with rates that are double compared with children who are 5 to 15 years old. In the true determination of deaths associated with abuse, what is considered difficult is that routine postmortem examinations are not always conducted. The three most common abuse injuries that lead to childhood deaths are injuries to the head, followed by injuries to the abdomen, and then intentional suffocation (Kirschner and Wilson, 2000; Reece and Krous, 2001). According to The National Center for the Review and Prevention of Child Deaths, the most common causes of childhood deaths associated with abuse were head trauma, shaking deaths, burns, drowning, and smothering (2013).

PREVENTION OF CHILD ABUSE

Preventing child abuse before it occurs is the ultimate goal of reducing the incidence of child maltreatment. An essential component of child abuse prevention is readily available and affordable positive parenting classes in which skills are taught and reinforced. Good communication, knowing when to respond to a child's physical and emotional needs, and appropriate discipline are all parts of positive parenting strategies (CDC, 2013). Programs that set out to improve the parent-child relationship, and those that provide social support and role modeling, have been successful in reducing the incidence of child abuse.

PATIENT TEACHING GUIDELINES

Three ideas to communicate to parents struggling with positive parenting include:

- Count to 10 before responding to a child or disciplining a child.
- Understand how to match the discipline with the child's developmental stage. Know what can be expected from each child and do not expect more than the child is cognitively, emotionally, or physical able to do.
- Take care of oneself; to be a good parent means to take care of oneself so that stress, anger, and short temper responses can be minimized.

Preventing many child abuse cases starts with early reporting of the evidence of suspected abuse or neglect. If a health-care professional suspects a child is being maltreated or threatened to be maltreated, he or she should call the National Child Abuse Hotline at 1-800-4-A-Child (1-800-422-4453).

For a list of CDC activities that promote child abuse prevention strategies see the CDC Web site.

MEDICAL AND NURSING MANAGEMENT OF CHILD ABUSE

In managing child abuse, it is imperative that a comprehensive treatment plan be developed that includes a variety of team members using a family-focused care model. First and foremost, the child should be protected from further abuse. The abuse perpetrator needs to be identified quickly. The authorities must be notified to begin this process of identification, and careful documentation of all that is heard, seen, and done is imperative. The entire health-care team's role is to protect the child, provide safety, offer support, and begin to conduct assessments and diagnostics to confirm abuse. CPS' role is to identify the perpetrator and ensure the child's continued safety.

Child abuse does not affect the genders equally. Males are known to suffer greater emotional harm from incest than female victims do. Overall, female children are now being reported as suffering child abuse more often than male children.

THERAPEUTIC COMMUNICATION

The child must understand that the abuse was not his or her fault. The pediatric health-care team, as they are establishing a trusting relationship and rapport with the child, must emphasize that the child did not cause the abuse, nor are they responsible for the abuse that has occurred.

The following steps are those that the care team should use in the care and protection of a child who has been a victim of child abuse:

1. **Stabilization:** The child's physical, physiological, and emotional health needs to be stabilized. The early identification and treatment of physical harm (eg, head trauma, shaken baby syndrome, spiral fractures, and bleeding) needs to be the first priority in the care of a child who has been abused.
2. **Protection From Harm:** The care team needs to set up circumstances to prevent further harm. The child may need a police hold, security may need to be involved, social services will need to talk to the family, and CPS may need to provide temporary medical foster care.
3. **History Taking:** The team must identify if there are inconsistencies between the injury and the parental-child history or description of the cause of the injury. The history must be carefully documented because records can be required in court.
4. **Collection of Laboratory Specimens:** The collection of specimens needs to take place as soon as possible using protocols that protect the evidence, such as the collection of semen and human hairs from the child's body.
5. **Securing of Photographs:** Many health-care environments will have a policy that guides the health-care team in how to document the visual evidence of abuse via photographs.
6. **Differentiation of Child Abuse From Other Medical Conditions:** One challenge for the health-care team, social services, and CPS members is to differentiate potential child abuse from other medical conditions or even childhood injury from normal activities and rigorous play.
7. **Determination of Spiral Fractures:** Spiral fractures are often associated with violent abuse, so meticulous radiography needs to be taken to determine if the child's fracture is a spiral fracture. This type of fracture is considered very rare in conditions or circumstances other than abuse.
8. **Rule Out Congenital Brittle Bone Disease:** A very rare condition, brittle bone disease must be ruled

out in the presence of multiple fractures found in a variety of healing stages.

9. **Distinguish Between Abuse and Cultural Care Practices:** Cultural care practices exist that can leave physical marks that resemble child abuse.

LABS & DIAGNOSTICS

Laboratory analysis and diagnostics that can aid the team in determining if abuse versus other medical conditions is present include the following:

- Skeletal bone surveys
- CT scan
- Ophthalmological examination
- Color photographs
- Examination of cerebrospinal fluid
- Pregnancy tests
- STD screening tests
- Evidentiary examinations of specimens per local coroner, CPS, or medical examiner

SAFETY *STAT!*

Do not wash or bathe a child who has been a suspected sexual abuse victim. Many specimens will be collected from the child's clothing and skin. It is important to obtain these specimens for the legal system.

TEAM WORKS

Do not use a personal cell phone for photo collection of child abuse evidence; contact the administration and follow the institutional protocol carefully. Team members do not want to be found with child abuse photographs on personal cell phones.

CULTURAL CONSIDERATIONS

There are some cultural healing practices (eg, coining and cupping) that leave physical markings on a child's skin that mimic physical child abuse. It is important for a pediatric nurse to understand these practices exist and be prepared to help the pediatric health-care team distinguish between forms of child abuse and cultural care practices that are believed to promote a child's healing. This is a delicate situation because cultural healing practices are very important to families and should be respected.

■ NURSING CONSIDERATIONS AND CARE

Child abuse identification and reporting are difficult aspects of being a pediatric nurse. Being able to identify when abuse has occurred when signs and symptoms are vague is difficult for even experienced nurses. Care must be given to protect the child from on-going abuse. If a child has infected wounds, infections, injuries, or disease processes where there was a delay in seeking treatment, or no treatment was sought, it is the nurse's responsibility to follow up, discuss the findings with the physician and social worker, and report as indicated. Reporting abuse to the appropriate authorities is essential in the prevention of escalating violence and continued harm.

SAFETY *STAT!*

Look for behavioral signs, as well as physical signs of abuse. If a child who is suspected of neglect, emotional abuse, or physical abuse displays fear, irritability, aggression, withdrawal, apathy, or a "radar gaze" (ie, child is constantly surveying the environment for the onslaught of further abuse), be caring and suspicious. Ask team members to assist you.

Using more experienced staff to help the process and maintaining a team approach can assist the new pediatric nurse through the difficult and emotionally-charged experience. It is important to understand that maintaining safety for a child who has been abused includes essential communication, teamwork, and the legal steps needed for protection. A new pediatric nurse should have the confidence to report suspected abuse. Discussing the case with the charge nurse, nursing supervisor, or nurse manager is appropriate to have support in the reporting process. All pediatric nurses must be familiar with institutional policies on reporting child abuse. Team members, child care custodians, and other mandatory reporters who do not report child abuse are at risk for legal consequences such as heavy fines and/or jail sentences. The consequences for the child of not reporting child abuse includes continued trauma and the continuation, and sometimes escalation, of the abuse. Families with an abused child will not secure help, such as child care and appropriate child discipline classes of abuse, if the abuse is not reported.

Team members who do not report child abuse are at risk for heavy fines and/or jail sentences. Using the nursing process to organize care for the abused child can also assist in the complexity of the situation for a child and family suffering abuse. Remember that child abuse crosses all cultures, all developmental stages, and all socioeconomic levels.

NURSING CARE PLAN for the Abuse Victim

Nursing Assessment:
- Do not conduct a physical assessment while alone with the child. You may be implicated for the cause of the abuse.
- During the assessment phase the nurse collects both subjective and objective information.
- Include the parent's description of the cause of the injury and circumstances surrounding the injury event such as supervision, witnesses, and other pertinent data. Objective data gathering includes collecting information about the injured child, such as taking pictures of the bruises and documenting the number, size, color of bruises, extent of injury, and any associated factors.

Physical Indicators:
- Include the description of each and every sore, bruise, rash, and burn. Note whether your physical findings match the history of what the parents say is the cause of the injury.

Behavioral Indicators:
- Include descriptions of the parent-child interactions, noting what is said and how the family interacts, including nonverbal communication.
- Note any identified delays in seeking medical care for the child; ask the parents why they did not seek care earlier in the injury.
- Assess for suspicious injuries; assess for injuries where the history does not match the physical evidence.

Nursing Diagnoses:
- There is a risk for injury related to intentional physical and emotional abuse.
- The child expresses fear related to an unsafe home environment.
- There is altered parenting related to a poor understanding of a child's cognitive and developmental abilities and needs.
- There is altered parenting related to use of violence.
- Risk exists for post-trauma syndrome, related to repeated episodes of physical and emotional harm or abuse.
- There is anxiety related to the uncertainty of parent-child interactions and physical and emotional abuse.

Planning:
Create patient-centered goals during the planning phase of the nursing process that have these five components:
1. Child-centered
2. Future-oriented
3. Measureable
4. Realistic
5. With a timeframe

The child will gain 0.5 kg of weight per week while hospitalized by experiencing a quiet, supportive, and supervised eating environment with the child's selected favorite foods.

Implementation:
- Protect the child from further abuse, regardless of which type of abuse the child has experienced.
- Meet the child's immediate psychological and physical needs first.
- Gain the child's trust and then work on gaining the parents' trust in your nursing care; do not demonstrate any signs of judgment but be professional, supportive, and engaged.
- Minimize child's fear and anxiety by providing a quiet, supportive, supervised environment with access to play therapy.
- Engage the child in play that encourages his or her expressions of anxiety, fear, and, especially, guilt.
- Foster positive parenting by demonstrating appropriate care for the child and providing positive reinforcement for their attempts at good care.

Expected Outcome:
- The child remains free of harm and is able to heal his or her injuries in a caring and supportive environment.

Continued

NURSING CARE PLAN for the Abuse Victim—cont'd

Evaluation of Outcome:
- The child shows no evidence of physical neglect.
- The child shows no evidence of emotional neglect.
- The child experiences less fear and anxiety.
- The child learns to tell parents about abuse by others.
- The parent demonstrates positive parenting behaviors.
- The parent demonstrates positive interactions with the child.

Key Points

- Global perspectives, historical perspectives, and legal aspects of child abuse, including the development of laws aimed at protecting abused children, are continuing to demonstrate how prevalent child abuse is worldwide and across all socioeconomic levels and cultures. It is important for the pediatric nurse to possess strong assessment skills and follow-through to protect children of all ages.
- The various types of abuse include physical abuse, physical neglect, emotional abuse, emotional neglect, and sexual abuse.
- Child-related factors that influence child abuse include children who are unplanned for, have difficult temperaments, have chronic diseases, or are seen as "different" from their siblings. Parental factors that influence child abuse include experience with severe punishment when they were children, poor impulse control, accepting a free expression of violence within the home, social isolation, a

lack of parenting mentors, little or no respite care, low self-esteem, and substance abuse.
- Classic symptoms and clinical presentations of the various types of abuse include low birth weight; poor weight gain; a lack of normal growth and development, including language delay; vacant eyes and/or gaze aversion; radar gaze; an expressionless face; infrequent smiling; anxiousness; subdural hematomas; fractures; bruises; retinal hemorrhages; bruises in various stages of healing; thermal injuries; traumatic hair loss (ie, alopecia); spiral fractures; STDs; and evidence of physical neglect, such as very poor hygiene.
- Maintaining safety for a child who has been abused includes essential communication, teamwork, and taking the legal steps needed for protection. Health-care team members who do not report child abuse are at risk for heavy fines and/or jail sentences.

REVIEW QUESTIONS

1. Child abuse, or maltreatment of a child, is defined in most states in the United States as:
   1. Lack of economic resources within a home
   2. Domestic violence between family members
   3. Intentional harm directed at a child
   4. Negligence in providing safe living conditions

2. Child neglect is defined as all of the following *except:*
   1. Lack of physical care to the child, such as inadequate food and feedings
   2. Absence of emotional care and stimulation that allows a child to develop normally
   3. Denial of education to a child, such as not enrolling a young child into an appropriate school
   4. Preventing a child from participating in extracurricular activities within a school setting

3. Within the six categories of child abuse or maltreatment, the following are listed as types: *(select all that apply)*
   1. Physical violence
   2. Sexual abuse
   3. Emotional abuse
   4. Emotional neglect
   5. Physical restraint
   6. Physical neglect

4. While assessing a young school-aged child for the potential of sexual abuse, all of the following would be taken into consideration except:
   1. Seductive behaviors demonstrated by the child
   2. Inappropriate knowledge or interest in sexual activities or acts
   3. Fear of a particular family member, neighbor, or friend
   4. Obsession with masturbation in privacy

5. One of the first steps in confirming that a child has experienced abuse is which of the following?
   1. The nurse hears the stories of abuse from a younger sibling.
   2. The nurse identifies there is a discrepancy between the injury present and the reported history of the injury.
   3. The nurse identifies a history of substance abuse in one of the parents.
   4. The nurse assesses a history of a difficult and prolonged labor for the mother of the child.

6. Priority assessments of a young child suspected of being a victim of child abuse include:
   1. Tests for STDs in a child with suspected sexual abuse
   2. Developmental assessments to determine the level of cognitive processing
   3. Skeletal radiographs of a child with a suspected glove burn
   4. Assessment of relationships with siblings and the order of birth

7. What is the name of the situation where a child presents with rare, recurrent, unexplained, prolonged, and often unsubstantiated illnesses or conditions?
   1. Intentional child abuse
   2. Munchausen's syndrome
   3. Child abuse syndrome
   4. MSBP

8. The pediatric nurse working in a clinic admits a child with a fading ecchymotic ring around his left eye. What is the most appropriate question to ask the child?
   1. "Did you get that black eye during sports?"
   2. "Who did this to you?"
   3. "Have you been bullied at school?"
   4. "How did you get the black eye?"

9. Which of the following burn marks would cause the pediatric nurse to become the most concerned?
   1. Burns around both feet with edges marked in a line above the ankle
   2. Splash marks on the child's anterior chest and abdomen
   3. A small round burn on the side of thumb
   4. Large fluid-filled vesicles with erythema on both shoulders

10. As long as the pediatric nurse is told that a child abuse report has been filled out by team members who cared for an abused child before his or her shift, the nurse will not need to fill out a report.
    1. True
    2. False

CRITICAL THINKING QUESTIONS

1. What steps are most appropriate for a new pediatric nurse to take when he or she suspects a child has been physically or emotionally abused?

2. What family resources are available in your community to assist families with undue stress, lack of resources, or those who have social isolation?

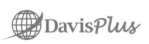 **DavisPlus**

For additional resources and information, visit **www.DavisPlus.com.** Post-Conference Questions and Activities, Answers, and References can be found on DavisPlus.

unit EIGHT

Deviations in Pediatric Health

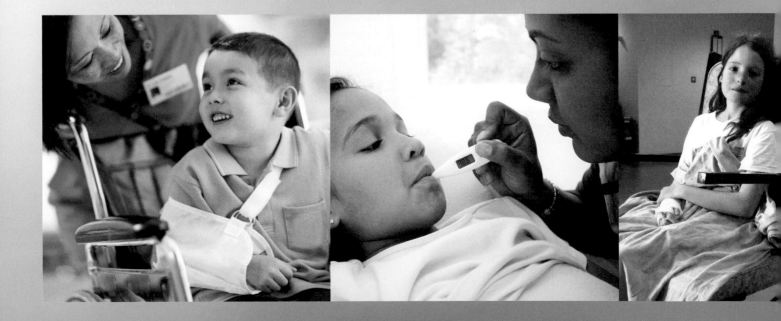

29

Child With a Neurological Condition

KEY TERMS

cranial nerves
encephalopathy
grand mal seizure
increased intracranial pressure (ICP)
ketogenic diet
meningitis
myoclonic
Reye's syndrome
status epilepticus (SE)
tonic-clonic seizure

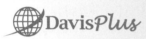 **DavisPlus** For audio pronunciation guide, visit www.DavisPlus.com

CHAPTER CONCEPTS

Assessment
Inflammation
Neurologic Regulation
Oxygenation
Perfusion
Trauma

LEARNING OUTCOMES

1. Define the key terms.
2. Describe the anatomy and physiology of the peripheral nervous system (PNS) and central nervous system (CNS).
3. Discuss each of the senses and describe the developmental process of sensory organs at birth.
4. State the components of a holistic nervous system assessment, including the 12 cranial nerves and rapid neurological checks.
5. Analyze the clinical presentation and various functioning levels of children with varying degrees of cognitive impairment (CI).
6. Discuss the phenomenon of and the clinical outcomes of a child who experiences "near drowning."
7. State the serum value of lead that denotes lead poisoning in children.
8. Define the various types of seizure disorders and describe the assessments, nursing care, and treatments for each.
9. Analyze the consequences of various nervous system pathologies, including hydrocephalus, neural tube defects, meningitis, Reye's syndrome, and intraventricular hemorrhage (IVH).
10. Describe factors associated with a diagnosis of a traumatic brain injury.
11. Discuss the clinical phenomenon of childhood migraine headaches and describe the various treatment options for this condition.
12. Describe issues of safety relative to a child with a neurological disorder or condition, including safe environments, safety precautions, rapid assessments for changes in clinical status, and safety around medications for neurological conditions.

REAL-WORLD CASE STUDY

Randal

■ Randal, a 16-year-old patient presented to the emergency department (ED) with severe headache, fever for 4 days, moderate dehydration, and a large lesion on his right toe that was not healing. The parents described how worried they were about his level of illness and quickly brought him in to the ED when he became confused at the dinner table. After laboratory specimens, wound culture, and blood culture were all taken, and after a 20 mL/kg 0.9% normal saline (NS) bolus was administered, the teen became lethargic. The child was admitted into the pediatric intensive care unit (PICU) with an initial diagnosis of bacterial meningitis and was prepared for a lumbar puncture. His cerebral spinal fluid (CSF) was cloudy and his temperature increased to 39.3°C. Broad spectrum antibiotics were started STAT. Randall demonstrated focal seizure activity within 1 hour of being admitted to the PICU, and was immediately placed on seizure precautions. An appropriate safe dose of lorazepam was administered through his IV to stop his seizure activity. Randal was placed on droplet precautions with constant supervision in the PICU. Randal's parents were very frightened and expressed great concern about his rapid decline. The nursing supervisor came and spoke to them, educated them about the condition, oriented them to the unit, and offered them a sleeping room so they could stay overnight and keep updated.

1. What are standard assessment tools that are used to monitor a child with a suspected neurological condition?
2. How does the team secure seizure precautions?
3. What are the side effects of antiseizure medications?
4. How can family-centered care be implemented for this teen's parents so they feel they are engaged with the health-care team?

CONCEPTUAL CORNERSTONE

Sensory Perception
The child's perception of sensory stimulation is produced by the nerve tissue of the PNS and CNS. The concept relates to all neurological structures that take in and process sensory information. The neuron, being the central component of the sensory experience, is protected by a myelin sheath. When a child experiences a sensory stimulation, either pleasure, pain, or other sensory information, the stimulus is transformed into an electrical current that runs between afferent nerve fibers (ie, toward the brain) to the area of the brain that corresponds to interpretation. The brain then processes the sensory stimuli. Efferent nerve fibers (ie, away from the brain and toward the body) then respond to the brain's interpretation with a motor movement. Sensory perception is key to safety. If a child experiences a pain or sensation, the brain will process the information and cause the child to move away from, let go, or recoil from the uncomfortable sensation. Young infants, with nerve fibers yet to be myelinated, respond with primitive reflexes that are replaced with purposeful movement as the nerves mature cephalocaudally (ie, head down to inferior extremities).

Before one can provide care to a child with a neurological disorder, it is important to review the anatomy of the neurological system. The two main divisions of the nervous system consist of the CNS and the PNS. Each of these two systems has unique functions to regulate all of the systems of the human body. The autonomic nervous system (ANS) provides bodily functions without conscious effort and includes the motor and sensory nuclei in the brain and spinal cord.

THE DEVELOPMENT OF THE NERVOUS SYSTEM

During early embryonic development, the nervous system is beginning to develop. During the later intrauterine developmental period, the fetus has been shown to respond to stimuli. After birth, the neonate's nervous system continues to develop and, within the first year of life, the infant moves from primitive reflexes to purposeful movement and on to the beginning of fine motor movement. The pincer grasp, with an average age of first presentation at age 7 to 8 months, is an example of the steady development of the infant from reactive movements, such as reflexes, to fine motor movements, such as being able to pick up a small object with the fingers (Fig. 29.1).

Central Nervous System

The CNS is composed of the brain and the complete spinal cord. The brain contains the cerebrum, which is the center of consciousness, and the two cerebral hemispheres. The frontal lobe controls speech, voluntary muscle movements,

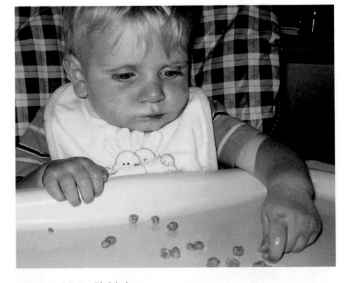

FIGURE 29.1 Child showing a pincer grasp.

center for personality, and areas for behavioral, autonomic, and intellectual functions. The brain also contains the temporal lobe for taste, hearing, and smell; the parietal lobe for sensory coordination and interpretation; and the occipital lobe for visual stimuli interpretation. Other anatomical components of the brain are the diencephalon, which houses the thalamus (sensory relay for pain, pressure, and temperature), the hypothalamus (controls the ANS; regulates emotion, behavior, hunger, and thirst; and secretes antidiuretic hormone and oxytocin), the cerebellum, and the brainstem.

Peripheral Nervous System

The PNS is composed of the 12 pairs of cranial nerves and the 31 pairs of the spinal nerves. **Cranial nerves** are numbered by order they contact the brain; they originate in the cranial cavity and innervate the head (Fig. 29.2). This system connects the brain to the remote areas of the child's body. The PNS has both afferent neurons (ie, sensory) that

transmit information from the organs, skin, and tissue to the brain, and efferent neurons (ie, motor) that transmit regulatory and control information from the brain to the body. Figure 29.3 depicts the nerves of the spinal cord and vertebral structures.

TEAM WORKS

Team Assessment of a Child's Cranial Nerves

The pediatric health-care team will work together to assess a child's cranial nerves.

I Olfactory: Provides the ability to transmit a sense of smell to nasal cavity (tested with a cotton ball soaked with stimulus such as vanilla oil)

II Optic: Provides the ability to transmit visual signals from the retina of the eye to the brain (tested with various visual cues)

III Oculomotor: Provides the ability to perform most eye movements (tested by requesting the patient follow finger commands)

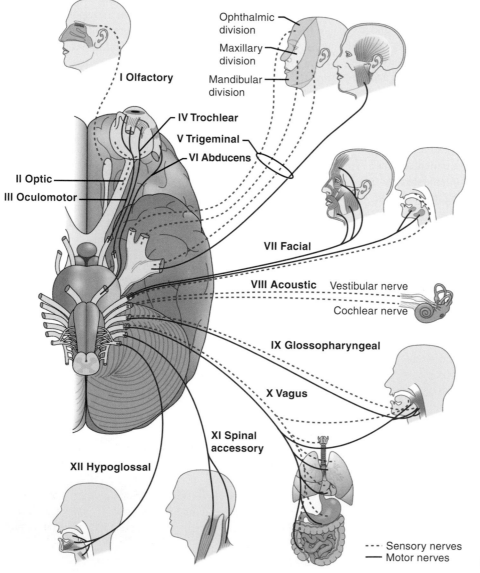

FIGURE 29.2 Cranial nerve origins.

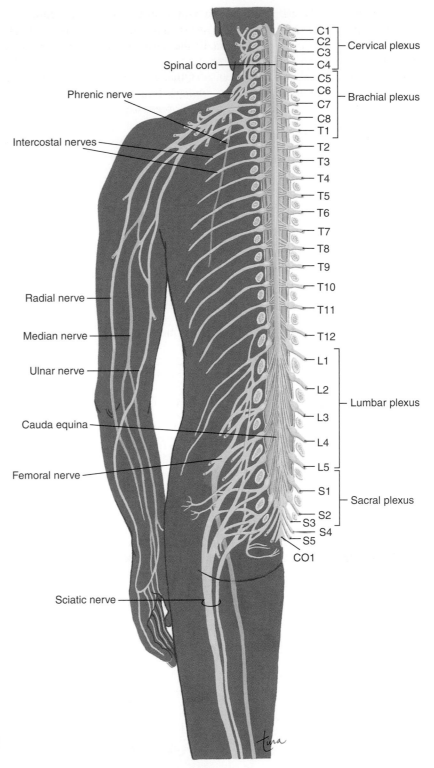

FIGURE 29.3 The spinal cord and vertebral body.

IV Trochlear: Provides the ability to laterally rotate the eyeball (tested by asking the patient to rotate the eyeball inward, down, up, and outward)

V Trigeminal: Provides the ability to feel sensations in the face and perform mastication (tested by requesting the patient to perform chewing movements on command and testing the patient's response to cotton ball sensations to the full face)

VI Abducens: Provides the ability to perform abducted movements of the eye (tested by requesting that the patient follow commands to move eyes left and right)

VII Facial: Provides the ability to demonstrate motor movements of facial expressions and taste of anterior 2/3 of tongue (tested by requesting the patient to move her face in various expressions, and by testing taste on the front of the tongue)

VIII Acoustic: Provides the ability to detect sound, body rotation, and gravity (tested by assessing the patient's ability to hear bilaterally, close the eyes, and know where his or her body is in relation to gravitational pull)

IX Glossopharyngeal: Provides the ability to taste in the posterior 1/3 of the tongue (tested by providing the patient with various tastes by providing stimuli such as salt, sugar, and bitters)

X Vagus: Provides the ability to vocalize and swallow effectively (tested by assessing the ability of the patient to vocalize and the effectiveness of the patient's ability to swallow)

XI Spinal accessory: Provides the ability to use the sternocleidomastoid and trapezius muscles (tested by asking the patient to shrug and move the head effectively side-to-side and up-and-down)

XII Hypoglossal: Provides the ability to move all muscles of the tongue (tested by requesting the patient perform bolus swallowing and speech articulation)

The following is a common mnemonic that helps to remember the cranial nerves:

On Old Olympus' Towering Tops, A Finn And German Viewed Some Hops

Autonomic Nervous System

The ANS is responsible for involuntary body functions. The ANS regulates salivation, digestion, respiration, perspiration, urination, cardiovascular function, and sexual arousal by way of the hypothalamus, which supervises the sympathetic nervous system (SNS) and the parasympathetic nervous system.

Sympathetic Nervous System

The SNS provides the emergency responses the body needs to respond to stimuli. This includes the "fight or flight" response, which entails decreased peristalsis, increased heart contractions, peripheral blood vessel constriction, increased perspiration, bronchiole dilation for effective breathing, and dilation of the heart and peripheral blood vessels. All of these contribute to a response to physical or emotional stress.

The Brain

The brain, which includes the three protective membranes—dura mater, arachnoid membrane, and pia mater—provides the coordination of the entire nervous system (Fig. 29.4). CSF forms in the brain's lateral ventricles and flows through the third and fourth ventricle to circulate to the subarachnoid space of the spinal cord (Fig. 29.5). Excessive CSF is absorbed by the arachnoid membrane to keep a fluid and pressure balance.

After a child's skull bone fuses and can no longer provide a means of adapting to increased pressure (eg, with an abscess, a tumor, or brain injury), the ICP balance is maintained by three homeostatic mechanisms:

- Production or absorption of CSF within the brain
- Blood vessel dilation or constriction within the brain
- Production and circulation of hormones that cause increased or decreased production of urine (ie, aldosterone)

The child's age and developmental level provide guidance about how to assess functioning of the CNS. Although the CNS is one of the first systems to form within uterine fetal development, it is actually one of the last to fully mature during childhood. Myelination needs to take place throughout the brain for motor control and coordination, as well as for cognitive maturity. The ability of infants' cranial sutures and fontanels to respond to pressure allows for compensation when increased ICP is occurring. **Increased intracranial pressure (ICP)** is increased pressure within the brain's ventricles that

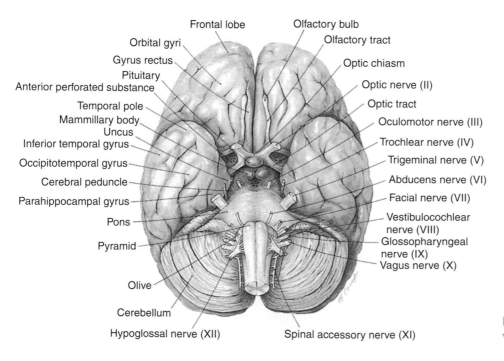

FIGURE 29.4 Brain structures as viewed from the ventral surface.

Frontal lobe
Orbital gyri
Gyrus rectus
Pituitary
Anterior perforated substance
Temporal pole
Mammillary body
Uncus
Inferior temporal gyrus
Occipitotemporal gyrus
Cerebral peduncle
Parahippocampal gyrus
Pons
Pyramid
Olive
Cerebellum
Hypoglossal nerve (XII)

Olfactory bulb
Olfactory tract
Optic chiasm
Optic nerve (II)
Optic tract
Oculomotor nerve (III)
Trochlear nerve (IV)
Trigeminal nerve (V)
Abducens nerve (VI)
Facial nerve (VII)
Vestibulocochlear nerve (VIII)
Glossopharyngeal nerve (IX)
Vagus nerve (X)
Spinal accessory nerve (XI)

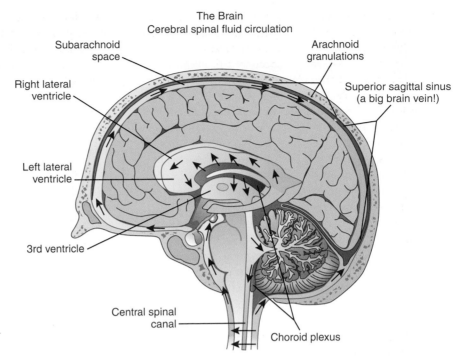

The Brain
Cerebral spinal fluid circulation

FIGURE 29.5 CSF circulation and corresponding structures.

is caused by either an overproduction or a lack of absorption of CSF. The ability of the cranial sutures to open, if needed, and the ability of the fontanels to bulge under pressure, abruptly stops when the bones completely fuse.

COMMON NEUROLOGICAL DISORDERS DURING CHILDHOOD

CNS disorders are a varied group affecting one or more of the intricate components of the system: the brain, spinal cord, CNS, PNS, and ANS. Trauma, injuries, accidents, infections, tumors, and congenital anomalies can all contribute to the development of CNS disorders. Figure 29.6 illustrates the major locations of brain infections.

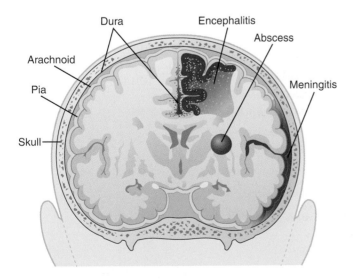

FIGURE 29.6 Major brain infection locations.

Nursing care of children with CNS diseases or disorders requires rapid assessments, followed by comprehensive workups and diagnostics examinations, then careful monitoring for changes in clinical status or the development of complications. Complications associated with CNS diseases or disorders can have devastating effects, leading to permanent brain damage or lasting motor or sensory dysfunction. Nurses must have a foundation of knowledge about how to conduct assessments and then know what to report to whom so the child can be stabilized. Medications are an important part of caring for a child with a neurological disorder.

The pediatric nurse must master developmentally-focused neurological assessments to report deviations or changes rapidly to the health-care team. It is imperative that these assessments be practiced so that when faced with an emergency, CNS injury, brain infection, or suspected child abuse case, including shaken baby syndrome, the nurse can identify changes in normal or expected neurological health and report them to the appropriate team member for further diagnostics or interventions. Mastery of neurological assessments will save lives by decreasing morbidity and mortality.

TEAM WORKS

Interdisciplinary Neurological Assessments
Pediatric nurses assist the health-care team in providing complete health histories and rapid physical examinations. When a child presents with a neurological concern, the team works together to determine factors that influence the condition and to identify all clinical presentations of the disorder.
Health History
• Risk factors for neurological system injury (eg, accidents, intentional injuries such as child abuse)

- Risk factors associated with perinatal period such as injury, infections, maternal toxic exposures, illicit drug use, alcohol use, and prematurity
- Familial history of seizures, cranial deformities, mental illness, neural tube defects, and chromosomal anomalies

Physical Examination

- Rapid visual assessment: Rapid assessment of the level of consciousness, skin color for cyanosis, and ability to breathe effectively
- Further inspection of child including level of consciousness (ie, full, confused, disoriented, lethargic, obtunded, coma) and posturing (ie, decorticate and decerebrate), as well as abnormal movements such as tremors, seizure activity, or tics
- Vital signs (VSs) assessing for hypertension or hypotension, widening pulse pressure, bradycardia, and dyspnea/apnea. Temperature should be taken to assess for abnormal core body temperatures. (Do not attempt oral temperatures in a neurologically impaired or seizing child.)
- Remember! A fixed and dilated pupil is a serious neurosurgical emergency!
- Remember! A brainstem herniation presents with opisthotonos, nuchal rigidity, poor PERRLA (ie, Pupils Equal, Round, and Reactive to Light and Accommodation), bradycardia, abnormal respiratory patterns, and increased blood pressure reading for age with widening pulse pressure (ie, widening systolic and diastolic readings)!

When a child first presents with concerns, rapid examinations are conducted to quickly assess the status of the child's neurological system. A rapid neurological examination includes a quick assessment of the child from head to toe:

- Overall level of consciousness and ability to respond to verbal and tactile/pain stimuli
- Short- and long-term memory
- Ability to speak without slurring, delay, or regression
- Ability to swallow effectively
- Use of accessory muscles
- Strength of hand grip and strength of movement of legs
- Incontinence in a potty-trained child
- Cerebellar status of balance, coordination, and gait

Other assessments are important for a pediatric nurse to review to be prepared for a child who presents with suspected or confirmed neurological concerns. For the newborn and young infant, primitive reflexes are assessed to investigate neurological health. Primitive reflexes occur in the infant's brainstem or areas of the spinal cord. The absence of reflexes in the developmental period of a newborn or young infant does not confirm the presence of neurological disease, injury, or concern. The assessment of reflexes is part of a holistic neurological assessment and gives basic information about the communication pattern between the CNS and the PNS, and the health of the system. Exaggerated primitive reflexes may demonstrate a condition of the CNS whereas diminished primitive reflex responses

may indicate a condition of the PNS. Most newborn and infant primitive reflexes are gone by the first few months of life.

The following neonate and young infant reflexes are assessed:

- **Moro's:** Movement with a change in equilibrium, such as a sudden movement down that causes the child to reach his or her arms up and grasp with the fingers
- **Sucking:** Ability to demonstrate effective sucking movements when an area around infant's mouth is touched
- **Startle:** Movement when exposed to a loud sound, with pulling of the arms and legs in toward the trunk
- **Fencing/Tonic Neck:** Movement of arms with a rapid, small movement of head; child will pose in fencing position with the arm extended and the fist opened on the side the head is turned toward, bringing in the arm on the opposite side while clenching that fist
- **Dancing/Step:** Small stepping motions when the child is held carefully up by the trunk (not under the arms); child demonstrates small steps when the sole of the foot touches a surface

Assessment of infant's fontanels is also part of a neurological assessment. The infant should be in an upright position for the assessment. The health-care provider assesses for a recessed fontanel, which could indicate dehydration, or a bulging fontanel, which could indicate increased ICP.

LABS & DIAGNOSTICS

- Laboratory studies that may be ordered to assess a child's neurological health include:
    - Electrolytes to rule out disturbances such as hypernatremia or hyponatremia
    - Complete blood cell count (CBC) to rule out signs of infection
    - Serum lead level to assess for lead exposure or toxicity
    - Blood culture to rule out severe infections
- Diagnostic tests that may be ordered to assess a child's neurological status include:
    - Lumbar puncture to collect CSF and cultures for infections
    - Electroencephalogram (EEG)
    - Urinalysis to rule out toxic exposures

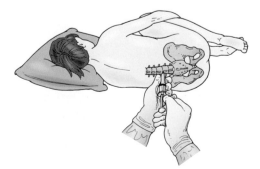

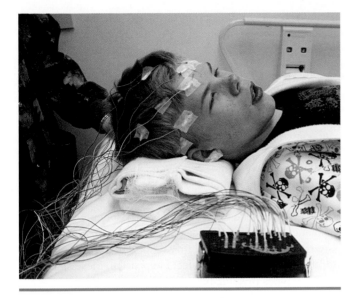

Neurological disorders in childhood often require long medical treatment plans and care. The degree of disability and restoration of function depends on the location of the disorder, the amount of damage that has occurred, and the quality and timeliness of medical interventions. Frequently, children are required to be on medications that promote stability of the neurological disease. See Table 29.1 for a list of common medications pediatric nurses should be aware of.

THE FIVE SENSES

Infants are born with some intact sensory organs, and others that must mature with time and exposure. For instance,

hearing is considered fully intact at birth after the amniotic fluid is removed from the external ear canal. Olfactory (ie, smell) is also considered fully intact at birth. Visual acuity is dependent on nerve maturation. An infant's visual acuity is thought to range between 20/200 and 20/300 and is not fully intact until close to the child's fifth birthday. Touch is thought to be fully intact at birth, but the sense of taste must develop.

CONGENITAL NEUROLOGICAL DISORDERS

A congenital disorder is one that exists from birth. These disorders can take place during fetal development or during the pre-, intra-, or immediate postbirthing process. There are a number of conditions that affect a child's neurological health that can be linked to either fetal development or the birthing process. The following outlines the most prevalent congenital conditions within the neurological system.

Cerebral Palsy

Cerebral palsy (CP) represents a group of disorders that involves the functioning of the nervous system and brain. CP is considered a birth accident from anoxia before, during, or after the birth process up to the second year of life. Premature infants have a higher risk of developing CP because of the higher incidence of bleeding in the brain, brain infections, severe jaundice, and head injuries. CP is a nonprogressive injury of the brain and nervous system directly related to a low level of oxygen to the CNS structures, which is termed *hypoxia*. Symptoms of CP can be mild to very severe. The degree of disability relates to the severity of the hypoxia episode.

There are five types of CP:

1. **Ataxic:** Poor muscle coordination, poor equilibrium, and unsteady gait with possible wide-based gait
2. **Spastic:** Hypertonicity with poor posture control, legs scissoring, altered quality of speech, persistent primitive reflexes, and persistent muscle contractions with potential development of contractures
3. **Hypotonic:** Generalized poor muscle control with muscle dystrophy
4. **Dyskinetic:** Also called *dyskinetic-athetoid*, this type involves constant involuntary wormlike movements that diminish during sleep and that affect facial musculature
5. **Mixed:** Child presents with a variety of CP clinical presentations

Assessments of Cerebral Palsy

The child may have CP involving one or both sides of the body. CP may affect both arms, both legs, or only one arm or leg. Symptoms, if severe, may be detectable at 3 months of life. The child with CP will demonstrate delayed motor growth and mastery of first year skills such as rolling over, sitting up, crawling, standing, and walking.

TABLE 29.1 MEDICATIONS COMMONLY USED IN NEUROLOGICAL DISORDERS

Purpose	Drug Used
Anticonvulsants to prevent or manage seizure activity	• Gabapentin (Neurontin) • Clonazepam (Klonopin)
Diuretics to decrease increased ICP	• Mannitol (Osmitrol) • Furosemide (Lasix)
Neuromuscular blockers to prevent resistance to mechanical ventilation and agitation	• Pancuronium (Pavulon) • Rocuronium (Zemuron)
CNS stimulants to treat attention deficit hyperactivity disorders	• Methylphenidate (Concerta, Ritalin) • Dextroamphetamine (Adderall)

Assessments for CP include identifying the presence of one or more of the following signs:

- Tight muscles that do not stretch, possibly worsening over time
- "Scissors" movements of arms and legs
- Joint contractures in which the joints do not open and do not have full range of motion (ROM)
- Paralysis or muscle weakness
- Determination if the motor symptoms are present bilaterally or unilaterally
- The presence of tremors
- Floppy extremities or overextension of joint areas
- Ability to suck, swallow, and manage secretions
- The presence of pain
- Effectiveness of airway for ventilation, airway clearance, and the containment of saliva

Interventions for Cerebral Palsy

There are no treatments or cure for CP. The pediatric health-care team provides support, symptom management, and interventions to promote mobility and socialization, and to reduce injuries. Medications exist that assist with spasticity, drooling, and tremors. Surgical procedures exist to reduce joint contractures and severe gastroesophageal reflux.

 DRUG FACTS

Treatment for motor spasticity and excessive drooling includes the administration of the botulinum toxin. Baclofen is a pharmaceutical agent that has been effective in reducing spasticity and tremors.

Nursing Considerations for Cerebral Palsy

Nursing considerations focus on assisting the pediatric health-care team to reduce complications for the child with CP. Teaching the family how to maintain a clear airway is imperative. Demonstrating how to perform passive ROM exercises helps to slow the process of contractures. Pediatric nurses need to monitor for the development of poor nutrition, failure to thrive (FTT), constipation, bowel obstruction, and osteoporosis.

Safety is a key component to the care of a child with CP and includes all aspects of the child's life, including the prevention of aspiration, falls, and contractures. Maintaining safe equipment for mobility and preventing pressure ulcers is paramount.

Neural Tube Defects

Neural tube defects are considered a group of disorders within the CNS system related directly to birth defects. The inappropriate closure of the neural tube during embryonic development can lead to one of several neural tube defects. Each defect has varied levels of clinical symptoms and disability associated with the severity of the deficit. Although the origin of a neural tube defect is considered multifactorial, there is a strong association with the lack of sufficient maternal folic acid consumption at the time of conception. The following list represents the several types of neural tube defects found in childhood.

- **Anencephaly:** The child is born with a severe brain anomaly that is associated with the absence of both hemispheres and the presence of a brainstem and cerebellum only. If the newborn survives, the child's condition is incompatible with life and death will occur in time.
- **Encephalocele:** The child is born with an abnormal sac of fluid that causes the brain tissue to herniate through an abnormal defect in the skull. The brain tissue may be found within this sac.
- **Spina Bifida:** The child is born with a defect within the spinal column. Spina bifida occulta means there are no signs other than the possibility of skin dimpling at the site of the defect. When the defect is apparent, there are two general types of spina bifida:
  - **Type 1: Myelomeningocele:** The child is born with a portion of the vertebral column not closed, leading to the protrusion of a sac containing not only CSF but also the meninges and a portion of the child's spinal cord.
  - **Type 2: Meningocele:** The child is born with a defect in the bony spinal column resulting in an abnormal protrusion of a CSF-filled sac located externally to the child's spinal column.

Assessments of Neural Tube Defects

Assessments of neural tube defects, including spina bifida, start with appropriate and early fetal assessments. Ultrasounds should determine the presence of the abnormality and a Cesarean section for safe delivery is a must.

The pediatric nurse should assess for neurological disabilities below the level of the deficit. Frequent head circumferences will be ordered to assess for hydrocephalus. Because nerves for bowel and bladder innervate below the site of the defect, the nurse should assess bowel and bladder function.

Interventions for Neural Tube Defects

After birth, the abnormal sac should be handled with care and the nurse assesses for leaks, rupture, and infection around the sac area or infection in the CNS in general. The sac should be kept moist by carefully applying NS-soaked gauze. The family will need support and interdisciplinary team teaching to better understand the consequences of the surgery and possible long-term deficits.

The child will have routine postoperative care that focuses on fluid balance, preventing infection, and special care to the skin at the operative site. The child should be provided early ROM and support for the lower extremities that may have neurological deficits. The bladder may need intermittent catheterization.

Nursing Considerations for Neural Tube Defects

Nursing considerations for neural tube defects include paying special consideration to the development of latex allergy because this population has a much higher incidence in the development of this allergy.

Families need to understand that the child with neural tube defect can have a healthy and productive life but that they will need to be aware of associated motor limitations and the possibility of bladder catheterization. Pediatric nurses must teach the public about the importance of taking folic acid starting before conception and continuing during pregnancy as part of healthy eating and adhering to prenatal vitamins.

NEUROLOGICAL INJURIES

Across the developmental period, children can experience severe injuries that affect the health and function of the neurological system. Injuries can be to the child's PNS or CNS. Many of these devastating injuries can be prevented with appropriate supervision, teaching the child safety, and by providing anticipatory guidance to caregivers and parents. The following section outlines several neurological injuries.

Drowning and Near Drowning

Injuries remain the most common cause of death during childhood beyond the first few days of the newborn's life. Primary prevention of injuries is an important part of a pediatric nurse's family education responsibilities. Averting an injury reduces childhood morbidity and mortality. Drowning ranks high overall as the cause of unintentional injuries throughout childhood (CDC, 2015). The two peak periods for drowning or near drowning are in the preschool period and during later adolescence.

Drowning is defined as a submersion in a liquid medium followed by suffocation and asphyxia. With submersion, rapid and irreversible multisystemic injuries occur, which can lead to death. When a child dies with the 24-hour time period after submersion, it is titled *drowning*. If the child lives beyond 24 hours, even if the child later recovers or dies, it is titled *near drowning*. Toddlers and preschoolers are at risk when they are unsupervised, which typically occurs in residential pools and bathtubs, and around buckets or trashcans of water. Adolescents are at risk, especially boys between 15 and 19 years of age, for drowning or near drowning at natural bodies of water such as lakes, ponds, rivers, and oceans. In the United States, 90% of all drownings and near drownings for children younger than age 5 occur at home pools (CDC, 2015). Gender distribution for near drowning has a ratio of males to females of 4:1.

Degrees of disability associated with drownings and near drownings are related to the victim's clinical course. The outcome of the event relates to duration of submersion, circumstances surrounding the event, rapid response of the rescue, and how effective the postsubmersion resuscitative efforts are. The pathology of near drowning can be summarized as a multiorgan effect of hypoxemia. Cardiopulmonary resuscitation (CPR) should start at the scene to rapidly restore oxygenation, ventilation, and circulation. Close to 80% of all childhood near drowning victims survive, and close to 92% of those make a complete recovery (CDC, 2015). If a child requires transfer to a tertiary PICU, the survival rate with neurological recovery drops to approximately 50%; up to 35%

will perish; and up to 27% will suffer severe brain damage (Behrman, Kliegman, et al, 2001).

Assessments of Drowning and Near Drowning

Assessments for a child brought into the health-care arena for postsubmersion injury involve assessing the airway, ventilation ability, quality of respirations, presence of effective heart rate and blood pressure, arterial blood gases (ABGs), and level of hypothermia. Level of neurological intactness and level of consciousness should be assessed.

Interventions for Drowning and Near Drowning

Interventions for drowning victims include rapid and effective advanced resuscitation, including ventilator support using oxygen, restoration of cardiac rhythm, correction of hypercapnia and hypoxia, correction of shock (signs are altered mental status, cool extremities, and slow capillary refill), and IV fluid administration with boluses of a nondextrose-containing solution such as lactated Ringer's (LR) solution or NS. It is common for the child to suffer extensive volume depletion because of severe pulmonary edema and intracompartmental fluid shifts. Wet clothes must be removed, the environmental temperature must be very warm, and the child should be wrapped in warmed blankets.

Nursing Considerations for Drowning and Near Drowning

Nursing considerations include supporting the team during the resuscitative efforts. They also include supporting the family, who will be in great distress and emotional shock. Initiating a rapid referral for a social worker, clergy, or other spiritual support system and offering to call extended family should be considered.

Intraventricular Hemorrhage (IVH)

IVH is a very severe diagnosis within the CNS. In IVH, the child experiences a rupture of the vascular network of the circulation within the germinal matrix and a bleed within the brain develops. Depending on severity of the bleed, the child may have full recovery or may experience severe brain damage or death from the anoxia associated with the bleed and pressure. The most common age group for an IVH is prematurity, when the infant is less than 32 weeks' gestation. IVH can develop secondary to severe neonatal respiratory distress, birth asphyxia, metabolic disorders, or congenital vascular structural anomaly. Close to 90% of cases develop not at birth but within 3 days of birth.

Assessments of Intraventricular Hemorrhage

The child with suspected IVH will have an MRI or a CT scan to confirm the bleed. Serial hemoglobin and hematocrit levels will be drawn to assess the severity and continuation of the bleed. ICP will be measured and assessed on a regular basis. The child with IVH will show somnolence, very poor muscle tone, and the absence of Moro's reflex. In very severe cases, the child may demonstrate bulging and tense fontanels.

Interventions for Intraventricular Hemorrhage

Interventions for IVH include providing a reduced stimuli environment and minimal handling of the child. Care is taken to keep the head midline and relaxed to decrease hydrostatic pressure changes, which cause further ICP. The child may require transfusion therapy while being treated for ICP and acidosis, which is provided with catheter placement (ie, ventriculostomy) and removal of the subdural fluid collection.

Nursing Considerations for Intraventricular Hemorrhage

One of the most important nursing considerations for a child receiving care for IVH is to keep the child's head midline, comfortable, and supported. Any movement of the child's head should be done with great caution and should require the assistance of two staff members. Any stimulation that would produce discomfort or crying should be minimized.

Lead Poisoning

Lead is everywhere. Lead is a commercially used substance that appears as a heavy, soft, and gray-blue metal substance; it can be a naturally occurring substance. Lead poisoning is particularly tragic in children because undetected high levels of lead can lead to encephalopathy, poor school performance, and lower intelligence levels. **Encephalopathy** is a generalized brain dysfunction of varying degrees that causes an impairment of arousal, orientation, speech, and cognitive processing.

Lead is considered highly toxic because of its affinity for a group of proteins called sulfhydryl (SH). After binding to this protein group, lead irreversibly impairs brain function. This impairment causes the brain tissues to become affected, leading to acute encephalopathy. This encephalopathy is often preceded by behavioral changes such as attention disorders, intellectual disabilities, hyperactivity, colic, constipation, and severe abdominal pain. The ensuing encephalopathy leads to ataxia, papilledema, seizures, impaired consciousness, and coma. A child with significant lead poisoning must be rapidly removed from the source of exposure and then hospitalized for treatment of the lead poisoning.

Lead poisoning continues to be a national concern. Children are exposed to lead in their environments through contaminated soils in play areas, contaminated clothing worn by parents who work in lead dust environments, exposure to lead-based paints in older homes, and imported candy, jewelry, and pottery that were processed with lead. Although lead paint was banned from consumer use in 1977, lead can be released into a child's home environment via peeling or chipped paint, chalking procedures, or renovation activities of older homes. Lead-contaminated household dust from paint remains the number one lead exposure source for American children (National Institutes of Health [NIH], 2015). See Box 29.1 for a summary of cultural practices that have the potential to cause increased lead level exposures in children.

Box 29.1 Cultural Practices that May Increase Lead Exposure

Families need education about the potential exposure to lead from their culturally based health-care practices. Pediatric nurses have the responsibility to identify when complementary or alternative health-care practices or substances are being used to treat a child's health-care condition, and rapidly report such use to the health-care team. All alternative, naturopathic, and complementary medical practices should be reported to the pediatric health-care team so that the team can assess their indications, dosing, and side effects for safety. Families should be approached with respect so that full disclosure can be secured. The following bulleted lists provide cultural pediatric health-care remedies that may expose children to lead if consumed.

- Lead-containing remedies used by some Asian communities include:
  - *Bali goli*
  - *Chuifong*
  - *Ba-baw-san*
  - *Ghasard*
  - *Tokuwan*
  - *Kandu*
- Lead-containing remedies used in Mexico to treat colic-like illnesses (referred to as *empaco*) include:
  - *Rueda*
  - *Liga*
  - *Coral*
  - *Alarcon*
  - *Maria Luisa*
- Lead-containing cosmetics and remedies used by various Middle Eastern cultures include:
  - *Saoott*
  - *Cebagin*
  - *Alkohl*

Lead can also be consumed by children through the following sources:

- Root vegetables that uptake lead from contaminated soil
- Imported cans that contain food processed in other countries
- Pottery or ceramic when the layer of protective glaze wears off
- Brass fixtures, lead pipes, solder, and older plumbing in homes built before 1986
- Candies such as the chili-based sweets imported from Mexico

Degrees of disability are related to toxic lead exposure. The Centers for Disease Control and Prevention (CDC) offers guidelines (CDC, 2014) for recognizing when a serum lead level shows potential toxicity in children. See Table 29.2 for the CDC's serum blood lead levels and recommended subsequent actions.

DRUG FACTS

Medical Treatments for Lead Poisoning and Associated Lead Encephalopathy

Indications: Medical interventions and treatments are initiated when the child is symptomatic or when the child's blood lead levels are above 19.

Medication: **Dimercaprol (BAL)**, 75 mg/m² every 4 hours for a total daily dose of 450 mg/m²

- Side effects: Serious side effects include hypertension and nephrotoxicity.
- Precautions: Do not administer to a child who is currently taking iron supplements because the combination of the two can cause severe nausea and vomiting.
- Administration guidelines: Assess if the child has a peanut allergy. Dimercaprol may contain peanut oil.
- Nursing considerations: Causes significant pain on intramuscular (IM) injection. Check with the pharmacy to see if lidocaine or procaine may be added to the IM shot to minimize the pain on injection. May cause burning sensations in throat, mouth, and lips. May cause tachycardia and feelings of restlessness and anxiety.

Medication: **Edetate calcium-disodium (EDTA)**, 1,500 mg/m²/24 hours by continuous infusion

- Side effects: Serious side effects include renal tubular necrosis.
- Precautions: Child may develop cerebral edema from rapid increase in ICP during IV infusion. IM route may be preferred. Pregnancy and lactation safety have not been established. A child with known kidney problems, low blood pressure, or low urinary output (UOP) should not be given EDTA.
- Administration guidelines: 35 mg/kg twice daily IM every 12 hours for 3 to 5 days. If a second dose is required, at least 4 days should pass between doses.
- Nursing considerations: Because EDTA is excreted in the urine, secure the patient's IV and establish UOP before infusing. For accuracy, wait 1 hour after administration before drawing postinfusion serum lead blood samples. Warn the family that the child may have allergy-like symptoms of a runny nose. Chills and fever are common.

Assessments of Lead Poisoning

Initial assessments of a child with suspected lead poisoning include a thorough and accurate assessment of the child's environmental history, including the year the home was built and the type of paint used. Lead-containing paint places a child at high risk for exposure. It is imperative to assess the child's age and participation in teething on window sills or doorways, or the child's participation in pica behaviors. A nickel-size lead-based paint chip will cause blood levels to rise.

TABLE 29.2 CENTERS FOR DISEASE CONTROL AND PREVENTION LEAD LEVELS RECOMMENDATIONS

Blood Level (micrograms/dL)	Actions Recommended
0–9	No immediate concerns for the child, follow-up needed
Greater than or equal to 10	Considered "lead poisoned"
10–14	Conduct a survey of the environment; if many children are found, then survey the community for the source of lead exposure
15–19	Conduct a survey of the environment, and provide education to families about lead exposure and increased health risks with exposure
20–24	Remove the child from the source of the lead and bring the child to the medical facility for a workup
25–54	Remove the child from the source of lead, conduct testing, and, if positive, treat
55–69	Remove the child from the source of lead and treat with EDTA or DMSA
Greater than or equal to 70	Rapidly provide emergency hospitalization and treat with BAL and EDTA

Children may present with the following symptoms of lead poisoning:

- Metallic taste in mouth
- Gastrointestinal (GI) upset, including abdominal cramping
- Decreased UOP
- Alteration in mentation
- Parents describing their child as having a "personality change"
- Black-blue discoloration or line along the gums
- Paresthesia or abnormal sensations

Interventions for Lead Poisoning

Interventions for lead poisoning begin with the confirmation of the child's blood level. All symptomatic children, regardless of their measured lead blood level, are medically treated in a hospital environment. Emergency treatment for symptoms may include a pediatric intensive care stay.

Nursing Considerations for Lead Poisoning

Nursing considerations while caring for a child with suspected or known lead poisoning begin with assessing for changes in normal behavior for the child's developmental stage and age, and then promptly reporting any new signs or symptoms. Children with mild lead exposure require the provision of a safe home, school, and play environment with education for the whole family about the hazards of lead exposure. Children with higher levels of lead poisoning require medical treatments during a hospitalization. Children should be monitored for the side effects of medical therapy, including following clinical nursing protocols about monitoring the child's blood pressure during infusions.

Health-care institutions may have a policy to not discharge or release a child to his or her family home if the home is the suspected source of the lead poisoning. The child and family may need temporary housing until the house is inspected and considered lead-free and environmentally "clean."

PATIENT TEACHING GUIDELINES

There are nationwide family education programs created to promote the awareness of lead poisoning in communities. These programs can help communities identify high-risk homes and buildings, as well as contaminated community spaces. Accurate and reliable home test kits are available. Because lead poisoning has potential long-term consequences for children, the public must continue to have widespread education programs to teach lead exposure prevention. Pediatric nurses should contact their local public health department to ask how they can become involved with educational programs. Health fairs, lectures to parent meetings at schools, and other community awareness programs exist and must continue.

Meningitis

Meningitis is a condition of inflammation of the membranes of the brain or spinal cord, often caused by an infectious process. This inflammation can be caused by bacteria, viruses, or chemical agents that enter the bloodstream and spread through the CSF. When exposed, the pathogen causes severe inflammation of the meninges and possible cerebral edema. Causative organisms include *Escherichia coli* and group B streptococcus (GBS) for newborns and infants, and *Haemophilus influenzae* type B, *Streptococcus pneumoniae,* and *Neisseria meningitidis* for older children. If bacterial or viral in nature, meningitis can be spread by droplets of mucus during sneezing, coughing, or nasal congestion. The organisms that cause meningitis can enter the child's body via the nasal cavity, via the middle ear if the tympanic membrane is injured, via neurosurgery, or via trauma. The incidence of meningitis has been greatly reduced in the public via the administration of the childhood vaccine for *H influenza.*

Meningitis can be found in all ages across childhood but is much more common in infants and toddlers.

Prognosis with meningitis is dependent on the age of the child during infection, which organism is the etiology, and the response to treatment. The younger the child, the greater chance of acquiring bacterial meningitis, which can be fatal if not identified and treated promptly. If the child has acquired viral meningitis, no treatment is warranted other than supportive care with an expected duration of illness of 6 to 10 days. Without treatment, complications include thrombi, brain abscesses, blindness, deafness, seizures, and paralysis.

The most dangerous form of meningitis is meningococcal meningitis. This type of bacterial meningitis is caused by *N meningitidis* and leads to a sudden, rapid, fulminate infection, resulting in disseminated intravascular coagulation (DIC), a life-threatening critical condition; massive adrenal hemorrhages; and purpura; and carries a high mortality rate of 90% or more. If a child of any age presents with abrupt eruption of a purplish rash or petechial rash, the health-care team must suspect meningococcemia and initiate immediate medical attention. Meningococcal meningitis must be identified rapidly with immediate antibiotic administration to save the child's life.

Assessments of Meningitis

Assessments for meningitis include early identification of the following symptoms:

- Poor feeding habits
- Fever
- Irritability, high-pitched cry, and inconsolable when held
- Lethargy
- Bulging fontanels
- Opisthotonos positioning: Hyperextension of the child's neck and back, or nuchal rigidity where the child holds the neck very still
- Kernig's sign: Resistance and sudden pain with knee extension when child is in a supine position with knees flexed up (Fig. 29.7)
- Brudzinski's sign: When the child's neck is flexed during supine position, the child will suddenly flex the knees and hips (Fig. 29.8)

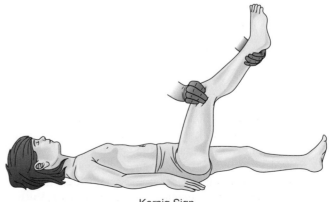

Kernig Sign

FIGURE 29.7 Kernig's sign.

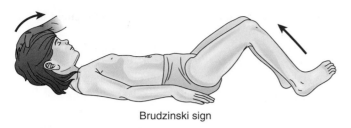

Brudzinski sign

FIGURE 29.8 Brudzinski's sign.

Interventions for Meningitis

After laboratory specimens are rapidly collected for accurate urinalysis, including CBC, CSF culture, and blood culture, antibiotics are started immediately. The antibiotic administered must match the causative organism for the best prognosis and rapid recovery. Corticosteroids may also be administered to prevent cerebral edema and anticonvulsants may be required if the child is seizing from the infection or toxin.

Nursing Considerations for Meningitis

Nursing considerations for meningitis include meticulous maintenance of a patent IV catheter for antibiotic therapy, symptoms management, and fluid as needed. Care should be taken to keep antibiotics administration on time and therapeutic serum values of antibiotics on target. The nurse should keep the child's condition guarded and, until the causative agent is identified, the child should be on strict airborne and contact isolation. The combination of these two forms of isolation is often termed *respiratory isolation* and should be left in place for 24 to 48 hours after the administration of antibiotics begins. Some institutions require no less than three doses of antibiotics to be administered before respiratory isolation is discontinued.

The pediatric nurse should monitor the child for ICP and increasing head circumferences. If there is a change in head circumference, the child may be experiencing the complication of meningitis called *obstructive hydrocephalus.*

Reye's Syndrome

Reye's syndrome is a nonspecific, noninflammatory encephalopathy with organ involvement, including the liver, spleen, kidney, pancreas, and lymph. Death, although rare, can occur because of brain tissue herniation in association with severe cerebral edema, sepsis, and shock. Reye's syndrome is strongly associated with the use of salicylates (ie, aspirin) to treat symptoms of varicella infections or influenza. The Academy of Pediatrics has issued warnings to parents and health-care professionals to avoid using salicylates in children with possible infections of varicella or influenza types A or B. Nevertheless, Reye's syndrome can occur without the use of salicylates.

Assessments of Reye's Syndrome

Early symptoms of Reye's syndrome may be irritability, diarrhea, and rapid breathing. As the condition progresses, Reye's syndrome is associated with six major clinical presentations. Not all of the clinical presentations below may be present, but

the pediatric team will assess for the following in a child with suspected Reye's syndrome:

- Encephalopathy
- Increased ICP
- Metabolic dysfunction
- Hepatic dysfunction
- Renal damage
- Fatty infiltration of the viscera

Interventions for Reye's Syndrome

A team approach is needed to provide interventions and treatment for Reye's syndrome. Interventions include:

- Monitoring the child carefully for progression through the stages of Reye's syndrome (Table 29.3)
- Monitoring the child for changes in neurological status and immediately reporting any slight change in neurological status, including the level of consciousness, confusion, and neurological deficits
- Assessing the child for symptoms of GI bleeding, pancreatitis, or liver failure
- Providing hydration with a source of glucose (mainly IV fluids)
- Implementing seizure precautions to keep the child safe if seizures occur
- Monitoring the child's respiratory status and immediately reporting any signs of dyspnea
- Checking the child's Glasgow Coma Scale (GCS) score
- Assessing for the presence of increasing ICP
- Elevating the child's head of bed (HOB) by 30 to 45 degrees
- Keeping the child free of discomfort and pain, and helping the child to avoid crying
- Providing a quiet environment to rest
- Reinforcing the patient/family teaching session about the importance of follow up, including auditory, speech, and potential motor and/or intellectual deficits

Further medical treatments are dependent on the child's clinical status and the severity of the syndrome. The administration of diuretics for improved fluid balance, plasma and vitamin K to prevent bleeding, and airway support, including ventilation, may be required treatments.

Nursing Considerations for Reye's Syndrome

Nursing assessments and interventions for Reye's syndrome include:

- Symptoms of hypoxia
- Presence of seizures
- Hypoglycemia
- Coagulopathies
- Electrolyte imbalances
- Hyperthermia
- Care of a wound after liver biopsies are performed

The staging of Reye's syndrome is a process performed by the pediatric medical team. See Table 29.3 for a listing of the five stages associated with Reye's syndrome and the corresponding symptoms.

TABLE 29.3 STAGES AND SYMPTOMS OF REYE'S SYNDROME

Stage	Symptoms
I	Lethargy, vomiting, sleepiness, normal posture, brisk pupil reaction, and purposeful response to pain stimuli
II Follows 5–7 days after stage I	Combative, stuporous (ie, not fully conscious), and disoriented, with a normal posture, a sluggish pupil reaction, and purposeful or non-purposeful response to pain stimuli
III	Coma, decorticate posture, and sluggish pupil reaction
IV	Coma, seizures, decerebrate posture, and sluggish pupil reaction
V	Coma, apnea, limpness, and no pupil reaction

Source: National Institutes of Health, www.nih.gov

Spinal Cord Injury (SCI)

The causes of SCI include trauma, tumors, infections, and congenital disorders. Motor vehicle accidents (MVA) account for more than 50% of SCIs. Previous conditions such as trisomy 21, spina bifida, rheumatoid arthritis, and degenerative disc disease put a child at greater risk for SCI. The cervical area of the child's anatomy is the most frequent site of an SCI. Traumatic fracture dislocation is the most common form after the 11th birthday. There are three types of SCI:

1. Complete SCI, which causes a complete loss of sensorimotor and reflex activity below the site of injury.
2. Incomplete SCI, which causes the preservation of some motor and/or sensory function below the site of injury.
3. Sacral sparing of the SCI, in which motor/sensory activity at the anal mucocutaneous border exists.

The degree of disability depends on the location of the injury and immediate spinal cord stabilization after injury.

Assessments of Spinal Cord Injuries

Assessments of SCIs will depend on the severity of the accident. Typically, the initial emergency team will perform a complete neurological examination followed quickly by either a CT or an MRI. Because the initial injury may have caused swelling of tissues at the site, it is important to continue to assess a child's neurological status at appropriate time intervals to monitor for changes in symptoms. Orders will be written to conduct a variety of neurological examinations at specific intervals. It is imperative that any change in the assessments be reported immediately to the neurologist.

Interventions for Spinal Cord Injuries

The child must be placed on a straight back board with neutral head and neck alignment. A cervical collar is often applied. Respiratory stabilization is imperative because respiratory insufficiency may be delayed after injury. The child is monitored for neurogenic shock, which presents as bradycardia and hypotension. The treatment often includes high-dose methylprednisolone, which is administered within 8 hours of the injury.

Nursing Considerations for Spinal Cord Injuries

Nursing considerations when caring for children with SCIs include caring for their elimination needs. The child with an SCI may need to be catheterized and the child and/or family may need to be taught how to catheterize using clean technique for long-term care. Teens should be encouraged to have a frank discussion with his or her pediatric nurse about sexuality and sexual function.

Traumatic Brain Injury

Head injuries are the most common type of injury across childhood. Approximately 5% of severe head injuries are fatal and another 20% have long-term disabilities, including personality changes. The complications of head injury that lead to severe outcomes relate to both increased ICP and cerebral edema. Minor closed head injuries typically have no change in mental status, no evidence of skull fracture, and no abnormal findings on a neurological examination. Even with a minor head injury, the child may demonstrate a brief loss of consciousness, headache, lethargy, and vomiting. A major head injury is more complicated because the brain tissue is injured and the symptoms and outcomes are more severe.

Primary brain injuries develop at the time of trauma when the brain tissue suffers initial damage. For instance, a coup-contrecoup injury, which results from accelerated or decelerated motor vehicle movements, is a bruising of the brain within the bony cranium that can lead to increased ICP, apnea, and a loss of consciousness.

Secondary brain trauma develops as the child's body is responding to the injury. Here brain damage occurs secondary to developing cerebral edema, hypoxia, hypotension, increased ICP, and hemorrhage. Secondary brain trauma can develop hours or days after the injury with irreversible consequences if not treated.

SAFETY *STAT!*

Head injuries are often caused by young children falling. Falls take place from high chairs, changing tables, allowing an infant to sleep on an adult bed, when a child using a walker falls down stairs, shaken baby syndrome, and many forms of child abuse. Older children suffer brain injury from sports and MVAs, especially when the child is not required to wear protective equipment, such as a snug-fitting helmet with the *straps buckled!*

HEALTH PROMOTION

Protecting the Head From Injury Across Childhood

Parents, especially first-time parents, need instruction about how to handle their infant safely. Early safe practices can support a neonate and young infant's head and neck, therefore preventing injuries.

Neonate
- Carefully handle the head; the neonate's head should be supported by one's hand or should lay on one's arm while carrying
- Carefully handle the head during dressing, especially with clothes with sleeves
- Maintain head and neck alignment while sleeping or being held
- Never shake the newborn

Infant
- Use car seats correctly; a car seat should be set up facing the rear to prevent coup-contrecoup head injuries
- Use head support cushions with an infant car seat to prevent a young infant's head from sagging or drooping
- Prevent falls after an infant masters rolling from front to back or back to front
- Do not use baby walkers, especially in the presence of stairs (walkers are not recommended by the AAP)

Toddler
- Use an appropriate forward-facing car seat with a secure chest harness
- Prevent falls; child is still head-heavy
- Prevent falls into buckets of water or water-filled trashcans, which pose a risk because the child is too young and too weak to keep his or her head pushed up and out of the water
- Prevent injuries on tricycles; the toddler must be supervised and must wear a helmet

Preschooler
- Ensure the use of safety devices and protective equipment when participating in any sports or cycling
- Teach preschoolers to never go into the street; preschoolers must be supervised at all times during play
- Prevent falls from play structures; provide supervision and the use of foam padding

School-Aged Child
- Teach bike safety skills and the need for consistent helmet use with the *chin strap buckled*
- Use snug-fitting sports safety devices and protective equipment
- Prevent head injuries from playing with piñatas at parties; keep children back and do not use devices such as a golf clubs or baseball bats, from which children can experience a severe facial, skull, and brain injury. Use only plastic bats or plastic tubes.

Adolescent
- Insist on proper seat belt use in cars and the importance of not texting while driving
- Teach teens about head injuries when diving into natural water sources
- Teach about using protective equipment at all times when skating, skateboarding, skiing, and participating in contact sports

Types of Traumatic Brain Injuries

Children are vulnerable to the development of traumatic brain injuries (TBIs). Neonates and young infants are considered to be at particular risk because of their large head size and weight-to-body ratio. Beyond infancy, children who participate in contact sports or those who take physical risks during unsafe play or unsafe activities are prone to head injuries. The following sections present common brain injuries that occur anytime during the developmental period.

CONCUSSION. Also called a *mild traumatic brain injury,* this condition is associated with a transient loss of consciousness from shearing and/or compression of the brain's nerve tissue. Children with concussions tend to have what is called *postconcussion syndrome,* in which they have headaches, difficulty with memory, problems at school, photophobia (ie, extreme sensitivity to light), and possible personality changes. If a child experiences a concussion with a contact sport such as football, protocols must be followed to seek health care immediately.

THERAPEUTIC COMMUNICATION

Families whose child suffers a concussion need support. Concussions can be mild, with few symptoms, or a concussion can be a temporary but serious injury that affects the child's thinking process and academic performance. Families need education about what to expect for symptoms, rest, and treatments. Family members might feel traumatized and experience fear, grief, remorse, and sadness. Suggesting a visit from a social worker or a clergy member who can provide support is recommended. Staying with the family and providing professional presence, silence, or listening is very therapeutic.

CONTUSION. A contusion is considered a bruising of the brain tissue. It is typically associated with blunt trauma, which causes tears to the vasculature and tissue. Both head concussions and head contusions are serious. A concussion represents more wide-spread injury and can be in more than one location, while a contusion is considered a localized bruising occurring in one area of the brain tissue.

Assessments of Traumatic Brain Injuries

The nurse must assist the health-care team with preparing to implement rapid neurological assessments for a child who has experienced a traumatic brain injury. These assessments include:

- Assessing airway for patency and effective breathing patterns
- Monitoring VSs and neurological checks frequently to look for signs of shock, poor perfusion, and increased

ICP; Cushing's triad is considered a late sign of ICP and presents as a widening pulse pressure, an irregular breathing pattern, and bradycardia
- Monitoring level of consciousness (LOC) with the GCS; children who demonstrate a GCS of 8 or less have significant poorer outcomes, including significant disabilities (Fig. 29.9)
- Assessing cranial nerves as ordered

🗨️ LEARN TO C.U.S.

A school nurse is watching a football game in which a freshman student experiences a contact injury to the head and loses consciousness briefly. The child asks the coach if he can continue playing. The school nurse intervenes in the situation and uses the Learn to C.U.S. method of communication to express his concerns:

C: "I have a **concern** that your player wants to return to the game after this head injury.

U: I am **uncomfortable** that a "second hit" to the head can cause serious brain injury.

S: We have a **safety** issue here. The child cannot continue to play and, because of the loss of consciousness, needs to be seen by a health-care provider now."

Interventions for Traumatic Brain Injuries

Medical treatments for a TBI depend on the seriousness of the injury and the presenting complications. Complications include brain hypoxemia with swelling, increased ICP, enlarging hematomas, seizures, and hyperthermia. Airway management is the priority intervention. Typically, after diagnostics are undertaken to determine the location, severity, and associated complications of the injury, the child will be monitored in a PICU for severe injuries or on the pediatric unit for milder injuries. The child will rest, may be sedated, and will be provided a low-stimulation environment. Steroids might be ordered. Intubation and airway support on a ventilator may be required. TBI can cause post-traumatic hyperthermia, so the child's core body temperature must be managed. The child will need the HOB raised to help decrease ICP. In severe cases, the child will have ICP monitoring through cranial bolts and a transducer. This equipment allows the neurologist to monitor the child's ICP readings as a waveform on a monitor. Research continues about the use of hyperosmolar saline (ie, hypertonic 3% saline) given via IV to shift water from intracellular to extracellular compartments, thus reducing cerebral edema and pressure (Su, Huh, et al, 2013).

TEAM WORKS

Assessment with the GCS is imperative for a child with a TBI. Severe scores (ie, 3 to 8) require life support. The pediatric health-care team members work together to determine the child's GCS score and assess for subtle changes in clinical status.

Nursing Considerations for Traumatic Brain Injuries

Nursing considerations for TBIs include monitoring for very subtle signs of changes in clinical presentation and then

Pediatric Modification of the Glasgow Coma Scale		
Eye Opening		
1 year 4 Spontaneously 3 To verbal command 2 To pain 1 No response	**0–1 year** 4 Spontaneously 3 To shout 2 To pain 1 No response	
Best Motor Response		
>1 year 6 Obeys 5 Localizes pain 4 Flexion withdrawal 3 Flexion abnormal (decorticate) 2 Extension (decerebrate) 1 No response	**0–1 year** 6 Normal spontaneous movements 5 Localizes pain 4 Flexion withdrawal 3 Flexion abnormal (decorticate) 2 Extension (decerebrate) 1 No response	
Best Verbal Behavior		
0–2 years 5 Coos, babbles 4 Irritable 3 Cries to pain 2 Moans to pain 1 None	**2–5 years** 5 Appropriate words 4 Inappropriate words 3 Cries/screams 2 Nonspecific sounds 1 None	**5 years** 5 Oriented, converses 4 Disoriented 3 Inappropriate words 2 Incomprehensible sounds 1 No response
Scoring: • 13–15: Mild head injury • 9–12: Moderate head injury • <8: Severe head injury; intubation may be required		

FIGURE 29.9 Glasgow Coma Scale. *(Modified from Jennet, B. and Teasdale, G.: Aspects of coma after severe head injury. Lancet 1:878, 1977; James, H.E.: Neurologic evaluation and support in the child with an acute brain insult. Pediatric Ann 15:16, 1986; Siberry, G., and Iannone, R.: The Harriet Lane Handbook, 15th ed. St. Louis, Moseby, 2000, p. 14; and Andreoni, C. and Klinkhammer, B.: Quick Reference Guide for Pediatric Emergency Nursing. Saunders, Philadelphia, 2000.)*

rapidly reporting them to the health-care team. Managing the airway is always the top nursing care priority for a child who presents with a traumatic head injury.

The parents will be in great distress not knowing what the final outcome will be for their child. Upon discharge, the nursing staff must teach the family what clinical signs or symptoms to look for with increasing ICP and how to prevent further head trauma injuries. The child is typically admitted for observation and diagnostics, placed on NPO status until a thorough neurological evaluation is performed (ie, swallowing, choking, and aspiration risks evaluated), and then treated as medically indicated for the specific injury. If the child is unconscious the nurse must maintain an NPO status to prevent aspiration, establish turning schedules to keep the child's skin free from pressure ulcers, provide suctioning prn, and provide other supportive nursing care as needed.

Treatments for TBIs include meticulous monitoring for symptoms of ICP; medications to reducing swelling of brain tissue, such as diuretics and corticosteroids; and anticonvulsants if warranted. Children may require a stay in the intensive care unit on a cerebral pressure monitoring device such as subarachnoid bolts, intraventricular monitoring systems, or subdural monitoring systems.

OTHER NEUROLOGICAL DISORDERS

Although less common than brain injuries associated with trauma and injuries, children can present with other neurological disorders that require medical attention and nursing care. The following section represents those disorders that are not trauma-related but whose prevalence in children warrants an understanding of the condition, assessments, and required care.

Brain Tumors

Brain tumors are the most common solid malignancy during childhood, with a frequency only second to leukemia. Tumors are classified according to their physical location and grade. Tumor locations include the supratentorial regions, the subtentorial region, the temporal lobe, and the posterior fossa. The most prevalent brain tumor in children under 7 years of age is the medulloblastoma. Cerebellar astrocytoma is the most common subtentorial tumor of childhood and has a 5-year survival rate of 90%. Brain tumors are graded as either low grade, or localized, or higher grade, which denotes invasive properties.

Assessments of Brain Tumors

In general, the child will present with both signs and symptoms of ICP and focal neurological signs that are associated with the size and location of the tumor. It is quite common that the child will have demonstrated behavioral or personality alterations for as long as weeks before the tumor is identified. These behaviors can include poor school performance, irritability, hyperactivity, forgetfulness, and lethargy. Many brain tumors cause nausea, vomiting, visual acuity changes, and headaches.

Interventions for Brain Tumors

Interventions for brain tumors are dependent on the size, location, and age of the child. Typical treatment includes surgery, irradiation, and chemotherapy. Complications of a tumor growing within the bony cranium include ICP, the compression of vital brain structures, hydrocephalus, brainstem herniation, and the complications associated with the negative effects of radiating the brain. These long-term effects include endocrine, intellectual, and motor deficits.

Nursing Considerations for Brain Tumors

Nursing considerations for a child with brain tumors include providing a great deal of support for the family. A diagnosis of cancer causes fear, anxiety, sadness, and bewilderment. Families need information about the diagnosis, treatment, follow-up care, and long-term prognosis only as they can process the information. It is important to repeat answers to their questions as many times as necessary.

Nursing care focuses on the assessment of changes in clinical presentation preoperatively and postoperatively. Care should be taken to follow all orders carefully for each neurological assessment ordered. Assess VSs frequently before and after brain surgery for tumor removal and report signs of increased ICP.

Cancer treatment is often prolonged, with untoward associated symptoms. Cancer treatment can cause nausea, hair loss, bone marrow suppression, neutropenia, pain, life-threatening infections, and emotional distress.

PATIENT TEACHING GUIDELINES

If the child requires brain surgery to remove or debulk (ie, surgically make smaller) the tumor, the child's postoperative clinical presentation may worsen at first and then improve as the postoperative cerebral edema decreases with healing.

Childhood Migraine Headaches

Children as young as infants can get the same types of severe headaches as adults. The symptoms associated with childhood headaches may present differently than adult symptoms because children frequently encounter bilateral pain whereas adults experience unilateral pain. Children who are young and developmentally unable to describe location and severity pose extra challenges in managing headaches. As the child grows, his or her headaches may also evolve and present differently than they did during earlier periods. Because children engage in rigorous play and sports, it is imperative that significant head injuries are ruled out, such as those that cause intracranial bleeding and ICP.

Migraine headaches may cause nausea, vomiting, severe head pain, and sensitivity to sound and light. These headaches are associated with feelings of pulsation and throbbing, are sometimes relieved by sleep, and are often triggered by caffeine, menses, and stress.

Types of Childhood Migraine Headaches

Not all migraine headaches are the same. Children may present with one of the four types of childhood migraine headaches: chronic daily headaches, cluster headaches, tension headaches, and psychogenic headaches.

CHRONIC DAILY HEADACHES. Chronic daily headaches can cause symptoms similar to migraines but are presented in increasing frequency. If a child experiences headaches for more than 15 days per month and for at least 3 consecutive months, then further diagnostics are warranted to rule out infection, abscess, or head injury.

CLUSTER HEADACHES. Cluster headaches are uncommon for children who are school-aged and younger. The sensory experience can be described as "stabbing, sharp pain" unilaterally that can last anywhere from 15 min to as long as 3 hours. Children with cluster headaches often experience associated symptoms of agitation, congestion, runny nose, and teary eyes (www.mayoclinic.org, 2015).

TENSION HEADACHES. Causing a feeling of tightness around the head or on both sides of the child's head, tension headaches present as a dull ache rather than throbbing. Children with tension headaches often become more symptomatic with physical exercise and play. Tension headaches are differentiated by their pain presentation, as well as a lack of nausea and vomiting, which are so often associated with migraines.

Sleep deprivation headaches are a type of tension headache associated with obese children who have sleep apnea or those with conditions that cause chronic hypoxia.

PSYCHOGENIC HEADACHES. Psychogenic headaches may be difficult to diagnose. They are associated with a mental health issue, such as conversion disorder, also called *functional neurological symptom disorder,* in which an individual experiences stress in physical symptoms that do not have a physical cause. Psychogenic headaches require treatment because pain is a subjective experience and requires professional assessments, interventions, and an evaluation of the effectiveness of the interventions.

Assessments of Childhood Headaches

Assessments for childhood headaches must include the following:

- A health history of previous headaches in younger years, a family history that indicates a genetic predisposition, and any neurological disorders, deficits, birth trauma, or vision disorders
- Risk factors such as extreme sports that cause dehydration and previous head injury
- A physical examination, including the location, severity, intensity, and description of pain, as well as associated symptoms such as nausea, vomiting, behavioral changes, photophobia, sound phobia, and congestion
- Assessment for any clinical signs of infection, including fever, a stiff neck, or a pertinent history of recent communicable diseases
- A head CT scan if the child demonstrates neurological symptoms such as seizures, pain upon rising in the morning, headache associated with vomiting, or any change in mental status, such as personality, mood, or school performance

Interventions for Childhood Headaches

Interventions for childhood headaches depend on the type, severity, and associated disability. Treating any infections, especially chronic sinus infections, meningitis, or encephalitis, is paramount. If the child has experienced a significant head injury, then treatment may include hospitalization for observation and treatment of the injury. Stress can be a contributing cause of tension headaches. Eyesight should be checked because eye strain may contribute to the headache experience. If the child is experiencing bullying or relationship difficulties with peers, teachers, or parents, then referring the family for counseling may be warranted as part of a holistic approach to managing headaches. There are many medications currently being used to treat migraine headaches in childhood. The family will work with a pediatrician or pediatric neurologist to create a holistic treatment plan based on the location and severity of the headaches, and the level of disability.

Nursing Considerations for Childhood Headaches

Headaches can be frustrating for both the child and the parent. Parents may be reluctant to offer young children pain medication for their headaches, and young children may be reluctant to take oral medications. It is important to take a holistic approach to identifying triggers and offering suggestions for symptom management.

The child's diet should be looked at as research has shown that foods and beverages that contain the preservative nitrate may be a trigger for the headaches. Nitrates are found in hot dogs, cold cuts, bacon, and commercially prepared foods and food mixes. Although used to treat some headaches in adults, caffeine can be a trigger for headache in children. Any foods or beverages that contain chocolate, as well as coffee, tea, and many sodas, may contribute to the child's headaches and should be avoided.

It is important that the pediatric nurse find meaningful and effective ways to help alleviate symptoms, including prescribed medications, rest and relaxation, stimulation reduction, massage, warm or cold packs to the forehead, and other means of complementary therapy. Children may respond to sleep, resting in a dark and quiet room, nonsteroidal anti-inflammatory drugs, antiemetics, and the headache medications sumatriptan succinate, isometheptene, and ergotamine. If the headaches continue, stronger medications, including propranolol, cyproheptadine, verapamil valproate, and several of the antidepressants may be used.

NURSING CARE PLAN for Children with Neurological Conditions

For children who experience a neurological condition that affects the CNS, the following nursing diagnoses should be considered:

Nursing Diagnoses:
1. Ineffective cerebral tissue perfusion related to injury is present.
2. There is ineffective airway clearance related to impaired neurological status.
3. There is impaired gas exchange related to impaired breathing patterns.
4. The child exhibits acute confusion related to brain tissue/cerebral injury.
5. There is risk for vascular trauma related to brain injury.
6. There is risk for ineffective family coping related to the traumatic injury of a child.
7. The child exhibits nausea related to brain tissue damage.
8. There is impaired comfort related to head injury.
9. There is impaired memory related to head trauma.
10. There is risk for delayed growth and development related to the long-term consequences of a CNS disorder.

Cognitive Impairment

The term *cognitive impairment* has replaced *mental retardation*. CI is considered a disability because it involves significant limitations in intellectual functioning and adaptive behaviors. During the developmental period (ie, birth to age 22), CI is perceived as limitations that have developed in the child's social, conceptual, and adaptive skills.

There are varying degrees of CI. The assessment of degree with which a child presents includes the assessment of the IQ, or intelligent quotient:

- **Mild:** IQ of 50 to 55 and up to 70; most prevalent, at 80% of those with CI. Considered educable to a mental age of 12 to 13 years old, mostly independent.
- **Moderate:** IQ of 35 to 40 and up to 50 to 55, and found in 15% of those classified with CI. Most Down's syndrome children function at this level. Considered "trainable" to the mental age of an 8- to 10-year-old.
- **Severe:** IQ of 20 to 25 and up to 35 to 40. Considered the mental age of a toddler, this status requires complete custodial care for safety and activities of daily living.
- **Profound:** IQ below 20 to 25. Considered having a mental age of an infant; requires complete care, supervision, and protection.

Assessments of Cognitive Impairment

The pediatric health-care team should focus on the child's developmental status and not on the child's chronological age. The team should participate in assessing the ability of a child with a CI to perform motor and psychosocial tasks. A true determination of the child's level of functioning and limitation is performed over time and the child should have at least two testing periods.

SAFETY *STAT!*

The interdisciplinary pediatric health-care team who suspects a child has CI will conduct assessments for toxic exposures, environmental hazards, genetic disorders, and any other chronic conditions that may have interfered with the child's development.

Interventions for Cognitive Impairment

Interventions for a child with CI start with ensuring the child is safe and cared for. Using Maslow's hierarchy of needs, the pediatric nurse can assist the family with basic support for nutrition, safety, and socialization. Goals should be made that are realistic for the child's level of functioning. Each goal should be broken down into distinct tasks that can be mastered over time with practice. Participating in activities of daily living, appropriate socializing, and safety precautions are all possible goals that can be worked on.

PATIENT TEACHING GUIDELINES

The child with CI and their family need to have measures of success acknowledged as goals are accomplished. When a moderately or severely cognitively impaired child learns the steps of a task and masters the task in completion, such as oral hygiene or hand washing, the entire family should feel successful.

Nursing Considerations for Cognitive Impairment

It is important that the pediatric health-care team encourage families of cognitively impaired children to become active in national, state, regional, and local support organizations. Special Olympics, the American Association on Intellectual and Developmental Disabilities, and county-run developmental centers are three examples of organizations that can provide support and assistance.

Hydrocephalus

Hydrocephalus is a condition that presents with an increased production, a decreased reabsorption, or an obstructed flow of CSF within the ventricles and subarachnoid spaces of the brain. An obstructed flow of CSF is also called *noncommunicating hydrocephalus,* whereas impaired absorption of CSF is called *communicating hydrocephalus.* In the presence of tumors, structural abnormalities, trauma, or hemorrhage, noncommunicating hydrocephalus can develop, causing significant CNS symptoms and impairment. With scarring, hemorrhage, or the presence of congenital anomalies, communicating hydrocephalus can develop.

Assessments of Hydrocephalus

Assessments of suspected or actual hydrocephalus include frequent measurements of the circumference of the child's head. These measurements should take place directly above the eyebrow, on the widest part of the child's head. The child's fontanel should be palpated for the presence of a full and possibly tense bulge. In infants, the skull's suture lines may widen in the presence of increasing pressure and the child's scalp veins may become distended and prominent (eg, "cracked pot" appearance; Fig. 29.10). The nurse should assess the child's affect and mood, looking for a high-pitched cry, irritability, and/or lethargy. The child should also be assessed for "sunset eyes," in which the white sclera is visible above and around the iris as the eyes appear to be looking down (Fig. 29.11). In severe hydrocephalus, the child may not have the neck and upper back strength to hold their head up or support the weight of the head for any period of time. If the child with hydrocephalus demonstrates acute vomiting, especially after rising in the morning, severe ICP associated with the child's diagnosis of hydrocephalus must be suspected and immediately reported for intervention.

Interventions for Hydrocephalus

The main intervention for the development of hydrocephalus is the placement of a ventral-peritoneal (VP) shunt, which

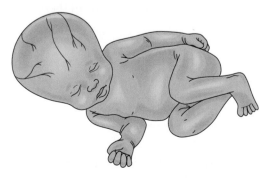

FIGURE 29.10 The cracked pot look (Macewen's sign) on an infant's scalp because of increased cerebral pressure.

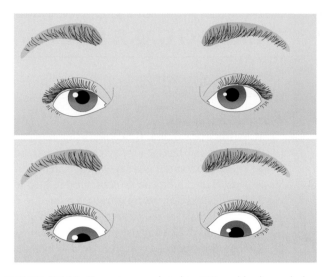

FIGURE 29.11 Sunset eyes related to ICP and hydrocephalus.

is placed surgically (Fig. 29.12). This shunt is used in the presence of increasing pressure; it allows the flow of CSF to descend from the ventricle through the shunt tubing into the child's peritoneal cavity, where it is absorbed and eliminated. The shunt must be monitored over time for malfunction. Shunt malfunction can occur with the blockage of biological material or may become ineffective as the child grows and develops to the point that the shunt is too short for the child's size. The parents must be taught how to assess for changes in clinical presentation associated with sudden increased ICP. They must also learn how to manually pump the shunt to ensure patency. This procedure is dependent on the type of shunt used, and postoperative and long-term care should be individualized based on the shunt manufacturer's recommendation.

Nursing Considerations for Hydrocephalus

The pediatric nurse must support the child and the family because there may be CIs or other associated neurological deficits associated with hydrocephalus. With shaken baby syndrome, the child may have other severe neurological sequelae other than ICP, such as retinal hemorrhages and subsequent CI with learning disabilities (see Chapter 28, The Abused Child). Families need support as they learn to care for the child whose head may be abnormally large and heavy. The child may need to have constant head support. If sitting in a high chair, the child's head may need to rest on a pillow, or if sitting in a car seat, extra padding may be necessary to keep the child's head in a neutral central position.

The pediatric nurse must know how to manage an obstruction in the shunt and teach the family this management. Signs and symptoms of infection should be discussed because the presence of the shunt places the child at risk for sepsis.

Increased Intracranial Pressure

Within the rigid cranial vault of the child's skull, any increased pressure can cause significant symptoms and injury.

Ventriculoperitoneal (VP) Shunt

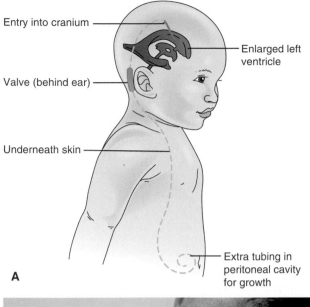

Entry into cranium

Enlarged left ventricle

Valve (behind ear)

Underneath skin

Extra tubing in peritoneal cavity for growth

A

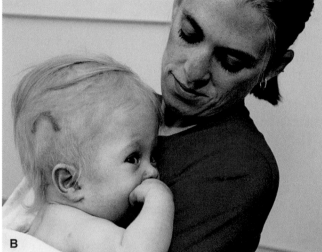

B

FIGURE 29.12 VP shunt.

Increased ICP can result in the child's brain being herniated, which results in progressive deterioration of the brainstem, and, without treatment, causes apnea and death. A history associated with ICP includes head trauma, bleeding disorders, extensive fevers, and overhydration of a child with diabetic ketoacidosis (DKA) and syndrome of inappropriate antidiuretic hormone (SIADH). ICP that is caused by cerebral edema can be caused by abscesses, meningitis, tumors, water intoxication, hypoxia, hydrocephalus, and other causes.

Assessments of Intracranial Pressure

Assessments of ICP include identifying associated clinical signs and symptoms of occipital headache, vomiting (eg, projectile vomiting in older children), altered mental status, visual disturbances, and generalized neck pain. Assess the child for hypertension, bradycardia, and bradypnea. A young

child may demonstrate increased head circumference and a bulging anterior fontanel. Further assessments include:

• **Sunset Eyes:** The white of the sclera is present above the iris
• **Posturing:** Can be decerebrate (ie, damage to nerve pathway between the spinal cord and the brain, which is typically found with brainstem injuries) or decorticate (ie, caused by a stroke, another anterior brain injury, or brain hemorrhages within the cerebral hemispheres) (Fig. 29.13)
• **Seizures:** May be generalized or focal
• **Macewen's Sign:** "Cracked pot," with enlarged bluish scalp veins
• **Diplopia:** Double vision
• **Unequal Pupils:** PERRLA should be performed to assess for this condition
• Sudden change in feeding habits
• Irritability, restlessness, and crying with holding or cuddling

Interventions for Intracranial Pressure

Nurses should be able to assist the team in an emergency response to increasing ICP. Immediate interventions for acute increased ICP include:

• Stabilizing the airway by administering CPR as needed
• Maintaining a patent airway
• Providing a source of oxygen to maintain stable oxygen saturations and ABGs
• Suctioning the child carefully and only if needed (suctioning can cause rebound increased ICP)
• Monitoring the child's pediatric GCS score; if the team determines the value is 8 or less, the child will need to be rapidly intubated
• Elevating the HOB
• Treating the child's presenting seizure activities if needed
• Turning down the lights and providing an environment with low visual and auditory stimulation

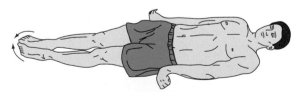

Abnormal Extension (decerebrate posturing)

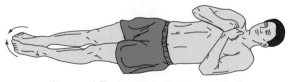

Abnormal Flexion (decorticate posturing)

FIGURE 29.13 Posturing with severe head injury: decerebrate and decorticate.

- Preparing to assist the team in transferring the child to the highest level of care, such as the PICU
- Assisting in the rapid transfer to a diagnostic department, such as MRI or CT scanning
- Carefully managing the child's IV to maintain a portal for emergency medications such as diuretics and anticonvulsants
- Administering diuretics, corticosteroids, or both

Nursing Considerations for Intracranial Pressure

ICP can be life-threatening. The role of the pediatric nurse is to support an interdisciplinary team in stabilizing the child and then to monitor the child for any sudden change in clinical status. Any new symptoms or changes must be reported immediately to prevent brain tissue anoxia and brain damage. The child may demonstrate signs of diabetes insipidus (DI) in which the child produces large quantities of very dilute urine with a low specific gravity, or SIADH, in which the child's UOP is grossly diminished.

Seizure Disorders

A seizure is a disruption of the electrical communication among the neurons within the child's brain. Recurrent seizures are commonly known as *epilepsy.* A seizure may also be called a *paroxysmal involuntary brain disturbance.* Seizures do not actually constitute a medical diagnosis but rather are a symptom of an underlying CNS injury or disorder.

During a seizure, the child's brain either fires electrical stimulation between the neurons when it is not supposed to or it does not fire when it should. The result is a disruption in the expected patterns of electrical current between the neurons, which leads to an excitatory or inhibitory mechanism and causes a seizure. The manifestations of the seizure may include a loss of consciousness, abnormal motor movements, behavioral abnormalities, autonomic dysfunction, and sensory disturbances.

The definition of a seizure disorder is when a child experiences an unprovoked seizure two or more times within a 24-hour period. Close to 40% of all childhood seizures are partial. Table 29.4 provides a description of types of seizures found in childhood. The cause of a seizure disorder is often unknown. Likewise, the cause of most neonatal and infant seizures remains unknown. Seizure disorders may have familial tendencies, may be associated with brain injuries, or may be caused by an infectious process. Full body seizures are called **grand mal seizures.** Common causes of seizures in pediatric clients include:

- Trauma
- Hemorrhage
- Brain malformations

TABLE 29.4 TYPES OF CHILDHOOD SEIZURES

Type of Seizure	Description	Characteristics	Treatment
Infantile Spasms	Uncommon, generalized seizure presenting between 3 and 12 months of age; peaks at 4–8 months.	Sudden stiffening, then jerking; child flings arms out, bends body forward, and bends knees up; called *jackknife seizures.* Child may lose some motor skills after onset of diagnosis.	Treated with anticonvulsants and steroid therapy.
Simple Partial Seizure	Type of partial seizure only occurring in part of the child's brain. Symptoms depend on location of electrical activity in brain.	Child presents with clonic or tonic movements involving extremities, neck, and face. May experience sensory sensations such as pain or numbness. Only lasts on average 10–25 sec. Child experiencing simple partial seizure will remain conscious during process with no postictal state. Some children verbalize during a simple partial seizure.	Treatment varies. May include anticonvulsant therapy based on the location within the brain and the severity of symptoms.

TABLE **29.4**   **TYPES OF CHILDHOOD SEIZURES—cont'd**

Type of Seizure	Description	Characteristics	Treatment
Complex Partial Seizure	Often starts with the motor activity associated with simple partial and then progresses to other body sites with a loss of or altered state of consciousness.	Sometimes preceded by an aura, this common type of partial seizure does impair consciousness. In children, motor movements are complex and mimic purposes such as picking, pulling, or rubbing objects, or running in a repetitive nondirective way. In infants, child will demonstrate chewing, lip smacking, salivation, and excessive swallowing movements.	Treatment consists of anticonvulsant therapy.
Grand Mal or Tonic-Clonic Seizure	A type of severe seizure that crosses over the brain's hemispheres and causes full-body neuromuscular seizure activity. This generalized dramatic seizure is associated with an aura, a loss of consciousness, a shrill and piercing loud cry, and tonic presentation followed by tonic-clonic movements of the entire body that alternate with the relaxation of muscles.	Child may experience pronounced saliva secretion, cyanosis because of apnea, and loss of bladder and sometimes bowel sphincter control. Will demonstrate a postictal state of deep sleep or may be semi-comatose, in which he or she only responds to painful stimuli. This may last up to 2 hours with an average of 30 min. Child will be confused but will not recall seizure activity.	Airway must be supported after seizure activity. Do not force any object in mouth to maintain airway during seizure (eg, no tongue blades or oral airway insertion). Place the child in a side-lying position after the seizure activity stops to facilitate saliva drainage and the child's tongue to fall forward.
Absence Seizure	Generalized seizure more often found in girls; tends to develop after the fifth year. Formally titled *petit mal seizure.*	Often identified in a classroom setting because the child suddenly "checks out" with blank stare, flickering eyelids, and lack of general body movements. May demonstrate facial twitches or myoclonic movements. Lasts approximately 30 sec or less. Child may have many in one day. No postictal state.	Treated with anticonvulsant therapy.

Continued

TABLE 29.4   TYPES OF CHILDHOOD SEIZURES—cont'd

Type of Seizure	Description	Characteristics	Treatment
Myoclonic Seizure	Type of generalized seizure involving the brain's motor complex.	Child will demonstrate sudden whole-body or limited body part massive jerking. Child may or may not lose consciousness. Often accompanies other forms of seizures.	
Miscellaneous Seizures			
Febrile Seizure	Type of generalized seizure associated with a rapid rise in core body temperature. Febrile seizures are considered age dependent and are rarely seen before 9 months of age or after the fifth birthday. They are the most common seizure noted during childhood and they spontaneous remit without the use of specific anticonvulsant therapy. Incidence rate is 2%–5% of the population.	Previously healthy infant or young child presents with generalized seizure activity, often following bacterial or viral infections. Febrile seizures do not last more than 5 min, are generally not associated with brain damage, and are considered harmless for most children. Febrile seizures are not considered a seizure disorder, and the child may not be treated with long-term anticonvulsants unless the seizure is prolonged, focal, or recurs within 24 hours of the first one.	Treatment focuses on finding the source of the rapid rise in temperature and treating infection. Child should be monitored for repeated febrile seizures with every infection after first presentation. Child should receive antipyretic medications with first signs of infections to prevent further febrile seizures.
Status Epilepticus (SE)	Defined as a continuous seizure that lasts longer than 30 min or the occurrence of serial seizures with no regained consciousness between. The most common form of seizures associated with SE are generalized tonic-clonic. The causes of SE include fever, sudden withdrawal of antiepileptic medication, electrolyte disturbance, hypoxia/ischemia, infection, or trauma. Considered a neurological emergency, a child in SE requires a finely orchestrated medical team approach to prevent the child's death.	Characterized by back-to-back seizure activity of clustered seizures where the child does not regain consciousness or recover between seizures.	Children in SE need to be transferred to an intensive care environment for airway support and possible intubation if ventilation via bag valve mask is not successful. Diazepam or lorazepam should be administered immediately to manage the seizure activity. Treatment is life support and rapid administration of anticonvulsants to stop the continuing seizure activity. Oxygenation, stabilization of blood glucose, and stabilization of electrolytes should be aggressively managed to prevent morbidity and mortality.

- Genetic disorders
- Brain dysmaturity (ie, small brain size and function related to fetal development)
- Infection, such as meningitis
- Fever
- Electrolyte abnormalities, especially related to sodium, and the presence of hyperglycemia or hypoglycemia
- Inborn errors of metabolism
- Drug-related injuries or significant exposures (eg, cocaine, chemotherapy, alcohol, lead, and cyclic antidepressants)
- Structural CNS lesions

PATIENT TEACHING GUIDELINES

Febrile seizures are the most common convulsive event in the childhood period, with an incidence rate of 2% to 5% of all children between 6 months and 5 years of age.

The degree of disability associated with a seizure disorder depends on the type of seizure and the location of the origins of the seizure within the child's brain. If the child experienced an anoxic event that prevented brain tissue perfusion, the degree of disability may be mild to severe. Many children with seizure disorders also have accompanied brain injuries or insults. The degree of long-term disability depends on the etiology and severity of the seizure disorder.

Assessments of Seizure Disorders

The child presenting with seizure activity should have a complete health history, with associated risk factors identified. The nurse should gather the following health history information from the family of a child who recently experienced seizure activity:

- Any family history of seizures or neurological impairments
- Complications associated with the prenatal, perinatal, and postnatal period
- Documented delays in the child's developmental motor milestones
- Exposure to environmental toxins, infectious diseases, or physical trauma, especially to the head
- A history of domestic abuse, child abuse, or any form of nonaccidental injury
- Age of child at the time of the first seizure

The nurse should gather the following information related to the seizure event:

- Precipitating factors surrounding the seizure event or seizure disorder
- Description of the child's clinical presentation during the seizure (helps to determine the possible type) such as grand mal or **myoclonic** (spasmodic jerky movements)
- The presence of an aura, a loss of consciousness, injury during seizure (ie, head injury with a fall) and the postictal state
- Current medications, including past or current anticonvulsant therapies
- Compliance with the current medication regimen

Interventions for Seizure Disorders

The nursing care of a child with a seizure disorder begins by securing a safe environment. Assess the child's mobility and the need for safety devices. Some children with a severe seizure disorder must wear helmets to keep their heads safe from injury when the seizure causes a fall. Seizure precautions should be maintained while the child is hospitalized. This includes padding the side rails, providing constant supervision while the child is ambulating in the halls or playing in the playroom, and maintaining safety while the child is being transported via gurney or wheelchair. Suction and oxygen should be available at all times.

If a child experiences a seizure, the child should be kept safe during the seizure activity: no one should try to stop or control the motor movements; no one should try to place a tongue blade or any object in the child's mouth; and make sure to move objects that might cause bodily harm during the seizure. The child should be wearing a medical alert bracelet (Fig. 29.14).

Adherence to the seizure medications regimen prevents seizure activity associated with a sudden drop in anticonvulsant therapy serums. Families need to be reminded about the importance of exactly following the prescribed medications and participating with monitoring routine serum blood levels of the anticonvulsant therapy to ensure therapeutic blood levels. The family should also be reminded that if the child becomes ill, vomits, or experiences any health deviation, they should report the symptoms to their primary health-care provider for guidance. GI illnesses, vomiting, and dehydration can affect the anticonvulsant therapy. If a helmet is ordered for protection of the child with frequent **tonic-clonic seizures**, the family must be educated about having the child wear the helmet when awake. The family should also conduct an assessment of their home and remove furniture with sharp edges and make any other home environment changes. Parents must realize that sleepiness and slow reaction times may be generalized side effects of seizure medications.

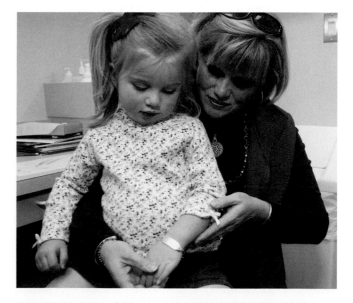

FIGURE 29.14 A child wearing a medical alert bracelet.

If a child's seizure disorder remains uncontrolled despite the use of various anticonvulsant therapies, surgery may be warranted to remove the area of tissue causing the electrical activity, or at least surgically disrupt the area of brain tissue causing the seizures.

A cluster of seizures that are back to back are dangerous. This is called **status epilepticus (SE)** and can cause both significant injury as well as death from hypoglycemia.

Research continues to provide innovations in seizure therapies. One technology being used to treat seizures is vagal nerve stimulation, which is a treatment to reduce the frequency and intensity of seizures by placing a small electric stimulator in the neck around the vagal nerve. While sending intermittent electrical signals to the brain, this technology interrupts a seizure that is just starting to develop. The vagal nerve stimulator is used for children who continue to have loss of consciousness during generalized or complex partial seizures when not controlled by medications.

LABS & DIAGNOSTICS

Tests for Seizure Disorders

Although there is no one test to diagnose childhood seizures, several diagnostics may be completed to put together what is referred to as a "constellation of information" to determine the type, location, and severity of the brain's abnormal electrical activity.

Laboratory Studies

- Serum electrolytes, including calcium levels and glucose levels, to rule out metabolic disorders, hypoglycemia, and hypocalcemia
- Anticonvulsant serum drug levels: These drugs must be kept in a therapeutic range because low levels may cause seizures to occur and high levels can lead to toxicity. Report immediately any subtherapeutic or toxic levels. Common laboratory safe ranges are the following:
  - Diazepam: 0.2 to 1.5 mcg/mL
  - Carbamazepine: 4 to 12 mcg/mL
  - Phenobarbital: 15 to 30 mcg/mL
  - Phenytoin: 10 to 20 mcg/mL
  - Valproic acid: 50 to 125 mcg/mL
  - Primidone: 7 to 10 mcg/mL
  (Van Leeuwen, Poelhuis-Leth, et al, 2011)
  Diagnostic Studies
- EEG to identify the location and type of seizure; this testing may be a 24-hour video monitoring EEG
- CT or MRI to rule out injury, brain tissue abnormalities, tumors, abscesses, and intracranial bleeds
- Skull x-rays if trauma is identified or suspected

Special Considerations for Seizure Disorders

There are several special considerations in managing seizures. These include recording seizure activity, providing anticonvulsant medications, and having the child with seizure disorders follow a ketogenic diet.

RECORDING SEIZURE ACTIVITY. One of the most important aspects of caring for a child with a seizure disorder is to teach and reinforce the need for the caregivers, guardians, or family members to document each seizure event. A log should be maintained for health-care professionals to review. The log should document the date; time; precipitating events; type of seizure activity, including motor movements; the length of time of the seizure; and any associated events, such as loss of consciousness, bladder or bowel incontinence, nausea or vomiting, and the postictal state, including periods of drowsiness and complaints of headache.

KETOGENIC DIET. The **ketogenic diet** is a special diet that has been widely studied and provides relief from seizures for some children. First developed in the 1920s and further investigated in 1976, the ketogenic diet is a special high-fat, low-carbohydrate diet that is thought to help control seizures in some people who have a documented history of epilepsy. The term *ketogenic* means that the diet produces ketones within the body as the high-fat primary source of energy is processed and broken down. The theory behind the diet is that the process of ketone breakdown leads to a higher ketone blood level, thereby improving seizure control.

Most physicians who encourage the ketogenic diet do so when the patient has not had success in seizure control, even with several anticonvulsant therapies. It is offered as an adjunct therapy to children, but is rarely suggested for adults. The diet helps to control seizures in certain cases, but does not provide an immediate seizure-free status. The overall diet includes a 4:1 or 3:1 fat to protein ratio. Research has shown that children who begin and continue following a ketogenic diet can demonstrate between a 50% and 90% reduction in the number of their seizures. Conditions for which a ketogenic diet is suggested for seizure reduction include:

- Focal seizures
- Infantile spasms
- Dravet's syndrome
- Doose's syndrome
- Rett's syndrome
- Glucose transporter 1 (GLUT-1) deficiency

PATIENT TEACHING GUIDELINES

Foods that are encouraged for consumption during the ketogenic diet include:
- Heavy whipping cream
- Butter
- Canola oil
- Olive oil
- Mayonnaise
- Coconut oil
- Bacon
- Peanut butter
- Sour cream
- Cheese

The child must not ingest carbohydrates. This diet highly restricts carbohydrates, and includes avoiding starchy fruits and vegetables, breads, pasta, grains, and all sugars; the child must be 100% compliant. Families should work closely with a dietician to learn about the food selections and restriction. Because the diet is so restricted, the child will need to take vitamin and mineral supplements, including folic acid, vitamin D, calcium, and iron. Most ketogenic diets are initiated within a hospital environment over the course of 3 to 4 days to monitor the child's ketones and responses to the change in diet.

COMMON ANTICONVULSANT THERAPY. Common anticonvulsant therapy for long-term seizure management includes many drugs. Table 29.5 provides examples of commonly used medications to control childhood seizures (Rudd and Kocisko, 2014; Van Leeuwen, Poelhuis-Leth, et al, 2011; www.nih.gov).

SAFETY *STAT!*

For SE, anticonvulsant therapy will be for short-term emergency management and includes the following medications:
- Diazepam (Valium or Diastat) per rectum
- Phenobarbital (Solfoton)
- Fosphenytoin (Cerebyx)

Nursing Considerations for Seizure Disorders

When teaching families about how to care for their child with a seizure disorder, the nurse should provide the following information about anticonvulsant therapy:

- Adolescents must be seizure free for 1 year to obtain their driver's license. They may be on anticonvulsant therapy to be eligible for license.
- Parents must understand the importance of following the therapeutic serum levels of anticonvulsant therapy.
- Teens should avoid alcohol because it reduces the threshold of seizures.
- Families should never abruptly stop administering anticonvulsant therapy to their child as doing so may cause seizures.
- Caregivers must understand the importance of medication administration, proper hydration, and promptly reporting any side effects, illness, or change in cognition or well-being.

Remind families to treat their child with a seizure disorder as they would any of their children. Children with chronic illnesses need play opportunities, social activities, outings, and school engagement. Any restrictions on sports activities, swimming, or physical education will be determined by the neurology team and are based on the type and severity of the seizures.

TABLE 29.5 ANTICONVULSANT MEDICATIONS

Medication	Dosage	Side Effects	Precautions
Phenytoin (Dilantin)	0.2 mg/kg	Gum hyperplasia, ataxia, gastric distress, anemia, sedation, nystagmus, hirsutism, and depressed myocardial function	If given IV, must only be mixed with dextrose; NS causes crystallization
Valproic acid (Depakene)	10–60 mg/kg (titrating doses)	Hepatic failure, scalp hair loss, thrombocytopenia	Can cause vomiting, which will lower therapeutic levels
Carbamazepine (Tegretol)	10–35 mg/kg (titrating doses)	Hepatic toxicity, potentially fatal hematological and cardiovascular complications	Monitor for liver dysfunctions throughout use
Primidone (Mysoline)	15–20 mg/kg at bedtime; starting dose increasing to 250 mg three times a day	Nausea and vomiting, nystagmus, fatigue, and vertigo	Contraindicated in patients who are hypersensitive to phenobarbital; abrupt withdrawal may lead to SE
Clorazepate (Tranxene)	Initial dose up to 15 mg daily divided doses, up to 60 mg per day as needed	Increased salivary secretions or dry mouth, tremors, blurred vision	Typically used for children more than 9 years of age
Clonazepam (Klonopin)	25 mcg/kg, titrating up to 1–2 mcg/kg/day	Irritability, appetite changes, ataxia, increased salivary secretions	Monitor for depression

Continued

TABLE **29.5** ANTICONVULSANT MEDICATIONS—cont'd

Medication	Dosage	Side Effects	Precautions
Ethosuximide (Zarontin)	7.5 mg/kg per day up to 45 mg/kg; maximum dose is 1.5 g/day	Irritability, anorexia, abdominal pain, anemia, and weight gain	Monitor CBC for anemia every 6 months
Phenobarbital (Solfoton)	3–5 mg/kg in infants; 5–8 mg/kg/day for young children; up to 40 mg/kg in older children	Hyperactivity, temper tantrums, attention deficit, Stevens-Johnson syndrome, rash, GI distress, irritability	Monitor for impaired cognition

Key Points

- The two main divisions of the nervous system consist of the CNS and the PNS. Each of these two systems has unique functions that regulate body systems.
- The brain, which includes three protective membranes—dura mater, arachnoid membrane, and pia mater—provides the coordination of the entire nervous system.
- The child's age and developmental level provide guidance about how to assess functioning of the CNS. Although the CNS is one of the first systems to form within uterine fetal development, it is actually one of the last to fully mature during childhood.
- Neurological disorders in childhood often require long medical treatment plans and care. The degree of disability and restoration of function depends on the location of the disorder, the amount of damage that has occurred, and the quality and timeliness of medical interventions.
- Children are at risk for a number of neurological disorders or injuries. CI, CP, seizure disorders, and lead poisoning are a few disorders that a pediatric nurse must become familiar with to help the health-care team identify early

the signs and symptoms and expedite interventions to maximize the potential for treatment and management. Children, especially adolescents, are at an increased risk of TBIs and SCIs.
- Teaching communities to insist that children wear protective equipment when playing sports, riding in a car, and playing at home or in parks is an important part of preventing head injuries and any lasting neurological deficits that may result.
- Families need a tremendous amount of support and education when they have a child with a neurological disorder. Many disorders carry a lifetime of care, and families need the guidance to learn how to care for their child. They also need to receive information about support available from regional and national organizations.
- Preventing complications of many neurological disorders, such as cerebral edema, increased ICP, and contractions, are a priority for pediatric nurses. It is essential that the nurse establish a therapeutic relationship that supports collaboration and teaching, and that provides emotional support.

REVIEW QUESTIONS

1. A mother brings her toddler into the pediatric public health clinic stating that his "personality has changed." The mother states the child has regressed developmentally and is, at times, hyperactive and very emotional. The pediatric nurse should include the possibility of which of the following:
   1. Intentional child abuse with a possible head injury
   2. Early signs of an emotional or cognitive disturbance
   3. Meningitis or another brain infection
   4. Possible exposure to lead

2. A father calls the pediatric clinic stating their local laboratory called to say their 4-year-old child who has a seizure disorder had a serum blood level of phenobarbital of 52 mcg/mL. What should be the next action of the nurse receiving the call?
   1. Ask the father to bring the child into the clinic for an appointment right away.
   2. Ask the parents to take the child back to the laboratory for a second draw to recheck the value.
   3. Tell the primary caregiver the laboratory value and await instructions.
   4. Tell the family to skip the next dose of the medication and then continue as ordered.

3. Lead is a:
   1. Commercially used substance
   2. Heavy, soft, and gray-blue metal substance
   3. Naturally occurring substance
   4. All of the above

4. Which cranial nerve would be assessed if a child who was in an MVA was brought in with a facial droop?
   1. III
   2. V
   3. VII
   4. XII

5. Of all of the following listed below, which is *not* considered a potential source of lead exposure to children?
   1. Glazed ceramics
   2. Treated building construction lumber
   3. Jewelry
   4. Imported cosmetics and particular remedies for health conditions

6. When reinforcing parental teaching about febrile seizures, the pediatric nurse includes the following:
   1. It is considered a seizure disorder and will require anticonvulsant therapy.
   2. It is associated strongly with genetic predisposition; all other siblings should be monitored.
   3. It relates to how rapidly the child's fever rises during an infectious process.
   4. It is considered a one-time event and requires no further medical attention or treatments.

7. What is the current CDC guideline for recognizing when a serum lead level shows potential toxicity in children?
   1. 5 mcg/dL
   2. 10 mcg/dL
   3. 25 mcg/dL
   4. 50 mcg/dL

8. Which of the following are associated with the administration of the anticonvulsant therapy phenytoin? *(select all that apply)*
   1. Gum hyperplasia
   2. Ataxia
   3. Gastric distress
   4. Anemia
   5. Sedation
   6. Weight gain
   7. Nystagmus
   8. Hirsutism

9. The child with migraines should have his or her diet investigated because research has shown foods and beverages that contain the preservative nitrate may be a trigger for the headaches. Nitrates are found in hot dogs, cold cuts, bacon, and commercially prepared foods and food mixes.
   1. True
   2. False

10. The licensed vocational nurse (LVN) is working with a pediatric registered nurse (RN) who is giving care to a child suspected of having meningitis. The LVN must immediately report which of the following symptoms to the RN?
   1. A headache described with a pain scale score of 4
   2. A sudden increase in thirst
   3. A change in energy level
   4. An abrupt eruption of a purplish rash or petechial rash

CRITICAL THINKING QUESTIONS

1. A 3-year-old child presents to the ED in postictal state after a generalized seizure. The parents report the child has been fussy, hitting the side of her head with her fists, and intermittently crying. What do you suspect has occurred in this clinical situation? What priority nursing care should be initiated and what short- and long-term teaching should be offered?

2. The ketogenic diet was first presented in 1920. Discuss the components of a ketogenic diet and how research studies have shown it to work for some children. Discuss the debate behind the ketogenic diet and analyze the long-term consequences for the child. Does the multidisciplinary pediatric health-care team in your area support the use of this diet? Why or why not?

3. Lead poisoning remains a serious national public health concern. What current initiatives are taking place on a nationwide level to increase the public's and health-care professionals' awareness of the concerns? How can a pediatric nurse become involved in public health initiatives?

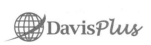

For additional resources and information, visit **www.DavisPlus.com.** Post-Conference Questions and Activities, Answers, and References can be found on Davis*Plus*.

30

Child With a Sensory Impairment

KEY TERMS

amblyopia
astigmatism
cataract
cerumen
color blindness
conductive hearing loss
deafness
decibel
enucleation
esotropia
exotropia
glaucoma
hard of hearing
hyperopia
legal blindness
leukokoria
myopia
nystagmus
otitis media
refractory errors
retinoblastoma
retinopathy of prematurity (ROP)
school vision
strabismus

DavisPlus For audio pronunciation guide, visit www.DavisPlus.com

CHAPTER CONCEPTS

Assessment
Development
Promoting Health
Safety
Sensory Perception
Trauma

LEARNING OUTCOMES

1. Define the key terms.
2. Describe the most common causes of visual impairment during childhood and differentiate between the care of a child with eye trauma, eye disease, and eye tumor.
3. Analyze common reactions when a family is told their infant or young child will be sensory impaired.
4. Discuss the national organizations that provide support to families who have a child with a visual or hearing impairment.
5. Differentiate between blindness and visual impairment, and between hard of hearing and deafness.
6. State the diagnostic examinations, assessments, treatments, and clinical outcomes of children with a confirmed diagnosis of retinoblastoma.
7. Discuss the resurgence of ROP and the care that can be provided to premature infants to reduce the possibility of developing this pathology.
8. State the definitions of the various visual impairments or visual disorders, including strabismus, amblyopia, and nystagmus.
9. Describe the various types and causes of congenital and acquired hearing impairments during childhood.
10. Outline a plan of care for a child with a new diagnosis of hearing impairment and describe the new technologies available to assist a child with a hearing impairment.

REAL-WORLD CASE STUDY

Lauren

■ Lauren, a 13-year-old girl, was attending a Fourth of July celebration with her family at their local community park. While standing with her family and a group of her peers, a bystander lit a large firework that malfunctioned and sprayed Lauren's face with burning chemicals. She was taken to a local emergency room and received treatment for her facial wounds. Because of the extent of the burn on

REAL-WORLD CASE STUDY *continued*

her eyes, she was required to wear bilateral eye dressings for no less than 3 weeks while her eyes healed. The only time the dressings were to be removed was during her ophthalmic assessments by her pediatric eye specialist, who was monitoring her visual sensory impairment carefully, or by her parents, if the dressing became wet or soiled. Lauren progressed from being very frightened that she could lose her vision to being very angry at her dependence on her mother for her daily care, her loss of socialization throughout her summer vacation from school, and decreased visits from her peer group.

1. Considering Lauren's developmental level, how would one expect her to react to her condition?
2. How might nursing staff assist the family in preparing a safe home for her while she is blind from the bilateral eye dressings that will be on for 3 weeks?

CONCEPTUAL CORNERSTONE

Safety

Early identification of a visual impairment or a hearing impairment allows for interventions to be initiated that provide for speech development, socialization, growth and development, and academic success. Visual and hearing impairments that are not found early can cause delays in a child's development and cause challenges in the school environment and for academic success. Even with a slight hearing loss (ie, the child needs to have greater than 15 to 24 decibel loss) creates the need for professional assistance with speech therapy, special academic accommodations, and possibly auditory training (Shargorodsky, Curhan, et al, 2010). Once identified, there are numerous new procedures, technologies, and devices that can be used to improve the child's sensory function. National organizations now provide families with support and education. Nurses are instrumental in facilitating the relationships between health-care centers, academic settings, and national organizations.

Children must have their sensory organs protected from injury and trauma. Vigorous play can result in eye injury, and loud noises (ie, approximately greater than 85 decibels) can result in hearing impairment. Pediatric nurses must provide anticipatory guidance for families to learn about protecting their child's sensory organs, and teaching adolescents about protecting their hearing.

Sensory impairments in childhood are a serious national concern. Both visual and hearing impairments can have significant consequences on a child's cognitive, social, and emotional development, sense of well-being, and academic success. Early detection through screenings and prompt interventions will assist the child and family in adapting to the effect of a diagnosis of a congenital or acquired sensory impairment.

Nurses are uniquely positioned to be integral in the early identification of sensory impairments. Nurses need to support and participate in national efforts to screen all early school-aged children for hearing and visual acuity, and help any affected child to secure a referral for interventions and/or treatments. Nurses also have the opportunity to educate families on risk factors for sensory impairments such as proper nutrition, injury prevention, anticipatory guidance, and adherence to well-child checkups and school screenings.

The incidence (ie, new cases) and prevalence (ie, existing cases) of sensory impairments are difficult to determine because they are not considered reportable conditions. Current literature states an estimate of between 3% and 11% of children have a sensory impairment that needs an intervention. Worldwide, it has been determined that the leading cause of visual impairment throughout childhood is the underidentified need for a child to simply wear corrective glasses (Powell, Wedner, et al, 2011).

Noise-induced hearing loss (NIHL) can occur over a period of time or can be immediate. NIHL can be permanent or it can be temporary. Sometimes it is not apparent that hearing damage is occurring. Most hearing loss associated with NIHL can be prevented. Approximately 16% of teenagers 12 to 19 years of age have reported some hearing loss related to loud noises (Centers for Disease Control and Prevention [CDC], 2010). School screenings are highly effective in identifying children at risk, although these screenings are limited to developing countries and are not administered worldwide. The most common cause of hearing impairment is **conductive hearing loss,** which is associated with repeated cases of otitis media (OM).

Unfortunately, when a child experiences a sensory impairment, his or her academic success becomes at risk. Children in the classroom who are suffering visual impairments may complain of headaches and squint regularly during class. For example, nearsightedness, or **myopia,** is a major form of visual impairment and has a profound effect on a child's ability to follow teachers' written instructions. According to a Cochrane review of research on the value of early school screenings, it was determined that variances exist in screening settings, training of personnel, threshold of passing or failing a screening test, frequency of screenings, and referral of the child to an appropriate health-care provider. Nurses need to continue to be involved with the process of screening children for sensory impairments and they need to rapidly report suspected deviations.

THE DEVELOPMENT OF VISUAL ACUITY

The human eye develops during embryonic growth starting in the third week of life. As the fetus grows, the optic nerve extends from the growing neuroepithelium, as does the retina, iris, and ciliary body. Newborns are born with very poor vision even though their eye anatomy is fully intact. With 2 million nerve fibers that need to connect the eyes to the brain, the first few weeks of life the newborn has very poor vision with recognition of light and dark only. It is not until 3 months of life that an infant acquires the level of visual acuity to recognize a face. Nurses should encourage parents to hold their newborn close to their faces as part of the bonding process (Fig. 30.1).

Structures of the Eye

The anatomy of the eye is very complex (Fig. 30.2). In general, the eye has three layers: the inner retina; the middle layer, which includes the iris, choroid, and ciliary body; and the outer sclera, including the cornea. There are two major cavities in the eye; the anterior cavity (ie, small cavity in front of the lens) and the posterior cavity (ie, the larger cavity). The anterior section is filled with aqueous humor and the posterior cavity is filled with vitreous humor. Communication between the eye and the brain takes place along the optic nerve (ie, the second cranial nerve).

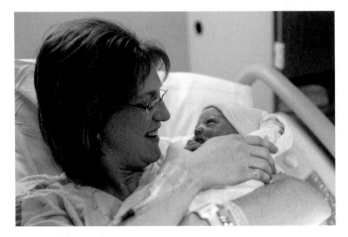

FIGURE 30.1 Mother holding newborn close.

VISUAL IMPAIRMENT

Visual disturbances in young children are a common problem. The American Optometric Association (2011) estimated that 25% of all children have a visual disorder requiring screening and follow-up care. The term *visual impairment* is used to describe those impairments that most prescription lenses will not correct and may require surgical interventions. Wong (2007) estimated that approximately 30 to 64 children out of every 100,000 within the population will demonstrate a visual impairment. Visual impairments during childhood can be either congenital or acquired. Congenital visual impairments include those associated with hereditary conditions, genetic anomalies, and consequences of exposure to a toxin, infectious disease, or early prematurity. Acquired visual impairments are associated with a traumatic injury to the eyes, brain damage from anoxia or shaken baby syndrome, or a disease process whose consequence is an effect on the child's visual acuity.

TEAM WORKS

Using Correct Terminology

It is important that the health-care team members use the correct terms when differentiating between visual impairment and blindness. When a child is considered blind, there is no visual sensory experience. *Visual impairment* is a term used to denote that a child's vision is reduced or impaired, but some sensory experience is taking place. This is the same with the terms *deafness* and *hard of hearing*. When a child has **deafness**, there is no processing of acoustic stimuli, whereas the term **hard of hearing** is used to denote some processing of acoustic stimuli. The terms should not be used

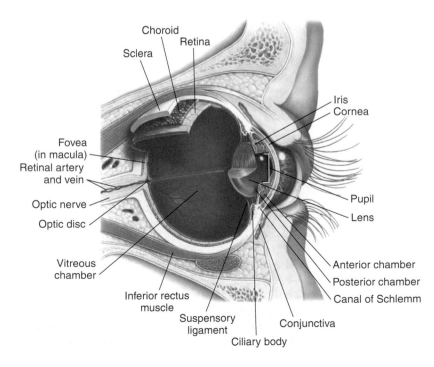

Choroid
Retina
Sclera
Iris
Cornea
Fovea (in macula)
Retinal artery and vein
Optic nerve
Optic disc
Pupil
Lens
Vitreous chamber
Anterior chamber
Posterior chamber
Canal of Schlemm
Inferior rectus muscle
Suspensory ligament
Conjunctiva
Ciliary body

FIGURE 30.2 Anatomy of the human eye.

incorrectly, especially around families. When in doubt, confirm the child's past medical history and use the correct term to reduce a parents' fears. A visually impaired child should not be called blind unless confirmed.

The etiology of visual impairment in children can be a genetic predisposition or cause, a prenatal exposure such as to a toxin or interuterine infection, or it can be associated with postnatal conditions. Postnatal conditions include conditions such as trauma, juvenile rheumatoid arthritis, albinism, or a condition that affects the vasculature of the retina such as **retinopathy of prematurity (ROP)** (ie, retinal damage for premature infants associated with high oxygen levels and environmental factors) or sickle cell anemia. Worldwide, the World Health Organization (WHO) estimates that 13.8 million children have some degree of severe visual loss or eye damage because of a vitamin A deficiency (www.ncbi.nlm.nih.gov, 2011).

Trauma to the eye structures continues to be a major concern in the pediatric population. Trauma to the eyes can be from vigorous play that causes an instrument such as pencil or scissors to enter the eye, or it can be caused from a severe injury associated with fire, car accidents, exposure to chemicals, or exposure to prolonged sunlight. Corneal abrasions are one of the most common causes of mild trauma to the eye during childhood. See Box 30.1 for a presentation on corneal abrasions.

PATIENT TEACHING GUIDELINES

Protection of Sight

Use of sunglasses for children who are exposed to intense sunlight for long periods of time must start at a young age and be required by parents or guardians. Sunlight can be very damaging to the eyes because of ultraviolet (UV) exposure. The most damaging exposure takes place when sunlight reflects off snow, water, pavement, or sand. Cumulative damage over childhood can have a lasting effect on vision because the human eye lens cannot repair itself. The lens of the child's eye transmits approximately 70% more UV than the eye of an adult. Appropriate sunglasses should be worn consistently from young childhood throughout the lifespan (Jones, 2012).

Box 30.1 Concerns About Corneal Abrasions

Most corneal abrasions are caused by the irritation and inflammation associated with a foreign body on the eye. Children can have a foreign body enter their eye structures and experience considerable discomfort, resulting in deep rubbing or scratching around or on the eyes. Patching of the eye for at least 24 hours to provide for comfort and the administration of sterile antimicrobial eye drops may be warranted.

The most common type of visual disturbance leading to visual impairment is a refractory error. When a child experiences this type of condition, the light rays bend as they pass through the lens and therefore do not fall directly on to the child's retina. A refractory error leaves a child either nearsighted because the light rays fall in front of the retina (ie, myopia), or farsighted because the light rays fall beyond the retina (ie, **hyperopia**). Table 30.1 provides a list of visual impairments found in children.

Assessments of Visual Acuity

Routine vision screening is an important part of a well-child visit, even when the child is an infant. Many visual abnormalities are treatable or correctable if they are discovered early and promptly. If left untreated, a child's visual impairment may lead to progressive visual loss and eventual blindness. It is important to screen early school-aged children so a visual disorder or disturbance does not affect their scholastic performance.

The term *school vision* is used when a child is considered to be partially sighted with a measured or approximate visual acuity of 20/70 to 20/200. *Legal blindness* is a term used to note that a child's visual acuity is measured or approximated to be below 20/200.

Children should be routinely screened for not only visual acuity, but also, if warranted, assessed for strabismus, refractory errors, and amblyopia because these are the three most commonly found visual impairments of all preschoolers. The most important aspect of screening is to make sure parents are notified, a referral is made, and a follow-up appointment with a visual specialist is carried out. The American Optometric Association supports mass screening of all early school-age children, both in public and private schools, to ensure a child's quality of life and achievement of full potential (www.AOA.org, 2011).

HEALTH PROMOTION

National School-Aged Child Screening Guidelines for Sensory Impairments

The following are common guidelines implemented by state initiatives for early detection of visual and hearing impairments:

- Should be done within first few months of entering public or private early childhood education, such as kindergarten, beginning at 4 years of age and older. Should be conducted on any first-time school entrants from 4 years of age through 12th grade.
- Ideally, visual and hearing screening is repeated in first, third, fifth, and seventh grade.
- Documentation should be collected on each child and should include the child's name, type of screening test done, date of screening, screener, and screening results.

Visual Screening

Visual screening tests should include: a distance acuity for both eyes (eg, 20/20, 20/30) with approved charts such as Snellen's "tumbling E," Snellen's alphabet, or Sloan's letter chart; HOTV crowded test set; and a muscle balance test,

TABLE 30.1   VISUAL IMPAIRMENTS FOUND IN CHILDHOOD

Impairment	Description
Amblyopia	Unilateral or bilateral decrease of best corrected vision in an otherwise healthy eye often because of asymmetric refractive error (ie, deflection from a straight path or change in direction of light) or the presence of strabismus.
Astigmatism	A visual disorder where the refraction of a ray of light is spread over a diffuse area rather than sharply focused on the retina. This is because of a difference in the curvature of the cornea and lens of the eye
Cataracts	An opacity (ie, cloudy appearance) of the eye lens, often caused by trauma, aging, metabolic or endocrine disease, or the side effects of certain medications such as steroids
Esotropia	Inward deviation of the eye laterally
Exotropia	Outward deviation of the eye laterally
Glaucoma	A group of eye diseases that leads to increased intraocular pressure and eventually the atrophy of the optic nerve
Color Blindness	An inability to distinguish certain colors or any colors at all
Nystagmus	Involuntary back-and-forth movements of the eyes, most often noticeable when the patient gazes at rapidly moving or fixed objects
Refractory Error	A common eye disorder where the eye bends light and is unable to focus because of an abnormal shape of the eye
Strabismus	Abnormal alignment of the eyes that interferes with binocular vision; both eyes do not properly align with each other (also called *cross-eye* or *wall-eye* in lay terms)

such as Hirschberg's corneal light reflex test or the cover-uncover test.

Hearing Screening

Hearing screening tests should include: a pure tone sweep-check screen recorded for both ears conducted at an intensity level less than or equal to 25 decibels.

(Check with your state's Department of Health Services to find guidelines for children at various ages and to find documentation on your state mandates.)

Nurses will be participating in a variety of assessments for visual acuity based on the setting in which they practice and based on the availability of equipment. The following list describes assessments that are commonly used.

- **Snellen's test** (for 6 years of age through adolescence): This form of visual testing uses a chart with numbers, letters, or figures. The child covers one eye, stands back 20 feet, and vocally describes the letters, shapes, or figures to the testing personnel. The child typically starts with large letters, reads across to the end, and then reads the next line that is smaller. This continues until the child is unable to accurately read a line. Each line denotes a level of visual acuity.
- **LEA symbol chart** (ages 3 to 6, preschool): The purpose of this chart is to check for visual acuity of children who

do not yet know the alphabet. Visual acuity is screened with the child at a distance of 10 feet using what is known as LEA symbols; common symbols that can be matched by this age group on a response card. The child either stands or sits and is instructed to match the symbols on a response card being shown.

- **Unilateral cover test for infants or young children:** Here an infant or young child is assessed for their ability to follow an object when one eye is covered. A small toy can be used to entice a young child to follow the object with his or eyes. Each eye is then assessed. If an older infant or young child becomes fussy during the examination, this may indicate they are frustrated that they cannot see the desired toy through the eye that is uncovered.
- **Corneal light reflex test:** Here a light is directed toward the bridge of the nose and the light reflex is then examined for symmetry and to make sure the light shines in the same spot on both of the child's eyes. A misalignment is suspected if the light reflex is not symmetrical or is off-centered in both eyes.

Visual Impairment or Blindness in Infants

Identifying visual impairment in infants is more challenging than an older child who can demonstrate cues of squinting, eye-rubbing, or vocalizing complaints of difficulty focusing. Visual impairments in infants require a different set of assessment techniques. In young infants, certain disturbances of vision would have to be identified by inspection of the inner eye such as ROP, cataracts, or glaucoma. In older infants, if the parent or nurse identifies a lack of tracking an object that would normally be interesting to this developmental stage, then an impairment would be suspected. For instance, if an infant does not find pleasure in tracking a colorful toy across visual fields, turn to visually inspect a musical toy or interesting auditory stimuli, or if they do not focus on the caregiver's face when close, an impairment should be suspected.

Eye Infections

Children are especially prone to eye infections. Eye infections can be viral or bacterial and many are highly contagious. Two common infections are conjunctivitis and neonatorum eye infections.

Conjunctivitis

When a child presents with inflammation of the conjunctiva, "pinkeye" must be ruled out. The conjunctiva is normally clear, smooth, and moist. If this lining, which covers both the eye and under the lids, becomes inflamed, the eye should be evaluated for an infection, allergy, foreign body, or trauma. When the drainage is purulent, bacterial contamination must be suspected and antibiotic eye drops are ordered. If the culprit is bacterial, this eye condition is considered a highly contagious infection.

Nursing considerations include preventing the spread of the bacterial infection. Teaching should include how to cleanse the purulent drainage with a warm, moist cloth used only once. Proper hand washing followed by a "no touch" rule needs to be reinforced for both the caregiver and the child. When eye drops are instilled, the top of the medicine bottle should never touch the child's tissues because this will contaminate the medicine dropper and could lead to continued re-infection. If an antimicrobial ointment is ordered, the family should be taught to instill the ointment from the inner cannula to the outer cannula by dispensing a thin, steady stream into the lower eyelid.

PATIENT TEACHING GUIDELINES

Care of a Child With Bacterial Conjunctivitis

Questions frequently asked by parents include the following:

1. *What are the most common causes of conjunctivitis in childhood?*
   Conjunctivitis is an inflammation of the conjunctiva that is usually caused by infection or allergy. It is frequently referred to as *pinkeye* and is the most common acute eye disorder seen by pediatricians and pediatric nurse practitioners. It may be viral or bacterial. Bacterial conjunctivitis is found to be twice as common as viral conjunctivitis. Common organisms causing bacterial conjunctivitis are *Streptococcus* and *Staphylococcus*.
2. *What are the characteristics of an infectious conjunctivitis?*
   Typically, in bacterial conjunctivitis, the eye is very red; there is a purulent (ie, pus) discharge; the affected child is often a preschool child; and there may be an associated OM (ie, ear infection).
3. *Why is there a need to determine if the cause is viral or bacterial?*
   Viral conjunctivitis does not require antimicrobial eye drops or eye ointment treatment. The child should not receive prolonged periods of topical treatment if the cause is viral.
4. *What is the treatment for bacterial conjunctivitis?*
   The pediatrician or nurse practitioner will order antibiotic treatment to speed healing and eradicate the bacteria. This allows children to return to daycare centers and schools within 24 hours of treatment. The child should have both eyes treated even if only one eye appears red. Treatment with eye drops is usually needed 4 times a day for no more than 5 days.
5. *Are there any home treatments for bacterial conjunctivitis?*
   There is no safe substitute for seeking a diagnosis and treatment from a primary health-care provider. It is most important to finish all of the antibiotic eye drop or ointment treatment. At home, make sure you wash your hands before and after applying the medication to the child's eyes. Remember, the infection is contagious. Applying warm, moist compresses to the child's eyes will help with the removal of the pus drainage and will feel soothing. Do not cross-contaminate the cloth between the eyes; use a separate cloth for each eye and do not reuse the cloth again without thoroughly washing the cloth in hot water. Throw away any tissues used, make sure siblings or others in the home do not have contact with the cloths used for cleaning the infected eye, and wipe down counters and surfaces with a disinfectant cleaner. Have the child wash his/her hands frequently.
6. *How do I apply the eye drops or eye ointment?*
   Applying eye drops or ointment 4 times a day for up to 5 days can create a battle between you and your child. Try to solicit help from another adult. One adult will need to have the child lean their head back and the adult will need to open the eyelid with one hand while instilling the medication with the other hand. The child will blink, sometimes excessively. Do not let the child rub their eyes after the instillation. Do not let the medication bottle tip touch the child's eyes because this may cause trauma and may contaminate the medication bottle. If possible, have the child stay lying down for a minute or two with the eyes closed. The entire medication dose must be completed unless instructed otherwise by the health-care provider.

   Call your child's health-care provider IMMEDIATELY if you find:
   - The child's outer eyelids have become very red or swollen
   - The child complains that his or her vision has become blurred or changes in any way
   - Your child has a fever, vomits, or **starts** acting very sick

---

SAFETY *STAT!*

Contact Lenses and Eye Infections

If the child usually wears contact lenses, make sure the child wears glasses until the infection is gone and the health-care provider says it is safe to return to the use of the contacts. Do not allow a child to apply makeup. Throw away mascara if the child has used it during the infection.

Neonatorum Eye Infections

Also called *neonatal conjunctivitis* or *ophthalmia neonatorum,* this type of eye infection occurs as a newborn passes through a birth canal infected with a bacterial infection of either *Neisseria gonorrhoeae* or *Chlamydia trachomatis.* Treatment includes eye drops containing erythromycin. It is imperative that the nurse teach the family to cleanse the eyes of the infant with a clean cloth soaked in warm water. The cloth must not be reused or re-infection may occur. If left untreated, the infant may experience complete blindness.

Nursing Considerations for a Child With a Visual Impairment

Children of all ages who experience either a congenital, primary, or acquired visual disturbance need support and education. A traumatic event that leads to the sudden loss of vision affects the child both emotionally and developmentally. It is important to provide special care based on the etiology of the visual impairment and the child's developmental needs. Children who sudden lose their vision based on traumatic injury or accident need support when initially learning they are going to be impaired. The nursing supervisor and spiritual leader, as well as the Child Life, social services, child psychology, pediatric ophthalmology, and pediatric surgical services should provide support, rapid assessments, and interventions for the child and family who present with a significant eye trauma.

If a child is going home after eye surgery with bilateral eye dressings in place, the family should be instructed to create a safe home environment. Removing clutter, placing needed objects within reach of the child, providing verbal guidance for moving around the home, and supervising the child in activities of daily living are all important to secure safety.

THERAPEUTIC COMMUNICATION

Families who present to the pediatric health-care setting with a child who has just suffered a traumatic loss of vision or hearing will need special support. The fear and anxiety associated with the potential loss of vision or hearing is profound and each member of the family needs support. The health-care team should:

- Acknowledge each family member's feelings.
- Request backup from other members of the nursing staff so you can stay with the family.
- Provide presence; do not walk away unless necessary.
- Allow the parents to express their feelings, ask questions, and feel supported.

After a child recovers from eye surgery or treatments, the child might benefit from assistive devices to improve comprehension of his or her environment, socialization, and success at school. There are six general forms of assistive devices available for a child with a visual impairment within a health-care setting:

- Signage and information presented in Braille
- Information and books in large print suitable for the individual child's need
- Audio tapes
- Computer speech output
- Computer screen readers that enlarge print
- Adaptive keyboards

DISORDERS OF THE EYE

During the developmental period of childhood, there are several conditions or pathologies that can be acquired in the sensory organs. Generally, disorders of the eye remain uncommon. Some are very uncommon, such as the rare malignant tumor of the eye called a *retinoblastoma,* and others are increasing in incidence, such as ROP.

Retinoblastoma

When a child suffers from a cancerous tumor of the eye, a **retinoblastoma** (ie, a malignant tumor of the retina) must be ruled out. The retina is made up of nerve tissue that is able to sense light as it comes through the lens and then sends visual signals to the brain via the optic nerve. In approximately half of all cases of retinoblastoma, the gene mutation causing the tumor of the retina to grow develops in a child with no family history of eye cancer. Generally affecting children between the ages of 1 and 2 years, this cancer presents with a whitish glow as light falls on the affected eye's retina. The phenomenon is know as *leukocoria,* also called cat's eye reflex. Other symptoms the child might present with include double vision, "crossed eyes," misalignment, eye pain, redness, and overall visual impairment. The tumor may affect only one eye or both eyes (Fig. 30.3).

Assessments for the presence of retinoblastoma include dilation of the pupil with an eye evaluation. A magnetic resonance image (MRI) or computed tomography (CT) scan will be ordered to evaluate for the presence of metastasis, especially around the bony orbit.

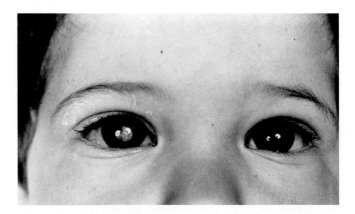

FIGURE 30.3 Retinoblastoma.

Treatment of retinoblastoma includes laser surgery or cryotherapy for small tumors. Radiation, chemotherapy, and possibly **enucleation** (ie, eye removal) may be warranted for aggressive or larger tumors. If the tumor spreads to the bones around the eye, or spreads to the brain via the optic nerve, more aggressive therapy is needed to control the metastasis. As long as there is no evidence of the cancer spreading beyond the retina, the cure rate for early retinoblastoma is very high.

Retinopathy of Prematurity

ROP is an eye disease of the premature infant. When an infant is born prematurely, the retina is not fully vascularized. At the birth of the premature infant, the development of the vascularity arrests, and then begins to proliferate abnormally. Retinal blood vessels branch out excessively and increase in number, and a small hemorrhage may occur, leading to scarring. Sometimes the fibrovascular proliferation extends into the vitreous humor. The scarring process pulls the retina away from the basement membranes, resulting in impaired vision or blindness in the infant. Excessive oxygen use and quantity in premature babies has been associated with the development of ROP. Infants born weighing less than 1,250 g are at the greatest risk.

SAFETY *STAT!*

Improved survival of infants born weighing 1,000 g or less, considered extremely low birth weight (ELBW), is causing an increase in the incidence of ROP. Children who are born at or less than 28 weeks' gestation are a particular risk (Sahin, et al, 2014).

Assessment for the presence and severity of ROP begins with an eye examination, often performed in the neonatal intensive care unit (NICU). Location of disease within the three zones of the retina (zone 1 extends from the center of the retina, followed by zones 2 and 3 extending around and out from zone 1) is followed by severity, listed as stage 1 to 5. Zones are centered around the optic nerve, with zone 1 being the most posterior zone of the retina. Although stages 1 and 2 do not indicate blindness, progression of disease can occur.

Preventing ROP begins with the judicious use of oxygen and very careful monitoring of newborns receiving oxygen therapy. Using transcutaneous measurement devices and starting with low-flow oxygen therapy have been found to decrease incidence and severity.

Recent research has demonstrated that oxygen levels administered in excess of 40% were most concerning in the development of ROP. Furthermore, the absence of protective measures to reduce premature newborns' exposure to light also contributes to the development and severity of ROP. Nurses must be aware of the possibility of ROP because there is now a resurgence in its incidence. Careful administration of oxygen, early screening, and rapid interventions are required to reduce the incidence and severity of ROP. Although the cause of ROP is still not fully understood, the goal is to prevent the newborn from developing early ROP.

Treatment for ROP consists of cryotherapy. This procedure is recommended for both of the infant's eyes whenever there is a stage 3 ROP or higher. Stage 3 is when half of the circumference in zone 1 or 3 is present. Further studies are being performed to identify the efficacy of anticoagulation therapy and laser photocoagulation therapy.

In most infants with ROP, the disease spontaneously subsides. Premature infants with severe forms of ROM may have complete and permanent blindness. Nursing considerations include preventing the use of indiscriminate amounts of oxygen for premature and ELBW infants, preventing exposure to light, and increasing stability after early birth.

PATIENT TEACHING GUIDELINES

National Organizations That Provide Support for Children With Visual Impairments

- Lions Clubs International: Information on free eyeglasses, regional and local visual screening tests (low cost or free)
- National Association for Parents of Children with Visual Impairments: Information on different visual disorders and pathologies
- American Printing House for the Blind: Information on providing written materials for the blind
- American Council of the Blind: Information for families with a blind child; resources and educational materials

---

THE DEVELOPMENT OF HEARING

The sense of hearing begins during early fetal development, with intact hearing acuity achieved between the 22nd and 23rd week of gestation. The sounds of the mother's heart, digestion, blood flow, and other normal anatomical sounds are heard by the fetus. Research has shown that the fetus, starting at approximately 19 weeks' gestation, will demonstrate movement when exposed to sound (Hepper and Shahidullah, 1995).

Structures of the Ear

The human ear processes sound through a six-step process (Fig. 30.4). Disease, damage, infection, or inflammation to any part of the six-step process can cause hearing impairment. The six-step process, in order of occurrence, is:

1. Sound waves enter the outer ear and pass through the ear canal.
2. The ear drum vibrates and sends the vibrations to the three ear bones (ie, malleus, incus, and stapes).
3. The three bones change the sound vibrations to fluid vibrations in the cochlea of the inner ear.
4. A travel wave forms along the basilar membrane, and the inner ear hair cells (ie, sensory cells) then respond to the wave.
5. The tiny hairlike projections on top of the hair cells move to an up-and-down motion and hit against the

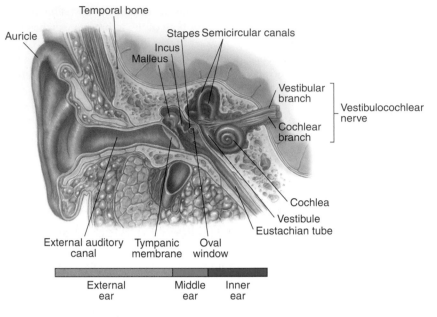

FIGURE 30.4 Structure of the human ear.

overlying structures. This process changes the motion into an electrical signal.

6. The electrical signal then is sent via the auditory nerve to the brain for processing and recognition.

HEARING IMPAIRMENT

A child's hearing impairment can be just as devastating to parents as a visual impairment. Hearing impairments, one of the most common disabilities in the nation, are categorized as any condition that interferes with the child's ability to receive auditory information from the environment or verbal communications taking place around them. The incidence of hearing impairments is estimated to be 3 out of every 1,000 well infants and 2 to 4 out of every 100 neonates admitted into NICUs (Wong, 2008). Nurses need to be advocates for children with hearing impairments and need to provide play, stimulation, and services that maximize the child's developing language and socialization.

NIHL in childhood can be caused by sounds during hunting, snowmobiling, attending concerts, and with the consistent use of ear buds with music being played too loud (National Institutes of Health [NIH], 2015). Nurses must provide screening and education to help prevent hearing impairments in early and late childhood. Promoting the use of noise reduction devices such as ear plugs and over-the-ear headphones can help prevent NIHL.

Three Main Types of Hearing Impairment

Children can present with a hearing loss defined by three distinct types: conductive, sensorineural, and combined. The following list describes the differences between the three.

• **Conductive hearing loss:** A condition that interferes with the ability of the child to receive auditory communications from their environment; this occurs when the tympanic membrane cannot vibrate after sound passes through the ear canal. Cerumen buildup, OM, or foreign bodies can all be the causes of conductive hearing loss.

• **Sensorineural hearing loss:** This condition is directly related to damage to the auditory nerve or the cochlea. This condition may be congenital, such as with rubella syndrome, or acquired, such as exposure to ototoxic drugs. The damage to the eighth cranial nerve causes the inner ear to malfunction.

• **Combined conductive/sensorineural hearing loss:** Also called *mixed hearing loss,* this condition involves the combination of conductive and sensorineural hearing loss.

DRUG FACTS

Exposure to ototoxic drugs, such as the antibiotic category of aminoglycosides, can be a significant source of hearing impairments. When administering aminoglycosides, the pediatric health-care team must administer the drug within the safe dose range and, when indicated, follow serum levels of the antibiotic (ie, peaks and troughs) to make sure the child is not exposed to toxic quantities of the drug. Other ototoxic drugs include the chemotherapy drug cisplatin and certain IV diuretics, such as furosemide (Lasix), when pushed too rapidly.

SAFETY *STAT!*

Sound with decibels sustained or repeated at 85 or above are likely to cause hearing damage. Older children who listen to loud electronic music through ear buds at full volume are exposed to approximately 105 decibels, which causes damage to the inner ear structures. The louder the sound in decibels, the shorter period of time is required to cause significant hearing damage.

Assessments of Hearing Impairment and Ear Structures

Hearing screening should begin early to promote optimal development for the infant (Fig. 30.5). Hearing impairments can affect a young child's communication ability by interfering with his or her ability to talk and interact with others. Visual inspection and audiography should both be performed to rule out any hearing impairment.

Hearing acuity is often expressed in a unit of sound called a *decibel.* See Box 30.2 for a summary of the intensity of sounds as measured by decibels. If a child is unable to hear at a certain level of decibels, then they are considered hearing impaired up to that number.

Visual assessment of a child's ears should begin during early well-child checkups during infancy. When visualizing the tympanic membrane of children under 3 years, the pinna should be pulled straight out and down. For children older than 3 years, the pinna should be pulled straight out and up. These gestures allow for the maximal visualization of the ear drum. The younger child has a different position of the eustachian tube than an older child, which results in decreased drainage of fluids.

Early infant behaviors indicating hearing impairment include the lack of a startle reflex to loud noises. If an infant does not turn his or her head to identify a noise, a hearing impairment should be suspected. For toddlers and preschoolers, a hearing impairment should be suspected if the child participates in gestures to communicate his or her needs and has little or no speech skills, or if speech is garbled and unintelligible. School-aged children and adolescents who sit closer than expected to speakers, turn the TV louder than others, or who demonstrate declining school performance and fewer social interactions should be worked up for an acquired hearing impairment.

Many states now require mandatory newborn hearing screening. Before a newborn is discharged from the hospital,

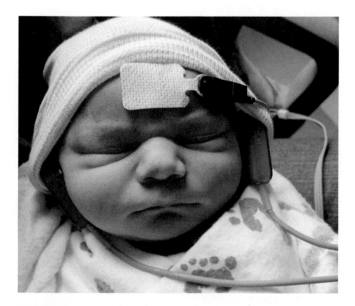

FIGURE 30.5 Newborn having a hearing screening test.

Box 30.2 Sound Intensity Expressed as Decibels

0 = Softest sound a healthy and normal human ear can hear

10 = Sound of a heartbeat or the rustling of leaves

20 = Sound of a person whispering at 5 feet away

30–45 = Normal conversation between two people

60 = Noise found at a typical restaurant

70 = Noise found on a typical city street

80 = Sound of a loud radio played inside a room

90–100 = Sound of a passing train

105 = Sound of electronic music through ear buds at full volume

120 = Sound of loud music (ie, inside rock concert) or the sound of thunder

125 = Sound of sirens up close

140 = Sound of a jet plane taking off while standing near by

150 = Sounds of firecrackers and firearms at close range

Greater than 140 = Considered the human pain threshold

a screening procedure takes place while the infant sleeps. Electrodes are placed on the neonate's scalp and mandible. Light sounds are transmitted via headphones, and brain electrical activity is assessed. If the newborn is not screened before discharge from the postpartum period, screening can take place during a well-neonate visit.

Nursing Considerations of a Child With a Hearing Impairment

Pediatric nurses must adapt their care to provide holistic care to a child with a hearing impairment. Providing technology that increases the child's acoustic processing and understanding of what is going on around him or her is very important. When prescribed, the nurse should provide positive reinforcement for wearing hearing aids. Anticipatory guidance should include protecting the child from harm, how to care for utilized hearing assistive devices, and the promotion of a normal childhood with play, socialization, and academics.

SAFETY *STAT!*

It is imperative that children wear devices that are prescribed and made for them to enhance their sensory experiences. Wearing hearing aids at all times when awake and keeping a child's prescription glasses on increases development and improves socialization and academic success.

DISORDERS OF THE EAR

There are several disorders of the ear that can be found in pediatrics. Some of the disorders relate to congenital defects and others are acquired. The following represent select common disorders of the ear found in children.

Buildup of Cerumen

Cerumen, or ear wax, is a natural substance produced within the auditory canal to provide an antibacterial action. Cerumen can be produced in a variety of colors from golden, light yellow to a dark brown. Often quite viscous, ear wax can build up in some children and be a contributing factor to hearing impairments. Upon assessment, it may be found that a wall of ear wax is present and needs to be gently removed by irrigation with warm tap water or carefully removed with an ear wax removal tool by a trained health-care professional. Parents and caregivers should be discouraged to provide these interventions because damage to the tympanic membrane can occur.

SAFETY *STAT!*

Neither parents nor children should ever try to remove ear wax by using any instrument, including pencils, sticks, or any sharp object; this may perforate the tympanic membrane. The use of commercially made ear wax removal devices remains controversial. Tell the parents not to use any instrument in their child's ear without discussing it with their primary health-care provider.

If a family seeks consultation for cerumen buildup, an over-the-counter product for ear wax removal may be successful in cleaning out simple accumulation. The family should be instructed to have the child lie down with the affected ear up, and then instill the prescribed amount of drops per the product label. A cotton ball can be placed in the auricle of the ear to prevent rapid drainage of the medication. If an over-the-counter medication is not successful in cleansing the ear, then a trained health-care professional should be notified and the child should be brought in for irrigation.

Otitis Media

Otitis media (OM) is either a viral or bacterial infection that causes the buildup of inflammatory fluids or pus behind the tympanic membrane. OM is often accompanied by discomfort. OM is one of the most common childhood illnesses, with the greatest incidence between 6 and 36 months of age. The most common cause of conductive hearing loss is multiple episodes of OM. Parents need to understand as their child grows, the angle and position of the eustachian tube will change, facilitating drainage and the repeated episodes of

OM will decrease. Children, in general, have a greater slant in their eustachian tubes that can collect fluids and contribute to the development of OM.

The pathology behind OM is a dysfunction within the eustachian tube. The eustachian tube is meant to provide drainage and ventilation of the middle ear. If a child is experiencing an upper respiratory infection, the eustachian tube becomes edematous and blocks the draining of inflammatory fluids. The presence of the inflammatory fluids acts as a medium for bacterial growth and viral multiplication, and a middle ear infection develops. Children who are born with malformations of the head and neck, such as Down's syndrome or cleft palate, are more susceptible to episodes of OM. Common causative organisms for OM include *Neisseria catarrhalis, Haemophilus influenza,* and *Streptococcus pneumoniae.* OM with effusions is the buildup of inflammatory fluids or pus behind the tympanic membrane. OM without effusions is the presence of inflammation within the inner ear without the presence of inflammatory fluids or pus.

Infants should never be put to bed with a bottle. Infants who fall asleep with a bottle in the mouth can have a collection of fluids enter the eustachian tube and contribute to the development of OM.

SAFETY *STAT!*

Lack of a complete set of childhood immunizations is associated with the development of one or more bouts of OM. The administration of the annual influenza vaccine and the pneumococcal conjugate vaccine (PCV) have been shown to be useful in preventing acute OM because there is a direct association between influenza and S pneumoniae.

Assessments for OM include irritability, pulling at ears, hitting the side of the head, diarrhea, vomiting, and fever. Some children are asymptomatic. A confirmed diagnosis comes from the visual inspection with an otoscope to identify a red, bulging, and nonmobile tympanic membrane. Treatment for an ear infection may or may not include oral antibiotics. If the physician identifies the infection as being viral in nature, then the child's symptoms will be addressed, but no antimicrobial treatment will be offered. Ear infections are more common in children and adolescents who have Down's syndrome (Fig. 30.6). Both dysfunction in the immune system of a child with Down's syndrome and the abnormal anatomical structure of the child's face contribute to more frequent ear infections (Rudd and Kocisko, 2014).

Repeated OM may require surgical interventions. The placement of tympanostomy tubes through a procedure called a *myringotomy* can be performed in a day-surgery setting. A small incision is cut into the ear drum and small tubes are placed. The tubes allow the drainage of inflammatory

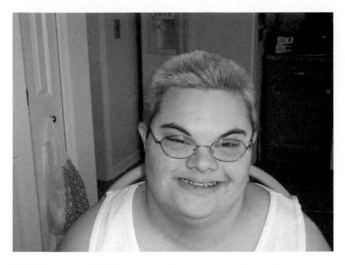

FIGURE 30.6 Children and adolescents with Down's syndrome are more at risk for ear infections.

fluids and reduce the pressure buildup that is causing discomfort. Parents need to understand that the tubes will come out on their own by spontaneously extruding through the ear drum into the ear canal and falling out. No surgical removal of the tubes is warranted. Typical preoperative and postoperative care is required, including teaching the family about the operative process, anesthesia, and the reduction of symptoms after the fluids and pressure are released by the tubes. Postoperative care instructions include the signs and symptoms of on-going infection, reporting of postoperative fevers, and understanding that the tubes will fall out on their own. Securing follow-up appointments after surgery is also an important part of teaching.

PATIENT TEACHING GUIDELINES

Tympanoplasty
Tympanoplasty is usually offered in an out-patient or short-stay surgery environment.
- Preoperative guidelines:
  - Your child will be put to sleep with anesthesia prior to the procedures. He or she must not eat or drink after midnight the day before (but follow specific institutional policy). Any preoperative fevers, infections, cough, or respiratory infections must be reported to the surgical department. Any allergies the child may have should be reported.
- In the postoperative period the child may experience:
  - Mild pain in the ear and neck
  - Drainage from the ear for 48 hours
- Guidelines for home care after myringotomy for tympanoplasty tube insertion include:
  - Avoid getting water in the ear and be careful while bathing.
  - No swimming until cleared by the surgical team.

- If the drainage is pus or if there is an odor with any drainage, report this finding immediately.
- If ordered, follow instructions for ear drops and complete the entire amount of the prescription as ordered, even if the child feels better.
- Use acetaminophen for postoperative pain.
- Resume normal activities the day after surgery.
- If the tubes fall out too early, or if there is increased discomfort in the ear, call your provider.

Nursing Considerations for Otitis Media
Parents may need to be taught to use ear plugs for their children who have repeated episodes of OM that require tympanostomy tube placement to prevent bath water or pool water from entering the ears.

A sudden relief of pain associated with OM may mean that the tympanic membrane has ruptured and the pressure buildup behind the ear drum has been relieved. The nurse should assist the health-care team to look in the auditory canal for clear, cloudy liquid or pus draining from the ear and carefully remove the drainage.

One of the most important components of nursing education concerning OM is to explain to the parents that if the infection is bacterial, they must administer the entire dose of antibiotics. Some prescriptions are for 5 days, and others may be for 10 to 14 days of therapy.

If the health-care provider diagnoses the child with viral OM, then the parents need to understand that antibiotics will not be effective in treating the infection. Whether the OM is from a viral or a bacterial infection, children can be given an antipyretic and anti-inflammatory to reduce symptoms of pressure and discomfort.

Smoking around a child has been correlated with the development of OM. Breastfeeding helps to reduce the incidence of OM during infancy and toddlerhood (Fig. 30.7).

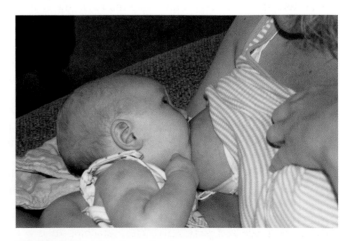

FIGURE 30.7 Infant breastfeeding.

NURSING CARE PLAN for the Child With Sensory Impairments: Sudden Hearing Loss and Care in the Hospital

Assessment:
- Assess the child's hearing acuity using a health-care team approach.
- During the assessment phase, the nurse collects both subjective and objective information.
- Engage the child in play using medical toys and dolls to decrease his or her stress and to provide distraction during the assessment.
- Include the parent's description of the cause of the injury and circumstances surrounding the sudden loss of hearing event.

Physical Indicators:
- Assess the child's outer ear structures and inner ear structures with an appropriately sized otoscope with attached light; use appropriate technique for the child's age (ie, pull the pinna down and back for young children to maximize the visualization of the tympanic membrane).

Behavioral Indicators:
- Include the parent-child interactions, noting what is said and how the family interacts, including nonverbal communication.
- Note any identified maladaptive responses displayed either by the child or the family toward the sensory impairment.

Nursing Diagnoses:
- There is a risk for injury related to decreased auditory cues of the environment (eg, inability to hear traffic).
- The child is exhibiting fear related to the sudden loss of auditory cues of the environment.
- There is altered parenting related to depression and sadness from the child's loss of sensory perception.
- There is a risk for post-trauma syndrome.
- There is anxiety related to thoughts of the child's future and academic success.

Planning: Create patient-centered goals during the planning phase of the nursing process that have the five components: Child-centered, future-oriented, measureable, realistic, and with a time frame.
- The child will learn to navigate his or her home environment in such a way that no harm or injury will be experienced within 1 month of discharge.
- The child will demonstrate peer interactions and play.

Implementation:
- Provide immediate support and referral to a mental health specialist if the child has a traumatic loss of hearing; be present and therapeutic during the shock phase.
- Protect the child from physical harm as they learn to navigate the environment
- Meet the child's immediate psychological and physical needs first.
- Provide family support and education concerning socialization and healthy peer interactions.
- Minimize the child's fear and anxiety by providing a quiet, supportive, supervised environment with access to play therapy.
- Engage the child in play that encourages his or her feelings and expressions of anxiety, fear, and especially guilt.
- Foster positive parenting by demonstrating appropriate care for the child and providing positive reinforcement for active involvement in providing for the sensory impaired child.
- Use assisted listening devices for hearing impairment:
  - Assistive listening devices (ALDs) help amplify the sounds the child will want to hear.
  - Augmentative and alternative communication (AAC) devices help children with a hearing impairment to express themselves; these utilize a simple picture board or a computer program that synthesizes speech from text.
  - Use of alerting devices that connect to a doorbell, telephone, or alarm; these emit a loud sound or blinking light to let someone with hearing loss know that an event is taking place or that communication is needed.

NURSING CARE PLAN for the Child With Sensory Impairments: Sudden Hearing Loss and Care in the Hospital—cont'd

Evaluation of Outcome:
- Child remains free of harm and is able experience a caring supportive environment
- Child shows no evidence of physical harm from dangerous navigation
- Child shows no evidence of emotional neglect or social isolation
- Child experiences less fear and anxiety
- Child and family members demonstrate positive interactions
- Parent demonstrates positive parenting behaviors

 ## CULTURAL CONSIDERATIONS

Family Responses to the Sudden Loss of Visual or Hearing Sensory Perception

Upon learning that a child has experienced a sensory loss, a family will have a response based on their coping strategies, support systems, and cultural perspectives. Visual impairment or loss carries with it an intense traumatic response for many family members and can be classified as a crisis. Considering all disabilities, the loss of sight in a child is associated with the greatest fear (Hockenberry and Wilson, 2007). Regardless of the family constellation or the cultural background, when a child loses his or her sight, the family needs education, support, and counseling. Early interventions and adherence to a plan to support the child's growth and development become a paramount goal for all family members.

OVERALL NURSING CONSIDERATIONS FOR A CHILD WITH A SENSORY IMPAIRMENT

Interference in the normalcy of the child's physical features and sensory perceptions may cause stress in the family's functioning. When a child becomes deaf or blind, or suffers from significant sensory loss, the family may experience a sense of loss toward the child's productive future. It is important to assess the severity of the effect on the family's cultural values and ensure there is a referral made to a mental health professional who can assist the family in coping. The child should never be socially isolated or kept from experiencing a healthy, stimulating childhood with socialization, cultural involvement, and play. Adequate communication skills and independent self-help skills must be fostered and parents need to be encouraged to "let go" and allow their child to develop independent skills.

Preventing a sensory impairment is the most important aspect of the nursing care of high-risk children. Teaching families and children of all ages how to protect their sensory organs should begin in early educational levels; reinforcement of information should continue throughout adolescence.

PATIENT TEACHING GUIDELINES

Preventing Noise-Induced Hearing Loss

NIHL is the only type of hearing loss that can be prevented. Nurses must teach children and families prevention practices, such as:
- Know what noises can produce hearing impairments (eg, loud and sustained).
- Wear protective devices made to reduce sound, such as ear plugs, ear muffs, and headphones
- Reduce exposure to loud and sustained sounds; step back and away from loud sounds such as amplifiers.
- Prevent exposures to harmful sounds; be aware of potential sources.
- Protect the ears of children too young to protect their own ears.
- Participate in screening.

National organizations can assist the family in adapting to the change in the child's sensory experiences and provide professional and peer support. These organizations include:

- National Federation of the Blind
- National Association for Visually Handicapped
- American Council of the Blind
- National Association for Parents of Children with Visual Impairments
- National Institute on Deafness and Other Communication Disorders (NIDCD)

Key Points

- Early identification of a visual or a hearing impairment allows for interventions to be initiated that provide for speech development, socialization, growth and development, and academic success.
- Nurses need to support and participate in national efforts to screen all early school-aged children for hearing and visual acuity and enable children to secure a referral for interventions and/or treatments.
- The most common cause of hearing impairment is called *conductive hearing loss* and it is associated with repeated cases of OM that lead to scarring.
- Routine vision screening is an important part of a well-child visit, even when the child is an infant. Many visual abnormalities are treatable or correctable if they are discovered early and promptly.
- Common reactions when a family is told their infant or young child will be sensory impaired include fear and anxiety associated with the potential loss of vision or hearing. These reactions can be profound, and each member of the family needs interdisciplinary team support.
- Screening efforts are important during childhood so that visual and auditory impairments can be found early. Common vision screening techniques include Snellen's

test, LEA symbols, and the unilateral cover test. Newborn hearing screening, which is mandated in many states, also allows for early identification of hearing impairments.
- Eye infections are common in children and include viral or bacterial conjunctivitis and ophthalmic neonatorum. Families need to learn specific care techniques to prevent the spread of eye infections.
- Retinoblastoma generally affects children between the ages of 1 and 2 years; this cancer presents with a whitish glow as light falls on the affected eye's retina.
- ROP is an eye disease of the premature infant. ROP causes a scarring process that pulls the retina away from the basement membranes, resulting in impaired vision or blindness. Excessive oxygen use and quantity in premature babies and a birth weight of less than 1,250 g are associated with the development of ROP.
- A traumatic event that leads to the sudden loss of sensory processing affects the child both emotionally and developmentally. It is important to provide special care based on the etiology of the impairment and the child's developmental needs.
- Children who suddenly lose their vision or hearing based on traumatic injury or accident need support when first learning they are going to be impaired.

REVIEW QUESTIONS

1. While assessing the ears of a 2-year-old for possible OM, how would the nurse pull the pinna for maximal visual assessment of the tympanic membrane?
   1. Up and out
   2. Down and out
   3. Do not pull at all
   4. Straight out

2. What are the most common causes of ROP?
   1. Bright lights and prematurity
   2. Bright lights and oxygen therapy
   3. Oxygen therapy and loud noises
   4. Prematurity and oxygen therapy

3. What is the name of the visual appearance of the retina in children with a confirmed retinoblastoma?
   1. Opacity reflex
   2. Cataract opacity
   3. Cat's eye reflex
   4. Cloudy reflex

4. While teaching new parents about the need to protect their premature infant's hearing in the NICU setting, which of the following would be included in the teaching session?
   1. Keep the noise level down to prevent the startle reflex.
   2. Keep the isolette covered to prevent exposure to florescent lighting.
   3. Monitor the infant's temperature to assess for a fever.
   4. Immediately notify a nurse if you hear your infant's IV or cardiorespiratory (CR) monitor's alarm.

5. What is one of the most effective means to prevent a hearing impairment during early childhood?
   1. Participate in school screenings for hearing deficits.
   2. Participate in well-child checkups throughout childhood.
   3. Ensure the child has all of his or her immunizations.
   4. Ensure that child completes his or her full prescription of antibiotics for OM.

6. Infants and young children have a higher risk for OM because of:
   1. Their genetic immune dysfunction
   2. The natural sugars that are present in milk, formula, and breast milk
   3. The anatomical location of the eustachian tubes
   4. The natural slant of the eustachian tube

7. The sticky natural substance that is found in the outer ear canal is called:
   1. Cerumen
   2. Wax
   3. Serum
   4. Mucus

8. The most common pathological microbes associated with pediatric OM are: *(select all that apply)*
   1. *N catarrhalis*
   2. *H influenza*
   3. *S pneumoniae*
   4. *Corynebacterium diphtheriae*
   5. *Staphylococcus*

9. While reinforcing teaching to parents of young children, the licensed vocational nurse (LVN) describes the importance of completing all childhood immunizations. One immunization is especially important to prevent OM. The LVN would be correct in stating that this immunization is which of the following?
   1. Pertussis vaccine
   2. PCV
   3. Rubella vaccine
   4. Mumps vaccine

10. The signs and symptoms of OM include which of the following? *(select all that apply)*
    1. Irritability
    2. Pulling at the ears
    3. Hitting the side of the head
    4. Diarrhea
    5. Vomiting
    6. Fever

CRITICAL THINKING QUESTIONS

1. What is the relationship between a young child not having his or her immunization requirements completed and the development of hearing impairment? Which childhood infectious or communicable diseases contribute to the risk for or actual development of a hearing impairment?

2. What are the controversies around the national recommendations concerning the prescription of antibiotics for a young child with OM?

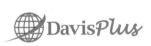

For additional resources and information, visit **www.DavisPlus.com.** Post-Conference Questions and Activities, Answers, and References can be found on DavisPlus.

31

Child With a Mental Health Condition

KEY TERMS

addiction
depression
lethality of attempt
mental illness
neuroleptic
neurotransmitter
personality disorders
schizophrenia
suicidal ideation
suicidal thinking
suicide
suicide attempt
tardive dyskinesia

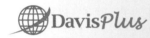 **DavisPlus** For audio pronunciation
guide, visit
www.DavisPlus.com

CHAPTER CONCEPTS

Addiction
Cognition
Development
Mood
Safety
Self

LEARNING OUTCOMES

1. Define the key terms.
2. Describe current trends in the incidence and prevalence of mental health issues across the span of childhood.
3. Analyze the effect of a mental health diagnosis on the child's interactions with family, school, social networks, and society as a whole.
4. State the goals for therapeutic communication between the nurse and the child and/or family when interacting with an acute exacerbation of a mental health condition.
5. Describe commonly used assessment tools for anxiety, depression, and mood disorders.
6. Analyze the effect of a diagnosis of attention-deficit hyperactivity disorder (ADHD) on a child's interaction with family and school.
7. Describe the clinical presentation and pharmacological management of schizophrenia in childhood.
8. Analyze the effect of bullying on a child's well-being and describe the relationship between bullying and childhood depression.
9. Differentiate between anorexia nervosa and bulimia eating disorders and discuss the assessment, clinical presentations, and therapeutic management of each.
10. Describe the types of suicide behaviors (ie, gestures, attempts, and successful suicide) and state the effect of suicide on those left behind.
11. Review the most common categories of psychiatric pharmacological treatments for the management of a mental health diagnosis in childhood and state the common side effects and therapeutic ranges for each drug.
12. Analyze the development of substance abuse during childhood and state the consequences and safety factors associated with substance abuse on the child's mental health, family interactions, social network, and school performance.

Charlie

■ Charlie, an 11-year-old boy with a diagnosis of autism, attends a sibling camp for children with oncology conditions. Charlie's sister has leukemia. Because of Charlie's special needs, one young adult counselor was selected to be Charlie's counselor in a 1:1 ratio. This decision was made for safety and because it was his first time at camp and away from his family.

Upon checking in the first morning, it was apparent that Charlie was at risk for being unfocused and wandering. The slightest movement in the forest or anything of interest that caught Charlie's eyes would cause him to quietly move toward the stimulus and leave the group. He needed constant supervision. Charlie participated in masturbation on a regular basis and needed frequent guidance that it was not appropriate around others. Avoiding unnecessary touch was important to Charlie and members of the crew knew to talk to him but not try to touch him, even in a friendly manner.

The week was successful and Charlie was able to attend all 6 nights and 7 days of the pediatric oncology sibling's camp. His sister showed increasing social engagement and it was apparent how much she valued this time of play while having her brother there with her at camp.

1. What aspects of autism can be seen in Charlie's behaviors at camp?
2. What is the relationship between touch and autism?
3. What would have been important talking points from the camp nurse to help the camp counselors prepare for Charlie's participation in the overnight camp?

CONCEPTUAL CORNERSTONE

Safety

Children who have been diagnosed with a mental health condition are at greater risk from safety issues. Children with mood disorders such as depression and anxiety, or children and teens with eating disorders, are at risk for self-harm. It is imperative that the concept of safety be in the forefront of the minds of pediatric health-care team members. Any indication of self-harm or suicide risk must be taken very seriously and the child must be provided with a safe environment and immediate referral to a comprehensive psychological support program. Every suicide-related comment, or any outward signs of self-harm such as cutting, participation in violence, or suicide idealization or attempts, must be acted on immediately. Pediatric nurses have the ethical and legal responsibility to provide safety to children with mental health issues; not every pediatric health-care setting is set up to provide for the needs of children with mental illness. Knowing what to screen for in all children, what to look for in high-risk children, and when to call for help are important aspects of maintaining safety and securing prompt interventions for children with mental health conditions and illnesses.

Occurring in about 20% of the U.S. population, childhood mental illness is a serious social concern. In any given year, more than 5 million children have a mental illness that significantly interferes with the daily life of the child and the family. Using the term *mental illness* can be considered inadequate because there are often significant physical factors associated with the disorders. Heredity and brain chemistry are thought to be involved with the development of a childhood mental disorder.

Because children are naturally going through physical, emotional, and social growth and development, it is important to identify what is considered "normal" for the child's age. Children can demonstrate a range of abilities and behaviors. When ruling out a mental illness, health-care providers must first determine how the child copes, adapts, and relates to others and the world within the context of his or her developmental stage and age. Because there is not a known cause of a mental illness, a combination of factors such as parenting, family dynamics, heredity, stressors, biological chemistry, and psychological trauma must be investigated. Health-care professionals need to determine if the behaviors that are being displayed are causing a significant disruption to the family's and child's life. Tests are then conducted to evaluate for mental illness. When identified early and treated with psychotherapy and medications, many children with a mental illness are able to live full, productive lives.

One challenge for health-care professionals is to provide holistic care for a child who presents in an acute phase of a mental disorder. The team needs to quickly identify what the underlying mental diagnosis is, identify the severity of the child's presenting symptoms, intervene appropriately, and then secure follow-up with a mental health expert. Children may present to any health-care setting in an acute phase, but will most likely present in an emergency room or clinic setting. An assessment of history, medications currently prescribed, precipitating factors, and current mental state are all imperative and require a team approach.

 ## THERAPEUTIC COMMUNICATION

Establishing a rapport with a child who presents to a health-care setting for medical care or who presents with an acute exacerbation of a mental illness or condition is a priority action. Establishing a trusting rapport using a pattern that works for the child's ability to communicate is challenging. Without appropriate therapeutic communication techniques, the team will have more challenges with assessment, diagnosis, and treatment. Even just taking vital signs, collecting specimens, administering medications, providing safety, and providing basic care can be challenging during an acute exacerbation of a childhood mental illness.

Unfortunately, most research in mental health issues has historically focused on the adult. Researchers are investigating how factors associated with childhood development may have an effect on the child's mental health. Determining and defining emotional and behavioral problems across childhood is not an easy or straightforward process. Risk factors, hereditary influences, and medication effectiveness continue to be central issues for continued research.

CULTURAL CONSIDERATIONS

Some cultural groups view mental illness as something that should be hidden, not discussed or disclosed. The pediatric health-care team working with diverse cultural groups should communicate their support in disclosing mental health issues with extended family to gain support and help. Health-care team members, such as a Child Life Specialist or social worker, can assist a family in formulating comfortable ways to share the news with others.

ATTENTION-DEFICIT HYPERACTIVITY DISORDER

ADHD is a neurobehavioral disorder and is one of the most common mental disorders currently diagnosed in both children and adolescents. ADHD persists to adulthood (Centers for Disease Control and Prevention [CDC], 2014). Research has not been able to determine why the incidence of this disorder is steadily increasing. Children suffer from difficulty focusing on schoolwork and activities at home, difficulty in controlling their behavior, and difficulty relating to family members throughout the day. The prevalence of ADHD is now at 11% (ie, 1 in 10) of school-aged children and is found to be more prevalent in male children (1 in 5 boys and 1 in 11 girls) (CDC, 2014). ADHD used to be thought to be solely associated with environmental factors and inconsistent parenting. Through the use of brain imaging technology, scientists have observed that ADHD may be associated with how the brain is neurologically wired and physically structured. In some regions of the brain, a significant developmental delay, as much as 3 years, is found related to ADHD. The delay has been found in the frontal cortex, where one normally suppresses inappropriate actions, displays focused attention, and controls moment-by-moment memory. Research continues internationally to determine the intricacies of this disorder and the best treatments across the lifespan.

To maintain safety for the child with ADHD, it is important that members of the health-care team understand the types of ADHD so that they can anticipate a child's behavior. This is especially true when the team is attempting a medical procedure or trying to explain important topics to the child while in the clinic or hospital. There are three main types of ADHD:

• Predominately inattentive; it is challenging for the child to concentrate, finish a task, or follow another person's conversations or academic instructions

• Predominately hyperactive-impulsive; the child struggles to sit still, keep his or her hands to himself or herself, and interrupts others frequently
• Combined presentation that includes behaviors listed in both of the above types

TEAM WORKS

Pediatric health-care team members need to understand when ADHD is most commonly diagnosed. For mild ADHD, the average age of diagnosis is 8 years of age. For moderate ADHD, the average age of diagnosis is 7 years, and for severe ADHD, it is 5 years (CDC, 2014).

Children who are diagnosed with ADHD display three clinical characteristics: impulsivity, inattention, and hyperactivity. Because ADHD often affects both school and home behavior, children with this disorder need a combination of therapies, including pharmacological therapies with central nervous system (CNS) stimulants, structured school environments, family counseling, and home behavior management plans to reduce impulsive behaviors (Fig. 31.1).

DRUG FACTS

In 2011, the average percentage of children with ADHD who are taking medication was 6.1%. Medications for ADHD include amphetamine (Adderall), methylphenidate (Ritalin), dextroamphetamine (Dexedrine), and pemoline (Cylert).

Assessments of Attention-Deficit Hyperactivity Disorder

According to the *Diagnostic and Statistical Manual of Mental Disorders* (Fifth Edition) (DSM-V) criteria for diagnosis of ADHD in children, at least six of nine symptoms must be

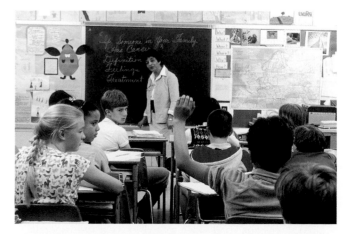

FIGURE 31.1 A structured classroom helps children with ADHD to learn. *(Photo from the National Cancer Institute; by Michael Anderson.)*

identified in the child's presentation (CDC, 2015). The following list describes the symptoms the child would display that represent ADHD:

- Fidgets with fingers, hands, objects
- Often leaves his or her seat in the classroom when expectations are to stay seated
- Experiences forgetfulness at school, with homework assignments, and at home with daily activities
- Becomes easily distracted and excited when distracted
- Seems to not listen and does not follow through with explained expectations of desired actions
- Talks excessively and blurts out answers before called upon in class
- Interrupts, intrudes on others, and does not have the capacity to wait for his or her turn
- Cannot pay attention to detail and makes frequent mistakes that are considered careless
- Has difficulty playing quietly and has problems with focusing on play without frequent changes in play activities

The above symptoms must be present for longer than 6 months' duration. The mental impairment must be present in at least two settings and must occur before the child's seventh birthday. In making the diagnosis of ADHD, serum lead levels should be assessed and phenylketonuria and other diagnoses should be ruled out.

As children suffer with ADHD, they often experience a host of negative feedback about their behaviors. They also often experience a lack of patience from family, teachers, and others who interact with them. Parents need to be taught how to structure the child's day to increase routines, and must be given clear instructions and expectations. Social skill training includes group settings and can focus on problem-solving skills. Psychosocial treatments include behavior modification with positive reinforcements such as a token economy (eg, receiving a coin or marble to place in a jar and, once filled, the child receives a prize or privilege) for both the home and school environments.

Interventions for Attention-Deficit Hyperactivity Disorder

Interventions for ADHD are generally pharmaceutical in nature. There are alternative and complementary interventions for children with ADHD (eg, structured and frequent exercise), but the standard of medical care is the use of medications to help the child focus and be successful in school. The following represents a list of common medications prescribed for children with ADHD.

- Methylphenidate (Ritalin)
- Dextroamphetamine and amphetamine (Adderall)
- Methylphenidate (Concerta)
- Lisdexamfetamine dimesylate (Vyvanse)
- Dexmethylphenidate (Focalin)
- Guanfacine (Intuniv)
- Atomoxetine (Strattera)
- Bupropion (Wellbutrin)
- Pemoline (Cylert)

Nursing Considerations for Attention-Deficit Hyperactivity Disorder

Parents need support and education when they have a child with ADHD. When in the hospital, the parents might find controlling their child's behaviors especially difficult because their routines and familiar processes are thrown off. Families should be given education about local and national support groups and organizations that specialize in locating resources and offering ideas for behavior medication. Pediatric nurses need to display patience when a child with ADHD is hospitalized because his or her symptoms can progress, leading to mood swings and aggression.

Nurses need to assess for the side effects associated with the use of psychostimulant therapy. These include decreased appetite, nervousness, insomnia, weight loss, tics, headaches, and stomachaches. Families must be taught not to allow their child to consume caffeine and decongestants, and to instruct that ADHD medications are contraindicated with monoamine oxidase inhibitors (MAOIs), which are a group of antidepressant drugs. If the child is taking pemoline, liver function tests must be conducted because this drug is associated with life-threatening liver failure. Pemoline is not considered a first-line (ie, often prescribed first before other drugs) drug for the treatment of ADHD.

PATIENT TEACHING GUIDELINES

Parents might express concern about administering medications to help control symptoms of ADHD. It is important to teach the family about the importance of the medications and the side effects. Parents should know that side effects of psychostimulant therapy include restlessness, headache, tremors, fever, blurred vision, and tachycardia. Concerns about these side effects should be addressed to the prescribing physician.

The pediatric nurse should assess if there is a complete multimodal approach to the child's care, including behavior modification, parental education and hands-on training, classroom accommodation, social skills training, and the family's active participation in local, region, and national organizations.

AUTISM SPECTRUM DISORDER

Autism is a pervasive developmental disorder found in greater frequency than historically documented. Current data demonstrate a prevalence rate of 3 to 4 per 10,000 children. Autism is more common in males, with a ratio of female to males of 3:4.2.

Considered one of a spectrum of conditions, this disorder is included with conditions such as Rett's syndrome (ie, brain, communication, motor, and growth disorder) and Asperger's syndrome (ie, milder form of autism). There is no known cause for autism but it is known to exist from birth, with early symptoms noted as early as late infancy. Genetics, irregular brain regions, and environment most likely play roles in the development of autism (ninds.nih.gov, 2015). Autism consistently develops before the child is 30 months of age. The condition is characterized by a pervasive and severe impairment in the child's communication skills and social interactions, and may be accompanied by repetitive and restrictive behaviors. The child will not relate comfortably with others and does not want to be touched, cuddled, or comforted by others.

TEAM WORKS

Tips to working with autistic children in a health-care setting include the following:

- Minimizing touch and explaining to the child when touch is needed
- Giving the autistic child time to prepare for the next activity
- Understanding that autistic children may be withdrawn and quiet
- Acknowledging that autistic children may have trouble with interpersonal relations, including avoiding eye contact and having unusual language disturbances
- Stressing to the parents that the autistic child might feel overwhelmed in a new environment

Assessments of Autism

Based on a spectrum, this disabling mental condition can be found at varying levels of disability. The child should be tested for intelligence because many autistic children fall into a functional, cognitively impaired range on conventional psychological tests. An autistic child will present with the following symptoms and behaviors:

- Minimal interaction with others, as well as being withdrawn and needing solitary play; may not respond to his or her name (Fig. 31.2)
- A desire for very limited touching, cuddling, or molding into the body (eg, clinging or hugging closely or tightly) of their caregivers or family members
- A minimal display of anticipatory behaviors; the child does not respond to acknowledgment of others, such as a parent coming home from work and approaching the child

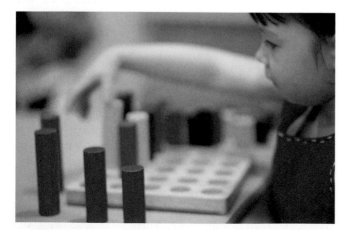

FIGURE 31.2 An autistic child prefers to play alone.

- Lack of anxiety in a young child when separated from his or her parent
- The use of peripheral vision instead of focused eye contact, and the avoidance of direct eye contact
- Minimal meaningful speech and repetition, such as repeating words he or she has heard over and over; this is a condition known as *echolalia*
- Pronoun reversal (ie, mixing up grammar) and nonsensical rhyming
- Possible appearance of being deaf but, in actuality, not being hearing-impaired; may wander off and not hear others calling his or her name
- Lack of startle responses to some stimuli and heightened responses to others; overall, seeming to lack focus
- The performance of what is seen as socially unacceptable behaviors such as self-stimulating behaviors (ie, open masturbation), as well as repetitive and rhythmic motions such as rocking
- A display of distress and resistance to changes in daily routines
- A marked need for sameness and attachment to an object with tantrumlike rages if routines are disrupted

Interventions for Autism

There are no treatments or cures for autism. It is a lifelong behavioral and emotional disorder. Therapy should begin at a young age and should focus on speech and language, parent bonding and training, and the securing of a special education classroom with knowledgeable and experienced teachers. Older children and adolescents should have behavioral therapy, psychotherapy, cognitive theory, and may benefit from pharmacotherapy if the associated symptoms of anxiety, depression, or obsessive-compulsive symptoms are present.

Nursing Considerations for Autism

The nursing care of autistic children can prove to be very challenging. Hospitalized autistic children may become very agitated because their routines are disrupted and they cannot process information to understand their need to be hospitalized. The best way to approach a hospitalized autistic child is to work with the child one-on-one, giving directions without rationales and minimizing touching the child to prevent emotional outbursts. The child's environment should be calm and nonstimulating. The nurse should be very supportive and empathetic to the parents, who may be distressed over their child's upset behaviors during hospitalization.

TEAM WORKS

When needing to provide an autistic child with medical interventions, the pediatric health-care team needs to plan ahead and work as a team. Bringing a member of Child Life to the treatment room or area where the procedure will take place so that they can provide distraction and recovery with praise right after the painful procedure is helpful. Appropriate pain-reducing techniques such as numbing cream, a cold pack over the site, and deep breathing should be used. Depending on the autistic child's reaction, a therapeutic hold might be necessary to accomplish the task but should be done rapidly and for the shortest time possible. The team should expect the child to be frightened and to possibly display behaviors associated with autism such as resisting touch and language disturbances.

EATING DISORDERS

Eating disorder incidence and prevalence is on the rise. Both male and female genders are afflicted by these common disorders. Eating disorders may be serious, dangerous, and fatal if not identified early and medically treated. Often associated with poor self-image, poor self-esteem, and very poor perception of physical self, eating disorders are a result of an unrealistic attitude toward body size and a distorted view of being "fat" when the child or teen can be very emaciated. According to the National Institutes of Health (NIH), people with eating disorders have a tremendous fear of gaining weight, and can continue to lose more weight even when it is considered to be unhealthy for their height and age (2015).

Assessments of Eating Disorders

Assessment for eating disorders should be comprehensive to include the child's physical status, clinical presentations, emotional state, and laboratory analysis. The following list shows assessments that should be performed (www.mayoclinic.org, 2015; nih.gov, 2015):

- The child should have his or her weight and height plotted on a national growth chart to determine the severity of the weight loss.
- Metabolic and electrolyte panels should be drawn to determine if there are imbalances, including metabolic alkalosis from vomiting.
- An assessment of cardiac function should be conducted, including orthostatic blood pressures for evidence of true hypotension, and electrocardiogram (EKG) for dysrhythmias associated with severe electrolyte imbalances.
- Evidence of malnutrition such as thinning hair and hair loss, brittle fingernails, dry skin, enamel loss on teeth, amenorrhea, mood changes, bradycardia, hypothermia and cold intolerance, and loss of libido is appropriate to assess. "Russell's sign" might be present, which is bite marks on fingers and knuckles from the child inducing vomiting.
- An assessment of the child's use of laxatives, diuretics, enemas, and diet pills should be conducted and reported immediately to the primary care provider.

Interventions for Eating Disorders

Like many of the mental health conditions found in childhood, treatment for eating disorders is considered multimodal and requires lengthy interventions. Psychotherapy is the mainstay of theory and includes behavior modification to decrease the manipulative behaviors associated with food restriction, purging, and binging. Measures are carefully used to slowly remove the anxiety surrounding eating, and the child or teen must be involved with planning healthy meals that include adequate calories. Medications may be required to support the child, such as antidepressants or appetite stimulants.

Nursing Considerations for Eating Disorders

The pediatric nurse needs to understand the anxiety associated with eating for a child with an eating disorder. They may become angry, disruptive, and manipulative in pleading to not be forced to consume calories. Close attention should be given to make sure the child does not have an opportunity to purge and vomit after meals. Teens have been known to find creative ways to engage in purging while hospitalized. The nurse must carefully monitor eating habits and document carefully what is eaten, when it was eaten, and how long it took to consume. It is important for the nurse to be a healthy role model for both the child and family.

Nurses should be aware that not all children with bulimia will have a documented reduced weight. These children may consume several thousand calories in a short period of time followed by purging or extreme exercise that leads their weight to be within an expected range. The goal for nursing interventions when caring for children with eating disorders will include securing a weight within 10% of expected for age and height, resolving underlying emotional and psychological problems, correcting malnutrition, preventing severe consequences such as electrolyte and cardiac dysfunction, and assisting with a treatment plan to restore the child's perception of health and healthy body image.

Because eating disorders can be fatal, it is imperative that early identification and treatment be secured. If not treated, eating disorders can result in multibody system failure, leading to death. Parents must be educated on the need to participate fully in therapy. Pediatric nurses can be instrumental in becoming involved with adolescent education and prevention through community action.

Common Eating Disorders

The most common eating disorders include anorexia nervosa, bulimia, and binge eating disorders, restrictive eating disorders, and pica. The symptoms vary among the various disorders, and there is overlap among them.

Anorexia Nervosa

One of the most frequently encountered eating disorders in children is anorexia nervosa. The cause of the development of this disorder is not known. There are diagnostic criteria that aid in the diagnosis of the eating disorder. Risk factors have been identified and include negative self-image, problems eating during the infancy developmental period, anxiety disorder, abundant focus on rules and achievements, and trying to be "perfect" (nlm.nih.gov, 2015).

Diagnostic criteria for anorexia nervosa include four main attributes. Children will have a voluntary refusal to maintain a normal body weight at or above a minimally anticipated weight for their age, height, and size at 85% or less than expected. They will have a tremendous fear of gaining weight, viewing themselves as "fat" even when demonstrating the characteristics of being significantly underweight. They will have a denial of their condition, viewing their body with a disturbing sense of poor image, and not recognizing the seriousness of their condition. Lastly, for females, there will be amenorrhea, defined as the absence of three periods in a row.

Bulimia and Binge-Eating Disorders

Another type of eating disorder is binge eating/purging, also called *bulimia*. Bulimia is when the child eats a great deal of calories and follows with purging behaviors of enemas, laxatives, diuretics, or self-induced vomiting behaviors, or a combination. Bulimia is characterized by an excessive appetite and insatiable eating. Bulimia nervosa is defined as when a child has recurrent episodes of binge eating followed by guilt, humiliation, shame, and then self-induced vomiting, dieting, and exercise.

The child will try to cover up the behaviors associated with bulimia by sneaking food, hiding food, taking laxatives, vomiting, or over-exercising.

Restrictive Eating Disorders

Another type of eating disorder is the restricting type, where the child participates in episodes of food restriction and severe calorie reduction. Also defined as avoidant/restrictive food intake disorder (ARFID) per the DSM-V, this disorder prevents food consumption.

Pica

When a child is persistently consuming materials that are not food substances (ie, non-nutritive), the child is experiencing an eating disorder called *pica*. This disorder is more common in young children; about 10% of children under 6 have some pica behavior. Developmental disability and cognitive impairment have been associated with the development of pica behaviors. Complications occur when the child eats dangerous substances such as paint chips, toxic plant materials, and sharp or hard objects. Medical conditions such as intestinal obstructions from nonfood items and anemia should be considered as complications of non-nutritive eating. Pica behavior must be present for no less than 30 days to be considered a diagnosis (nlm.nih.gov, 2014).

Treatment for pica is complicated because the pediatric health-care team must rule out any physiological pathologies before addressing the emotional or affective component

---

NURSING CARE PLAN for the Adolescent with Anorexia Nervosa

Nursing Diagnosis: There is imbalanced nutrition; less than the body's requirements is being ingested because of food-restrictive behaviors.

Patient Goals:
- The teen will consume adequate calories on a daily basis to gain weight and have adequate growth by a designated date determined by the medical team.
- The teen will participate in an eating-based behavior modification plan constructed by an interdisciplinary team.

Interventions:
- Nutritional services and a certified dietician will construct a meal plan with increasing daily calories until adequate daily calorie consumption is attained
- Nursing staff will ensure the child is consuming the high-calorie diet and not participating in self-induced vomiting after eating or excessive exercising
- Nursing staff will monitor for the use of enemas, laxatives, or diuretics
- Nursing staff will weigh patient once weekly to monitor progress toward weight goal and will monitor for child placing weighted materials in clothing to increase weight measured
- Interdisciplinary team will meet in conference with family to explain goals of care and discuss the pathology and severity of the eating disorder
- Nursing staff will work with interdisciplinary team to develop a realistic behavior modification plan, including participation in counseling
- Nursing staff will be alert for clinical signs of depression

Expected Outcomes:
- The child will demonstrate a higher self-esteem and demonstrate adequate progressive weight loss toward the medically ascribed goal.
- The family will participate in care with a nonjudgmental attitude and reinforce the need for active partnership in the medical plan of care, with follow-up.

to pica. Treatment follows after lead poisoning and anemia are assessed for. Treatment then consists of treating the behavior through rewards and mild aversion therapy (nlm. nih.gov, 2014).

PERSONALITY, ANXIETY, AND MOOD DISORDERS, AND SCHIZOPHRENIA

Children can suffer from personality, anxiety, and mood disorders, and schizophrenia. **Personality disorders** disrupt a child's daily life but can further be the cause of severe behaviors that manifest in all aspects of the child's life, including socialization, academics, preparation for adulthood, and intimate relationships. Mood disorders are those conditions in which the child experiences emotional or "mood" fluctuations that can be very disruptive to the child's daily functioning and overall quality of life. A commonly found mood disorder during the childhood period is depression. Depression is linked to many older child and adolescent suicidal behaviors.

Anxiety

Worrying, fearfulness, and feelings of anxiety are normal and regularly found throughout childhood as an expected developmental experience. When the state of anxiety is no longer attached to a specific event, or when the feelings of anxiety become disabling for the child, then the anxiety is considered pathological and requires treatment. Infants experience a form of anxiety when they are only 7 to 8 months old. As they experience the understanding that they are separate from their caregiver, they experience separation anxiety and then stranger anxiety. This a normal and expected first experience of anxiety. If anxiety is experienced repeatedly throughout childhood and interferes with social, academic, and normal cognitive development, then the child should be evaluated.

Although some anxiety is expected during childhood, childhood anxiety disorders are becoming more common for children across all ages. Many attribute this increase in mood disorders to stress in our society and environments. Anxiety disorders can cause a child to feel overwhelmed, feel a sense of dread, and can be triggered by everyday activities such as going to school, facing homework and peer interactions. Feelings of irrational, persistent fear and worry take over the child's thinking and affect most aspects of the child's life; school, home, and relationships (Anxiety and Depression Association of America [ADAA], 2015).

Several subtypes of anxiety disorders exist within childhood. These subtypes differentiate the experience of anxiety and have particular feelings associated. The subtypes are included below:

1. **Separation anxiety disorder:** This disorder differs from the separation anxiety an older infant commonly experiences in that the older child has unrealistic anxiety and persistent worry that harm will befall him or her if separated from the primary caregiver. This includes resistance to attend school or social events, or even going to sleep.

2. **Generalized anxiety:** With this disorder, children worry excessively about future events, competence, or previous behavior. Often, generalized anxiety is demonstrated through somatic (ie, related to the body rather than the mind) complaints and great difficulty relaxing.

3. **Panic disorders:** With panic disorders, children feel an overwhelming sense of worry and panic. They may present with physical symptoms of an increased heart rate, sweating, and increased blood pressure.

4. **Phobias:** Phobias are a type of anxiety that is experienced only under a specific condition that the child will try to avoid.

5. **Post-traumatic stress disorder (PTSD):** In this disorder, anxiety results from an external traumatic event that was perceived by the child or adolescent as very dangerous and/or life-threatening; intrusive and recurrent recollection of the event occurs, which causes the child extreme distress. This distress may be demonstrated through sleep disorders, sadness, and feelings of helplessness and vulnerability.

6. **Obsessive-compulsive disorder (OCD):** OCD is marked by a child's persistent repetitive thoughts, repetitive rituals, or repetitive movements that do not contribute to a level of social integration (ie, social acceptance with family, peers, and members of society).

Assessments of Anxiety Disorders

Pediatric nurses working with a team of health-care providers can provide assistance in conducting assessments for anxiety disorders. This is especially important with the increase of anxiety disorders in children. Assessments for anxiety disorders should include:

- Biophysical assessments of vital signs for tachycardia and tachypnea with shortness of breath
- Gastrointestinal (GI) symptoms of nausea and stomachache
- Neurological symptoms, such as headache and body pains
- Sleep disturbances; nightmares
- Poor school performance and decreased participation in age-appropriate activities
- Poor self-esteem
- Use of drugs and alcohol to dull the sensations of anxiety

Interventions for Anxiety

Children need professional counseling to deal with their anxiety disorder. The goal is to increase their self-esteem and to teach them relaxation exercises and self-regulated interventions to address the feelings of anxiety. School-aged children and older age groups may be able to conduct self-help exercises to reduce their anxiety. These include verbalization of feelings, exercise, deep breathing, visualizations, relaxation techniques, and problem-solving techniques. When moderate anxiety exists, the child will need a referral for cognitive-behavioral interventions. If severe, the child will need therapy and may need to be placed on anxiolytic (ie, antianxiety) medications.

Nursing Considerations for Anxiety

When a child or teen enters the health-care arena, their anxiety symptoms may surface and become an important part of the child's care. For instance, a child who has an anxiety disorder and who must be hospitalized for an impending surgical procedure may have a sudden increase in symptoms that warrant professional interventions. Child Life Specialists and staff pediatric psychologists should be called in to work with the anxious child. Anxiety causes suffering and the child should be provided with care that reduces his or her symptoms when he or she becomes ill.

When in a specific anxiety moment, the nurse can assist the child by staying right with the child, maintaining a calm and relaxed approach, and offering the child positive reinforcement for describing their feelings. Young children may not be able to express themselves clearly but will respond to a calm environment and soothing support. Meditation, prayer, and alternative therapies can also be tried to assist with anxiety symptoms.

PATIENT TEACHING GUIDELINES

Passion flower, theanine (ie, an amino acid in green teas), and valerian have been reported to decrease the symptoms of anxiety (www.mayoclinic.org, 2014). Since dietary supplements are not regulated by the U.S. Food and Drug Administration (FDA) they are not required to run extensive tests for safety and efficacy. The amount of the herb within a supplement, side effects, and warnings may not be fully understood. Always inform patients and their families to check with their physician or primary care provider before starting herbal remedies to avoid complications and unwanted interactions while taking other medications.

PTSD is a type of anxiety disorder in which the child has suffered a severely traumatic event or life-threatening event. This includes such things as a car accident, witnessing a homicide or suicide, national disaster, rape, or war. The child may re-experience the traumatic event over and over again in her thoughts or dreams. The child may act out the event through play or express his or her experience through his or her behaviors. In severe cases, the child becomes hypervigilant (ie, overexcited or overstimulated), believing the incidence could occur again, and therefore experiencing severe sleep deprivation, exhaustion, rapid heart rate, and elevated blood pressure. Nurturing and compassionate nursing care is imperative. A trusting relationship should be a major focus for the nurse and the child. The child must be referred for professional counseling so that healthier, more effective coping behaviors can be developed.

Bipolar Disorder

Bipolar disorder is characterized by alternating mania and depression, or a rapid cycling of mood particular to children. Children may experience grandiose thoughts, pressured speech, extreme irritability, emotionality, distractibility, and high levels of activity, often at bedtime.

Treatment for bipolar disorder is lithium carbonate. This medication is known to prevent or decrease the incidence of acute manic episodes. Therapeutic levels of this medication must be tracked by serum blood levels, with the ideal level being 1 to 1.2 mEq/L for initial treatment followed by 0.5 to 0.8 mEq/L for maintenance. The most common side effects associated with the administration of lithium are fatigue, headache, impaired memory, ataxia, abdominal pain, dry mouth, and tremors. Once the medication is started, the therapeutic effects can take up to 5 to 7 days to occur.

Dysthymic Disorder

Dysthymic disorder is characterized by periods of major depression and periods of what is considered normal mood lasting several days or several weeks. The feelings of depression, also called *dysphoria,* are less intense than a persistent major depression, but depression is classified as a chronic disorder. A genetic link is suspected with this disorder. Children may present with a pre-existing disorder such as somatization disorder, anxiety disorder, or anorexia nervosa. Some children with dysthymic disorder will appear passive, dependent, and lonely, while others will be aggressive, angry, and negative. Because of the cyclic pattern of this disorder, children are at risk for developing substance abuse. Treatment consists of antidepressants.

Depression

Depression is not a state of sadness; it is a serious medical illness that affects young children and teens. The incidence of depression in children is increasing and it is imperative that a pediatric nurse can identify symptoms, assist with a formal assessment, and secure treatment. According to Barclay (2010), 37% of girls and 20% of boys in the 9th to 12th grade levels indicated that their depressive symptoms were severe enough to impair the teen's daily functioning (Fig. 31.3). The highest rates of depression are reported in minority groups. Less than 25% of these children are receiving any treatment for depression. The best way to identify depression in children and teens is to regularly screen for the symptoms. The Depression

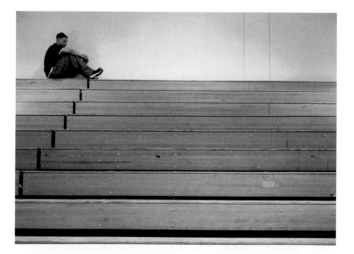

FIGURE 31.3 Children and adolescents experience depression.

Scale for Children takes only 3 to 5 min to administer and is considered quite sensitive in detecting depression.

The cause of depression in children is unknown. There may be an association with an imbalance of brain chemistry, such as a deficit of a **neurotransmitter** (ie, a chemical that is released at the axon of a nerve that inhibits or excites a target cell), such as serotonin, dopamine, or norepinephrine. Depression has a hereditary link; it may be also associated with another illness, substance abuse, or environmental influences. Stressful events such as a death, a move of the family, or severe illness may trigger depression. Childhood depression is not considered normal or associated with life's experiences. It is a medical diagnosis with severe symptoms and consequences that require immediate medical attention. Early treatment may help avoid the depression getting worse, extending for a long period of time, or becoming a lifetime challenge.

A medical diagnosis of major depression in childhood occurs after the child has displayed symptoms nearly every day for 2 weeks straight or longer. The child feels hopeless, sad, and angry, and demonstrates a loss of interest in activities that he or she usually enjoyed. It also includes a spiraling down in academic performance. Depression also includes physical symptoms such as fatigue, sleep disturbances, appetite disturbances, muscle aches, and headaches. Children may display frequent crying spells.

Depression is also called *clinical depression, major depressive disorder, dysthymic disorder,* and *unipolar depression.*

Assessments of Depression

Childhood depression is complicated and requires professional training. Childhood depression presents with a variety of clinical signs and symptoms. There are many reliable and validated tools available for professionals to use to confirm the diagnosis of depression in children across the developmental period and across ages. The following lists the most common symptoms children display:

• Preschool children may demonstrate weight loss and a lack of interest in play normally expected of their age group.
• School-aged children may have trouble concentrating at school, paying attention, making decisions, and recalling information. School-aged children may be less confident in their academic performance and state that they "can't do anything right."
• Adolescents may demonstrate poor hygiene, stop communicating with their friends and family, and lose interest in teen life activities. Teens are at risk for suicidal thoughts. Depression is more common in adolescent girls than boys.

Interventions for Depression

If a child is diagnosed with mild or moderate depression, professional counseling is imperative and may be enough. For more severe depression, the child will require professional counseling and antidepressant medications. Current research supports this combination of treatments for 2 years to have a less likely incidence of the depression reoccurrence. Psychotherapy for children can last between 8 and 20 sessions.

When medications are ordered for a child with depression, the pediatric nurse must know the common side effects and precautions. The purpose of antidepressant medications is to help balance some of the natural chemicals in the brain called *neurotransmitters.* When neurotransmitters are deficient, the child's mood and affect are considerably altered. Antidepressants are based on restoring the imbalance of serotonin, dopamine, and norepinephrine. The most commonly prescribed antidepressants are the selective serotonin reuptake inhibitors (SSRIs), including:

• Sertraline (Zoloft)
• Paroxetine (Paxil)
• Escitalopram (Lexapro)
• Fluoxetine (Prozac)
• Citalopram (Celexa)

SAFETY *STAT!*

A child who is placed on an SSRI antidepressant must see a mental health specialist weekly for at least the first 4 weeks to assess for an increased risk of suicidal tendencies.

Other pharmacological substances for antidepressant activity are the serotonin and norepinephrine reuptake inhibitors (SNRIs), including venlafaxine (Effexor) and duloxetine (Cymbalta). The medication that works on the neurotransmitter dopamine is bupropion (Wellbutrin) and does not fit into any specific drug type. Children may also be ordered tricyclic antidepressants (commonly referred to simply as *tricyclics,* or *TCAs*), MAOIs, or tetracyclic antidepressants (commonly referred to simply as *tetracyclics,* or *TeCAs*).

LABS & DIAGNOSTICS

Serum Levels of Psychiatric Drugs

Several psychotropic medications require a steady-state plasma concentration (ie, a steady serum level of the drug). Monitoring the serum levels of these drugs helps to ensure the child is receiving an adequate dose but not a toxic dose. Research shows that the most accurate monitoring of serum levels of psychotropic drugs occurs when a child is being treated with only one drug, not multidrug treatments. After a serum level is ordered, check with the health-care team when to administer the next dose. Watch for orders that change the child's doses in response to the serum drug levels.

The following drugs may be observed by serum levels:
• Haloperidol
• Chlorpromazine
• Fluphenazine
• Perphenazine
• Sulpiride
• Thioridazine
• Thiothixene
(www.ncbi.nlm.nih.gov/pubmed/2868820)

The new series of antidepressants have fewer side effects in children than do older medications. Side effects should still be monitored for and reported immediately to the prescribing primary care provider. The side effects of SSRIs and SNRIs include nausea, headache, drowsiness or sleeplessness, and agitation with jitters. If tricyclic antidepressants are ordered, the side effects to monitor for include constipation, dry mouth, blurred vision, and drowsiness. With MAOIs, families need to be aware of the danger of having the child ingest foods that contain tyramine. Tyramine is found in some cheeses, pickles, and wine, as well as in several over-the-counter (OTC) decongestants. When a child ingests tyramine while on an MAOI, risks include a sharp increase in blood pressure, which has been associated with cerebral vascular accidents.

Children who are placed on antidepressants must not stop them without follow-up by the prescribing care provider. If the child's depression symptoms subside and the child feels better and performs better in his or her social life and academic performance, the family should not stop the medications without direction. If a first-prescribed medication is not considered effective to help with the child's depression symptoms, a second line of antidepressants will most likely be ordered. This process has been well researched and is called *Sequenced Treatment Alternatives to Relieve Depression (STAR*D)* (www.nimh.nih.gov, 2015).

Some families may want to discuss herbal remedies for their child's mild-to-moderate depression. Patients' families commonly ask about the herbal medicine Saint John's wort, which was not deemed more effective to treat severe depression versus a sugar placebo pill in a 2002 clinical trial sponsored by NIH (nccih.nih.gov, 2014). According to the National Center for Complementary and Integrative Health (NCCIH) (nccih.nih.gov, 2014), the Saint John's wort plant and flower have been shown to help some types of depression. Saint John's wort is widely used internationally as a first-line herbal alternative for mild depression. For children with mild-to-moderate depression, more clinical trials are needed to determine the effectiveness of this herbal substance. Pediatric care providers must question the use of herbal substances used by families, such as Saint John's wort, because it has been known to interact with several other medications, including medications for HIV, some chemotherapies, and organ transplant antirejection medications.

The use of Saint John's wort herb can have dangerous side effects and should not be a replacement for antidepressants in children. Serotonin levels can increase to dangerous levels with symptoms ranging from tremors, diarrhea, confusion, hypothermia, muscle stiffness, and even death. Families must discuss their intention of using Saint John's wort with their primary caregiver before administering it to a child (NCCIH, 2014).

HEALTH PROMOTION

Sunscreen and Psychotherapeutic Medications

Several mental health disorders require the use of psychotherapeutic medications that make a child photosensitive. The medication may enhance ultraviolet (UV) light absorption of the skin. Children on the following medications should be monitored for sunburn and skin damage:

- Chlorpromazine (Thorazine)
- Fluphenazine (Prolixin)
- Trifluoperazine (Stelazine)
- Perphenazine (Trilafon)
- Mesoridazine (Serentil)
- Thioridazine (Mellaril)

An antianxiety medication that causes photosensitivity is Alprazolam (Xanax). Antidepressant medications that can cause photosensitivity include:

- Amitriptyline (Elavil)
- Nortriptyline (Pamelor)
- Paroxetine (Paxil)
- Sertraline (Zoloft)
- Fluoxetine (Prozac)
- Mirtazapine (Remeron)
- Venlafaxine (Effexor)

Preventing photosensitivity and burns should include the following measures:

- Wearing adequate protective clothing when in the sun, even on cloudy days
- Wearing light-colored, lightweight, and loose-fitting clothes
- Wearing a brimmed hat
- Applying at least an SPF 30 sunscreen on a daily basis, while also limiting sun exposure
- Choosing a waterproof or sport sunscreen if very active, sweating, or swimming

Nursing Considerations for Depression

A child with depression needs astute nursing care. Nurses caring for a child who is admitted with a diagnosis of depression should monitor the child for social isolation, increasing symptoms with hospitalization, and the potential for self-harm. Engage the Child Life department to provide distraction and support for the child during your care. Ensure that the health-care team has a plan for the child and that the family is engaged in the care required. Children with depression should have their regular antidepressant medications administered on time, according to the child's regular schedule. Inquire if serum levels are required to monitor the appropriate blood serum levels.

A family's culture may influence how they view their circumstances, whether or not they seek assistance and treatment, and how they follow through with treatment plans. It is very important for the pediatric health-care team to identify the child's family views about a diagnosis of childhood depression because not all families will recognize or acknowledge that their child is demonstrating depression. Some families have cultural values that influence their attitudes about mental illness in children. Certain cultures may see mental illness as being possessed by spirits, or they may see the child's mental illness as a punishment for something the child or the parents did. Some cultural groups will be reluctant to disclose the child's mental illness with others. It is important to educate all members of the family about the cause and treatment of child-hood mental illness, stressing that no one, especially the child, is to blame. Depression may prove a difficult diagnosis for families to recognize and acknowledge because some family members may feel shame, guilt, or fear. Families need support when their child is diagnosed with a mental illness, and depression has a unique set of challenges when cultural values and beliefs intertwine with the child's clinical presentation.

General guidelines for families to help a child who experiences depression include the following:

- Do not isolate the child. Keep him or her associated with extended family members.
- Make sure the child is seen by professionals who can help through counseling and medications.
- Make sure the child takes medicines that are ordered. Families should also know the common side effects to watch for.
- Do not blame anyone for causing the depression, especially the child. Depression is not caused by another person.
- Know that as the depression is treated and the feelings lift, the child will have less negative feelings and better expectations for themselves.
- Encourage the child to set small goals for himself or herself that he or she can work on each day. This may include building a craft over time, increasing time spent on homework each day, or planting a garden.
- Provide healthy foods and snacks, and have family members be role models of good nutrition.
- Assess the child for drug and alcohol use because these substances are dangerous when taken with antidepressants.
- Provide activities that make the child feel good. Engaging in conversation or playing with the whole family may improve the child's feelings.
- Be aware that depressed children are often targets of bullying at school. School officials must be notified of all bullying episodes so that the child can be protected during treatment.
- Call the National Suicide Prevention Lifeline as soon as the child displays thoughts or actions of suicide.
- Do not give up on the child or yourself in caring for the child. Do not get discouraged and do not feel you and your family are alone. Do not feel embarrassed—seek and secure help early.
- Talk about the depression as a family and seek clergy or traditional healers to provide support while receiving professional help as well.

Suicide in Childhood

Suicide is defined as death by taking one's own life. Suicide in children has become much more common than in previous years. Suicide rates are estimated to be close to 157,000 deaths per year (CDC, 2014), with males outnumbering females (81% versus 19%). Suicide has been reported to be the third-leading cause of death in youth ages 10 to 24 (CDC, 2014). The three main causes of death associated with suicide are guns, poisoning, and strangling. Suicide attempts in children are far more common than lethal suicides, with up to 2% to

6% of children trying to kill themselves throughout their childhood. With every 300 suicide attempts in childhood, 1% are successful. There is a strong association between suicide and a major depressive disorder. Up to 22% of children with a suicide attempt have an underlying psychiatric disorder.

Families who have marital difficulties, child abuse, or substance abuse are more likely to have an adolescent with a suicide risk. In addition, in one-third of adolescent suicide cases, a parent, sibling, or other first-degree family member has expressed suicidal thoughts or suicidal gestures, or has committed suicide.

TEAM WORKS

Using the most current and appropriate terms associated with mental illness and suicide is crucial (Box 31.1). The term *suicide gesture* has been defined as an attempt at suicide but without the means to take one's life, and also as a nonfatal act of deliberately causing harm or injury to oneself. This term is being phased out because it is seen as possibly dismissive of a very serious attempt, which could place the child at risk.

Suicide is considered a threat or an attempt to end one's life. Because of this, during childhood, the child may not be at a developmental level of cognition to understand the finality of death, but may attempt or commit suicide. All threats must be taken very seriously. In the United States, suicide is the

Box 31.1 Common Terms Associated With Suicide

Suicidal thinking: When a child or teen is thinking about suicide but has no plan; this is not uncommon, with about 3% of the general teen population reporting suicidal thinking at one point in their development.

Suicidal ideation: Children and teens who have thought out a plan but have not carried out any behaviors toward suicide. An example would be a teen who is collecting pills but has not made a plan or a gesture toward taking his or her life.

Suicide attempt: Suicidal attempts are very dangerous; the child or teen takes actual steps to ensure death. However, either the child is found by another person in time to secure emergency health care and resuscitation or is unsuccessful and lives through the attempt. Jumping off a high bridge, with full intention of death, but living through the jump and being rescued is one example.

Lethality of attempt: This refers to the determination of the potential threat of death per the patient's description of plans, methods, reasons, and availability of rescue.

Suicide: This means death via taking one's own life.

fourth-leading cause of death for children from 10 to 14 years of age, and the third-leading cause of death for children from 15 to 19 years of age. About one-third of childhood suicides involve the ingestion of an abused substance. When trauma is involved in a suicide, the health-care team must also consider intoxication or drug abuse. Males are more likely to use violent means and firearms as the major method of death.

ASSESSMENTS OF SUICIDE.   Any threats of suicide must be taken seriously. The child's seriousness, impulsivity, desperation, and degree of premeditation should all be taken into account. With suicide threats or gestures, the precipitating event should be identified. In addition, whether the child intended to be found and stopped or intended to have a serious injury or death should be assessed.

Some hospital and clinic settings will automatically assess an older school-aged child or a teenager for suicidal thoughts. Check with institutional policy to see if there is a standard assessment tool or an assessment question that is used to solicit the child to share if they have had or are having suicidal thoughts.

INTERVENTIONS FOR SUICIDE.   There is one main area for interventions for a child who shows evidence of suicidal thoughts or actions. The child must be taken seriously, supervised constantly, and supported immediately. This may mean the child is transported to an in-patient hospital or psychiatric unit for further assessments and treatments. Treatments will include medications to stabilize the child and can include the following (www.mayoclinic.org, 2015):

• Fluoxetine (Prozac) for children 8 years old and older
• Escitalopram (Lexapro) for children 12 years old and older
• Sertraline (Zoloft)
• Fluvoxamine (Luvox)
• Clomipramine (Anafranil)

The use of antidepressants in children requires careful monitoring. Antidepressants used in children have a black box warning (ie, an FDA warning concerning severe side effects that can occur; therefore caution must be used when administering). Some individuals under 25 years of age have shown to have increased suicidal behaviors when on antidepressants (www.mayoclinic.org, 2015).

SAFETY *STAT!*

If a pediatric nurse suspects that a child is at risk for a suicide while he or she is in the hospital or the child speaks about suicide thoughts while in a clinic, the nurse must report this concern immediately and mobilize a team to provide safety. While hospitalized the child will be placed on a suicide watch and staffing will be assigned to provide observations. Hospital and clinic rooms must be secured from any dangerous instrument or device that might be used, and opening of the window must be prevented. Constant supervision may be required for children with suicide risk, no matter what the clinical setting.

NURSING CONSIDERATIONS FOR SUICIDE.   The nursing care of a child or teen with a suicide attempt requires immediate stabilization and hospitalization with round-the-clock observation. Both Child Protective Services and the police or other law enforcement department must be contacted. The child's home may be searched for weapons, drugs, and access to medications. The following nursing care should be considered:

• Evidence of self-inflicted trauma should be accompanied by C-spine stabilization (cervical spine), cardiorespiratory monitoring, and the collection of serum and/or urine toxicology screens.
• If the use of poisonous substances is suspected, the health-care team will need to contact the American Association of Poison Control Centers to discuss appropriate medical treatments. The child will require cardiorespiratory monitoring and any other emergency response needed to support the airway and circulatory system. A serum toxicology screen must be collected.
• Because 90% of adolescents who attempt or are successful in committing suicide have a diagnosable psychiatric illness such as major depression, mood disorder, substance abuse, or schizophrenia, the child must be evaluated by a child mental health specialist for appropriate treatment. The pediatric nurse should ensure a timely consultation during early hospitalization.

Schizophrenia

Childhood **schizophrenia** is a chronic, severe, and disabling psychiatric disorder characterized by delusion, hallucination, and thought disorder. The affected child appears to be in a chaotic state, with paranoid delusions, hebephrenia (ie, a characteristic of schizophrenia marked by inappropriate affect, such as silliness and inappropriate laughter and mannerisms), alternating moods, aggressive behaviors, and social withdrawal. This severe, chronic, and debilitating mental illness affects about 1% of the population, affecting 1.5 times more males than females (National Institute of Mental Health, 2015). The typical age of the initial diagnosis of childhood schizophrenia is late adolescence or early adulthood, with gradual onset. Eighty percent of children with schizophrenia demonstrate auditory hallucinations. (National Institute of Mental Health, 2015).

The child suffers while experiencing thinking that is completely out of touch with reality. The child hears voices that are not there, sees people who are not present, may suffer physical symptoms of "bugs crawling on the skin," and displays behaviors and feelings that have no basis in reality. Adolescents and young adults may experience paranoia and feel as though people are plotting against them.

Types of Schizophrenia

Five subtypes of schizophrenia are diagnosed based on the primary symptoms the child is experiencing:

1. **Paranoid schizophrenia:** This type of schizophrenia is the most common type. The child displays preoccupation with one or more delusions or auditory

hallucinations, and experiences feelings of paranoia associated with the experience.

2. **Disorganized schizophrenia:** In this type, the child displays disorganized speech and behaviors.

3. **Catatonic schizophrenia:** The child has resistance to movement, exhibits abnormal movements, demonstrates repeating behaviors, or cannot move.

4. **Undifferentiated schizophrenia:** In this type, the child displays two or more of the following symptoms: disorganized speech, catatonic behaviors, negative thoughts, and delusions.

5. **Residual schizophrenia:** The child displays a lesser form of schizophrenia without delusions, paranoia, or heightened sensitivity, but is withdrawn, speaks very little, is disinterested in most activities, and exhibits a decrease in function.

Assessments of Schizophrenia

The assessment of schizophrenia in children is complicated and must be done by professionals who are experienced and trained in this area. Because of the severity of the brain disorder, assessments include behavior and emotional aspects. Combinations of delusions, disordered thinking, disordered speech, hallucinations, and an impaired ability to function are all evaluated. If the child is young, early symptoms to assess for include late crawling and late walking, delays in language development, and abnormal motor movements such as arm flapping and persistent rocking.

Interventions for Schizophrenia

There is no single treatment for schizophrenia. Treatment must continue for the child's lifetime. The child may benefit from a **neuroleptic** medication (ie, class of psychiatric medications used to treat several mental illnesses, including bipolar disorder and schizophrenia) therapy to manage some of the symptoms of this disorder, such as hallucinations and psychotic delusions. Family involvement and a commitment to the child's taking his or her medications are imperative.

Nursing Considerations for Schizophrenia

Children with schizophrenia need strict follow-up to ensure that the medications are adhered to. It is important for the nurse to assist in managing the care of the child and family.

The pediatric nurse should carefully assess the child for side effects from psychiatric medications used to manage the symptoms of schizophrenia. Neuroleptic medications can cause sedation and anticholinergic (ie, inhibiting the neurotransmission of acetylcholine) side effects. When antipsychotics interfere with the cholinergic neurons, they produce side effects at the organ system where the neurons are located. For instance, if the GI tract is affected, there is dry mouth, cramping, and constipation. When muscles of the eyes are affected, side effects include blurred vision. When the bladder is affected, associated side effects include difficulty urinating. When antipsychotics are taken with tricyclic antidepressants, there can be significant anticholinergic activity, resulting in delirium, confusion, and poor attention.

Tardive dyskinesia is a serious side effect of neuroleptics and is characterized by choreoathetoid movements (ie, involuntary movements such as twisting and writhing) of the facial musculature, limbs, and trunk. Dyskinesia can develop in as many as 20% to 30% of children treated long-term with neuroleptics. Dyskinetic symptoms are reversible if they occur during the withdrawal or discontinuation of the medications, but may not be reversible if they develop during drug therapy. Neuroleptic malignant syndrome is a rare side effect of neuroleptic therapy and is characterized by what is called a "lead pipe" stiffness of the extremities and high fevers. It is imperative to check in with families concerning the development of early side effects.

Other Types of Mental Health Disorders

Mental health disorders in children include commonly known mental health diagnoses. Children can suffer emotionally from their mental health state and use drugs to cope with their condition. This type of coping is considered negative behavior; substance abuse, widespread across older childhood, is a major concern for pediatric health-care providers. Another condition that has recently received a great deal of media attention is severe bullying. Bullying has been directly linked to anxiety, depression, and suicide. Pediatric nurses must develop skills to quickly assess for children and teens who are abusing substances and who are victims of bullying.

Substance Abuse

The NIH states that there is a cumulative decline in drug involvement in children since the mid-1990s. Nevertheless, the use of illegal and illicit substances in children and teens is very concerning. About 13% of children in the eighth grade report the use of at least one illicit drug in the prior 12 months. About 40% of adolescents report they have been "drunk" within the last year. Some teens try illicit substances only a few times, and others develop cravings and urges that lead to abuse. The most commonly claimed substances used are tobacco, marijuana, alcohol, stimulants, hallucinogens, inhalants, prescription drugs, opiates, cocaine, "club drugs" like ecstasy, and steroids. Alcohol and marijuana remain the two most often tried substances across childhood. Inhalants cause serious brain damage (Fig. 31.4). See Table 31.1 for a list of common drugs currently being abused during childhood.

Children who live in homes where substance abuse is taking place are at a much higher risk for developing a serious drug or alcohol abuse problem. Children who are experiencing depression are at greater risk; children who do not feel valued by their parents have a higher tendency to experiment with illicit substances and have a greater risk for abuse.

Complications associated with substance abuse in childhood and adolescents include feelings of hopelessness, alienation, and depression. Injuries, accidents, unplanned pregnancy, violence, drowning, and suicide are also associated with substance abuse.

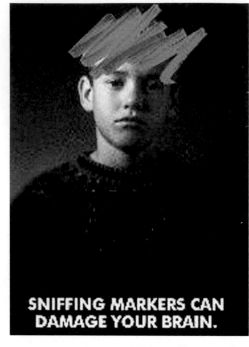

SNIFFING MARKERS CAN DAMAGE YOUR BRAIN.

FIGURE 31.4 Substance abuse includes inhalants. *(Reproduced with permission of the National Inhalant Prevention Coalition, 1991.)*

PATIENT TEACHING GUIDELINES

Assessing for Signs of Alcohol and Drug Abuse in Children and Teens

Parents need to be taught how to assess for substance abuse in their children. The following are behaviors or symptoms to be aware of:

- General changes in overall attitude
- Sudden personality changes that disrupt school work, school attendance, grades, and quality of work
- Sudden outbreaks of anger, aggression, nervousness, and jitteriness
- Increased secretiveness
- Engagement in a new social circle of friends who have no interest in meeting the family
- Withdrawal from responsibility
- Red eyes and complaints of being overly tired
- Loss of interest in previously engaged hobbies, activities, and sports
- Loss of interest in personal grooming, hygiene, and personal appearance to others
- Borrowing of money or stealing of money or objects to sell
- Association with known substance abusers

TABLE 31.1 COMMON DRUGS ABUSED BY YOUTH

Street Drugs	Prescription Drugs
• Marijuana	• Barbiturates
• Cocaine	• Methamphetamine (Desoxyn)
• Crystal meth (methamphetamine)	• Cough and cold medicines: dextromethorphan
• Ecstasy	• Sleeping pills
• Heroin	• Antianxiety medications (anxiolytics)
• Acid (LSD)	• Fentanyl (Duragesic)
• PCP (phencyclidine)	• Hydrocodone (Vicodin)
• Mushrooms (psilocybin)	• Oxycodone (OxyContin)
• Peyote plant (mescaline)	• Oxymorphone (Opana)
• Nitrous oxide	• Hydromorphone (Dilaudid)
• Crack	• Meperidine (Demerol)
• Speed (ice)	• Diphenoxylate (Lomotil)
• Gamma hydroxybutyrate (GHB; Xyrem)	• Alprazolam (Xanax)
	• Diazepam (Valium)
	• Dextroamphetamine (Dexedrine)
	• Methylphenidate (Ritalin or Concerta)
	• Amphetamine and dextroamphetamine (Adderall)
	• Bath salts
	• Ketamine (Special K)
	• Benzodiazepines

Source: www.doitnow.org, 2015; www.drugabuse.gov

• Secretive behavior around possessions and suspicious behavior such as frequent trips to the bathroom, storage areas, basement, and places where drugs or alcohol could be stored

ASSESSMENTS OF SUBSTANCE ABUSE. Assessing whether or not a child or teen is abusing substances can be difficult. Many youth use drugs "recreationally" out of curiosity and peer pressure, and do not consider themselves as abusing drugs. According to Robinson, Smith, et al, use does not always lead to abuse; what is important is not how much a person is using but how the use is causing problems with health, school, home, and relationships (2015). There may be outward signs such as needle marks and symptoms of use, and there may be affective signs of depression, guilt, shame, and drug-seeking behaviors. Other signs of substance abuse that should be assessed are academic performance, problems with relationships at home, social isolation, and whether another family member has or has had **addiction** problems. Pediatric nurses must be astute in looking for physical signs of substance abuse and addiction behaviors, such as uncontrollable cravings (Box 31.2) (Robinson, Smith, et al, 2015).

There are three known categories of substance abuse for children:

• **Use:** This is where a child or teen participates in the drug use very occasionally. There is no evidence of withdrawal if the drug is not used and there is no evidence of the development of tolerance (ie, the need for increasing quantity to achieve the same results).

• **Abuse:** The child or teen continues to use the substance even though there are social, academic, physical, and psychological problems created by the use of the drug.
• **Dependence:** This is when the substance is progressively taken in higher quantity to achieve the same desired results. The child or teen has a persistent desire but lack of success in controlling the illicit substance use, and there are frequent periods of intoxication. The child may also experience withdrawal symptoms and may take the substance to relieve the withdrawal symptoms.

INTERVENTIONS FOR SUBSTANCE ABUSE. Treatment for substance abuse across childhood includes identifying if there is a dual diagnosis, such as depression, and treating the mental health disorder. Factors associated with treatment include the child's age, gender, values and culture, family factors, and the presence of a coexisting mental health disorder. Medications may be ordered that help to treat the addiction. For instance, naltrexone may be given for alcohol or opiate dependency, bupropion may be given for marijuana or tobacco abuse, and methadone may be given for heroin addiction. After detoxification in either an outpatient or inpatient setting, treatment can include addressing the mental health issue, psychotherapy, behavior modification, cognitive therapy, 12-step programs, or, if needed, residential treatment. The child or teen will be frequently tested for drug use. Many children addicted to substances benefit from peer group therapy (Fig. 31.5).

Interventions and treatments for substance abuse in children should be thought of as threefold: (1) the child's physical needs, which must be immediately met, including addressing the detrimental effects of substance abuse and symptoms of withdrawal; (2) the child's cognitive and emotional needs, as affected by the addiction; and (3) the child's family dynamics, if trust has been broken or the addiction has had severe consequences on family relationships. In general, children cannot stop the substance abuse without treatment and emotional support. Families must be aggressive in their interventions to help their child.

NURSING CONSIDERATIONS FOR SUBSTANCE ABUSE. Pediatric nurses need to teach parents the signs and symptoms of

---

Box 31.2 Physical Signs of Substance Abuse and Addiction in Children

Assessment of physical signs of addiction should take place during well-child visits and any other health-care interactions. Nurses should never assume that a child is not taking drugs and should screen for clinical signs and symptoms with each encounter.

• Physical signs of depression, such as being withdrawn
• Physical signs of abuse, violence, or injuries
• Pregnancy and sexually transmitted infections
• Nausea, vomiting, diarrhea, and other GI problems
• Insomnia and poor quality of sleep
• Sweating, shaking, and tremors
• Bloodshot eyes, pupil dilation or pupil constriction, and flushed face
• Poor personal grooming and body odor
• Poor oral hygiene and bad breath
• Impaired speech and coordination
• Lethargy, drowsiness, or inattentiveness

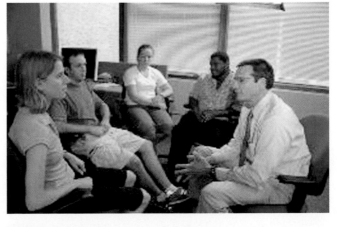

FIGURE 31.5 Teens can benefit from peer group therapy. *(Photo from NIH.)*

substance abuse in children. Families need to understand the laws surrounding children and tobacco and alcohol. Helping families secure professional interventions is key. Teach parents that if they suspect substance abuse, they should immediately contact their physician or pediatrician and contact an educational consultant to help find the right program and treatment for their child. Securing an educational advocate can also provide assistance with navigating the child's or teen's school situation. Encourage parents to talk frequently about drugs and the risks and dangers of illegal substances to their children; to communicate family values and meaningfulness of their relationship with their child or teen; and to set rules and consequences of breaking the family rules.

It is very important to teach parents not to leave prescription narcotics where children can find them. There is increasing abuse of prescriptions drugs, such as acetaminophen and hydrocodone (Vicodin), diazepam (Valium), oxycodone (OxyContin), and even methylphenidate (Ritalin), which is used to help control ADHD. Some children abuse OTC medications such as cough syrup or cold pills. Medications should be locked and kept away from children and their peers (Fig. 31.6).

Parents must acknowledge that their child is suffering from substance abuse and seek help for the entire family. Community-based organizations can be of vital assistance in supporting parents and family members in realizing the severity of the situation and making referrals to local support systems for treatment of the addiction. Organizations that can provide education and support for families who have a child participating in substance abuse include:

1. Alcoholics Anonymous (AA) World Services
2. National Institute on Alcohol Abuse and Alcoholism (NIAAA): The Cool Spot
3. KidsHealth
4. National Institute on Drug Abuse (NIDA), NIH
5. Partnership for Drug-Free Kids

Bullying

Bullying has become a national concern. Bullying takes many forms, including physical force and violence, spreading rumors about others, social exclusion, severe teasing, "ganging up" on others, and using social media to send insulting messages or pictures. Victims often display low self-esteem, loneliness, anxiety, depression, poor academic performance, and suicidal thoughts. Victims can experience poorer physical health, including headaches, sleeping problems, GI distress, and other inflammatory processes. Bullying is known to cause long-lasting emotional scars and life-long memories. Children who witness bullying also suffer with fear, guilt, and distraction in school work.

Bullying can begin as early as the later preschool period. Bullies may choose their victims at random or they may persecute other children who have a "different" look such as obesity, small stature, or unique features. Sometimes bullying victims have special learning needs, cognitive impairment, or mental health issues.

ASSESSMENTS OF BULLYING. Assessing for bullying is important and may save lives. Children need to have the opportunity to talk about the bullying without fear of retribution or increased torment. Try using questions, such as: "Are there any kids at your school who tease you in a mean way?"; "Are there kids at your school who you really do not like? Why?"; "Have you been harassed on social media?"

The pediatric nurse must look for physical and emotional signs of bullying. Obvious signs can be cuts, bruises, black eyes, torn personal belongings, or damaged school supplies. Other signs may be extreme school aversion, frequent absences, symptoms of depression, somatic complaints, and poor school performance. Bullies choose victims based on their perception of power over others and those who are deemed "different" from them.

INTERVENTIONS FOR BULLYING. Bullying must be stopped before a child is hurt or hurts themselves. Interventions for immediate bullying scenarios should include the following:

- Stand between the children involved
- Block eye contact between the bully and the victim
- Do not try to sort out the facts at that moment; do not discuss the reasons at the time of the incident
- Do not let bystanders walk away; they need to witness the intervention
- State out loud the behaviors that you saw and heard
- State clearly that bullying is against the rules and will not be tolerated

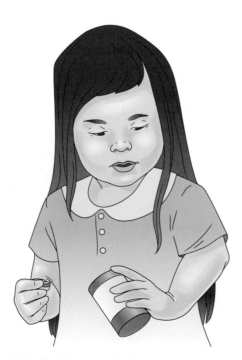

FIGURE 31.6 Child finding leftover narcotics.

SAFETY *STAT!*

Bullycide is a new hybrid term used to describe a suicide directly related to a child experiencing severe bullying.

Cyberbullying has superseded physical bullying as the reason for bullycidal behaviors. Bullycidal behavior has been linked to feelings resulting from chronic bullying: persistent emotional pain, reliving embarrassing moments over and over again, and bullying by a figure of authority (www.bullyingstatistics.org, 2015).

The bullied child needs to feel safe and supported. Never question the child in front of others. Do not allow the bullying to escalate or the situation to happen again. Increase supervision to prevent a repeat situation. Make sure there is guidance given to the bystanders; they should know that they can help by telling the bully to stop and immediately getting an adult to handle the situation. The bully needs consequences. These include the loss of a privilege and enforced "watching" them for a period of time.

NURSING CONSIDERATIONS FOR BULLYING.   Under no circumstances can bullying be allowed within a health-care setting. Whether hospitalized in an acute care setting or a long-term facility, children must behave respectfully to each other. Any bullying witnessed within a health-care setting must be stopped and interventions implemented.

Pediatric nurses need to keep aware of how to assess for bullying and how to provide support and interventions. Bullying is very serious and can lead to depression, anxiety, and suicidal behaviors. The child needs to have support from the school where he or she is enrolled. The health-care team, including Child Life services, can place a call to the school to describe the child's reported experiences. The child should be told that bullying is never to be tolerated and that it takes adult interventions to stop the bullying from continuing between children and teens. Although the hospital cannot provide services, a social worker should be notified. Requesting a referral for a child psychologist is appropriate. A child who has been bullied needs to be referred for help. Make sure the family knows to contact the school authorities, who should have protocols for intervening.

Key Points

- Current trends in the incidence and prevalence of mental health issues across the span of childhood help health-care professionals become prepared to care for children and teens. Trends include an increase in autism, ADHD, depression, and other mood disorders. An awareness of risk factors can assist health-care professionals to screen, identify issues, and intervene.

- A mental health issue has a serious effect on the child's interactions with family, school, social networks, and society as a whole and requires a holistic approach through counseling or therapy, medication, and follow-up care.

- Goals for therapeutic communication between the nurse and the child/family when interacting with an acute exacerbation of a mental health condition include establishing rapport, building trust, and communicating the importance of interventions to help the child cope and recover.

- Many professional assessment tools exist to aid in diagnosing anxiety, depression, and other mood disorders. These tools are administered by mental health-care professionals and the results guide treatments and therapy.

- ADHD has a serious effect on a child's interaction with family and school. Early identification and initiation of treatment can assist the child in demonstrating improved behavior in the classroom and greater achievements in academic performance.

- Anorexia nervosa and bulimia eating disorders have distinct patterns of behavior. Often associated with a child's poor self-image, poor self-esteem, and very poor perception of his or her physical self, the prevalence of these disorders in current society is increasing for both genders. The nurse needs to understand the differences between the diagnoses and assist the team with interventions to prevent poor outcomes, including death.

- There is no known cause for autism but it is known to exist from birth, with early symptoms noted as early as late infancy. Genetics, irregular brain regions, and environment most likely play a role in the development of autism.

- Bullying is a very serious experience for a child and can lead to depression, anxiety, and suicide. Bullying must be identified and interventions must take place to provide for the child's safety and well-being. Bullying can manifest as threats of physical violence, actual violence, or emotional pain from ridicule, meanness, or social isolation.

- Substance abuse during childhood is a major concern. Pediatric nurses need to be able to identify the physical and affective signs of substance abuse and addiction. Parents need to first acknowledge that their child has a substance abuse problem and seek information, help, and treatment for their child.

REVIEW QUESTIONS

1. A teenage girl is seen in the pediatric clinic for a routine physical examination required for her to play high school sports. Her weight is plotted on a national growth chart and is within a normal range. Her mother expresses concern that her daughter may be experiencing an eating disorder. Which of the following could she be experiencing?
   1. Anorexia nervosa
   2. Anxiety disorder
   3. Mood disorder
   4. Bulimia

2. While teaching the family of a child who has just been placed on a SSRI antidepressant, the nurse tells the family to make sure the child avoids all of the following foods *except:*
   1. Aged cheese
   2. Pickles
   3. Blackened meats
   4. Dishes cooked with wine

3. Which of the following medications causes photosensitivity and an increased chance of severe sunburn?
   1. Lorazepam (Ativan)
   2. Doxycycline (Acticlate)
   3. Lithium (Lithobid)
   4. Chlorpromazine (Thorazine)

4. A high-priority assessment for a child admitted into the hospital for complications associated with substance abuse is:
   1. Dynamics of family and parent interactions
   2. Child's social structure
   3. Thoughts of suicide
   4. Academic performance

5. A father brings his 30-month-old daughter in to the pediatric clinic for a check-up. He explains that she has not begun to talk and is often found sitting watching a window ornament for long periods of time. He expresses concerns that his daughter may be autistic. What would be an appropriate question to ask this father?
   1. "Does your child cuddle up to you when you hold her?"
   2. "Does your child have an older sibling who 'talks' for her and share her needs?"
   3. "Does your child attend a childcare facility where she may not be getting enough attention and play?"
   4. "Does your child have temper tantrums more than you would expect?"

6. Which medication is the first-line antagonist for a suicide attempt with an overdose with acetaminophen (Tylenol)?
   1. Acetylcysteine (Mucomyst)
   2. Activated charcoal
   3. Ice water gastric lavage
   4. Narcotic action

7. Medications may be ordered to help treat addiction in children. While helping the pediatric health-care team assess a child with a known substance abuse problem, the nurse knows that all of the following are true *except:*
   1. Naltrexone may be given for alcohol or opiate dependency
   2. Bupropion may be given for marijuana or tobacco abuse
   3. Methadone may be given for heroin addiction
   4. Antabuse may be given for methamphetamine addiction

8. For a child with schizophrenia, neuroleptics may be prescribed. Tardive dyskinesia is a serious side effect of neuroleptics and is characterized by which of the following?
   1. Choreoathetoid movements of the facial musculature, limbs, and trunk
   2. Grand mal seizures without loss of consciousness
   3. Copious salivation and drooling
   4. Fatigue and lethargy

9. A father of a child recently diagnosed with ADHD is expressing concern about putting his child on medications. The pediatric nurse would be correct in stating that what percentage of children, on average, takes medications for this condition?
   1. 100%
   2. 50%
   3. 6%
   4. 22%

10. The pediatric nurse has been invited to give a presentation to staff working at a public health clinic. While presenting on current health concerns for children, the nurse describes the effects of bullying. The nurse would be correct in saying that bullying comes in many forms including: *(select all that apply)*
    1. Physical force
    2. Violence
    3. Spreading rumors
    4. Social exclusion
    5. Severe teasing
    6. Using social media to send insulting messages or pictures

CRITICAL THINKING QUESTIONS

1. A 12-year-old girl presents with syncope and severe abdominal pain. All diagnostic and laboratory tests come back negative. Her mother describes that she is experiencing severe bullying in her school; she has very limited English language skills and has been targeted by a group of teen girls. Both the mother and the child are requesting to remain in the hospital until her symptoms improve. How would you go about referring her for counseling? What does this child need from a pediatric nurse? Can a hospitalization provide this child an avenue for recovery and skill building? What are potential outcomes of a bullying situation that is not resolved at the school level?

2. Suicide is an important concern for children who have mental health issues, depression, and social isolation. How can a pediatric nurse assist with suicide prevention education and early interventions when a child has been noted to be at risk for suicidal behaviors?

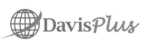

For additional resources and information, visit **www.DavisPlus.com**. Post-Conference Questions and Activities, Answers, and References can be found on Davis*Plus*.

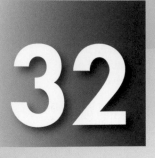

32

Child With a Respiratory Condition

KEY TERMS

adventitious breath sounds
alveolar sacs
alveoli
atelectasis
bronchodilation
crepitus
cyanosis
eustachian tubes
hemoptysis
inhaler
laryngitis
nasopharyngeal
nebulizer
pneumothorax
rales
respiratory syncytial virus (RSV)
rhonchi
stridor

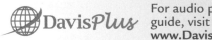 **Davis**_Plus_ For audio pronunciation guide, visit www.DavisPlus.com

CHAPTER CONCEPTS

Inflammation
Oxygenation
Perfusion
Safety
Sleep, Rest, and Activity

LEARNING OUTCOMES

1. Define the key terms.
2. Review the differences between the anatomy and physiology of a newborn's and a child's respiratory system and an adult's.
3. Describe the breathing patterns, adventitious breath sounds, and symptoms one may encounter in respiratory distress.
4. State the assessments conducted in the physical examination of an infant or child with a respiratory condition.
5. Review the care required for a child with croup, including possible causative factors and developmental groups most vulnerable to this disease.
6. Discuss the various methods of intervention for a child with a respiratory condition, including the different oxygen delivery systems.
7. Compare the pathophysiology, diagnostic methods, and treatment for tonsillitis and epiglottitis.
8. Compare and contrast sudden infant death syndrome (SIDS) and apparent life-threatening event (ALTE), including risk factors, monitoring, and possible causes.
9. Describe the pathophysiology of asthma, treatment protocols administered across childhood, and teaching required for the patient and family to minimize adverse effects.
10. Review the effect of respiratory diseases on a family and the teaching needs of the family to safely care for a child hospitalized for treatments or who is being cared for at home.

REAL-WORLD CASE STUDY

Heather

■ A 5-year-old girl has been admitted to the pediatric unit of the hospital with severe asthma for her third inpatient visit within the last 12 months. Her father, who only speaks Cantonese, is her primary caregiver and her mother works long hours during the week. During her last hospitalization, the family was given a prescription for a short-acting asthma rescue inhaler, a nonsteroidal anti-inflammatory inhaler, and antibiotics because her x-ray demonstrated a secondary pneumonia. The father states he was unable to fill all of the prescriptions because of limited family resources and chose to fill the antibiotic only. The child received 6 hours of continuous nebulized albuterol in the emergency room and then was admitted for every 2-hour interval of nebulized medication administration of albuterol and ipratropium (Atrovent) inhalation treatments.

1. What challenges does this family face while trying to care for a preschool child with severe asthma?
2. How will her triggers be identified? What are common triggers for an asthma attack?
3. What are the educational needs of this family?

CONCEPTUAL CORNERSTONES

Oxygenation

A child with a serious respiratory condition or infection will be at risk for *ineffective gas exchange* because of poor *oxygenation*. Acute respiratory illnesses such as bronchiolitis cause a young child to be significantly distressed. The concept of oxygenation concerns the ability to adequately take in sufficient amounts of oxygen to provide for the body's cellular demands. Without sufficient oxygenation and gas exchange, the child will become hypoxemic, hypoxic, and cyanotic. These three serious signs of inefficient oxygen intake and gas exchange can become life-threatening. The responsibility of the pediatric nurse is to understand the symptoms associated with poor oxygenation and provide immediate relief through the administration of supplemental oxygen and medications that improve gas exchange.

Children who experience acute and chronic respiratory conditions require specially trained health-care personnel who are knowledgeable about the underlying pathophysiology and the treatments, equipment, and medications necessary to care for this pediatric subset. Diagnosis of these diseases relies strongly on history-taking and physical assessment, making comprehension of these data essential. The possible severity of the illnesses may require practitioners with critical care backgrounds because routine symptoms can rapidly become life-threatening.

It is imperative for families of these patients to have a clear understanding of the disease process and treatment parameters. Often the child is cared for at home, either upon discharge from the hospital or if the symptoms do not warrant hospitalization.

THE DEVELOPMENT OF THE RESPIRATORY TRACT

Immediately after birth, the newborn infant's lungs progress through a rapid developmental period. The immediate time period after birth requires that the infant's lungs progress from a fluid-filled environment to independent oxygenation and ventilation.

The Development of the Lungs at Birth

Before birth the fetus' lungs are not inflated, but are filled with amniotic fluid. Oxygen and carbon dioxide are exchanged via the mother's circulation through the placenta and umbilical cord. When the newborn takes its first breath a few seconds after birth, oxygen flows into the lungs, starting inflation and reducing blood-flow resistance to the lung. Amniotic fluid drains, is suctioned, or absorbs. When the lungs begin the work of respiration, oxygen moves into the blood vessels and carbon dioxide is exhaled.

Alveoli Development

The exchange of the gases oxygen and carbon dioxide occurs in microscopic sacs within the lung tissue called *alveolar sacs* or *alveoli* (plural). At full-term birth (ie, 40 weeks' gestation), the neonate has approximately 20 to 50 million alveoli. These gradually increase in number as the child grows until reaching the total, adult amount of 300 million by the age of 8. As the number of alveoli increases, the alveolar surface area also increases, allowing the gas exchange to become more efficient and explaining the progressive slowing of the normal respiratory rate.

Anatomy of the Respiratory Tract of a Child Versus an Adult

The respiratory system consists of the following organs: the nose, pharynx, larynx (ie, voice box), trachea (ie, windpipe), bronchi, bronchioles, and lungs. These are involved in taking in oxygen upon inspiration and expelling carbon dioxide upon expiration. Upper respiratory tract anatomy includes the nose, nasal cavity, ethmoidal air cells, frontal sinuses, maxillary sinus, larynx, and trachea. Lower respiratory tract anatomy includes the lungs, bronchi, bronchioles, and alveoli. The lungs themselves are a pair of conical organs made up of spongy, pink-gray tissue. The lungs are encased in a membrane called the *pleura*. The pleura contains the only nerves in the respiratory system; hence it is the only site for pain. The right lung has three lobes; the left has two lobes. Therefore the right lung is somewhat larger and sits higher in the chest. The main-stem bronchi lead to the right lung and the left lung. In the lungs, the main-stem bronchi divide into smaller bronchi, and then into smaller bronchioles. The bronchioles terminate in the microscopic air sacs called *alveoli*.

A child's nose is relatively narrower than an adult's, causing it to become obstructed more easily. It contains no cilia to prevent the introduction of micro-organisms to the lower airways and is richer in blood supply, which can cause an increase in inflammation. These factors can lead to mouth-breathing and more difficulty breathing. The maxillary sinus is not well-developed until the age of 6, and the frontal sinus not until the age of 12, resulting in fewer incidences of sinusitis. The **nasopharyngeal** and palatine tonsils gradually develop between the ages of 1 and 10 years, at which point the tissue starts to shrink. In those years, the occurrence of tonsillitis is much more prevalent. The **eustachian tube** runs between the middle ear and the pharynx. It is wider and shorter than in the adult and acts like a conduit, bringing micro-organisms from the pharynx to the middle ear, causing otitis media (OM). The throat is longer and narrower, with soft cartilage that results in increased congestion, edema, obstruction, and difficulty breathing. The trachea and bronchi have soft cartilage, a smaller lumen, a lack of elastic tissue, and poor ciliary movement. The lungs do not develop their total number of alveoli until age 8. This causes more breathing difficulty and cyanosis; they are less compliant than an adult's, causing the child to have to work harder to breathe. The pulmonary tissue is rich in vasculature, resulting in more inflammation.

SAFETY *STAT!*

Because the trachea and bronchi have soft cartilage, a smaller lumen, a lack of elastic tissue, and poor ciliary movement, these characteristics can work together to cause an increase in the occurrence of respiratory infections. The small lumen and poor ciliary movement also cause young children to have more difficulty clearing secretions, making them more at risk for the development of viral and bacterial infections caused by pooled secretions.

HEALTH HISTORY

The pediatric nurse should work with the health-care team to conduct a health history on a child who presents with a suspected respiratory condition. Questions concerning the child's health and environment include the following:

• Chronic lung disease (CLD) in family members
• Other acute or chronic conditions experienced by the child
• Smoking by family members or caregivers of the child
• Respiratory conditions at birth
• Exposures to environmental toxins such as mold, pesticides, or pollution

PHYSICAL ASSESSMENT

When encountering a child who presents with a respiratory condition, a thorough assessment is warranted. Assessments should include the full variety of techniques: auscultation, percussion, olfaction, palpation, inspection of breathing effort, and assessment of the chest wall configuration.

General Respiratory Assessments

The pediatric health-care team will want to be notified immediately if a child presents in respiratory distress. Any difficulty with ventilation or abnormal positioning to maximize air exchange should be reported immediately so that rapid interventions can take place. After viewing the child to assess for distress, the nurse should support the assessment of the child's breath sounds.

Auscultation

Auscultation of the chest will serve to assess the characteristics of respiratory sounds, identify abnormal sounds, and evaluate vocal resonance (Fig. 32.1). A pediatric stethoscope will help to localize abnormal sounds. The stethoscope diaphragm transmits high-pitched sounds more effectively. Auscultate the breath sounds over the entire chest, alternating between the two sides for comparison of the anterior and posterior. Breath sounds can best be heard when the child is at rest, but the deep breath taken between cries can be effective, too.

Percussion

Percussion evaluates the lungs' resonance and density. As with auscultation, a pattern of alternating sides will allow comparison. Indirect percussion is done by placing the middle finger of the nondominant hand in an intercostal space and tapping with the fingers of the other hand. Direct

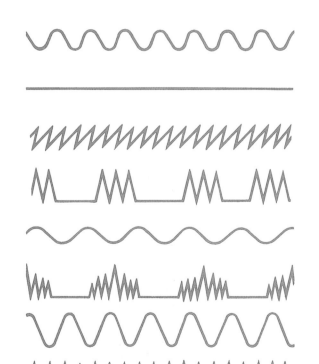

FIGURE 32.1 Normal and abnormal breathing patterns: eupnea, apnea, apneustic, Biot's, bradypnea, Cheyne-Stokes, hyperventilation, Kussmaul's, and tachypnea.

percussion involves tapping with the fingertips and is used for examining infants.

Olfaction

Olfaction is the sense of smell and the ability to distinguish different odors. This sense is easily altered in pediatric patients because they frequently have nasal congestion.

Palpation

Palpation is performed to evaluate chest movements, respiratory effort, abnormalities of the chest, and tactile fremitus. It is done with open palms and outstretched fingers. Placement of the palm on the chest can help determine the depth of retractions and the use of accessory respiratory muscles. Lightly touching the skin with the fingertips can locate **crepitus** (ie, a crackling sound heard in the lungs) or subcutaneous emphysema, small pockets of air under the skin caused by trauma or fractures. Tactile fremitus is the vibration caused by talking or crying. Having the child repeat words while alternating his or her hands over the chest and back aids in evaluating the quality of the vibrations.

Inspection

Inspecting the child's respiratory effort includes the respiratory rate, chest movements, signs of distress, and presentation of an emotional state such as anxiety. See Table 32.1 for a summary of expected respiratory rates per minute for children.

TEAM WORKS

Breathing Patterns

It is imperative that all members of the pediatric health-care team can identify when a child demonstrates a change in respiratory pattern or displays respiratory distress. It is also important that each team member uses the same title of the breathing pattern so there is no confusion. The following lists the common breathing patterns:

- **Kussmaul's breathing:** Slow, deep, labored respirations, often caused by metabolic acidosis
- **Bradypnea:** A respiratory rate slower than normal (normal range depends on age)
- **Tachypnea:** A respiratory rate faster than normal (normal range depends on age)
- **Cheyne-Stokes breathing:** A cycle of respirations with rapid, deep breathing, followed by a gradual slowing of breathing, and finally a period of apnea in a crescendo/diminuendo pattern
- **Hyperventilation:** Respirations that are deeper and more rapid than normal and result in a low carbon dioxide level
- **Hypoventilation:** Respirations that are more shallow and slower than normal and result in a high carbon dioxide level
- **Apnea:** A period of time without breathing

Assessment of Chest Movements

Normal chest movement is bilaterally symmetric, rising and falling with inspiration and expiration. The chest movement

TABLE 32.1 PEDIATRIC RESPIRATORY RATES PER MINUTE

Age	Respiratory Rate per Minute
Birth–12 months	30–60
1–2 years	20–40
2–5 years	20–30
6–9 years	16–22
10–16 years	16–20
17+ years	12–20

of infants and young children is less pronounced than the abdominal movement. The abdomen rises as the chest does with inspiration. The diaphragm is the key respiratory muscle in all children younger than 6 years old.

Chest Configurations

An infant's chest is normally considered rounded: the lateral diameter is approximately equal to the anteroposterior diameter. This should disappear by the age of 2, when the lateral diameter is greater than the anteroposterior diameter by 2:1. The following list demonstrates chest configurations that are considered abnormal:

- **Barrel chest:** Chest is rounded in appearance; after the age of 2, the cause may be a chronic disease such as asthma or cystic fibrosis
- **Pigeon chest (ie, pectus carinatum):** The presence of a protuberant sternum, which causes an increase in the anteroposterior diameter; it is genetic in origin
- **Funnel chest (ie, pectus excavatum):** Depression of the lower sternum, which causes a decrease in anteroposterior diameter; it is genetic in origin

Assessments of Respiratory Distress

A child who is experiencing difficulty breathing will look extremely anxious in response to hypoxia. A child who is in respiratory distress will assume a position that will maximize the ability to draw air into the lungs:

- In the *tripod position,* the child will sit or stand leaning forward with the arms resting on the knees. This increases the ability to use the thoracic and neck muscles as accessory respiratory muscles.
- The *sniffing position* involves tilting the head back to maximize the effort to draw air into the lungs via the nose.

Any child who displays signs of respiratory distress needs to have his or her condition reported so that he or she receives immediate interventions to help alleviate distress and increase oxygenation.

Evaluation of the Energy and Effort to Breathe

A child will show physical signs of increased effort to breathe. The following list describes the physical signs that a child will display when he or she is experiencing air hunger and is trying to maximize oxygen intake:

- **Use of accessory muscles:** A child under 6 years of age uses the diaphragm as the primary muscle for breathing. Use of the thoracic muscles for breathing indicates respiratory difficulty and may result in chest contractions.
- **Chest retractions:** The soft tissue of the chest shows a visible depression beneath the breastbone (substernal), above the collarbone (supraclavicular), between the ribs (intracostal), or beneath the ribcage (subcostal). The use of accessory muscles is an attempt to pull in more oxygen.

RESPIRATORY ABNORMALITIES

Children in respiratory distress will often display abnormal clinical symptoms. These symptoms will include signs of hypoxia and hypoxemia. When seen, the pediatric nurse must report the findings immediately to the health-care team.

Types of Respiratory Distress

A number of signs and symptoms may indicate that a child is not getting sufficient levels of oxygen. Hypoxia describes a state of insufficient oxygen in general that can result in insufficient oxygen in the blood (ie, hypoxemia). These signs and symptoms may include:

- **Cyanosis:** Bluish coloring on the lips, around the mouth (ie, circumoral), in the nail beds, or pale or gray skin
- **Nasal flaring:** Nares open wider with each inspiration to pull more oxygen into the lungs
- **Diaphoresis:** Increased sweat, particularly on the head, while the skin is cool or clammy rather than warm to the touch; this may accompany tachypnea
- **Head bobbing:** With insufficient oxygen levels, the infant thrusts his or her head forward with each inspiration; this is because of the neck muscles being too weak to hold the head stable with lung retractions

Adventitious Breath Sounds

Abnormal breath sounds in a child are the same as in the adult. Common abnormal breath sounds, also called *adventitious breath sounds,* are found when a child has a condition that is interfering with normal oxygenation and ventilation. In young children, adventitious breath sounds are loud and may be heard without the use of a stethoscope.

- **Wheezing:** A whistling noise with inspiration and/or expiration that may be audible or only heard with auscultation; this may indicate the airway is narrowed because of swelling and/or bronchoconstriction
- **Crackles/rales:** A high-pitched, intermittent sound caused by air passing through fluid in the lungs; it

sounds like rubbing hair through one's fingers in front of the ear
- **Sibilant rhonchi:** A musical, hissing, or squeaking sound heard louder on expiration that is caused by bronchospasm or narrowing of the airways
- **Sonorous rhonchi:** A coarse, snoring sound on inspiration or expiration that is caused by secretions causing a partial obstruction of the airways
- **Stridor:** A high-pitched sound on inspiration usually accompanied by gasping in an attempt to draw in air past a severe airway obstruction. Stridor is considered a severe symptom.
- **Grunting:** A grunting sound with each expiration may indicate the body's effort to improve oxygenation by trying to keep the alveoli open so that they are better able to fill with air

OVERALL INTERVENTIONS FOR A CHILD WITH RESPIRATORY DIFFICULTIES

A child experiencing respiratory distress requires immediate support. Through interventions designed to reduce poor oxygenation and ineffective gas exchange, the pediatric health-care team provides the child with emergency interventions that reduce the child's symptoms and improve the child's respiratory status. Emergency interventions to support the airway include oxygen delivery, suctioning, and airway management.

Emergency Interventions

The American Association of Pediatrics (AAP) established guidelines for emergency treatment in pediatric emergencies in their Pediatric Advanced Life Support (PALS) course. Included is supplemental oxygen therapy, airway management, foreign body (FB) aspiration, cardiopulmonary resuscitation (CPR), tracheostomy, endotracheal intubation, and mechanical ventilation.

SAFETY *STAT!*

Pediatric nurses, regardless of the clinical setting in which they practice, must be confident in their ability to respond to a child who presents with or develops respiratory distress. Knowing how to rapidly identify a child in distress, having the ability to select the most effective oxygen delivery system, and knowing how to support a child's compromised airway are some of the most important skills a pediatric nurse needs to master and practice on a regular basis.

OXYGEN THERAPY GUIDELINES BASED ON SEVERITY

When a child presents with a respiratory condition, oxygen therapy is often prescribed. There are a variety of means to improve a child's oxygenation through supplemental oxygen (Fig. 32.2).

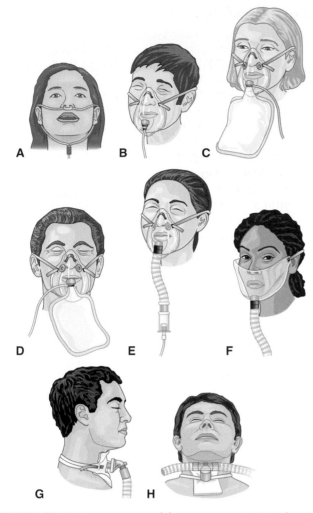

FIGURE 32.2 Various oxygen delivery systems. A, Nasal cannula. B, Simple face mask. C, Partial rebreathing mask. D, Nonrebreathing mask. E, Venturi mask. F, Face tent. G, Tracheostomy collar. H, T-piece.

The following list describes the most common interventions used to improve oxygen delivery:

1. **Oxygen hood:** A transparent plastic cylinder that encloses the neonate's head in a humidified, oxygen-rich environment. It allows freedom of movement and no attachment of a plastic apparatus to the face, which may induce crying and therefore further oxygen consumption. It may produce cold stress, if unheated.

2. **Oxygen tent:** This device provides a transparent, plastic-enclosed, humidified, oxygen-rich environment for a pediatric patient too large for a hood.

3. **Blow-by oxygen:** This device consists of corrugated oxygen tubing that "blows" oxygen and/or nebulizer medication by an infant's nose, allowing inhalation without the attachment of a plastic apparatus to the face. This can be used by a family member with the child held on the lap or lying down.

4. **Nasal cannula:** This device consists of two soft, plastic prongs attached to oxygen tubing that allows

low-flow oxygen to flow into the nasopharynx. It is contraindicated in nasal obstruction and is not recommended in neonates.

5. **Simple face mask:** This device includes a plastic reservoir system that fits over the mouth and nose, which is attached to oxygen tubing and fitted to the head with an elastic strap. Holes on either side of the mask allow carbon dioxide to be exhaled and not trapped in the mask. Possible aspiration of emesis is a consideration. It is not appropriate for neonates.

6. **Nonrebreather mask:** A plastic bag at the base of the mask provides an additional reservoir of oxygen. One-way valves on the reservoir bag and the side of the mask prevent expired carbon dioxide from mixing with the oxygen supply and room air from entering the mask and diluting the oxygen concentration. This enables a higher concentration of oxygen to be delivered than with simpler devices. It is not appropriate for neonates.

7. **Venturi masks:** This device consists of a simple mask with a valve that allows a precise percentage of oxygen to be delivered rather than as measured by liter flow. It is not appropriate for neonates.

See Table 32.2 for information about oxygen delivery devices.

TABLE 32.2 OXYGEN DELIVERY DEVICES AND CORRESPONDING OXYGEN DELIVERY

Device	Size for Children	Size for Infants
Nasal Cannula	0.5–4 LPM	0.25–2 LPM
Simple Mask	6–10 LPM	5–8 LPM
Partial Rebreather	10–12 LPM	Varies depending on newborn or infant size
Venturi Mask	Liter flow indicated for specific FiO_2 device	Liter flow indicated for specific FiO_2 devices
Nonrebreather Mask	10–15 LPM	n/a
Aerosol	8–12 LPM	Depends on size and age of newborn or infant

Abbreviations: FiO_2, Fraction of respired oxygen; LPM, Liters per minute.

INTERVENTIONS TO ASSIST A CHILD WITH RESPIRATORY DISTRESS

A child with respiratory distress may require supplemental oxygen as well as other interventions to ease effort to breathe. Suctioning is a gold standard for young children with conditions that produce increased secretions; other interventions that assist in the removal of secretions and aid in breathing, and assessments that provide key information on the status of the child's distress, are also utilized.

Chest Physiotherapy

This intervention involves the use of gentle percussion via cupped hands or a vibratory device to mobilize respiratory secretions to promote expectoration. This is followed by repositioning from side-to-side and with the head dependent to optimize the drainage of secretions.

Nasal Suctioning

This process involves gently extracting oropharyngeal and nasopharyngeal secretions by a suction catheter or a bulb syringe, as is age-appropriate. This may be preceded by flushing with minute amounts of normal saline to facilitate loosening and thinning of secretions.

Breathing Exercises

Expectoration of secretions and promotion of respiratory activity can be facilitated by having the child take a few deep breaths and then cough forcefully several times. This helps to mobilize secretions and optimize respirations by forcing the alveolar sacs to open and thus better fill with oxygen. The same effects can be obtained by the use of an incentive spirometer (IS), a plastic device that uses deep inspiration to exercise the lungs and airways.

Apnea Monitors

An apnea monitor is a device that can be sent home with an infant who has had one or more episodes of respiratory arrest, periods of apnea greater than 20 sec, or an ALTE. It is attached to the infant by chest electrodes or a belt and monitors dysrhythmias as well. Apnea monitors have not been proven to reduce mortality in SIDS.

Oxygen Saturation Machines

Oximeters use fiberoptic science to measure the concentration of oxygen in the surface capillaries in the fingers, toes, or earlobes. It is a noninvasive method that measures the oxygen as a percentage.

COMMON RESPIRATORY DISORDERS

There are several common respiratory disorders or conditions frequently found in the childhood period. Children, from infancy through adolescence, can be exposed to respiratory pathogens that cause common ailments. The following sections present the most common respiratory conditions found during childhood.

Nasopharyngitis

Nasopharyngitis is otherwise known as the common cold. It is a viral infection caused by 1 of more than 200 viruses, but is most commonly caused by a rhinovirus. Preschool and grade school children are the developmental groups most frequently affected by this infection. The symptoms may include coughing, sneezing, fever, nasal and upper airway congestion, sore throat, watery or itchy eyes, headache, and chills. Contagion from one person to another is by droplet method.

Assessments of Nasopharyngitis

The cold virus attaches itself to the lining of the nose and upper airway, causing the release of histamine, which causes swelling and congestion. Symptoms usually improve after 4 to 5 days and are gone by 10 days to 2 weeks.

Symptoms of nasopharyngitis are based on the severity of the inflammation located within the nasopharyngeal space. Feelings of pressure, fullness, congestion, coughing, sore throat, headache, and sinus pressure pain can all be experienced and should be assessed for.

Interventions for Nasopharyngitis

There is no test that detects the cold virus. A throat culture may be done to diagnose a possible bacterial infection, such as strep throat caused by one of the *Streptococcus* bacteria.

A child with a cold is more susceptible to bacterial infections such as sinusitis, OM, and strep throat. Antibiotic therapy may be used to treat the secondary infection. Otherwise, symptomatic treatment is given, such as antipyretics for fever, antidecongestants, analgesics for a sore throat or headache, antihistamines for itchy eyes, or a cough suppressant. Other methods of treatment may include increasing fluid intake to thin secretions, a cool-mist humidifier for congestion, adequate rest, using a nasal aspirator to remove secretions from an infant, and avoiding smoking or second-hand smoke.

Nursing Considerations for Respiratory Infections

As small children are more susceptible to viruses, family members need to be instructed in transmission, symptomatic treatment, hand washing, and covering mouth and nose while coughing and sneezing. Many parents request treatment by antibiotics and need education that this is not necessary unless there is a secondary bacterial infection as well. If the child is diagnosed with strep throat, adherence to oral antibiotic therapy is essential. The child may return to school 24 hours after the last fever and after the child has had a minimum of 24 hours of antibiotics.

Tonsillitis

Tonsillitis is an inflammation of the tonsils. The tonsils are parts of Waldeyer's ring, a group of different bodies of lymphatic tissue encircling the pharynx. This tissue is separated into the palatine tonsils, the pharyngeal tonsil (ie, adenoids), and the lingual tonsils. The purpose of the tonsils is not known but is presumed to support immunization. Increased numbers of bacteria are found in the tonsils, but this number decreases with increased age. Tonsillitis is usually caused by the bacteria *Staphylococcus aureus* and beta-hemolytic *Streptococcus*. The disease occurs more frequently in children under 6 years and some experience it much more frequently than others.

Assessments of Tonsillitis

The most common symptom of tonsillitis is throat pain exacerbated by swallowing. This may prevent the child from taking a sufficient amount of oral intake or oral medications. Other complications can include adenoiditis, recurrent OM, middle ear fluid, peritonsillar abscess, and nasal obstruction with mouth breathing and snoring. Assessment focuses on inspection of the throat, ears, and vital signs, especially an accurate temperature. A complete blood cell count (CBC) may be done to determine the degree of infection based on the white blood cell count (WBC), and to make sure a prospective surgical patient has a sufficient red blood cell count (RBC).

Interventions for Tonsillitis

Treatment of a streptococcal pharyngotonsillitis usually includes some form of penicillin for 10 days. Palatine tonsils must be removed after a peritonsillar abscess occurs, but otherwise the decision to perform a tonsillectomy depends on the frequency of infections and the child's age. Symptomatic treatment with liquid acetaminophen for pain and fever is common.

Nursing Considerations for Tonsillitis

The nurse's responsibility includes symptom management, prevention of complications, preparation for surgery, if indicated, and patient and family teaching. Pain and fever can be treated with over-the-counter (OTC) medications and sufficient fluid intake. Because swallowing is often painful, it is important to provide the child's favorite fluids, including ice cream and popsicles, which may prove soothing to an irritated throat. Fluid intake is also important to prevent dehydration, a more prevalent occurrence in the pediatric population. If a tonsillectomy is planned, the nurse must ensure NPO status, arrange for signed parental consent, and fill out a preoperative checklist. The parents and the child, appropriately for his or her age, should be informed of each aspect of interventions and be allowed to ask questions.

SAFETY *STAT!*

A child in the postoperative period after a tonsillectomy must be monitored for frequent swallowing because this could indicate a postoperative bleed.

Infant Respiratory Distress Syndrome (Hyaline Membrane Disease)

Hyaline membrane disease (HMD) occurs when there is insufficient **surfactant** (ie, a lipid-based substance secreted by the alveoli in the lungs) in a (usually) premature infant's lungs. Surfactant is a substance made of protein, neutral lipids, and phospholipids that is produced by the cells in the infant's airway between 24 and 28 weeks' gestation. HMD strikes about 60% to 80% of all infants younger than 28 weeks. Caucasian males are particularly at risk. By 35 weeks' gestation there is usually enough surfactant present to assist adequate respirations. This substance serves to keep the alveoli open during inspiration and expiration to ensure adequate oxygenation and the exhalation of carbon dioxide. Without sufficient surfactant, the alveoli collapse a little more with each breath, producing damaged cells, called *hyaline membranes,* into the airway, damaging lung tissue, and causing progressively more difficulty breathing. This may result in the need for mechanical ventilation. Without this help, the infant will work harder and harder to breathe as the oxygen levels in the blood drop and the rising carbon dioxide levels in the blood cause acidosis.

The most common complications that can result from HMD are caused by air leaking from the lung tissue. *Pneumomediastinum* is air leaking into the mediastinum or the space between the two pleural sacs. *Pneumothorax* is air leaking into the chest cavity. *Pneumopericardium* is air leaking into the sac surrounding the heart. *Pulmonary interstitial emphysema (PIE)* is air leaking and becoming trapped between the alveoli. The infant may also develop a chronic condition called *bronchopulmonary dysplasia (BPD)* (see "Bronchopulmonary Dysplasia").

Assessments of Respiratory Distress Syndrome

HMD can be determined by a number of means, including physical assessment, to observe cyanosis, tachypnea, shortness of breath, working hard to breathe, flaring nares, grunting, and chest retractions. Symptoms may peak by the third day of life. A gastric aspirate shake test is performed within 30 min after birth to determine the amount of surfactant present. A lecithin/sphingomyelin ratio less than 2:1, a bubble stability test indicating lung immaturity, or the absence of phosphatidylglycerol can also determine HMD. A chest x-ray (CXR) will show a glassy pattern in the lungs and increased opacity. Arterial blood gas (ABG) will show oxygen, carbon dioxide, and acid-base readings. Lung function studies quantify how well the lungs are working. An echocardiogram shows the lung volumes. An upper abdominal ultrasound can show the extent of the opacity in the lungs.

Interventions for Respiratory Distress Syndrome

Prevention involves delaying birth as long as it is safe for the mother and infant to give the lungs sufficient time to produce enough surfactant. The mother can also be given corticosteroids before delivery to reduce the risk and severity of the disease. Artificial surfactant (Exosurf) can be given directly to the infant's lungs prophylactically for prematurity or therapeutically if mechanical ventilation is required.

Nursing Considerations for Respiratory Distress Syndrome

All procedures and treatments related to the assessment and treatment of respiratory distress syndrome must be explained to the family. Any invasive procedures require written, informed consent. The nursing staff will assist with any diagnostic procedures, intubation, administering oxygen and medications, and maintaining ventilation. Close monitoring of the child in distress for signs and symptoms of complications is required and should be conducted by the entire pediatric health-care team. A child's condition can rapidly deteriorate and therefore should be closely monitored.

Epiglottitis

The epiglottis is made of cartilage and is at the base of the tongue. Epiglottitis is a serious, possibly life-threatening bacterial infection that causes inflammation and swelling of the throat. This can cause breathing problems that may progress rapidly, triggering obstruction of the airway. This can cause an emergency so quickly that the diagnosis itself necessitates immediate admission to a hospital. It is caused by either *Haemophilus influenzae* type B (HIB) or group A beta-hemolytic streptococci and primarily affects 2- to 8-year-olds.

Assessments of Epiglottitis

The symptoms of epiglottitis may resemble the symptoms of an upper airway infection. These may include sudden onset of a severe sore throat, fever, hoarse voice, and a cough. Worsening symptoms may also involve drooling, no voice, leaning forward in the sitting position (ie, tripod), and keeping the mouth open (Fig. 32.3).

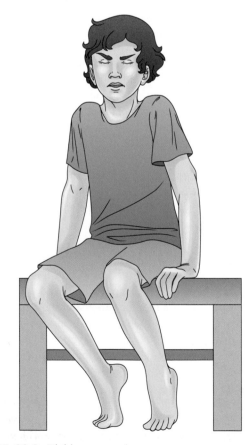

FIGURE 32.3 Child in a tripod position.

The diagnosis is usually made by physical examination and history of the symptoms. The child's primary caregiver may also order a neck x-ray, an ABG, and a CBC. In extreme circumstances, a surgeon may perform a visualization of the airway in the operating room.

SAFETY *STAT!*

Do not use a tongue blade to visually assess the throat of a child who presents with symptoms of epiglottitis. When inflamed, the use of a tongue blade on the infected tissue might result in further swelling and inflammation, potentially closing off the child's airway completely.

Interventions for Epiglottitis

In an emergency, the child's airway and breathing may be assisted with intubation and mechanical ventilation. Close monitoring of the breathing will determine when this is necessary. An IV line will be started to administer antibiotics. Steroids will be given to reduce and prevent swelling in the airway. IV fluids will be given if the child is unable to swallow. HIB vaccines are recommended at the ages of 2, 4, 6, and 15 to 18 months, which significantly decreases the possibility of acquiring the disease. All members of the family and those in close contact with a child diagnosed with epiglottitis are treated prophylactically with rifampin.

Nursing Considerations for Epiglottitis

Epiglottitis is a potentially critical condition that can be very frightening for the patient and family. It is the nurse's responsibility to explain all procedures and treatments and lend emotional support. The nurse will monitor the patient's airway and breathing very closely and treat as needed. The nurse will administer oxygen therapy, IV fluids, and medications (Fig. 32.4). Maintain the child on a pulse oximeter (Fig. 32.5).

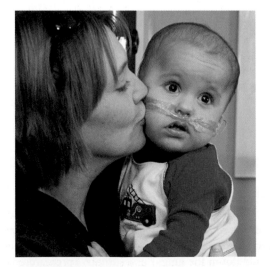

FIGURE 32.4 Child on oxygen therapy.

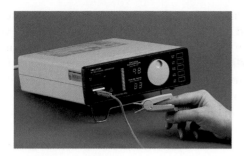

FIGURE 32.5 Pulse oximetry.

 LEARN TO C.U.S.

You are assisting a nurse practitioner in care of a toddler with suspected epiglottitis. He asks you to get a tongue blade to hold the child's tongue down to better visualize the airway structures and obtain a culture. You can use the C.U.S. method of communication to express your concerns:

C: "I have a **concern** about your request.

U: I am **uncomfortable** using a tongue blade in the throat because this may cause complete obstruction.

S: I think we have a **safety** issue here."

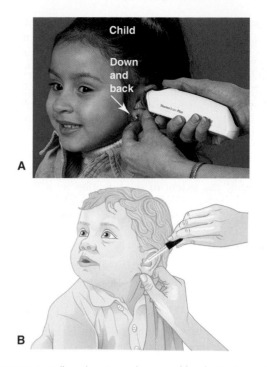

FIGURE 32.6 Pulling the pinna down and back. A, Assessing the tympanic temperature reading of a child. B, Administering medications in the ear canal of a child younger than 3 years old.

Otitis Media

Acute OM is a middle ear infection usually caused by bacteria or a virus. It occurs more frequently in infants and toddlers because the eustachian tubes are straighter and shorter and act as a conduit for respiratory infections to the ear. Inflammation or infection of the adenoids may also result in infection of the middle ear. These types of infections may resolve spontaneously or may require antibiotic therapy. Risk factors include children age 6 months to 2 years, secondhand cigarette smoke, childcare in a group setting, American Indian or Inuit ethnicity, drinking from a bottle while lying down, winter, and a family history of ear infections.

Persistent fluid in the middle ear, or persistent or frequent ear infections in children, may lead to a loss of hearing, learning disabilities or developmental delays, delayed speech because of a temporary hearing loss at a significant developmental stage, or a permanent hearing loss. The infection may also spread to the mastoid bone or, rarely, to the brain. Symptoms may include ear pain, especially when lying down; pulling at an ear; excessive crying; irritability; a loss of balance; fever greater than 38°C; poor eating; and drainage from the ear.

Assessments of Otitis Media

Diagnosis is made via history and physical examination, including inspecting the ears with an otoscope. It is easiest to perform the examination with the child sitting on the parent or caregiver's lap, facing away, and encircled in his or her arms. This serves to calm the child as well as provide some gentle restraint. For young children, the pinna must be pulled down for an ear assessment, medication administration, or tympanic temperatures (Fig. 32.6).

Interventions for Otitis Media

Treatment of the infection is considered controversial as it may include antibiotics only if it is deemed that bacteria may be the cause of the ear infection or the underlying respiratory infection. Otherwise the treatment is symptomatic: administering antipyretics for fever and/or analgesics for pain, encouraging fluids, or administering eardrops to treat the pain directly. If the infection occurs frequently or is draining pus, a surgical procedure called a myringotomy, which is an incision of the ear drum, is performed, followed by the insertion of a small tympanostomy tube to help facilitate drainage. This tube will fall out on its own as the child grows.

Nursing Considerations for Otitis Media

A nurse may need to reinforce to the family the reasons that antibiotic therapy is not usually given for this infection: it is usually caused by a virus or may resolve on its own. Symptomatic treatment must be explained as well as the reasons to call the child's primary caregiver if the symptoms recur.

Croup

Croup is a disease caused by a viral infection that causes swelling of the airway. This results in stridor upon inspiration. The most common virus that causes croup is the parainfluenza virus, but it can also be caused by **respiratory syncytial virus (RSV),** influenza virus, measles, adenovirus, or enteroviruses. Infection occurs through direct contact with secretions, starts in the upper airway, and descends to the larynx. Croup is most common in infants and children aged 3 months to 5 years because their smaller airways occlude more easily with swelling. It affects boys more than girls and is seen more in winter.

Assessments of Croup

The symptoms are related to the presence of an infection and a swollen airway. The child may have a congested nose or throat, fever, **laryngitis,** and stridor. What may start out as a mild cough will progress to a harsh, "barking" cough that is the distinguishing feature of the disease. The symptoms are typically worse at night and usually improve within 3 to 7 days.

Croup is usually diagnosed via history and physical assessment. Neck and chest x-rays may be done, as well as a CBC to determine the extent of the infection by a WBC. Pulse oximetry is a noninvasive method of measuring oxygen in the blood and can be monitored continuously, if need be.

Interventions for Croup

If the child's breathing is sufficiently compromised, hospitalization may be necessary. Breathing treatments with steroids and/or bronchodilators may be given to open the airway. Steroids may also be given by mouth or IV to reduce swelling in the airway. Treatment at home includes a cool-mist humidifier, encouragement of fluid intake, and bedrest to minimize respiratory effort.

Nursing Considerations for Croup

Croup is usually treated at home and the family needs to know what to watch for to decide whether it is necessary to take the child to the doctor's office or emergency room. Clinical signs of respiratory distress include restlessness, increased respiratory rate, and difficulty breathing. If there is no cool-mist humidifier in the home, the same effect can be reached by taking the child outside in the cold, night air.

Apnea

Apnea is a period of more than 20 sec without any breathing. In pediatrics, most babies who experience apnea are premature by at least 35 weeks' gestation. The apnea usually occurs during rapid eye movement (REM) sleep. The apnea may occur during the first week of life, but is considered more serious when it occurs immediately after birth or after the second week of life. It is also more serious the longer it lasts, if the infant turns blue, or if it is accompanied by a slower heartbeat (ie, bradycardia). Apnea accompanied by bradycardia is referred to as "As and Bs." Some possible causes of apnea are an immature central nervous system (CNS), blockage, bleeding or damage in the brain, infection, gastric reflux, metabolic abnormality, stimulation of reflexes such as hyperextension of the neck, or hyperthermia or hypothermia.

Assessments of Apnea

A careful assessment is important to determine whether there might be some other cause for apnea other than prematurity. A complete physical examination will be done to rule out any physical disorders. Blood tests such as a CBC and metabolic panel will be performed to check for infection, blood glucose abnormalities, electrolyte imbalance, or hypercalcemia or hypocalcemia. Chest and abdominal x-rays will be done to check for anatomical abnormalities.

An apnea study will be done to test breathing effort, heart rate, and oxygenation.

Interventions for Apnea

Periods of apnea can be stopped by stimulating the infant by massaging or patting the skin. Possible causes should be determined and treated to prevent further incidents. The breathing rate and patterns, as well as heart rate, will be closely monitored. Caffeine or theophylline may be given as CNS stimulants. A continuous positive airway pressure (CPAP) breathing machine may be used to keep the airway open through a continuous flow of oxygen.

Nursing Considerations for Apnea

Witnessing a child's apnea episodes can be very frightening for parents and other family members. Nurses need to explain what apnea is, how it can be treated, and the parameters the infant must meet to be discharged. Parents' fears about a possible reoccurrence once the infant is discharged home must be addressed. If the infant will be using an apnea monitor once home, the family must be instructed in its use.

Apparent Life-Threatening Event

An ALTE is a collection of symptoms that usually occurs in children under 1 year of age (ie, infants). The symptoms may include cyanosis, apnea, coughing, gagging, and a change in muscle tone. This may have a digestive, neurological, cardiac, metabolic, or respiratory origin, but 50% of all cases are idiopathic. Risk factors include premature birth, prematurity with RSV, prematurity with general anesthesia, rapid feeders, and male gender.

In the 50% of causes that have an underlying etiology, treatment may alleviate the possibility of recurrence. Outcomes depend on causative factors and the prompt recognition and treatment given.

Assessments of an Apparent Life-Threatening Event

A thorough history, including family history and physical assessment, needs to be performed to attempt to determine possible physiological causes. Causes include seizures, CNS infection, intussusception, gastroesophageal reflux, swallowing abnormalities, respiratory infection, sleep apnea, FB obstruction, cardiac dysrhythmias, or metabolic or electrolyte disorders. Some diagnostic tests done to determine the underlying cause may include CXR, electrocardiogram (EKG), CBC, metabolic panel including electrolytes, ABGs, urinalysis and culture, stool culture, blood culture, RSV nasal swab, and lumbar puncture.

Interventions for an Apparent Life-Threatening Event

Treatment depends on the underlying cause, if any has been determined. Once treatment for the cause has been carried out, the event tends not to reoccur. For an event significant enough to merit CPR, hospitalization with cardiac and oximetry monitoring is indicated.

Nursing Considerations for an Apparent Life-Threatening Event

If there has been no specific underlying diagnosis, home cardiopulmonary monitoring with event monitoring capabilities may be indicated. This is controversial because it may give families false reassurance; no decrease in mortality in the case of SIDS has been documented with such monitoring. The family must be educated about the treatment of a subsequent event that progresses from gentle to more vigorous stimulation to CPR.

Asthma

Asthma is a chronic, inflammatory disease with symptoms triggered by exposure to substances causing an allergic reaction (ie, allergens). Those symptoms are swelling and inflammation of the airway, tightening of the muscles around the airways, and increased mucus production. These symptoms result in a narrowing of the airway, making it more difficult to breathe. Causes of asthma are not entirely understood but may include a familial tendency for the disease, infections, a reaction to environmental substances, and exercise. Asthma is most commonly seen in children younger than age 5 years and children with a family history, allergies, and exposure to secondhand tobacco smoke.

Assessments of Asthma

Symptoms of asthma may include coughing, either constantly or intermittently, but especially at night time. The child may complain of chest tightness, chest pain, or fatigue, and may display anxiety. Shortness of breath may occur, especially with increased activity. Wheezing, which sounds like whistling or a musical sound, may be heard with inspiration and/or expiration.

Asthma is diagnosed by physical assessment with particular attention paid to the existing symptoms and a history, including family history. Spirometry will measure and monitor oxygen levels, quantify the severity of the episode, and determine the effectiveness of treatment. Peak flow monitoring (PFM) measures the speed of the air exhaled to determine the severity of the patient's incapacity. A CXR will show consolidation in the lungs caused by infection or abnormalities of the airway passages. ABGs will show oxygenation and the ability to exhale carbon dioxide. A CBC will show the presence of infection in the WBC and the ability to transport oxygen on the hemoglobin (Hgb) molecule. Allergy tests may be done to try to determine possible causes of an exacerbation of the asthma.

Interventions for Asthma

Asthma therapy is intended to promote adequate oxygenation, improve the size of the airway, facilitate the removal of secretions, and alleviate anxiety. Supplemental oxygen may be given if levels are below normal. Steroids given orally or via IV and inhaled bronchodilators and breathing treatments will reduce swelling and enlarge the airway to allow easier passage of air and breathing. Suctioning will remove excess secretions from the airway, as will encouraging coughing. Increasing fluid intake will help to thin secretions. Sedation may be given for anxiety to facilitate treatment and procedures. Table 32.3 provides a list of common asthma medications, and Fig. 32.7 depicts the most appropriate method to administer asthma medication inhalers.

Nursing Considerations for Asthma

It may be as frightening to be in the hospital as it is to have difficulty breathing for a child and his or her family. The

TABLE 32.3   TYPES OF ASTHMA MEDICATIONS

Category	Purpose	Medication Types
Long-term asthma control medications	Taken regularly to control chronic symptoms and prevent asthma attacks; the most important type of treatment for most people with asthma	• Inhaled corticosteroids • Leukotriene modifiers • Long-acting beta agonists (LABAs) • Theophylline • Combination inhalers that contain both a corticosteroid and a LABA
Quick-relief medications (ie, rescue medications)	Taken as needed for rapid, short-term relief of symptoms; used to prevent or treat an asthma attack	• Short-acting beta agonists such as albuterol • Ipratropium (Atrovent) • Oral and IV corticosteroids (for serious asthma attacks) • Racemic epinephrine
Medications for allergy-induced asthma	Taken regularly or as needed to reduce the body's sensitivity to a particular allergy-causing substance (ie, allergen)	• Allergy shots (immunotherapy) • Omalizumab (Xolair)

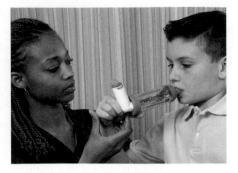

FIGURE 32.7 The appropriate method to administer asthma medication inhalers.

nurse can help to relieve this fear by calm explanations of procedures and treatments, making sure not to overwhelm them with too much information. The child will most likely need to use an **inhaler** (ie, a device used to breathe inhaled medications into the lungs) and a **nebulizer** (ie, a device that aerates respiratory medications) at home, and the family, or the child if he or she is old enough, will need to be instructed in their use.

Many primary care providers caring for children with asthma provide a written guideline on how to respond to a child with asthma symptoms. The guideline includes a color-coded system to guide the parents of the child in interventions, dependent on the child's daily peak flow.

PATIENT TEACHING GUIDELINES

Color-Coded Zones for Asthma Assessments and Interventions

Peak flow measurements are conducted on a device that measures how fast air is moved from the lungs. The color-coded areas on the device provide information like a signal on a traffic light, representing safe (green), caution (yellow), and danger (red) zones.

Children over the age of 5 years will be requested to perform peak flow measurements on a regular basis. Children with severe asthma will be asked to perform peak flow measurements at least once or twice a day. The following peak flow findings will indicate to the family what interventions are needed:

- Green Zone:
  - This is considered the safety zone.
  - Peak flow measurements are between 80% and 100% of the child's personal best when not experiencing asthma symptoms.
  - The child is instructed to take his or her daily medications and participate in all normal activities.
- Yellow Zone:
  - This is considered the caution zone.
  - Peak flow measurements are between 50% and 80% of the child's personal best when not experiencing asthma symptoms.
  - The child experiencing asthma symptoms in the yellow zone is now instructed to slow down, take his or her fast-acting inhaler now, and keep his or her inhaler available throughout the day.

- Red Zone:
  - This is considered the danger zone.
  - Peak flow measurements are below 49% of the child's personal best when not experiencing asthma symptoms.
  - The child is experiencing a severe asthma attack and should be seen by his or her primary health-care professional, be taken to the closest emergency room, or the parent should call 911 if needed. All medications should go with the child for evaluation.

HEALTH PROMOTION

Tips to Reduce Asthma Triggers in the Home

1. Determine air quality for the day by checking the local weather report for mold, pollen, pollution, and high ozone levels; avoid or adjust physical activity and exercise on days of poor air quality.
2. Dust all hard surfaces throughout the home on a weekly basis using a damp cloth with soap.
3. Never smoke around a child, especially in the home or car.
4. Put dust covers on mattresses and pillows, and wash weekly.
5. Replace heating and cooling appliance filters on a regular basis.
6. Assess the home every season for the buildup of mold, water leaks, and home damage caused by water to prevent exposure to various mold growths.
7. Vacuum carpet, floors, and any fabric-covered furniture on a weekly basis using a HEPA filter vacuum system that is cleaned after each use.
8. Check the home for pests, especially cockroach evidence, and seal all openings found along walls, plumbing openings, and cracks to prevent infestations. Keep the home clean and free of trash. Place screens on windows. Use insect traps (sticky tapes) instead of spraying pesticides.
9. Remove pets from the home that have fur and keep small caged animals (eg, birds, gerbils, hamsters) in their clean cages as much as possible.
10. Know the child's triggers and monitor for their presence!

(Adapted from Top 10 Ways to Reduce Asthma Triggers at Home; retrieved from www.in.gov/isdh/reports/breatheasyville/athome/toptenhome.html.)

Bronchiolitis

Bronchiolitis is a lower respiratory infection caused by a virus, most likely RSV, but can also be caused by the parainfluenza virus, rhinovirus, or adenovirus. Possible bacterial causes are mycoplasma pneumonia and chlamydia pneumonia. Bronchiolitis usually affects infants who have immature immune systems and lack cilia in their airways to block infections. The infection starts in the upper airways and then progresses to the lower airways, causing inflammation that obstructs breathing. Risk factors include winter, male gender, secondhand smoke, lack of breastfeeding, older siblings, and attendance in daycare.

Symptoms may include nasal or upper respiratory congestion, wheezing, cough, loss of appetite, increased crying, fever, and irritability. The infant may start breathing harder or faster than normal.

Assessments of Bronchiolitis

Diagnosis is usually made by history taking and physical assessment. A nasopharyngeal swab will be done to test for RSV or other viruses. To rule out other illnesses, other tests may be performed, such as a CXR, sputum culture, blood cultures, or a pulse oximeter to measure oxygen saturation levels.

Interventions for Bronchiolitis

Treatment of bronchiolitis is symptomatic and will depend on the specific symptoms displayed. Gentle bulb syringe aspiration of nasal oral secretions, antipyretics for fever, and nebulizer treatments with bronchodilators may be performed. In more severe cases, the infant may need to be hospitalized for IV therapy to treat dehydration, or for oxygen therapy for hypoxia or dyspnea. High-risk or premature infants may receive an immunization injection called palivizumab (Synagis) or respiratory syncytial immune globulin (RSV-IGIV) to prevent contracting the infection.

SAFETY *STAT!*

A young infant with RSV bronchiolitis may experience severe respiratory distress very suddenly. Rapid suctioning in both nares of the thick mucus produced by this condition may be enough to ease the infant's distress. Instilling saline drops right before suctioning may decrease the thickness of the mucus and allow more efficient suctioning.

Nursing Considerations for Bronchiolitis

If the infant is stable enough to be treated at home, the family may need instruction in caring for him or her. Encouraging fluids to thin secretions and for adequate hydration, giving nebulizer treatments for **bronchodilation** (ie, a means of opening the airway), suctioning by bulb syringe, and other medications may be ordered.

Bronchopulmonary Dysplasia

Bronchopulmonary dysplasia (BPD), also known as *chronic lung disease (CLD),* is the term used for long-term respiratory problems in premature infants. It is caused by damage to the lungs from mechanical ventilation and prolonged oxygen treatment that causes scarring in the lung tissue. Specific causes may be underdeveloped alveoli, insufficient surfactant, the prolonged use of high-concentration oxygen, the pressure from a ventilator, suctioning, or the trauma of intubation. Risk factors are less than 34 weeks' gestation, less than 2,000 g or 4 pounds and 6.5 ounces birth weight, HMD, PIE, patent ductus arteriosus (PDA), Caucasian male, a family history of asthma, and chorioamnionitis (ie, infected maternal uterus).

Assessments of Bronchopulmonary Dysplasia

The symptoms of BPD include respiratory distress, flaring nares, tachypnea, and chest retractions. Diagnosis is made when mechanical ventilation and/or oxygen is still necessary after the infant has reached 36 weeks' gestation. A CXR will show a spongy appearance of the lungs.

Interventions for Bronchopulmonary Dysplasia

Treatment includes supplemental oxygen, mechanical ventilation until the lungs mature, bronchodilators and steroids to maximize airway clearance, fluid restriction and diuretics to diminish excessive fluid in the lungs, and good nutrition to promote healing and growth. Several months of mechanical ventilation may be required in the most severe cases. The infant may require home oxygen upon discharge from the hospital but will usually be weaned off it by the age of 1 year.

Nursing Considerations for Bronchopulmonary Dysplasia

Families with an infant on mechanical ventilation will need a great deal of support and teaching. They may have to learn about administering oxygen, breathing treatments, and medications at home. They must be taught to guard against respiratory infections after discharge because the child is at higher risk. The possibility of rehospitalization must be considered.

Cystic Fibrosis

Cystic fibrosis is an autosomal recessive genetic disorder caused by a mutation in the protein cystic fibrosis transmembrane conductance regulator (CFTR) gene that regulates sweat, digestive juices, and mucus. It causes scarring and cysts in the pancreas. The gene initiates excessive sodium absorption in the lungs, turning usually thin secretions to thickened secretions. While similar changes occur in the gastrointestinal and reproductive systems, this chapter focuses on the effects of the disease on the respiratory system. Approximately 1,000 babies are born with the disease each year and are primarily Caucasian.

Thicker respiratory secretions are harder for the child to clear, which predisposes him or her to pneumonia. The bacteria *Pseudomonas aeruginosa* is the most prevalent cause of infection, followed by *S aureus* and *H influenzae*. Frequent infections may cause a chronic cough, wheezing, **hemoptysis** (ie, blood in respiratory secretions or mucus), **atelectasis** (ie, collapsed or airless lung) secondary to **pneumothorax** (ie, a collection of air or gas in the pleural cavity), and apnea. The cough worsens in the morning or after exertion. Nasal polyps may form and may need to be surgically removed. A high rate of sinusitis may occur.

Assessments of Cystic Fibrosis

Cystic fibrosis can be diagnosed by genetic testing for the abnormal gene, either via a blood sample or buccal swab, and a sweat test for excessive sodium and chloride. A CXR will show consolidation from thick mucus and any chronic damage to the lungs, as will pulmonary function tests. A sputum culture and sensitivity will identify any bacterial source of an infection and antibiotics to treat the infection effectively.

LABS & DIAGNOSTICS

An infant with a sweat chloride test of greater than 60 milliequivalents demonstrates a positive value for a diagnosis of cystic fibrosis.

Interventions for Cystic Fibrosis

Treatment is specific to the symptoms the child displays and focuses on decreasing their severity and decreasing progression. Physical therapy and exercise help to loosen secretions and induce coughing to expectorate them. Chest percussions do the same. Mucolytic agents break up secretions, causing them to become easier to remove. Nebulization is an effective way to provide medications. In the most critical cases, bilateral lung transplantation or a heart-lung transplantation may be necessary.

Nursing Considerations for Cystic Fibrosis

As cystic fibrosis is an autosomal recessive trait, the family may have questions about the risk of other children having the disease. A nurse not conversant with genetics will need to arrange a referral to an organization or person who can provide information. Family members will need to learn how to provide nebulizer treatments and chest percussions, and will need to learn about the importance of ridding the lungs of sputum.

Foreign Body Aspiration

FB aspiration accounts for 3% of all deaths in children younger than 15 years old, with toddlers consisting of 77% of this group. Toddlers' developmental characteristics cause risk factors such as putting objects into their mouths, learning to walk and run, poor dentition, supervision by a sibling, and immature swallowing coordination. Most objects are organic, with 54% of FB aspirations caused by peanuts.

After an FB is aspirated, there are three distinct clinical phases:

1. In phase one, the child may exhibit choking, gagging, coughing, hoarseness or aphonia, wheezing, stridor, and circumoral cyanosis. The possibility of death is very high.
2. The second phase is the asymptomatic period that can last up to several months after the aspiration, depending on the location, the amount of airway obstruction, and the aspirant.
3. The third phase shows renewed symptoms. Airway inflammation or infection from the FB may cause cough, wheezing, fever, sputum production, and hemoptysis.

Assessments of Foreign Body Aspiration

Diagnosis can be based on history and a focused physical assessment. A chest or neck x-ray may reveal the location of the FB or trapped air. A child may present with adventitious breath sounds such as stridor and wheezing. The child should be assessed for respiratory distress and adequate air exchange.

Interventions for Foreign Body Aspiration

If the child is still able to breathe and cough, he or she should be closely monitored while attempts are made to spontaneously expel the FB. If there is apnea, back blows and chest thrusts are recommended by the AAP and the American Heart Association (AHA). Blind finger sweeps are not recommended because this might force the FB further into the airway. Rigid bronchoscopy may be necessary for visualization of the airway and removal of the FB. After the object is removed, treatment is focused on the prevention of complications, including the prevention of infection, the reduction of swelling, and opening the airway. Antibiotics will be given for signs and symptoms of infection, such as increased mucus production with fever. Steroids and bronchodilators will be given to maintain the airway.

Nursing Considerations for Foreign Body Aspiration

Education is needed for the family to ensure only developmentally appropriate foods are given to a child. After the FB is removed, further education will show what symptoms to observe for in a swollen or compromised airway. Instruction about discharge medications may be needed.

Sudden Infant Death Syndrome

SIDS is the sudden, unexpected death of an infant less than 1 year old with no apparent cause discernible on the history, physical assessment, or postmortem examination. It used to be called "crib death" because the infants are commonly found after being presumed to be asleep. There is no known specific cause, but many contributing and risk factors have been documented. There may be a correlation with the infant sleeping too deeply or with a buildup of carbon dioxide in the infant's lungs. Contributing causes may include the infant sleeping on his or her stomach, drug use or smoking by the mother, a teenage mother, a sibling with SIDS, secondhand smoke, soft bedding, and close-together pregnancies. Risk factors include male gender, age 2 to 6 months, Native American or African American, birth in fall or winter, prematurity, lower-income family, late or no prenatal care, and a multiple birth.

Assessments of Sudden Infant Death Syndrome

There are no symptoms, treatments, or diagnostic tests. An autopsy may be required by law but typically will not show the cause of death.

Interventions for Sudden Infant Death Syndrome

While there is no treatment available for this disorder, there are many preventive measures that can be taken and need to be explained to the families of newborns. Since the AAP's initiation in 1994 of the "Back to Sleep" campaign, the recommendation to have infants sleep on their backs has significantly reduced the number of SIDS deaths. Another campaign to

NURSING CARE PLAN for the Child With Foreign Body Obstruction

Pathophysiology:

Suffocation and death may occur with FBs in the airway. Children under the age of 5 years are at the greatest risk for FB aspiration and obstruction, peaking between 1 and 2 years of age. When the child places something in his or her mouth and then inhales deeply or chokes while running, the object becomes lodged in the trachea. FB obstruction is also a higher risk in children who have few or no molar teeth, leaving larger pieces to swallow, and in children who do not chew their food well. Very young children may not have a completely coordinated mouth and tongue, and may aspirate while eating. The age of the greatest risk begins at 7 months, when an infant is quite mobile and able to use the pincer grasp to pick up small objects and place them in the mouth, through 4 years of age, when children still place small objects in their mouths. Most objects are aspirated into the right-sided airway because this is the direct entry from the trachea. The objects at greatest risk for aspiration are the following:

- Seeds
- Grapes
- Popcorn
- Nuts
- Hot dogs
- Pebbles
- Coins
- Toy parts, such as plastic car wheels
- Watch batteries
- Buttons
- Hardware (eg, pen caps, paperclips, and pins)

Assessments:

1. Choking or gagging when a small object or food is first swallowed and then inhaled
2. Stridor (ie, high-pitched sound of an obstructed airway); sudden coughing and wheezing
3. Inability to speak or hoarse voice
4. Not breathing, becoming blue (especially around the lips), and then becoming unconscious

Nursing Diagnoses:

1. There is ineffective airway clearance related to FB aspiration and choking.
2. The child has experienced aspiration, with risk related to age, ineffective coordination of chewing and swallowing, rapid respiration rates, and the absence of a full set of molar teeth.
3. The child's breathing pattern is ineffective because of aspiration, obstruction, and choking.
4. The child's gas exchange is impaired related to the presence of FB and asphyxiation.

Interventions:

1. Maintain a patent airway.
2. Prevent further episodes of aspiration; keep the child NPO until further notice.
3. Position the patient for comfortable and effective breathing.
4. Administer oxygen as needed to promote effective gas exchange.

---

eliminate maternal smoking, the pregnant mother's exposure to smoke, and the infant's exposure to secondhand smoke are all believed to reduce the occurrence of SIDS.

Nursing Considerations for Sudden Infant Death Syndrome

The loss of a child to SIDS is a traumatic event for both the family as a group and for the individual members of the family. The recommendation of a support group such as a SIDS support group may offer solace to a grieving family by giving them the opportunity to benefit from communication with others in the same situation.

 CULTURAL CONSIDERATIONS

Prevention of Sudden Infant Death Syndrome

Ethnic groups with the highest rate of SIDS include African Americans, Native Americans, and Alaskan natives. Although teaching, modeling, and reinforcement should include all ethnic groups, those identified as high-risk need astute nursing care and health promotion teaching.

Elements that increase the risk of having a SIDS baby include the following:

- Bed sharing with parents or others and the infant
- Soft bedding or pillows in the crib

- Multiple birth infants (ie, twins or more)
- Male babies
- African-American, American-Indian, or Alaskan-native infants
- Premature infants
- Infants with a sibling who died of SIDS
- Mothers who smoke or use illegal drugs
- Teenage mothers
- Short time between pregnancies
- No prenatal care or late prenatal care
- Families living in poverty

(Source: American Lung Association)

PATIENT TEACHING GUIDELINES

Eight Tips to Lessen the Risk of Sudden Infant Death Syndrome

There is no 100% way to prevent SIDS.

1. Put your baby on his or her back to sleep each and every nap and night. Tell anyone who helps to take care of the baby to make sure this is done consistently. Rebreathing carbon dioxide is a risk factor.
2. Never smoke around the baby or in the home. Babies who are exposed to smoke are three times more at risk to die of SIDS. Smoking during pregnancy is also a major risk factor for SIDS. Secondhand smoke also places a baby at risk for SIDS.
3. Place the baby on a firm mattress with no toys, stuffed animals, or bedding to prevent suffocation and smothering, and to reduce the incidence of SIDS. The baby should be dressed in a sleeping outfit that provides sufficient warmth without the use of blankets.
4. Breastfeed the baby as long as you can. Babies that are breastfed have a 50% reduced chance of dying of SIDS.
5. Do not sleep with the baby in your bed but keep your young baby in the same room. Although it is dangerous to sleep with an infant, the chance of SIDS is decreased when the baby sleeps in the same room as the parents.
6. Immunize your baby. Infants who have participated in the AAP and Centers for Disease Control and Prevention (CDC) immunization guidelines are 50% less likely to die of SIDS.
7. Prevent overheating.
8. Do not give honey to an infant under 12 months of age. Honey can be contaminated with *Clostridium botulism* (ie, botulism), which may be linked to SIDS.

Key Points

- There are distinct differences between the anatomy and physiology of a newborn's and a child's respiratory system, and that of an adult. These differences are important to review to evaluate, interpret, and teach to prevent complications. Differences include the size of the airways, respiratory rates, total tidal volumes, and others.
- Adventitious breath sounds during respiratory distress include stridor, rales, and rhonchi. The nurse must be able to distinguish when a child is demonstrating an increased work of breathing, dyspnea, and respiratory distress to quickly intervene to reduce complications.
- Assessments conducted in the physical examination of an infant or child with a respiratory condition are holistic and include both the respiratory system and the cardiac system. Gas exchange and oxygenation are the two main concepts associated with the respiratory system. Assessments of overall respiratory status include palpation, olfaction, percussion, and inspection.
- Young children are particularly vulnerable to contract respiratory infections because of their limited immunity, increasing social exposure to community acquired infections, and their small airways and shorter tracheas. Young children can also have increased symptom severity and

worse adventitious breath sounds. A child who is demonstrating shortness of breath or respiratory distress requires immediate interventions, which may include bronchodilators, steroids, antibiotics, racemic epinephrine, oxygen, and fluids.
- There are various methods of intervention for a child with a respiratory condition, including various oxygen delivery systems. These include infant crib tents, simple face masks, partial rebreather masks, nonrebreather masks, and ventilators. Each has a particular function and flow of oxygen.
- Epiglottitis is considered a respiratory emergency and requires experienced health-care team members to carefully manage the child's airway. Neither culture swabs nor a tongue blade should be used for assessment or specimen collection because rebound inflammation can occur and occlude the child's airway. Epiglottitis is a severe condition that has a high mortality rate. Rapid diagnosis and the implementation of antibiotics are required. HIB is often the bacterial culprit.
- SIDS is associated with many risk factors including sleeping prone, smoking in the home, male gender, winter season, and previous SIDS in a sibling. Nurses need to be confident in teaching the "Back to Sleep" principles to reduce the incidence.

REVIEW QUESTIONS

1. Which of the following are used to treat or relieve the effects of infant respiratory distress syndrome (ie, HMD)? *(select all that apply)*
   1. Delay birth as long as possible to allow the lungs more time to mature
   2. Antibiotics
   3. Inhaled synthetic surfactant
   4. Mechanical ventilation
   5. Inject the neonate with steroids

2. Which of the following may occur in a child with cystic fibrosis? *(select all that apply)*
   1. Wheezing
   2. Nasal polyps
   3. Hemoptysis
   4. Collapsed lung
   5. Apnea
   6. A barking cough

3. What physical examination sign/symptom is most worrisome in terms of degree of airway compromise?
   1. Fever
   2. Wheezing
   3. Cough
   4. Stridor

4. A 3-year-old presents to the emergency department with signs of respiratory distress. The child has epiglottitis associated with high fever, is apprehensive, and is drooling. It is imperative that the nurse avoid which of the following?
   1. Listening to the child's lungs
   2. Assessing the child's vital signs
   3. Weighing the child
   4. Inspecting the child's mouth and throat with a tongue blade

5. Which statement by the mother indicates understanding of the nurse's teaching related to a newborn?
   1. "I should expect my baby to breathe more slowly than I do."
   2. "I should use a blanket to cover my newborn when he sleeps."
   3. "I should give all of the pills in my baby's prescription to my baby even if the symptoms have gone away."
   4. "I should call my doctor if my newborn breathes fast while he's sleeping."

6. While the pediatric health-care team is teaching parents of a child who has just been diagnosed with cystic fibrosis, the mother asked if there was something she did to cause this illness. The team would be correct in responding that:
   1. There is no known cause for the condition of cystic fibrosis.
   2. The development of cystic fibrosis is directly related to the child's immune system.
   3. Cystic fibrosis is a trait passed on to the child by the father's genes exclusively.
   4. Cystic fibrosis is an autosomal recessive trait from both parents' genes.

7. While discharging a family from the pediatric clinic, the mother of a young child with strep throat asks when the child can return to preschool. The nurse would be correct in stating: *(select all that apply)*
   1. 24 hours after the last fever
   2. 24 hours after the first dose of oral antibiotics
   3. 24 hours after consuming 1 L of oral fluids
   4. 24 hours after the last complaints of throat pain
   5. 24 hours after the last dose of pain medication

8. While at school, a school-aged child with a history of asthma develops feelings of a tight chest and cough. The school nurse would be correct in administering which of the following medications?
   1. Oral steroids
   2. Inhaled beta agonist
   3. Inhaled steroids
   4. Oral leukotriene modifiers

9. A child presents with RSV bronchiolitis. The team provides treatments and comfort measures to the child. What treatments are included?
   1. Suctioning, oxygen, and rest
   2. Albuterol, oxygen, and steroids
   3. Racemic epinephrine, rest, and IV fluids
   4. Suctioning, steroids, and rest

CRITICAL THINKING QUESTIONS

1. What is the controversy over treating OM with antibiotics?
2. Your patient has a highly contagious respiratory infection. Explain the precautions that would be taken to prevent spreading the infection to other patients in the pediatric department.
3. What are the five methods of respiratory examination? Describe how you would perform each one.

DavisPlus

For additional resources and information, visit **www.DavisPlus.com.** Post-Conference Questions and Activities, Answers, and References can be found on Davis*Plus*.

Child With a Cardiac Condition

LEARNING OUTCOMES

1. Define the key terms.
2. Describe the overall anatomy and physiology of the cardiovascular system in the fetus, newborn, and child.
3. Differentiate between the most common congenital cardiac conditions found in infants and children.
4. Identify general relationships between cardiac and pulmonary functions.
5. Describe nursing observations and assessments of the child who presents with a potential cardiac disorder.
6. Describe the nursing care of the child with a cardiovascular disorder.
7. Identify culturally significant issues related to children with cardiac conditions.
8. Describe infectious sources of cardiac malfunction found in children.
9. Describe the educational needs of a child with a cardiac disorder and his or her family using a developmentally-appropriate approach.
10. Describe how to safely administer cardiac medications to a child, including the correct steps to administer medications, the evaluation of medication effects, and appropriate patient and/or parent teaching.

REAL-WORLD CASE STUDY

Janisha

■ Janisha, a twelve-day-old, previously healthy infant girl, is brought to the emergency room by her parents. She exhibits irritability, difficulty breathing, poor appetite, sweating when feeding, and dusky (ie, slightly cyanotic or bluish in color) lower extremities. Jasmine, the mother, shares that her pregnancy and delivery were normal. On assessment the baby has a heart rate of 160 bpm, a respiratory rate of 44 breaths per minute, an axillary temperature of 36.8°C, a heart murmur, and a delayed capillary refill of 4 sec. Her weight is 30 g above her birth weight. After performing four extremity blood pressure readings, the nurse informs the pediatric health-care team that the baby

continued on page 546

KEY TERMS

cardiopulmonary
cardiovascular
fetal
hypoxemia
left-to-right blood flow shunt
oxygenation
right-to-left blood flow shunt

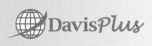 DavisPlus For audio pronunciation guide, visit **www.DavisPlus.com**

CHAPTER CONCEPTS

Comfort
Communication
Family
Medication
Nutrition
Oxygenation
Perfusion
Safety

has lower blood pressures and weaker pulses in her lower extremities than in her upper extremities. The nurse connected the baby to a cardiorespiratory monitor and a pulse oximeter. On auscultation there were bilateral fine crackles to the bases. An echocardiogram is ordered along with a chest x-ray and a 12-lead electrocardiograph (EKG). The diagnostic tests reveal a coarctation of the aorta and a patent ductus arteriosus (PDA).

The infant was transferred immediately to the pediatric intensive care unit (PICU) where IV access was obtained and an infusion of prostaglandin E1 (PGE1) was started. Her parents were visibly upset. The mother was in tears and the father, Jonas, was asking for a second opinion as the baby was prepared for surgery. A family conference was called with all health-care providers in attendance to address the parents' questions and concerns. The nurse asked what support the parents had access to from family, friends, and faith communities. She then notified the hospital chaplain, at the parents' request, to provide increased support to the family as they begin to cope with their daughter's diagnosis and treatment.

1. What vascular event precipitated the decompensation of the baby after 12 days of life?
2. What could cause the infant to have poor feeding patterns?
3. What would the pediatric health-care team members explain to the parents of this infant when asked about the duskiness of the lower extremities?

CONCEPTUAL CORNERSTONE

Growth and Development

An infant who is born with a congenital heart defect (ie, developed during fetal development and existing since birth) is at risk for delayed growth and development. The inadequacy of the oxygenation of tissues and subsequent poorer perfusion, and the complications of obtaining the required amount of daily calorie intake, put the infant at risk. Many infants will require longer feeding periods because of fatigue and shortness of breath. Most infants will be placed on a higher calorie per ounce formula to ensure adequate caloric intake. Taking precise weights, early reporting of weight loss or a lack of increase in weight, and patience with feeding the infant and teaching the infant's caregiver will assist the newborn or infant with a congenital heart defect to grow and develop.

The vast majority of children are born with healthy cardiovascular systems and do not experience pathology in this system. A congenital cardiovascular condition (ie, existing since birth) is rare and complex, requiring a pediatric health-care team approach and a long period of follow-up and surveillance. Congenital conditions require a child to endure many diagnostic procedures, often followed by surgical repair. Acquired cardiovascular conditions are much more common across the developmental period. Whether congenital or acquired, the pediatric nurse must have a thorough understanding of the anatomy and physiology of the cardiovascular system. This includes fetal and newborn heart anatomy and physiology.

The concepts of oxygenation and ventilation affect the child's cardiovascular system because the heart's main function is to distribute oxygenated blood throughout the child's tissues. While learning the structures of fetal and newborn circulation, reviewing the effect of adequate ventilation and subsequent oxygenation on the cardiovascular system is imperative.

THE DEVELOPMENT OF THE CARDIOVASCULAR SYSTEM

To grasp the often complex nature of cardiac conditions in children, it is important to start with an understanding of how the heart circulates blood, or perfuses the tissues in the body, in a child without cardiac disease. In the most basic of terms, the heart and blood vessels form a pump-driven circulation system. The heart contains specialized muscle, the myocardium, which is electrically sensitive. When it contracts in response to electrical impulses from natural pacemakers, it sends blood pulsing through the circulatory and pulmonary vascular system. The objective of the cardiac pump is to circulate oxygen-carrying blood out to the body and receive the deoxygenated blood to begin the cycle of sending the blood to the lungs for reoxygenation. Key principles of cardiac function are as follows:

- The atria, ventricles, heart valves, and cardiac vessels are formed and functioning around the eighth week of pregnancy.
- The right atrium and ventricle circulate deoxygenated blood to the lungs; then the oxygenated blood cycles back to the left atrium and ventricle to be pumped to the rest of the body.
- The precisely timed cardiac cycles of contraction (ie, pumping) and relaxation (ie, refilling) are driven by a complex system of electrical conduction pacemaking nodes and myocardial (ie, cardiac) muscle fibers located throughout the heart.
- Assessing heart rate, pulses, capillary refill, and blood pressure provides basic but essential assessment data points of how well the heart can perfuse the tissues. The level of mentation (ie, mental status and alertness) and quantity of urine output can also indicate the cardiac output of blood to key organ systems. Signs of hypoperfusion that require immediate intervention and notification of health-care providers may include:
  - Prolonged capillary refill time greater than 3 sec
  - Weak or absent pulses

- Pale or cyanotic skin color to the nail beds, mucosa, and circumoral area (ie, the area around the mouth)
- Decreased mental status
- Decreased urine output of less than 1 to 2 mL/kg/hour
- Cool extremities
- Tachycardia
- Hypotension or near-normal blood pressures initially
- Basic blood pressure readings reflect the pressure during the cardiac contraction phase (ie, systole) and relaxation phase (ie, diastole).
- **Oxygenation:** The stages of getting oxygen to the cells for use by the body consist of:
  - Oxygen content in the blood after respiration occurs
  - Oxygen delivery to the tissues
  - Gas exchange, including tissue uptake of oxygen

Differentiating Hypoxia From Hypoxemia

Hypoxia, which is a lowered oxygen saturation (ie, less than physiological levels, usually less than or equal to 90%), is an acute and potentially life-threatening situation in which insufficient oxygen is delivered to the tissues. Immediate action must be taken to improve oxygen delivery. Oxygen therapy and the resolution of circulatory issues that restrict the flow of blood to the tissues are key. Oxygen delivery issues are often **cardiovascular** (ie, relating to the heart and entire blood vessel system in nature). **Hypoxemia** (ie, abnormally low level of oxygen in the blood) can be a cause of hypoxia. Hypoxemia and hypoxia are not interchangeable concepts. *Hypox* (low oxygen) + *emia* (blood) refers specifically to low concentration of the oxygen being carried by the hemoglobin (Hgb) on red blood cells (RBC). Hypoxemia tends to be more chronic in nature and can have a respiratory or cardiovascular etiology.

Fluid and electrolyte balance is critical to monitor, manipulate, or maintain optimal blood pressures and perfusion. Fluid overload can lead to congestive heart conditions. A lack of adequate fluid in the cardiovascular space can lead to low blood pressure and shock. Electrolytes such as sodium, potassium, and chloride, as well as other blood chemistries, are important in cardiac function.

- Renal (ie, kidney) function is an essential part of maintaining fluid and electrolyte balance. Urine output can be a major indicator of how effectively the heart is perfusing important organ systems because the kidneys are very sensitive to poor blood flow and will slow down or stop making urine if they are not well-perfused.

Findings to immediately report to the health-care provider are decreased perfusion, unanticipated weight gain, an increased respiratory rate, and noncompliance with the medication plan. These assessment findings can be signs of impending heart failure.

Fetal Cardiac Structures

The formation of the heart is a complex series of twists and turns of a "heart tube" into the final configuration of great vessels, atria, and ventricles. Errors in the twisting of the heart tube are the source of many structural abnormalities found in congenital heart defects. Before birth, a fetus has blood flow pathways that allow the delivery of oxygen and nutrients to the baby without the use of the lungs. Because of the early development of the heart and vascular structures, cardiac defects can be present before the woman knows of her pregnancy. At delivery, the pathways change to allow increased blood flow to the newly expanded lungs and respiration begins.

Three Fetal Shunts

The three **fetal** (ie, pertaining to a fetus) shunts provide blood flow pathways that allow oxygenated blood to mix with deoxygenated blood. This mixing ensures oxygen delivery to the fetus. The shunts normally close at birth or soon after. These shunts are:

1. **PDA:** A vessel outside the heart that connects the descending aorta and the left pulmonary artery; allows for the bypass of the majority of blood to the fetal lungs and directs the oxygen-rich blood to the fetus's body (ie, systemic system).
2. **Ductus venosus:** A vessel outside the heart that connects the umbilical vein to the fetal inferior vena cava; this structure allows the oxygen-rich blood from the placental circulation to bypass the liver and be directed right to the fetal heart.
3. **Foramen ovale:** An opening between the two atria of the fetal heart; this structure is present to bypass the majority of oxygen-rich blood to the lungs and redirect the oxygen-rich blood to the left side of the heart for rapid distribution to the fetus's systemic system.

Fetal Cardiac Blood Flow

Fetal blood flow is strongly influenced by the pressures found in the lung vasculature and the systemic system in relationship to the blood pressures in the remainder of the baby's body.

- The systemic system has low pressure and lower resistance to rapid fetal blood flow.
- The pulmonary system has high pressure and resistance within the fetal pulmonary vasculature as the vessels are vasoconstricted and the structures for breathing are engorged with amniotic fluid, causing the resistance. (Blood must be bypassed or redirected through the shunts to preserve the fetal pulmonary vasculature from injury.)
- The placental system of vasculature has low pressure and resistance in order for a large quantity of fetal blood to be oxygenated rapidly and carbon dioxide to be released rapidly (the fetus has a high heart rate).

These three pressure areas help the blood flow through the fetal shunts so that the oxygenated blood is mixed with deoxygenated blood rapidly and effectively. This mixing results in the necessary oxygenation and tissue nourishment to allow fetal development to continue. To better understand how the shunts work, it is helpful to select a starting point, such as the placenta, and trace the flow arrows through the cardiovascular system shown in Fig. 33.1.

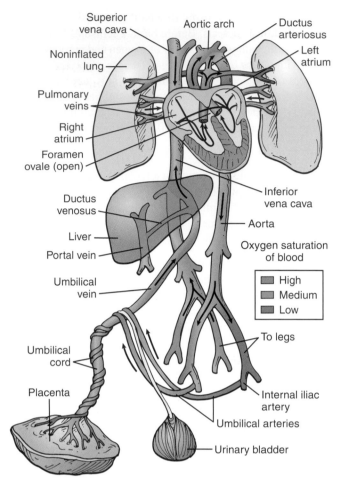

FIGURE 33.1 Fetal cardiac blood flow.

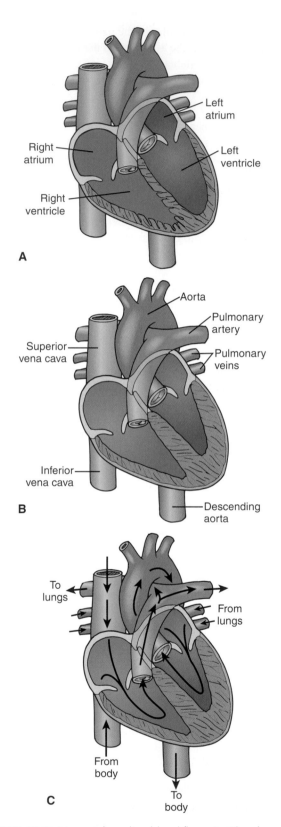

FIGURE 33.2 Neonatal cardiac blood flow. A, Chambers of the heart. B, Vessels of the heart. C, Normal blood flow.

Postnatal Blood Flow

Once delivery is complete and blood flow from the placenta stops, a brief period of change to extrauterine life occurs. This process is termed *transition.*

Typically, the majority of the transition process happens in a matter of minutes and continues through the first several months of life (Fig. 33.2). This move from oxygenation via the maternal/placental route to the respiratory system is primarily dependent on the infant's ability to close the fetal shunts and shift the pressures to a point where the high pulmonary vascular pressures are lower than the baby's systemic vascular pressures. This shift in blood flow and a complex cascade of chemical changes allows the newborn's newly expanded lungs to exchange the gases necessary for successful respiration. Eventually, the fetal shunt structures seal shut and/or become ligaments. If there are issues with the closure of the fetal blood flow pathways or interruptions in the shifting of the intracardiac and extracardiac pressures, the infant will not be able to perfuse tissues and may experience significant respiratory distress. Most shunts close spontaneously, but those that persist may require surgical repair.

Heart Rate and Blood Pressure

Heart rate and blood pressure are related measurements of cardiac function. They vary according to the age of the child,

with normal heart rate values decreasing with age and normal blood pressure values increasing with age (Table 33.1). It is important to assess all vital signs accurately, including blood pressure, heart rate, respiratory rate, temperature, and oxygen saturation. There is evidence that hypertension is

TABLE 33.1 NORMAL BLOOD PRESSURES AND HEART RATES FOR CHILDREN

Age	Systolic Blood Pressures (in mm Hg)	Diastolic Blood Pressures (in mm Hg)	Heart Rates (in bpm)
Premature	55–75	35–45	120–170
0–3 Months	65–85	45–55	100–150
3–6 Months	70–90	55–65	90–120
6–12 Months	80–100	55–65	80–120
1–3 Years	90–105	55–70	70–110
3–6 Years	95–110	60–75	65–110
6–12 Years	100–120	60–75	60–95
Greater Than 12 Years	110–135	65–85	55–85

Sources: (Rudd and Kocisko, 2014; Linnard-Palmer, 2010)

underdiagnosed in the pediatric population, even over extended periods of time. This underdiagnosis is attributed to two things: (1) a knowledge deficit in health-care practitioners about pediatric blood pressure norms, and (2) a lack of awareness of the patient's earlier blood pressure measurements (Hansen, Gunn, et al, 2007).

Electrical System of the Heart

The conduction system of the heart regulates the precise timing of atrial and ventricular contractions. Opening and closing of heart valves begins with the first of three areas of specialized intrinsic conductive tissues:

1. Near the top of the right atrium is a small plexus of electric-generating tissue called the *sinoatrial (SA) node.* The SA node generates an electrical impulse about 60 to 100 times per minute. As this impulse traverses the conduction system, the atria contract first, pumping blood into the ventricles, and then, almost immediately, the ventricles contract.
2. The electrical impulse continues to travel down the sinus node to the atrioventricular (AV) node.
3. The conduction stops very briefly and then continues down the conduction pathways via the bundle of His into the ventricles, which contract and send blood out to the body or to the lungs. The bundle of His divides into right and left pathways to provide electrical stimulation to both ventricles via Purkinje's fibers found in the walls of the ventricles themselves.

Almost all heart tissue is capable of initiating an electrical impulse and a resulting contraction, in effect becoming the pacemaker. Arrhythmias (ie, abnormal heart beats) occur when:

• There is an interruption in the normal conduction pathway.
• The SA node (ie, the primary pacemaker) generates an abnormal rhythm or rate.

• Another node (ie, AV node) or tissue (ie, Purkinje's fibers) becomes the primary pacemaker.

The conduction of the impulse throughout the heart is cyclical and can be documented in the form of a waveform shown on an EKG machine. The basic segments of the waveform are reflecting the timing of the contraction, relaxation, and rest (ie, recharging) phases of the cardiac cycle, as well as the valve function (Fig. 33.3).

The first upward curve of the EKG tracing is the *P wave.* The P wave indicates that the SA node has fired an impulse and the atria are contracting to pump blood into the ventricles. This is called a *sinus rhythm.* Next, there is a short downward section connected to a steep upward spike and then a steep downward spike, called the *QRS complex.* This indicates that the ventricles are contracting, sending blood to the body and lungs. Next, there is a short upward

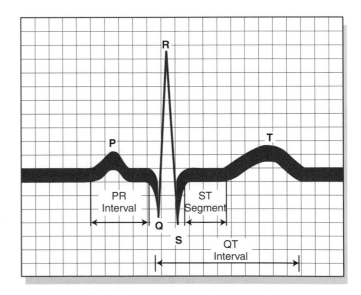

FIGURE 33.3 EKG waveform.

segment called the *ST segment*. The ST segment reflects the time from the end of the ventricular contraction to the beginning of the rest period before the next ventricular contraction. The final upward notch is the *T wave*. The T wave indicates the resting period necessary for the heart to start the next beat.

Each segment of the EKG waveform has specific measurements that are considered normal. Variations in timing, the shape of the different segments, or the speed of the heart rate are analyzed by health-care practitioners as a diagnostic tool.

INTRODUCTION TO CARDIAC CONDITIONS

Children with heart disease are born with the disorder (ie, a congenital heart defect) or have acquired it sometime after birth. Heart disease can affect the actual structures in the heart and/or can alter circulatory function. Cardiac conditions can adversely affect health through hypoxemia and impaired tissue perfusion because of heart failure. They are a leading cause of death from birth defects in the first year of life. Almost 1% of babies born in the United States, about 40,000 births annually, have congenital heart defects, making it the most common type of birth defect (Centers for Disease Control and Prevention [CDC], 2011). Some characteristics of women who have a higher risk of having a baby with a heart defect are women who are obese, have diabetes, or smoke (CDC, 2014; National Center on Birth Defects and Developmental Disabilities, 2011).

To identify the presence of a cardiac condition in children, the pediatric health-care team works together to identify classic symptoms and clinical presentations. The following section describes the information needed to make a differential diagnosis of heart disease or cardiac pathology during childhood. Table 33.2 provides an overview of types of congenital heart defects in children.

Health History

A thorough health history of a child who presents with a cardiac condition, either congenital or acquired, is a priority nursing action. The history should include:

- Past medical history of the child, including the presence of known congenital anomalies and conditions associated with cardiac malformations, such as Down's syndrome, fetal alcohol syndrome, and Turner's syndrome
- Maternal history of characteristics associated with an increased risk of heart disease in children, including diabetes, rubella, obesity, alcohol use, smoking, and previous pregnancy losses
- Current and past medications, including over-the-counter products and holistic remedies
- Signs in infant: The following may be present: cyanosis that worsens with activity or feeding, heart murmur, low weight for stature, diaphoresis (ie, sweating), fatigue when feeding, and a weak, irritable cry
- Signs in older children: Older children (ie, toddler, preschool, school-aged, and adolescent) may also exhibit decreased activity levels, dizziness or syncope, a thin build, and chest pain

TABLE 33.2 TYPES OF PEDIATRIC CONGENITAL HEART DEFECTS

Heart Defect	Description and Usual Shunt
ASD	A passage between the left and right atria that results in increased blood flow to the lungs (ie, left-to-right shunt)
VSD	A passage between the left and right ventricles that results in increased blood flow to the lungs (ie, left-to-right shunt)
Pulmonary Stenosis	Narrow pulmonary artery or valve that obstructs blood flow coming out of the ventricles
Aortic Stenosis	A constriction at or around the aortic valve
Coarctation of Aorta	A narrowing of the aorta at or around the location of the ductus arteriosus that obstructs blood flow out of the ventricles
TGA	The pulmonary artery is connected to the left ventricle versus the right ventricle and the aorta is connected to the right ventricle versus the left ventricle (survival is dependent on PDA until surgical repair is done)
HLHS	Incomplete development of the aorta, aortic valve, left ventricle, and mitral valve that necessitates the right ventricle to circulate blood to the body as well as to the lungs
PDA	Occurs when the fetal shunt between the pulmonary artery and the aorta does not close; increased blood flow to the lungs (ie, left-to-right shunt)
Tricuspid Atresia	Complete obstruction of the tricuspid valve (ie, right-to-left shunt)

Physical Assessment

Keen observation skills will be needed to care for the child with heart disease as the child's condition can decompensate rapidly with only subtle signs of warning. Unlike adults who have slightly higher resuscitation results if they become pulseless (with success because of immediate defibrillation), a child has a dismal survival rate if the heart completely stops versus if her heart rate is dangerously low (ie, bradycardic) (Donoghue, et al, 2009). Early intervention and prevention of the circumstances that would contribute to **cardiopulmonary** (ie, relating to both the heart and the lungs) compromise are required. Key observations for a child with a known cardiac condition include:

- A complete set of vital signs, including an oxygen saturation (ie, pulse oximeter) reading and a pain score
- Auscultation of heart sounds: It is important to develop the skills, honed by frequent practice, to identify heart sounds and to describe them accurately when charting. Two typical heart sounds are heard as a "lub-dub" for systolic-diastolic sounds and are labeled S1 and S2. Abnormal heart sounds can be murmurs, which are sounds that result from turbulent blood flow in the heart. They have different characteristics, depending on the defect. These are the characteristics of the heart sounds that should be noted:
  - Location: The anatomic location where the sound is best heard
  - Frequency: Either a high pitch (best heard with the diaphragm of the stethoscope) or a low pitch (best heard with the stethoscope's bell)
  - Timing: The time during systole, diastole, or both phases during which the sound is heard
  - Intensity: Loudness, which is graded on a scale of 1 to 6, which corresponds from faint to very loud
  - Quality: In charting, use descriptive terms such as *musical, click, swish, blowing, harsh,* or other suitable terms
  - Duration: Early, mid, late, or pan (ie, across the whole sound); long or short
  - Radiation: Other areas of the body where the heart sound may be heard
- Observe for signs of chronic hypoxemia, such as cyanosis, clubbing of fingers, poor weight gain, rapid respiration (ie, tachypnea), dyspnea (ie, labored breathing), and polycythemia (ie, high RBC count).
- Assess for signs found in children with heart failure, such as tachycardia, heart murmurs (including extra heart sounds S3 and S4), cool extremities, weak pulses, sluggish capillary refill, anorexia, generalized paleness, mottling, fatigue, poor urine output, diaphoresis, cardiomegaly on chest x-ray, and poor growth (ie, failure to thrive [FTT]).
- Look for signs of systemic venous congestion found in heart failure, such as peripheral edema, enlarged spleen and liver, neck vein distention (except in babies), and ascites (ie, abdominal fluid collection).
- Observe for signs of pulmonary congestion associated with heart failure, such as exercise intolerance and recurrent respiratory infections. The health-care team must also investigate for tachypnea, stridor, grunting, nasal flaring, retractions (ie, accessory muscle usage), and abnormal lung sounds such as crackles, which indicate extra fluid and dyspnea.
- Evaluate the social and cultural structure and support of the patient and her or his family members. Assess anxiety levels and reached developmental milestones to plan teaching and emotional support for the patient and the patient's family.

LABS & DIAGNOSTICS

Common Diagnostic Procedures and Laboratory Tests for Pediatric Cardiac Conditions

Common Diagnostic Procedures
- Electrocardiography (ie, 12-lead EKG)
- Chest radiography (ie, x-ray)
- Echocardiogram
- Cardiac catheterization

Common Laboratory Tests for Children With Cardiac Conditions
- Complete blood cell count (CBC) with differential
- C-reactive protein (CRP)
- Blood cultures
- Antistreptolysin-O (ASO) titer and throat cultures if *Streptococcus* infection is suspected
- Hgb
- Hematocrit (Hct)
- Serum electrolytes
- Arterial blood gas (ABG)
- Erythrocyte sedimentation rate (ESR)

GENERAL NURSING CARE OF THE CHILD WITH A CARDIAC CONDITION

Comprehensive nursing care that includes psychosocial, cultural, and emotional aspects, as well as physiological components, for children who live with a cardiac condition is key to optimizing the quality and length of life. Comprehensive nursing care can prevent complications and includes involving parents and caregivers in every phase of diagnosis, treatment, and recovery. The child's developmental stage and level should be taken into consideration so the child can continue to develop and grow as expected cognitively and emotionally. Child Life services must be included in the child's care. The following aspects of nursing care will support a child with a known or suspected cardiac condition:

- Offer effective care to reduce fatigue and discomfort: Provide frequent rest breaks and small, frequent meals; cluster care to allow time between interventions; bathe as needed; and soothe and console the child to keep crying to a minimum, especially in the presence of cyanosis.
- Provide empathetic care by providing respite care for the parents, private time to hold their child, and a calm and soothing environment.

- Monitor daily weights and intake and output (I&O) to track nutritional and fluid status.
- Track vital signs, laboratory tests (including serum electrolytes), and renal function to evaluate for developing complications.
- Share developmentally appropriate resources and provide support for children and family to continue the child's growth and maturation.
- Administer prescribed medications and monitor for effects and untoward responses.
- Monitor the coping of the child and family, and provide culturally and spiritually appropriate care.
- Include interdisciplinary involvement with social services, Child Life Specialists, and academic support for older children.
- Create a nursing care plan that reflects holistic care.

SAFETY *STAT!*

It is imperative that the nursing team obtain accurate weights as ordered. Weights should be done when the child is naked,

and at the same time each day on the same scale. Any change in weight must be reported right away. The child needs calories to continue to grow and many cardiac conditions cause the child to hold fluids and gain water weight. Changes in weight must be reported because an antidiuretic may be ordered. Specifically, several conditions could be causing an infant with a congenital heart defect not to grow and gain weight as expected and desired. These situations are:

- The infant becomes fatigued during feedings and does not finish the nursing or bottle session.
- The cardiac condition is causing the child to become short of breathing while eating and therefore the child does not take in the full amount of calories.
- The parents may be concerned with the child's condition, and in focusing on that, are not aware of the child's calorie needs.
- The cardiac condition might be causing oxygenated blood flow to return to the lungs, increasing pressure on the pulmonary vasculature and causing fluids to build up. If the child has crackles or rales, the child might not be able to finish a meal because of shortness of breath.

NURSING CARE PLAN for the Child With a Congenital Heart Defect

Potential Nursing Diagnoses:
- Altered cardiac function related to abnormal anatomy of the heart
- Altered oxygenation related to abnormal blood flow, decreased cardiac output, hypoxemia, and hypoxia
- Risk for infection because of accumulation of fluids in the lungs (eg, acyanotic heart defects)
- Potential for altered nutrition related to increased metabolic demand, shortness of breath during feedings, or fatigue during feedings
- Knowledge deficit related to the congenital defect and subsequent care for the child
- Risk for altered parenting related to a child with a chronic health condition because of stress, worry, anxiety, and fatigue
- Risk for pain because of operative, postoperative recovery, repeated phlebotomy, and diagnostic procedures

Expected Outcomes:
- The child will experience minimal discomfort and distress from diagnosis and treatment of their congenital heart defect.
- The family will learn to assess for complications associated with congenital heart defects, including learning how to take an apical pulse, learning the symptoms of respiratory distress, learning the symptoms of infection, and learning how to identify the signs of fluid accumulation in the lungs and tissues.
- The child will not experience an injury associated with a condition of the cardiovascular system.
- The child will maintain adequate nutrition and calorie intake for growth and development throughout the diagnosis, treatment, and subsequent care needed for a cardiovascular condition.
- The family will maintain safety while administering the required doses of medications needed for the child's cardiovascular condition.

Interventions:
Assist the pediatric health-care team to teach the family to provide safety for the child with a cardiovascular condition including:
- How to assess their child for discomfort and distress and provide comfort measures
- How to assess for tachycardia, bradycardia, respiratory distress, evidence of infection, edema, and respiratory distress from fluid accumulation
- When and how to report concerning conditions or developments to the appropriate primary care provider

NURSING CARE PLAN for the Child With a Congenital Heart Defect—cont'd

- How to provide for adequate nutrition including high calorie formula, breastmilk with human milk fortification, or high calorie foods for older infants and toddlers
- How to maintain safety while drawing up and administering medications needed for the child's cardiovascular condition

Evaluation of Outcome:
- The child experiences minimal distress and discomfort.
- The child demonstrates incremental growth and development.
- The family maintains safety in all aspects of care and medication administration.

CULTURAL CONSIDERATIONS

A family's cultural background can influence the parent's care of the infant with a cardiac condition, and has implications for the nursing care of the child as well. When a family is faced with the devastating news that their child has heart disease, either congenital or acquired, it is no surprise that cultural practices can affect all aspects of care from the onset of symptoms to long-term care requirements. When faced with the diagnosis and treatment of cardiac disease in their child, families may strive to adhere to their cultural norms with care and treatments that are specific to their cultural population. Examples of some cultural practices that may require careful attention and creative problem-solving include the following:

- Hispanic families may view good health as a reward for living a good life by working hard, avoiding misbehavior, and eating healthfully. They may view illness as a punishment for wrongdoing.
- Islamic Muslim families may refuse assessments of their female children by male health-care practitioners. They may also refuse pain medications with narcotic components, as well as any medications that might be addictive or have alcohol as a component.
- Hindu families may require extra time for cultural rituals before consenting to surgeries, treatments, or diagnostic procedures. They may also refuse medical products that have beef-based components.
- Chinese families may seek to practice Chinese medicine, such as herbal medicine and acupuncture, before pursuing help from modern medicine. Many hold superstitious beliefs regarding health and illness. Social interaction is very polite and modest.
- Native American families have tight community bonds and may look to tribal leadership for approval of medical interventions and surgeries for their children. Traditional tribal medicine does not validate asymptomatic disease, so the family may not comply with routine screening. Medicine and spiritual practice are intertwined, so holy rituals, songs, and herbs are often desired. Disease may be perceived to be a result of a breech against a prohibition or taboo.

- The best nursing care includes an assessment of the family's cultural beliefs and practices. Questions can include:
  - What is your cultural and religious background?
  - Do you have cultural or religious practices that the team should be made aware of so we can provide you with time and space?
  - Do you have an elder or leader of your cultural or religious community we can contact for you?
  - Is there anything our team can provide your family and extended community to make this situation easier for you? (Linnard-Palmer, 2006)

SYSTEM-FOCUSED NURSING CARE

System-focused nursing care includes providing for the complicated components of the cardiovascular system. Nursing care should be provided related to the pediatric patient's cardiac conduction, circulation, and perfusion:

- Ensure fluid and electrolyte balance:
  - Sodium restriction, if ordered
  - Fluid restriction, if ordered
  - Potassium supplementation, if indicated (may be contraindicated if child is taking angiotensin-converting enzyme [ACE] inhibitors)
- Increase tissue oxygenation:
  - Check the pulse oxygen saturation readings every 2 to 4 hours and PRN.
  - Maintain clear airway by suctioning the child as needed.
  - Give humidified, cool oxygen by hood, mask, or nasal cannula as ordered.
- Ensure adequate nutrition:
  - Provide increased caloric density by offering an increased-calorie formula.
  - Supplement breastfeeding with a high-calorie formula or fortified breast milk.
  - Follow oral feeds with gavage (ie, tube) feeding if unable to take enough feeding for growth.
  - Allow rests with feedings; complete feeds within a half hour.

- Position the infant in a semi-upright position.
- If nipple feeding, consider a soft preemie or regular nipple with a cross-cut to allow a faster flow of milk with less effort.
- Schedule small, frequent feedings; in infants, feed every 3 hours or consider continuous gavage feedings at night.
- Decrease cardiac workload:
  - Ensure bedrest and a low stimulation environment; keep lights low and noise level down.
  - Elevate the head of the bed (ie, semi-Fowler's position at 45 degrees) or ensure that the infant is held upright; an infant or toddler car seat can be used to provide an elevated head of bed as well.
- Teach the family about the care of the child according to the family's preferred method of learning. The pediatric health-care teams must first determine who will be involved in the teaching session and determine their readiness to learn. The types of teaching can include:
  - Oral presentation
  - Visual materials that are printed
  - Visual materials via video
  - Demonstrate/return demonstration
  - Written materials (different languages may be required)
  - Online resources from professional and reputable organizations

---

SAFETY *STAT!*

Do not give a child with a cardiac condition oxygen without consulting with a pediatric cardiology team. The indiscriminate use of oxygen can place a child at risk for complications associated with cardiac shunts and subsequent perfusion.

CARDIAC DISORDERS

Disorders of the cardiovascular system include both cyanotic and acyanotic heart defects. Although the presence of a congenital heart defect is rare, the following section outlines the specific anatomy, physiology, and care concerns for children with these defects (Fig. 33.4 and 33.5). Far more commonly, infectious processes occur that can influence the integrity and function of the cardiovascular system. They include rheumatic fever, Kawasaki's disease, and subacute bacterial endocarditis (SBE).

Cyanotic Heart Defects

Cyanotic heart defects are a group of heart malformations or lesions that have **right-to-left blood flow shunts.** Right-to-left blood flow shunts are cardiovascular conduits through which blood flows from the left side of the heart, which usually perfuses the systemic circulation, to the right side of the heart, which usually perfuses the pulmonary circulation. Cyanotic heart defects produce some level of cyanosis. This cyanosis may not be readily visible on assessment, so pulse oximetry,

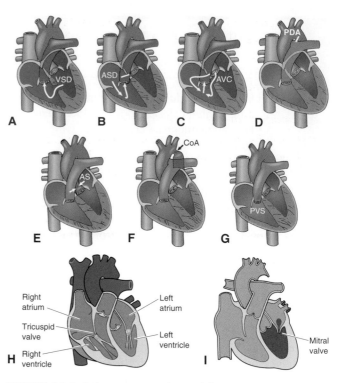

FIGURE 33.4 Select acyanotic heart defects. A, VSD: Opening between ventricles. B, ASD: Opening between atriums. C, Atrioventricular septal defect (ie, atrioventricular canal): Low ASD continuous with high VSD and cleft of mitral and tricuspid valves. D, PDA: Fetal ductus does not close at birth. E, Aortic valve stenosis: Narrowing or stricture of the aortic valve. F, Coarctation of the aorta: Narrowing of aorta at the insertion of the ductus arteriosus. G, Pulmonic valve stenosis: Narrowing of the entrance of the pulmonary artery. H, Tricuspid stenosis: Failure of the tricuspid valve to develop. I, Mitral stenosis: Failure of the mitral valve to develop.

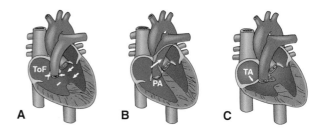

FIGURE 33.5 Select cyanotic heart defects. A, TOF: Includes VSD, pulmonic stenosis, overriding aorta, and right ventricular hypertrophy. B, Pulmonary atresia. C, Tricuspid atresia.

which measures oxygen saturation without a blood sample, is valuable. The routine use of pulse oximetry in the care of newborn infants to detect congenital heart disease, particularly severe heart disease, has been supported (Mahle, et al, 2009). It is not unusual to confirm low oxygen saturations between 50% and 90% in infants with varying degrees of defect severity. Normal saturations typically are greater than 92%. Four characteristics that are also found in this class are:

- Defects that allow the mixing of oxygenated and deoxygenated blood

• An infant or a child who is ductal dependent (a neonate needs a PDA for survival in the initial period of life)
• Low pulmonary blood flow
• High pulmonary blood flow

Transposition of the Great Arteries

In transposition of the great arteries (TGA), the great vessels of the heart are anatomically switched. The pulmonary artery is connected to the left ventricle (versus the right ventricle) and the aorta is connected to the right ventricle (versus the left ventricle). The infant's survival is dependent on a PDA until surgical repair can be done. The signs and symptoms that are seen with this disorder include:

• Heart murmur
• Cyanosis that becomes severe in hours to days as the PDA closes
• Heart failure
• Cardiomegaly (ie, enlarged heart on chest x-ray)

A critical and life-preserving intervention includes the immediate administration of an IV drip of PGE1, which chemically maintains the patency of the ductus arteriosus.

DRUG FACTS

The action of PGE1 includes dilation of vessels and the inhibition of clotting. This allows a patent flow of blood through the ductus arteriosus and maintains perfusion before a surgical intervention is performed to re-route the blood flow and repair the PDA.

Tetralogy of Fallot

Tetralogy of Fallot (TOF) includes a set of four defects that result in mixed blood flow throughout the newborn's cardiovascular system. Without the presence of anatomical defects allowing for mixed blood flow, the fetus would not have survived fetal development. This life-threatening condition requires a series of surgical repairs and can be diagnosed by echocardiogram, cardiac catheterization, or both. The four defects that make up the diagnosis of TOF include:

• Ventricular septal defect (VSD)
• Pulmonary stenosis
• An overriding aorta
• Right ventricular hypertrophy

Signs and symptoms seen with the TOF defect are:

• Prominent heart murmur
• Growth retardation/FTT
• Polycythemia and clotting disorders
• Cyanosis (not affected by oxygen therapy), severe difficulty breathing, clubbed fingers, and acidosis

SAFETY *STAT!*

Interventions for Tet Spells

• For tet spells, also known as *hypercyanotic spells*, the immediate intervention is to have the child flex his or her knees to the chest to lower venous return.
• Have the child squat to decrease venous return, which can temper hypercyanotic spells, or place the infant in a knee-to-chest position to increase venous return.
• Administer morphine to calm the child and slow down tachypnea.
• Administer 100% oxygen, which easily dilates the pulmonary vessels, allowing more blood flow to the lungs, which in turn can help resolve the hypercyanotic spell.

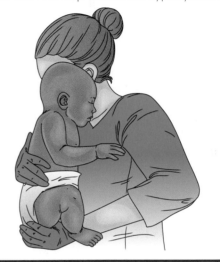

If oxygen saturations are very low, the cardiologist will consider ordering the registered nurse to administer PGE1 to preserve the blood flow through the PDA and provide some oxygenated blood via mixing. Surgical repair for the TOF is completed when the child is about 6 months old. Long-term issues include pulmonary valve leaking, arrhythmias that necessitate a pacemaker, and periodic evaluation via echocardiogram, a Holter's monitor, or an exercise stress test.

Hypoplastic Left Heart Syndrome

Hypoplastic left heart syndrome (HLHS) is a severe, complex heart condition that consists of incomplete development of the aorta, the aortic valve, the left ventricle, and the mitral valve. The condition necessitates that the right ventricle compensate by circulating blood to the body as well as to the lungs. Signs and symptoms of HLHS include:

• Weak pulses to all extremities
• Low pulse oximetry readings that do not increase with the administration of oxygen
• Critical, life-threatening hypotension and shock when the ductus arteriosus closes

If possible, plans are made to deliver the infant in a high-level care facility that can provide aggressive treatment immediately. Surgical repair must be staged in three steps to be completed by 3 years of age. Heart transplantation is also considered because of multiple long-term sequelae such as blood clot formation, rapid fatigue with exercise, arrhythmias that necessitate pacemaker placement, and cardiac failure.

Tricuspid Atresia

Tricuspid atresia is when the tricuspid valve is missing or not developed properly; this results in a right-to-left shunt. There is an absence of the normal blood flow from the right atrium to the right ventricle. A three-part, staged surgical repair is required. These children present with:

• Severe cyanosis a few hours after delivery that worsens as the ductus arteriosus closes
• Heart failure
• Growth retardation/FTT

As with other ductal-dependent cardiac malformations, PGE1 is indicated to keep the blood flow through the ductus arteriosus. These infants are often placed on a ventilator very soon after birth. This defect is severe, and children with it are critically ill and are at risk for arrhythmias and sudden death. Cardiac transplantation is considered an option if a donor heart is available for an infant.

Acyanotic Heart Defects

This group of heart malformations or lesions is composed of those that have a **left-to-right blood flow shunt** (cardiovascular conduit through which blood flows from the left side of the heart, which usually perfuses the systemic circulation, to the right side of the heart, which usually perfuses the pulmonary circulation). Acyanotic heart defects rarely produce initial cyanosis, but can leave the body undersupplied with blood flow. The defects in this group can flood the lungs with excess blood flow, leading to congestive heart failure (CHF).

Patent Ductus Arteriosus

PDA is a defect that occurs when the fetal shunt between the pulmonary artery and the aorta does not close. The defect causes increased blood flow to the lungs in a left-to-right shunting pattern. Premature infants are especially susceptible to PDAs. A PDA can be asymptomatic. If symptoms are present, the signs and symptoms of this disorder are:

• Labile oxygen saturations and blood pressures as the PDA intermittently opens and closes
• Systolic heart murmur (sounds like a machine hum)
• Wide pulse pressure (ie, the difference between the systolic and diastolic blood pressures)
• Bounding pulses
• An active chest wall to the left of the sternum above the heart

The PDA can be closed surgically, but efforts are usually made to support the infant until the PDA closes spontaneously or an attempt is made to chemically close it with a course of indomethacin, which inhibits prostaglandins and promotes constriction of the ductus arteriosus.

Ventricular Septal Defect

Ventricular septal defect (VSD) is the most common congenital heart defect according to Hoffman and Kaplan (2002). This defect is a passage between the left and right ventricles that increases blood flow to the lungs, resulting in a left-to-right shunt, which can lead to CHF. The signs and symptoms associated with a VSD are:

• Being possibly asymptomatic (without obvious signs and symptoms) if the defect is very small
• Heart failure
• FTT
• A delayed, harsh, loud murmur usually not heard until pulmonary pressures decrease between 4 and 8 weeks of age

Treatment for CHF that results from a VSD can include diuretic therapy to decrease fluid in the lungs and digoxin to strengthen the contractions of the heart. Symptomatic VSDs require surgical closure of the defect.

Atrial Septal Defect

An atrial septal defect (ASD) is a passage between the left and right atria that results in increased blood flow to the lungs, creating a left-to-right shunt. The ASD can be a residual opening remaining from the foramen ovale fetal shunt. Signs and symptoms of an ASD are:

• Possibly being asymptomatic
• A harsh, loud murmur
• Potential for an enlarged right atrium
• Mild CHF

If the defect is large or symptomatic then surgical repair is needed. In some cases, minimally invasive repairs can be accomplished during a cardiac catheterization.

Aortic Stenosis

Aortic stenosis consists of a constriction at or around the aortic valve. If the aortic valve is constricted, then the left ventricle must pump harder to eject blood out into the body. An aortic stenosis is associated with the following signs and symptoms:

• Heart murmur
• Chest pain; weak, thready pulses; intolerance to exercise; hypotension; syncope; and dizziness
• An enlarged left ventricle

An EKG will be normal, but the defect is seen on an echocardiogram. Exercise stress tests give information about the severity of the restriction and the reduction in tolerance to activity. Repair can be done through a cardiac catheterization procedure in which the constricted valve is dilated. If the catheterization is not successful in restoring normal aortic blood flow, open heart surgery with possible valve replacement is needed. If the valve is replaced, antibiotic prophylaxis will be necessary.

Pulmonary Stenosis

Pulmonary stenosis consists of a narrow pulmonary artery or valve that obstructs the blood flow coming out of the ventricles. This condition necessitates surgical repair. EKG tracings are normal. Diagnosis is best made by echocardiogram, and cardiac catheterization will be considered to measure the degree of stenosis. Signs and symptoms of pulmonary stenosis are:

• Systolic heart murmur, often with a "click" quality
• If narrowing is severe, cyanosis is apparent
• Intolerance to exercise
• Enlargement of the right ventricle

If possible during cardiac catheterization, the stenotic valve may be dilated (ie, widened) to relieve the obstruction. If the defect is too complex, open heart surgical repair will be necessary.

Coarctation of the Aorta

Coarctation of the aorta consists of a narrowing of the aorta at or around the location of the ductus arteriosus that obstructs blood flow out of the ventricles. Diagnosis is made by echocardiogram. Pulse oximetry can be very useful to help detect a coarctation because of the tendency for higher oxygen saturations in the upper limbs than in the lower extremities. More than a 3% difference between upper and lower extremity saturations is cause for further investigation. Often, infants who are diagnosed with a coarctation were discharged home within a few days of birth only to be readmitted within a few weeks of life. Those infants begin to have difficulty breathing and eating, have an increased heart rate, and may show signs of congestive heart disease because of the natural closing of the PDA. The PDA can mask the effects of the reduced blood flow distal to the coarctation so that when it begins to close, the infant can become extremely ill very quickly. Depending on the severity and location of the defect, surgical repair may be indicated. Signs and symptoms of this condition are:

• Heart murmur to the left sternal border area
• Tachycardia
• An enlarged heart as evidenced on chest x-ray
• Tachypnea, particularly with feeding or crying
• Difficulty eating because of shortness of breath from extra blood flow to lungs and fatigue
• Weak or absent lower extremity pulses, which result from decreased cardiac output
• Lower blood pressures to the lower extremities than to the upper limbs
• CHF may develop as the PDA closes
• Hepatomegaly from fluid overload associated with CHF
• Vertigo, headaches, and leg pain
• Increased oxygen saturation and blood pressures in the upper extremities as compared with the lower extremities
• Low weight or slow weight gain because of inability to finish feeds

---

SAFETY _STAT!_

Pediatric nurses must take blood pressures on all four extremities to identify if there are increased results in the upper extremities as compared with lower extremities; there is greater blood flow out of the aortic arch to the upper extremities versus the lower extremities.

PGE1, which causes vasodilation of the ductus arteriosus and allows it to temporarily remain open, may be indicated to reduce the development of heart failure. Postoperative complications may include renal damage, which results from clamping the descending aorta during surgery. Prophylaxis with antibiotics may be needed if aortic valve malformations are diagnosed.

SAFETY _STAT!_

Hypertension is also a common complication associated with coarctation of the aorta and may necessitate antihypertensive therapy. Meticulous assessment of blood pressures is important. Do not take a blood pressure when an infant or young child is crying because the result will not be accurate.

Congestive Heart Failure

CHF is a major complication of cardiac disease. Generally, if CHF develops before 1 year of age, it is because of a congenital defect. If developed after 1 year of age, the etiology most likely is from an acquired cause.

Assessment of CHF

The endpoint of undetected or untreated CHF is death, so strong assessment skills and early detection are key. The cardinal signs of CHF include:

• Tachycardia
• Cardiomegaly
• Tachypnea
• Hepatomegaly

Interventions for Congestive Heart Failure

Treatment of CHF is focused on improving cardiac output. Treatment includes the following:

• Preventing, when possible, congenital heart defects by minimizing maternal risk factors such as obesity, diabetes, and smoking
• Reducing cardiac workload
• Using diuretics to treat symptoms of fluid overload
• Supporting nutrition for maximal growth and development
• Providing cardiac surgery to repair the defect if it is progressing

Medications can be used to manage the symptoms of CHF. Medications include digoxin to strengthen the contractions of the heart, diuretics such as furosemide (potassium wasting) or chlorothiazide (potassium sparing) to increase urine output and reduce fluid overload. Drugs such as an ACE inhibitor (eg, captopril or enalapril) are potentially used to reduce the systemic resistance (ie, afterload) that the heart must pump against.

PATIENT TEACHING GUIDELINES

Digoxin Administration Guidelines for Parents Giving Home Medications

- Take the child's pulse for a full minute before giving a digoxin dose and if the pulse is lower than the specified rate for the child's age (ie, 90 bpm for infants) do not administer the dose. The cardiologist will determine the minimal heart rate for administration. Call the health-care provider before giving any medication if the heart rate is lower than the minimal specified rate.
- Administer digoxin every 12 hours.
- Watch closely for signs of digoxin toxicity or overdose. Notify the health-care provider immediately if any of the following signs are noted:
  - Decreased heart rate
  - Nausea and vomiting
  - Loss of appetite
- If a dose is missed, do not give an extra dose or increase the dose.
- If the dose is vomited, do not repeat.
- Give water after the dose to prevent tooth decay.
- Keep digoxin in a locked cabinet and in the original package.

Nursing Considerations for Congestive Heart Failure

Nursing considerations for a child with congestive heart disease include:

- Close monitoring of fluid and electrolyte levels, including an assessment of heart sounds, the presence of swelling, and lung sounds (eg, crackles or rales), all of which indicate increased lung congestion
- Observing for worsening CHF despite the current treatment plan
- Reducing the cardiac workload
- Providing supplemental oxygen as ordered
- Meticulous observations of daily weights

SAFETY *STAT!*

Whenever possible, an infant or a young child with CHF should be weighed on the same scale, without clothes or a diaper, to identify weight changes. Increasing weight indicates the child with CHF is retaining fluids, which causes further stress on the diseased heart.

Some children with heart failure, especially if the failure is from cardiomyopathy or congenital heart disease, require cardiac transplantation. The nursing interventions for cardiac transplantation include:

- Maintaining a plan of care per the health-care practitioner's order for pharmacological support, fluid and electrolyte management, and infection control
- Preparing for surgery and providing postoperative care
- Providing the child and family with developmentally appropriate and culturally and spiritually sensitive support
- Providing instructions on maintaining the essential medication regimen post-transplant
- Instructing the patient and family regarding signs and symptoms of organ rejection

Rheumatic Fever

Rheumatic fever is an inflammatory disease that affects children from 6 to 12 years of age. Rheumatic fever can occur after a throat infection or scarlet fever caused by *Streptococcus*. If a child is partially treated or untreated for these infections, rheumatic fever can result. The disease can cause permanent heart damage to heart valves; adequate treatment requires long-term antibiotic therapy.

Assessment of Rheumatic Fever

Presenting signs and symptoms of rheumatic fever include:

- A recent history of a respiratory infection
- Throat pain
- Nontender nodules under the skin over bony prominences
- Pink, flat, nonitching rashes on the trunk and the surfaces of the extremities next to the body that appear and disappear rapidly
- Enlarged joints that have painful swelling, indicating inflammatory changes; intermittent periods of pain that resolve without treatment and return to a different joint
- Cardiac changes, including an enlarged heart, tachycardia, changes in heart rhythm, a new heart murmur, chest pain, and faint heart sounds
- Fever
- Fatigue
- Poor appetite
- Intolerance to activity
- Neurological changes, including chorea (ie, involuntary muscle movements, weakness, involuntary facial motion, a labile emotional state, and random movements of the arms and legs)
- Irritability, behavioral issues, and decreased ability to concentrate

Interventions for Rheumatic Fever

Rheumatic fever can be prevented by mandating complete antibiotic treatment for streptococcal throat infections and scarlet fever. Management of the disease includes:

- Laboratory tests, including throat cultures and blood samples for an elevated or rising serum ASO titer, an elevated CRP level, and an ESR that reveals a response to inflammation

- 12-lead EKG
- Long-term treatment with penicillin or erythromycin

SAFETY *STAT!*

Parents need to understand the importance of long-term oral antibiotic therapy and that the medications to treat rheumatic fever can last from 5 to 18 years of age.

Nursing Considerations for Rheumatic Fever

Nursing considerations for the care of a child with rheumatic fever include:

- Assisting with procedures
- Providing developmentally appropriate patient education regarding treatments and disease management
- Reassuring the patient and family about the self-limiting nature of the chorea symptoms (ie, involuntary muscle movements, weakness, involuntary facial motion, a labile emotional state, and random movements of the arms and legs)
- Monitoring the heart rate, rhythm changes, and the presence of murmurs for cardiac decompensation
- Preparing for a surgical valve replacement and postoperative care
- Providing patient and family education regarding medical follow-up care
- Administering antibiotic therapy
- Providing patient and family education about completing the antibiotic therapy regimen as well as adhering to long-term medication, prophylactic antibiotics before dental work, and follow-up appointments every 5 years

Kawasaki's Disease

Kawasaki's disease is an inflammatory disease that affects the skin, mucous membranes, blood vessels, and lymph nodes. The disease occurs mainly in male children of Asian descent under the age of 6. The condition can affect children of all ages and races. The cause of Kawasaki's disease is unknown, but there may be an association with a viral or an autoimmune factor. Most children recover completely but will need medical follow-up to monitor for progressing intravascular inflammation. Inflammation of the coronary arteries (ie, blood vessels that supply the heart muscle itself) and aneurysms can result from the inflammation and cause significant complications. Healing and recovery from Kawasaki's disease may take weeks.

Assessment of Kawasaki's Disease

Signs and symptoms of this disease include:

- A high, persistent fever of 38.9°C to 40°C that lasts 5 days or longer and that may not respond to antipyretics such as acetaminophen or ibuprofen

- Extremely red and swollen eyes without drainage
- Skin and mucous membrane changes such as red membranes in the mouth; dry, cracked, red lips; a bright red tongue (ie, strawberry tongue) with a white coating; red and peeling skin on the genitalia, hands, and soles of the feet; and flat rashes on the trunk
- Joint changes, including painful, swollen hands and feet on both sides of the body
- Swollen lymph nodes (or sometimes a solitary node) in the neck
- Potentially, associated symptoms of irritability, cough, runny nose, diarrhea, vomiting, and abdominal pain

Interventions for Kawasaki's Disease

Treatment for Kawasaki's disease involves the immediate administration of IV gamma immunoglobulin (IVIG). Significant improvement is usually seen within 24 hours. Aspirin therapy is also used.

SAFETY *STAT!*

In general, children should not be given aspirin because of the association with Reye's syndrome. Kawasaki's disease is one of the only conditions in which a child receives aspirin therapy.

Nursing Considerations for Kawasaki's Disease

Care for a child who presents with Kawasaki's disease includes the following:

- Monitoring for signs of developing coronary artery inflammation, myocarditis, pericarditis, meningitis, and arthritis
- Administration and maintenance of IVIG therapy
- Pain management
- Developmentally appropriate patient and family teaching related to Kawasaki's disease and treatment
- Administration of high-dose aspirin therapy for anti-inflammatory and blood-thinning action

If recognized and treated early, children can recover fully from Kawasaki's disease, but a small number do succumb to the disease and some develop coronary artery disease anyway. Because of this, follow-up care with an echocardiogram every 1 to 2 years is recommended.

SAFETY *STAT!*

Children who have been diagnosed with Kawasaki's disease need to have scheduled follow-up appointments. Parents need to understand the importance of these subsequent appointments to monitor heart function.

Subacute Bacterial Endocarditis

SBE is an infection in the lining of the heart. Early diagnosis, while the symptoms are subtle and relatively mild (ie, suba-cute), is important to prevent severe disease. The cause of bacterial endocarditis is turbulent blood flow or other factors that damage the lining of the heart, which allows circulating bacteria, inflammatory cells, and clots to adhere to that area and proliferate. A few strains of streptococci and staphylo-cocci are common infectious organisms.

Assessment of Subacute Bacterial Endocarditis

Risk factors for SBE include the following:

- Congenital cyanotic heart disease
- The presence of central venous catheters
- IV medication use
- Residual postoperative defect or cardiac catheterization
- Rheumatic fever (ie, *Streptococcus* infection)

Interventions for Subacute Bacterial Endocarditis

If the infection is caught early and the bacterial infection is sensitive to treatment by penicillin, then the cure rate is almost 100%. If diagnosed late or if the infection is not sensitive to treatment by penicillin, the mortality rate is up to 25%. This makes preventative measures in susceptible children a high priority. Preventive antibiotic therapy before invasive proce-dures and dental work is essential.

The primary symptoms of SBE, which are flu-like symp-toms that last more than 2 weeks, are more common in those with heart defects.

This contrasts with acute bacterial endocarditis, which is more common in those with a normal heart configura-tion. Patients with acute bacterial endocarditis typically present with the following symptoms, which last less than 2 weeks:

- Fever
- Fatigue, sweats, chills, loss of appetite, joint pain, confu-sion, headache, malaise, and cough
- May have a positive history of IV drug use

Nursing Considerations for Subacute Bacterial Endocarditis

Nursing considerations for children at risk for SBE are:

- Administering IV antibiotics for about 8 weeks to treat SBE
- Providing developmentally appropriate patient and family teaching for mandated antibiotic prophylaxis for dental and surgical procedures that involve the respiratory and gastrointestinal mucosa
- Teaching the patient and family about the prophylactic administration of antibiotic therapy
- Providing patient and family teaching about the signs and symptoms of SBE and the need to contact the health-care provider immediately if SBE is suspected

SAFETY *STAT!*

It is imperative to reinforce teaching for parents about pro-phylaxis oral antibiotic therapy before dental procedures. The family must contact their pediatric health-care provider ahead of time to ensure that a prescription for antibiotics can be obtained and filled before dental cleaning or procedures take place. Stored antibiotics might expire; therefore a new prescription should be requested.

Key Points

- A nurse practicing in the pediatric specialty will come into contact with children with cardiac conditions intermittently and will care for children who have cardiac compromise related to other disease processes frequently. Overall, the development of a pediatric cardiac anomaly is rare.
- There is a direct relationship between the pulmonary sys-tem and the cardiovascular system. Without an effectively functioning heart, the oxygenation process carried out by the lungs will not be effectively distributed.
- Congenital heart defects are categorized into two large groups: those that produce cyanosis (ie, right-to-left shunt-ing) and those that do not produce cyanosis (ie, acyanotic left-to-right shunting).
- Children will also present with infectious processes within the cardiovascular system. These include Kawasaki's dis-ease, SBE, and rheumatic fever.
- CHF is a major complication of cardiac disease. Gener-ally, if CHF develops before 1 year of age, it is because of a congenital defect. If CHF develops after 1 year of age, the etiology is most likely from an acquired cause.

- The cardinal signs of CHF in children with cardiac condi-tions include tachycardia, cardiomegaly, tachypnea, and hepatomegaly.
- Culture has implications for the nursing care of children with a cardiac condition. When families are faced with the devastating news that their child has heart disease, either congenital or acquired, it is no surprise that cultural practices can affect all aspects of care from the onset of symptoms to long-term care requirements. Perceptions on causes of illness and how to care for the child are influenced by the family's culture.
- Educating parents about the care of their child with a car-diac infection or anomaly is very important to maintain safety. Correct medication administration, adequate caloric intake, and prevention of infections are all important areas of nursing education.
- A holistic approach to nursing care, with awareness of the developmental tasks and emotional and social needs of the child and family, will positively affect the quality of life for patients with heart disease.

REVIEW QUESTIONS

1. A 22-month-old toddler squats intermittently when walking. She is irritable, cyanotic, and is now appearing listless and progressively more unresponsive. The most likely cardiac malformation is
   1. Tricuspid atresia
   2. TGA
   3. TOF
   4. Pulmonary stenosis

2. Oxygenated blood mixes in the fetal heart through a shunt between the pulmonary artery and the aorta. What is the name of the shunt?
   1. Hepato-aortic shunt
   2. Ductus arteriosus
   3. Ductus venosus
   4. Foramen ovale

3. Select the disease state that increases the risk of delivering a baby with a congenital heart defect.
   1. Chronic hypertension
   2. Anorexia
   3. Diabetes
   4. Renal disease

4. Which of the following cardiac conditions found in children arise from malformations in the fetal development of the heart?
   1. Rheumatic heart disease
   2. Congestive heart disease
   3. TGA
   4. Hypoxemia

5. A 7-year-old boy has returned from a cardiac catheterization. Postoperative nursing interventions include: *(select all that apply)*
   1. Assessing pulses for symmetry and strength
   2. Assuring continuous cardiac monitoring and pulse oximetry to monitor for dysrhythmias, bradycardia, hypotension, hypoxia, and hypoxemia
   3. Maintaining the affected extremity in a flat position for 4 to 8 hours to prevent postprocedure bleeding
   4. Checking for allergies to shellfish and/or iodine
   5. Assessing I&O closely for sufficient urinary output, dehydration, or hypovolemia
   6. Assessing for the pain level using a developmentally appropriate tool for the age of the child

6. A term newborn is diagnosed with TGA. Which priority nursing intervention should be instituted immediately?
   1. Administering an echocardiogram
   2. Providing oxygen via nasal cannula at 2 liters per minute
   3. Preparing for intubation and placement on a ventilator
   4. Establishing IV access and initiating a PGE1 drip

7. When assessing the conduction system of the heart by looking at an EKG strip, the P wave indicates that which of the following areas in the heart has fired an electrical impulse?
   1. Purkinje's fibers
   2. AV node
   3. Bundle of His
   4. SA node

8. Pediatric heart failure is most common in infants with congenital heart disease but can present in older children because of which of the following:
   1. Myocarditis
   2. Excessive exercise and a thin body frame
   3. Rhinovirus infections
   4. Severe nausea and vomiting

9. Coarctation of the aorta causes the infant to struggle to feed because of shortness of breath. The cause of the shortness of breath is directly related to the infant's lung's inability to ventilate and provide the body with oxygen.
   1. True
   2. False

10. You must take a pulse for a full minute before giving a digoxin dose, and if the pulse is lower than the specified rate for the child's age (ie, 90 bpm or infants), the dose is administered because the medication is working.
    1. True
    2. False

CRITICAL THINKING QUESTIONS

1. Describe how neonatal cardiac blood flow shunts from left to right and right to left affect cardiac output and pulmonary blood flow, and what symptoms are associated with each circumstance.

2. Recall assessments for adequate tissue perfusion that reflect good cardiac function and compare this with poor tissue perfusion.

3. A 5-year-old, previously healthy boy is seen in the pediatrician's office with irritability; extremely red eyes; dry, cracked, red lips; red palms and soles of his feet; joint pain; and fever for a week. His heart rate is 118 bpm, and his blood pressure is 116/80 mm Hg. What diagnosis could be made and what nursing care should take priority?

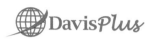

For additional resources and information, visit **www.DavisPlus.com.** Post-Conference Questions and Activities, Answers, and References can be found on DavisPlus.

Child With a Metabolic Condition

LEARNING OUTCOMES

1. Define the key terms.
2. Review the functions of the endocrine glands and the hormones secreted by each.
3. Discuss the location of each of the following endocrine gland: pituitary, thyroid, parathyroid, adrenal, pancreas, testes, and ovaries.
4. Analyze the effect of a metabolic disorder across the lifespan of a child including alterations in growth and development.
5. Review the complications associated with hyposecretion or hypersecretion of the various endocrine glands.
6. Differentiate the pathology between type 1 (ie, insulin-dependent DM) and type 2 (ie, non-insulin-dependent DM).
7. Review the various inborn errors of metabolism including the assessments, treatments, and nursing care associated with each.
8. Discuss the need for long-term care and follow-up for children who are diagnosed with a metabolic disorder.
9. State the conditions associated with the development of syndrome of inappropriate antidiuretic hormone (SIADH).
10. Recognize the need for rapid assessment and identification of a metabolic disorder during childhood to provide treatment that provides appropriate support for growth, metabolism, and nutrition for child health and development.

REAL-WORLD CASE STUDY

Valerie

■ A 3-year-old child was brought to the community pediatric clinic by her father. After being seen by a pediatrician, the child was immediately sent to a pediatric endocrinologist. The young girl presented with fine pubic hair and the father was concerned about her health. The endocrinologist performed a thorough health and physical assessment and could not find any further signs of early puberty. Laboratory evaluation was inconclusive for a medical diagnosis of precocious

continued on page 564

KEY TERMS

acanthosis nigricans
acromegaly
Cushing's syndrome
diabetes insipidus (DI)
diabetes mellitus (DM)
diabetic ketoacidosis (DKA)
exophthalmos
gigantism
glucagon
goiter
Graves' disease
Kussmaul's respirations
lipodystrophy
polydipsia
polyphagia
polyuria

DavisPlus For audio pronunciation guide, visit www.DavisPlus.com

CHAPTER CONCEPTS

Assessment
Development
Female Reproduction
Metabolism
Stress

puberty. Upon further discussion, the nurse heard the father tell the team that he rubs testosterone cream on his chest each night. Upon further questioning, the father stated he did not wash his hands and did indeed hold his daughter to his chest most nights during their playful bedtime ritual of reading, talking, and cuddling in bed.

1. What is the definition of precocious puberty?
2. What concerns does the team have about her early presentation of pubic hair?
3. What teaching components are needed from the pediatric health-care team to the father?

CONCEPTUAL CORNERSTONE

Metabolism

The concept of metabolism is very complex. The human body relies on a fine balance of hormones in very minute amounts to be accurately secreted from 10 endocrine glands. When balanced, the child should grow and develop as expected, experience puberty as expected, and be able to reproduce. Any disruption of this fine balance produces a host of complications, including disruptions in growth, energy, storage of glucose, fluid balance, responses to stressful stimuli, sodium and electrolyte balance, and sexual development. Medical science now provides advanced assessment techniques, advanced laboratory evaluations, and medical treatments through hormone replacement that have moved the field of endocrinology to advanced levels. Pediatric nurses work in teams to assist families in adjusting to hormone imbalances and endocrine dysfunctions.

The metabolic system includes seven endocrine glands: pituitary, thyroid, adrenal, parathyroid, testes, ovaries, and pancreas. Each of these glands has an important function to regulate various aspects of a child's growth and development, sexual reproduction, metabolism, fluid balance, and the body's response to stress stimuli. Hormones are secreted in very small amounts in the bloodstream but provide powerful metabolic regulation throughout the body. When the balance is off and there is hyposecretion or hypersecretion of hormones, endocrine dysfunction occurs and pathological conditions can develop.

ENDOCRINE GLANDS

The metabolic system is made up of several glands, each secreting hormones with a specific purpose to maintain the child's growth and development, sexual reproduction, metabolism, fluid status, and response to stress stimuli. There are 10 glands total, including the hypothalamus, thyroid, thymus,

adrenal, ovaries, testes, pancreas, parathyroid, pituitary, and pineal (Fig. 34.1).

The endocrine system has three parts: (1) the gland in which the hormone is produced; (2) the target cell where the chemical messenger (ie, the hormone) is needed; and (3) the transport system in which the chemical messenger (ie, the hormone) travels (ie, the blood). Each gland secretes minute amounts into the bloodstream to then influence the action of distance cells. Endocrine glands are found in many areas of the body.

Hormones are complex chemical substances released by endocrine glands that have a physiological controlling effect on other target cells all around the body. An integral system of feedback regulates the production and secretion of hormones based on the body's long-term needs (eg, growth) or short-term needs (eg, fluid balance). The pituitary is considered the master gland of the endocrine system.

Pituitary

The pituitary is a round, pea-size gland located in the brain; it is attached to the hypothalamus. The pituitary has an anterior and a posterior lobe. The pituitary's anterior pituitary lobe is often referred as the "master" gland as it controls the release of the other hormones from the endocrine glands located throughout the body. The pituitary secretes a number of hormones, each with an essential purpose.

• *Somatotropin* is a growth hormone that regulates bone and soft tissue growth and blood glucose.

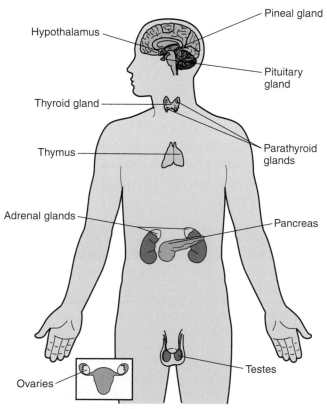

The Endocrine System

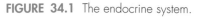

FIGURE 34.1 The endocrine system.

- *Follicle-stimulating hormone (FSH)* stimulates the secretion of estrogen and progesterone in females by the ovary, and stimulates the seminiferous tubules to produce sperm.
- *Luteinizing hormone (LH)* stimulates ovulation in females and the secretion of testosterone.
- *Gonadotropin hormone* stimulates the gonads to mature and produce sex hormones and germ cells.
- *Prolactin hormone* produces and maintains milk production after childbirth.
- *Thyroid-stimulating hormone (TSH)* stimulates the thyroid gland to synthesize and release thyroxine.
- *Adrenocorticotropic hormone (ACTH)* stimulates the adrenal cortex to convert cholesterol into adrenal steroids.
- *Melanocytes-stimulating hormone* promotes the skin's pigmentation.
- *Luteinizing-releasing hormones* stimulate the release of LH and FSH by the pituitary gland.
- *Oxytocin* is a hormone that stimulates uterine contractions and the let-down effect for breast milk release.
- *Antidiuretic hormone (ADH or desmopressin)* stimulates the kidneys to reabsorb water and sodium, causing the child's body to retain fluids.

One of the most common endocrine experiences of later childhood is puberty. If a young patient presents with evidence of early puberty, the medical diagnosis of precocious puberty may be made. Precocious puberty is caused by the premature release of gonadotropin hormones from the pituitary gland. This condition can also be related to an ovarian malignancy or other rare medical conditions in children.

SAFETY *STAT!*

When administering desmopressin to a child, such as when conducting a DDAVP challenge in which desmopressin is administered and monitored via serial blood levels to investigate the uptake, make sure they do not drink fluids for up to 6 hours after the medication is administered as they may experience overhydration and the dilution of serum electrolytes.

PATIENT TEACHING GUIDELINES

It is important to know that teens progress through puberty at variable rates. Some progress more slowly than others and this experience is not considered abnormal or part of a pathological situation. Pediatric nurses should explain this to both patients and their parents to reduce concerns and answer questions.

Thyroid

The thyroid gland is a reddish-brown soft mass with right and left lobes. It is located between the sides of the cricoids and thyroid cartilage at the sixth tracheal cartilage just posterior to the larynx. The thyroid gland secretes triiodothyronine (T_3), thyroxine (T_4), and calcitonin. The thyroid gland hormones help regulate blood calcium concentrations, and the processing of protein, fat, and carbohydrate catabolism. The thyroid gland has the major role of regulating the basal metabolic rate by influencing body heat, appetite, heart rate and cardiac output, and the utilization of oxygen and carbon dioxide.

Parathyroid

The parathyroid gland is located next to the thyroid gland. The main function of the parathyroid is to regulate and maintain calcium levels. The gland also influences potassium, phosphate, and magnesium levels in the body. The parathyroid gland secretes the parathyroid hormone (PTH). If there is an excess of PTH, hyperparathyroidism and hypocalcemia occur. If there is a deficiency of PTH, hypoparathyroidism occurs, leading to hypercalcemia.

Adrenal

The adrenal glands, located superior to the kidneys, are responsible for the production and release of substances called mineralocorticoids, also known as *aldosterone*. The adrenal glands also produce the three sex hormones: progesterone, estrogen, and androgens (such as testosterone). The sex hormones regulate the child's sexual maturity. The medulla of the adrenal gland produces epinephrine (ie, adrenalin) and norepinephrine for the child's stress response, as well as the glucocorticoids cortisol and corticosteroid.

SAFETY *STAT!*

If a child has adrenal gland dysfunction that leads to an overproduction of adrenalin, they may experience tachycardia, tremors, restlessness, hypertension, and nausea/vomiting.

Pancreas

The pancreas has many functions. The endocrine portion of the pancreas secretes the hormone insulin from the β cells located in the ductless cluster of islets of Langerhans; it also secretes the hormone **glucagon** from the α cells. Glucagon is stored in the liver and is used to regulate blood glucose levels should the child experience hypoglycemia. Damage to the α and β cells results in poor control of blood glucose. α and β cells have the following functions:

- **α *cells:*** α cells produce and secrete glucagon, which accelerates glycogenesis to increase blood glucose. Glucagon is considered an antagonist to the hormone insulin.
- **β *cells:*** β cells produce and secrete insulin, which promotes glucose, protein, and fatty acid transport into cells. β-cell secretions promote the movement of potassium and phosphate ions across cell membranes, carrying glucose molecules into cells.

Ovaries

Located in the pelvis below and the behind the fallopian tubes, the ovaries are the size of a large almond. The ovaries are the female gonad and are responsible for sexual reproduction. These gonads secrete progesterone and estrogen. Estrogen stimulates overall RNA and protein synthesis, pubic and axillary hair growth, breast development during puberty and pregnancy, and pelvic enlargement, and it promotes the epiphyseal closure of bones. Estrogen also causes fluid retention by influencing the action of the renal tubules to absorb more water and sodium. Progesterone helps prepare the uterus for a fertilized ovum. During pregnancy, progesterone helps to keep the uterine smooth muscle calm.

Testes

The testes are the male gonad and are responsible for reproduction and sexual maturity. The testes secrete testosterone, which stimulates the testes to produce spermatozoa, the closure of epiphysis, muscle development, body hair growth, and the enlargement of external genitalia. Located in the scrotum, the two testes each have, within its own compartment, ducts that emerge from the top of the gland and attach to the epididymis.

COMMON ENDOCRINE GLAND DISORDERS

When a gland experiences dysfunction, the body's metabolic status is interrupted. The pediatric nurse must be able to identify situations in which metabolic dysfunction is so rapid that treatment can begin. Even small disruptions in hormones secreted by the various glands can have a large effect on the child's homeostatic state.

Syndrome of Inappropriate Antidiuretic Hormone (SIADH)

When a child experiences shaken baby syndrome (SBS), head trauma, a brain tumor, brain surgery, or an infection of the brain, he or she is at risk for developing SIADH, which is a syndrome of inappropriate ADH. The overproduction and excretion of ADH from the posterior pituitary results in the kidneys absorbing more water, which results in decreased urine output and increased fluid retention. The child's fluid volume expands in the vessels and the extra fluid results in hyponatremia. Hyponatremia is the condition of diluted sodium concentrations within the blood. If the child experiences an insult to the brain, such as trauma or surgery, the fluid retention from SIADH can contribute to increased intracranial pressure, a dangerous condition that can be fatal.

Assessments of Syndrome of Inappropriate Antidiuretic Hormone

Assessments of SIADH include clinical symptoms of hyponatremia. Hyponatremia symptoms include weakness, confusion, and anorexia. Acute SIADH will also present with symptoms of fluid overload and decreased urine output. Checking for urine specific gravity may be required to identify the development of SIADH.

Interventions for Syndrome of Inappropriate Antidiuretic Hormone

Interventions for pediatric SIADH are aimed at controlling fluid retention and balancing low serum sodium levels. Treatments for SIADH include:

• Fluid restrictions
• The administration of IV solutions of 0.3% normal saline
• IV administrations of furosemide (Lasix)

Nursing Considerations for Syndrome of Inappropriate Antidiuretic Hormone

The nurse must be aware of the risk of developing SIADH. Any signs of fluid retention, reduced urine output, or changes in the child's neurological system should be reported to the appropriate primary care provider. The nurse must be able to identify symptoms of dilutional hyponatremia such as weakness and confusion. It is important that the nurse can distinguish between SIADH and **diabetes insipidus (DI).** In DI, the opposite of SIADH occurs. In DI, there is a reduced production of posterior pituitary secretion of SIADH and the child's urine has a very low specific gravity. DI causes the child to produce copious urine (ie, uncontrolled diuresis).

Deficient Anterior Pituitary Hormone: Pituitary Dwarfism

Pituitary dwarfism occurs in early in utero development, when the growing fetus's pituitary secretes too little quantity of growth hormone. The cause of dwarfism is unknown but may be related to lesions or trauma. When a child is born with dwarfism, the child will demonstrate growth with normal body proportions, but within a shorter overall stature. A child deficient in growth hormone typically demonstrates a growth pattern of less than 2 in. annually until the preschool period, when an even more apparent delayed growth is demonstrated. Because of the appearance associated with growth failure, young children may appear to be overweight. When growth hormone deficiency (GHD) is suspected, the child will have an analysis of his or her bone age (ie, an x-ray of wrist and hands), the blood serum level of growth hormone, and previous growth plots.

Assessments of Pituitary Dwarfism

As the child grows, he or she will appear younger than his or her age. Intelligence is normal with dwarfism and the child displays an expected mental age and cognitive processing. The child with dwarfism will have a delayed but normal development of puberty. Assessments include both a laboratory evaluation of GHD and radiographic evaluation of bone age.

Interventions for Pituitary Dwarfism

Dwarfism does not have any treatment that is considered 100% effective. Once diagnosed with GHD, the child will be given injections of human growth hormone. Some children will respond to this treatment and others will not. The earlier the treatments are started, the greater chance of response. Children need to be emotionally supported to embrace their size and be given positive reinforcement about their accomplishments.

Nursing Considerations for Pituitary Dwarfism

Nursing care of the child with pituitary dwarfism includes a thorough assessment for dental anomalies because the child's jaw may have growth retardation. This delay leads to challenges in the permanent teeth's eruption. The child and family will need emotional support to help cope with the dwarfism state. The pediatric nurse should provide information about local and national support groups and information about dwarf-related growth patterns. (Further information can be found at the Human Growth Foundation and the MAGIC Foundation.)

THERAPEUTIC COMMUNICATION

Parents of children with growth hormone deficiencies may be very stressed and emotional. The nurse should provide therapeutic communication to support the feelings of the family and diffuse the fears. Acknowledge the parents' fears and worries, reinforce teaching about medical advances and hormone replacement, and reassure the parents that their child will be followed closely, but will grow, develop, and thrive.

Hypersecretion of Anterior Pituitary Hormone: Gigantism

Gigantism is a condition of high linear bone growth that results from the excessive production and secretion of insulin-like growth factor (IGF-1). The clinical presentation of hypersecretion of the anterior pituitary hormone results in gigantism (ie, large overall size) or **acromegaly** (ie, long extremities). The pituitary cells may have experienced hyperplasia or a pituitary tumor may be present. The disease of acromegaly is severe, is often diagnosed late, and has complications associated with cerebrovascular, respiratory, and cardiovascular disease. Bone malignancies are also associated with this condition.

Assessments of Gigantism

If the hypersecretion of the anterior pituitary gland occurs after the child's epiphyseal growth plate has sealed, then the symptoms may manifest as enlarged hands, feet, jaw, tongue, and nose. The child may also present with thickening of the skin on the body and coarseness of the facial features. The condition is complex and is also associated with:

- Mild to moderate obesity
- Visual changes
- Soft-tissue hypertrophy
- Peripheral neuropathies, such as carpel tunnel syndrome
- Osteoarthritis
- Endocrinopathies
- Headaches
- Oily skin and acne
- Excessive sweating

Interventions for Gigantism

After laboratory studies are conducted to diagnose growth hormone excess, other tests include magnetic resonance imaging (MRI) to assess the pituitary gland for adenomas, and x-rays to assess the severity of skeletal malformation. There is no single treatment for gigantism or for the complication of acromegaly. Surgical interventions for pituitary adenomas may be required and research continues on medications for growth hormone excess.

Nursing Considerations for Gigantism

Nursing care of the child with gigantism includes psychological support for possible altered body image. The child will be dealing with an overall larger size than expected and will be larger than his or her peers, or he or she may have larger sizes of certain body parts. As the child enters the preteen and teenage years, extra support is needed to cope with the features and overall presentation.

Hyposecretion of Thyroid Gland Hormone

A child's basal metabolism rate is regulated by the hormones secreted by the thyroid gland. The thyroid depends on a consistent source of dietary iodine and tyrosine. Hypothyroidism can be congenital and can be caused by a spontaneous gene mutation. Children whose diets or drinking water are deficient of iodine are at risk for developing hypothyroidism. Hypothyroidism may also be caused by decreased gland development over childhood or from medications that suppress the production of thyroid hormones. This condition occurs in approximately 1:4,000 live births and is two times more common in girls. Congenital hypothyroidism, which is present at birth, will progress to cognitive impairment if not identified and treated early.

Assessments of Hypothyroidism

The child should be assessed for an enlarged tongue; short, thick neck; short stature; and possible hypotonia. For acquired hypothyroidism, the child should be assessed for the presence of a **goiter** (ie, an enlargement of the thyroid gland) as well as for signs and symptoms of a slowed metabolic rate, including:

- Hypothermic skin temperatures
- Slow pulse
- Easy weight gain
- Decreased appetite
- Constipation
- Unexpected tiredness and fatigue
- Delayed mental processing
- Decreased perspiration on exertion

Assessment for hypothyroidism occurs during state-mandated routine neonatal screenings of T_4. The optimal time for screening is between 2 and 6 days of life via a heelstick. Early testing is problematic as an early test may demonstrate a falsely high TSH level. There is a natural increase in TSH shortly after birth. If the T_4 level is found to be decreased, then the child's TSH level should be drawn. A T_4 level under 3 mcg/100 mL and a TSH level greater than 40 mcg/100 mL are considered indicative of primary hypothyroidism.

Priority nursing diagnoses for a child with hypothyroidism include constipation, fatigue, a risk for altered health maintenance, hypothermia, and altered nutrition (less than body requirements).

Interventions for Hypothyroidism

Treatment for hypothyroidism includes following the child's T_3 and T_4 blood levels and appropriately administering thyroxine and thyroid hormones as replacement for low blood levels. The child should have a source of vitamin D as part of the treatment.

Nursing Considerations for Hypothyroidism

Nursing care for the child with hypothyroidism should focus on teaching the family that medication compliance for life is essential, and that regular checkups and blood levels are important for the child's care. The child will be placed on a thyroid hormone replacement therapy such as levothyroxine (Synthroid, Levothroid). These medications can be crushed and placed in a small amount of formula, food, or water.

Hyperthyroidism

When the thyroid hormone levels are increased, the child will be diagnosed with hyperthyroidism. One form of hyperthyroidism is an autoimmune destruction of the gland called *Graves' disease.* The highest incidence of Graves' disease is found in adolescent girls, but it may be found in young children if their mother has Graves' disease. The female-to-male ratio for the development of Graves' disease is 4:1. Signs of Graves' disease include an increased production of T_4, enlargement of the thyroid gland, and ocular signs, including protrusion, stare, and eyelid lag.

Assessments of Hyperthyroidism

The assessment of hyperthyroidism includes screening for T_3 and T_4 blood serum levels. Clinical signs and symptoms include tremor, muscle weakness, nervousness, irritability, fatigue, weight loss, diarrhea, excessive perspiration, and protrusion of the eyeballs called *exophthalmos.* The child may present with a nontender enlarged thyroid gland called a *goiter.* Many children experience heat intolerance, sweating, and weight loss despite increased appetite.

SAFETY *STAT!*

Newborns undergo blood screening for inborn errors of metabolism. Blood screening should not take place after 24 hours because there is a natural rise in TSH.

Interventions for Hyperthyroidism

Medications for hyperthyroidism are focused on decreasing and limiting the thyroid gland's secretion of thyroid hormone.

Medications include propylthiouracil or methimazole (Tapazole). If the child demonstrates a "thyroid storm," which is a state of excessively high levels of thyroid hormone, the child may require the administration of a β-adrenergic blocking agent such as propranolol to reduce the symptoms of adrenergic hyper-responsiveness.

Nursing Considerations for Hyperthyroidism

Nursing care includes teaching the family that the child may display an inability to stay seated at school, a short attention span, and problems with academic success. The family needs to understand that medication therapy will be started to decrease the secretion of the thyroid hormone and will be required for the rest of the child's life. Because of the increased metabolism, the family should be encouraged to provide the child with five meals a day that are high in protein and calories. Body weight should be monitored on a regular basis. If the child has gastrointestinal complaints such as cramping and frequent defecation, supportive care such as effective comfort means should be presented. If the child's condition is severe and there is eye protrusion, the family must be taught how to instill moistening drops (gtt is the unit of measurement in drops) into the conjunctiva.

SAFETY *STAT!*

If a child with hyperthyroidism is demonstrating significant eye protrusion, the family must be taught how to safely prevent eye injury. The eyes must be kept moist and the child needs to wear protective eyewear and sunglasses.

Hyperfunction of the Adrenal Gland: Cushing's Syndrome

Cushing's syndrome, also called *hyperadrenocorticism,* occurs when there is an overproduction and a hypersecretion of adrenal hormones, leading to a prolonged exposure to corticoid hormones. High levels of cortisol are produced, which result in a decreased secretion of ACTH. Cushing's syndrome is often associated with a tumor growth in the adrenal gland, or with the excessive or prolonged use of corticosteroids for the management of inflammatory illnesses.

Assessments of Cushing's Syndrome

The patient with hyperfunction of the adrenal gland is assessed for evidence of hypersecretion of the adrenal gland hormones, including:

- Central obesity (ie, adipose tissue on the chest, face, and abdomen)
- Decreased glucose tolerance
- Poor wound healing
- Muscle weakness and atrophy from increased glucogenesis
- Easy bruising
- Osteoporosis
- Acne
- Hirsutism (ie, abnormal amounts of facial hair)

- Hypertension
- Mood disorder
- Decreased linear growth

Interventions for Cushing's Syndrome

With the chronic use of steroid hormones, a gradual tapering down and discontinuing of the medication may improve the syndrome. Surgery may be required if there is an adenoma that causes the syndrome. Before the child or teen has surgery, the medical team may prescribe medications that inhibit cortisol production, such as mitotane, along with medications that help to reduce the side effects of high blood pressure and high blood glucose.

TEAM WORKS

Many team members are required to care for a child with a new diagnosis of type 1 DM. The following list demonstrates typical team membership:

- Endocrinologist
- Nutritionist
- Diabetic Educator
- Diabetic Nurse Practitioner
- Hospital Staff Nurse
- Endocrinology Clinic Staff
- Child Life
- School Nurse
- School Teacher
- School Administrator

Nursing Considerations for Cushing's Syndrome

Nursing care includes ensuring that there is an order for slowly tapering corticosteroids if the child is on these medications. Fast withdrawal or abrupt discontinuation of corticosteroids results in Cushing's syndrome. The nurse should also be aware of the need to help the child's immune function and should monitor the child for the development of infections. Families need to understand that mood swings are expected with the hypersecretion of ACTH and that the mood disorder may last weeks to months after treatment is discontinued.

DISEASE PROCESSES OF THE METABOLIC SYSTEM

The metabolic system is associated with several complex disease processes. Because the metabolic system is made up of many glands with various essential functions, disease of any one of the glands can interfere with the child's growth, nutrient metabolism, body temperature, sexual maturity and function, and sense of well-being. The two common pathologies are type 1 and type 2 diabetes.

Type 1 Diabetes Mellitus

Previously called *juvenile diabetes,* type 1 **diabetes mellitus (DM)** is a chronic metabolic disorder marked by hyperglycemia.

In type 1 DM, no insulin is produced. Insulin, the essential hormone produced by the β cells, allows glucose to enter into cells for energy, growth, and all types of cellular function. Insulin is essential for life.

Type 1 DM is classified as insulin-dependent because the child requires daily and lifelong insulin injections or the use of an insulin pump. Most commonly diagnosed between 10 and 14 years of age, type 1 DM can be diagnosed anytime between infancy through young adulthood. The incidence rate of type 1 DM is 15 per 100,000 people in North America, with a peak onset of 10 to 12 years of age for girls and 12 to 14 years of age for boys. Type 1 DM is only now being surpassed by type 2, non-insulin-dependent DM (NIDDM) because of increasing rates of childhood obesity.

There is a genetic association with the human leukocytic antigen in approximately 20% of cases. Further etiologies for type 1 DM include an autoimmune response or an environmental factor that includes an exposure to a significant viral infection.

Type 1 insulin-dependent DM is caused by an autoimmune attack on the β cells of the pancreas. This may occur approximately 1 week after a significant immune insult, such as an upper respiratory illness. Autoantibodies, which cause β cell destruction, have been found to be present as long as 9 years before the clinical symptoms of type 1 DM start. As the child's body begins to starve for glucose, fatty acids from converted triglycerides are created, forming ketones. The presence of ketones denotes metabolic acidosis.

The child often first presents with **diabetic ketoacidosis (DKA)** when the diagnosis of type 1 DM occurs. DKA is a dangerous toxic state that requires intensive care. A lack of available glucose to the body's cells results in adipose and muscle tissues being broken down to make glucose available for energy use. As the fats are converting to energy, the liver produces a byproduct of ketones. Ketones cannot be used by the cells in the absence of glucose, so ketones accumulate in the body, spilling into urine, and cause a metabolic acidotic state. The child's body will attempt to compensate by ridding the body of ketones through excreting more carbon dioxide through the respiratory system. The increased depth and rate of respirations is called *Kussmaul's respirations.* As the body loses its ability to compensate and ketones continue to increase, the child experiences severe dehydration, severe acute renal failure, and eventually coma and death. DKA must be managed by a health-care team within an intensive care environment. Serum potassium levels, pH, PO_2, PCO_2, and blood urea nitrogen are all followed closely to evaluate the management of DKA. Children typically present with very high blood glucose levels when they have developed DKA. A minimal level would be greater than 200 mg/dL, but most of the time the child presents with blood sugars much higher.

One of the greatest concerns for a child with type 1 DM is the severe experience of low blood sugar, hypoglycemia, because severely low blood sugar can be dangerous and even lethal.

HEALTH PROMOTION

Avoiding Hypoglycemia

Hypoglycemia is defined as a blood glucose level of less than 70 mg/dL (American Diabetes Association [ADA], 2009). Note the following information related to hypoglycemia:

- May be caused by too much insulin administered or from not eating enough
- Occurs anytime in the life of a child with DM
- Symptoms develop rapidly and need to be identified quickly for treatment
- Can be life-threatening because of a lack of or a very decreased level of blood glucose to brain tissues
- The child needs to have a standard protocol for hospitalization, home, and school experiences
- Hospitalized patients may experience severe hypoglycemia with:
  - NPO status
  - Reduced oral intake because of illness or surgery
  - Discontinuation of enteral feedings
  - Insulin given with meal followed by a subsequent lack of oral intake or food
  - A rapid transport of a hospitalized child who needs a diagnostic examination before the child has chance to finish the meal, leaving too much insulin circulating for a too small amount of food intake
  - A sudden reduction in oral or IV corticosteroid therapy

Treatment for hypoglycemia includes:

- Rapidly administering 15 to 20 g of a carbohydrate
- Reassessing the child's blood glucose within 15 min
- Giving second dose of carbohydrates if needed
- Monitoring the child's vital signs
- Keeping the child quiet and supervising the him constantly until his blood glucose level is stable
- If the child has a decreased level of consciousness, giving dextrose 50% via IV per ordered and following up with IV glucagon if ordered

Assessments of Type 1 Diabetes Mellitus

Assessments of type 1 DM are multifold and include a variety of clinical presentations within different body systems. The pediatric nurse needs to assess all body systems if type 1 DM is suspected. Assessments for type 1 DM include the following:

- Excessive blood glucose leading to glycosuria (occurs when blood glucose levels exceed the renal threshold of 160 mg/dL)
- Elevated 8-hour fasting blood glucose levels
- Osmotic diuresis with the presence of high blood glucose, leading to large amounts of urine, dehydration, hypotension, and eventual kidney shutdown
- Excessive hunger (ie, **polyphagia**), increased and excessive thirst (ie, **polydipsia**), and excessive urination (ie, **polyuria**)
- Thin appearance; may look malnourished and complains of feeling fatigued

- Fruity breath
- Dry and flushed skin
- Blurred vision
- Yeast infections in females
- Confusion

A diagnosis of type 1 DM consists of one serum blood plasma glucose level of greater than 200 mg/dL or two blood plasma glucose levels of greater than 126 mg/dL. An insulin-dependent child with diabetes who is experiencing an illness or experiencing stress can have hyperglycemia and may need to have their insulin temporarily adjusted.

Interventions for Type 1 Diabetes Mellitus

Treatment of type 1 insulin-dependent DM consists of care priorities. The first priority is to assess for and treat DKA. This requires that the child's acidotic metabolic state be stabilized and serum electrolytes be normalized. Typically, a child with DKA presents to the emergency room and then is rapidly transferred to the pediatric intensive care unit for close monitoring and treatment. The child is treated with normal saline boluses until the blood glucose level is at 250 to 300 mg/dL, and then IVF are switched to D51/2ns to prevent hypoglycemia rebound. Insulin infusion (ie, insulin drip) is initiated and titrated to prevent the blood glucose level from dropping more than 50 mg/dL per hour.

After stabilization, the child is then weaned from IV regular insulin to subcutaneous injections before being transferred to the pediatric unit for intensive family teaching about managing diabetes. Under no circumstances should the child receive IV solutions with potassium until the child's urine output is well-established. Adding potassium supplementation to the IV puts the child with an already existing electrolyte imbalance at risk for hyperkalemia and possible heart arrhythmias. Specific care protocols will exist (often stored electronically) at each health-care institution to rapidly guide the health-care team in treating a child's DKA state.

Nursing Considerations for Type 1 Diabetes Mellitus

After the first priority of stabilizing the DKA is performed, the next priority is to engage the family in the child's care by having them check the child's blood glucose and draw up the insulin. Teaching should begin right away and must include all members of the child's family. The Drug Facts feature lists typical insulins that can be ordered for a child with type 1 DM. See the Patient Teaching Guidelines feature for a teaching plan for a newly diagnosed child with type 1 DM and a summary of a nursing process for a newly diagnosed child with type 1 DM.

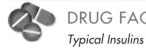 **DRUG FACTS**

Typical Insulins

- Lispro (Humalog) is a rapid-acting, clear insulin with an onset of 5 to 15 min, a peak of 30 to 90 min, and a duration of less than 4 hours.

- Regular insulin is a short-acting, clear insulin with an onset of 30 min, a peak of 2 to 3 hours, and a duration of 6 to 8 hours.
- Neutral protamine Hagedorn (NPH) (Humulin) is an intermediate-acting, cloudy insulin with an onset of 1 to 2 hours, a peak of 6 to 12 hours, and a duration of 18 to 26 hours.
- Glargine (Lantus) is a long-acting, clear insulin used for basal needs only with an onset of 4 to 6 hours, a peak of 14 to 24 hours, and a duration of 28 to 36 hours.

PATIENT TEACHING GUIDELINES

Patient and Family Teaching for a Child Newly Diagnosed With Type 1 Diabetes Mellitus

Mixing Insulins

1. Draw up the clear insulin in an insulin syringe first, and then draw up the cloudy insulin so that the clear insulin does not appear contaminated with the cloudy insulin if any enters the clear insulin vial.
2. Do not shake any vials of insulin. Gently rotate the vial in your hand and treat it carefully. The amino acid chains can break with vigorous handling.
3. Rotate the child's injection sites to prevent **lipodystrophy** (ie, a complication of insulin injections where there is a change of subcutaneous fat under the skin; either atrophy or hypertrophy). Include the child in the process of selecting sites.
4. Make sure the child has eaten before the injected insulin peaks. This is especially important if the treatment plan includes a rapid-acting insulin such as lispro.
5. Seek the assistance of the primary care provider to adjust the insulins if the child is sick, stressed, is starting a new exercise plan, or is experiencing a growth spurt. More or less insulin may be required.
6. Insulins may be given by a specific insulin syringe and needle, an insulin pen with adjustable quantities for injection, or a subcutaneous insulin pump.
7. Do not mix rapid-acting insulin lispro (Humalog) into the same syringe with long-acting insulin glargine (Lantus).

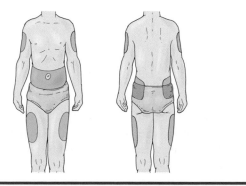

Nursing care for a child with a new diagnosis of insulin-dependent type 1 DM consists of the following:

- In the early stages of diagnosis and care, the child must have his or her blood glucose checked qid with a home blood glucose monitor (Fig. 34.2).

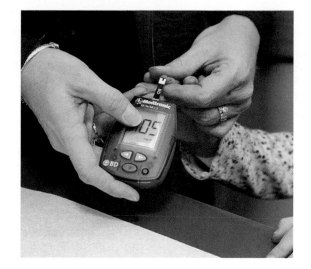

FIGURE 34.2 Blood glucose monitor for home use.

- The pediatric endocrinologist will follow the child's case closely for several weeks after the initial diagnosis and will adjust the child's rapid-acting and long-acting insulins for the best control. Meticulous documentation by the nursing staff of all blood glucose checks and insulin administration, including the site, is essential.
- Carbohydrate counting for all meals and snacks is now the universal gold standard. Carbohydrate counting should begin immediately and should involve the child and family in the food selections, as well as in calculating the total carbohydrates per meal or snack. The child's rapid-acting insulin will be calculated based on the total amount of carbohydrates the child anticipates eating and is typically one unit of rapid-acting insulin for every 15 to 30 g of carbohydrates.
- Insulin pumps may be used after the child's diabetes is well-controlled with injections (Fig. 34.3).

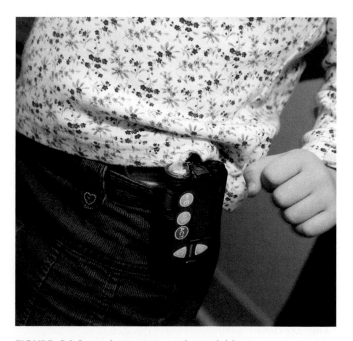

FIGURE 34.3 Insulin pump worn by a child.

- Long-term control and compliance with blood glucose monitoring and injections is monitored by blood levels of hemoglobin A1c (HbA1c). This laboratory value measures the average amounts of blood glucose over 90 days, with the goal being an HbA1c level set by the child's specific age.

The child's digestive system converts carbohydrates (CHO) into glucose (ie, blood sugar). Usually, as the blood sugar rises, the pancreas secretes more insulin. In type 1 diabetes, the child lacks insulin, which requires him or her to reduce carbohydrate intake. Carbohydrate counting is an important tool to determine how much insulin a child will need to take and is an important means of reducing spikes in blood glucose. Almost 100% of carbohydrates consumed rapidly becomes blood glucose. Carbohydrate counting is a meal-planning approach to reduce postprandial (ie, after meals) glycemia responses.

Foods high in carbohydrates include the following:

- Breads, pastas, cereals, and grains
- Rice, starchy vegetables, beans, corn, peas, and potatoes
- Fruit, fruit juices, and fruit smoothies
- Milk and flavored yogurts
- Candy, soda, jelly, cakes, and cookies

The grams per category of food are the following:

- One fruit serving = 15 g of CHO
- One milk serving = 12 g of CHO
- One starch serving = 15 g of CHO
- One vegetable (nonstarchy) = 5 g of CHO

Most children should have a goal of 45 to 60 g of carbohydrates per meal, with each 15 g of carbohydrates requiring one unit of regular or rapid-acting insulin (to be determined by the endocrinologist and catered individually for each child). Families must be taught to read food labels and predetermine what a child's meal CHO component will be.

- Age 0 to 3: Daily goal is 210 g of CHO
- Age 4 to 7: Daily goal is 240 g of CHO
- Age 8 to 12: Daily goal is 270 g of CHO
- Girls age 13 to 17: Daily goal is 255 g of CHO
- Boys age 13 to 17: Daily goal is 300 g of CHO
  (Source: Dartmouth-Hitchcock Children's Hospital at Dartmouth)

The following organizations provide online sites for carbohydrate counting assistance:

- Children With Diabetes: A Resource Guide for Families and Schools (www. http://www.health.ny.gov/publications/0944.pdf)
- Cultural and Ethnic Foods and Nutrition Education Materials (https://fnic.nal.usda.gov/sites/fnic.nal.usda.gov/files/uploads/ethnic.pdf)
- Diapedia (www.diapedia.com)

LABS & DIAGNOSTICS

Understanding Hemoglobin A1c

Hemoglobin A1c is a measure of glycosylated hemoglobin. It is followed as a routine check of the overall blood glucose level during the previous 90 days.

Blood Serum Values: (according to the DCCT % known as the Diabetes Control and Complications Trial)

- Less than 6 years old: 7.5 to 8.5 DCCT %
- 6 to 12 years old: Less than 8 DCCT %
- 13 to 19 years old: Less than 7.5 DCCT %

Teaching is the most important part of caring for a child with diabetes. Families need to be taught to safeguard their child from periods of hyperglycemia and hypoglycemia. Hypoglycemia is dangerous and symptoms of this condition must be acted upon immediately. See the Patient Teaching Guidelines feature for a summary of symptoms of hyperglycemia and hypoglycemia. The child should always wear a medical alert bracelet so that if hypoglycemia or hyperglycemia occurs, the condition can be identified and help can be summoned quickly.

Families need to understand the phenomenon of the "honeymoon phase" that can occur shortly after a child is diagnosed. They need to understand that even though there may be a short period of time when the pancreas produces a small amount of insulin after the DKA is resolved, the child will need insulin injections for life. When a child is diagnosed with type 1 insulin-dependent diabetes, a "honeymoon phase" may occur as the remaining functioning insulin-secreting cells of the pancreas attempt to provide adequate amounts of insulin. Typically, 90% of these cells are destroyed, and the remaining 10% are stimulated to produce insulin. The child demonstrates a period of time where blood glucose levels are moderately controlled. When the remaining percentage of cells suffers damage or auto-destruction, the child's blood glucose levels rise again. It is important for families to understand that both hypoglycemia and hyperglycemia are concerns. The pediatric nurse should teach the family how to recognize values that are associated with each, what causes the values and what the symptoms are for each. Table 34.1 provides information about what is important for families to understand about hypoglycemia and hyperglycemia.

Complications related to type 1 insulin-dependent DM should be discussed and include the following:

- A life expectancy shortened by up to one-third
- Nephropathy (ie, kidney disease) as the primary cause of death
- Comorbidities that include renal failure, premature atherosclerosis, heart disease, and stroke
- Retinopathy, which commonly develops sometime during the lifespan
- Poor wound healing that requires specialists to intervene

TABLE 34.1 CHARACTERISTICS OF HYPOGLYCEMIA AND HYPERGLYCEMIA

	Hyperglycemia	Hypoglycemia
Blood Glucose Range	Greater than 200–250 mg/dL	Less than 70 mg/dL
Blood pH	Greater than 7.2	Normal
Causes	Injecting too little insulin	Eating too little, eating later than usual, more exercise than usual, illness or injury or stress, medication interaction
Symptoms	Fatigue Flushed appearance to skin Dry skin Dehydration Polyuria Polyphagia Ketones in urine Dark-colored urine	Pale Diaphoresis (ie, sweaty) Confusion Slow thinking Decreased level of consciousness Tremors Poor coordination Dizziness Weakness Nervousness Irrational behavior/personality change Blurred vision
Interventions	Give rapid-acting insulin such as lispro, as ordered Provide fluids Do not add potassium until urine output is restored	Give a fast-acting source of carbohydrate Give 4 ounces of orange juice Give 4 ounces of apple juice Give a small gel tube of cake icing Give an over-the-counter glucose product made for a child with diabetes

Families need to understand that diabetes is a labor-intensive and lifelong chronic illness that is best managed by competent family members at home with the support of a specialized health-care team. See the Patient Teaching Guidelines feature for information about instructing a family with a child newly diagnosed with diabetes. Managing a chronic disorder from early childhood on can be a significant stressor and families need support to be successful. The Team Works feature provides a list of national organizations for childhood diabetes support.

PATIENT TEACHING GUIDELINES

Home Care Instructions for Children of All Ages With a New Diagnosis of Diabetes

Staff instructions: At time of discharge, make sure that all teaching has occurred and that areas of confusion or weakness have been reviewed.

The child's family should be educated about the medications, monitoring glucose, high and low blood glucose values, supplies, and when to call for professional help.

Medication Information

1. Home medication list, including trade and generic names
2. Home medication indications, timing in relation to meals and bedtime, and action of each of the insulins ordered for the child (ie, how rapid the insulin's onset time is)
3. How to interpret the insulin dosing based on carbohydrate counting and sliding scale coverage (ie, insulin coverage that changes based on the child's routine blood glucose level)
4. How to draw up insulins using the proper syringe, and double-checking the level drawn up by holding the syringe at eye level
5. How to prepare the injection site by washing hands with soap and water and drying thoroughly, or using an alcohol prep pad and allowing the alcohol to completely dry
6. How to inject the insulin at either a 45- or 90-degree angle (based on the injection site and the amount of subcutaneous adipose)
7. How to check the expiration date of the insulin and how to store it
8. Safe lancet and syringe disposal
   Monitoring Glucose
1. Importance of washing the child's hands before the finger-stick blood glucose check
2. How to use the glucometer the family will have at home
3. How to keep a log of all blood glucose values for the pediatric endocrinologist to monitor

High and Low Blood Glucose Values

1. Signs and symptoms of low and high blood glucose levels
2. Testing the child's blood glucose if the level is greater than 240 mg/dL
3. Testing the child's urine for ketones if the measured glucose level is greater than 300 mg/dL

Supplies

1. Keeping supplies safe at home and out of the reach of younger children
2. Keeping a "to-go" kit when traveling
3. Keeping a checklist of needed supplies for home care (ie, lancets, syringes, monitoring strip if needed, insulin(s), alcohol pads, ketone slips, and an interventional source of carbohydrate if the child is hypoglycemic)

When to Call for Professional Help

1. Two blood glucose levels of 70 mg/dL, or greater than 300 mg/dL
2. Low blood glucose levels that require glucagon
3. Any level of ketones found in the urine
4. Emergency numbers posted by the home phone, on the refrigerator, and with the parents at all times

Type 2 Diabetes Mellitus

Non-insulin-dependent diabetes, known as type 2 DM, is typically seen in overweight and obese children. This disease process is increasing to epidemic proportions because of childhood obesity rates across the nation. Fifty to eighty percent of children with type 2 diabetes have a genetic predisposition to the disease. Environmental factors for type 2 DM include moving from a low-incidence area to a higher incidence area, being in colder climates, and exposure to viral infections (ADA, 2014). Type 2 DM is now considered the biggest cause of morbidity (ie, disease) and mortality (ie, death) for the next generation of adults. Type 2 non-insulin-dependent DM can progress to type 1 insulin-dependent DM in as little as 5 years. Type 1 diabetes is a chronic, immune-mediated condition characterized by a loss of insulin-producing β-cells in the pancreatic islets in those who are genetically susceptible. Type 2 DM is caused by a developed insulin resistance, as is insulin deficiency. Insulin resistance causes diminished liver, adipose tissue, and muscle tissue sensitivity to the small amount of insulin that is produced. Type 2 DM is diagnosed via laboratory analysis of hyperglycemia (Knip, Veijola, et al, 2005).

NURSING CARE PLAN for the Juvenile With Type 1 Insulin-Dependent Diabetes

Assessments and Observations:

1. Physical assessment to check weight loss or weight gain
2. Adherence to insulin therapy
3. Knowledge of the disease process, signs and symptoms of hyperglycemia and hypoglycemia, and checking for ketones
4. Skills performance on a glucometer, calculations of carbohydrate counting, and drawing up and injecting insulin
5. Ability to manage diabetes at school
6. Collaboration with and involvement of the endocrinologist and diabetic nurse educator regarding the child's care
7. Level of coping with the disease process
8. Support and involvement of family

Nursing Diagnoses:

1. There is a knowledge deficit regarding disease process and self-management of disease.
2. The child is experiencing an alteration of metabolism related to hyperglycemia or hypoglycemia.
3. There is an alteration in the child's nutrition.
4. The child is experiencing pain or discomfort with fingerstick blood glucose checks.
5. The child is experiencing anxiety related to the disease process.
6. There are inadequate coping skills related to management of the disease.

Expected Outcomes:

1. The patient and parents will demonstrate acceptance of the disease process and the care required to manage the disease.
2. The patient and parents will demonstrate an understanding of the disease process and potential complications associated with insulin-dependent diabetes in childhood.
3. Blood glucose levels will remain in the range set by the pediatric endocrinologist and will be measured by the desirable level of HbA1c drawn every 90 days.
4. The patient will demonstrate adequate nutrition level by maintaining an appropriate weight set by a nutritionist.
5. The patient will demonstrate comfort with fingerstick blood glucose level checks.

NURSING CARE PLAN for the Juvenile With Type 1 Insulin-Dependent Diabetes—cont'd

Interventions:

1. Refer the patient to a social worker within 24 hours of a new diagnosis to assess coping strategies.
2. Involve the diabetic nurse educator within 24 hours of the diagnosis.
3. Identify all caregivers and determine their roles in managing the child's disease process.
4. Provide education for all caregivers and the child according to his or her developmental level.
5. Repeat the teaching session about managing the child's disease process over the course of the first few days.
6. Thoroughly explain all test procedures and be available to answer questions.
7. Collaborate with the Child Life Specialist to provide support, medical play therapy, and distraction.
8. Monitor the child's response to metabolic control.
9. Check the child's neurological status at regular intervals to ensure there is no evidence of cerebral edema.
10. Monitor the patient's weight and record it.
11. Initiate an age-appropriate pain management protocol and use a pain scale appropriate to the child's age and developmental level.

Assessments of Type 2 Diabetes Mellitus

Because type 1 and type 2 DM disorders differ, it is important that the pediatric nurse communicate his or her concerns to the health-care team rapidly. If a child displays clinical signs or symptoms of either form of DM, the health-care team needs to be informed. The following assessments can be found when a child presents with type 2 (ie, non-insulin-dependent) DM:

• The presence of hyperglycemia as indicated by the levels of blood glucose in fingersticks or the laboratory values of serum after phlebotomy
• The child may also demonstrate a darkened and thickened pigmentation, called *acanthosis nigricans,* around the skin at the base of the neck at the flexural area
• Hypertension
• Sleep apnea
• Hyperlipidemia

Interventions for Type 2 Diabetes Mellitus

Treatment for type 2 DM consists of exercise, weight loss, oral hypoglycemic medications, insulin if unable to be controlled by medication, and metformin (Glucophage) medication to decrease glucose production by the liver.

Nursing Considerations for Type 2 Diabetes Mellitus

Nursing considerations for type 2 DM in childhood include supporting the child and educating all members of the family about the disease process and the goal of preventing the conversion of type 2 (ie, non-insulin-dependent) DM to type 1 (ie, insulin-dependent) DM. It is important to teach the family about the importance of lifestyle changes to prevent periods of hyperglycemia. It is also important that families understand that weight management and blood glucose control both assist with reducing the chance of developing complications associated with the disease process.

TEAM WORKS

National Organizations for Childhood Diabetes Support

It is imperative to provide families with information about how to connect with other families experiencing the challenges of caring for a child with DM, other health-care facilities that provide diverse disease management, other health-care providers that are conducting research, and other professionals such as diabetic educators. National organizations that provide support include the following:

• Juvenile Diabetes Research Foundation/TypeOneNation
• American Diabetes Foundation
• American Academy of Pediatrics

INBORN ERRORS OF METABOLISM

Inborn errors of metabolism represent a large class of genetic diseases and are caused by multiple conditions of altered biochemistry. These alterations include abnormal enzyme accumulation, some with toxic effects. The four major categories are disorders of carbohydrate metabolism, disorders of amino acid metabolism, disorders of organic acid metabolism, and lysosomal storage disease.

Inborn errors of metabolism are rare autosomal genetic disorders. The disorders are recessive in nature, meaning that the child has a 50% chance of being a carrier, a 25% chance of having the disease, and a 25% chance of not having the disease or being a carrier. The incidence of inborn errors of metabolism ranges from 3.5 to 40 per 100,000 births in the United States. The most important aspect of the disease is to identify the symptoms of the pathology as early as possible and rapidly begin to make dietary changes to prevent complications. The development of severe neurological deficits, such as developmental delay, low IQ, and seizure disorders, must be prevented by impeding the accumulation of toxic byproducts (ie, enzymes and food not metabolized and stored) in the body (www.nlm.nih.gov, 2013).

Types of Inborn Errors of Metabolism

There are more than 100 types of inborn errors of metabolism for which testing can be performed. The most commonly encountered types include:

- **Phenylketonuria (PKU):** PKU is a congenital autosomal recessive disease marked by an inability to metabolize phenylalanine. The liver has a deficient amount of the enzyme phenylalanine hydroxylase, which normally breaks down phenylalanine into tyrosine. Phenylalanine is an essential amino acid found in most natural sources of protein. The buildup of phenylalanine causes brain damage. The child will demonstrate a musty-smelling urine. Decreased levels of tyrosine will cause a deficiency of the pigment melanin. Most children with PKU are blonde and have blue eyes. Their fair skin is prone to the development of eczema and photosensitivity. Testing for PKU should take place after the newborn has digested adequate amounts of breast milk or formula.
- **Galactosemia:** This defect is caused by deficiency of the galactose enzyme. This deficiency results in liver failure, renal tubular damage, and cataracts.
- **Maple Syrup Urine Disease (MSUD):** MSUD is caused by a deficiency of decarboxylase, whose purpose is to degrade several amino acids. Without decarboxylase, the child may experience altered tonicity and seizures. The child will demonstrate a maple syrup odor to their urine.

Assessments of Inborn Errors of Metabolism

Assessments of inborn errors of metabolism are through newborn blood screening panels, which should take place after the first 24 hours of feedings in the immediate neonatal period. All newborns should be screened to identify biological markers. New technologies such as electrospray ionization and tandem mass spectrometry have allowed very sensitive screening for asymptomatic newborns. Rapid and accurate testing reduces morbidity (ie, illnesses) and mortality (ie, death) rates in newborns. Most infants with inborn errors of metabolism will show symptoms within a few weeks of life. In older infants, failure to thrive, lethargy, and neurological toxicity will be seen. Rapid assessments and diagnoses save lives (Raghuveer, 2006).

If the child has had a home birth or an early discharge from the maternity ward, it is important to conduct a rapid analysis of the newborn screening specimen. This analysis can be done by having a home care nurse draw the newborn's blood or by having the child seen in a pediatric clinic. Symptoms to watch for include:

- **PKU:** Elevated phenylalanine in the blood builds up to harmful levels and can cause intellectual disability, seizures, behavioral problems, and psychiatric disorders. Key indicators will be a musty body odor, poor weight gain, and delayed growth.
- **Galactosemia:** The inability to process the simple sugar galactose leads to life-threatening complications in just a few days after birth. Infants present with feeding difficulties, lethargy, poor weight gain, jaundice, liver damage, and bleeding.
- **MSUD:** The inability to process certain proteins (ie, amino acids) is characterized by vomiting, poor feeding, lethargy, seizures, developmental delay, and, if left untreated, coma and death. The name comes from a distinct sweet odor of the infant's urine.

Interventions for Inborn Errors of Metabolism

There are many different types of inborn errors of metabolism. In general, interventions for inborn errors should start as early as possible, when the child is first diagnosed. The child might present in metabolic acidosis, which will need to be immediately corrected with sodium bicarbonate. If the child presents with seizures, anticonvulsants will need to be administered. The gold standard for treating inborn errors of metabolism is through dietary therapy, enzyme replacement, and, when applicable, organ transplantation (Raghuveer, 2006). Specific treatments for common inborn errors of metabolism include:

- **PKU:** This disorder is treated by eliminating dietary phenyl ketones, such as high-protein foods. Milk, eggs, meat, beans, and nuts should be highly reduced or avoided. If infant formula is used, a formula with an enzymatic hydrolysate of casein is substituted for milk (such as Lofenalac or Pregestimil). As the child grows, eggs, flour, fish, legumes, nuts, breads, cheese, poultry, meats, and food with phenylalanine-type sugars must be avoided.
- **Galactosemia:** This disorder is treated by eliminating dietary galactose (not lactose). Galactose makes up approximately 50% of the sugars found in milk. Most infants with galactosemia cannot tolerate human or animal milk, or any form of foods that contain galactose. Soy-based, lactose-free, or meat-based formula such as Nutramigen must be administered.
- **MSUD:** This is treated by restricting branched-chain amino acids in the diet, which are found in high-protein foods.

Key Points

- The functions of the endocrine glands and the hormones secreted by each are essential for regulation of various aspects of a child's growth and development, sexual reproduction, metabolism, fluid balance, and the body's response to stress stimuli. The endocrine glands are the pituitary, thyroid, parathyroid, adrenal, and pancreas.

- The effects of a metabolic disorder across the lifespan of a child include alterations in growth and development. Many disorders have devastating effects, such as neurological sequelae, and therefore must be identified early and rapidly so that treatments can be initiated.

■ Complications associated with hyposecretion of the various endocrine glands include hypothyroidism and type 1 and type 2 diabetes. Diseases of hypersecretion of endocrine glands include hyperthyroidism (ie, Graves' disease), hyperadrenal activity (ie, Cushing's syndrome), and hypoglycemia.

■ Type 1 (ie, insulin-dependent) and type 2 (ie, non-insulin-dependent) DM differ in clinical presentation but both require hypoglycemic drugs to maintain normal blood glucose levels. Type 2 DM can progress to type 1 during childhood, requiring the child to have subcutaneous shots and frequent fingersticks for blood glucose monitoring.

■ Inborn errors of metabolism are autosomal recessive in nature and are caused by multiple conditions of altered biochemistry, including abnormal enzyme accumulation of a reactant, some with toxic effects.

■ Children with metabolic disorders need long-term care and follow-up to assess for complications; learning disabilities and challenges; and compliance with diets, medications, and treatments. Most metabolic disorders are followed by laboratory analysis, which provides information to the pediatric health-care team on needed care, education, and encouragement.

REVIEW QUESTIONS

1. SIADH causes a decreased release of ADH that results in the kidneys reabsorbing water.
   1. True
   2. False

2. The endocrine system is responsible for: *(select all that apply)*
   1. Regulating the child's metabolism
   2. Growth
   3. Fluid and electrolyte balance
   4. Digestive processes
   5. Stress response
   6. Sexual reproduction

3. A father brings his 13-year-old son to the pediatric clinic, concerned that the teen has minimal body hair and a high voice. The most appropriate response the nurse should say to the father is:
   1. "Your son will need a visit to the lab for a venipuncture."
   2. "Your son is very delayed in puberty and will need testosterone injections."
   3. "There is no concern at this time. Teens progress through puberty at various times."
   4. "A computed tomography (CAT) scan of the brain to assess his pituitary gland will be ordered for your son."

4. An infant was born 36 hours ago. Laboratory tests have just been ordered for the neonatal screenings, including hypothyroidism. The nurse knows this is not the optimal time to draw an infant's blood for laboratory tests because:
   1. The baby is becoming active and will therefore be difficult to draw via a heelstick.
   2. The baby needs to digest formula first before the labs are drawn.
   3. After 24 hours, there is a natural rise in the TSH.
   4. T_4 levels fluctuate the first week of an infant's life.

5. Which of the following are initial symptoms of a new diagnosis of type 2 DM? *(select all that apply)*
   1. Fruity, sweet odor on breath
   2. Sudden weight loss
   3. Extreme thirst
   4. Frequent urination
   5. Increased appetite

6. A 17-year-old teen male asks the pediatric nurse why he has to learn how to inject insulin rather than just take the pill his grandmother takes for her diabetes (oral hypoglycemic). The best response by the nurse would be:
   1. "Your grandmother's diabetes has improved so she moved from injections to pills."
   2. "You will be able to take pills also as you grow older and manage your blood sugars well."
   3. "You have a different type of diabetes that needs to be controlled by insulin injections."
   4. "Let's ask the doctor if you can take pills while you are in school and injections at home."

7. Precocious puberty is a term used to describe which of the following:
   1. Puberty that occurs at least 2 years after what is the national average
   2. Puberty that occurs when a child has experimented with drugs and alcohol
   3. Puberty that occurs as young as 8 years
   4. Puberty that occurs as young as 10 years

8. The pediatric nurse is teaching a 17-year-old teen about his injections for type 1 diabetes. The nurse is correct in teaching the teen that a laboratory test will be drawn every few months to check on his adherence and compliance with insulin coverage. The laboratory analysis is called:
   1. Insulin serum levels
   2. Trending of blood glucose levels
   3. Pancreatic enzyme levels
   4. Glycosylated hemoglobin

9. While discussing the best way to continue playing on the football team with a 16-year-old high school junior with type 1 diabetes, the nurse would be correct in saying that before exercising the teen should:
   1. Take an additional three units of fast acting insulin
   2. Eat a high carbohydrate snack to ensure an increase of calories
   3. Drink two 8 ounce bottles of electrolyte sports drink
   4. Eat a high-protein snack of cheese, crackers, and turkey slices

10. While teaching an 11-year-old about rotating injection sites for her insulin, the nurse states that complications can occur with using a single site repetitively. This is true because of the chance of developing:
    1. Infection at the sites of repeated injection
    2. Scar tissue that leads to reduced absorption
    3. Vasodilation leading to rapid acting insulin effects
    4. The development of lipodystrophy

CRITICAL THINKING QUESTIONS

1. Children who present with head trauma are at risk for SIADH. When this occurs, the child is at risk for fluid overload and increased intracranial pressure. What nursing observations are required to identify the clinical presentation of SIADH and what precautions should be taken to provide safe nursing care for these children?

2. Families often ask questions about the differences in growth and maturity that they see in their teen children's friends compared to their child. With the diversity in growth, body hair distribution, sexual maturity, and voice maturation, devise an appropriate response to concerns expressed.

3. A teenager with DM can have problems adhering to his or her diet of counted carbohydrates and low concentrated sweets. What are the current recommendations for helping a teen with diabetes control his or her blood glucose levels? Can he or she go a little "crazy" with the diet once in a while, such as at a birthday party?

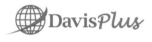

For additional resources and information, visit **www.DavisPlus.com**. Post-Conference Questions and Activities, Answers, and References can be found on Davis*Plus*.

Child With a
Musculoskeletal Condition

LEARNING OUTCOMES

1. Define the key terms.
2. Discuss the normal anatomy and physiology of the musculoskeletal system throughout childhood.
3. Describe nursing care of a child with a musculoskeletal disorder related to the developmental stage the child is in.
4. Critique holistic assessments conducted to rule out a musculoskeletal disorder in childhood.
5. Define various childhood injuries that lead to traumatic musculoskeletal injuries or disorders.
6. Differentiate the laboratory values that are used to identify and monitor disease progression for a child with a musculoskeletal disorder.
7. Describe the various bone fractures potentially experienced in childhood and the associated traction and/or therapy used for each.
8. Discuss the principles behind traction and the psycho-social-biological needs of a child who is required to undergo a period of time in traction.
9. Analyze various childhood disease processes of the musculoskeletal system such as congenital clubfoot, JRA, scoliosis, and muscular dystrophy.
10. Describe safety imperatives while caring for a child in traction.

KEY TERMS

compartment syndrome
epiphyseal plates
kyphosis
lordosis
osteomyelitis
pressure ulcers
scoliosis
traction

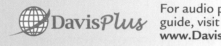 **DavisPlus** For audio pronunciation guide, visit www.DavisPlus.com

CHAPTER CONCEPTS

Comfort
Infection
Inflammation
Mobility
Nutrition
Perfusion
Trauma

REAL-WORLD CASE STUDY

Noah

■ A 14-year-old middle school student was playing football with an afterschool league in his home town. During a game, he suffered a compound fracture of his left tibia and fibula. The wound was immediately stabilized by paramedics at the athletic field, but was considered to be a serious "dirty" or contaminated wound because considerable amounts of dirt were introduced into the site during the injury. Paramedics irrigated the wound with 0.9% normal saline and the teen was immediately placed on broad-spectrum antibiotics upon arriving at the emergency room (ER). The wound required three surgical debridements

continued on page 580

REAL-WORLD CASE STUDY *continued*

before the placement of metal hardware to stabilize the fractured bones. The child experienced a 5-week hospitalization because of the nature of the complicated wound and subsequent site infections. Both parents expressed concern about the teen's school absence and his hospitalization in a pediatric health facility more than 125 miles from home.

1. What pain assessment tool would best be used for this teenager's developmental stage and condition?
2. What concerns would the health-care team have about this type of wound?
3. With the length of time required for this complicated compound lower leg fracture and subsequent absence from school, what resources can be offered to this child to maintain his academic requirements?

CONCEPTUAL CORNERSTONE

Teaching and Learning

One of the most important concepts related to the musculoskeletal system and associated disorders during childhood is teaching and learning. Families need teaching and anticipatory guidance from infancy through adolescence concerning the prevention of significant injury and trauma. Fractured bones, soft-tissue injuries, and associated conditions are common during the developmental period of childhood. Teaching and reinforcing about protective pads, helmets, sports safety, motor vehicle safety, pedestrian safety, and more must start during young childhood and continue through adolescence. Nutrition is also an important part of teaching and learning concerning the musculoskeletal system. Children need adequate calcium, vitamins, and protein to maintain musculoskeletal health. Many congenital and acquired disorders of the musculoskeletal system require a family to learn about the care of the child and how to anticipate complications. Surgery, casting, and immobility all require significant and holistic pediatric health-care team teaching to prevent complications and maximize the healing process.

Active children are very prone to injuries of the musculoskeletal system. Providing supervision during play for young children, appropriate guidelines and protective equipment throughout childhood, and early intervention after injury are all important aspects of care. Children most prone to injuries are those who are obese, are risk-takers, are inadequately supervised by adults, and who participate in sports activities before they have acquired the appropriate motor skills and coordination.

THE DEVELOPMENT OF THE MUSCULOSKELETAL SYSTEM

The musculoskeletal system is developed during fetal development and is structurally intact at birth. All of the 206 bones are present at birth but are more cartilage than bone material. This allows the infant to be flexible during the birthing process. The other components of the musculoskeletal system are all present at birth, including bone marrow, where blood cell production (ie, hematopoiesis) occurs; joints; and muscle. The development of the musculoskeletal system is complex in that the functions of body structure, protection, blood cell production, joints for mobility, and muscles for movement, are all interrelated and included.

Bones

The musculoskeletal system comprises two distinct components: skeletal muscles and skeletal bones. Made up of 206 bones, all existing from birth, the skeletal system grows and develops across childhood. Bone growth in length occurs in the cartilage area of the bones called the *epiphyseal plates* (considered the "growth plate" of long bones, where new bone growth, or ossification, occurs). When the epiphyseal plates close, growth stops. Children who have bone injuries heal much faster than adults because their bones are still growing. On average, a child's bones heal at a rate of 1 week for every year of life up to age 10 (Selekman and Jakubik, 2007). Long bones are the sites of most orthopedic musculoskeletal disorders and fractures.

Children's rapid growth and active status requires nutrition that supports the musculoskeletal system. A child's nutrition highly affects the bones' ability and effectiveness of producing the blood cells in the long bone's marrow. Iron, vitamins B_{12} and folate, and protein are required for adequate production of bone marrow cells (Mayo Clinic, 2015). Table 35.1 outlines pediatric daily nutritional requirements for muscle and bone health throughout the developmental stages.

Blood Cell Production

Blood cells are produced in the marrow section of long bones. Red blood cells, white blood cells, and megakaryocyte cells that produce platelets for clotting are all formed within this marrow. A double protective layer of connective tissue called the *periosteum,* rich with nerves and blood vessels, covers the long bones. A child's nutrition highly affects the ability of the child's bones to grow at expected rates and to heal after injury, as well as the effectiveness of the blood cell production in the long bone's marrow.

Joints

Joints are another large component of the musculoskeletal system. A joint is a location where two or more bones join together for structure and function. The function of joints is to provide either a fixed attachment of bones, or provide mobility. Some joints are in positions for movement, such as the hip joint, with its structure of a ball and socket. Others are between structures to hold them firmly, such as the cranial

TABLE **35.1** **DAILY NUTRIENTS FOR BONE HEALTH DURING CHILDHOOD**

Developmental Stage	Protein Requirements	Calcium Requirements	Vitamin D Requirements	Vitamin C Requirements	Iron Requirements
Infancy	Newborn: 2.4 g/kg/day Infant: 1.75 g/kg/day	500 mg	7–8.5 micrograms	25 mg	11 mg
Toddlerhood	13–15 g	500 mg	200 IU	15 mg	7 mg
Preschool-Aged	19–21 g	800 mg	200 IU	25 mg	10 mg
Early School-Aged (ages 6–10)	34 g	1,300–1,500 mg	200 IU	45 mg	8 mg
Later School-Aged (ages 11–13)	35 g	1,300 mg	200 IU	45–50 mg	8–10 mg
Adolescence	45–52 g	1,300–1,500 mg	200 IU	60–75 mg	11–15 mg (Teen girls may require more based on menstrual cycles and heaviness of flow.)

Sources: Agriculture and Consumer Protection Agency, 2014; CDC.org; NIH.org

sutures or the symphysis pubis. There are three major categories of joints:

1. *Synovial joints* are between long bones and provide motion.
2. *Fibrous joints*, such as those between cranial sutures
3. *Cartilaginous joints* provide cartilage cushions, for example the symphysis pubis, rib attachments, and vertebral discs.

Muscles

The muscles of the skeletal system are also an integral component of the entire musculoskeletal system. The striated muscles of this system provide voluntary contraction and relaxation at the command of the central nervous system. The muscles that provide the mobility of the musculoskeletal system are attached to the bones by tendons. Ligaments either hold bones to each other at the site of the joint or they provide an attachment of organs to bones. Unlike tendons, ligaments are nonelastic; yet like tendons they have a small blood supply and require long periods of time for healing after an injury.

COMMON CHILDHOOD INJURIES

Four common types of childhood injuries within the musculoskeletal system are soft-tissue injuries, specifically strains or sprains; dislocations; contusions; and fractures. A strain is an injury from the excessive use of a body part, such as trauma to muscles and tendons from a forcible stretch or violent contraction. A sprain is a painful trauma to ligaments that ranges from a pull to a tear. A dislocation is a temporary displacement of a bone from its normal position. A contusion is a bruise or bruising of a musculoskeletal structure, such as a "bruised bone." A fracture is an injury directly to bone material. *Soft-tissue injury* is a phrase used to capture many types of injuries within the musculoskeletal system that do not include the child's bones.

Soft-Tissue Injuries

Strains are injuries to muscles or tendons. Sprains are injuries to the ligaments. Dislocation occurs between long bones when joints are not limber. Shoulder dislocation occurs when the shoulder joint capsule, which has limited muscle padding for protection and only the rotator cuff for ligament support, becomes stretched and then dislocates. Contusions occur when there is an impact injury and the tissues tear, leading to hemorrhages in soft tissue, resulting in a significantly ecchymotic and tender area. Football is a high-impact sport in which the most significant contusions take place in the thigh. With a collision type of impact, the contusions can be so significant that the child becomes temporarily disabled with the trauma, bleeding, pain, and swelling.

When a child experiences a soft-tissue injury within the musculoskeletal system, health-care providers can use the RICE mnemonic to foster a more rapid healing process (Fig. 35.1):

- **R = Rest** the limb to prevent further trauma or injury. Especially with active young children, providing rest will slow down the child and prevent the child's activity from causing more harm.
- **I = Ice** the site of the injury with careful consideration to application intervals that will not cause tissue damage from the intense cold. The ice should be applied for no longer than 10 to 15 min intervals with 30-60 minutes between applications, should have a towel or layer of cloth between the ice and the skin, and should be used for up to 36 to 48 hours after the initial time of the injury.
- **C = Compress** the site with bandages such as the ACE bandages to help prevent swelling through edema and to provide support and immobilization of the injured site.
- **E = Elevate** the injured limb to prevent edema buildup and drain existing edema.

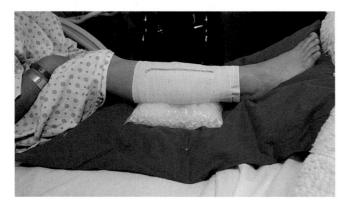

FIGURE 35.1 Application of RICE.

Fractures

Fractures are common during childhood and the two most common fractures are clavicular (ie, collarbone) and greenstick fractures. Clavicular fractures are common because many athletic injuries are to the upper chest area. Children who fall from a distance are at risk for clavicular fractures, and they are common during birth for infants with cephalopelvic disproportion (ie, larger newborn head and body than the mother's pelvic size can withstand). Greenstick fractures are fractures of the long bones caused by a side bend of the long bone, which leads to a fracture on the tension side of the bend. There are many types of fractures, including transverse, spiral, oblique, greenstick, comminuted, and compression (Fig. 35.2). Box 35.1 provides a list of common fracture types seen in children.

CHILDHOOD SCREENING FOR MUSCULOSKELETAL CONDITIONS

Screening of children for injuries or musculoskeletal disorders should begin in early childhood. During well-child checkups, the health-care provider should ask parents about any injuries or evidence of trauma. The child should be assessed for normal gait, full range of movement, and pain or discomfort in the joints. School-aged children should be assessed for the development of **scoliosis** (ie, lateral curvature of the spine). Children across all developmental periods should be assessed for the risk, development, or presence of being overweight or obese. Being overweight or obese causes a child to be more prone to injuries. Screening children is important as orthopedic anomalies, disorders, or injuries may interfere with development within the musculoskeletal system, may interfere with the functioning of other organs, and may prevent the child from participating in sports activities and social events.

While assessing a child with a skeletal injury, child abuse must be ruled out. With an estimated 25% of all fractures in

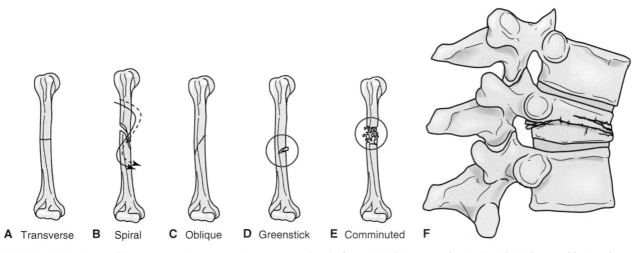

A Transverse   **B** Spiral   **C** Oblique   **D** Greenstick   **E** Comminuted   **F**

FIGURE 35.2 Types of Fractures: A, Transverse: Line crosses the shaft at a 90-degree angle. B, Spiral: A diagonal line coils around the bone; caused by a twisting force. C, Oblique: A diagonal line across the bone. D, Greenstick: Bone is bent, but not broken; more common in children. E, Comminuted: Three or more fracture fragments. F, Compression: Bone becomes wider and flatter; usually seen in the spine.

Box 35.1 Common Types of Fractures in Children

1. **Bend fracture:** A child's bone may bend up to 45 degrees without breaking. The consequences of this bending include slow straightening, some degree of deformity, and possible slow healing.
2. **Buckle fracture:** Also called *torus*, this fracture consists of a raised projection.
3. **Greenstick fracture:** This fracture is considered incomplete and will extend only partially through the affected bone.
4. **Commuted fracture:** This is a fracture in which the bone is splintered or broken into pieces.
5. **Complete fracture:** This is a fracture in which a complete divide exists within the bone, splitting the bone into two pieces.
6. **Growth plate fracture:** When the fracture is within or extends through a growth plate, called the *physis*, the child may suffer bone growth deformities, including shorter limb lengths. Growth plate fractures are also called *impacted fractures*.
7. **Complicated fracture:** This is a fracture in which the fractured bone impairs, damages, or complicates the function of another body part or organ, such as a rib fracture that extends into lung tissue.
8. **Compound or open fracture:** This is a fracture that is so severe that the bone extends through the muscles, fat, and tissues, protruding through to the skin's surface.
9. **Spiral fracture:** This is a fracture that follows a helical line along and around the course of a long bone; may be associated with child abuse injuries.

children 3 years old and younger found to be caused by child abuse, it is imperative that the pediatric health-care team be aware of this possibility. The most important part of this assessment is an incongruence between the reported history of the child's injury by the parent and the injury the child presents with. Within the musculoskeletal system, distinguishing intentional fractures from unintentional fractures can be a challenge.

Spiral fractures are of particular concern. A spiraling fracture injury (ie, helical line along and around the course of a long bone) caused by childhood play activities is rare. A clinical finding of a spiral fracture warrants further child abuse assessments. The medical team may order a variety of diagnostic examinations and laboratory values to determine if there are other injuries present such as fractured ribs, especially in various stages of healing. They will also assess any other possible cause of the fracture, such as bone disease, calcium deficiencies, or underlying pathologies. Safety must be maintained. The team should protect the child from further harm. If confirmed, the child's case must be referred to the local Child Protection Services.

SAFETY *STAT!*

Multiple fractures in various stages of healing should raise high suspicion of child abuse. A social worker should be contacted immediately to help coordinate reporting efforts and Child Protection Services must be notified. Furthermore, infants who present with femur, midshaft, metaphyseal, humerus, radius-ulna, and tibia-fibula fractures should raise suspicion for child abuse because these fractures are not a common finding in this age group.

CULTURAL CONSIDERATIONS

Care of a Child in Traction for a Spiral Fracture

Katrina, a 2½-year-old, was admitted via the ER for a suspected child abuse case resulting in a right femur spiral fracture. Her mother, a young Hispanic woman, brought Katrina into the ER midmorning with concerns that her child would not stand; had a persistent, whimpering cry; and wanted to be held at all times. The mother reported that the young child had fallen down a flight of cement stairs located in the front of their home the day before. No other medical history was offered and the child had had no significant childhood illness or injuries, was up-to-date on her immunizations, and had had nothing but two chest colds and two bouts of bilateral otitis media since her uncomplicated birth.

The mother is a single parent but stated that her boyfriend, an older man, was very involved with the child's care, watched Katrina while the mother worked part-time, and was the only one present during the fall. The child presented in the ER with a significant new closed femur fracture, with a clearly identified spiral shape extending the entire length of the right femur. In the ER, the child was medicated for pain with a narcotic analgesia and a muscle relaxant to reduce muscle spasms around the site of injury. The child was evaluated by a pediatric orthopedic surgeon, placed in skin traction, and transferred to the unit for further evaluation and full 90/90 traction.

The child will require at least 5 weeks of hospitalization for traction. The mother, tearful, admits that she did not witness the fall and is concerned about her daughter's safety. The pediatric social worker came to the bedside midafternoon and interviewed the mother, provided support, and initiated a child abuse report. The mother and child were visited frequently during the hospitalization by a large supportive family, food was brought in daily for the mother and child, and the child was accompanied by the mother at all times. Child abuse was suspected for this injury and the mother's boyfriend was charged with child abuse and child endangerment.

General Assessments of Musculoskeletal Deviations

The pediatric health-care provider should conduct a thorough holistic assessment of the child's site of pain, injury, or potential disorder. The following list provides a guideline for this assessment:

- Assess function in the affected part:
  - Determine the ability of the child to perform range of motion (ROM) of the affected body part, the ability of the child to perform fine and gross motor movements, the amount of weight the child can bear on the affected limb, whether or not the injury or affected area is bilateral, and the presence of inflammation and pain.
  - Palpate the bone and joints under question for warmth, alignment, and any abnormal nodules, lumps, or unusual findings.
  - Assess the child's affected limb for muscle tone, the degree of weakness, the presence of deep tendon reflexes, the quality of pulses, and the presence of abnormal sensations.
- Assess the child's body size and weight in relation to the deficit, disorder, or injury and plot the measurements on a standardized growth chart (can be found on the Centers for Disease Control and Prevention [CDC] Web site).
- Assess the child's autonomy of movement and ambulation, and independence in terms of mobility and fine or gross motor skills.
- Request a final summary of the child's x-ray assessment of the amount of ossification and the presence of a fracture or other injury.
- Assess the child's laboratory studies related to the musculoskeletal system for the presence of deficiencies.

LABS & DIAGNOSTICS

Tests Related to the Musculoskeletal System During Childhood

Blood Tests for Bone and Muscle Health:

- **Complete blood cell count (CBC):** Used to assess the degree of anemia associated with a significant bleed after a musculoskeletal trauma
- **Elevated white blood cell count:** Used to determine the presence of infection in conditions such as **osteomyelitis** (ie, inflammation of the bone tissue and the marrow caused by an infection)
- **Erythrocyte sedimentation rate (ESR):** If prolonged, the sedimentation rate will indicate the presence of inflammation and may be elevated in the presence of Ewing's sarcoma.
- **C-reactive protein (CRP):** A protein produced by the liver that becomes elevated in the blood plasma in the presence of inflammation
- **Bacterial cultures:** Cultures drawn from the blood to assess for the presence of an organism-causing infection in conditions such as osteomyelitis
- **Rheumatoid factor (RF):** An antibody present in 10% of children with juvenile rheumatoid arthritis (JRA)
- **Antinuclear antibodies (ANA):** A serum test that does not confirm the presence of JRA but that may indicate the presence of this disease

Diagnostic Tests for Bone and Muscle Injuries, Disorders, or Diseases:

- **Prenatal ultrasound:** An assessment for the presence of musculoskeletal disorders, such as congenital clubfoot
- **Radiograph:** An x-ray or other image used to assess for the location and severity of fractures
- **Periodic radiograph:** An x-ray or other image used to assess the effectiveness of treatments and the rate of bone healing
- **Computed tomography (CAT) scan:** Imaging used to determine the presence and extent of injury, infection, tumors, nodules, bleeding, and inflammation
- **Bone scan:** An imaging test used to determine the presence of tumors, nodules, abscesses, and overall bone health
- **Salter-Harris fracture classification system:** A system used to identify the severity of growth plate injures; graded between I and V
- **Bone scintigraphy:** A nuclear scanning test used to assess bone images through a radioactive isotope injected into the body to illuminate injury, disease, or a condition
- **Magnetic resonance imaging (MRI):** Medical imaging used to visualize the exact location and severity of an injury
- **Arthrography:** X-ray imaging done under general anesthesia that allows determination of the best position of the femoral head for healing

Interventions for Orthopedic Injuries

Immobilization, casts, braces, and **traction** (ie, a therapy used to help in the healing process of a fracture often using two lines of pull for extension and stabilization) are considered the cornerstones of treatment for orthopedic injuries and fractures. Allowing the site to rest, stabilizing the injury site with casts and braces, and providing a line of pull via traction are required for significant injuries.

A child with a musculoskeletal injury often requires a period of time in which the injury is immobilized so that healing of the affected fracture, degenerative disease, bone infection, or spinal cord disorder can be promoted. Immobilization is the complete opposite of the natural state of movement and exploration of a child. It is considered a stressful event and may have lasting consequences on the child's developmental maturity process. Immobilization works by resting the affected site, decreasing muscle spasms that may interfere with healing, providing an opportunity for traction, and promoting bone growth. Box 35.2 provides information about ten of the potential negative consequences of immobilization.

Casts

Children who experience common simple fractures are often placed in a cast and sent home for recovery. After radiographic confirmation that the fracture is present, where it is, and its severity, a child may be casted in an outpatient or emergency setting. Casting materials may be plaster or synthetic. Synthetic casts are typically made out of a polyester-cotton tape or a knitted fiberglass tape permeated with a resin made of polyurethane. While the material is drying or setting, the nurse should only handle the cast with the palm of the

Box 35.2 Ten Consequences of Immobilization During Childhood

The following are concerns the pediatric nurse should keep in mind while caring for a child who must undergo a prolonged bedrest for immobilization of a musculoskeletal injury or disorder:

1. Bone demineralization and the release of calcium into the blood; the condition mimics osteoporosis; hypercalcemia and the potential for development of renal stones (ie, renal calculi)
2. Decreased joint mobility and the potential for the development of joint contractures
3. A decrease in muscle mass called *disuse atrophy,* which is a decrease in the size, endurance, and strength of muscle tissue
4. An accumulation of respiratory secretion, which leads to the potential of respiratory infections
5. The development of a weak cough as abdominal, back, and respiratory muscle strength diminishes
6. A decreased rate in metabolism with a reduced overall daily caloric intake
7. The development of orthostatic hypotension from venous pooling that leads to syncope/dizziness
8. Decreased cerebral blood flow
9. The development of feeding issues (caused by eating supine), decreased appetite, and constipation
10. Decreased circulation of blood to the skin, reducing healing, and promoting skin breakdown and the development of pressure sores/ulcers

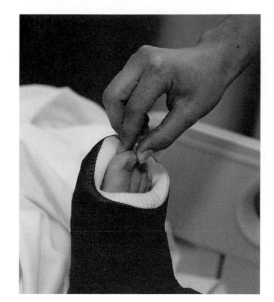

FIGURE 35.3 The nurse assesses CRT.

hand because finger manipulation may cause indentation. The child's affected area inferior or distal to the site must be checked for neurological, sensory, and circulatory status. The family should be taught how to assess the child's affected limb, assess for cast integrity, and be taught when to report a change in status (Fig. 35.3). If the fingers, toes, or skin below the cast are pale, cool, and without pulse, the nurse should report this finding immediately so that the chance of injury can be diminished.

A severe complication of a bone fracture is the development of **compartment syndrome.** This syndrome occurs when the traumatic injury causes pressure to build up in a confined space, such as in the rigid fascia surrounding the muscles. Muscle tissue bundles are surrounded by a sheath of connective tissue that does not adapt to increasing pressure. If a bleed occurs or there is a buildup of inflammatory fluids, the pressure building up within the muscles can lead to ischemia and necrosis, causing severe tissue damage. If a child who is casted complains of increasing feelings of pain and pressure, the situation should be reported immediately so the cast can be removed to assess for pressure and tissue

damage. Tight dressings, tight casts, bleeding episodes, inflammatory fluid buildup, burns, trauma, and surgical procedures all place a child at risk for severe tissue damage from compartment syndrome.

A cast should be snug but free of irritation. The cast material should be kept free of moisture. The application of tape in a petaling design helps to reduce irritation around the cast edges; in addition, many casts have cushioning within the casting material. If a child experiences pain or feelings of pressure under the cast, it may be removed for an assessment of the affected site and re-casted as needed. Because of an infant's rapid rate of growth, a cast may have to be removed and re-casted to account for the limb lengthening. This will be influenced by how long the cast must remain for healing.

There are a variety of types of casts used for fractures or injuries during childhood (Fig. 35.4 and 35.5). Spica casts are used for infants and toddlers to provide stability and immobility during bone healing.

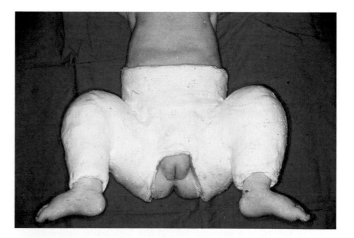

FIGURE 35.4 Child in a spica cast.

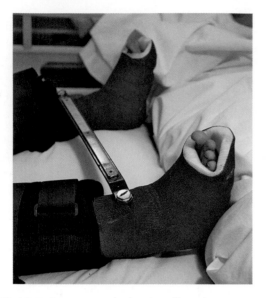

FIGURE 35.5 A cast is applied to the affected extremity to keep it immobile while healing.

PATIENT TEACHING GUIDELINES

Care of an Infant With a Hip Spica Cast for Congenital Hip Dysplasia

For a child with a cast, teach the family:

- While drying, use only the palms of the hands to turn or lift a child. Never use fingers, which can indent the cast.
- After application, maintain taped petals to prevent the cast edges from causing skin irritation or breakdown.
- Maintain a dry cast at all times. Wrap the cast during bathing with plastic and tape.
- In children with severe skeletal injuries that require surgical interventions, check for circulation, color, sensation, movement, and temperature. To prevent injury, teach the family to report any changes to their primary care provider immediately.
- Never pick up the child via the crossbar between the abducted legs as this could lead to breakage and the need to re-cast.
- For young children, use a disposable diaper under the edges of the cast to prevent the cast from getting wet or soiled.

Braces

Braces are appliances used to assist a child in his or her mobility and posture. Braces are individually made for each child's size, height, and need, and are constructed of leather, metal hinges, and/or plastic shells. For instance, a child with scoliosis may wear a thoracic-lumbar-sacral-orthotic (TLSO) brace to help the lateral curvature of the spine realign during the adolescent growth period.

Assessments of a child wearing a brace include the following:

- Skin integrity around the site of the brace should be assessed. For instance, a child in a TLSO brace for scoliosis should have the skin around the superior and inferior brace edge checked for skin breakdown or irritation.
- Proper fit should be assessed as the child grows.
- Any complaints of discomfort or pain experienced while in a brace should be reported.

Traction

The use of traction during childhood has three distinct purposes. First, traction is used to provide a realignment of a body part after injury or surgery. Second, it is used to provide a decrease in muscle spasms through pulling, stretching, and fatiguing the muscles during the healing process. Third, it is used to provide immobilization of the fracture site during the healing process. Traction has three components:

1. Forward force, which is conducted by the child's pulling his or her body forward
2. Counter traction, which is a backward pull accomplished by the use of weights (eg, sandbags or waterbags) typically over the side or the end of the hospital bed
3. Friction, which is provided by the child's body weight lying on the sheets, helping to keep the child's body in alignment and counter traction in place

All three components of traction are necessary to heal a significant fracture in a child who is immobile for a period of time.

There are two types of traction: skin traction and skeletal traction. Skin traction is provided by bandages constructed of elastic bandages, moleskin, or adhesive wrapped around the injured limb and providing a pull on the skin during traction. Skeletal traction provides a direct pull on the skeleton and includes the surgical placement of metal hardware, such as pins, wires, bolts, and rods. Care must be taken to assess for inflammation and infection at the sites of the metal hardware used to maintain skeletal traction. Pediatric nurses must have a plan to provide wound care to the sites of the pins.

During traction, it is the health-care provider's responsibility to ensure the child stays in alignment. This can be challenging because children are in constant motion. The child should be checked frequently to make sure the child is centered on the bed and in alignment with the traction, with the weight hanging freely over the side of the bed. If the weights are found on the floor, this should be reported because further injury to the site may have occurred. If the child requires realignment or needs to be readjusted, the weights should be left freely hanging. During traction, the use of the weight should never be interrupted, such as by placing the weights on the bed for transport. The child's family needs to understand the type and function of traction so they can assist in caring for the child, maintaining traction, and reporting problems.

For both skin and skeletal traction, a thorough skin assessment is warranted as the child is at risk for impaired skin integrity. A child in traction should have slight changes in position on a regular basis to prevent the development of **pressure ulcers.** Also referred to as *decubitus ulcers,* pressure ulcers are skin wounds that result from impaired circulation or inadequate perfusion from pressure. Position changes and turning schedules should be every 2 hours and should be documented. For skeletal traction, the pin site should be checked for problems with healing, such as the presence of draining, pus, or redness not associated with healing. Check for neurovascular integrity by assessing CCSMT:

- **C = Circulation** should be assessed by pressing on the skin and observing for capillary refill time (CRT). CRT should be brisk in a healthy child without pre-existing cardiovascular disease.
- **C = Color** should be assessed. Look for any deviation, such as pale skin or blue skin.
- **S = Sensation** should be assessed by asking the child if he or she is experiencing any abnormal feelings of buzzing, burning, or tingling. These may indicate nerve regeneration or nerve damage.
- **M = Movement** should be assessed by asking the child if he or she can wiggle toes or fingers, or move the extremity below the site of injury.
- **T = Touch** should be assessed by asking the child if he or she can feel the presence of the caregiver's fingers on the skin below the site of the injury.

SAFETY *STAT!*

So that immediate interventions can take place that will ensure perfusion, the health-care team should check the injured site for the presence of the five Ps of ischemia:

- P = Pain
- P = Pallor
- P = Pulselessness
- P = Paresthesia
- P = Paralysis

For skin traction, the edges of the bandages should be checked for skin breakdown. If the child is required to use a bedpan and urinal, the skin should be checked for breakdown related to the presence of urine and/or feces. It is imperative that a child in traction receive frequent skincare, meticulous hygiene after toileting, and daily sponge baths.

TYPES OF TRACTION. Various types of traction are used for the same purpose: to stabilize the bone and fracture site for healing and to provide a line of pull to maintain the position of healing. The following list describes various types of traction used in childhood bone injuries:

- **Buck's extension:** Buck's extension is a type of skin traction applied to the child's leg in a fully extended position. This traction is used for shorter-term periods of immobilization and healing. With complete stabilization, the child may be able to turn to a side-lying position.
- **90/90 traction:** This is a type of skeletal traction in which the child's lower leg is supported by a sling or a boot while the distal section of the fracture is pinned or wired. 90/90 traction allows the child more movement of the central part of the body, thus facilitating greater movement for toileting, hygiene, skin integrity assessment, and play (Fig. 35.6).

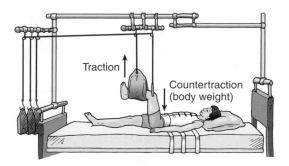

FIGURE 35.6 The 90/90 femoral traction is most commonly used to treat femur fractures and complicated femur fractures.

- **Bryant's traction:** Bryant's traction is the only skin traction available for a young child, aged 2 or younger, with a lower-extremity fracture. Bryant's traction allows the child to provide his or her own countertraction by lifting the buttocks up and off the crib, or by dangling the legs in the air, with the traction pulling up and over the end side of the crib (Fig. 35.7). The legs are straight and the body is in a 90-degree angle toward the ceiling. Although only one leg may be affected, both legs are suspended in the same way.
- **Ilizarov external fixator:** Using a system of telescoping rods, pins, and wires, the Ilizarov device promotes limb lengthening by consistently and gently providing tension to lengthen bone tissue. After an osteotomy is performed in surgery, the device provides tension to grow new bone tissue by acting like a new growth plate. The device, brought to the United States by a Russian scientist, also allows for the correction of rotational or angular defects and immobilization for childhood bone fractures. These devices can be as small as thumb-size, or as large as is needed for a lower extremity. Special care is given to preventing infection at the various pin sites. Because of the

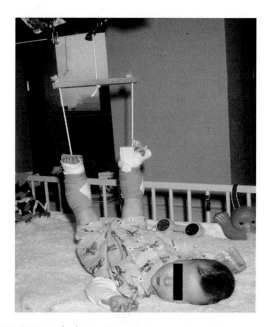

FIGURE 35.7 A baby in Bryant's traction.

length of time required to benefit from wearing the device, families must be taught how to provide aseptic pin care.
• Other traction setups used in children include Dunlop's and Russell's (Fig. 35.8 and 35.9).

SAFETY *STAT!*

Neither the health-care team nor the family should ever disrupt the line or pull of traction or the weight of the sandbags because the site might become reinjured.

HAZARDS AND COMPLICATIONS OF LONG-TERM TRACTION.
While caring for a child with traction, all members of the pediatric health-care team must be observant for complications.

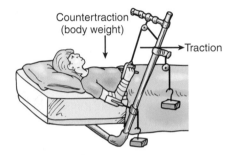

FIGURE 35.8 Dunlop's traction is used in the treatment of a supracondylar fracture of the humerus.

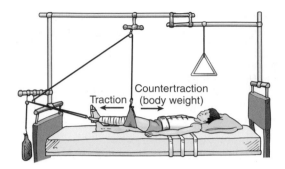

FIGURE 35.9 A child in Russell's traction (with trapeze).

Maintaining safety for the child is the highest priority while in traction. Children may require extended lengths of time in traction, which inherently puts the child at risk for a number of concerns.

• **Skin breakdown:** Prevent skin breakdown by assessing frequently to provide early identification. Cleanse the skin frequently and remove all urine, feces, and sweat daily. Provide meticulous skin care after each toileting episode. Use a mirror to assess for the development of redness or pressure ulcer formation when the child is lying supine. Assess the bed for small toys, such as crayons, jacks, and Legos, because the child may have decreased skin sensation while at prolonged bedrest and may not know there is an object under his or her skin. Use tools to assess severity of any confirmed redness or skin breakdown. Implement

---

NURSING CARE PLAN for a Child in Traction

Assessments:
1. Assess the child for discomfort or pain at the surgical site or at the site of fracture.
2. Assess the child for alignment in bed, especially when he or she is mobile.
3. Assess the traction setup, including assessing that the weights are hanging freely over the bed.
4. Assess that the child consumes adequate nutrition and hydration, and assess for the presence of constipation.
5. Assess the child for skin breakdown, using a mirror if needed to check the skin (posterior).
6. Assess the child's lungs for increasing secretions or the development of a respiratory infection.
7. Assess the child's emotional state and coping strategies associated with being in traction.

Nursing Diagnoses:
1. There is a risk for injury related to traction as evidenced by prolonged bedrest.
2. There is a risk for constipation related to prolonged bedrest and decreased fluid intake as evidenced by hard and infrequently passed stools.
3. There is a risk for impaired skin integrity related to pressure points of traction or casting as evidenced by the development of decubitus ulcers.
4. There is a risk for ineffective coping related to prolonged bedrest as evidenced by child's behaviors demonstrating regression toward behaviors found in earlier developmental stages (eg, thumb sucking, wanting a diaper, tantrums).

Expected Outcomes:
1. The child will not develop constipation while at prolonged bedrest during traction.
2. The child will not develop stage I pressure ulcers while in traction during hospitalization.
3. The child will engage daily in social activities and appropriate play activities for his or her developmental stage.

NURSING CARE PLAN for a Child in Traction—cont'd

Interventions:

1. Calculate the child's fluid maintenance and provide a variety of favorite fluids to ensure the child takes in more than a minimal amount of fluids.
2. Engage the dietary office and nutritionist to plan a diet that will provide high fiber via fruits and vegetables to prevent constipation.
3. Turn the child frequently on a specified schedule to prevent pressure ulcer formation.
4. Post a turning schedule to communicate between shifts and carefully document all repositioning and turning.
5. Provide for the child's emotional state and promote coping strategies (eg, toddlers and preschoolers will become very distraught if parents need to leave; parents should explain to the child why they need to leave and how long they will be away).

Evaluation of Outcome:

1. Has the child produced a soft, formed stool daily?
2. Has there been a development of impaired skin integrity, such as the presence of a stage I pressure sore?
3. Has the child engaged daily in productive and satisfying social encounters? Does the child demonstrate effective coping strategies?

and document a rigorous turning schedule to make sure pressure ulcers are not forming.

- **Constipation:** Prevent constipation by providing adequate fluids and a fiber-rich diet. Be creative in how the fiber content of the diet is increased. Involve the family and provide favorite and familiar fruits and vegetables, smoothies, or fiber additives (eg, powder).
- **Boredom and decreased stimulation:** Prevent regression and behavior problems from boredom by eliciting the assistance from members of the Child Life staff and the volunteer staff to provide a program of developmental stimulation. Provide activities, music, homework, arts, socialization, and reading to stimulate the child on a regular basis. Find stimulating activities that are appropriate for the child's developmental stage.
- **Pain:** Assess the child's pain level by using a valid pain assessment tool such as the Wong-Baker FACES pain rating scale.
- **Respiratory congestion and complications:** Prevent the buildup of pulmonary secretions from prolonged bedrest during traction by using an incentive spirometer and blowing games, such as blowing bubbles and keeping up a cotton ball by blowing through a straw.
- **Bone health:** For a child in traction, it is imperative to maintain a diet rich in protein and vitamins for bone health and bone healing. Nutritional disorders, vitamin or protein deficiencies, and failure to thrive can all affect a child's bone health and the ability of bones to heal.

Child Life Specialists are excellent and highly skilled at creating a play and simulation program for children who are hospitalized for long periods of time in traction. The play should include all of the child's senses; be focused on the child's developmental stage, not the child's chronological age; keep the child's attention; be creative; and maximize their learning.

PATIENT TEACHING GUIDELINES

Parents must understand the importance of play and stimulation for their unique child. The child should be provided activities, creative art projects, and learning opportunities appropriate for their developmental stage. For instance:

- Toddlers may experience great stress by not being able to move, so activities should maximize their ability to move, provided safety is maintained. Tossing a large soft ball, playing with building blocks in bed on the overbed table, and playing with large trucks or dolls are recommended.
- Preschoolers will need a variety of art projects, and games that include make-believe are often well-accepted.
- School-aged children will benefit from games, board games, cards, and appropriate media. School-aged children must be given the opportunity to feel industrious and complete their homework.
- Teenagers will want intellectually stimulating and peer-focused games, as well as limited appropriate screen time with video games and social media. Homework must continue in this age group.

COMMON MUSCULOSKELETAL DISORDERS

Children may present with congenital or acquired disorders within the musculoskeletal system. Congenital disorders, which are those that exist from birth, are conditions that are found in the early infancy period, or the condition may not surface until the child is older and ambulatory. Acquired disorders may be caused by traumatic injuries.

Clubfoot

Congenital clubfoot (ie, *talipes equinovarus*) is an abnormal deformity of the foot that causes the heel to turn inward and the entire foot to be in a plantar flexion (ie, downward position) and a rigid adduction. The condition may be identified in utero via a prenatal ultrasound. This condition is typically unilateral, but may be found bilateral (Fig. 35.10).

Assessments of Clubfoot

At birth, the delivery team notes the deformity during the initial newborn assessment. The deformity is identified and the parents are provided support and education concerning the treatment plan for nonsurgical correction.

Interventions for Clubfoot

The infant will undergo a series of casting procedures to stretch and move the deformity to alignment. Serial casting is performed as the young infant grows rapidly and the deformity moves into place. It is not uncommon to have the child's foot re-casted every 2 weeks.

PATIENT TEACHING GUIDELINES

Parents may have concerns with needing to bring their infant back to the casting clinic at frequent intervals for the removal of a cast for clubfoot and the application of the next one. It is important to explain to the family members that as the infant is rapidly growing in length and weight, serial casting is the safest way to ensure that that cast will be effective and not cause pressure.

Nursing Considerations for Clubfoot

Clubfoot is a painless disorder, so the infant does not suffer. The goal is to correct the disorder as much as possible before the older infant begins to bear weight in standing and attempting to walk. Families will need support as they may feel anxiety and despair that their newborn is not "perfect." Reassure the family that the condition will start to be treated within days to weeks of birth.

Congenital Hip Dysplasia or Dislocation

Congenital hip dysplasia, also called *developmental dysplasia of the hip (DDH),* is considered the most common congenital musculoskeletal disorder in infants and children. During a well-child assessment of a newborn, evidence of an abnormally shallow acetabulum of the hip is noted and the femoral head may move slightly or a have a significant "slip" out of the socket. The hip joint is unstable and requires intervention. Risk factors for hip dysplasia include breech presentation, large birth weight, multiples, oligohydramnios (ie, low levels of amniotic fluid during fetal development), female gender, first-born children, and family history.

Assessments of Congenital Hip Dysplasia or Dislocation

Physical examinations performed on a newborn to confirm the presence of a shallow hip socket and the slipping of the femoral head within the acetabulum include the following:

- **Ortolani's click maneuver:** With the child in the supine position, the caregiver slowly manipulates the hip joint from behind to assess for a slip forward of the femoral head into the acetabulum (Fig. 35.11).
- **Barlow's maneuver:** In the supine position, the caregiver assesses for the audible "clunk" sound when manipulating the entry or exit of the femoral head into or out of the acetabulum while applying pressure from the front.
- **Shortened leg on the affected side:** The caregiver lays the child supine with the knees bent up, assessing for an apparent shortening of the femur; the affected hip demonstrates a lower knee.
- **Asymmetrical skin folds in the gluteus:** During assessment of the newborn, there is asymmetry of the skin folds on the affected hip (Fig. 35.12).
- **Trendelenburg's sign in the older child:** While standing, the older child lifts his or her leg on the unaffected side, demonstrating an elevated hip joint from the posterior angle.

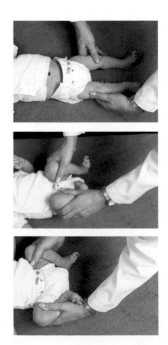

FIGURE 35.11 Barlow's and Ortolani's assessment techniques.

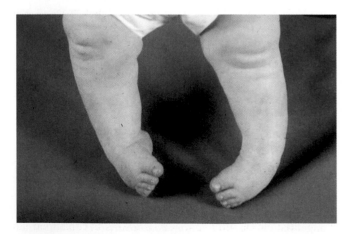

FIGURE 35.10 Congenital clubfoot.

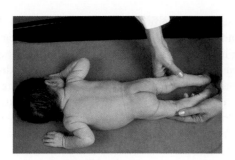

FIGURE 35.12 Inspecting an infant's gluteal folds for congenital hip dysplasia.

Interventions for Congenital Hip Dysplasia or Dislocation

After DDH is confirmed via radiographic examination, the severity of the shallowness of the acetabulum is determined. Immediate treatment is started to stop the progression of the deformity. In young infants, the femoral head is placed into the acetabulum and the child is splinted in a flexed and abducted position, using one of a variety of abduction devices, such as the popular Pavlik harness. Use of an abduction device must continue for up to 6 months. Parent education is vital and frequent assessments with strap length adjustments are warranted as the infant is experiencing rapid growth.

Nursing Considerations for Congenital Hip Dysplasia or Dislocation

Early newborn screening is an essential aspect to early identification of DDH. With screening of all newborns, early identification and rapid placement of an abduction device will allow up to a 95% cure rate without the need for surgical interventions.

HEALTH PROMOTION

Parental education is essential because the family must understand the importance of 24-hour-a-day use of the harness and the assessment of the child's skin and circulation around the sites of the straps.

PATIENT TEACHING GUIDELINES

The family needs to understand how to assess for the integrity of the abduction device and what complications are associated with a poor fit, slipping of the straps, or a loss of skin integrity under the strap contact sites. Assessments that need attention include straps that are not snug enough to keep the infant in an abducted position (ie, knees up and out), straps that easily fall away from their required position, and skin that is red, raw, or open. It is important to keep a layer of cotton under the straps to prevent skin chaffing and skin sores from developing. If these complications are found, the family should report them to their care provider for assistance and skin care treatments.

For older children with DDH, immobilization using traction or surgical interventions to produce a reduction may be needed. The surgical procedure of an osteotomy has an aim of reconstructing an acetabulum with a shallow angle so that the femoral head stays in place. A period of time in postsurgical casting may also be needed.

Legg-Calve-Perthes Disease

A child who presents with an aseptic necrosis of the femoral head is diagnosed with Legg-Calve-Perthes disease. Confirmed via radiography, the child is typically between the ages of 2 and 12 upon diagnosis. The pathophysiology behind the disorder remains unknown but the basis of the problem stems from a disrupted circulation pattern to the tissues of the femoral head. Occurring over a period of several months to years, there is a slow disruption to the blood supply to the tissues, including to the femoral head, the acetabulum, and the growth plate (ie, epiphysis).

Assessments of Legg-Calve-Perthes Disease

The disorder is one of the older child; preschool-aged and school-aged children may present with a limp hip joint, discomfort, or hip joint stiffness, especially after joint manipulation. The child may or may not have a history of a trauma in the area. The most effective method of confirmation is via radiography or a CAT scan.

Interventions for Legg-Calve-Perthes Disease

The child is put on rest because activity may further exacerbate the disorder by causing microfractures to the femoral head's epiphysis. Traction, bracing, and surgical interventions may all be warranted to restore hip ROM and assist with the revascularization of the affected area. Treatments are most effective for children younger than age 10; older children may develop a significant degenerative arthritis without treatment.

Nursing Considerations for Legg-Calve-Perthes Disease

Pediatric nurses should be aware of the need for long treatment programs that require parents to adhere to treatment plans. Families need support when the treatment plan calls for long periods of reduced activity for healing. Working with the child's school personnel to adapt a physical education and play program will assist with the adherence needed for appropriate healing.

Slipped Capital Femoral Epiphysis

Also known as a *coxa vara,* a slipped femoral capital epiphysis occurs as a spontaneous displacement of the most proximal epiphysis of the femoral head in an inferior and a posterior direction. Occurring most commonly during an active accelerated growth episode, the child presents with either a sudden or a progressive slip of the functional joint, causing a hip disability, a limp, and complaints of hip pain.

Assessments of Slipped Capital Femoral Epiphysis

Considered to be idiopathic, the diagnosis is confirmed via radiography with an accompanied ruling-out of endocrine, hormonal, and renal dysfunction or disorders. An obese child is at a greater risk for this disorder. Radiographs will demonstrate the presence of a displacement of the femoral head, an abnormally wide femoral growth plate, and a "slipping" of the femoral neck within the acetabulum, causing trauma on the blood vessels feeding the epiphysis.

Interventions for Slipped Capital Femoral Epiphysis

Slipped femoral capital epiphysis requires a 100% non-weight-bearing status, bedrest, and surgical intervention of the placement of metal pins or metal screws to correct the deformity.

Nursing Considerations for Slipped Capital Femoral Epiphysis

The most important aspect of assisting the child toward a cure is early identification and reporting of the symptoms of this disorder so that immediate bedrest, immobilization, non-weight-bearing status, and surgical interventions can be initiated.

Scoliosis

Scoliosis is typically not identified until a child is 10 years of age or older and is considered idiopathic in most cases. The disorder may be considered congenital, associated with a neuromuscular disorder that encompasses weakness or neuron disease, or associated with a progressing muscular dystrophy. The disorder involves three distinct vertebral presentations: a lateral curvature of the spine, a thoracic hypokyphosis (ie, upper posterior rib protrusion), and a degree of spinal rotation that causes the apparent rib asymmetry so often noted in a screening assessment. Rarely complaining of pain, the child will typically present in their preadolescent growth spurt, with a report of improperly fitting clothing or one shoulder being higher than the other.

deformity. Once identified, scoliosis is then further evaluated to rule out pathology of other diseases or accompanied disorders (Fig. 35.13).

Scoliosis is then assessed for the degree of deformity, which will determine the treatment plan. Bracing and exercising is the preferred method of treating mild spinal curves while the child is experiencing a growth spurt. Bracing is never considered curative because, without the growth spurt, the brace could not guide the spine into alignment as the skeleton is maturing. Surgical interventions are required when the spinal lateral curvature is greater than 40 degrees.

Interventions for Scoliosis

Bracing is conducted by individualizing an apparatus that is well-fitted and worn 23 hours a day. A popular brace constructed of leather and metal is called the *Milwaukee Brace* or *CTLSO* (ie, cervical-thoracic-lumbar-sacral orthosis). Thoracic-lumbar-sacral-orthotics (TLSO) are large, plastic, snug-fitting braces that extend from the underarm down to the below the waist. These braces are also constructed individually for each child and are worn for the entire length of the predicted adolescent growth spurt. They may be required to be worn for 2 to 3 years to be effective.

Surgical procedures for severe lateral curvatures require straightening and realignment using internally fixated metal rods, wires, and/or pins with or without spinal bony fusion. Metal instruments include Harrington's rod, Luque's wires, Dwyer's instrumentation, and other devices that provide solid support and fusion. The surgical procedure requires an extensive hospitalization stay that includes monitoring the child closely for pain and neurological integrity, log-rolling the child while changing positions until mobilization is re-established, and preventing a postoperative spinal injury.

Considerable pain is expected from the surgical manipulation of bone and tissue trauma occurring with surgical procedures.

PATIENT TEACHING GUIDELINES

Two other conditions that an adolescent may present with are **kyphosis** and **lordosis**. It is important to distinguish these conditions from scoliosis:

- **Kyphosis:** A condition of exaggerated angulation of the posterior curvature of the thoracic (ie, upper) spine; in lay language, kyphosis is also referred to as "humpback" or "hunchback" in nature
- **Lordosis:** A condition of anterior convexity of the lumbar spine.

Assessments of Scoliosis

Children should be participating in school-wide screenings or scoliosis screenings during well-child checkups. Typically, the most common and rapid early identification is made by simply having the child lean forward at the hips and the screening personnel visually inspects the child for a rib hump

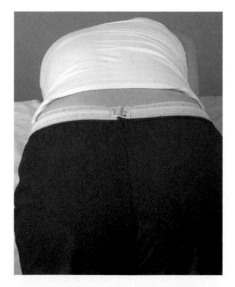

FIGURE 35.13 Assessment of scoliosis includes having the child bend forward to see unevenness of ribs.

Therefore narcotic pain control measures should be administered around the clock, not just PRN, and should be accompanied by muscle relaxers for spasms to assist the child in mobility and surgical recovery.

DRUG FACTS

If a patient-controlled analgesia (PCA) machine is going to be used for postoperative pain control in a child having scoliosis surgery, it will be imperative that the child learns how to use the machine before surgery when learning can take place without the distraction of the pain experience.

Nursing Considerations for Scoliosis

The prepubescent and adolescent child is often concerned with body image. Not only does the disorder cause distress, but the bracing and orthotics required can lead to difficulties with adherence to the treatment plan and the consistent use of braces and orthotics. It is important for the pediatric nurse to consistently remind the teen that if the brace is not worn during the greatest growth spurt, the scoliosis may progress, causing further body image concerns.

Postoperative care of the child undergoing surgical correction for significant scoliosis requires meticulous nursing care focused on safety. This care should focus on keeping the child in the immediate postoperative period controlled for pain, free of injury, flat on his or her back, and carefully log-rolled. The pediatric nurse should request assistance from at least one other caregiver and/or a physical therapist (PT) to prevent injury. A PT can be instrumental in motivating and supporting a child in adhering to the treatment plan, as well as in providing safe tips for early mobility (as early as the day after surgery).

TEAM WORKS

Child Life Specialists should be involved in the child's presurgical preparation and teaching. They can be instrumental during the highly symptomatic postoperative healing phase by providing distraction, play, and pain adjuncts, such as visualization and guided imagery.

Osteogenesis Imperfecta

A very uncommon disorder with devastating consequences is the genetically linked, autosomal dominant, heterogeneous disease called *osteogenesis imperfecta (OI)*. This disease is commonly known as "brittle bone disease" because the child suffers from fractures and skeletal deformity. This disorder may be so severe that the infant does not live through the birthing process. The child's entire life is affected by this disorder, with a decrease in life expectancy, multiple fractures, and the use of a wheelchair for mobility.

The pathology of this disease is a defect in the genes that produce the precursor of collagen. Without healthy collagen, the major component of the structure of bone, the bone is fragile and susceptible to faulty bone mineralization, fractures, and very abnormal bone growth architecture, which leads to deformities. The child may or may not present with a bluish discoloration of the eye sclera, hearing loss, joint laxity (ie, looseness or increased flexibility), and poor structure of the bones that support the child's teeth.

Assessments of Osteogenesis Imperfecta

Prenatal screening typically is not performed for this rare disorder, so early identification is by death in utero or a newborn suffering several fractures during the birthing process. If prenatal diagnostics are performed and the disease is identified in utero, then the infant must be born by Cesarean section for the greatest chance of safety and survival.

Interventions for Osteogenesis Imperfecta

OI cannot be treated medically. The child and family are offered supportive care and genetic counseling. Research continues in the area of bone marrow transplantation. Goals of supportive care are to reduce the possibility of further fractures, prevent the development of contractures, promote safety, and reduce injury.

Nursing Considerations for Osteogenesis Imperfecta

Newborns, infants, and young children require special physical handling to prevent injury. Very specific guidelines are needed about restricting activities while promoting play, socialization, education, and development. Much education is required for family members to understand the severity of the disease and how it is genetically linked. Families should be encouraged to find further education and support by seeking guidance from the national organizations for OI, including The National Organization for Rare Diseases and the Osteogenesis Imperfecta Foundation.

Juvenile Rheumatoid Arthritis

JRA, also known as *juvenile idiopathic arthritis (JIR)*, is a group of idiopathic chronic inflammatory joint diseases that first manifest during the early childhood period. The disorder may be linked to an autoimmune dysfunction after an exposure to a viral or bacterial infection followed by an acute attack of the joint tissue by the immune system. The rheumatic process leads to the destruction of the child's synovial tissue layers, which line the joints and secrete a lubricating material for ease of joint motion. The chronic nature of the disease leads to very painful joint destruction and fibrosis of the joint cartilage. Joints appear enlarged, abnormally shaped, and larger than normal. They may feel warm during periods of inflammation exacerbation.

Assessments of Juvenile Rheumatoid Arthritis

Upon presentation of a child with painful, swollen joints, confirmation of the disease is by laboratory assay and clinical presentation. Laboratory values include an elevated ESR, leukocytosis, possible positive ANA test, low hemoglobin and hematocrit levels, and elevated CRP levels. Clinical presentation includes the onset of the disease before the child's 16th birthday and the presence of inflammation in more than one joint that lasts for at least 6 weeks.

Interventions for Juvenile Rheumatoid Arthritis

Because there is no cure for JRA, the plan of treatment consists of decreasing the inflammation, reducing pain, and preventing severe joint erosion and joint dysfunction from the acute inflammatory process. The child's ROM and normal growth patterns should be supported both during an acute exacerbation and during periods of decreased inflammatory processes. A team approach should be used to provide the child with physical, social, educational, emotional, and spiritual support. Box 35.3 provides information about the classifications of medications used to treat JRA.

Antirheumatic medications are effective in suppressing the inflammatory process and include NSAIDs, slower-acting antirheumatic drugs (SAARDs), corticosteroids, cytotoxic medications (eg, methotrexate, abatacept, chlorambucil, and cyclosporine), tumor necrosis factor inhibitors, and intramuscular gold and biological agents.

Physical management includes working with an occupational therapist and a PT at regular intervals to improve muscle strength, ROM, splinting, pain reduction, and child development through the mastery of self-care and independence.

Nursing Considerations for Juvenile Rheumatoid Arthritis

Nursing care consists of focusing on the prevention, education, and the management of discomfort; balancing rest and activity; supporting normal growth and development; decreasing the change or disfigurement; and facilitating adherence to treatment plans and frequent outpatient visits. The pediatric nurse should help the child find what level of joint pain is acceptable using a developmentally appropriate pain scale and then provide pain-relief measures with the acceptable level of discomfort as stated by the child as the goal.

Duchenne's Muscular Dystrophy

Duchenne's muscular dystrophy (Duchenne's MD), also referred to as *pseudohypertrophic muscular dystrophy,* is part of a group of 30 genetic diseases that causes progressive weakness and degeneration of skeletal muscles. Duchenne's MD is the most common form found in childhood, occurring in approximately 1 out of every 3,500 male births. This progressive disorder of the voluntary neuromuscular system is X-linked and therefore is almost exclusively a male-dominated disorder. The protein dystrophin, produced in the skeletal muscle, is greatly reduced by a mutation in the gene that encodes dystrophin. Children who present with Duchenne's MD demonstrate an unusually high blood level of creatinine kinase.

Box 35.3 Medication Classifications Used to Treat Juvenile Rheumatoid Arthritis

- **Nonsteroidal anti-inflammatory drugs (NSAIDs):** NSAIDs can reduce inflammation and relieve pain. These are over-the-counter medications and include naproxen sodium (Aleve), ibuprofen (Motrin, Advil), and others. Side effects include gastrointestinal (GI) distress, gastric ulcers, tinnitus, higher levels of bruising, bleeding into the stomach, fatigue, and liver damage.
- **Steroids:** Medications in the corticosteroid category relieve pain and reduce inflammation by slowing the damage occurring to the joint tissues. Examples of steroids include prednisone and methylprednisolone. Serious side effects can occur and include thinning of the bones, weight gain with a round face, cataracts, diabetes, and easy bruising.
- **Immunosuppressants:** This classification of drugs includes azathioprine, cyclophosphamide, and cyclosporine. The most concerning side effect of immunosuppressants is their effect on the immune system, which is an increased susceptibility to infection.
- **Disease-modifying antirheumatic drugs (DMARDs):** Methotrexate, hydroxychloroquine, minocycline, and leflunomide are examples of DMARDs and are known to cause bone marrow suppression, severe lung diseases, and liver tissue damage.
- **Tumor necrosis factor-α (TNFα):** This factor, naturally produced in the body, is administered to produce an anti-inflammatory process that helps to reduce painful joints, swollen joints, morning stiffness, and overall pain.

Assessments of Duchenne's Muscular Dystrophy

Around the third to fourth year of life, during or after the child begins to walk, the child presents with progressive muscle weakness that produces difficulty in performing normal childhood activities. First symptoms include difficulty in running, skipping, climbing stairs, or riding a tricycle or bicycle. As time progresses, the child will demonstrate a waddling gait and difficulty in rising from a squatting or sitting position on the floor, referred to as the Gowers' sign. As time progresses and the muscles are infiltrated with fatty tissue, the child's muscles feel firm or, as some describe, "woody" on palpation. During the later stages of the progressive disease, the child's muscles experience profound dystrophy. Gait becomes impossible and the child may progress to respiratory failure from wasting of the thoracic and diaphragm muscles. Mortality is associated with respiratory disease, failure, and arrest.

To confirm the diagnosis, blood and urine tests are performed. Serum aldolase, creatinine kinase, and myoglobin are measured for abnormally high levels. Serum electrophoresis is also performed to determine how much of various proteins are present in the child's DNA. Muscle biopsies are also conducted to monitor the child's presentation of symptoms by determining the severity of nerve disease, muscle wasting disease, inflammation, and overall myopathy.

Interventions for Duchenne's Muscular Dystrophy

There are no known treatments for this progressive disease. Research continues in the use of corticosteroids. The child and family are supported through the slow declining process. Care is focused on promoting optimal functioning as long as possible, treating respiratory infections early, and delaying the debilitating process for as long as possible using positive-pressure ventilation, tracheostomy, and mechanical ventilation. Family-centered care is always used to support the family to enable them to give their child care and empowerment by including the family in all treatment discussions, treatment plans, and end-of-life care. Soliciting the assistance of occupational therapists to help the child with the progressive weakness has been shown to be of great assistance.

Nursing Considerations for Duchenne's Muscular Dystrophy

The pediatric nurse should focus on three aspects of the child's care: injury prevention, normal growth and development, and the preservation of self-help skills, such as activities of daily living (ADL). The nurse can be instrumental in providing emotional support, spiritual support, and interdisciplinary care communication. Nurses should be assessing the child and family for symptoms of social isolation, depression, stress, and anger, and evaluating overall quality of life.

Research continues in the areas of gene replacement therapy to investigate if the defective dystrophin gene can be replaced with a more functional gene. Cell-based therapies are also being investigated to promote the production of critical proteins, such as dystrophin, by specific muscle cells.

Families should be encouraged to seek state-of-the-science information and support from national organizations such as the Muscular Dystrophy Family Foundation, the Muscular Dystrophy Association, and Parent Project Muscular Dystrophy (PPMD).

Osteomyelitis

Children under the age of 10 years are at the greatest risk for the development of a bone infection from trauma, injury, or an infection found elsewhere in the body that migrates as an infected hematogenous emboli and sequesters (ie, stays put or wedges) in the child's bone marrow. Osteomyelitis has a developmental influence; neonates present with group B streptococci, infants can present with *Escherichia coli* bone infections, and older children may present with *Salmonella, Staphylococcus aureus,* and *Neisseria gonorrhoeae* as the causative organism. Puncture wounds, otitis media infections, dental abscesses, pyelonephritis, open fractures, and contamination from surgical procedures can all lead to the development of osteomyelitis in childhood.

Osteomyelitis develops as the causative organism is trapped in the vasculature of the bone, causing inflammation, edema, sequestration, and vascular congestions (Fig. 35.14). Because of the inflammation and growing infection, the bone tissue may become destroyed, causing great discomfort. In young infants, the infection may cross from the bone vasculature into the joint space, spreading the infection.

Assessments of Osteomyelitis

Osteomyelitis should be suspected when a child presents with a history of a puncture wound or infection that now produces pain, warmth at the site, guarding, refusal to use the extremity, fever, and leukocytosis. Isolating and identifying the causative agent is imperative to match the correct antibiotic. Cultures of aspirated fluids, serum blood cultures, or sinus drainage through the skin should all be collected and sent to the laboratory for antibiotic susceptibility testing. Assessing for risk factors for osteomyelitis can help with the differential diagnosis. Risk factors include puncture with a foreign body, bone trauma or injury, immunosuppression, and malnutrition.

Treatments for Osteomyelitis

After cultures are collected, empiric antibiotics are started immediately, with the most likely coverage for the suspected organism. Immediately upon return of the culture findings, the antibiotics are adjusted to cover the exact microbe. With the enclosed bony structure of the skeleton, antibiotics are often required for a period of 3 to 4 weeks. A child might benefit from the use of a peripherally inserted central catheter

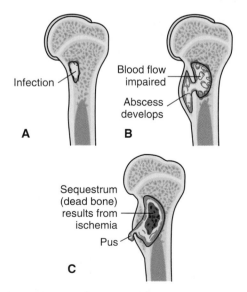

FIGURE 35.14 Sequence of osteomyelitis development. A, Infection begins. B, Blood flow is blocked in the arc of infection and an abscess with pus forms. C, Bone dies within the infection site and pus continues to form.

instead of trying to maintain sequential peripheral IVs. If antibiotics are not effective, surgical interventions to remove the infection may be required.

Nursing Considerations for Osteomyelitis

Nursing concerns focus on the accuracy of antibiotic administration and the control of discomfort. Febrile states should be reported and antipyretics administered. If an open wound is present, such as with an osteomyelitis-related surgical wound or a puncture site, standard precautions should be used to prevent the cross-contamination to other patients. Children can experience poor appetite and poor oral intake; the nurse should monitor for appropriate caloric and fluid intake to promote healing.

Key Points

- The musculoskeletal system comprises 206 bones, all existing from birth, and contains two distinct components: skeletal muscles and skeletal bones. The skeletal system grows and develops across childhood. Bone growth in length occurs in the cartilage area of the bones called the epiphyseal plates and when the epiphyseal plates close, growth stops.
- Red blood cells, white blood cells, and megakaryocyte cells that produce platelets are formed within the bone marrow. A double protective layer of connective tissue, called the *periosteum,* which is rich with nerves and blood vessels, covers the long bones.
- A child's nutrition highly affects the bones' ability and effectiveness in production of blood cells in the long bone's marrow. Iron, vitamins B$_{12}$ and folate, and protein are required for adequate production of bone marrow cells (Mayo Clinic, 2015).
- Childhood injuries that lead to musculoskeletal traumatic injuries or disorders include strains, sprains, contusions, and fractures of various types.
- Laboratory values that are used to identify and monitor disease progression for a child with a musculoskeletal

disorder include CBC, ESR, blood cultures, RF, and ANA.
- Bone fractures experienced in childhood may require immobilization, casting, or traction therapy. Traction uses lines of pull to immobilize, provide stability, and create tension on the fractured site. Examples of traction include Bryant's traction, Buck's extension, cervical, 90/90 traction, Ilizarov device, and Russell's traction.
- Children undergoing immobilization and/or traction for an extended period of time require interdisciplinary care that includes physical therapy, occupational therapy, the support of Child Life Specialists, and the dietary office. The child's developmental level should be considered as holistic interventions and play are created.
- Congenital childhood disease processes of the musculoskeletal system include congenital clubfoot, JRA, scoliosis, congenital hip dysplasia, OI, and Duchenne's muscular dystrophy.
- Maintaining a safe environment is imperative while caring for a child in traction. Complications such as discomfort, constipation, skin breakdown and pressure sores, and boredom and monotony should be anticipated and addressed.

REVIEW QUESTIONS

1. All of the following are risk factors associated with the development of osteomyelitis: *(select all that apply)*
   1. Foreign body
   2. Bone injury
   3. Female gender
   4. Immunosuppression
   5. Malnutrition
   6. Infancy

2. You are the bedside nurse for a young boy admitted for r/o fracture of the femur. While the child has been transported off the unit for an x-ray of his affected limb, the parents come to you and state that they are leaving the unit for the night to care for their other siblings and will be back in the early morning to visit before work. The best response the pediatric nurse should say is:
   1. "That is fine; we will see you in the morning."
   2. "I will tell your son what your plans are for you so he understands why you are not here."
   3. "I think it would benefit your son if you wait to say good night to him before you leave and explain when you will return."
   4. "I will call a member of Child Life to come and sit and play with your son so he is not in distress."

3. Before surgery, priority nursing care for an adolescent boy with scoliosis includes:
   1. Teaching the parents how to use an age-appropriate numerical pain scale
   2. Discussing with the child how to use a PCA machine
   3. Verbalizing what an "advancing diet" will be, starting from NPO and progressing to a regular diet
   4. Assessing the child's knowledge base of the pathology of severe scoliosis

4. The nurse has been notified that she will be admitting to the pediatric floor a child with complications associated with Legg-Calve-Perthes disease. In preparing for the admission, the nurse knows that this diagnosis is congenital and involves:
   1. Bilateral phalanges
   2. A slipped femoral head
   3. The entire vertebral column
   4. The head of the femur

5. While assessing a child who is hospitalized in a spica cast, the nurse performs frequent checks to the interior aspects of the affected casted limb. Each are included in the assessment except: (select all that apply)
   1. Circulation
   2. Color
   3. Movement
   4. Touch
   5. Sensation
   6. Pain
   7. Strength

6. The percentage of fractures for children under 3 years old suspected to be child abuse is:
   1. 15%
   2. 25%
   3. 40%
   4. 100%

7. When assisting a school-aged child who had a soft-tissue injury while playing soccer, the pediatric nurse suggests to the parents to do the following immediately: (select all that apply)
   1. Apply ice to the site of the injury.
   2. Have the child lie down or sit down and rest the injured extremity.
   3. Offer the child an appointment to see an orthopedist.
   4. Apply compression to the site to reduce the chance of swelling.
   5. Administer an opioid pain medication to immediately control pain.
   6. Elevate the extremity.

8. While answering questions from the parents of a child with a new diagnosis of JRA, the pediatric nurse is asked why the child has so much pain. The nurse would be correct in stating that:
   1. "Adherence to anti-inflammatory medications will reduce overall pain."
   2. "The pain is directly related to the child's developmental stage; the older the child, the more pain the diagnosis will cause."
   3. "The severe pain is related to immobility because the child will hold their affected joint still for an extended period of time."
   4. "The rheumatic process leads to the destruction of the child's synovial tissue layers, which secrete a lubricating material for ease of joint motion."

9. While assisting the pediatric health-care team of an orthopedic clinic, the licensed vocational nurse (LVN) knows that the highest priority in caring for a child with a newly placed spica cast is to:
   1. Report any changes in discomfort
   2. Report any changes in circulation, sensation, and movement
   3. Confirm parents' understanding of the purpose and care of the cast
   4. Determine if the fracture was caused by intentional injury

10. Laboratory values that are used to identify and monitor disease progression for a child with a musculoskeletal disorder include which of the following? (select all that apply)
    1. CBC
    2. ESR
    3. Potassium
    4. RF
    5. ANA
    6. Serum protein levels
    7. Blood cultures

CRITICAL THINKING QUESTIONS

1. What are various holistic interventions that a pediatric nurse can provide to a child who is experiencing a prolonged hospitalization and period of time of bedrest in traction? Which departments or professionals can provide support, distraction, play, and assistance in preventing common side effects or untoward reactions to the experience of prolonged traction?

2. How should the health-care team initiate care and treatment for a child with a confirmed spiral fracture? What might be a suspected cause of the injury? What steps would be taken to rule out intentional injury on a child who presents with a spiral fracture?

3. How would a pediatric nurse intervene for a family whose early school-aged child refuses to eat fruits and vegetables during a prolonged hospitalization for a significant femur fracture that requires 6 to 8 weeks of bedrest with traction? What are ways to prevent skin breakdown and constipation for this child? Develop a care plan for this child to prevent complications.

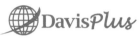

For additional resources and information, visit **www.DavisPlus.com**. Post-Conference Questions and Activities, Answers, and References can be found on Davis*Plus*.

Child With a Gastrointestinal Condition

LEARNING OUTCOMES

1. Define the key terms.
2. Review the growth and development of the gastrointestinal (GI) tract from the newborn period through adolescence.
3. Describe the components of a health history for a child who presents with a GI disorder.
4. Review assessment techniques when caring for a child who presents with dehydration, vomiting, diarrhea, constipation, or abdominal pain.
5. Describe the pathophysiology and clinical presentation of common intestinal infections such as *Clostridium difficile (C diff.)*, viral gastroenteritis such as rotavirus, and parasitic infections in the GI tract.
6. Interpret data that would need to be reported immediately associated with various congenital or acquired GI abnormalities.
7. State common diagnostic tests used to rule out specific GI infections or disorders.
8. Describe the care of a child who has been hospitalized for surgery to correct a congenital or acquired GI disorder including perioperative assessments, symptom management, and diet progression.
9. Recognize the teaching needs of a family whose child presents with an infectious GI disorder. Include providing safety to others to prevent cross-contamination through effective communication, use of infection control measures, and evidence-based practices to control spread.

KEY TERMS

Clostridium difficile (C diff.)
Crohn's disease
emesis
fistula
gastroenteritis
gluten intolerance
intussusception
Salmonella food poisoning

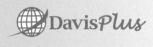 For audio pronunciation guide, visit **www.DavisPlus.com**

CHAPTER CONCEPTS

Bowel Elimination
Comfort
Development
Digestion
Nutrition

REAL-WORLD CASE STUDY

Gabriel

■ An 8-year-old has been admitted to the pediatric unit of the hospital with a new diagnosis of Crohn's disease. The child has been losing weight over the last 6 months and presents with a growth chart plot finding for weight in the 25th percentile. She has had a history of slightly bloody watery stools off and on over

continued on page 600

REAL-WORLD CASE STUDY *continued*

the last 3 months and was seen by her community-based pediatrician on several occasions. Today she is admitted for an upper GI series by radiology for a nutrition consultation and she is to start a new IV medication, infliximab (Remicade). She was placed on the oral anti-inflammatory mesalamine (Asacol) 4 weeks ago but continues to complain of abdominal pain, bloating, flatulence, and bloody stools.

1. How prevalent are inflammatory bowel syndromes in the pediatric population?
2. What other symptoms might this 8-year-old display with the diagnosis of Crohn's disease?
3. What foods might she be intolerant of and what foods should she avoid?
4. What are the side effects of immunosuppressant drugs such as infliximab (Remicade)?

CONCEPTUAL CORNERSTONE

Elimination

The primary responsibility of the GI system is to digest and absorb foods and fluids, and provide for colon elimination. Congenital, acquired, and infectious GI conditions affect the elimination process. They require meticulous attention to the potential rapid loss of fluids and electrolytes, acid-base imbalances, and poor nutritional intake. During the absorption, digestion, and elimination process, the GI system is prone to infectious pathogens. Acute and chronic abdominal pain is often associated with GI conditions. Children can present with abdominal pain that can be nonspecific with no identifiable pathology or etiology. Children can also present with acute abdominal pain that represents serious conditions such as acute appendicitis, severe food poisoning, or intussusception. The pediatric nurse must evaluate the child's overall elimination process, fluid balance, and discomfort, and report the findings.

GI conditions may present as either acute disorders with bacterial, parasitic, or viral etiologies, or they may present as congenital or acquired structural disorders. Both may cause inflammatory responses and/or problems with motility of the GI tract. Some disorders present with constipation and others with diarrhea. The term *gastroenteritis* is defined as an inflammatory process that occurs in the stomach, small intestine, or large intestine. Clinical signs and symptoms include nausea, vomiting, anorexia, abdominal distention, abdominal pain, and diarrhea.

It is imperative that the nurse assesses the degree of dehydration and reports the severity of the child's condition promptly.

SAFETY *STAT!*

Many GI disorders and infections cause the child to experience significant diarrhea. Diarrhea can lead to loss of body fluids rapidly if the stool loss is continuous. The loss of fluids from the intestinal tract can lead a child to experience mild, moderate, or severe dehydration.

THE DEVELOPMENT OF GASTROINTESTINAL ABNORMALITIES

Many GI disorders can have their origins traced to the child's fetal development. The disorder may or may not be first detected during the newborn period. As the child grows and matures, the disorder may appear with the introduction of solid foods and the further advancement of the child's diet. A thorough health history should include questions about the child's food habits, known food allergies, the use of vitamins or supplements, cultural practices concerning food and eating, bowel habits, and at least a 3-day diet history. An investigation concerning any symptoms associated with daily nutritional practices should include questions concerning the child's ingestion, digestion, absorption, and elimination.

Maturity of the Gastrointestinal Tract in Infancy

Neonates are born with what is considered a sterile gut. This implies that the entire intestinal lining must be introduced to normally expected bacteria to aid the infant in the process of digestion and elimination. Normal exposure to the environment, including the mother's breast tissue, will assist with the introduction of microbes that make up the digestive system's normal flora. Vitamin K cannot be processed without the presence of this normal flora; thus newborns receive a shot of vitamin K to assist with the production of clotting factors.

The newborn has only a small stomach capacity of approximately 15 to 20 mL. As the infant grows quickly during his or her first year of life, so does the volume capacity of the child's stomach. By the end of the second week of life, the newborn's stomach capacity expands to 90 mL.

SAFETY *STAT!*

It is imperative that the pediatric nurse knows the volume capacity of the stomach during the newborn period because overfeeding can lead to distress, bloating, distension, and regurgitation of breast milk or formula.

HEALTH HISTORY

The nurse should take a thorough health history of a child who presents with either an acute GI disorder or a structural

GI disorder. Components of this health history should include:

- Food habits, including the typical daily intake of foods consumed, daily calories consumed, the estimated amount of fluids consumed daily, and levels of appetite
- Elimination habits and patterns
- Problems associated with each step of the digestive/ elimination process, including refusal, dysphagia, evidence of heart burn, delayed stomach emptying, spitting up, wet burps or regurgitation of food, abdominal pain, abnormal stooling patterns, and excessive flatulence
- Past medical history related to the GI system, including illnesses, injuries, accidents, surgeries, and significant family history

PHYSICAL ASSESSMENT

The nurse assists with the physical assessment of the child and prepares by placing the child in a comfortable supine position. Young children do not tolerate GI assessments as well as older children. If tickling is a problem, place the child's hand on the abdomen and then gently place your hand over the child's hand. Have the child slowly pull his or her hand away and this will reduce the sensation of tickling. The following are included in a GI assessment and should be conducted in this order:

1. Assess weight and height.
2. Ask about bowel elimination routine and last bowel movement, including normal frequency and consistency.
3. Determine the hydration status, including mucous membrane moisture, turgor, the presence or absence of tears, and peripheral pulses.
4. Inspect the abdomen for contour, rashes, lesions, asymmetry, masses, and pulsations.
5. Palpate light and deep, and assess for rebound tenderness.

While assessing a child's abdomen, the nurse should follow a specific order to prevent the child from refusing or guarding his or her abdomen if pain or discomfort is elicited: Start with auscultation, proceed to percussion, and then perform light to deep palpation. Further assessments may be needed and include laboratory evaluation and further diagnostic testing. All abnormal findings should be reported immediately.

LABS & DIAGNOSTICS

Common Diagnostic Tests Performed for Gastrointestinal Function

- Laboratory tests
  - **Chemistry panels:** Demonstrate the blood levels of electrolytes that are affected by fluid loss, dehydration, persistent diarrhea, and persistent vomiting.
  - **Complete blood cell count (CBC):** Demonstrates the level of anemia by showing the hematocrit and hemoglobin

levels; anemia can be caused by nutritional deficiencies, GI bleeds, and chronic inflammatory processes.
  - **Liver profiles:** Demonstrate the involvement of the liver in inflammatory processes and other liver-related pathologies.
  - **Lipid profiles:** Demonstrate the levels of triglycerides and lipids in the blood.
  - **Erythrocyte sedimentation rate (ESR):** Demonstrates the level of inflammatory chemicals found in the blood. Elevated ESR can denote the severity of the inflammatory bowel process.
  - **Thyroid function:** Demonstrates the functioning of the thyroid gland, which helps to regulate metabolism.
  - **C-reactive proteins (CRP):** Demonstrates the presence and severity of inflammation.
  - **Fecal fat collection (72 hour):** Collecting a timed sample of feces for fecal fat can demonstrate how the body is processing dietary fat. Elevated findings are indicative of the bowel mucosa being unable to process, breakdown, and prepare for the digestion of oral fats.
  - **Stool examination:** Demonstrates the presence of ova and parasites, and for culture.
- Diagnostic tests
  - Bowel and abdominal radiograph
  - Abdominal and pelvic ultrasound
  - Upper GI series
  - Barium enema
  - Rectal biopsy
  - Rectosigmoidoscopy

COMMON GASTROINTESTINAL DISORDERS

Children will present to health-care providers with a variety of mild to severe GI disorders. These disorders can affect the consumption of fluids and can also affect nutrition, digestion, and elimination. The following sections describe common GI disorders found across childhood.

Enteral Feeding

In pediatrics, there are many reasons a child may need to receive enteral feedings. This includes congenital intestinal function disorders; oral malformations; conditions that cause dysphagia; failure to thrive (FTT), which requires additional calories; and neurological disorders that disrupt adequate calorie consumption. Caloric need will be determined by a nutritionist working with the health-care team to ensure a child will respond adequately with weight maintenance or weight gain. Daily weights, hydration, adequate stooling, and tolerance of the feedings will determine if the procedure is successful.

There are several means of administering enteral feedings to children. The placement of a nasogastric tube (NGT) is the primary means to administer nutrition for short-term requirements. If a child needs extended feeds, a gastrostomy tube may be placed surgically, extending from the external abdominal wall to the stomach. This is called a *PEG tube* or *percutaneous endoscopic gastrostomy tube.* When the gastrostomy tube is at the skin level, it is often referred to as a "button" (Fig. 36.1).

Children with incompetent cardiac sphincters, neurological impairment, inadequate cough, or poor motor control may be at risk for aspiration of the tube feeding solution and should be monitored closely to assess for signs of aspiration pneumonia. The prevention of aspiration pneumonia can be accomplished by positioning a child in an upright position and checking for the amount of residual formula still present within a child's stomach before starting the feeds. Follow orders meticulously to assess for remaining, or residual, stomach contents and hold feeds if the amount exceeds recommendations. Typically, the primary care provider will order how frequently to assess residual and how much residual will be allowed before the administration of an NGT feeding. For instance, if an older infant has more than 30 cc of residual feed in the stomach before starting the next bolus feed, the feeding may be held for an hour or more to allow the stomach to empty.

SAFETY *STAT!*

The determination of residual feed in a newborn, infant, or young child's stomach helps to prevent overfeeding, which may result in vomiting and the potential aspiration of vomitus.

Parents or caregivers should be taught how to care for their child with a feeding tube from the beginning of therapy. The involvement of family in the care of the child's tube and feeding will empower the family to care for their child. The family should be instructed how to care for all aspects of the process, including how to appropriately mix the feeding solution, safely administer the solution, and monitor for untoward effects such as bloating, diarrhea, constipation, or vomiting.

PATIENT TEACHING GUIDELINES

Family Education for the Administration of Enteral Feeds Via a Nasogastric Tube

1. Interpret the order for the feeding procedure.
2. Wash hands to prevent contamination of the feeds.

3. Mix feeding powder correctly with clean water for a correct amount of feed (may be continuous or bolus feeds).
4. Attach the feeding bag to the connecting tubing (some products come commercially attached).
5. Position the child in a safe, upright position, if able.
6. Check the placement of the feeding tube.
7. Check for the presence of residual feeding solution in the stomach by slowly aspirating stomach content for the volume remaining in the child's stomach.
8. Flush tubing with 3 to 10 mL of clean water to ensure the entire tube is patent.
9. Double-check the setup from the bag to the tubing to the child's nares to ensure that there are no kinks or knots.
10. Slowly start feeds to ensure tolerance.
11. Monitor the child for potential or actual aspiration pneumonia (ie, assess for coughing, vomiting, signs of distress, or a change in condition).
12. When feeding is complete, remove the tubing from the NGT in the child.
13. Clean the bag and the tube with tap water and save them for the next feeding.
14. Change the bag and the tubing at ordered intervals to prevent contamination or problems with feeding solution buildup and clogging.

The nurse's responsibility with enteral feedings encompasses the accuracy of the procedure, clinical improvement, and safety. The following information provides nursing care checklists for pre-, intra- and postenteral feedings.

- **Prefeeding**
  1. Ensure a complete order, including the feeding solution type, the amount to be administered, the time period for administration (either bolus or continuous), the frequency and length of time of the feeds required, the quantity of residual allowed before feedings are held, and whether or not the child's medications may be administered via the feeding tube.
  2. Obtain feeding solution and mix with ordered fluids if in a powder form. Ensure the formula has not expired. Double-check the accuracy of the mixture because too-dilute feeding solutions may cause weight loss over time if the child does not receive

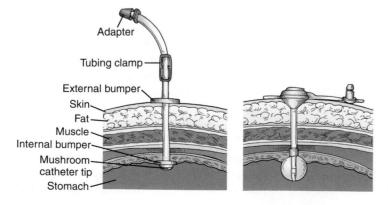

FIGURE 36.1 Types of enteral feeding devices.

the ordered calories, and solutions that are too concentrated may lead to diarrhea or stomach distress.

3. Set up equipment and ensure that the tubing and bag are clean. The tubing and bag should be changed every 24 hours.
   a. NGTs stiffen when left in place for a long period of time. Make sure there is no presence of irritation of the skin around the nares caused by this process.
   b. If inserting the tube for the feed, make sure the wire stylet used only for inserting the tube has been removed.

- **Intrafeeding**
1. Confirm placement by attaching a small syringe to the end of the NGT and aspirating for stomach content.
2. Ensure patency by flushing the tube with 3 to 5 mL of clean water. Do not force the flush if resistance is encountered because this could damage the tubing or cause perforation.
3. Begin feeds and monitor for tolerance and aspiration. The infusion may be delivered by gravity or by pump.
4. Continue feeds as ordered, either bolus or continuous.
5. If the child is an infant, provide non-nutritive sucking during the infusion. This has been noted to decrease restlessness, improve weight gain, and increase states of alertness (Selekman and Jakubik, 2007).

- **Postfeeding**
1. When the infusion is complete, disconnect the tubing and flush the NGT/GT well with 3 to 10 mL of water, depending on the age of the child. Use smaller amounts for infants.
2. Assess the child's tolerance and monitor for distension, abdominal discomfort, and diarrhea.

SAFETY *STAT!*

Do not leave NGT/GT feeds hanging for any extended period of time. Feeds left at room temperature for over 4 hours are at risk for the development of bacterial contamination.

Vomiting

Vomiting, or **emesis,** is defined as the forceful expulsion or emptying of stomach content caused by either a GI disorder or by a non-GI disorder, such as increased intracranial pressure, food allergies or intolerances, the ingestion of a toxic substance, or the administration of chemotherapy. GI disorders that cause a child to vomit include reverse peristalsis from a pyloric sphincter blockage, esophageal reflux, overdistension from increased intake, or severe gastroenteritis. The vomiting experience is controlled by the emetic center of the medulla, called the *chemoreceptor trigger zone.* Antiemetic medications effective in preventing or reducing nausea and vomiting work by influencing this center.

The pediatric nurse must identify if the child is experiencing true emesis or wet burps. Wet burps or the simple spitting up of undigested breast milk, formula, or food is caused by an increase in pressure in the stomach, especially immediately following a forceful burp. True vomiting is characterized by rapid expulsion of most or all of the stomach content. Vomiting is a well-coordinated and well-defined process, unlike spit-up, which is passive.

Assessment of Vomit and Associated Symptoms

Vomiting is a common pediatric experience and is associated with many conditions. Vomiting may indicate pathology is present and needs to be assessed for a number of factors. The following list provides guidance on the assessment of vomiting in children.

- Differentiate vomiting from wet burps or simple spitting up in the infant.
- Assess the frequency, consistency, and precipitating factors.
- Identify the characteristics of the vomit, such as the presence of blood, bile, mucus, or undigested foods, sometimes produced long after consumption, which may indicate a slow gastric emptying.
- Determine if the vomiting is associated with fever, diarrhea, or headaches.
- Assess the abdomen for the presence of distention, pain, and bowel sounds.
- Measure the girth of the abdomen using a clean paper measuring tape, placing the tape directly over the child's umbilicus.
- Assess the child's overall nutritional status, feeding schedule, and any other associated factors.
- During infancy, assess the feeding position, the quantity of food taken in, and the type of formula used and the recipe for mixing it.
- Assess for metabolic alkalosis, which results from large losses of acid-rich stomach contents.
- Check for clinical signs of dehydration such as skin turgor, a low moisture level of the mucous membranes, thirst, and tachycardia.
- Assess for conditions that produce vomiting, such as the presence of an associated infectious illness.
- Assess the child's psychological status because emotions and rising adrenaline levels with stress both may trigger the chemoreceptor trigger zone.
- Assess for the experience of projectile vomiting, which is associated with pyloric stenosis.
- Assess the child for self-induced vomiting or rumination.

NONRETRACTABLE NAUSEA AND VOMITING. When a child is experiencing nonretractable symptoms, such as vomiting, even with the use of antiemetics, it is important to assist the team in ruling out other severe conditions. Pyloric stenosis, obstructions, tumors, foreign bodies, and the ingestion of poisonous materials should be considered.

Interventions for Vomiting

When a child is experiencing vomiting, safety is imperative. Children with decreased consciousness may be at risk for aspiration of the vomit into their pulmonary system. The following guidelines provide tips on how to keep a vomiting child safe.

- Place the child in an NPO status and maintain until there has been no vomiting for 12 to 24 hours.
- Ensure safety for the child by preventing the aspiration of stomach content: Place the child in an upright position and maintain a patent airway.
- Ensure the presence of suction; either wall suction or a bulb syringe.
- Introduce fluids, such as an oral electrolyte solution, first; progress the diet as tolerated. Young children tolerate an oral solution such as Pedialyte and older children do well with low-sugar, noncarbonated beverages.
- Medications should be withheld or, if essential, should be given in a rectal or parenteral form.
- Maintain strict intake and output (I&O) and monitor the stool status for possible accompanied diarrhea.
- Instigate good oral hygiene after vomiting.

Nursing Considerations for Vomiting

The child who has had an extended period of time vomiting should be monitored for dehydration, aspiration, sore throat, and weight loss. Persistent vomiting can be detrimental to the child's teeth and oral hygiene should be provided after each vomiting episode.

Gastroesophageal Reflux

The return of stomach content through the esophagus can be caused by either a poorly developed or an incompetent cardiac sphincter. Premature infants and children with conditions that cause decreased muscle tone are especially prone to the development of gastroesophageal reflux (GER), also called *gastroesophageal reflux disease (GERD)*. The acidity of stomach content causes the child to experience pain and, in severe cases with repeated exposure, can cause the esophagus to erode. Symptoms appear immediately after the child consumes food as levels of stomach acid increase. If a child with GERD experiences an aspiration of the acidic stomach contents, they are at risk for developing pneumonia. Most cases of reflux resolve before the end of the infant developmental period (by 1 year of age), but complicated cases will need surgical interventions.

Assessment of Gastroesophageal Reflux

The child with a confirmed diagnosis of GER should be assessed for severity and esophageal tissue damage from the stomach acid reflux. Important assessment considerations include the following:

- The child's GER behaviors in relation to eating/feeding patterns
- The onset of GER in relation to the child's positioning
- The pH of the stomach content
- Coexisting weight loss or FTT
- Severity of discomfort in the chest area, described as inconsolable crying in infancy or adultlike patterns of heart burn seen in older children

Prepare the child for diagnostic assessment procedures, including barium swallow or an upper GI series of x-rays.

Interventions for Gastroesophageal Reflux

A child with GER needs to be supported to prevent complications. The following list addresses the most important aspects of care.

- Place the child in an upright position for the pre-, intra-, and postfeeding time periods.
- Provide small meals, feed slowly, and assess for tolerance.
- Burp frequently to prevent a buildup of swallowed air.
- Administer ordered GERD medications as directed at least 30 min before eating.
- Pharmacology may include medications that reduce the amount of stomach acid produced (eg, famotidine, cimetidine, and ranitidine), increase the timeframe of stomach content emptying, and increase gastric peristalsis (eg, metoclopramide). The prevention of esophagitis is imperative to reduce the child's discomfort.
- If the child is an infant, work with the nutritionist to determine the feasibility of thickening the formula. This may require an alternative nipple because thicker formula may not flow through a traditional nipple. This can become a safety hazard and should not be done unless the child has been assessed by a nutritionist or a speech therapist has evaluated the child's swallowing reflex.

Nissen's fundoplication surgery may be required for a child with persistent and severe GERD that leads to growth problems and esophageal tissue damage from stomach acid. This surgical procedure provides for the establishment of an intra-abdominal segment of the esophagus by creating a lower esophageal sphincter that significantly reduces the reflux of stomach acid into the esophagus. The surgical procedure includes creating an antireflux valve made up of a portion of the fundus of the stomach, thus creating a high-pressure zone. The surgical procedure leads to an increased opening pressure required to cause reflux.

Nursing Considerations for Gastroesophageal Reflux

Not only does a diagnosis of GERD cause significant discomfort, frequent regurgitation of acidic stomach contents places the child at risk for developing esophageal erosion and scar tissue that can lead to strictures or narrowed lumen. It is imperative that the pediatric nurse identify GERD early, differentiate it from other pain such as indigestion or more severe problems such as heart pain, and provide pharmacological and nonpharmacological interventions such as positioning after eating and sleeping positions with the head of the bed elevated.

Diarrhea

When a child is experiencing diarrhea, there is an increased frequency and decreased consistency of stool. Water increases in the bowel because of an osmotic pull, an electrolyte imbalance, and poor water absorption with an inflammatory process or when peristalsis is increased. Many causes contribute to the development of diarrhea, including infectious processes, food allergies, and exposure to toxins or malabsorption conditions. Diarrhea is a common outcome of many childhood illnesses, including both GI and respiratory disorders, and may accompany the administration of antibiotic therapy. Great caution should be taken to assess for the development of metabolic acidosis with extended periods of diarrhea; with stool loss, there is a loss of alkaline.

Dehydration is also associated with stool loss. Monitoring a child during periods of diarrhea is important to determine overall fluid loss. Careful assessment of I&O allows the nurse to determine if a child will need further fluids either orally, if the child can, or if an IV will need to be placed to provide parenteral fluids. Report any change of condition rapidly to prevent complications of dehydration. Diarrhea can cause severe fluid loss that progresses to electrolyte imbalances, hypovolemic shock, and even death in the pediatric patient. See Table 36.1 for information about levels of dehydration.

Culture plays a large role in how families view health conditions for their children. When a child presents with a history of GI problems, such as vomiting or diarrhea, when and how a family addresses the child's symptoms may have a cultural influence. See the Cultural Considerations feature for information about introducing a diet to a child with a GI disorder.

 ## CULTURAL CONSIDERATIONS

Introduction of a Diet to Children With Acute Gastrointestinal Disorders

Cultural preferences play a large part in how families feed their children. Many cultural and ethnic groups have preferences for foods when their child is ill. When a child has a GI disorder and associated symptoms such as diarrhea, vomiting, and nausea, families may wish to conform to their cultural norms and treat their child with diets or care that is specific to their cultural group. The following are several examples of these cultural practices:

- Chinese families may wish to provide *jook*, a warm rice and broth soup that is a soothing nutritional meal.
- Vietnamese families may wish to apply the concepts of hot and cold foods to the child's diet to influence balance and harmony within the body.
- Russian families may wish to provide homemade foods, including broths and steamed vegetables.
- Mexican families may wish to provide homemade foods and abstain from any commercial or cafeteria-prepared foods.

Assessment of Diarrhea

The pediatric nurse should conduct a series of assessments for a child with diarrhea because significant losses can become an acute situation rapidly. The nurse should assist the healthcare team by providing meticulous and accurate assessments of the child's stool output. Make sure there is a diaper scale handy or place a hat in the toilet or commode to measure accurate stool losses. All abnormal findings should be reported immediately.

- Measure the overall stool loss and the duration of symptoms.
- Measure the overall I&O, assessing for significant imbalances.
- Check the color and consistency of the stool.
- Weigh the patient daily.
- Assess pain and cramping.
- Check for the presence of frank or occult blood.
- Assess the relationship of diarrhea stooling with feeds.
- Check the skin integrity around the anus.
- Check the patient's hydration status.
- Assess the abdomen for bowel sounds, and palpate for masses and distention.
- Check for the presence of accompanying fever.
- Assess for the presence of causative factors such as stress, inflammatory bowel disease, food sensitivities or intolerances, allergies, and medications.

SAFETY *STAT!*

Pediatric nurses must be aware that there are three types of dehydration associated with fluid loss:

- *Isotonic,* in which water and sodium losses are proportional (ie, sodium is normal, between 130 mEq/L and 150 mEq/L)

TABLE 36.1   LEVELS OF DEHYDRATION

Levels of Dehydration	Estimated Weight Loss	Clinical Presentation
Mild	Up to 5%	Dry mucous membranes, elevated pulse, capillary refill at 2 sec, slightly increased thirst, urine specific gravity over 1.020
Moderate	Up to 10%	Irritability, great thirst, mild orthostatic blood pressure (BP), capillary refill between 2 and 4 sec, decreased tears, oliguria, moderate thirst, increasing urine specific gravity
Severe	10–15% or more	Extreme thirst, tachycardia, orthostatic BP, sunken anterior fontanel, anuria, lethargy to comatose state in infants

- *Hypotonic,* in which serum sodium levels are below expected values (ie, sodium is low, less than 130 mEq/L)
- *Hypertonic,* in which there is a greater water loss than sodium loss (ie, sodium is high, more than 150 mEq/L)
  In severe diarrhea, the most common dehydration states are isotonic and hypotonic (London, Ladewig, et al, 2011).

Interventions for Diarrhea

Diarrhea can cause significant discomfort for a child, regardless of the child's age. Not only should the following list of interventions for diarrhea be followed, but special attention to the child's anal skin integrity should be given as copious diarrhea can lead to skin breakdown and further discomfort. Requesting interventions for a soothing and protective cream should be considered.

1. Place the child on NPO status for a bowel rest until fluids are ordered and can be tolerated.
2. Begin oral rehydration fluids; for infants, administer an electrolyte solution as ordered.
3. Avoid fruit juices or any fluids with concentrated sugars.
4. Introduce foods slowly and monitor for tolerance.
5. Use BRAT or BRATTY diets: bananas, rice or rice cereal, applesauce, and toast; or bananas, rice or rice cereal, tea, toast, and yogurt.
6. Administer antidiarrheals, antiprotozoals, or antibiotics as ordered.
7. Cleanse the diaper area carefully, especially the rectal area, after each stool to prevent breakdown. Apply topical ointments for protection and soothing. Do not use commercial baby wipes because these may contain alcohol, which causes further skin breakdown.

SAFETY *STAT!*

All components of a BRAT or BRATTY diet should be low in sugar as the introduction of foods with sugar can cause fluids to shift to the bowel, increasing fluid loss.

Nursing Considerations for Diarrhea

When the etiology of a child's diarrhea is unknown, contact precautions should be initiated. If there is a suspicion that the etiology of the child's diarrhea is *Clostridium difficile (C diff.),* then expanded contact precautions should be initiated and only hand washing should be conducted. *C diff.* is not inactivated by alcohol-based hand sanitizers.

Families need education on the prevention of serious GI illness from food that is contaminated by infectious pathogens. Teaching families about safe food preparation, appropriate disinfection of kitchen surfaces, and hand washing before and after handling food will help reduce the incidence of food poisoning.

SAFETY *STAT!*

Salmonella *Food Poisoning*

Salmonella food poisoning is not an uncommon GI illness. This type of illness is caused by the pathogenic *Salmonella* bacilli that produce a range of reactions from mild gastroenteritis to fatal food poisoning. The incubation period is approximately 6 to 72 hours (Hockenberry and Wilson, 2013). There are more than 1,400 species. Safe food handling and washing, cleaning food preparation surfaces, cooking food thoroughly, and hand washing all help to reduce the incidence of this infection.

THE USE OF ENTERIC PRECAUTIONS. Until the etiology of the diarrhea is identified, it is important to maintain precautions to prevent the potential spread of an infectious disease. Contamination of stool with *C diff.* or parasites can spread the disease to others. Use contact precautions and enteric precautions to prevent cross-contamination.

Constipation

Constipation is an increased consistency and decreased amount of stool when compared to the child's normal and expected stooling pattern. Constipation is the most common complaint during childhood, causing 5% of all clinic visits (Ball, Bindler, et al, 2014). Although children each have unique stooling patterns, including some who do not stool every day, constipation is considered an abnormal state of dry, hard, and infrequent stooling. Constipation may be associated with straining, but the presence of straining does not mean the child is constipated.

Childhood constipation can be categorized as either acute or chronic. There are several etiologies of each one. Acute, or infrequent and resolvable, constipation can be associated with a diet low in liquids, which leads to a decreased amount of fluid in the GI system, producing hard, drier stools. Often, pushing fluids and providing a high-fiber diet rich in fruits and vegetables is all that is needed for a child with infrequent constipation.

With chronic constipation, interventions are needed to produce a normal stooling pattern. Chronic constipation is not uncommon and may relate to poor fluid intake, decreased activity levels, or poor nutrition. See the Health Promotion feature for further information about childhood chronic constipation.

HEALTH PROMOTION

Chronic Constipation

- Differentiate between acute recurring episodes of constipation versus chronic episodes via a complete history and physical examination; determine if there a history of a meconium plug.
- Mild constipation will resolve with diet manipulation.
- Chronic constipation will require the restoration of the child's regular evacuation pattern.
- The distended rectum will need to be shrunk to its normal size.

- The child will need an organized, planned toileting routine supported by the family and the family's lifestyle.
- Suppositories, enemas, and possibly GoLYTELY (ie, a polyethylene glycol electrolyte solution) may need to be used to empty the child's bowel as the toileting routine is initiated.
- Increasing the child's daily intake of fiber is an important addition to the toileting routine.
- A timer can be used to encourage the child to stay on the toilet for a predetermined time twice a day to get a routine established; usually 5 to 10 min, depending on the child's age, is sufficient.
- Positive reinforcement, counseling, and education should all be part of the bowel retraining routine.

Assessment of Constipation

Although constipation does not frequently require medical interventions other than home interventions, the nurse should assess for the frequency of, precipitating factors related to, and the severity of a child's constipation. Whether the constipation is situational or chronically experienced should be differentiated.

- Note the frequency of passing hard, dry, and infrequent stools. Assess how long the situation has been present.
- Ask for a sample of the stool and perform the guaiac test for the presence of frank or occult (ie, hidden) blood.
- Measure the patient's abdominal girth and document it daily (Fig. 36.2).
- Assess the level of pain during stooling and any accompanying abdominal pain.
- Assess the child's perirectal area for the presence of rashes, inflammation, bleeding, and fissures on the anal area.
- Question the child and caregiver about the child's reluctance to use the toilet in public, at friends' or families' homes, or at school. Assess if the child is demonstrating the withholding of stooling for a period of time.

Interventions for Constipation

Interventions for constipation range from simply modifying the child's diet with fluids and fiber, to requiring daily medications that soften stool or increase peristalsis. A regular pattern should be established using the least invasive measures first. Adding fresh fruits and vegetables to a child's diet when these foods have been limited or absent may be enough to produce a regular stool pattern.

- Teach the family to add fiber to the child's diet with each meal.
- Provide an opportunity for the child to try new high-fiber foods such as prunes or other dried or fresh fruit he or she may not have tried before.
- Provide stool softeners, such as glycerin suppositories, oral mineral oil, or docusate sodium (Colace).
- If appropriate, add a small amount of corn syrup to the infant's formula to increase the osmotic load and help liquefy hard stools (discuss with the primary care provider before initiating this intervention).
- Lubricate the anal area to allow easier passage of hard stools.
- If appropriate, digitally remove the stool very gently.

Nursing Considerations for Constipation

If these interventions are not successful in treating a child's constipation, it may be appropriate to discuss with the primary care provider the initiation of prescribed laxatives. Unlike stool softeners that provide lubrication via increased water to the stool, laxatives increase peristalsis and increase water to the stool.

If a child presents with chronic constipation, it is important to refer the child for further work-up. The child may have an obstructive condition, **encopresis,** or another diagnosis that requires in-depth diagnostics and careful follow-up (Box 36.1).

Cleft Lip and Cleft Palate

Cleft lip occurs during fetal development in approximately the seventh week of gestational growth. This congenital condition occurs because of the failure of the tissues to fuse completely and may be partial or complete, and unilateral or bilateral (Fig. 36.3). Cleft lip is more common in boys than in girls. The family may experience shock and grief after birth, and bonding may be affected. It is imperative that the nurse discuss the newborn's other positive features and promote the bonding experience. One serious complication may be the risk of aspiration during feedings or with wet burps because there is incomplete closure of the mouth. Effectiveness of the child's sucking ability must be assessed and a feeding device may need to be used to ensure adequate nutritional intake.

Cleft palate also occurs during fetal development but during a different time (see Fig. 36.3). The defect takes place during the 9th and 10th weeks of fetal development. The incidence of cleft palate is double in girls versus boys. The severity of the incomplete fusion of the bone and tissue of the upper jaw and the palate will determine the complexity of the long-term care. In severe cases, not only are the soft and hard palates involved, but portions of the maxilla. Aspiration is common and the child with cleft palate is at risk for more frequent respiratory infections and bouts of otitis media. Natural defenses against bacterial infections are decreased with the increased open spaces in the oral cavity.

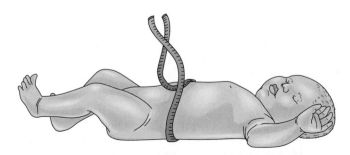

FIGURE 36.2 Measurement of abdominal circumference.

Box 36.1 Case Study

A Preschooler With Encopresis

Encopresis is a form of chronic constipation that requires a bowel retraining routine. A preschool boy presents with frequent incontinence of stool during the late afternoon. The mother complains that the child has "dirty" underwear every day and every few days will produce a large stool in his pants with the child seemingly not aware or bothered by the presence of the stool and the smell of feces. The parents finally bring the child in after hiding their concerns from friends and family for almost a year. The child is shy and cautious in his interactions. Diet history demonstrates a well-rounded, age-appropriate diet complete with fruits and vegetables.

After an emotional discussion with the pediatrician, a diagnosis of encopresis is made. Recommendations included a commercially prepared enema on day one followed by time on the toilet reading books for no less than 10 min three times a day. The child was to produce at least a "half cup" of stool per day. The family was to not punish the child in any way for accidents and they were to find ways of identifying and decreasing stress in the child's life. Dietary modifications included increased oral fluid consumption, more fresh fruits, and a high-fiber cereal daily. After 6 weeks of the program, the child's encopretic episodes decreased and the family reported much less distress.

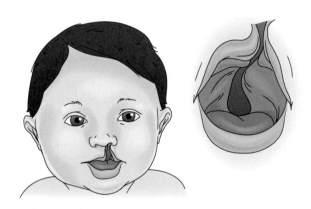

FIGURE 36.3 Infant with cleft lip and cleft palate.

The surgical repair of cleft lip usually takes place when the infant is at least 10 weeks of age and weighs 10 pounds. Surgical repair of cleft palate is much more complex, may take serial surgeries for extensive surgical fusions, and will not take place until the infant is older than 10 months and weaned from the bottle.

Assessment of Cleft Lip and Palate

Initial assessments for cleft lip and/or cleft palate take place in utero during routine ultrasonic evaluations of the fetus. If the condition was not noted during prenatal care, then the condition(s) should be assessed for during the immediate postbirth assessment. The following list provides guidance for assessing for the presence and severity of cleft lip and/or cleft palate:

- The infant must be assessed for respiratory distress during feedings.
- Assess for the ability of the infant to produce a complete and quality suck and swallow; assess for the presence of an air-tight seal around the nipple.
- Assess for the development of abdominal distention during feedings and burp the baby frequently.
- Assess for bonding issues and provide support during the early newborn period.

Interventions for Cleft Lip and Palate

Interventions for cleft lip and palate include preoperative and postoperative interventions.

PREOPERATIVE INTERVENTIONS. Preoperative interventions include the following:

- The infant should be fed smaller, more frequent feedings slowly in an upright position; care should be given not to increase the chance of aspiration with feedings.
- Feedings should be stopped frequently to provide thorough burping and to prevent wet burps that are associated with aspiration.
- Provide preoperative interventions to improve the infant's nutrition: a cleft lip nipple with a palate flap, medicine droppers, syringe feedings, or manual compression of the nipple.
- Request gavage feedings if nipple feedings do not demonstrate a successful growth pattern and weight gain.
- Administer a small amount of sterile water to the infant after feedings to remove residual formula or breast milk from accumulating in the open palate area; in addition, sterile water reduces the medium for bacterial growth.
- Provide emotional support and education to the family to improve bonding behaviors and to increase holding and touching.
- Provide preoperative education about the surgical procedure for cleft lip (ie, cheiloplasty) and/or cleft palate (ie, staphylorrhaphy), and the postoperative care they can anticipate.

POSTOPERATIVE INTERVENTIONS. Postoperative interventions include the following:

- Maintain an airway free of the accumulation of secretions and monitor for edema or any narrowing that places the infant at risk for airway compromise; assess for distress, cyanosis, tachycardia, or restlessness.
- Monitor for postoperative infections; no oral temperatures should be taken after surgery to prevent tissue damage.
- Treat pain promptly and thoroughly; reevaluate at regular intervals and provide distraction/diversion.
- Prevent trauma to the suture line by avoiding crying, and use arm restraints to prevent rubbing of butterfly closures or fine sutures.

- Introduce feedings cautiously and monitor for dysphagia.
- After cleft lip repair (Fig. 36.4) on an older infant, care must be taken to prevent trauma to the suture line; only soft toys should be offered and any item that is pointed or stick-shaped should be avoided.
- To prevent further trauma, no straws or suction devices should be used.
- Clean the suture line carefully after feedings and prn to keep the site clean.
- Do not brush the child's teeth after palate surgery until ordered (ie, at least 2 weeks).

Nursing Considerations for Cleft Lip or Palate

Nurses caring for children in the postoperative period can use the acronym ESSR for interventions for an infant with surgically corrected cleft palate: *E*nlarged nipple, *S*timulate sucking by rubbing the nipple on the lower lip, *S*wallow, and *R*est after each swallow to allow for complete swallowing (Hogan and White, 2003). It is imperative that nursing care be focused on the prevention of suture line injury. Do not allow the infant to rub the suture line. Position the child supine or side lying to prevent injury to the surgical site (Kyle and Carman, 2013).

Nurses should be aware that the corrected cleft lip or palate rarely leads to issues in poor self-esteem or poor self-image. With new surgical procedures, suture lines are barely visible and typically do not cause emotional distress to either gender. Uncorrected cleft palate places the child at risk and families must be assessed for the competency of care during feedings when the newborn is discharged home before surgery. Long-term follow-up is imperative for cleft palate care, and families should be offered professional counseling if warranted during the period of waiting until the surgery is performed. Dental and orthodontic follow-up care is imperative as faulty dentition is a potential complication of surgical correction of cleft palate. Nursing diagnoses for a child with cleft lip and/or palate can be found in the Box 36.2. Using nursing diagnoses can help the nurse determine priority goals and interventions for safe care of children after surgery.

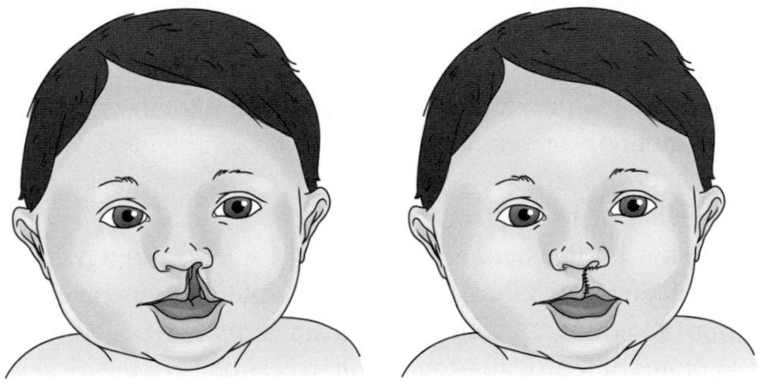

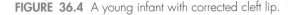

Cleft lip   Cleft lip repair

FIGURE 36.4 A young infant with corrected cleft lip.

Box 36.2 Nursing Diagnoses for Cleft Lip and Palate

- Risk for infection related to decreased infection fighting potential
- Risk for injury related to aspiration potential
- Breastfeeding ineffective related to lip or palate integrity alteration
- Altered nutrition is less than body requirements; related to poor oral intake
- Infant feeding pattern ineffective related to unrepaired congenital defect
- Knowledge deficit related to congenital defect
- Pain related to surgical procedure and postoperative period
- Home maintenance impaired related to required feeding procedures in preoperative period
- Parenting at risk for impairment because of bonding issues

Esophageal Atresia

The word *atresia* refers to an anatomical abnormality where a passageway terminates. Where a normal anatomical opening should be, an atresia is a pathological closure of the passageway. An esophageal atresia (EA) is when a newborn presents with an abnormal termination of the esophagus, alone or in association with other congenital defects. The presence of the esophageal blind pouch at the proximal end of the esophagus prevents the passage of breast milk, formula, or any fluids. Food does not enter the stomach and the newborn is at risk for aspiration of the fluids from the pouch. One needs to differentiate between an EA and a tracheoesophageal fistula (TEF) (Fig. 36.5). A TEF is another anatomical abnormality. Here the defect links the trachea and esophagus with an abnormal opening. Special care needs to be taken to prevent aspiration pneumonia in the period before surgical repair of the opening.

Assessment of an Esophageal Atresia

An infant may present with respiratory distress after the first introduction of breast milk or formula. If the anatomical anomaly allows for the passage of oral fluids, the child might become acutely distressed as the fluids pass into the infant's lungs. Assessment of EA and TEF includes checking for the following:

- The presence of excessive oral secretions
- Coughing, choking, and respiratory distress
- Possible intermittent cyanosis associated with fluid intake or excessive oral secretions
- The presence of an esophageal/tracheal fistula, as well as the presence of tracheal irritation from the infant's gastric acid passing from the esophagus into the trachea.

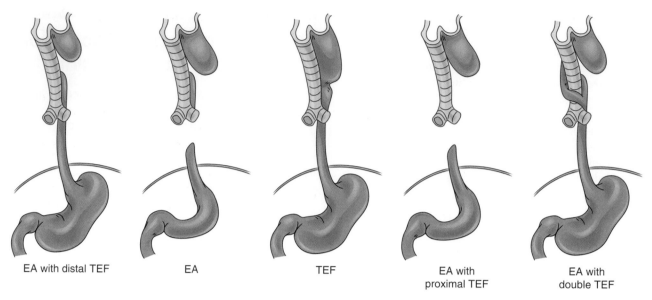

EA with distal TEF   EA   TEF   EA with proximal TEF   EA with double TEF

FIGURE 36.5 Illustration of EA and TEF.

Interventions for Esophageal Atresia

If suspected, the nurse should immediately report the findings to the pediatric health-care team and stop any further feedings. The nurse should also:

1. Maintain NPO status until a PEG tube is passed for feeds.
2. Suction frequently to prevent aspiration and periods of respiratory distress.
3. Prepare the child for surgery to repair the anatomical defect.

Nursing Considerations for Esophageal Atresia

A nurse should feed infants suspected of having an anatomical defect a very small amount of fluids for the first feed to assess for the presence of these anatomical defects. If a newborn tolerates a small amount of sterile water, then further feedings or breastfeeding can be initiated.

Tracheoesophageal Fistula

Infants with a confirmed TEF are born with a congenital defect of an abnormal opening, called a *fistula,* between the trachea and the esophagus. There are many combinations of defects that can be present and syndromes should be ruled out. Cardiac defects may accompany the presence of combinations of structural anomalies. After feeding, the newborn suffers tracheal irritation as the stomach acid enters the trachea, causing inflammation and discomfort.

Assessment of Tracheoesophageal Fistula

Nurses need to perform a rapid and thorough assessment of a child's airway, paying special attention to the child's swallow and choking. Assess for the following:

1. Coughing, choking, and intermittent cyanosis caused by food passing through the fistula into the trachea

2. The presence of abdominal distention from air entering the stomach from the fistula
3. Pain or discomfort from the gastric acids refluxing across the fistula

Interventions for Tracheoesophageal Fistula

Once suspected, the nurse should assist the pediatric health-care team to initiate steps to prepare the child for surgical interventions. The team will request the following:

1. Maintain an NPO status until diagnostic examinations are completed and a definitive diagnosis is reached.
2. Maintain a patent airway for the infant and have suction available at all times.
3. Prepare for surgery to reconstruct a patent trachea and esophagus without the presence of the abnormal fistula opening.

Nursing Considerations for Tracheoesophageal Fistula

Parents will need to be reassured and educated about the impending surgical procedure to repair the fistula. Explain that the surgery involves ligating the TEF and then the reanastomoses of the ends of the esophagus. In certain situations, there may need to be staged repair that requires more than one surgery. Expect the child to be on gastrostomy tube feedings until he or she is well-healed.

Pyloric Stenosis

When the circular areas of muscle that surround the pyloric valve hypertrophy, the stenosis leads to blocked gastric emptying. Hypertrophy and hyperplasia are progressive, and symptoms of gastric distention and hypertrophy of the muscle appear over time. Pyloric stenosis is identified with classic episodes of projectile vomiting and the clinical finding of an olive-shaped mass during palpation (Fig. 36.6). The etiology

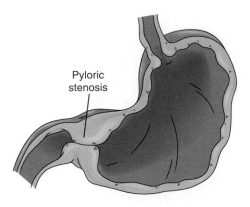

FIGURE 36.6 Pyloric stenosis.

of the development of the disorder is unknown. The male gender is affected five times more often and Caucasian children are at greatest risk. A surgical procedure called a *pylorectomy* is required and entails a small incision on the abdomen to split the hypertrophied tissue.

Assessment of Pyloric Stenosis

Parents are typically the first to identify that the infant has a significant deviation in the ability to pass food from the stomach to the intestines, noting the frequency and force of the infant's vomiting episodes. To narrow down the suspected cause of the vomiting, the following should be noted:

1. Progressively worsening projectile vomiting of nonbilious vomit in a previously healthy and thriving infant
2. Palpable, olive-shaped mass located in the infant's upper right abdominal quadrant
3. Clinical signs of dehydration, including decreased urinary output (UOP), decreased tears, poor turgor, sunken fontanels, and metabolic alkalosis from excessive vomiting
4. The child may resume feeds after projectile vomiting subsides.

Interventions for Pyloric Stenosis

Once identified via palpation and diagnostics tests, the child will need to be prepared for surgery. Guidelines for the child include the following:

1. Maintain an NPO status before pyloromyotomy surgery and prepare the family for postoperative care.
2. Before surgery, try to position the child on the right side to help prevent aspiration of vomitus.
3. After surgery, maintain NGT patency, flush as needed, and monitor strict I&O.
4. Correct any electrolyte imbalance.
5. Introduce clear fluids slowly and cautiously as ordered during the early postoperative period (usually within 6 to 8 hours after surgery).

Nursing Considerations for Pyloric Stenosis

Infants may present to the health-care facility with FTT and moderate to severe dehydration. Parents and caregivers may

not have recognized the severity of the vomiting. Assess the child for distress and report immediately any changes of clinical status.

Hirschsprung's Disease

When a child presents with poor passage of stool, infrequent explosions of stool, or ribbonlike stool, congenital aganglionic megacolon, or Hirschsprung's disease, is suspected (Fig. 36.7). Considered a megacolon disorder, this diagnosis is characterized by the absence of neuro tissue called *ganglia cells* in the lower colon. This condition is also called *congenital aganglionosis* and most commonly affects the rectosigmoid region of the child's bowel. The incidence is four times more common in the male gender.

Symptoms are associated with the inability of the aganglionic segment of colon tissue to produce peristaltic waves because of the lack of nerve innervations. This causes an accumulation of stool.

Assessment of Hirschsprung's Disease

This condition is usually diagnosed during early infancy but may not be severe enough to present until early toddlerhood. If a child has a history of infrequent stools, explosive stools,

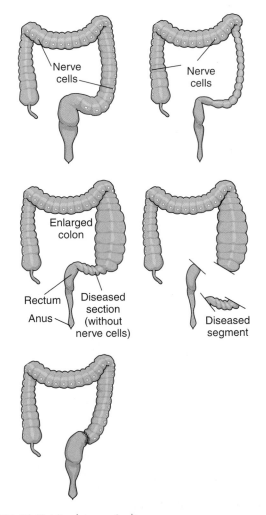

FIGURE 36.7 Hirschsprung's disease.

or stools that are thin and ribbonlike, a further assessment is warranted. The most common findings that lead the pediatric health-care team to suspect Hirschsprung's disease include the following:

- Failure of a newborn to pass meconium stool, followed by subsequent chronic constipation
- Evidence of FTT in the infant with possible hypoproteinemia and anemia
- Vomiting, constipation, episodic and explosive stooling, and abdominal distention and distress
- Reluctance to ingest feedings

Interventions for Hirschsprung's Disease

Care for the child with Hirschsprung's disease requires surgical intervention to remove the segment of bowel that does not have nerves and is causing the lack of peristalsis. The child will have diagnostics to confirm the disorder, including a tissue biopsy to identify the lack of nerves in the distal colon. Interventions for a child in the perioperative experience include the following:

- In the preoperative period, assess the child's stooling pattern and the characteristics of the stool passed.
- Prepare the family for the surgical procedure, including the possibility of a temporary placement of a colostomy (for non-pull-through surgical procedures).
- If an anal pull-through is performed, monitor for bleeding, edema, unusual drainage, fever, or any unexpected alteration in skin integrity.
- Postoperatively, provide meticulous skin care, antibiotics, pain control, and teaching/support for the family as they learn stoma care.
- After the return of bowel sounds and the passage of confirmed flatus, introduce feedings slowly and monitor for tolerance.

Nursing Considerations for Hirschsprung's Disease

During the preoperative period, as the child prepares for the surgical removal of the portion of the lower bowel that is aganglionic, the nurse should monitor for symptoms of electrolyte imbalances and dehydration. During the extended postoperative period, the family will need education and support to care for the temporary colostomy at home. Well-fitted colostomy appliances are required to reduce the chance of distressing leaks. Parents need to learn how to assess their child with a colostomy for complications of skin breakdown, obstruction, and emotional distress of their child.

Intussusception

Intussusception is an acute GI condition that is characterized by invagination or telescoping of one bowel segment into the other (Fig. 36.8). The most common site of the telescoping of the bowel is the ileocecal valve. Most commonly without an identifiable etiology, it has been known to be associated with hyperactive peristalsis, intestinal polyps, or an abnormal bowel lining. Unfortunately, this condition can

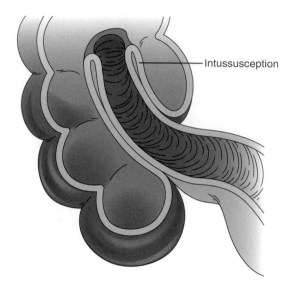

FIGURE 36.8 Intussusception.

recur and may lead to peritonitis. The child, typically between 6 and 24 months of age, presents in acute abdominal pain, guarding the abdomen and drawing the knees up toward the chest. Intussusception can become a life-threatening condition if the bowel becomes ischemic and necrotic from the edema and inflammation associated with the invagination. If gangrenous, the child will need immediate surgery with a temporary colostomy.

Assessment of Intussusception

The pediatric nurse assists the health-care team in assessing for the presence of this condition. The common assessments associated with intussusception include the following:

- Acute abdominal pain in a previously well child without previous GI symptoms
- Passage of red, blood-tinged stool referred to as *red currant jelly stool*
- Abdominal distention and tenderness
- Possible passage of bile-stained vomitus

Interventions for Intussusception

The pediatric health-care team will need to provide rapid interventions for a child who presents with an intussusception. Immediate reduction of the invagination is required to prevent severe tissue inflammation, injury, hypoxia, and death to the tissues.

1. A barium enema or water-soluble contrast enema will be performed to reduce the invaginated or telescoped bowel. In addition, air pressure may be used to confirm and then reduce the telescoped bowel.
2. Prepare the child and family for surgery if the enema is not successful.

Nursing Considerations for Intussusception

The family will need to be taught that the condition can recur and that immediate care must be sought to prevent complications. The family should state which symptoms should be monitored for so that they are confident about when to report the condition and come directly to the emergency room.

Imperforate Anus

An imperforated anus is a congenital condition in which the child is born with the absence of an anal opening. Requiring surgery, the child does not pass meconium or any stool substance. The nurse should identify this during the newborn's first assessment and immediately report the condition for consideration of surgery. The infants should be kept NPO until a complete evaluation is performed. New procedures allow for the reconstruction of the anal opening with active nerves by means of transplantation of nerve tissue.

Appendicitis

Appendicitis is the inflammation and often infection of the small lymphoid tissue called the *vermiform appendix.* The appendix is a tube-shaped blind sac located at the end of the intestinal cecum. If the lumen of the appendix becomes obstructed, usually by hard fecal material, parasites, or infectious bacterium, then the lumen becomes inflamed with the accumulation of mucus and subsequent distention. As the pressure increases, there is a higher risk of rupture. If the tissue becomes edematous or ischemic, which leads to perforation, the child is then at risk for sepsis and peritonitis.

The average age of onset of appendicitis is 10 years old; it is considered the most common cause of emergency abdominal surgery. It is imperative that a child is assessed rapidly by professional health-care providers if appendicitis is suspected; rupture can lead to peritonitis. Although rare, death can occur because of sepsis from peritonitis.

Assessment of Appendicitis

Appendicitis can mimic other abdominal conditions and therefore careful assessments to confirm this condition must be made. If suspected, no deep palpations should be conducted to prevent serious complications and increased pain. The pediatric health-care team will conduct diagnostic examinations and laboratory values to check for infection. The following should also be assessed:

• Progressive lower-right abdominal pain with associated nausea, vomiting, chills, and fever
• Elevated WBC count on laboratory evaluation
• Positive ultrasound findings of an enlarged or distended appendix
• A sudden stop of persistent and progressive abdominal pain, which should be reported immediately as it may mean perforation or rupture has occurred

Interventions for Appendicitis

Once confirmed, a diagnosis of appendicitis will need to be treated. Immediate surgery is warranted for children whose appendix has ruptured. Newer interventions include treating a milder, nonruptured appendicitis with nonsurgical means

and IV antibiotics. The following list should be considered when preparing a family for interventions:

• Prepare the child and family for a surgical appendectomy.
• Maintain NPO during evaluations and the preoperative period.
• Place the child in the semi-Fowler's position; this is often the position of comfort.
• Postoperatively, monitor the child for pain, bleeding, or wound infection.
• During the postoperative period of recovery for a child with a ruptured appendix, anticipate slower healing, more pain, and the need for an NGT and possible surgical drainage device.

Nursing Considerations for Appendicitis

Anticipate a difference in the postoperative period between children who experience appendicitis with rupture and those who experience it without rupture. When a child is postoperative without rupture, the child should follow an uncomplicated postoperative period with early ambulation and restoration of oral fluids with a rapid progressive diet. It is more complicated for children in the postoperative period following a ruptured appendectomy. Children may require days of antibiotics, may experience much more pain, and will resume ambulation at a slower time interval. Maintain close observation during the postoperative period for possible complications from the rupture, including obstructions, sepsis, and hazards of longer periods of postoperative bedrest.

The assessment of peritonitis associated with appendicitis rupture includes a high fever; a greatly increased WBC count; severe abdominal pain; the absence of bowel sounds; a rigid, boardlike abdomen; and the possible development of shock and death.

Inflammatory Bowel Syndromes: Ulcerative Colitis and Crohn's Disease

The most common pediatric inflammatory bowel diseases are ulcerative colitis and **Crohn's disease.** The cause of either of these two diagnoses is unknown but may be linked to dietary, infectious, or genetic causes. The human leukocyte antigen B27 (HLA-B27) and inflammatory bowel disease may be linked. Early in the child's disease experience, the two diseases look very similar and share similar clinical presentations and symptoms. The differentiation of the diseases requires careful consideration as both are characterized by remissions and exacerbations.

Ulcerative colitis is slightly more prevalent that Crohn's disease, with a peak incidence age range of 15 to 20 years old. One-third of children with ulcerative colitis have a family history.

Ulcerative Colitis

Ulcerative colitis primarily affects the large intestine, with continuous lesions involving the superficial mucosa. The bowel will demonstrate what is considered a "lead pipe" visual appearance as the bowel's muscle tissue hypertrophies with deposited fat and fibrous tissues.

ASSESSMENT OF ULCERATIVE COLITIS. A child with ulcerative colitis may have very mild or very severe symptoms. The following list of assessments is used for all children, regardless of the severity of their disease:

• Copious, frequent bloody stools, ranging from 3 to 20 per day
• After defecation, check if the child's abdominal pain is relieved
• Significant weight loss that usually occurs over just a few months' time
• Anemia, electrolyte imbalances, and an increased ESR
• Fever, tachycardia, pallor, and fatigue
• The presence of what is considered "extraintestinal symptoms," including joint tenderness, arthritis, and skin rashes

Diagnostics include a Hematest of stools, colonoscopy, barium enema, and biopsies.

INTERVENTIONS FOR ULCERATIVE COLITIS. Interventions for inflammatory bowel conditions will vary depending on the severity of the disease and include the following:

• Pharmacological interventions are initiated to reduce the inflammation and to support the child's nutrition, and include antidiarrheals, antiinflammatories, and analgesics.
• Modifications in the child's diet will be needed to help control the diarrhea.
• In severe exacerbations, the child will require IV hyperalimentation, IV steroidal anti-inflammatories, and the correction of acidosis and anemia.
• In 25% of the cases of ulcerative colitis, the child will require surgery to remove the diseased bowel segment.

Crohn's Disease

As with ulcerative colitis, Crohn's disease also causes ulcerations along the mucosal lining of the bowel but may affect any part of the alimentary tract, from the child's mouth to the anus. However, unlike ulcerative colitis, the lesions in Crohn's disease are called "skip" lesions because they are discontinuous with healthy bowel between lesions. Crohn's disease is known to cause fistulas, fissures, and thickened intestinal walls, with 50% of cases resulting in granulomas.

ASSESSMENT OF CROHN'S DISEASE. A child with Crohn's disease may have very mild or very severe symptoms. The child may have remissions and exacerbations of the inflammation in the bowel. The following list of assessments is used for all children, regardless of the severity of their disease:

• Diarrhea with frank or occult blood
• Moderate to severe cramping abdominal pain
• Weight loss with eventual growth retardation from nutritional deficiencies and electrolyte imbalances
• Abscess formation and perianal fissures and fistulas
• Extraintestinal manifestations of finger clubbing, arthritis, and amenorrhea, and delayed sexual development

INTERVENTIONS FOR CROHN'S DISEASE. Interventions for Crohn's disease include the following:

• Pharmacological interventions are similar to those for ulcerative colitis. Pharmacological interventions are initiated to reduce the inflammation and to support the child's nutrition and include antidiarrheals, anti-inflammatories, and analgesics.
• Nutritional deficiencies should be corrected.
• In 70% of cases, surgery occurs in childhood.

DRUG FACTS

Infliximab

Indicated for active moderate-to-severe Crohn's disease, infliximab (Remicade) neutralizes and prevents the activity of tumor necrosis factor-α, resulting in antiproliferative and anti-inflammatory activities. Nursing considerations during infusion include paying special attention to the child's reactions, such as fever, chills, pruritus, and urticaria, especially with the first and second infusions. Children can develop severe infections during the course of treatment, necessitating cessation of further treatment. Monitor for signs and symptoms of severe infections, including fever, sweats, cough, dyspnea, malaise, and weight loss.

Nursing Considerations for Inflammatory Bowel Diseases

It is imperative to follow the daily weight and fluid status of a child with an inflammatory bowel to identify disease progression or therapy responses. Nurses should promote the positive oral intake of fluids and foods that can be tolerated. With abdominal pain, the nurses should provide distraction, diversion, heating pads, frequent position changes, and, when needed, narcotic pain relief. Skin integrity is imperative when a child in an acute exacerbation is suffering frequent diarrheal episodes. When diarrhea is under control, slowly introduce low-residue, high-protein, high-calorie, and bland foods.

Nurses must be aware of the potential complications associated with inflammatory bowel diseases. Perforation, sepsis, hemorrhage, and obstructions should all be carefully monitored. With ulcerative colitis, it is imperative that families continue to bring their child in for follow-up visits because there is a 20% risk of colon cancer after the first 10 years. Surgical treatments are required if a child is not responsive to pharmacological interventions. Either an ileostomy or a colostomy may be performed. With education, guidance, and support, the child with an inflammatory bowel disease who has had surgery to remove the diseased portion of bowel can expect an active and engaged lifestyle.

Celiac Disease

When a child has the absence of an enzyme in his or her intestinal mucosal cells, the villi located in the proximal small intestine atrophy, leading to a decrease in intestinal absorption. The disease in response to this pathological process is called ***gluten intolerance,*** also known as *gluten-sensitive* *enteropathy.* The child is unable to fully digest the glutenin or gliadin protein components of certain grains. The child is unable to tolerate food products that include rye, wheat, oat, and barley glutens. The accumulation of the amino acid glutamine is toxic to the child's intestinal lining and chronic diarrhea results. The child may experience weight loss, foul-smelling stools, and increased flatulence (Rudd and Kocisko, 2014). Most infants will be symptomatic approximately 2 to 4 months after the introduction of foods that contain gluten. Some children do not present with symptoms until after 5 years old. Although the etiology is unknown, celiac disease is suspected to have an environmental influence. The child will require life-long dietary modification to prevent even the smallest exposure to glutens. Iron, folic acids, and fat-soluble vitamins are all malabsorbed because of the effect celiac disease has on the proximal small intestine (Ryan and Grossman, 2011).

Assessment of Celiac Disease

The assessment of celiac disease includes the following:

- Flare-ups and celiac crises associated with a precipitating event, such as gluten ingestion, infections, prolonged fasting, or exposure to anticholinergic drugs, which will present as acute abdominal pain, severe diarrhea, electrolyte imbalances, and possible metabolic acidosis
- The passage of steatorrhea or greasy, bulky, and very malodorous stools that appear frothy and full of fat
- Organic FTT, including weight loss or lack of gain, muscle wasting, and anemia
- Anorexia and abdominal pain, which are common

Anticipate laboratory studies of antigliadin antibodies (IgG and IgA) and a 72-hour quantitative fecal fat study. Also anticipate sending the child for a biopsy of the jejunum to assess for a flat mucosal surface with hyperplasia.

Interventions for Celiac Disease

Interventions for celiac disease include the following:

- Instruct the parents of the patient to provide the child with a gluten-free diet.
- Correct any electrolyte disturbances.
- Restore fluids if the child presents with dehydration from diarrhea, tachycardia, poor skin turgor, and elevated urine specific gravity.

Nursing Considerations for Celiac Disease

Nurses need to reinforce the plan for gluten-free diets, including a restriction of breads, pasta, and snacks that contain rye, wheat, oat, or barley. Many commercially prepared frozen food items and desirable childhood snacks contain a type of gluten, and families must become astute at reading and analyzing food labels. Unrestricted food items include eggs, fish, poultry, pork, beef, dairy, fruits, vegetables, rice, and cornmeal. With the increasing incidence of celiac disease in the general population, many wheat alternative breads and cereals are now available. The growing awareness of the disease is also prompting grocery stores and restaurants to provide gluten-free food and menu choices.

Support is available for families from the American Celiac Society, the Gluten Intolerance Group, and the Celiac Disease Foundation. Written instructions should be provided for families and follow-up is imperative to assess a child's risk for episodes of celiac crises. Research has shown that celiac disease–related antibodies are one way to closely monitor a child's clinical outcomes by looking at the long-term compliance with a gluten-free diet. As a child's antibody levels decrease, health-care professionals can be more confident that the child's diet is in compliance with the abstinence of glutens (Nachman, et al, 2011)

NURSING CARE PLAN for the Child With Celiac Disease

The following list of nursing diagnoses and goals can be used to determine the most appropriate interventions for a child with celiac (gluten intolerance) disease:

Nursing Diagnosis and Corresponding Goal:
- There is deficient fluid volume related to inflammation and excessive losses from GI tract as evidenced by loose stools and/or diarrhea.
- The child will demonstrate reduced diarrhea and equal I&O of fluids.

Nursing Diagnosis and Corresponding Goal:
- There is acute pain related to inflamed GI mucosa as evidenced by bloating and cramping.
- The child will demonstrate a 0 or a 1 on a subjective or objective pediatric pain scale.

Nursing Diagnosis and Corresponding Goal:
- There is a knowledge deficit related to necessary dietary changes as evidenced by gluten food choices and selection.
- The family will describe at least five meals that offer gluten-free items that are appropriate for the child's developmental stage.

Necrotizing Enterocolitis

An inflammatory disease of the intestinal tract that occurs primarily in premature infants or sick full-term infants is called *necrotizing enterocolitis (NEC)*. This condition is marked by varying degrees of dead or necrotic tissue in either the transmural or mucosal segments of the intestines. This life-threatening condition requires nursing and medical care in an intensive care environment. Several factors are involved in the development of NEC, including bacterial or viral infections, intestinal ischemia, and immaturity of the gut during feeds, which all lead to a damaged bowel with ischemia that develops into necrosis.

Assessment of Necrotizing Enterocolitis

The assessment of NEC includes the following:

- A history of prematurity, maternal pre-eclampsia or hemorrhage, umbilical catheters, cocaine exposure, sepsis, or asphyxia
- Free peritoneal gas and bowel inflammation that demonstrates dilated loops and thickening of the bowel

  Three stages may occur with the onset of NEC:

  1. **Stage 1:** Marked by fluctuating temperatures, hypoglycemia, abdominal distention, heme-positive stools, poor perfusion, lethargy, and recurrent apnea/bradycardia
  2. **Stage 2:** Marked by the above plus severe distention, grossly bloody stools, extreme abdominal tenderness, and absent bowel sounds
  3. **Stage 3:** Marked by the evidence of the beginning of septic shock, including the deterioration of vital signs, metabolic acidosis, severe edema of the abdominal wall, and disseminated intravascular coagulation (DIC)

Interventions for Necrotizing Enterocolitis

Interventions for NEC include the following:

- The child will require IV antibiotics, vascular support, and IV feedings in an intensive care environment.
- An ostomy may be required to remove the necrotic tissue and allow the bowel to rest and heal.

Nursing Considerations for Necrotizing Enterocolitis

NEC is a life-threatening disease with a long healing time. Associated with mortality, this condition requires an astute, high level of intensive care. Parents will need emotional support while their newborn or young infant is critically ill and will need to be taught how to care for the infant's ostomy.

Key Points

- The development of the neonate's GI system must go through a series of steps of maturation, including progressing from a sterile gut environment in the immediate neonatal period to intestinal lining that is colonized with active bacteria. This process is essential for healthy digestion.
- A pediatric nurse can expect to encounter a wide variety of GI disorders across childhood. Most take astute assessments and rapid interventions as the child may be at risk for severe fluid loss and subsequent dehydration, electrolyte imbalances, acid/base imbalances, and nutritional disorders.
- Acute GI infections require contact precautions to prevent the rapid spread of the disease to others. If *C diff.* is suspected or confirmed, the pediatric health-care staff must initiate expanded contact precautions that include hand washing with soap and water. Alcohol-based hand gel is not sufficient in inactivating the microbe.

- Chronic bowel diseases require a team approach with engaged follow-up care and continued teaching. Because of the relationship between nutrition and fluid balance and chronic bowel diseases, families need education for their child's care and support for ongoing follow-up care. Many chronic bowel diseases are marked with exacerbations and remissions, so families need to recognize when health-care interventions are required.
- Celiac disease is caused by gluten intolerance. With the increasing incidence of this chronic condition, pediatric team members need updated information to provide education about the dietary restrictions of foods that contain wheat, oats, rye, and barley.
- Offering emotional support for children with colostomies or ileostomies can positively influence the experience of a chronic GI disorder, especially for school-aged children and adolescents who have body image concerns.

REVIEW QUESTIONS

1. A 7-year-old girl was admitted on your unit for increasing lower-right quadrant abdominal pain with an admitting diagnosis of suspected appendicitis. Although her admission pain score was rated as a 9 to 10 on a numerical scale, she suddenly says her pain has subsided. What would your next action be?
   1. Report to the charge nurse that the child's pain is suddenly gone.
   2. Anticipate immediate surgery.
   3. Allow her to rest comfortably.
   4. Provide her choice of oral fluids.

2. Clinical findings associated with moderate dehydration demonstrate the severity of a child's condition. The following list includes findings that denote moderate dehydration. *(select all that apply)*
   1. Rapid pulse
   2. Dry mucous membranes
   3. Moderate thirst
   4. Normal fontanel
   5. 10% body weight loss
   6. Greater than 3-sec capillary refill

3. While helping a family make menu choices for their child with a new diagnosis of celiac disease, which food choices would the nurse support them ordering?
   1. Corn tortillas with melted cheese and a fruit salad
   2. Turkey sandwich on rye bread with a side of sliced apples
   3. Chili with Texas ten-grain toast and watermelon slices
   4. Spaghetti with meat sauce and grapes

4. After an infant returns from surgery to correct Hirschsprung's disease, the nurse should avoid:
   1. Introducing fluids when bowel sounds are definitively identified
   2. Positioning the infant supine
   3. Assessing the temperature rectally
   4. Providing a quiet environment to heal

5. What form of stool would the nurse explain to the parents of a child admitted with intussusception to expect?
   1. Ribbonlike brown stool in normal quantity
   2. Watery, light brown stool in large quantity
   3. Thick, greenish stool
   4. Scant stool appearing like red jelly

6. To help prevent diarrhea for a child taking oral antibiotics, the nurse would expect to also give:
   1. Pedialyte oral boluses
   2. A high-fiber diet
   3. Macrobiotic granules
   4. An NPO status and bowel rest

7. Symptoms of pyloric stenosis may include the following: *(select all that apply)*
   1. Severe abdominal pain
   2. Projectile vomiting
   3. Bilious vomiting
   4. FTT
   5. Lower intestinal cramping

8. A young child presenting to the emergency room with moderate dehydration associated with 5 days of vomiting may demonstrate clinical signs and symptoms of:
   1. Metabolic acidosis
   2. Metabolic alkalosis
   3. Respiratory acidosis
   4. Respiratory alkalosis

9. A nurse is caring for a school-aged child with FTT associated with cystic fibrosis who requires nasogastric feedings. The following may be used to check the correct placement before initiating the child's first nutritional feeding: *(select all that apply)*
   1. Demonstration of a high pH level in the NGT aspirate
   2. Aspiration of stomach contents
   3. Sound of air passing in the stomach via 5 cc of air through the tube
   4. Symptoms of coughing with flushing
   5. Placement of the end of a tube in a cup of water showing bubbling
   6. Radiography

10. A cardinal sign of a young diapered toddler having an intestinal parasite is:
    1. Nausea and vomiting
    2. Frequent diarrhea
    3. Persistent anal itching
    4. Perineal rash with satellite lesions

CRITICAL THINKING QUESTIONS

1. When a child presents to the emergency department in severe dehydration from intractable vomiting, what is the most accurate method of assessing the child's severity of dehydration if the health-care team does not have a baseline weight?

2. Describe the very best protective practices and isolation techniques that a nurse can use if he or she is taking care of a toddler with *C diff.* diarrhea.

3. If a child with severe lower-right quadrant pain and a mildly distended abdomen presents to the emergency room to rule out appendicitis and suddenly has a cessation of pain, what could this mean and what should the nursing team do as a priority form of care?

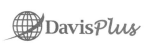 **DavisPlus**

For additional resources and information, visit **www.DavisPlus.com.** Post-Conference Questions and Activities, Answers, and References can be found on Davis*Plus*.

Child With a Genitourinary Condition

LEARNING OUTCOMES

1. Define the key terms.
2. Describe how a child's renal system affects fluid and electrolyte status, as well as acid/base balance.
3. Discuss the clinical presentation of a dehydrated child across childhood and discuss a plan of nursing care for a child in a dehydrated state.
4. Analyze the etiologies associated with a urinary tract infection (UTI) and discuss the risk factors associated with each age group.
5. Differentiate between glomerulonephritis and nephrotic syndrome in relation to assessments, medical treatments, and nursing care for each.
6. Describe various forms of congenital anomalies of the genitourinary (GU) tract.
7. Present a nursing care plan for a child with enuresis.
8. Describe various means to collect urine specimens for children of various ages.
9. Calculate fluid maintenance requirements for children of various weights in kilograms to safely maintain fluid status and prevent fluid overload.

KEY TERMS

acidosis
alkalosis
ascites
diurnal incontinence
epispadias
fluid maintenance calculation
glomerulonephritis
hemolytic uremic syndrome (HUS)
hyponatremia
hypospadia
mesoderm
nephrotic syndrome/nephrosis
nocturnal incontinence

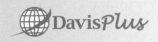 DavisPlus   For audio pronunciation guide, visit
www.DavisPlus.com

CHAPTER CONCEPTS

Urinary Elimination
Fluid and Electrolyte Balance

REAL-WORLD CASE STUDY

John

■ John, 4 years old, was admitted to the pediatric unit for evaluation of edema and massive proteinuria. Three weeks ago, he contracted an upper respiratory infection that his pediatrician believed to be of viral origin. A week ago, John began to wake up in the morning with puffy eyes. He has gained approximately 8 pounds in the last week. His mother reported that John has lost his appetite, is quite fatigued, and is experiencing diarrhea.

John's weight on admission was 19.27 kg (42.5 pounds). His height was 104 cm (41 in.). Physical examination revealed edema of his eyelids and face. Massive edema was also present in his extremities and scrotum. He appeared to have ascites. John's skin was pale

continued on page 620

and warm to touch, and shiny in appearance. His vital signs were within normal limits.

Urine analysis revealed 4+ proteinuria and a specific gravity (SG) of 1.030. His urine was dark and frothy in appearance. John's urinary output for 24 hours was 500 mL. His serum albumin level was 1.5 g/100 mL, his hematocrit was normal, and his serum sodium was 132 mEq/L. A diagnosis of minimal change nephrotic syndrome was suspected. A renal biopsy confirmed the diagnosis. John was started on high-dose corticosteroids and remained hospitalized in guarded condition.

1. Identify the three main clinical manifestations of nephrotic syndrome.
2. John was started on prednisone and a low-salt diet. Explain the rationale for this part of his treatment.
3. What are the side effects of long-term corticosteroid therapy in children?

CONCEPTUAL CORNERSTONE

Elimination

The genitourinary (GU) system is responsible for the removal of waste products from the blood and the formation of urine. Disturbances in the GU system can lead to an increased level of blood urea nitrogen (BUN) and creatinine in the blood and, ultimately, without treatment, renal failure. Through the elimination process, the GU system influences the regulation of the body's fluid and electrolyte balance. The kidneys respond to dehydration and hypotension with decreased urine output.

A child with an elimination condition such as an infection within the GU system often experiences pain and discomfort. Children with bladder infections and pyelonephritis often experience dysuria. Providing both pharmaceutical and nonpharmaceutical pain-reducing interventions is a primary nursing function. Pediatric nurses must report any concern with the process of urinary elimination, such as changes in quantity, color, clarity, and any symptoms experienced by the child. Meticulous care of children with complex urinary elimination conditions such as glomerulonephritis and nephritic syndrome requires teamwork and astute assessments.

Urology is the study of the normal and abnormal function of the kidney, renal, pelvis, ureter, bladder, urethra, and reproductive organs of both genders. Essential for life, the GU system provides a means to process and eliminate waste products from the blood, regulate body fluids,

regulate acid-base balance, and provide a means for reproduction. During the years of childhood, the GU system matures. In infancy, the child is poorly able to regulate fluid balance, concentrate wastes into urine, and eliminate waste byproducts of metabolism. As the child grows, the efficacy of this system develops. In the presence of disease or disorder, the child may experience fluid retention, hypertension, and the buildup of waste products called *uremia.*

Disorders of the GU system are common during childhood. Approximately 1.2 million children develop a UTI per year in the United States. According to the American Society of Pediatric Nephrology (2014), 300,000 children develop a disease in which protein and blood leak into their urine with conditions such as **hemolytic uremic syndrome (HUS)** or **glomerulonephritis.** Annually, renal dialysis will be required for 4,500 children and 2,000 infants will die because of diseases of this system. Although many GU disorders are present at birth, acquired disorders are common enough to warrant an understanding of signs and symptoms of infections, strictures, renal failure, and reproductive complications. The GU system is complex and many children with chronic disorders will have several specialists caring for them during the management of their disease. These can include pediatric urologists, pediatric nephrologists, pediatric surgeons, geneticists, transplant surgeons, pediatric nutritionists, social workers, and neurodevelopmental specialists.

There are many complex disorders of the GU system. Some disorders found during childhood are associated with kidney damage; others are associated with obstructions or blockages that prevent the elimination of urine from the bladder; and others are associated specifically with the male GU tract. Box 37.1 outlines examples of disorders associated with kidney damage.

SAFETY *STAT!*

A male child or teen who presents in acute pain in the testicle area may be experiencing testicular torsion. This is an acute condition of spermatic cord becoming twisted, which requires a surgical procedure to prevent damage to the tissues. Symptoms include sudden and severe pain, swelling, nausea, vomiting, and a lump in the scrotal sac.

SAFETY *STAT!*

All newborn infant males should be inspected for the condition of undescended testes. This condition occurs when one or both of the testicles fail to move into the scrotum before birth. Most infant males will have their testicles descended by 9 months of age. The nurse must communicate this abnormal finding so the child can be further evaluated.

Box 37.1 Disorders Associated with Kidney Damage

- **Glomerulonephritis:** A form of kidney inflammation (ie, nephritis) in which lesions are found in the glomeruli; noted for occurring after a *Streptococcus* infection
- **HUS:** A life-threatening acute condition of microangiopathic hemolytic anemia, thrombocytopenia, and acute nephropathy; often caused by eating contaminated raw or rare hamburger or other meats, or contaminated produce
- **Chronic and recurring UTIs:** UTIs that recur after treatment was completed; may be the same or a different microbe causing the infection
- **Hydronephrosis:** An obstruction of urinary outflow by any means, including kidney stones or bladder outlet obstruction
- **Polycystic kidney disease:** Any of several hereditary conditions where numerous fluid-filled cysts are found throughout the kidney and possibly other organs

Disorders associated with blockage of the elimination of urine from the bladder:

- **Neurogenic bladder:** Nerve damage resulting in abnormal retention or leaking of urine from the bladder
- **VUR:** Refluxing of urine up into the ureters before or after urination
- **Ureterocele:** Condition of a cystlike dilation of tissue near a ureteral opening into the urinary bladder caused by a congenital stenosis of the ureteral orifice
- **Megaureter:** Condition of an abnormally large ureteral lumen

Disorders associated with males only:

- **Hypospadia:** Abnormal positioning of the urinary meatus in various areas of the penis or base of the penis
- **Undescended testes:** Congenital disorder of lack of normal descending of the testes into the testicle sac
- **Cryptorchidism:** Absent or ectopic testes; failure of one or both testes to descend from inguinal canal into the scrotum
- **Testicular torsion:** Sudden twisting of the testicle structures (ie, processus vaginalis around the spermatic cord) leading to intense pain and damage if not surgically repaired; considered a surgical emergency
- **Micropenis:** Congenital disorder of an abnormally small penis
- **Priapism:** Unrelenting erection associated with sickle cell anemia; a large clot in the vessels of the shaft of the penis
- **Male hydrocele:** Fluid collections within the scrotal sac

THE DEVELOPMENT OF THE GENITOURINARY SYSTEM

The development of the urinary system begins during 11th to the 12th week of fetal development (Bowden and Greenberg, 2014). By the 13th week of fetal development, the kidneys are producing urine. Early **mesoderm** tissues (ie, the middle embryonic germ layer) give rise to embryonic structures that then form reproductive organs and the kidney. The newborn, experiencing immature kidney function, produces larger quantities of urine than in the later developmental stages, and produces urine that has a lower SG. This is because the immature kidney has a less efficient means to concentrate waste products. As the infant develops, the GU system matures and becomes effective in the process of removing waste products from the blood and forming urine.

RENAL FUNCTION

The function of the kidneys is five-fold and is essential for homeostasis. One function is to *eliminate liquid waste products* from the blood into the form of urine. This process of detoxification of the blood is essential for life. The kidneys also *produce erythropoietin* when the body is experiencing a state of hypoxia to stimulate the bone marrow to produce more red blood cells. The kidneys *produce rennin,* a powerful chemical that stimulates the production of angiotensin 1, which then stimulates the production of angiotensin 11, causing the peripheral vasculature to constrict in response to low total fluid volume. Angiotensin 11 also promotes the secretion of aldosterone, whose function is to promote reabsorption of water and sodium by the kidneys to raise blood pressure in response to low circulating volumes. The final responsibilities of the kidneys are to *regulate fluids and electrolytes,* and to *regulate acid/base balance.*

The body water percentage in infants is approximately 75% to 80%, whereas the body water percentages of teenagers is close to adults at approximately 55% to 65%. A premature infant's percentage of water is closer to 90%. The extracellular fluid percentage in a child is much higher than the extracellular fluid of adults—42% to 45% versus 20%. The infant cannot conserve a source of body water as well as an adult, and has less reserve than an adult to pull from the intracellular space. The infant has an extracellular fluid turnover rate of close to 50% per day, whereas adults have only a 20% daily fluid turnover rate. The higher extracellular fluid percentage and the higher turnover rate leave the infant at greater risk for dehydration. As the body grows and matures, adipose and solid body structures influence the total body water and reduce volume. Infants also have a larger total body surface area to body weight as compared with adults, causing greater fluid losses.

The child's renal immaturity affects the efficacy of the kidney's function. Developmental differences in children influence not only fluid and electrolyte balance, but also the process of waste elimination.

SAFETY *STAT!*

- Young children have a slower glomerular filtration rate. This slower rate leaves them more vulnerable to the effects of medications and toxins.
- Infant's kidneys do not concentrate waste products in the urine as well as adults, producing a lower urine SG of less than 1.010 (adult urine SG is 1.010 to 1.030).
- During stress, the infant's ability to regulate fluids and electrolytes diminishes.

Metabolism

Young children have a higher metabolism to provide energy for rapid growth. Their metabolism rate is approximately two to three times higher than that of an adult. This higher rate requires more water to remove the greater waste products associated with a higher metabolism. Because of higher respiration, heart rate, and peristaltic rates, the young child experiences more insensible water loss. Insensible fluids are lost normally through the pulmonary (ie, breathing), cutaneous (ie, evaporation, sweating) and gastrointestinal (GI) (ie, fecal) systems. If the child is experiencing a greater caloric expenditure, such as during high fevers, the insensible fluid loss is greater. (A child will experience about 30 mL of insensible fluid loss for each degree of temperature above 38°C.)

Body Electrolytes

The functioning and levels of electrolytes in the body have a major role in maintaining homeostasis. With fluid overload or severe dehydration, electrolyte imbalances occur, leading to potential pathology. Sodium, potassium, magnesium, phosphorus, and calcium all play an integral role in providing fluid balance, neuromuscular activity, bone growth stimulation, and the regulation of acid-base balance. Children become symptomatic when electrolyte imbalances are present, and treatment by replacement therapy may be required.

Sodium

Water follows the movement of sodium. Sodium highly influences the distribution of body water as it crosses back and forth between cell walls. Sodium is the principal cation of the child's extracellular fluid and provides the body's osmolarity (ie, fluid movement). Hypernatremia can be caused by either excessive loss of body water that is greater than a loss of body sodium, especially in conditions such as cystic fibrosis, improperly mixed infant formulas, an ingestion of seawater, or excessive salt intake. **Hyponatremia,** which is a decreased concentration of sodium in the bloodstream, can be caused by diuretics, vomiting, diarrhea, burns, third-spacing, tap water enemas, and an excessive intake of parenteral fluids, also known as *IV fluids.*

Potassium

Potassium plays a large role in neuromuscular excitability. Cardiac conduction depends on normal serum levels of potassium.

Potassium is the principal cation of intracellular fluid and therefore is the major determinant of cell membrane resting potential. Hyperkalemia can be caused by an excessive intake of parenteral potassium administration or an impaired renal excretory mechanism. Hypokalemia can be very serious because potassium regulates skeletal, smooth, and cardiac muscles. Hypokalemia results in electrocardiography changes.

SAFETY *STAT!*

Never administer a potassium replacement infusion without knowing that the child has an adequate urine output. Administering potassium with poor or no urine output can place the child in danger of cardiac dysrhythmias.

Magnesium

Nerve and muscle activity depend on a normal serum level of magnesium. Tetany, seizures, and tremors are associated with low serum magnesium. Hypomagnesemia can be caused by several malabsorption syndromes, hypoparathyroidism, prolonged IV therapy, diuretic use, and hypercalcemia. Hypermagnesemia is rarely observed and is directly related to decreased renal function, the overconsumption of magnesium-containing laxatives, IV fluids, antacids, or enemas.

Phosphorus

Phosphorus has two major roles: (1) to interact with calcium to provide adequate bone growth and (2) to provide crucial functions toward the production of energy for a child's rapid metabolism. A dysfunction of serum phosphorus can be demonstrated with the use of several cytotoxic (ie, chemotherapy) drugs.

Calcium

Serum calcium provides functions of regulating cell membrane permeability, supporting the clotting cascade, and determines bone and teeth health. Hypocalcemia is associated with vitamin D deficiency, malabsorption disorders, or nutritional deficiency. Hypercalcemia is associated with vitamin D intoxication, ongoing states of immobilization, malignancies, and the excessive use of thiazide diuretics.

Acid-Base Balance and Renal Regulation

The kidneys have a significant role to play in acid/base balance. If a child presents with metabolic or respiratory **acidosis** (ie, elevated acidity in the blood) or **alkalosis** (ie, reduced acidity in the blood), the respiratory system will be the first to contribute to achieving a state of homeostasis. This is done by either blowing off excess CO_2 to help correct acidosis, or by retaining CO_2 to help correct alkalosis. The renal system will also assist in the regulation of the acid-base imbalance but takes considerably longer than the respiratory system. The renal system will either retain HCO_3 (ie, for acidosis), or will release HCO_3 (ie, for alkalosis).

FLUID MAINTENANCE REQUIREMENTS

Monitoring for adequate fluid intake is an important role of the pediatric nurse. Young children who are ill may not take in oral fluids at the rate of consumption required to maintain fluid balance. Fever, infection, GI distress, and vomiting all contribute to extra fluid losses. Therefore the pediatric nurse calculates the child's daily fluid maintenance requirements and provides care with this in mind.

Fluid requirements can be conceptualized in three ways; the child may need fluid maintenance to provide what is needed for a balanced fluid level, the child may need fluid deficit replacement, or the child may need fluid replacement for ongoing fluid loses such as diarrhea, gastric fluid loss, or burn-associated fluid losses. The determination of fluid maintenance therapy is directly related to the child's metabolic rate.

Some medical conditions such as pediatric cardiac disease, cancer, or burns may influence the daily fluid maintenance needs and an order will be written to either give more or less than the basic fluid maintenance calculation. An order may state "provide one times maintenance" to provide for what is required to sustain adequate fluid balance, or an order may state "provide one-half maintenance" if the child is at risk for the consequences of fluid overload.

Information about **fluid maintenance calculation,** which is a calculation used in pediatrics to determine the daily maintenance of fluids that should be consumed or administered, is found in Table 37.1. To calculate more or less than one times maintenance, divide the total amount due for the 24-hour period by two for "half times maintenance," or double the total amount required for "two times maintenance."

Water Intoxication

Childhood deaths have been associated with the intake of large amounts of free water. The medical diagnosis associated with overhydration of water is called *water intoxication.* Children who have severe mental illness, low cognitive function, or pathologies associated with extreme thirst should be monitored for appropriate free water intake.

SAFETY *STAT!*

Deaths have been associated with water intoxication because of severe electrolyte imbalances, body fluid dilution, and cardiac arrest. Indiscriminate water intake should be avoided. Maintaining accurate intake and output (I&O) calculations, and documenting and reporting concerning findings should all be done to ensure safety.

Urine Output

As children grow and are better able to concentrate their waste products, the number of times they void their urine begins to reduce. A pediatric nurse will weigh a hospitalized infant's and young child's diaper on a scale in grams to determine a correct I&O. One gram of urine is considered 1 mL of urine. The weight of the diaper must be known and subtracted from the total weight of the urine and diaper together to only account for the urine. The following denotes the average urine output for different age groups:

- Newborns produce approximately 10 mL/hour
- Infants produce approximately 5 to 10 mL/hour
- Toddlers and preschool children produce approximately 15 to 20 mL/hour
- School-aged children produce approximately 10 to 25 mL/hour

Many conditions require an assessment of a child's urine. It is the pediatric nurse's responsibility to make sure the specimen is collected in an accurate manner as some tests require sterile technique, such as a urine culture, and others are clean-catch methods. Box 37.2 provides information about collecting urine. See Figure 37.1 for a photograph of an infant with a uro-bag in place.

TABLE 37.1 CALCULATING FLUID MAINTENANCE

Child's weight in kg	Multiply by mL/day	Subtotal	Divide by hourly need
First 10 kg (0–10 kg)	100 mL	X	Divide X by 24
Second 10 kg (11–20 kg)	1,000 mL plus 50 mL per each kg between 11 and 20	X	Divide X by 24
21–70 kg	1,500 mL plus 20 mL per each kg between 21 and 70	X	Divide X by 24

Examples of children weighing:

8 kg	100 mL X 8 = 800 mL/required per day or 800 divided by 24 = 33.3 mL/hour
12 kg	1,000 mL + (2 X 50 mL) = 1,100 mL/required per day or 1,100 divided by 24 = 45.8 mL/hour
26 kg	1,500 mL + (6 X 20 mL) = 1,620 mL/required per day or 1,620 divided by 24 = 67.5 mL/hr

Box 37.2 Urine Specimen Collection

Clean Catch: Cotton Balls Placed in Diaper

- Not suitable for a sterile specimen for culture and sensitivity but adequate for SG, pH, presence of blood and ketones
- Must obtain adequate volume to squeeze specimen into specimen container
- Do not use unless diaper is free of any stool
- Cleanse the child's perineum well before placing cotton balls to obtain specimen

Clean Catch: Uro-Bag: Female

- Placed on the labia majora under the diaper to catch the urine specimen

Clean Catch: Uro-Bag: Male

- Cut to fit, the bag is placed over the penis and testicles to catch the urine specimen

Clean Catch: Midstream Sample

- For older children sitting on the toilet or commode, urine is caught in specimen container as the child voids, midstream

Sterile Sample: In and Out Catheterization

- When an indwelling catheter is not required, this sterile procedure passes a small catheter into the child's bladder to obtain a sterile specimen, typically for culture and sensitivity

Sterile Sample: Indwelling Catheterization

- When a child has an indwelling catheter in place, a sterile syringe and needle are inserted in a cleansed rubber port located along the collection tubing to obtain a sterile specimen

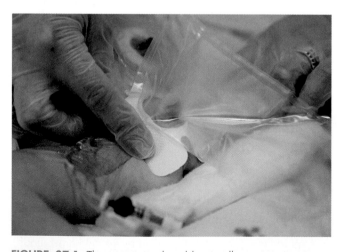

FIGURE 37.1 The nurse must be able to collect urine specimens in a bag that fits over the perineum in females or over the penis in males.

LABS & DIAGNOSTICS

Tests for Genitourinary Disorders

- Urinalysis
  - Checked for blood, glucose, ketones, protein, and pH
  - Conducted via dipstick
  - None of these substances are normally found in the child's urine; considered abnormal
- Urine Culture and Sensitivity
  - Collected for culture of bacteria or other infectious organisms
  - Placed in a culture tube and held in the laboratory
  - Specimen is checked over time for growth
  - Sensitivity of the bacteria grown out in the specimen is checked to match appropriate and effective antibiotic therapy (such as for a UTI)
- SG
  - Checked via machine to assess the concentration of urine
  - Normal values are 1.010 to 1.030
  - The lower the number, the more dilute the urine; water has an SG of 1.000
- IV Pyelogram
  - Checks the renal pelvic structures by radiography (ie, x-ray) following the administration of an IV injected contrast material (ie, dye)
- Voiding Cystourethrogram (VCUG)
  - Checks the bladder and surrounding structures during the process of voiding after the administration of contrast material (ie, dye), which is instilled into the child's bladder
  - Investigates the presence of reflux or strictures
- BUN
  - Checks the index of the glomerular filtration rate
  - BUN is a waste product of protein metabolism excreted via the kidneys
  - Normal values fluctuate with child's age, but are approximately 10 to 20 mg/dL
- Blood Creatinine
  - Checks the kidney function by measuring the waste product of energy metabolism from muscle
  - Normal values fluctuate with child's age, but are approximately 0.2 to 2.0 mg/dL
- Creatinine Clearance
  - Considered the best measure of kidney function in the child
  - Creatinine is the end product of energy metabolism from muscle
  - Collected over a period of time, such as 24 hours, and the specimen is kept refrigerated

DEHYDRATION

When a child's fluid intake is significantly reduced or there is a condition present that causes a loss of water and electrolytes, the child is at risk for developing dehydration. In very young children, severe dehydration can be life-threatening. Severe diarrhea, intractable vomiting, and prolonged diaphoresis (ie, sweating) can all cause a significant fluid imbalance by causing greater loss than intake. Hypovolemia ensues, followed by circulatory collapse and shock if not corrected in a timely manner. There are three types of dehydration, each of which needs unique corrective mechanisms.

Types of Dehydration

The three types of dehydration that can be found in childhood include isotonic, hypertonic, and hypotonic dehydration. The type most commonly found in dehydration is isotonic. Mild dehydration can be resolved with oral rehydration but moderate and severe dehydration will need IV solutions and monitoring.

Isotonic Dehydration

Isotonic dehydration is the loss of about equal parts water and electrolytes, leaving the child's serum sodium within normal values between 130 mEq/L and 150 mEq/L.

- **Causes:** Hemorrhages or slower significant bleeds
- **Treatments:** IV boluses of normal saline solution (0.9%) or, if tolerated, oral rehydration with oral electrolyte solutions such as Pedialyte

Hypertonic Dehydration

Hypertonic dehydration is when the loss of body fluids is found to be greater than the loss of electrolytes, leaving the child's serum sodium to be greater than expected, with values greater than 150 mEq/L.

- **Causes:** Loss of fluids such as poor PO intake, diarrhea, or vomiting
- **Treatments:** IV boluses of normal saline (0.45%) or, if tolerated, oral rehydration with diluted oral electrolyte solutions

Hypotonic Dehydration

Hypotonic dehydration is when the loss of electrolytes is found to be greater than the loss of fluids, leaving the child's serum sodium level well below normal, with values less than 130 mEq/L.

- **Causes:** Significant sodium loss, such as profuse sweating or as seen in children with cystic fibrosis
- **Treatments:** IV boluses of normal saline (0.9%) or infusions of lactated Ringer's solution with dextrose. The child may be supplemented with oral electrolytes to assist with correction.

Assessments of Dehydration

Assessing a child for dehydration is imperative. See Chapter 36, Child With a Gastrointestinal Condition, for a further discussion on assessing the child for dehydration. The pediatric nurse should inspect the child for the following:

- Strict assessment of I&O to monitor progression or management, including an hourly assessment of stool, urine, and vomit

- Determinants of severity of dehydration:
  - Mild is less than or equal to 5% body weight loss
  - Moderate is equal to 10% body weight loss
  - Severe is greater than or equal to 15% body weight loss
- SG and color of child's urine
- Daily weight to compare with baseline
- Dry skin and poor tissue turgor
- Dry mucous membranes
- Sunken fontanels and sunken eye sockets
- Pale skin and poor perfusion; delayed capillary refill and hypotension
- Decreased body temperature, rapid pulse, and tachypnea
- Lethargy, weak cry, and poor muscle tone

Interventions for Dehydration

Interventions for mild, moderate, or severe dehydration include oral fluid replacement if tolerated. When the child is suffering from an illness that causes significant vomiting, the child should be started on sips of fluid as tolerated when there has been no vomiting for 12 to 24 hours. The child with mild or moderate dehydration may be able to correct the dehydration with 30 to 50 mL of fluid per kilogram of weight for mild dehydration, and 60 to 90 mL of fluid per kilogram of weight for moderate dehydration. When severe dehydration or moderate dehydration with the inability to take in PO fluids is present, the child will require an IV placement for normal saline boluses (typically 20 mL/kg; repeated as needed) followed by at least the equivalent of a child's fluid maintenance calculation. Severe dehydration may need as much as 100 mL per kilogram of 0.9% saline to correct it.

Nursing Considerations for Dehydration

Children who are hospitalized with dehydration are typically quite sick and require close monitoring. It is imperative that the nurse monitor strict I&O, including weighing diapers (Fig. 37.2). If a child cannot tolerate PO fluid replacement therapy, IV therapy should not be delayed. If their cardiovascular system is affected and they demonstrate symptoms of poor perfusion, they may be moved to an intensive care unit (ICU) for closer monitoring. Children on the floor will have an IV placed for accurate and rapid fluid resuscitation. The pediatric health-care team who encounters a child in a clinic setting with dehydration will make a determination if the child can be rehydrated with oral rehydration fluids or needs to be sent to an emergency department for IV fluids.

SAFETY *STAT!*

Do not start any electrolyte solutions, especially potassium, until the child's urine output is restored to ensure appropriate elimination. If the child is in a critical state with renal failure, administered electrolytes can cause cardiac dysrhythmias.

If the dehydration is mild, the treatment orders may include starting the child on oral rehydration as tolerated. Provide commercial electrolyte solutions to infants and young children.

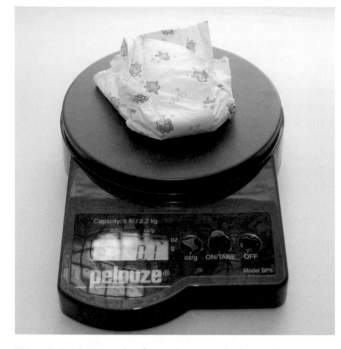

FIGURE 37.2 Example of a scale to weigh diapers for I&O.

It is acceptable to dilute the electrolyte solutions with water or a small amount of juice just to flavor the water. Check with the health-care team before implementing, and follow orders carefully. Do not try to rehydrate an older child with soda or sugary drinks as this will contribute to hypertonic dehydration. Milk should also not be used to rehydrate children.

It is important to think holistically and treat symptoms of discomfort, fever, and fatigue. The child should be provided mouth care with lemon/glycerin swabs. It is imperative that the child is closely monitored for strict I&O and any changes in clinical status, including changes in vital signs and mental status. Any change in mental status should be reported immediately as this may be a critical sign. Use the same scale with no clothes or diaper on to weigh the child for accuracy. If the child being treated for dehydration is an infant, provide a pacifier to allow sucking stimulation while receiving IV fluids.

COMMON GENITOURINARY DISORDERS

Across the developmental period, children can present with a variety of GU infections and disorders. Some infections are influenced by age, such as *Escherichia coli* infections in diapered infants and young children who are learning to toilet train. Nurses who are versed in common GU disorders and infections can assist the pediatric team in early and rapid diagnosis, preventing complications such as scarring, strictures, or infertility in the adolescent period or adulthood.

Urinary Tract Infections (UTIs)

UTIs are one of the most common childhood infections in which parents seek medical attention for their child. Females have more cases of UTI because of their shorter urethra, allowing bacteria to migrate more readily than in males. Most

commonly caused by bacteria, the infection can be located in three areas:

1. Bladder = cystitis
2. Urethra = urethritis
3. Kidney = pyelonephritis

UTIs can be caused by urine refluxing back into the ureters during or after urination, incomplete bladder emptying, or inadequate cleansing of the perineum after stooling. Diapered infants and toilet-training toddlers are at greatest risk for UTI from stool entering into the urethra.

Assessments of Urinary Tract Infections

Because of the fact that UTIs are so common in young children, the pediatric nurse must keep this in mind when interacting with families who are seeking care for children with fevers. The child with a suspected UTI should be assessed for:

- Frequency, urgency, and pain (ie, dysuria) associated with urination
- Odor of urine
- Color and clarity of the urine, noting the presence of red and white blood cells
- Fever
- Dehydration
- Hematuria and low pH
- Lethargy and poor feeding
- Abdominal, pelvic, or flank pain
- Number of occurrences of UTI in past

LABS & DIAGNOSTICS

Urinalysis

The key information provided by a urinalysis is the following: appearance, SG, pH, odor, glucose, protein, ketones, red blood cells, white blood cells, casts, nitrites, and leukocyte esterase.

Interventions for Urinary Tract Infections

Interventions for UTIs range from pushing oral fluids to IV antibiotics. Early identification can prevent complications such as urosepsis, a condition in immunocompromised children in which bacteria entering the blood stream from the urinary tract can be life-threatening. Interventions include:

- Providing favorite PO fluids or maintaining a patent IV for fluid replacement and fluid therapy to help wash out the bacteria from the bladder
- Pushing fluid consumption of more than 100 mL/kg/day
- Treating fever and discomfort
- Providing education on proper personal hygiene after toileting (ie, wiping front to back only)
- Teaching all family members how to clean female genitalia after stooling to ensure any fecal material is removed from the outer and inner labia
- Administered antimicrobials as ordered, including cephalosporins, sulfonamides, amoxicillin, or nitrofurantoin

DRUG FACTS

Antibiotics Used for Urinary Tract Infections

Antibiotics commonly used for the treatment of UTIs in children include:

- Amoxicillin (Amoxil)
- Ampicillin (Omnipen)
- Cephalexin (Keflex)
- Gentamicin (Garamycin)
- Sulfamethoxazole/trimethoprim, or co-trimoxazole (Bactrim, Septra)

Nursing Considerations for Urinary Tract Infections

When there is a history of UTI, it is important to teach the family prevention techniques, including the avoidance of strong detergents, soaps, bubble bath, or bath salts that may contribute to the formation of inflammation. See the Patient Teaching Guidelines feature for summary points for teaching families of children of various ages about personal hygiene for children.

PATIENT TEACHING GUIDELINES

Teaching Families About the Child's Personal Hygiene

UTIs are very common in young children. A large number of infants and children will be brought in for medical care for symptoms associated with UTI. Pediatric nurses are in a key position to teach prevention activities to decrease the incidence.

- Hand washing to prevent infection
  - Parents need to teach their children to wash their hands after every time they use the bathroom. If soap and water are not available, hand gel sanitizers should be used. Children should wash their hands after playing outside, in playgrounds, or at parks. Children should also wash their hands before and after helping to prepare foods, especially raw foods.
  - Hand washing can be presented as a fun game to young children. Singing the ABCs, *Twinkle, Twinkle Little Star*, or another short song while washing encourages the child to spend the time needed to be thorough.
- Girls wiping front to back
  - Because females have a shorter urethra than males, they are particularly vulnerable to UTIs.
  - Young girls must be taught how to wipe their perineum from front to back, not back to front, to prevent the contamination of stool into their meatus. This contamination is a common source of UTI.
  - Reinforcing this process is important. Young girls need reminders on a regular basis.
- Position for urination
  - Most young girls void with their legs together. This leaves them prone to urine refluxing into their vaginas, which can lead to vulvitis, vulvovaginitis, and infection.

- Diaper cleanup of stool
  - Parents need to wash their hands before changing a child's diaper if they have been handling contaminated substances.
  - Parents need to carefully remove all stool from a young child's perineum after each stooling.
  - Children should not have a delay in changing diapers with stool.

The Health Promotion feature provides information on how to prevent UTIs and sexually transmitted infections (STIs) in adolescence.

HEALTH PROMOTION

Preventing Urinary Tract Infections and Sexually Transmitted Infections in Sexually Active Teens

The development of UTIs in sexually active teens is not uncommon, especially in teenage girls. While conducting sex education classes, the pediatric nurse should include a discussion of prevention. The following information should be included in an adolescent sexual health curriculum:

- Teenagers should urinate before and after sexual intercourse. An empty bladder before sex reduces the friction associated with the development of bladder inflammation. The act of urine flushing the urethra helps to cleanse bacteria out from the opening of the meatus.
- If the teen participates in anal intercourse, the teen should take precautions to conduct personal hygiene immediately after sex to cleanse the perineum of bacteria harbored in the rectum. Vaginal intercourse after anal intercourse increases the chances of contracting infections.
- Teenagers should be taught to seek health care if they experience dysuria, blood in their urine, fevers and chills, discharge from the genitalia, or cloudy urine.
- Teenagers should be provided education and counseling about avoiding high-risk sexual behaviors and how to avoid unwanted sexual advances.
- Teenagers need to understand that they may be asymptomatic and need to seek medical attention for known contact with an infected sexual partner.
- Teenagers need to be taught about prevention of genital warts by the pre-exposure immunization against human papilloma virus.
- Teenagers need to be taught about the prevention of hepatitis A and B via pre-exposure immunization.
- Teenagers need to understand that with prompt identification and treatment, curative therapy is available for bacterial STIs.
- Females should be encouraged to have a Pap smear when they become sexually active and continue to have annual examinations (at a minimum).
- Teenagers need to know that their interactions with health-care professionals about topics associated with birth control, STI treatment, and related care are held confidentially.

Enuresis

Enuresis is a condition of voiding dysfunction. **Nocturnal incontinence,** the most common form, is the occurrence of involuntary voiding at night after the child has demonstrated a control of micturition. **Diurnal incontinence** is daytime incontinence and is mostly associated with a condition called *unstable bladder.* Although girls typically acquire bladder control at a younger age than boys, the overall occurrence of this condition is as high as 20% of children older than 5 years. Treatment is typically not offered until after the age of 6 in both genders because of how common this condition is.

Assessments of Enuresis

Assessment for the cause and severity of enuresis starts by a thorough medical examination and health history. Causes of urinary incontinence during childhood may be related to:

• Unstable (ie, uninhibited) bladder
• Holding on to urine or infrequent daytime voiding
• Cystitis
• Neurogenic bladder
• Bladder outlet obstruction
• Sphincter abnormality
• Trauma
• Overflow incontinence
• Iatrogenic causes

Interventions for Enuresis

Interventions for enuresis in children 5 and younger often involve reassuring the parents that the condition is considered self-limiting and the child should not be punished or scolded for the accidents. For young children, fluids should be restricted after the evening meal and the child must void before going to bed. Research has demonstrated a direct link between nocturnal incontinence and severe snoring associated with enlarged adenoids. If the parents report snoring, a referral to an otolaryngologist should be offered. An adenoidectomy may help cure some cases of nocturnal incontinence. For older children, active treatment consists first of motivation with activities such as a star chart and rewards. Older children may benefit from what is considered conditioning therapy with the use of an auditory alarm that detects wetness via electrodes in the linen or underwear. Medications can be used but are not considered curative. Desmopressin acetate, a synthetic form of an antidiuretic hormone, reduces urine production at night. Anticholinergic therapy with oxybutynin chloride may help during the daytime.

Nursing Considerations for Enuresis

Nursing considerations for childhood enuresis include role modeling empathy and a nonjudgmental, nonpunitive attitude toward the child. For parents of children younger than 5 years, the nurse must reinforce the need to provide emotional support, fluid restrictions in the evening, and bedtime voiding. For older children, the parents should be supported in initiating a plan of motivation with rewards. It may be helpful for the child to participate in changing their linens while hospitalized and

having the child carry clean underwear. The child should never be scolded, belittled, or made to feel bad by caregivers or parents because they are already at risk for peer humiliation and teasing. Often, simple steps to reduce the need to void at night are enough to assist the child and family with the stress of a child experiencing enuresis.

Nephrotic Syndrome/Nephrosis

Nephrotic syndrome/nephrosis is characterized by several symptoms that are associated with the development of pores along the final filtration membrane of the kidney and subsequent loss of serum proteins. Most nephrotic syndrome cases during childhood are considered idiopathic, meaning no known cause is found, with a good overall prognosis. Also called *minimal-change nephrotic syndrome,* the pathology is associated with relapses throughout childhood. Relapses are associated with poorer clinical outcomes and higher mortality rates. It is more commonly found in boys than girls. The cardinal symptoms of nephrotic syndrome are threefold (Fig. 37.3):

1. **Severe proteinuria:** Severe loss of protein through porous nature of the final urine filtration membrane, the glomeruli, into the urine
2. **Severe hypoproteinemia** (also called *hypoalbuminemia*): Severely low levels of protein left in the

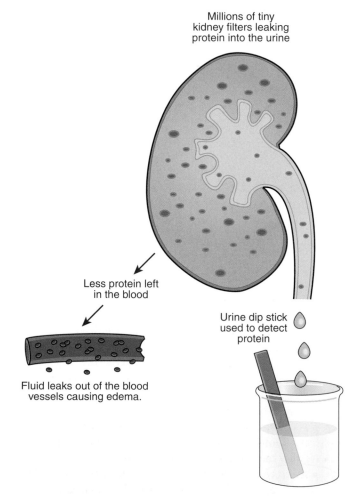

Millions of tiny kidney filters leaking protein into the urine

Less protein left in the blood

Fluid leaks out of the blood vessels causing edema.

Urine dip stick used to detect protein

FIGURE 37.3 Nephrotic syndrome.

serum, leading to generalized edema, especially noted in the abdomen (ie, **ascites**)

3. **Hyperlipidemia:** Elevated serum total cholesterol, triglycerides, and total lipids

Assessments of Nephrotic Syndrome/Nephrosis

Because of the complexity of a diagnosis of nephrotic syndrome, the pediatric nurse must be able to identify clinical signs and report changes in clinical status to the pediatric health-care team. Assessments for the development of nephrotic syndrome include:

- Fatigue
- Decreased appetite (ie, anorexia)
- Fluid accumulation (ie, edema)
- Weight gain with abdominal swelling
- Golden-yellow, foamy urine

Interventions for Nephrotic Syndrome/Nephrosis

Treatment is generally supportive. It is imperative that daily weights are conducted at the same time of day and on the same scale. Fluid retention is treated with diuretics, and hypertension, although not common, is managed. Corticosteroids are administered for a lengthy period of time; they have been shown to decrease the size of the pore through which proteins are lost. When the level of serum proteins is very low, the child may require IV administration of albumin. A nutritionist will follow the child and initiate a low-salt, high-protein diet. In severe cases, immunosuppressive therapy may be required.

SAFETY *STAT!*

When a child is on high dose corticosteroids for a lengthy period of time, the nurse must watch for signs of hypertension, hyperglycemia, immunosuppression, poor wound healing, emotional lability, and excessive hunger. All symptoms associated with long-term corticosteroid use must be reported.

Nursing Considerations for Nephrotic Syndrome/Nephrosis

Nursing considerations for a child with nephrotic syndrome include emotional support for the entire family. The appearance of the child can frighten the parents and support is needed to process and understand the pathology of the disease. The child will need to have vital signs and daily weights monitored carefully and any changes will need to be reported to the health-care team. The child's skin will need to be protected because edema causes the skin to become vulnerable to breakdown. Providing a low-sodium diet may assist in the increasing edema. Monitoring for problems with skin integrity, GI distress, poor nutrition, and fatigue are all nursing concerns. Families must be taught to look for symptoms of a relapse after the child is discharged. These symptoms include the appearance of albumin in the child's urine (ie, it is frothy, golden-colored, and viscous), as well as changes in the child's weight, fatigue level, and appetite.

PATIENT TEACHING GUIDELINES
Low-Sodium Diet

A low-salt diet may be ordered for a child who presents with nephrotic syndrome to decrease the fluid retention and third-spacing related to hyperalbuminemia. To prevent fluid effusions in the lungs, a low-sodium diet may be ordered; it assists in decreasing fluid retention and reducing the leakage of fluids from the intravascular space to the extravascular space.

DRUG FACTS
Medications for Nephritic Syndrome

Medications used in the care of a child with nephritic syndrome include:
- Diuretics for fluid overload
- Antibiotics if peritonitis occurs
- Corticosteroids for the reduction of the size of the pores on the glomeruli
- 25% albumin infusions to reduce edema and replace lost albumin (Rudd and Kocisko, 2014)

Acute Glomerulonephritis (AGN)

When a child experiences disease of the kidney's glomeruli, a condition called *acute glomerulonephritis* may occur. The glomeruli are small structures of the kidney that contain the blood vessels and the collection tubules, called *nephrons,* where urine is filtered from the blood. Glomerulonephritis often follows a severe infection such as a strep infection, where the larger immune/antigen complexes used to fight the infection become clogged in the nephrons, causing inflammation and impairment of the kidney's ability to filter urine. Streptococcal infections, inflammatory diseases of the arteries, and genetic dispositions are the most common causes of AGN. Glomerulonephritis may present 1 week to 10 days after a strep throat or strep upper respiratory infection. This disease primarily affects school-aged children and is rare in children under the age of 2 (Hockenberry and Wilson, 2013).

Assessments of Acute Glomerulonephritis

A child with AGN will present with classic symptoms that identify the disorder. Different from nephrotic syndrome in that serum proteins are not lost, AGN has clinical symptoms that represent renal failure as the final filtration membrane becomes clogged with antibody/antigen molecules.

Assessments of AGN include the following:

- Dark brown (ie, tea-colored) urine
- Low overall urine output
- Fatigue and lethargy
- High blood pressure
- Edema
- Sore throat
- Rash on buttocks and legs

- Joint pain
- Headache
- Increased breathing effort
- Seizures

Diagnostic evaluation for AGN includes throat, blood, and urine cultures to identify the presence of a streptococcal infection; urinalysis; chest x-ray for pulmonary congestion; renal ultrasound; and possibly renal biopsy. Laboratory findings that are inclusive of the pathology of AGN include:

- Mildly to moderately elevated BUN and creatinine
- Elevated antistreptolysin-O titer
- Elevated anti-DNase B titer
- Elevated erythrocyte sedimentation rate (ESR)
- Depressed complement C3 and complement C4 levels

Interventions for Acute Glomerulonephritis

Interventions for AGN center around the prevention of fluid overload and the prevention of further waste product (ie, urea) buildup. These interventions occur through the following:

- Administering diuretics
- Correcting electrolyte imbalances
- Treating the strep infection with antibiotics
- Managing associated hypertension
- Administering phosphate binders to reduce mineral phosphates in the blood
- Dialysis for the short-term management of the buildup of waste products in the blood

Nursing Considerations for Acute Glomerulonephritis

Nursing considerations for a child who presents with AGN include rapid interventions to prevent significant glomerular injury for the antigen-antibody deposits within the glomeruli. The nurse must rapidly identify any history of an infection anywhere in the body and report this significant information to the primary health-care provider. For instance, a typical latency period for AGN after an episode of acute pharyngitis is 10 to 20 days, whereas for a streptococcal skin infection, the latency period can be much longer, lasting up to 6 weeks.

The nurse must keep in mind that a diagnosis of AGN affects multiple systems. Headaches, GI disturbances, malaise, hypertension, and rapid weight gain are all associated with the disease and need meticulous nursing care.

Nursing diagnoses associated with AGN include:

- Excess fluid volume related to impaired renal function
- Impaired urinary elimination related to glomerular dysfunction
- Deficient knowledge regarding the pathology of AGN and its treatments and management

Hemolytic Uremic Syndrome

HUS is a rare and potentially lethal form of kidney failure in children who have developed an infection such as *E coli*. Outbreaks of HUS are more common in the summer and are closely associated with the consumption of inadequately

cooked meats, unpasteurized dairy products or juices, and contaminated swimming pools, water parks, day care facilities, and fast food restaurants. HUS can also be associated with certain medications. It is most commonly seen in young children between 4 months and 4 years of age. The presence of the bacteria in the blood damages red blood cells and causes massive lysis of the cells. Children who present with HUS and are experiencing seizures have a poor prognosis.

Assessments of Hemolytic Uremic Syndrome

A young child may present with vomiting, severe abdominal pain, and watery or bloody diarrhea. The child will appear quite ill, pale, fatigued, and dehydrated, and may demonstrate unexplained, small bruises visible only in the lining of the mouth. Because of the damaged red blood cells, the very small blood vessels of the kidneys become clogged and develop renal failure. As the kidneys are no longer able to eliminate waste products, uremia develops and the child experiences fluid retention. High blood pressure, edema, and fluid retention can occur, leading to the need for dialysis.

Interventions for Hemolytic Uremic Syndrome

The child will become quite ill during the hemolytic uremic process, often requiring an ICU stay. There is no known cure for HUS. The child's symptoms of initial dehydration followed by fluid retention will be treated, as well as electrolyte disturbances, anemia, and discomfort. IV nutrition may be required and antihypertensives may be administered.

Nursing Considerations for Hemolytic Uremic Syndrome

The child with HUS will present quite ill. The family will be experiencing stress and anxiety not knowing what is wrong with their child and will be concerned about the high level of care that will be required right after a confirmed diagnosis. Providing emotional support while answering all questions will be important to the well-being of the family. Because of the severity of the diagnosis, family members will be fearful of the potential of poor outcomes or the threat of death.

Teaching families about adequate food preparation and washing of fruits and vegetables can help prevent HUS. Part of anticipatory guidance for new parents is to remind them that adequate and safe food preparation reduces the likelihood of contamination and illness.

Congenital Genitourinary Anomalies

There are many GU disorders that are present since birth (ie, congenital). One important nursing consideration is to know the child's birth history and any surgical or nonsurgical procedures that were conducted to remedy the anomaly. Congenital anomalies can cause obstructions, strictures, an absence of anatomy, abnormal openings, or a delay in and/or inefficient urinary elimination, including urine reflux. One of the most common GU anomalies is vesicoureteral reflux (VUR) (Box 37.3).

Box 37.3 Congenital Anomalies of the Genitourinary System: Vesicoureteral Reflux (VUR)

VUR is a condition where urine flows back from the bladder into the ureters and often up into the kidneys during or after urination, causing urine to flow both directions. Damage to the kidney structures occurs because of scarring from recurrent UTIs. VUR is more common in young girls than young boys. As children grow, VUR is more common in boys because there is more pressure when voiding. The most common symptoms are urgency, dribbling of urine, UTI, and eventually high kidney damage (such as the presence of an abdominal mass from a severely swollen kidney) and hypertension. Identification of the disorder is by renal ultrasound and VCUG. VUR is graded on a scale of 1 to 5. If the child's reflux is considered 1 to 3, he or she may need no therapy and the condition will eventually resolve on its own. For 4 to 5, the child may require surgical interventions such as a flap-valve apparatus to prevent the reverse of flow, or if the child has had several UTIs, the scarred ureter and/or kidney tissue may need to be removed.

Assessments of Congenital Genitourinary Anomalies

Maternal-child nurses, as well as pediatric nurses, should assess a newborn for the presence of a congenital anomaly as part of a routine well-newborn assessment. Assessing the external genitalia, as well as assessing the first urine elimination, are important in the early identification of a GU anomaly. Visual inspection and palpation should be conducted as part of the initial assessment.

Interventions for Congenital Genitourinary Anomalies

Many congenital GU anomalies require surgical interventions. Depending on the severity of the condition, the pediatric surgical team may wait until the infant is less vulnerable to the complications of anesthesia, or until the family feels the child's psychosocial development may be affected by the anomaly. For instance, if a newborn boy is born with **hypospadia** (ie, an abnormal opening on the glans penis for the elimination of urine), surgery may be conducted before the child has concerns with body image. **Epispadias** is a congenital condition in which the meatus, the opening of the urethra, is located on the dorsum of the penis.

Another congenital anomaly is a neurogenic bladder associated with spina bifida. Anomalies that affect kidney function will require rapid diagnostic and medical/surgical interventions.

Nursing Considerations for Congenital Genitourinary Anomalies

Infants and young toddlers will not recognize that they have a congenital anomaly. Pediatric nurses must be available to answer questions concerning the child's anatomy and physiology related to the GU system, including any abnormalities. If the surgical correction can wait until the child is older, the family may feel strongly that the procedure should take place before the child recognizes that there are anatomical differences between himself or herself and other children. The decision about when the surgical procedure takes place may or may not be up to the parents' preferences, but, if so, the parents should be supported in their decision and given anticipatory guidance about body image perspectives for each of the developmental stages of childhood.

NURSING CARE PLAN for the Child With Neurogenic Bladder

Neurogenic bladder, also called *neuropathic bladder,* is a condition in which the signals along the nerves between the bladder and the brain are injured or damaged, resulting in the inability to regulate urinary elimination—essentially, from a paralyzed bladder. Neurogenic bladder is associated with spina bifida, spinal cord trauma, or central nervous system tumors. Neurogenic bladder causes urine leakage, retention, infections of the ureter and bladder, and possible kidney damage as the urine backs up, causing extra pressure.

Assessments:
1. There is urine retention or urine leakage.
2. Patient has an inability to empty the bladder when desired.
3. Patient experiences recurring UTIs.
4. There is a history of spinal cord trauma, tumors, injuries, or accidents.

Nursing Diagnoses:
1. There is impaired urinary elimination.
2. There is a risk for injury.

Continued

NURSING CARE PLAN for the Child With Neurogenic Bladder—cont'd

3. The patient is experiencing pain.
4. The patient is experiencing disturbed body image.
5. There is a knowledge deficit.

Goals:

1. The child will not experience urinary retention.
2. The child will not experience the development of a UTI.
3. The child will not experience complications associated with surgery during the postoperative period.

Interventions:

1. Insert an aseptic catheter to empty the child's bladder at regular intervals.
2. Administer prophylactic antibiotics to reduce the incidence of infection as ordered.
3. Teach all caregivers proper hand washing before performing catheterization and perineal hygiene care.

Evaluation of Outcome:

1. The child will have a frequent and regular elimination of urine from the bladder.
2. The child does not demonstrate hypertension or any injury or infection from the urine retention.
3. The family demonstrates independent care, understanding of the pathology associated with neurogenic bladder, and when to call for help or follow-up care.

Genetic or Congenital Reproductive System Disorders

In rare situations, an infant might be born with a genetic or congenital reproductive system disorder requiring assessments, diagnostic examinations, and surgical procedures. The following presents four types of rare congenital reproductive system disorders.

Types of Congenital Reproductive System Disorders

Some of the more common types of genetic or congenital reproductive or GU system disorders include ambiguous genitalia, exstrophy of the bladder, Turner's syndrome, and Klinefelter's syndrome.

AMBIGUOUS GENITALIA. Found in approximately 1:2,000 live births, this condition is associated with maternal or fetal hormonal imbalances. One such imbalance is congenital adrenal hyperplasia (Hockenberry and Wilson, 2013). Also called *hermaphroditism,* the condition is marked by the presence of both ovaries and testes, and/or the external genitalia varies between nearly fully developed female to nearly fully developed male anatomy.

EXSTROPHY OF THE BLADDER. Exstrophy of the bladder is a condition in which the lower portion of the abdominal wall and the anterior bladder wall are both missing, causing the child to be born with an exposed, or open, bladder on the abdomen. Occurring more frequently in boys than in girls, this condition appears as a red mass and demonstrates a continuous drainage of urine. The newborn's skin may become excoriated and the condition requires staging surgical repair soon after birth.

TURNER'S SYNDROME. Considered a female sex chromosome anomaly, Turner's syndrome is the loss of part or some of all of the sex chromosomes. This condition results in an abnormal short stature and underdeveloped gonads (ie, sex organs). The condition is noted at birth but demonstrated notably during childhood. Characteristics include a web neck, widely spaced nipples, a small mandible, epicanthal folds, a broad chest, and delayed sexual maturation during adolescence. Treatment includes growth hormone therapy.

KLINEFELTER'S SYNDROME. This condition is associated with an extra X chromosome (ie, XXY), producing a child who is relatively tall with delayed secondary sex development. Most are infertile, with azoospermia (ie, an absence of sperm count) and small testes. The condition is often not noted until adolescence, when puberty is absent. Klinefelter's syndrome is associated with behavior and psychiatric disorders, including aggression, antisocial acts, and anxiety. Treatment includes long-acting testosterone therapy.

Acquired Reproductive System Disorders

Acquired reproductive system disorders include a variety of conditions that develop during childhood. Acquired disorders refer to the development of a condition after birth, as compared with primary disorders that are present since birth.

Types of Acquired Reproductive System Disorders

Pediatric nurses must be knowledgeable about potential acquired reproductive or GU disorders. Foreign bodies, inflammatory conditions such as pediatric vulvovaginitis, and adhesion are three examples of acquired conditions. The pediatric health-care team must work together to identify the conditions rapidly to provide the child with treatment and comfort.

FOREIGN BODIES IN THE VAGINA. When a child presents with foreign bodies in the vagina, the health-care team will conduct an initial assessment for sexual child abuse. Some young children will place small toys or items in their ears, rectum, or vagina, but this must be weighed against the presence of a mental health problem. Manual removal of the item is attempted.

PEDIATRIC VULVOVAGINITIS. Vulvitis, or vulvar inflammation, is often associated with vaginitis from candidiasis (ie, fungal) infections. Young, prepubertal girls lack protective pubic hair and labial fat pads, and are therefore more susceptible to trauma and irritation. Chemicals in many soaps and commonly used bubble bath substances may also cause irritation and sensitivity to the vulvar skin and tissues.

LABIA ADHESIONS. There are a variety of etiologies associated with labial adhesions. These include scarring from surgical procedures, complications from female circumcisions still practiced in several countries, and scarring from chemical or thermal burns.

Sexually Transmitted Infections (STIs)

Infections passed from person to person during intimate genital contact or sexual intercourse are called *sexually transmitted infections*. The adolescent population has the highest risks for acquiring an STI and the highest rates of STIs in the general population. Adolescents who have unprotected sex with an infected individual, are younger than age 15, and who inject drugs are at the highest risk.

Assessments of Sexually Transmitted Infections

Sexually active teens may present with a variety of symptoms of STIs, including dysuria, lesions, odors, discharges, and discomfort. The pediatric nurse must feel comfortable in asking questions about health history, sexual history, the use of birth control (especially condom use), and the presence of symptoms of STIs. Assessments should be holistic and include a history and a physical examination, including inspection, palpation, and olfaction, and should be conducted with respect and privacy in mind. Some states allow underage (ie, 13- to 17-year-old) teenagers to seek medical care for birth control, Pap smears, and STI diagnosis and treatments without the consent or knowledge of a parent or guardian. Check your state's regulations before providing this confidential care to underage teens.

SAFETY *STAT!*

The early identification and treatment of STIs are imperative because, if left untreated, some infections can cause scarring of tissues, leading to difficulty becoming pregnant or to infertility.

SAFETY *STAT!*

Having confidence to talk to sexually active teenagers about condom use and the prevention of STIs is important to help teens prevent STIs. Condom use alone is not sufficient to prevent pregnancy and teens need to understand this fact.

Interventions for Sexually Transmitted Infections

Interventions for the treatment for STIs depend on whether the microbe is viral or bacterial. Oral antibiotics are often prescribed for STIs such as chlamydia and gonorrhea, whereas viral STIs such as herpes and genital warts have no cure. The use of antiviral medications has been shown to reduce the frequency and severity of genital herpetic lesions.

Nursing Considerations for Sexually Transmitted Infections

Education is required to prevent STIs by providing guidance for good perineal hygiene, education about condom use, and voiding before and after sex.

Types of Sexually Transmitted Infections

The most common STIs found during childhood include:

- **Chlamydia:** Caused by *Chlamydia trachomatis,* symptoms include dysuria (ie, burning on urination). It requires antibiotic therapy of a single dose of oral azithromycin.
- **Gonorrhea:** Caused by *Neisseria gonorrhoeae,* the symptoms include dysuria and purulent penile or vaginal discharge. It requires antibiotic therapy of a single dose of ceftriaxone.
- **Genital warts:** Caused by a variety of the human papillomavirus, it presents as visible warts on the labia, cervix, anus, or penis. It is without a cure. Cervical infections have an association with cancer.
- **Genital herpes:** Caused by the *Herpes simplex* virus type 1 or 2, it causes painful blisters. Itching, burning, and tingling may occur just prior to an outbreak. It is without a cure.

Key Points

- The GU system is a complex system composed of the kidneys, ureters, bladder, urethra, and reproductive organs.
- The kidneys have many important functions, including filtering water and solutes from the blood, and reabsorbing needed water, protein, electrolytes, glucose, and amino acids while allowing unwanted or unneeded substances to be secreted as urine.

- The kidneys regulate the acid-base system, which maintains homeostasis. The kidneys further produce and secrete rennin and erythropoietin hormones.
- Cardinal signs of a GU system dysfunction include fluid retention, fluid loss, dehydration, and electrolyte disturbances.

- Children can present with acquired GU disorders such as UTI, nephrotic syndrome, and glomerulonephritis, or they can present with complications associated with congenital GU disorders.
- Many congenital GU disorders require meticulous follow-up care and staging surgeries.

- The role of the pediatric nurse is to support a team effort in early identification, treatment, and follow-up care needed to assist a family whose child has a GU dysfunction.
- Education is required to prevent infections of the GU system.

REVIEW QUESTIONS

1. Ensuring that a young child hospitalized with nephrotic syndrome consumes adequate nutrition, the pediatric nurse monitors which type of diet?
   1. Low-sodium, low-protein
   2. High-sodium, high-protein
   3. Low-potassium, low-sodium
   4. Low-sodium, high-protein

2. A teenager admitted with acute renal failure is depressed and angry over her condition. The pediatric nurse spends time with the child reinforcing the need for continued social interactions and family support. Which of the following activities would be best for this child?
   1. Playing movies and video games in her room
   2. Attending an arts and crafts program in the playroom
   3. Ambulating the halls of the hospital for mild exercise
   4. Interacting on social media on a laptop in her room

3. Glomerulonephritis is marked by the deposition of immune complexes. Which of the following situations gives the most information about the development of this disease?
   1. A 1-year-old infant with bilateral ear infections
   2. A 3-year-old child, just entering preschool, with high fevers
   3. A 7-year-old with croup
   4. An 11-year-old with vulvitis

4. An infant presents to the urgent care clinic with tachycardia, no tears, sunken fontanels, and a serum sodium level of 139 mEq/L. Which type of dehydration is mostly likely occurring?
   1. Osmotic dehydration
   2. Hypotonic dehydration
   3. Hypertonic dehydration
   4. Isotonic dehydration

5. When reviewing the laboratory findings on a child hospitalized for a third relapse of nephrotic syndrome, which of the following results would be expected?
   1. Hypoalbuminemia and proteinuria
   2. Proteinuria and hyponatremia
   3. Hypoalbuminemia and hypernatremia
   4. Hypoalbuminemia and negative proteinuria

6. A newborn infant has been diagnosed with undescended testes. The health-care team assures the father that:
   1. Surgery is a safe option to bring the testicles down into the scrotal sac.
   2. Manual manipulation, although producing discomfort, is an option.
   3. No interventions are conducted at this time and the child will be reassessed.
   4. During circumcision, the neonatologist can perform a small procedure.

7. A teenage boy is brought into the hospital in severe pain to be tested for testicular torsion. He had been working out in the weight room at his high school. The parents express concern about their son's ability to be fertile after the procedure. The health-care team explains that:
   1. With a delay in treatment, the son may be infertile because of tissue ischemia.
   2. With prompt surgical correction, the teen should be fertile.
   3. Because of the removal of the testicles during surgery, infertility is an assumption.
   4. Without experiencing a relapse, the teen should remain fertile.

CRITICAL THINKING QUESTIONS

1. An 11-year-old female child presents to the urgent care clinic with a significant perineal rash, with itching and the sensation of burning on her labia. She also complains of a history of dysuria. Her father brings her into the clinic stating that she bathes in bath salts and bubble baths every day. What would your health history include? What key assessments would you conduct to further investigate this situation and clinical presentation? How would you conduct your assessments?

2. A mother calls the pediatric telephone triage line stating that her 8-year-old son has been wetting his bed every night for the last 3 weeks. She is concerned about his social life because he is preparing to attend a 2-week summer camp shortly. What would your history and assessments include?

3. A child is currently admitted for her fourth bout of nephrotic syndrome. What are your nursing care concerns for this child and her family?

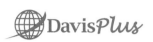

For additional resources and information, visit **www.DavisPlus.com**. Post-Conference Questions and Activities, Answers, and References can be found on Davis*Plus*.

38

Child With a Skin Condition

KEY TERMS

contactants
dermatological
exanthems
Lund-Browder classification tool
macular rash
papular rash
pustule
rule of nines
urticaria
vesicle
wheals

 **DavisPlus**   For audio pronunciation guide, visit www.DavisPlus.com

CHAPTER CONCEPTS

Development
Infection
Inflammation
Safety
Skin Integrity

LEARNING OUTCOMES

1. Define the key terms.
2. Review the special care needs of a newborn's and young infant's skin.
3. Determine best practices to manage the symptoms of skin disorders across childhood.
4. Differentiate among various rashes that can be found during childhood.
5. Analyze the care of a child with a first-, second-, and third-degree burn and prepare a holistic care plan for a child that requires sequential debridement of a significant burn.
6. Describe presentations of skin disorders that can be considered evidence of child abuse.
7. Review personal protective equipment that should be used to prevent the spread of various childhood skin infections.
8. Discuss the short- and long-term consequences of body piercing and tattooing.
9. Create a teaching plan for new parents to learn how to prevent burns during childhood, including electrical, immersive, contact, and heat burns.

REAL-WORLD CASE STUDY

Katrina

■ The father of Katrina, an 11-month-old infant, brought her to the public health clinic for a concern about a "growing, red, wet rash on her elbows and right face in the cheek area." The father said the child has been fussy lately, waking up during the night every 1 to 2 hours in tears, and sweating during long crying episodes. The rash appears to be raised; bright, beefy red; moist in the center; oval shaped in both locations; and about 3 to 5 cm wide, and 5 to 6 cm in length. The pediatric health-care team assesses the child and suspects the infant may have eczema on her arms and face. The team decides to do a thorough examination on the child, including laboratory assessments, and asks the father a series of health-related questions.

1. What is the cause of infantile eczema?
2. What are the classic signs and symptoms of childhood eczema?
3. What are other symptoms in other body systems that may be present when eczema is suspected?
4. What treatments can be used for eczema?
5. What can be done for the infant's symptoms?

CONCEPTUAL CORNERSTONE

Growth and Development

Skin, the largest organ of the body, has particular developmental aspects. Newborns are very susceptible to skin injury and their skin absorbs medications readily. Infants can experience a variety of rashes including contact dermatitis and candidiasis. Infants are particularly susceptible to food allergies with a skin component because of their expanding diets during the second 6 months of life. Toddlers and preschoolers, while exposed to more and more social environments, are particularly susceptible to acquire childhood communicable diseases and infections that may have distinct rashes (eg, measles, roseola, skin strep and staph infections, eczema). School-aged children may experience a variety of burns, such as electrical, contact, immersive, and heat burns, as well as sunburns. Adolescents can experience a variety of skin conditions from infections to burns to acne. A pediatric nurse should take a developmental approach to providing anticipatory guidance to families concerning skin issues. Prevention of skin breakdown, rashes, infections, and pressure ulcers is of primary importance to children across the developmental period if particularly vulnerable. Vulnerable children include those with immobility issues, immunosuppression, malnutrition, poor hygiene, and genetic predispositions.

The structure of the skin is composed of layers. The epidermis is the tough outer layer of the skin and the dermis is the highly vascular inner layer that provides support. The skin also includes a layer of subcutaneous fat. The accessory structures of the skin include sebaceous glands that provide sebum for the follicles of the hair, sweat glands that provide thermoregulation, nails for structure and the safety of the fingers, and hair. The skin itself is very sensitive to temperature, touch, pain, and pressure. Providing protection by supplying the body with the first line of defense from the invasion of infectious organisms, the skin protects the underlying tissues, organs, and vasculature from injury. Via pores, the skin helps the body to excrete salt and water. A major responsibility of the skin is to provide the body with the synthesis of vitamin D.

Common skin disorders found in childhood are classified as chemical, allergic, or microbial. Common microbial disorders include:

- Fungal skin infections
- Viral **exanthems** (ie, rashes)
- Viral skin infections
- Parasitic skin infections

Rashes (ie, exanthems) are very commonly associated with many childhood disorders and infections. Rashes lead to mild, moderate, and severe discomfort with pruritus (ie, itching) and can be caused by a variety of culprits, including:

- Food allergies (eg, citrus, strawberries, mango, papayas, wheat, and others)
- Contact with chemicals
- Skin allergies to a variety of causes
- Fungal infections
- Viral infections
- Bacterial infections
- Bites, mites
- Drug reactions

If a child's rash is of viral origin, instruct the parents not to give aspirin to the child for symptom management because of the correlation between aspirin and the development of Reye's syndrome.

SKIN AND CHILDHOOD

Although older adults have the greater risk in skin breakdown, injury, and delayed healing, the hallmark of quality nursing care across the lifespan begins with excellence in skin care from the newborn period. Skin breakdown, no matter the age of the patient, is now a measure by which hospitals evaluate their effectiveness. Tools exist to perform assessments and measurements of broken skin integrity, such as Braden's Q scale, which was adopted from the adult version of Braden's scale and was created specifically for pediatric patients. Pediatric nurses must keep in mind that even though their patients are small and young, skin problems do occur and a complete assessment of all skin surfaces is a must. In pediatrics, the causes of skin problems are classified as pressure ulcers (42%), those caused by frictional forces (23%), those caused by moisture associated with urine and feces (23%), and those caused by childhood activity (10%) (Suddaby, Barnett, et al, 2006).

TEAM WORKS

Taking precautions when caring for young children's skin is a team priority. Because an infant's epidermis is loosely bound to the dermis, they are susceptible to poor adherence of the tissue layers, and have greater chance of lesions and blisters when the skin is inflamed. Health-care team members should be thoughtful on how to keep newborn and infant's skin intact. Paper tape should be used rather than adhesive, which can cause tears when being removed.

Common areas of skin breakdown across childhood are different than those of adults (ie, sacrum, heels, and coccyx) and include the prevalence of breakdown on the occipital area, nose, buttocks, groin, back, chest, face, and ears.

Skin breakdown is staged by the following descriptions:

- **Stage I:** Nonblanchable erythema with skin intact
- **Stage II:** Partial-thickness tissue loss appearing as a superficial ulcer that involves the layers of the epidermis, dermis, or both
- **Stage III:** Full-thickness tissue loss appearing as a deeper ulcer that involves the subcutaneous tissue and extends down to, but not through, the fascia
- **Stage IV:** Full-thickness tissue loss with damage, destruction, or necrosis of underlying supporting structures, bone, and muscle; extending sinus tracts may be present

Neonatal Skin

The skin of the neonate is thin and covered with a fine, soft hair called *lanugo*. This thin layer of fine hair is shed within the first 28 days of life. Newborns have challenges with their skin because it is thin, has very little subcutaneous fat, allows rapid heat loss, and, because of newborns' greater percentage of body water as compared with adults, their skin allows for body water loss through evaporation. Infants are often born with clogged pores, called *milia*. All newborns should have 100% of their skin assessed shortly after birth for any unusual or common skin conditions or marks. Having this baseline will help the health-care team identify any deviations from the child's normal skin presentation.

SAFETY *STAT!*

Newborn skin is very thin. All topical medications should be assumed to be absorbed systemically. Only apply topical medications as ordered and in a very thin layer.

Infant Skin

The skin of young children is more sensitive and thinner than that of older children and adults. During the neonatal period, marks on the child's skin can be mistaken for birthmarks. Young infants bruise more easily and their skin is more reactive and sensitive to a variety of factors. Assessment of a child's skin should include the following considerations:

1. Assess rashes (Fig. 38.1):
   - Assess for the following types of rashes:
     - **Macular rash:** A flat rash with circumscribed boundaries and color changes
     - **Papular rash:** A raised, solid lesion with circumscribed boundaries and color changes
     - **Vesicle:** A rash with small, raised, clear, fluid-filled lesions with circumscribed boundaries
   - Note the distribution, size, shape, color, warmth, severity of the rash, and whether or not it is oozing fluids

2. Note any discomfort, tenderness, or pruritus. Pruritus can be severe enough to disrupt a child's quality and length of sleep.
3. Assess for the presence of hives, also called *urticaria,* which commonly accompanies symptoms of allergies or allergic reactions.
4. Assess the status of the child's hair shafts for evidence of infection, pus, or lice.
5. Assess the child's recent travel history, family history of skin conditions, and any associated systemic pathologies or illness, such as exposure to communicable diseases.
6. Assess the child's reported history of allergies to topical applications, foods, or environmental substances.
7. Assess an infant's recent exposure to new foods (eg, new exposures to citrus, protein, or formula).
8. Assess the child's recent skin exposure to soaps, detergents, lotions, medications, or any other **contactants** (ie, substances that cause an allergic or sensitivity response when the exposed to the skin).

TEAM WORKS

Wheals are round and elevated skin lesions, often temporary, that look white in the center and are surrounded by red inflammation. Wheals are often seen with insect bites and urticaria. The pediatric team may have to treat wheals for itching with an antihistamine topical cream, or oral or IV antihistamine.

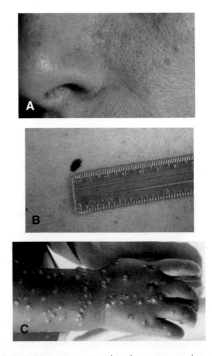

FIGURE 38.1 Lesions associated with various rashes. A, Macule. B, Papule. C, Vesicle.

SPECIAL CONSIDERATIONS FOR SKIN DISORDERS

Children are vulnerable to a variety of skin disorders and because of their age, they have special considerations associated with wounds, rashes, and infections. Because of their developmental perspectives, sometimes they have trouble describing their sensations, keeping their hands and fingernails away from a lesion or wound, and keeping their hands clean and preventing the spread of **dermatological** (ie, pertaining to the skin or study of the skin) infections from others. Children need parental assistance to manage rashes, lesions, infections, and their associated symptoms.

Special circumstances can make a child vulnerable to complications. If a young child has a surgical wound, he or she will need to have it covered securely so they do not become frightened or cause skin irritation or wound damage because of picking or manipulating the dressing, sutures, or staples. Wound healing needs to be viewed as a management responsibility for a pediatric nurse because children will not be able to verbalize the presence of drainage or a change in the appearance or integrity of a wound. Nurses and caregivers need to spend special attention to wound management, wound healing, preventing the spread of infections if the wound becomes contaminated, and childhood considerations (eg, infants scratching wounds, toddlers picking at wounds and pulling off dressings).

Heat Aggravation of Skin Disorders

Heat is often a source of irritation during a rash. Heat produces greater symptoms of discomfort on rash areas. Most rashes are soothed with the application of cool compresses, cool water baths, or cool water rinses. Do not apply warm packs to a child's lesions during hospitalization unless specifically ordered. Warm packs may be applied to promote healing if the child has an infectious rash such as pustules, cellulitis, or severe urticaria. Contact precautions should be used when caring for children with skin conditions in which warm packs are used.

The symptoms of discomfort associated with severe and persistent itching require nursing interventions. Children may benefit from baking soda paste applications, calamine lotion, oatmeal paste applications, or an oral antipruritic such as antihistamines. The child should be offered sources of playful distraction according to his or her development stage. Exposing the site of the discomfort to air may be beneficial. Neither powders, such as baby powder products, nor cornstarch should ever be applied to a rash because they may promote fungal or bacterial growth. Many young children experience worsened symptoms when commercially prepared baby wipes are used on sensitive skin because they may contain alcohol.

Preventing scratching takes creative interventions. Young infants may benefit from having their hands covered with clean socks to prevent scratching. Older infants may benefit from the use of elbow restraints, such as the application of bilateral "no-no's" (Fig. 38.2).

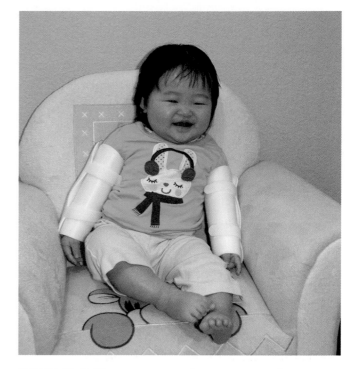

FIGURE 38.2 Elbow restraint used to prevent scratching or touching a wound.

SAFETY *STAT!*

Administering antihistamines to infants and young children can be dangerous. Do not administer oral or topical antihistamines to infants or young children without an order, and double-check medication calculations carefully to make sure the correct amount is administered. Oral antihistamines can cause severe sedation and death if given in inaccurate doses.

Wound Healing

The skin provides a normal protective barrier. When a child develops a lesion or wound, the barrier is not functioning properly. Healthy children's skin heals rapidly provided they are well nourished, well hydrated, kept clean, and are provided nursing care that promotes healing. Factors that delay wound healing are associated with dry wound beds (ie, moisture heals), nutritional deficiencies, issues with circulation, chronic illnesses, and infection. Wounds should not be treated with full strength chemicals such as povidone iodine (Betadine) or hydrogen peroxide as these solutions are cytotoxic (ie, preventing new growth of healing tissues) to children's wound healing.

HEALTH PROMOTION

Wound Healing in Children
Factors that influence wound healing in children include the following:

• **Dry wound base environments:** The health-care team should take measures to ensure that the base of the child's wound is moist but free of pus or exudates. Dry wound bases delay healing. Wet to dry dressing changes may be required to keep the wound base moist.

- **Nutritional deficiencies:** The health-care team should be alerted to poor intake of vitamins A, C, and B$_1$, as well as poor intake of adequate protein and zinc, all of which contribute to healthy skin and wound healing.
- **Issues with circulation:** Pressure ulcers, poor vascular circulation, and smoking can contribute to poor circulation, leading to a reduced supply of oxygen, fluids, and nutrients to the wound site.
- **Chronic illnesses:** Children who have pre-existing chronic illnesses such as diabetes, severe anemia, sickle cell anemia, or issues with peripheral vascular disease may experience delayed wound healing. Chronic mental health issues, chronic stress, and chronic anxiety may also contribute to aspects of delayed wound healing as poor self-care, poor hygiene, and stress hormones may influence wounds.

Preventing the Spread of Infection

The health-care team should make a rapid decision about the use of personal protective equipment during patient contact. The nurse must determine if contact isolation is warranted for anyone exposed to the child's skin, secretions, or personal belongings. It is better and safer to place a child immediately on contact precautions even before a diagnosis of the rash or lesion is made than to wait and cause exposures to families, visitors, and other health-care team members.

HEALTH PROMOTION

Hand washing equipment and signs should be made available to remind staff, families, visitors, and patients to wash hands frequently.

If the child is attending a childcare program, daycare, or school, it is important to determine if the child's skin condition warrants isolation from other children. Most childcare providers have a list of conditions that guide the decision to have the child stay at home until the rash or infection is considered no longer contagious. For instance, a child who contracts the varicella-zoster virus (ie, chickenpox) will need to stay home until the vesicle skin lesions are completely scabbed over and free of any oozing secretions. Check with professional Web sites such as the Centers for Disease Control and Prevention's (CDC) for information about isolation precautions and care guidelines to prevent the spread of an infectious skin disorder.

Clothing Suggestions During Skin Disorders

Families should be encouraged to dress their child with a skin disorder in loose, comfortably fitting, cotton clothing. Materials that are too tight or have synthetic materials may contribute to the level of itching and discomfort experienced by the child. Clothing that wicks perspiration and secretions away from the

rash or lesions may be helpful. Encourage the family to be careful with soiled clothing and bedding, washing it separately.

COMMON SKIN DISORDERS

It is very common to encounter children with skin conditions. Children can experience a variety of acquired skin conditions or have secondary skin infection superimposed on an existing wound. Skin conditions can have developmental influences such as infants in diapers, children new to preschool classrooms with close contact, and school-aged children exposed to *Streptococcus* and *Staphylococcus*.

Pediatric nurses must use meticulous precautions when handling children who have communicable skin lesions and infections. While in the health-care environment, children with known infections or those infections in which the microbe has not yet been identified should be placed on contact precautions (ie, gloves, gown). Families need to be reminded to wash their hands, wear gloves if indicated, and assist the team in preventing the spread of an infectious skin condition to others within the hospital or clinic setting. See Box 38.1 for common medications used for children's skin conditions and Box 38.2 for a list of common skin conditions in childhood, their clinical presentations, and common treatments.

Contact Dermatitis: Diaper Rash

Contact dermatitis is a common ailment of young children who are diapered. Contact dermatitis is related to the moist, warm environment contained by a plastic or synthetic diaper lining. Soaps, detergents, bubble baths, wool, tight clothes, and clothing dyes can cause this uncomfortable condition.

Box 38.1 Pharmacology for Common Pediatric Skin Lesions or Disorders

Topical Applications:

Anesthetics
Antibacterial
Antifungal
Antihistamines
Antipruritics
Antiviral
Tar preparations
Topical steroids (ie, hydrocortisone creams or triamcinolone)
Zinc oxide creams

Oral Medications:

Antibiotics
Antifungals
Antihistamines

Box 38.2 Common Childhood Rashes or Skin Conditions

- **Lyme disease:** This is the most common tick-spread illness in North America and Europe. The organism is spread by deer tick bites and may be difficult to diagnose without a blood test because many children do not display the potential signs and symptoms of a Lyme disease rash. The rash appears in association with fever, joint pains, mild sore throat, and a cough, and presents as a target with concentric circles of red next to clear areas.
- **Rocky Mountain spotted fever (RMSF):** RMSF appears as a rash that is caused by tick bites where bacteria is harbored in the tick's salivary glands. More common in the southeastern United States than in the Rocky Mountains, this rash appears as blanchable red spots on the wrists and ankles, spreading centrally toward the trunk. Later, the red rash will become raised and will have a nonblanching center.
- **Petechiae:** This is not a rash but rather a collection of small red or purplish flat lesions that do not fade when blanched and are caused by small broken capillaries in the skin. The presence of petechiae is associated with a viral illness or very low platelet levels.
- **Meningococcemia:** This is a life-threatening meningococcal sepsis caused by the bacterial invasion of the blood by *Neisseria meningitidis.* The rash appears as red or purple blotchy areas all over the child's body. Rapid antibacterial IV medication is required to save lives.
- **Kawasaki's disease:** Also called mucocutaneous lymph node syndrome (MCLNS), this disease usually affects children between 4 and 9 years of age. Without treatment, there can be serious effects on the child's heart. The child appears very ill, has high fevers, red eyes, red tongue (ie, strawberry tongue), cracked lips, and a rash with macules; papules appear very bright on the hands and soles of the feet.
- **Hemangioma:** A type of a benign tumor of the skin that presents as a birthmark with a vascular abnormality is a hemangioma. Also called a *port wine stain,* a *strawberry hemangioma,* or a *salmon patch,* a hemangioma can be a small single lesion or large, multisite lesions. When an infant is first born, the hemangioma may be invisible or very faint. As the infant grows, the lesion grows rapidly and deepens in color. Over time, the child's lesion may become smaller and fainter. If involution is to take place, it may take several years. Treatment may include steroids, embolization of the blood vessels by the injection of a material that blocks blood flow, laser treatments, or surgical removal. If a

child's hemangioma is causing breathing problems, bleeds regularly, impairs vision, or causes growth disturbances, it will require more aggressive medical and/or surgical treatments.
- **Warts:** Caused by the papillomavirus, warts are also known as *verruca.* Warts are typically roundish, elevated, firm papules. Treatment is focused on local destruction with curettage, cryotherapy with liquid nitrogen, or by application of a caustic solution. Warts in children can appear suddenly and disappear on their own without treatment.
- **Styes:** A localized infection and swelling of the glands of the eyelid. Styes typically present with inflammation followed by a raised tender lesion that may secrete purulent drainage. Pain, edema, inflammation, and conjunctivitis are common signs and symptoms. Treatment is focused on draining the stye. Warm packs to the area (a clean dressing or small towel must be used each time) several times a day for up to a week might be necessary to clear the stye.
- **Candidiasis:** Very common during infancy and early toddlerhood, *Candida albicans* is a form of yeast (ie, fungus) that causes severe diaper rashes. This fungus appears as a bright red and very uncomfortable rash with satellite lesions and grows readily in warm moist areas such as skin folds. Topical yeast infections require the application of an antifungal cream until clear.
- **Herpes simplex:** Herpes simplex is divided into two general categories: Type 1 produces "cold sores" in the mouth while Type 2 causes genital lesions (although lesions can be found on the cornea and face). Symptoms include a tingling, itching, then burning sensation on the skin, followed by an eruption of vesicles most often located directly on mucocutaneous junctions such as the lips, nose, and genitalia. The herpes virus is contagious and is treated with topical, oral, or IV acyclovir.
- **Frostbite:** A term used to denote severe tissue damage from freezing temperature or direct contact with frozen material. Two pathologies occur with frostbite; the intracellular fluids freeze within the tissues and the cold temperatures damage tissue that then block the blood supply. The frostbitten tissues are usually numb until treatment is initiated, then the tissue becomes very painful. Treatment includes total body warming, hydration with warm fluids, and then the body part is immersed in warm to tepid water. In extreme tissue damage, debridement or amputation may be needed.

When the child passes stool or urinates in the diaper, the condition is further irritated by the acidic level of the excrement or by the formation of ammonia from the urine within the diaper.

Assessments of Contact Dermatitis

Assessments of contact dermatitis include the following (Fig. 38.3):

- Characteristic bright red maculopapular rash within the area of contact between the skin and diaper
- Contiguous rash boundaries without satellite lesions that are classic for yeast infections
- Weeping of the skin rash
- Irritability or inconsolability of the infant, especially during diaper changes

Interventions for Contact Dermatitis

Interventions for contact dermatitis include keeping the skin under the diaper area clean and dry by changing the diaper immediately after soiling. Wash the skin very gently with a gentle soap and water, and apply a layer of vitamin A and D ointment, or a zinc oxide–based ointment after cleansing. The child should have the opportunity to have the skin exposed to air without any plastic or synthetic covering. A severe rash may require hydrocortisone 1% creme.

Nursing Considerations for Contact Dermatitis

The health-care team will determine if a child's severe diaper area rash is from contact with an allergen or a substance the child reacts to, or if the rash is yeast (Fig. 38.4). Family education about preventing and treating rashes in diapered children is found in the Patient Teaching Guidelines feature.

PATIENT TEACHING GUIDELINES

Preventing and Treating Severe Diaper Rash for Infants and Toddlers

Prevention

1. Thoroughly wash and dry the perineal area with each diaper change.
2. Change the infant's or toddler's diaper as quickly as possible after soiling.
3. Cleanse the skin folds, labia, and scrotum carefully after each fecal soiling.
4. Apply a thin layer of skin protective ointment such as a zinc oxide–based cream.
5. Remove foods from the diet that have been identified to exacerbate diaper rash (eg, strawberries, mango, citrus fruits such as oranges, lemons, limes, and grapefruits).
6. Use only cotton diapers or diapers with minimal synthetic material.
7. Use commercial diaper cleansing cloths sparingly as they may contain alcohol or other chemicals that cause drying of the skin. It is best to use a soft wash cloth and water.
8. Do not clothe the child in materials that contain aggravating dyes, harsh materials, or chemicals.
9. Use only mild soaps on the skin of young children to prevent chemical rashes.

10. Do not launder the infant's clothes or cloth diapers with fabric softeners as this may irritate skin.

Interventions

1. Promptly begin a regimen of quality skin care, including at least twice-daily washing of the affected area and application of recommended or prescribed medications; follow medication application instructions carefully to prevent an overdose of topical medications that may be absorbed systemically through an infant's thin skin. This type of washing allows for all layers of medications, creams, and excrement to be removed completely to enhance skin healing.
2. Allow the child's afflicted area to be in open air to help dry and heal the skin.
3. Provide for symptom management, including acetaminophen or ibuprofen, NEVER aspirin.
4. The provider should wash his or her hands thoroughly before and after caring for a rash to prevent secondary infections or transmission of the infectious agent to others.
5. Do not use plastic diaper covers; prevent the plastic diaper lining from contacting the rash.
6. Provide foods that increase the stool pH (more alkaline) such as fruits and vegetables and reduce fish, grains, and eggs.

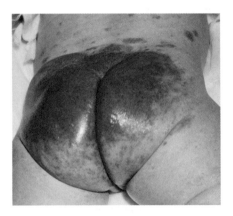

FIGURE 38.3 Infant with contact dermatitis.

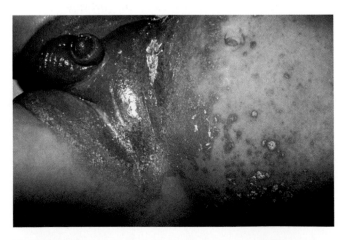

FIGURE 38.4 Infant with the fungal infection candidiasis.

Poison Oak and Poison Ivy

Children who have been exposed to the oily sap of a poison oak or poison ivy leaf can experience a delayed reaction (Fig. 38.5). The reaction is a hypersensitivity response of the immune system by the T cells. Exposure to the plant's leaves causes the child to come in contact with the sap on his or her skin. If the child has not been exposed previously, the delayed reaction is between 5 and 25 days after exposure. If the child has had a previous exposure, the response is noted within 1 to 2 days. The lesions found on the skin are not the source of cross-contamination or further spread. The inadequate removal of all of the oily sap is what causes further infection and more lesions. Animals, especially family dogs, are a source of infection because they carry the plant's oils to humans and shared environmental surfaces.

SAFETY *STAT!*

Children exposed to smoke from a fire where poison ivy, poison oak, or sumac (a shrub with the same active substance as poison ivy) is being burned can develop severe pulmonary inflammation and respiratory distress. Remind families who live in geographical areas where these plants are found not to burn them and, if needed, to keep children far from the smoke.

Assessments of Poison Ivy and Poison Oak

Assessments of rashes associated with poison ivy include severe pruritus, localized streaks of redness that extend from the site of exposure to the sap, and vesicles that break open and form crusts. Vesicles form in 24 to 72 hours after exposure and are very uncomfortable.

Interventions for Poison Ivy

A child who has a significant rash caused by poison ivy will need treatment to prevent discomfort from constant itching and irritation. Interventions for the rash caused by poison ivy include:

• Washing the skin carefully to remove all plant oils
  • The entire surface of the skin and scalp should be carefully washed to prevent further exposure to other skin surfaces or other family members. Poison ivy does not spread under the skin; only the plant's oil can cause the rash and is the sole source of spreading.
• Preventing the child from touching other body parts until a thorough cleansing has been completed
• Washing the child's clothing or any material the child touched before cleansing
  • The family should keep in mind that poison ivy's oil might remain on car upholstery and seat belts.
• Drying the skin carefully and then applying calamine lotion in two or three layers, letting each layer dry between applications
• Administering topical or oral antihistamines if ordered

Nursing Considerations for Poison Ivy

Nurses can be instrumental in teaching the public about poison ivy infection prevention and treatment. Posting a photograph for the public to view in areas where communities have poison ivy growing and where children play can help identify what the plant leaves look like. Families might believe that the rash is contained to just the area of irritated skin and not realize that the plant oil is what causes further lesions or spread to others, including any carried on pet hair.

Cellulitis

A child may present with an acute inflammation of the skin associated with a history of trauma, puncture wounds, sinusitis, impetigo, or a case of recent otitis media. Cellulitis is considered a deep bacterial infection of the skin. Several layers of skin can be affected, including the epidermis, dermis, and connective tissues. The infectious agent causes intense redness because of the spread of enzyme factors that break down networks of fibrin. The enzyme factors try to contain the spread of the infection. Usually found on the face, eye orbit, arms, and legs, the onset and spread of cellulitis can be quite rapid. The three most common infectious agents are group A β-hemolytic streptococci, *Streptococcus pneumonia,* and *Staphylococcus aureus.* Some children respond to oral antibiotics at home; those with more extensive infections require a hospitalization for IV antibiotic therapy. Complications of cellulitis include meningitis, glomerulonephritis, and septic arthritis.

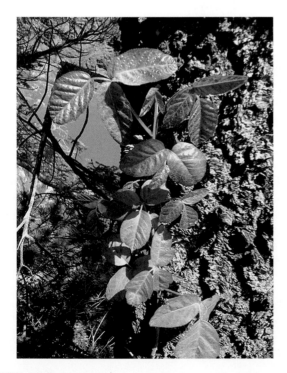

FIGURE 38.5 Poison oak.

Assessments of Cellulitis

Assessments of cellulitis include both inspection and palpation. Cellulitis can be superficial or it can cause a swelling of the afflicted area. Assessments include the following:

- Warmth, edema, tenderness around the affected site, and pitted edema over the affected site
- Possible presence of red "streaking" lines that extend from the site
- Febrile state and the presentation of appearing ill (eg, headache, chills, weakness)
- Enlarged regional lymphadenopathy
- Elevated white blood cell count
- High risk factors such as having an immunocompromised state or diabetes

Interventions for Cellulitis

Interventions for cellulitis include the following:

- A broad-spectrum oral antibiotic therapy for 8 to 10 days if cellulitis is contained and the infection is responsive within 2 days of therapy (oxacillin, sulfamethoxazole, or amoxicillin are common)
- IV antibiotic therapy if the cellulitis is extensive or invading structures such as the eye socket with periorbital cellulitis (nafcillin, dicloxacillin, or ceftriaxone are common)
- Warm packs, which can be soothing and can help reduce associated edema
- Nonocclusive dressings, which may be applied if the skin around the area is torn, ruptured, or oozing

Nursing Considerations for Cellulitis

When a child presents with cellulitis, contact precautions are instigated. Blood cultures may or may not be collected, depending on the severity of the infection, whether or not it is known what caused the puncture wound, and if the child presents with fevers from an associated systemic infection.

Eczema

Considered an autoimmune superficial inflammatory skin disorder, eczema is associated with a hereditary allergic tendency, sometimes called *atopic dermatitis*. Eczema can be part of a trio of conditions called *atopy*. Atopy is a hypersensitivity reaction from immunoglobulin E (IgE)-mediated reactions and is associated with asthma, eczema, and allergic rhinitis (ie, hay fever).

Eczema can present as a reaction to the emotion of stress, as atopic dermatitis, or as an allergic contact. Infant eczema appears on the face first with raised, red papules that then spread to the scalp and arms. The characteristic lesions appear raised, red, and with weeping vesicles.

The condition is associated with chronic relapsing pruritic lesions and may resolve by the time the child reaches adulthood. Most children with eczema present with severe itching (ie, pruritus), and most diagnoses (ie, 60%) occur in infancy. Commonly, both parents of a child with this disorder have a history of contact dermatitis, asthma, and hay fever. Dust mites remain the most common culprit of exacerbations in preschool and school-aged children's eczema outbreaks. There is no laboratory or diagnostic test for eczema (Fig. 38.6).

Eczema in a toddler appears as intense pruritus with a rash similar to the presentation of eczema in an infant. Some children might have continuous eczema from infancy through toddlerhood and others experience the onset in toddlerhood.

Adolescent eczema often appears as lichenification (ie, large, dry plaques or thickened lesions) typically on the face, neck, back, feet, fingers, toes, and dorsal aspects of the hands.

Assessments of Eczema

Assessments for eczema include the following:

- The child's history of allergies
- Red, scaling papules and vesicles with layers of crusting
- Common warm and moist locations, such as the popliteal and antecubital spaces
- Other common locations, such as the scalp, cheeks, wrists, neck, hands, and groin
- The presence of lichenification, which is indicative of chronic inflammation and which appears as thickened, deep lines

Interventions for Eczema

Treatments and care for a child with eczema need to be individualized for each child. Depending on the developmental level of the child, treatments will be implemented to decrease itching, provide symptom management, prevent infections, and minimize exacerbations. Overall, treatments include:

- Preventing secondary infections from persistent scratching and the resulting introduction of bacteria; keep the child's fingernails trimmed short
- Showering or bathing after sweating and then immediately applying a thin layer of over-the-counter emollient such as Eucerin cream or Lubriderm lotion
- Avoiding bath additives such as bubble bath concentrations or bath oils
- Applying a thin layer of steroid creams
- Applying topical immunomodulators as ordered
- Avoiding contact with wool, synthetics, or any fabrics that cause sweating and further itching
- Avoiding harsh detergents, soaps, and perfumes or lotions
- Avoiding wearing tight or constrictive clothing
- Preventing access to the rash: the child should not be able to lick, chew, or scratch the inflamed tissues. Soft gauze

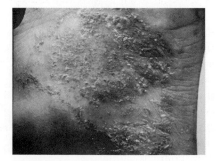

FIGURE 38.6 Child with eczema.

wraps may be needed to prevent the child from having access to the afflicted areas.
- Never scrubbing the inflamed site; wash with warm water at least once daily and pat dry

Nursing Considerations for Eczema

Families will need teaching concerning the care of a young child with eczema. Education must include the prevention of skin scarring at the affected site by preventing secondary infections. The family should try to identify if any foods cause exacerbations of their child's eczema and avoid any known allergens. Common allergens are pets, environmental allergens, and contact allergens. The family should be taught to avoid prolonged sun exposure and to apply sunscreen to prevent sunburns, which will highly irritate the site. Oral antihistamines and anti-inflammatory medications may be required if the pruritus is so intense that the child is experiencing sleep deprivation.

Thrush

Thrush is caused by a yeastlike fungus, *C albicans,* which is normally found throughout the vagina, gastrointestinal tract, and along the entire surface of the skin. The fungus proliferates in warm, moist areas and is common along the skin folds of obese persons. Thrush can also develop when a child is on oral antibiotic therapy. Chronic conditions such as hyperglycemia can also predispose a child to a *C albicans* infection.

Assessments of Thrush

Assessments for thrush should be started immediately upon identifying the classic symptoms of a skin or mouth yeast infection so that treatment can be started before the infection spreads. Assessments include the following:

- Complaints or signs of itching, burning, and irritation
- White plaques along the inside of the mouth with a bright red surface underlying the white patches
- Red and moist skin lesions that often present in characteristic "satellite" lesions, especially found in the perineum area, and that extend away from the center of the large fungal lesion

Interventions for Thrush

Interventions for infections with *C albicans* include the following:

- Topical application of a thin layer of antifungal cream on the skin
- A second application of antifungal cream with a healing skin ointment to the lesions to prevent body secretions from contributing further to the inflammation (eg, Aquaphor, Desitin)
- Administration of oral antifungal suspensions if the child presents with oral thrush
- Cool water soaks with clean, soft, cotton clothes or Burow's solution
- Loose-fitting cotton clothing
- Exposing the lesions to air

Nursing Considerations for Thrush

Many children with significant oral thrush have a change in their taste when eating. Some children will not want to eat during a thrush infection and the medication may take a few to several days to treat the infection. Warning families of this potential side effect of the infection and discussing possible alternative food choices, such as fruit smoothies, may be of assistance.

Cutaneous Fungal Infections: Ringworm

The term *tina* refers to a cutaneous (ie, skin) infection with a fungus. A skin infection with fungus is very common in school-aged children and is acquired through close personal contact and, on occasion, contact with infected pets. The term *ringworm* can be very misleading to families because cutaneous ringworm infections are not caused by "worms" (Fig. 38.7).

There are several types of ringworm infections. The location of the infection denotes the title of the ringworm infection:

- Tinea capitis involves the scalp and hair.
- Tinea pedis is the name of a common fungal infection, "athlete's foot."
- Tinea unguium is a fingernail or toenail fungal infection.
- Tina cruris is "jock itch," a common and noncontagious fungal infection in young athletes.
- Tinea corporis is a fungal infection involving the groin, extremities, and trunk.
- Tinea versicolor is a fungal infection of the skin characterized by darker and lighter varied patches on the child's back or chest, which causes uneven tanning. This condition is most commonly found in adolescence.

Assessments of Cutaneous Fungal Infections

Assessments for cutaneous fungal infections include the following:

- **Tinea capitis:** Patchy hair loss with an area of scaling on the scalp
- **Tinea pedis:** Intense itching between the child's toes with a characteristic erythematous rash that may include painful fissures that may weep
- **Tinea cruris:** After sweating, itching in the child's groin skinfolds with a characteristic red rash
- **Tinea corporis:** Cutaneous lesions that are ring-shaped can be found as one lesion or many and have a characteristic annular, scaling, erythematous, sharply marginated,

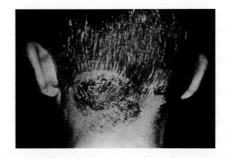

FIGURE 38.7 Child with ringworm.

indurated lesion with hyperkeratotic borders. The center of the ring may be clear or pink and the ring of the rash may consist of vesicles.

Interventions. for Cutaneous Fungal Infections

Interventions for the various cutaneous fungal infections include the following:

- **Tinea capitis:** Applying a thin layer of topical antifungal medication as ordered, using antifungal shampoos, and cleaning all potentially contaminated home and personal objects to prevent re-infection
- **Tina pedis:** Applying a thin layer of topical antifungal medication as ordered, antifungal powder, or antifungal spray to feet and between toes; having the child wear sandals in locker rooms and public showers
- **Tina cruris:** Applying a thin layer of topical antifungal medication as ordered to the affected area, changing underwear frequently when sweaty, showering immediately after exercise
  - Advise patients or the patient's parents not to store damp athletic clothes in a gym bag for any length of time as it contributes to fungal growth.
- **Tina corporis:** Applying a thin layer of topical antifungal medication as ordered to both the lesion and the skin around the circular lesion because the fungal infection spreads outward from the angular shape

Nursing Considerations for Cutaneous Fungus Infections

Adolescents who participate in group or team sports where pads or helmets are worn are at an increased risk for fungal infections. This age group should receive written information about how to cleanse sports pads on a regular basis, and should be encouraged to shower after practices or games to decrease the chance of contamination or transmission.

Scabies

When a child presents with severe itching and characteristic red lines with bright red patchy lesions, scabies must be suspected. Very contagious, a scabies infection is acquired by having close body/skin contact with an infected individual. Scabies mites are tiny insects that burrow deeply into the skin; females lay their eggs along the burrowing tract. Males die after mating. Females lay approximately 1 to 3 eggs per day and the eggs hatch every 30 days. After hatching, the larvae travel to the skin surface. Intense itching occurs because of movement, mite secretions, ova, and feces. The incubation period is considered 1 to 2 months after contact with an infected person.

Assessments of Scabies

Assessments of a scabies infestation include identifying classic clinical signs of red streaks where the mite burrows superficially under the skin and lays her eggs, as well as severe itching. Specific assessments for a scabies infection include the following:

- Intense itching that becomes worse at night, often interrupting a child's healthy sleeping pattern
- Skin "burrows" that appear linear, *S*-shaped, or curved, and that run along the superficial skin on the extremities, neck, legs, or trunk with a characteristic rash of macules, papules, and bright red erythema (may be 1 to 10 cm in length) (Fig. 38.8)
- Rashes that intensify between the child's fingers, wrists, buttocks, knees, elbows, and genitals
- The presence of rash and "burrows" on other members of the family
- Skin scrapings from burrow tract marks that reveal mites, ova, and feces under microscopic evaluation

Interventions for Scabies Infection

Interventions for a scabies infestation include treating the child and possibly other family members, and cleaning the surfaces and bedding of the child. Treatment for scabies includes the following:

- Apply a thin layer of scabicide, such as permethrin cream (Elimite); it is left on and then washed off after 8 to 10 hours (follow the instructions on the medication's package insert).
- The child may require scabicide to be applied on the entire body from the chin down to between the toes.
- The entire family may require treatment: Each member must have skin surfaces assessed or the infestation will continue within the family.

SAFETY *STAT!*

The medication Lindane lotion cannot be used on infants because of identified neurotoxicity and subsequent seizures. The family should discuss the age of the child with the pharmacist to make sure the medication is safe for the age of the child.

Nursing Considerations for Scabies

Although treatments are essential to rid a child of scabies, the infection must be treated keeping in mind the environment where the child lives and plays. The following guidelines should be discussed with the family to stress the importance to treating the child's living surroundings:

- Washing all clothing, linen, and blankets in a hot water cycle, with sheets and clothes changed and washed daily until all family members are free of mite infection
- Vacuuming furniture, floors, carpets, and car interiors carefully

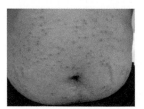

FIGURE 38.8 Classic rash on the abdomen caused by scabies.

- Storing nonwashable items in a tightly closed plastic bag for 3 to 4 weeks
- Notifying the child's school about infection and following the school district's requirements
- Understanding that the characteristic red burrow lesions may be present for 2 to 3 weeks after treatment as the epidermis heals
- Teaching the family that poor hygiene or unsanitary living conditions are not associated with a scabies infection
- Teaching the family not to share clothing, towels, bedding, or any personal hygiene items

Impetigo

Impetigo should be considered when a child develops a superficial infection of the skin that appears most commonly on the face and extremities, and is often demonstrated as round, oozing lesions (Fig. 38.9). Impetigo is a highly contagious superficial rash caused by staphylococci or, most commonly, by group A β-hemolytic streptococci. When an infection is identified as being caused by the microbe *S aureus,* it is often called *bullous impetigo.* The bacteria are usually carried in the child's nares and are passed between children by contact with sporting equipment, shared toiletries, toys, towels, or books. Impetigo accounts for more than 10% of all childhood rashes. The lesions can be spread over the body by the child's scratching and passing the bacteria on his or her infected fingernails and hands. This infection is very common in the toddler and preschool period (ie, children aged 2 to 5 years old).

TEAM WORKS

When a young child presents with classic, small, round lesions on the skin, the health-care team should assess if the lesions are impetigo, or if the child appears at risk for child abuse—assess if the lesions are cigarette burns. The two lesions look very similar and should be distinguished.

Assessments of Impetigo

Differentiating one rash from another during the developmental period is a challenge for the pediatric health-care team. Some lesions, such as impetigo, can mimic other infections. Assessments of impetigo include the following:

- Macular rash that progresses to a papular rash, and then to a **vesicular rash**, followed by a **pustule** (ie, a small

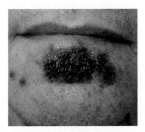

FIGURE 38.9 Teenager with impetigo.

raised skin lesion protruding above the skin line and filled with pus)
- Vesicles that rupture and ooze a honey-colored liquid
- Oozing lesions that are topped by honey-colored crusts
- Mild regional lymphadenopathy
- Various degrees of the feeling of burning and of pruritus
- Exposure to biting and stinging insects
- Others in the house infected with similar rashes

Interventions for Impetigo

Medication therapy includes topical and/or oral antibiotics. Common topical antibiotics include bacitracin ointment (Polysporin or Neosporin) or mupirocin ointment (Bactroban). Oral antibiotic therapy can include cephalosporins or erythromycin. The full course of antibiotics must be completed. After 48 hours from the beginning of antibiotic therapy, the child is no longer considered communicable and, if approved, may return to school.

Nursing Considerations for Impetigo

Nursing considerations for impetigo include soaking the lesions and then washing the site with warm compresses to remove the layers of crusts. The compresses or cloths should be immediately washed or discarded to prevent the spread of the bacteria to others. The child's nails should be cut short. Young children may need to have their hands covered to prevent scratching or digging at the lesions. If possible, lesions should be covered to prevent the spread of bacteria. All members of the family should use separate linens, towels, and wash cloths. Good hand washing techniques will reduce the chance of spreading the bacterial infection.

LABS & DIAGNOSTICS

Diagnostic Tests for Skin Disorders

- **Skin biopsies:** An invasive procedure that can produce discomfort, a skin biopsy is performed to obtain a small quantity tissue for histological analysis. Because of the invasive nature, informed consent must be obtained by the parent or legal guardian before the procedure is performed. It is best to obtain a skin sample in the treatment room; the discomfort potential should prevent the procedure from occurring in the child's bed (ie, safety zone). Ask for a topical anesthetic before the procedure and apply within a time frame that allows for a maximal anesthetic property.
- **Skin scraping:** A noninvasive procedure in which a sterile instrument or applicator is used to obtain epithelia cells for microscopic examination within a laboratory.
- **Skin cultures:** A noninvasive diagnostic procedure using a sterile applicator to identify the presence and type of bacteria, fungus, or virus within a lesion. Should be performed with gentle swiping gesture and quickly capped off and sent to the laboratory to prevent cross-contamination. Adhere to institutional policy as some culture applicators have color-coded designations for viral (may be green) versus bacterial (may be red) samples.

- **Skin sweat test:** This is a noninvasive diagnostic test to identify cystic fibrosis. A specially trained technician induces sweating on the arm via an electrode that then measures the sodium and chloride level of the sweat.

Lice

Lice infections are common during childhood. Lice are highly communicable parasites that are spread via combs, brushes, linens, coats, hooded jackets, play clothes, and hats. Lice can infest a couch, a bed, or car upholstery and therefore pose a communicable risk to others quite readily.

Lice do not fly or jump; rather, they need direct contact with another head of hair. The adult female louse prefers to lay her eggs at the very base of the hair shaft and uses a form of biological cement secreted by a gland next to her rectum to secure each egg sac, or nit, onto the base of the hair shaft. Only via direct contact does the adult louse leave the primary host and infect a new host.

The adult female louse can lay hundreds of eggs during her lifetime. The adult louse lives for 30 days and must eat almost daily. Adult lice can only live 48 hours away from a host. The adult louse has six legs and ranges in color from tan to black. The nits hatch every 10 to 14 days and, in their egg form, the nits can stay alive for 8 to 10 days away from a host. Lice are considered parasites because they feed on human blood. As a child scratches their scalp intensely, blood scabs form, which attract the feeding lice.

Symptoms of a lice infestation are marked by intense itching from three sources: the crawling behaviors of the six-legged adult louse, the feeding behaviors, and the presence of their waste products. When an adult witnesses a child with an intense head itch, lice should be suspected (Fig. 38.10).

Assessments of Lice

Assessments of lice infection include looking carefully for nits, empty egg sacs, and live adults on the move in several places on the child's scalp. Assessments should include the following:

- The presence of the adult lice in the hair; they may demonstrate rapid movement during assessment
- The presence of nits in the child's hair, which are typically 1 to 2 mm in diameter

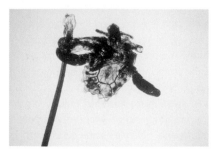

FIGURE 38.10 Adult louse and nit on a child's hair shaft.

- How long the child has been infected, which is determined by the distance between the scalp and the nits
  - Adult female lice lay their eggs next to the scalp so the newly hatched larvae can begin to eat immediately. The further away the nit is from the scalp, the longer the child has been infected.
- The severity of the symptoms associated with the lice infestation
- The emotional effect of the infestation to the child's well-being

Interventions for Lice

The treatment for lice is threefold:

1. The hair must be treated with a pediculicide.
2. Each nit egg sac must be removed meticulously one by one with great care and patience.
3. Lastly, the child's environment must be treated. Combs and brushes must be replaced or washed with hot water. Linens and clothes must be washed in hot water. Car upholstery must be treated, and carpets must be thoroughly vacuumed. All stuffed toys and items that cannot be washed must be placed in a tightly sealed plastic bag for 2 weeks to make sure the nits die.

SAFETY *STAT!*

The family must be taught to follow the pediculicide instructions carefully and not to extend the time the solution remains on the child's head because of toxicity.

Nursing Considerations for Lice

Because lice infestations are so common during childhood, there is plenty of opportunity to influence the education and knowledge of families, schools, and other institutions where children attend afterschool programs such as theatre, dance, and sports classes. Classrooms should not have coat racks where multiple clothes are hung on top of each other, and children need to be reminded not to share hats or hooded jackets. Children should have personal items kept in separate compartments, such as plastic tubs with lids that are marked with each child's name. Children must be reminded that although they want to share personal items with their friends, they should not do so to prevent lice infections.

Acne

Because of hormonal stimulation and increasing sebaceous gland activity, adolescents are especially at risk for acne. The increased stimulation and release of testosterone by circulating androgens is the main culprit of acne during teenage years; this goes for both genders. Normal bacteria found on the skin can contribute to the development of acne as the bacteria break down fatty acids and leave waste products. Most teenagers experience some degree of acne, and some cases are quite severe, requiring special skincare. A severe case of acne is called *acne vulgaris*.

The pathophysiology of acne concerns the clogging of the narrow channel of the sebaceous gland with sebum at the opening at the base of a hair follicle. The presence of trapped sebum is a medium for bacterial growth. As the hair follicles become infected by the presence of the bacteria, they expand into comedones (ie, classic white pimples). Noninflammatory blackheads (ie, open comedones) are also common and are caused by the comedo being exposed to air; the color changes as the trapped material oxidizes.

Common bacteria associated with acne include:

- *Propionibacterium acnes*
- *Staphylococcus epidermidis*

Assessments of Acne

Assessments of acne include the presence of clogged pores, as well as comedones (Fig. 38.11 and 38.12). Assessments should also include the presence of scarring and the emotional consequence of the child's or teen's acne on their self-esteem and self-perception.

Interventions for Acne

Care for a child with acne should begin with an honest conversation about how the child currently cares for his or her skin.

PATIENT TEACHING GUIDELINES

Acne Prevention and Care

Acne can present in mild or severe forms. Adolescents experience acne because of fluctuations in hormonal stimulations. These fluctuations increase the activity within the sebaceous glands, forming conditions for bacterial growth that break down fatty acids. There are two forms of acne: blackheads and pimples. Blackheads are clogged sebaceous glands and present as dark-colored clogged pores. The narrow channel between the gland and the surface of the skin becomes plugged with sebum and appears as brown, gray, or black "heads." Pimples are infected hair follicles that expand into comedones. When a child picks or tries to pop the comedo, the bacteria spread to surrounding tissues and the erythema and discomfort increases. Neither blackheads nor acne are caused by dietary intake of fat or greasy foods, poor skin hygiene, or emotional fluctuations. Nevertheless, these three phenomena can exacerbate existing acne conditions. Many lanolin-based cosmetics, the use of sports helmets, menses cycles, and sweating can also exacerbate an existing condition of acne. The most common areas of acne for older school-aged children and adolescents are the face, neck, back, and chest.

If isotretinoin (Accutane) is ordered for a child with severe acne, a sexually active teenage girl must be taught to use two methods of birth control for no less than 1 month before treatment begins to no less than 1 month after treatment is complete because this drug is considered highly teratogenic (ie, causing birth defects). In providing guidelines to a teen, the nurse should also address the child's self-esteem, self-image, and level of concern about his or her acne condition.

Guidelines for adolescent skincare include the following:

1. Wash the face twice a day with a mild soap.
2. During periods of severe exacerbation, use a product that contains 2% salicylic acid.
3. Do not reuse wash cloths; use a clean cloth for each wash to prevent the spread of bacteria.
4. Dry the face carefully.
5. Apply a thin layer of an antiacne cream, such as topical benzoyl peroxide. The adolescent may want to use a flesh-colored product.
6. Apply a very warm cloth to a pimple that is full of pus to promote drainage and provide soothing.
7. Keep hands away from the site and never "pop" or squeeze either closed or open comedones because this can cause inflammation, infection, and scarring.
8. Naturopathic remedies for acne include tea tree oil and aloe vera creams or ointments.
9. Take oral antibiotics in severe cases if there is no improvement with a strict daily skincare routine.

Nursing Considerations for Acne

Teenagers need to be reminded that acne is not caused by greasy foods or chocolate (ie, common myths), emotions, or poor hygiene, yet poor nutrition and oily skin can exacerbate acne. Pediatric nurses must communicate that the acne is caused by the opening of hair follicles becoming clogged with secretions, dead skin, and bacteria. Certain cosmetics, excessive sweating,

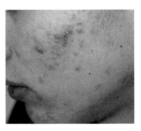

FIGURE 38.11 Teenage boy with comedones.

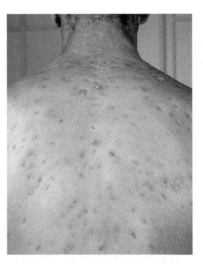

FIGURE 38.12 Teenager with inflammatory acne with pustules.

menstrual cycles, and the use of unclean athletic helmets can all exacerbate an existing acne condition.

Childhood Burns

Because most burns occur in children younger than 5 years old, parents need to assess the home environment for potential burn scenarios. Water heaters must be turned down below 48.9°C; matches, lighters, and candles should be placed out of reach; front burners on the stovetop should not be used; hot BBQ equipment must be kept out of reach; and flammable chemicals and liquids should be stored in locked cabinets out of children's reach. Burns are a very real threat to children; they are the third-leading cause of accidental death across all of childhood after motor vehicle accidents and drowning. Burns are the second-leading cause of death under the age of 14. Burn injuries can range from very mild redness and tenderness to massive tissue injury that causes life-threatening complications. Burns can be classified into four categories: electrical, thermal, chemical, and radioactive. Childhood burns may be caused by accident or may be a form of intentional child abuse, such as glove or sock burns, cigarette burns, or burns associated with a hot object. Glove or sock burns are considered submersion burns, which occur when a child's hand or foot is submerged into very hot scalding water, leaving a burn mark that appears on the hand or foot where a sock or glove would be.

- Electrical: Burns caused by electrical currents passing through the body; extent depends on strength and duration of current
- Thermal: Burns caused by contact, such as from hot metal in ovens or scalding hot water (also called heat burns); hot water causes third-degree burns in (burnfoundation.org, 2015):
  - 1 sec at 68.9°C
  - 2 sec at 65°C
  - 5 sec at 60°C
  - 15 sec at 56.1°C
- Chemical: Burns caused by exposure to highly caustic chemicals such as battery acids
- Radioactive: Burns caused by ionizing radiation or exposure to prolonged fluoroscopy procedures
- Immersive: Burns associated with a body part immersed (ie, fully extended into, such as the hand, arm, or foot) in scalding hot water

Assessments of Childhood Burns

An assessment of the percentage of the child's body burned is performed using a scale such as the **rule of nines** (ie, an assessment tool used to estimate the extent of a burn is used in late adolescence and adulthood) or the **Lund-Browder classification tool** (ie, an assessment tool that is used to estimate the percentage of body surface area [BSA] burned) (Fig. 38.13). Assessment tools have proven to be effective in accurately determining the size and severity of the child's burned BSA. The final percentage is then used to determine the fluid resuscitation status and the subsequent wound

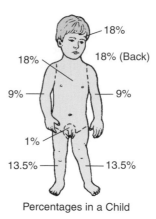

FIGURE 38.13 The modified rule of nines: BSA chart for estimating the percentage of the body burned.

interventions to promote healing. Minor burns are considered partial- or full-thickness burns that extend to less than 10% of the child's total BSA. Major burns are those that are considered full thickness and that constitute greater than 10% of the child's BSA, involve the respiratory tract, and/or that include associated fractures or soft-tissue injuries.

The first priority assessment conducted by the pediatric health-care team is the airway assessment of a child with a burn. Heat and smoke can cause serious upper and lower airway damage. The child may need to have oxygen, airway support, cardiopulmonary resuscitation (CPR) and possible intubation. Always inspect the child's lips and mouth for carbonaceous material, which can denote airway damage. A child with a significant burn or smoke exposure may have rapid pulmonary edema.

Assessments of burns include using a classification system that addresses both the depth and the degree of the burn (Table 38.1).

A team approach is needed to provide a thorough assessment of a child who has experienced a burn. Rapid assessment of the size, depth, and cause will guide rapid treatments:

1. Start with the child's airway and proceed through the steps of CPR as needed.
2. Assess the child's lips and mouth for evidence of carbonaceous material (ie, soot and smoke that causes severe lung involvement and tissue damage).
3. Assess the child for symptoms of shock.
4. Assess the child for hypovolemia.
5. Assess for the level of pain.
6. Assess for a fluid shift from intravascular to interstitial compartments, and assess for wound weeping.
7. Assess for renal function and urine output.
8. Assess the level of consciousness.
9. Assess for an infection that develops at a burn site after the first 24 hours, which is when infectious organisms have had time to multiply and invade wounds.

Box 38.3 provides the most common nursing diagnoses for children with burns.

TABLE 38.1 CLASSIFICATIONS OF BURNS

Burn Degree	Signs and Symptoms
First-degree burn (partial-thickness burn)	• Affects the epidermal layer only • Painful, dry, edematous skin appearing red • Appears as a sunburn; skin will peel off within 5 to 10 days • Damaged tissue heals within 3 to 7 days with evidence of scarring
Second-degree burn (partial-thickness burn)	• Extends through the epidermis into the dermis • Edematous with weeping of moisture • Very painful • Heals at various speeds depending on size and location • May require grafting
Third-degree burn (full-thickness burn)	• Extends through the epidermis, dermis, subcutaneous fat, and structures • Leathery dead tissue appearing dry and pale • Does not blanch because it is avascular • Most without pain • Heals at various speeds depending on size, complications, secondary infections, and grafting success
Fourth-degree burn (full-thickness burn)	Extends below the dermis and underlying structures to or through the bone

Box 38.3 Nursing Diagnoses for Children With Burns

1. Pain
2. Impaired skin integrity
3. Knowledge deficit
4. Anxiety
5. Risk for fluid volume deficit
6. Risk for altered nutrition
7. Risk for impaired circulation

Each developmental stage and associated age range has a type of burn associated with it. Parents must receive information about anticipatory guidance and burn prevention as the natural curiosity of a young child puts them at risk. The developmental stages of infancy through adolescence have classic burn types and severity:

• Infants: Sunburns, hot liquids spilled on the skin, standing infants pulling down hot cups of liquid, and death by home fires. Always test foods and fluids for level of heat before giving to child. Never hold an infant while drinking hot liquids.
• Toddlers: Contact with hot liquids, hot water in baths, pulling down hot pans or pots of liquid on the stove, and electrical burns. Keep pot and pan handles turned to the back of the stove. Keep toddlers out of the "traffic pattern" in kitchens to prevent spilling hot liquids while they play.
• Preschoolers: Same items as toddlers, plus playing with matches
• School-aged children: Experimenting with fire, chemical burns, electrical burns, and firecrackers. Teach school-aged children how to cook only when they are developmentally ready.
• Adolescents: Experimenting with fire and being burned by the flames

Parents need to know that most burns that occur with boys take place outside, and most burns with girls take place within the home. Anticipatory guidance about burn prevention, noting gender influences, should be discussed. Parents should always conduct assessments for areas of potential burns, and keep hot liquids, incense, candles, matches, hot BBQ equipment, and lighters out of reach of children. Scalding burns are the number one cause of burn in children and account for 17% of burn hospitalizations (burnfoundation.org, 2015).

Interventions for Childhood Burns

Treatment for burns includes an immediate stabilization of the child with special consideration to the child's airway and ventilation, fluid status, prevention of infection, and symptoms. With exposure to smoke and heat, the child's airway may be significantly compromised, which requires CPR. Immediate and longer-term treatment needs include the following:

1. Start by providing immediate CPR, using techniques from the American Heart Association, including an age-appropriate CAB (ie, compressions, airway, breathing) technique; maintain a patent airway following CPR and Pediatric Advanced Life Support (PALS) as needed.
2. Stop the burning process by removing the source of the burn.
3. Treat shock through fluid resuscitation therapy.
4. Use sterile technique at all times.
5. Relieve pain, including using morphine for major burns.
6. Elevate the burned body part.
7. Monitor serum electrolytes, protein status, and levels of hemoglobin and hematocrit.

8. Monitor fluid balance, including inserting a Foley's catheter and monitoring strict intake and output.
9. Restore serum protein loss through infusions of albumin.
10. Weigh the patient daily and use the daily weight for all medication, fluid, and nutritional calculations.
11. Transfuse blood products as needed for severe burns that affect hemoglobin.
12. Care for a burn wound by applying cool water (never ice as this may damage tissues further) and/or applying a cool, moist, clean cloth to prevent heat loss.
13. Apply topical medications to promote healing and provide protection (bacitracin ointment, silver sulfadiazine cream, or mafenide cream).
14. Provide developmentally appropriate support and education with explanations that the child can understand.
15. Assist with burn tissue debridement as needed (may be performed in a sterile unit OR in a specialized care unit as often as every 8 to 24 hours).
16. Provide a medication such as a histamine-receptor antagonist to prevent stress ulcers with major burns.

Complications associated with major burns must be anticipated and prepared for. Complications include:

- Airway compromise because of asphyxia from smoke and soot; severe edema of the respiratory tract
- Shock from fluid loss and fluid shifting
- Massive protein loss from weeping wounds
- Renal failure
- An excess buildup of serum potassium because of tissue destruction
- Extreme emotional reactions because of fear, anxiety, and stress

HEALTH PROMOTION

Preventing Sunburn in Children

Children are exposed to a large amount of sun during their childhood. Eighty percent of total lifetime sun damage occurs before a child's 18th birthday. Sun damage occurs throughout childhood during outside play and children's skin must be consistently protected from ultraviolet (UV) damage. Repeated sunburns that blister place a child at greater risk for the development of a type of aggressive skin cancer called *melanoma*. Repeated sun exposure places that child at risk for eye damage by affecting the cornea.

Parents and caregivers must be educated about the need to protect a child's skin. Skin protection from infancy through adolescence should be encouraged. From late preschool on, the young child should be encouraged to take part in his or her skin protection. The following list describes guidelines for protecting children's skin:

- Have the child avoid sun exposure between 10 a.m. and 4 p.m.
- Have the child wear protective clothing and a wide-brimmed hat.
- Wear sunscreen with at least a 30 SPF and reapply after swimming, exercising, and sweating.

NURSING CARE PLAN for the Child Who Requires Debridement

A holistic care plan for a child requiring sequential debridement is needed to assist the child with anticipatory and actual pain. Physical, emotional, and developmentally appropriate educational preparation is required as debridement of burns can be required as many as two times daily for days to weeks. Debridement includes the scrubbing and removal of dead tissue (ie, eschar) from the base of the area of the burn wound for the promotion of new epithelial growth and healing.

Nursing Diagnoses:
- There is fear related to repeated debridement sessions for burn wounds.
- There is pain related to manual scrubbing and removal of eschar.
- The child is experiencing powerlessness related to lack of control of and an inability to protest against repeated debridement sessions.

Expected Outcomes:
- Patient will demonstrate a progressive decrease in fear associated with debridement sessions as evidenced by decreasing protest.
- With subsequent debridement sessions, the patient will report a reduced pain scale score either through (1) subjective statements or a subjective pain scale score, such as a numerical pain scale, or (2) demonstrating behaviors associated with an objective pain scale, such as the FLACC pain scale score (**F**ace, **L**egs, **A**ctivity, **C**ry, and **C**onsolability of the patient).
- Patient will demonstrate an increased sense of power as evidenced by verbalizing that he or she feels like part of the team that is implementing the treatment plan for burn wound care.

- Do not allow an infant younger than 1 year of age to have any significant sun exposure.
- Do not apply sunscreen to infants younger than 6 months of age; their skin is thin and components are readily absorbed.
- Children with low melanin levels (ie, pale) are at greater risk and require more sun protection.

Nursing Considerations for Childhood Burns

The most important nursing consideration for burns is prevention. Prevention must be focused on providing information about the cause of burns for each developmental period. Anticipatory guidance for each developmental period must include family education on burn prevention.

PATIENT TEACHING GUIDELINES

Preventing and Treating Minor Burns

Burn Prevention
  Infants:
- Do not drink hot liquids around an infant, especially if holding an infant.
- Test the temperature of baby foods that have been microwaved before offering them to an infant.
- Do not microwave formula or breast milk; use a hot water bath away from the child.
- Do not apply hot packs to an infant's skin as this is a source of significant burns.
- Test the temperature of a bath before placing the infant into the water.
  Toddlers:
- Turn down hot water heaters to 48.9°C (120°F) or less.
- Test all bath water before allowing the child to climb into it.
- Do not allow toddlers around the stove, oven, or BBQ when cooking.
- Do not use front burners and turn pan handles away from the front of the stove.
  Preschoolers:
- Keep all matches away from young children.
- Do not allow preschoolers to help light fires or candles.
- Keep burning candles out of reach of preschoolers.
- Do not allow a preschool child to cook unsupervised.
- Teach preschoolers burn prevention safety through developmentally appropriate play.
- Lock all flammable chemicals and liquids.
- Clean the garage frequently, disposing of soiled rags exposed to flammable substances.
  School-Aged Children:
- Communicate family rules around burn prevention and frequently reinforce fire safety.
- Do not allow a school-aged child to cook unsupervised.
- Include the child in home fire safety inspections, such as having the child check the batteries in smoke detectors.
- Never allow children to use firecrackers or fireworks without direct adult involvement, guidance, and constant supervision.

  Adolescents:
- Teach teens regarding safety concerns around flammable chemicals and liquids.
- Teach teens about fire safety around cars and gas stations.
- Give positive reinforcement for safe behaviors.
- Some academic institutions recommend using "shock therapy" for education about fires by providing drama, movies, or media that convey worst-case situations and severe outcomes to teach teens appropriate safety measures and situations to avoid.
  Treatment of Minor Burns
  First-Degree to Second-Degree Burns:
- Prevent further burning. Take the child out of the sun and prevent subsequent sun exposure until fully healed.
- Place cool wash cloths on the skin.
- Dry by patting gently with a clean cloth.
- Apply a thick layer of burn cream with a topical anesthetic.
- Wear only loose cotton clothing over the burn.
- Do not allow the child to pull off sloughing tissue.

Tattoos and Piercings

Although tattooing laws and regulations may vary slightly from state to state, the application of a tattoo onto a child's skin, regardless of location, is illegal for a child under the age of 18 without a parent's permission. Adolescents, who are still developing critical thinking and learning about consequences of decision making, are at risk for not understanding the long-term consequences of tattooing. Because of access, some teens may be driven to find illegal sources of tattooing or they may have peers provide tattooing.

Every part of the skin on the body can be pierced or tattooed and may be done so on a child for cultural or ethnic reasons. The concern of the health-care team is to prevent infection after the piercing or tattooing has taken place.

The healing process for piercing and tattooing is directly related to the location. If a child has pierced ears, it may take up to 1 month for the piercing to heal. If the child has a navel piercing, the healing process may take upwards of a year to heal because of moisture, clothing irritation, or adipose layers of the stomach.

Assessments of Tattoos and Piercings

Piercing sites should be assessed for warmth, redness, pus, heat, and discomfort. If infection is suspected, a bacterial and fungal skin cultural swab may be warranted. The site should be thoroughly cleansed with a solution such as hydrogen peroxide, and a thin layer of antimicrobial cream should be applied. In the presence of an infection at the piercing site, the jewelry should not be removed during the treatment of the condition as this may cause an abscess to form. An allergic reaction to metals should be suspected if the rash or irritation does not heal with a regular skincare regimen. In this case, the jewelry should be removed in order for the allergic rash or lesion to heal. The child should take note of the particular metal that caused the allergy to avoid wearing any other jewelry of this type of metal.

Interventions for Tattoos and Piercings

Tattoo sites should be inspected for redness, an oozing of pus or sanguineous discharge, heat, swelling, and discomfort. It is important to teach the child about personal hygiene and hand washing. The tattoo site should be cleansed with mild soap and water daily. Solutions with hydrogen peroxide or alcohol should not be used as they may cause an interference with healing. A thin layer of antimicrobial ointment can be applied for the first few days to prevent infection and prevent scab formation. A child with a new tattoo should not swim, soak in baths, or use a hot tub until the skin of the tattoo is completely healed. Sunblock lotion or cream should always be applied to a tattoo.

Most states have laws concerning underage children (ie, less than 18 years old) obtaining tattoos. Know your state laws and provide appropriate information for teenagers interested in having a tattoo. Nurses can be very influential in the decision-making process for teens. If a teen is planning on having a tattoo placed, they need to know the laws, risks, and long-term consequences of tattooing.

Nursing Considerations for Tattoos and Piercings

Nurses should consider the effect of the tattoo or piercing on the child. A major concern is preventing or treating infections associated with the immediate time period after the tattoo or piercing is acquired; it is also important to prevent future infection of a piercing. Infectious diseases associated with tattooing performed without sterile technique and sterile equipment includes the contraction of:

- HIV
- Hepatitis B virus
- Hepatitis C virus
- *Mycobacterium haemophilum*
- *Mycobacterium tuberculosis*

Although seen as a form of body art by some, the potential negative long-term effects of tattoos placed during childhood or young adulthood may include regret, social shunning, and poor self-esteem. Tattoos placed on areas of the body that are hard to conceal (eg, face, neck, lower arms, and hands) may have detrimental consequences for the teen and may cause permanent discoloration, even with tattoo removal. Tattoos are applied with permanent inks administered through needles. It is imperative that safe precautions, sterile equipment, and skilled work be done to prevent short- and long-term consequences on the teen's health. Removing tattoos can be challenging depending on the size and darkness of the ink used to color the design. Surgical removal, laser technology, or skin grafting may be required. There may be considerable cost to remove a tattoo. Nurses are in a prime position to teach children and adolescents about the consequences of the decision to have tattoos.

Key Points

- The skin of newborns and young infants is fragile and special care should be given in providing nursing care. Special considerations are related to the rapid absorption of medications, from topical to systemic.
- A variety of rashes can be found during childhood. Being able to describe the size, depth, type, and look of lesions is an important nursing consideration. Differentiating among macules, papules, wheals, pustules, vesicles, and other lesions is a nursing standard of practice.
- A holistic care plan for a child requiring sequential debridement is needed to assist the child with anticipatory and actual pain. Physical, emotional, and developmentally appropriate educational preparation is required as debridement of burns can be required as much as two times daily for days to weeks.
- Some skin disorders can be considered evidence of child abuse. Being able to differentiate accidental burn marks from suspected child abuse burns such as sock burns, glove burns, and cigarette burns is important. Cigarette burns can mimic the look of impetigo. Burns with multiple degrees and thicknesses, as well as splash marks, need to be differentiated from submersion burns

or intentional burns (ie, child abuse) such as sock or glove burns.
- Part of anticipatory guidance is implementing a teaching plan for new parents on how to prevent burns during childhood, including electrical, immersive, contact, and heat burns. The nurse should provide information about lowering the home water heater to 48.9°C (120°F), keeping all pots on back burners with handles pointing away from the front of the stove, never drinking hot liquids while holding children, and keeping heaters or BBQ equipment safely away from all children.
- Personal protective equipment should be consistently used to prevent the spread of various childhood skin infections. The nurse must be able to quickly implement contact precautions to prevent the spread of viral, bacterial, and fungal skin infections. Hand washing equipment and signs should be made available for staff, families, visitors, and patients to use frequently.
- Body piercing and tattooing have short- and long-term consequences. Site infection, contraction of infectious diseases, regret, social shunning, and poor self-esteem are all possible consequences.

REVIEW QUESTIONS

1. Scabies is considered a highly contagious bacterial infection that causes extending streaks of bright red lesions across skin surfaces.
   1. True
   2. False

2. Parents must be taught to bathe their infant who has severe eczema with:
   1. Soap and cool water twice daily during an exacerbation
   2. Warm water only once a day with gentle pat drying
   3. Bath water as hot as the child can tolerate to soothe the skin
   4. Cold water soaks at least three times a day with air drying

3. A nurse providing teaching to the parents of a young child with a fungal diaper rash would need to provide more teaching and instruction if the parents were to state:
   1. "We will bathe the child in warm water with added hydrogen peroxide to treat the rash."
   2. "We will bathe the child's skin to remove all layers of medication, diaper cream, and urine at least once a day."
   3. "We will provide some diaper-free time to allow the skin to be exposed to air every day."
   4. "We will assess for extending satellite lesions and will report if they are not improving."

4. Calculate a Benadryl (oral antihistamine) order for a toddler with a severe pruritic rash. The order is for 0.5 milligrams per kilogram of weight by mouth every 6 hours as needed. The child weighs 22.5 pounds.

5. A new preschool teacher calls the pediatric clinic for guidelines on how to care for a child who presents with a large impetigo lesion. The pediatric nurse would explain that the most important action to prevent the spread is to:
   1. Keep the lesion covered with a large adhesive bandage.
   2. Teach the child and family good hand washing techniques.
   3. Cover the wound with a thick layer of zinc oxide to prevent the spread.
   4. Tell the family they will need to keep the child at home until the lesion is healed.

6. A mother of a 10-year-old boy asks about her son's warts located on several of the fingers on his right hand. The pediatric nurse's best response to her questions would include:
   1. Warts are precancerous lesions that need to be surgically removed by a physician.
   2. Warts are benign, not contagious, and will not spread anywhere else on your son's body.
   3. Warts are caused by a variety of infectious organisms including fungi, viruses, and bacteria.
   4. Warts are caused by the papillomavirus, can spread to other body parts and other people, and are treated with acids or freezing nitrogen.

7. Parents and caregivers are instructed not to give aspirin to a child who presents with a rash caused by a viral agent because of:
   1. The need to not mask a fever to best monitor if the child's condition is improving.
   2. To prevent the potentially serious risk of Reye's syndrome.
   3. To prevent the child from developing Kawasaki's disease.
   4. To encourage the child's fever to provide a natural pyrogenic effect that kills viruses.

8. While assisting in a class for new parents about injury prevention, the licensed vocational nurse/licensed practical nurse (LVN/LPN) would be correct in stating that second-degree burns are defined as: *(select all that apply)*
   1. Extending through the epidermis into the dermis
   2. Edematous with weeping of moisture
   3. Very painful
   4. Extending through the epidermis
   5. Healing at various speeds depending on size and location
   6. Possibly requiring grafting

9. Eczema is an autoimmune disorder that typically presents in red rash that is not communicable to others.
   1. True
   2. False

10. Children with significant burns requiring medical equipment may develop stress ulcers. A category of medications that can prevent stress ulcers is the H_2-receptor antagonists.
    1. True
    2. False

CRITICAL THINKING QUESTIONS

1. Children with mobility issues and challenges are at risk for the development of pressure ulcers. What illnesses, disease processes, or pathologies place children at risk? How are pressure ulcers assessed during childhood? Are the tools the same for children as for adults?

2. How do skin differences in young children (ie, infant BSA and the skin of a newborn/young infant) influence a pediatric nurse's care?

3. Permanent tattoo applications are not legal on children under the age of 18. Discuss the social, financial, and educational ramifications of teenagers having a tattoo placed on various parts of their body, especially their neck, arms, and face. How does the developmental stage of adolescence relate to their thought processes of tattoo placement? How are tattoos applied and how are they removed? What are the potential health consequences of having an illegally placed tattoo on a child?

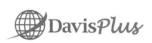 DavisPlus

For additional resources and information, visit **www.DavisPlus.com**. Post-Conference Questions and Activities, Answers, and References can be found on DavisPlus.

Child With a Communicable Disease

LEARNING OUTCOMES

1. Define the key terms.
2. Describe the purpose of vaccines and childhood immunizations and discuss the most common infections that children are immunized for.
3. Differentiate the purpose and use of various PPE used to prevent the spread of infection within health-care environments.
4. Differentiate between the various types of isolation techniques, including standard precautions, airborne precautions, contact precautions, droplet precautions, and reverse (also called *protective*) precautions.
5. Describe the most commonly encountered childhood infectious diseases and describe the transmission, incubation, common symptoms, and treatments or supportive therapy for each.
6. Describe basic safety precautions for preventing the spread of childhood communicable diseases.

KEY TERMS

acquired immunity
active immunity
antigen
communicable
epidemic
immunity
incubation period
passive immunity
personal protective equipment (PPE)
toxoids

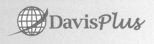 **DavisPlus** For audio pronunciation guide, visit www.DavisPlus.com

CHAPTER CONCEPTS

Assessment
Development
Infection
Safety

REAL-WORLD CASE STUDY

Philip

■ A child presents to his second grade teacher with a fever, nausea, and a severe sore throat. He said that he has been feeling sick for 2 or 3 days but today was the worse he has felt. The teacher calls the administrative office and has the child picked up from school by his mother. After taking the child to his community pediatrician, a call comes in later in the day that the rapid *Streptococcus* A test has returned positive and the child is to start on oral antibiotics immediately. The mother notifies the school. The administrative policy on contacting parents of all children within the classroom is initiated. The child stays home from school for 3 days and then returns to the classroom on day four.

1. What are the classic symptoms of *Streptococcus* A (ie, strep) throat?
2. What are the common antibiotics given to treat this condition?

continued on page 658

3. Why is there a protocol for notifying parents of the child's fellow classmates?
4. What are the guidelines that must be taught to the parents about oral antibiotic therapy for *Streptococcus* A?

CONCEPTUAL CORNERSTONE

Infection Control

Children with communicable illnesses are at risk for spreading their infections to others. Young children do not have the knowledge, skill, and capacity to prevent the spread of infections by controlling body fluids such as mucus, saliva, and stool. Infants easily transmit infections by placing their wet fingers into other's mouths; toddlers do not have the capacity to learn infection control measures without consistent teaching; preschool children share their items readily with their peers and can cause transmission of infectious pathogens; and school-aged children do not always participate in good hand washing techniques at school and after school. Pediatric nurses have the responsibility to provide parents with information on infection control measures so that other members of the family, and those in the community, do not acquire infections. Anticipatory guidance is a means to share information with parents concerning when and how to teach secretion control (eg, sneezing into sleeve, using tissues, washing hands independently). The concept of infection control includes measures implemented by health-care institutions, and behaviors performed by health-care team members, parents, and children. The two most important aspects of infection control are hand washing and the use of **personal protective equipment (PPE)**, which is equipment that is made available to health-care professionals to prevent the spread of infections or diseases. PPE includes the use of goggles, face shields, masks, gowns, and gloves.

One significant challenge of pediatric nursing is that young children may not be able to tell a parent, nurse, or primary provider what is wrong, or describe in depth what their symptoms are. The nurse's and health-care team's observation, recognition, and prompt treatment can make the difference in length and severity of a childhood illness. For example, symptoms such as decreased oral intake, diarrhea, abdominal pain, sore throat, rash, itching, and low-grade fever can indicate any number of childhood illnesses. Children with **communicable** (ie, capable of being transmitted from one individual to another) diseases often present with secondary conditions such as dehydration from prolonged poor oral intake or a lengthy bout of diarrhea. Sometimes the child will present in a critical state of sepsis and require immediate life-saving interventions. It is imperative that pediatric nurses are familiar with the most commonly encountered childhood communicable diseases so that containment, prevention of spread, rapid treatment, and prevention of complications can take place.

Many childhood illnesses, such as polio or smallpox, are no longer common because of vaccination programs and effective treatments. Ironically, the effectiveness of vaccines in eradicating or reducing the incidence of illness may cause parents to falsely believe they do not need to immunize for these serious, sometimes fatal diseases. Learning and staying current about childhood illness, infections, communicable diseases, vaccines/immunizations, and treatments is a very critical part of being an effective pediatric nurse.

Many governmental and medical university Web sites provide annual updates on childhood communicable diseases. The Web sites can be used to update a pediatric nurse's clinical practice by learning about current infections, care trends, and infection control measures associated with the infection. For instance, when *Ebolavirus* became an international concern, governmental Web sites such as that of the Centers for Disease Control and Prevention (CDC) provided infection-control guidelines based on the most current information. These resources can be used for quick reference, as well as family or community teaching. The resources also provide guidance on local or national reporting mandates as a few childhood communicable diseases are followed for **epidemic** (ie, the presence, or prevalence, of a disease within a particular region) and endemic (ie, the presence, or prevalence, of a disease within a widespread geographical area) patterns, such as pertussis, tuberculosis (TB), and measles.

Pediatric health-care providers are at risk for contracting childhood infectious and communicable diseases. It is the nature of working in health care while caring for children and having close contact with body secretions. Using PPE is mandatory when caring for a child with a communicable disease. Information on what to wear and how to implement infection control measures can be found in each health-care institution's policies and procedure manuals from the direction of the infection control nurse. When a child is hospitalized for complications associated with a communicable disease, it is important to post a sign on the patient's room to alert team members, family members, and visitors to take precautions. The child's condition should not be posted as that would breech patient confidentiality and privacy rules (ie, HIPAA). There are instances where health-care team members who are exposed to infectious diseases may have to take oral antibiotics to prevent a severe infection. For example, a health-care team providing emergency care for a young child who was camping around rat-infested ivy presented with the pneumonic version of the Bubonic plague. All health-care professionals who encountered the infected child and who were exposed to the child's respiratory secretions before wearing safe PPE masks had to take oral antibiotics to prevent infection. The local Public Health Department will dictate the condition and the medications required. Upon notification of an unusual microbe, such as the pneumonic version of the Bubonic plague, or upon notification of one of the mandatory reportable infectious conditions, such as measles and pertussis, the Public Health Department will work with the medical team of the clinic or hospital and provide guidelines about staff antibiotic use.

TEAM WORKS

Members of the pediatric health-care team must be knowledgeable about the use of PPE for specific isolation measures, which will help to prevent the spread of disease. The level of protection is dependent on the anticipated contact and exposure.

- **Standard precautions:** Hand washing, gloves, gowns, masks, eye protection, and facial shields as needed
- **Airborne precautions:** Private room with door closed, hand washing, masks, gowns, gloves, eye protection, and facial shields as needed
- **Droplet precautions:** Private room or room with patient with same organism, hand washing, mask if within 3 feet of patient, gown, gloves, and eye shielding as needed
- **Contact precautions:** Hand washing, gown, and gloves; may also be called *enteric contact precautions* when the transmission of a microbe is caused by the presence of the microbe in the stool.
- **Expanded contact precautions:** Hand washing only, no alcohol-based hand gels; gown and gloves
- **Protective precautions:** Also called *reverse precautions* or *neutropenic precautions*; the patient is protected from communicable diseases by a positive-pressure room. Here as the door opens, air is pushed out toward the hospital or health-care setting hallway to prevent airborne or droplet-transmitted microbes from entering the child's room

Only signs that clearly say the type of precaution required are allowed to be posted. A sign posted on a child's hospital door can say "Contact Precautions" but cannot say what disease or infection the child has. Most signage is now standardized and will list what PPE is required and will have pictures or illustrations of what is required.

VACCINES

An important aspect of childhood communicable diseases is the child's immune system's ability to respond. **Immunity** refers to the body's response of developing antibodies against specific bacteria, viruses, and toxins that, once developed, can prevent illness to future exposure of the organism. An **antigen** is a foreign substance such as bacteria, viruses, toxins, and foreign proteins that stimulates the formation of antibodies and therefore provides immunity. The effectiveness and duration of immunity depends on the strength of the immune response as well as the type of organism. Immunity to disease can be active or acquired. **Active immunity** results from the development of antibodies or sensitized T lymphocytes after being exposed to an invading organism. **Acquired immunity** is obtained by either exposure to a bacterium, virus, or toxin sufficient to stimulate an immune response by the body, or stimulating the body's immune response through vaccination or immunization. **Passive immunity** is the temporary immunity acquired by transfusing immune globulins or antitoxins either artificially from another human or from an animal that has been actively immunized against an antigen, or naturally from the mother to the fetus via the placenta.

In the case of vaccines, some types of lifelong immunity can be acquired through relatively few vaccines. Others, such as the flu vaccine, are seasonal and require yearly immunization. Vaccines that are not live-virus vaccines often require multiple doses to give complete immunity. Each dose of the vaccine gives only partial immunity; subsequent additional doses build on the prior immunity. In most cases the first dose of a vaccine gives 50% immunity, the second dose gives up to 75% immunity, and the third dose can give up to 90% immunity. Pediatric health-care team members provide children immunizations or vaccines on a time schedule to protect the child from developing an infection they have been exposed to. (See the Appendices for a childhood immunization schedule.)

PATIENT TEACHING GUIDELINES

How Immunizations Work to Fight Infections During Childhood

- A weakened form of the germ that causes disease is injected into a child's body via a needle and syringe. Sometimes the vaccine is made up of just part of the germ, but enough to start an important process.
- The child's body then produces antibodies in large numbers that can fight off the infection.
- Antibodies are a type of protein that are a part of the child's immune system and stand ready to fight infection. When the immune system recognizes germs have entered the body, these small proteins attach themselves to the germ and kill it.
- If the child is exposed to the germ that causes disease, there will be sufficient antibodies to fight off the germ so the disease does not occur.
- Not all childhood vaccines provide lifetime protection against disease.
- Childhood diseases that are found all over the world, and used to be common in this country, can be prevented by the completion of an immunization schedule.

It is important to understand the type of vaccine being given to understand what side effects may occur and provide education to parents and caregivers. The type of immunization can also determine if a particular vaccine is appropriate for certain populations; for example, live virus vaccines are not usually recommended for immunocompromised patients because of their inability to launch antibody production.

SAFETY *STAT!*

If a health-care provider suspects a child is having a reaction to an immunization, the child should be supervised at all times while calling for help. Allergic reactions, although rare, can be life-threatening because they can cause anaphylaxis (ie, bronchial constriction, throat swelling, and hypotension). If an allergic reaction occurs, it does not necessarily prevent the child from receiving other vaccines. Once the allergen is identified, such as eggs, a vaccine that does not contain the allergen will be administered.

Types of Vaccines

There are several types of immunizations available, with more than 30 types of vaccines and **toxoids** (ie, substances that are chemically modified to retain their antigen properties but are no longer considered poisonous; used to make immunizations) licensed for use in the United States. The main types of vaccines are described in Box 39.1.

Toxoids

Toxoids operate somewhat differently than other vaccines. Instead of producing antibodies against the actual organism, toxoids produce antibodies against toxins secreted by the bacteria.

To make the toxoid vaccine, the bacteria is grown in large amounts. The toxin is inactivated by chemical, heat, or other treatments, producing a nontoxic toxoid that can be given as a vaccination. After vaccination, the body stimulates the production of antibodies that will inactivate the bacterial toxin in the case of future exposure. This is the type of immunization used for diphtheria and tetanus.

Common Immunizations

Pediatric nurses should understand which are the most common immunizations administered to children. Being able to answer parents' questions and knowing where to locate accurate and up-to-date information is imperative to promote compliance to a complete immunization schedule. Immunization schedules may change on an annual basis. Both the CDC and the NIH provide information on the most current recommendations. Parents should receive an immunization handout with every immunization administered. Whenever a child is seen by the pediatric health-care team, immunizations should be discussed because adherence to the recommended schedule is important. Parents must be encouraged to keep track of each child's immunization document because this is needed for entrance into school. Table 39.1 provides a list of commonly administered immunizations.

Known Concerns About Vaccines

Over the last several decades, many individuals and organizations have expressed concerns over the increasing number of required or recommended vaccines. Although known for their life-saving qualities, there have been many concerns expressed widely via media, print, and the Internet. It is imperative that a

Box 39.1 Types of Vaccines

- **Polysaccharide conjugate vaccine:** Uses sugars from the bacteria and bonds them to portions of another germ. This type of vaccine does not contain live viruses and does not contain the whole microbe, so it will not cause the infection or disease.
- **Live virus vaccine:** This type of vaccine uses the whole virus, which has been manipulated in the laboratory in a number of ways to produce a weakened strain. These viruses mimic the natural virus so closely that the body can produce antibodies to provide immunity to the actual disease. The main benefit of a live virus vaccine is the strength of the immunity it produces. It is often effective with just one dose. The main deterrent to this type of vaccine is its ability, on rare occasions, to actually cause the disease, since it is a live virus. This is particularly important to note in immunocompromised patients. Examples of this type of vaccine are measles, mumps, rubella, chickenpox, rotavirus, oral polio, and the nasal flu vaccines.
- **Whole (inactive) virus vaccine:** This type of vaccine contains the whole, killed organism, which retains the surface and internal structures that are strong stimulants to the immune system. The virus is killed, or inactivated, by heat, phenol, formalin, or thimerosal. This kind of vaccine is effective, but there is the possibility of an allergic reaction. A limitation of this type of vaccine is the need for multiple doses to be given initially to produce sufficient immunity, and it often requires booster doses to maintain immunity. Examples of this type of vaccine are anthrax, cholera, whooping cough, rabies, inactivated polio, and typhoid.
- **Recombinant vaccine:** A newer form of vaccine-recombinant technology, this vaccine produces a genetically altered organism. It contains some manufactured proteins that match the germ's proteins closely, which stimulate the immune response in the body. These vaccines do not contain any part of the original germ so they do not have the risk of causing the disease. Examples of this type of vaccine are pneumococcal pneumonia and *Haemophilus influenzae*.

pediatric nurse be prepared to discuss concerns shared by family members (Box 39.2).

COMMON COMMUNICABLE DISORDERS

Children are susceptible to many infectious diseases or illnesses across the developmental period. Some children have mild cases that have no complications or long-term effects. Other children have complicated courses of illness that require hospitalization. Influenza, for example, is a common community-acquired illness; it is a disease process

TABLE 39.1 COMMONLY ADMINISTERED IMMUNIZATIONS

Vaccine Type	Schedule	Type	Common Side Effects	Serious Rare Reactions
Hepatitis B	Three doses: Birth–2 months; 1–4 months; 6–18 months	Inactivated virus	Low-grade fever, sore arm at site of injection (administer in the vastus lateralis muscle)	Serious allergic reactions, high fevers
MMR: Measles, Mumps, and Rubella	Two doses: 12–15 months; 4–6 years	Live virus	Fever, mild rash, swelling of the neck or cheeks, temporary stiffness and pain in joints, temporary low platelets	Seizures, serious allergic reactions, deafness, permanent brain damage
DTaP: Diphtheria *(C. diphtheriae),* Tetanus *(Clostridium tetani),* and Acellular Pertussis	Five doses: 2 months; 4 months; 6 months; 15–18 months; booster 4–6 years	Inactivated virus	Injection site reactions, nonstop crying for longer than 3 hours, tiredness, vomiting, low-grade fever	Seizure, fever greater than 40.6°C, and any tetanus-containing vaccine can, in very rare instances, cause a Guillain-Barré syndrome
Varicella	Two doses each at 12–15 months and 4–6 years, at least 2 months apart	Live virus	Fever, mild rash, and swelling of injection site	Seizures, lowered consciousness, permanent brain damage
Pneumococcal conjugate	Prevnar: Four doses at 2 months, 4 months, 6 months, and 15 months. One catch-up dose can be given through age 5 if any doses were missed.	Polysaccharide conjugate vaccine	Drowsiness, loss of appetite, redness or tenderness at the injection site	Life-threatening allergic reactions (very rare)
Haemophilus influenzae Type B (Hib)	Four doses: 2 months; 4 months; 6 months; and 15 months	Polysaccharide conjugate vaccine	25% of children experience redness, swelling, and pain at injection site. 5% may experience a moderate to high fever.	None known
Influenza	Annually from infancy through geriatrics	Inactivated virus	Soreness, swelling and redness at injection site, fever, body aches, fatigue, headache	Severe allergic reactions, Guillain-Barré syndrome (rare)

Box 39.2 Parental Concerns About Childhood Vaccines and Immunizations

- **Thimerosal**
  - Thimerosal is a water-soluble, crystalline powder used as an antiseptic that was used as a preservative in immunizations, but is no longer used, with the exception of some influenza vaccines. Concerns emerged because thimerosal is mercury-based and has been connected to minor reactions. Current science has not found a link between thimerosal and autism or any serious harm. Families can ask for influenza shots that do not contain thimerosal.
- **Aluminum**
  - Aluminum is added to many vaccines to improve the effectiveness. Combination vaccines may increase the amount of aluminum in a vaccine to make it optimally effective. It is unclear and insufficiently studied to determine how much aluminum may be toxic to infants and children and what effect it may have.
- **Guillain-Barré syndrome**
  - This disorder can be caused when the immune system, in response to a vaccine, also attacks the nervous system, causing temporary paralysis. This is usually temporary, lasting a few weeks, and can require intensive care. The most common vaccines this has been associated with are tetanus-containing vaccines and meningococcal vaccine, although it has been associated with other vaccines, including influenza. Parents need to understand that this is a rare complication and having a tetanus, meningococcal, or severe flu infection has much greater and more common risks.
- **Encephalitis/encephalopathy**
  - Encephalitis is inflammation and swelling of the brain. In rare cases infants will develop this postimmunization and have a high fever and intense screaming alternating with lethargy. The symptoms can last up to a few days. In a small number of cases this can progress to encephalopathy, a form of brain injury that causes permanent damage. This is associated with the old DTP vaccine, the MMR vaccine, and tetanus-containing vaccines.
- **Hypotonic/hyporesponsive episodes (HHE)**
  - HHE is a rare, sometimes serious reaction, associated with pertussis-containing (DTP) vaccinations. This reaction causes a sudden onset of hypotonia. The episode can last a few minutes to hours and it occurs in children less than 2 years of age. The reaction can be serious, sometimes requiring cardiopulmonary resuscitation (CPR). Frequently, children are hospitalized after an episode for observation even if symptoms have subsided.
- **Autism**
  - The medical and scientific community is clear there is no link between the immunizations and autism. Yet questions remain among the public and parents,

largely based on a report published in 1998 in the medical journal *The Lancet* that created controversy regarding vaccines, particularly the MMR, and a possible association to the development of autism. This article, as well as anecdotal stories and media coverage, has continued to serve as a source of controversy that has not subsided since the original publication of the paper. Dr. Wakefield, a gastroenterologist, treated 12 children with gastrointestinal symptoms who were also neurodevelopmentally delayed, eight of which had autism. The case study research retrospectively looked at the MMR immunization record of the children and determined that the children with autism had developed symptoms within a month of receiving an MMR vaccination. From this observation and parental history, he proposed the theory that the MMR vaccine might be the causative agent of the autism. His theory proposed the vaccine caused intestinal inflammation that led to permeability of the intestinal membrane, allowing neurotoxic proteins to enter the bloodstream, eventually affecting brain development and function. At least 20 epidemiological studies have been conducted that have shown no correlation between autism, the MMR vaccine, or thimerosal used in the vaccine.

- **Seizures**
  - Seizure activity has been found to be a rare reaction that children have experienced after any vaccine. Generally, seizures are considered to be secondary to fever. Febrile seizures are generally self-limiting and do not result in future health problems.
- **Autoimmune reactions**
  - Autoimmune reactions have been reported with some vaccines and are considered an overreaction of the immune system to the vaccine components. Reported vaccine associated autoimmune diseases have been rheumatoid arthritis, thyroid disease, Guillain-Barré syndrome, diabetes, and multiple sclerosis.
- **Other concerns**
  Religious objections
  - There are some religious faiths whose doctrines teach that medical procedures and treatments must be refused, limited, or delayed until prayer or clergy are counseled. Christian Scientists are one example of an international faith community that may refuse childhood immunizations.
  Fears about vaccine side effects
  - Some families may report that they are more concerned with the potential side effects (real or not) associated with childhood vaccines than they are concerned about their child acquiring the actual disease. This presents a teachable moment to describe the severity of potential complications associated with childhood infections such as pertussis, tetanus, varicella, and others.

that can present as a mild infection with an uncomplicated course of illness, or can be fatal. The child's health status at the time of becoming infected with a communicable illness will influence how the child presents and is treated. If a child has an underlying chronic illness such as asthma, cystic fibrosis, or a condition that causes immunosuppression, he or she may be more vulnerable to infections and require special consideration. The following section will outline the most frequently encountered communicable diseases in children.

PATIENT TEACHING GUIDELINES

If parents express concerns about immunizations, or if they have refused or delayed their child's immunizations, information the team should share to increase the understanding and improve adherence includes:

- Attempting to have both parents come to an educational session
- Educating the family about the importance of a complete immunization program for all children to prevent childhood diseases such as they are experiencing now
- Providing written information on the immunization schedule and on each immunization being administered
- Teaching them that there are catch-up schedules that can start right away
- Educating them about each of the diseases/infections and their complications
- Scheduling a follow-up appointment for after discharge so they can be seen right away by a pediatrician who will implement a catch-up immunization schedule

Influenza: The "Flu"

Influenza is a yearly occurring infection that occurs in the winter and has significant mortality and morbidity worldwide, particularly in the very young, the elderly, and immunocompromised patients. There are several strains of the virus with a different strain dominating each year. This makes developing the yearly vaccine challenging. Each year the flu shot is developed based on research that indicates which strains will be most prevalent during the upcoming year.

The flu can run a course for several days and patients can become quite ill. Dehydration is a major complication of the illness resulting from high fevers, nausea, vomiting, and diarrhea.

Severe muscle aches and pains are common with the influenza. Superimposed bacterial infections such as pneumonia are complicating factors that can compromise patients further and require antibiotics and hospitalization. School-aged children have the highest infection rate in the population and may be hospitalized because of the complications of this virus. Transmission of influenza is aerosol, requiring airborne precautions. The **incubation period,** which is the time interval between exposure to a communicable disease or infection and the presentation of the first symptoms, is between 24 and 72 hours.

Assessments of Influenza

Pediatric nurses must understand the common symptoms associated with influenza. The following summarizes common flu symptoms:

- **Generalized symptoms:** Rapid onset of fever, chills, conjunctivitis, headache, malaise, muscle pain (ie, myalgia), and sudden onset of rigor are common generalized symptoms.
- **Respiratory symptoms:** Inflammation of the larynx and trachea, cough, sore throat, nasal congestion, and retrosternal pain are associated with the flu. Children often develop croup, pneumonia, and bronchitis as secondary conditions.
- **Gastrointestinal symptoms:** Vomiting, abdominal pain, and diarrhea with secondary dehydration can occur with the flu and require fluid replacement therapy.
- **Central nervous system (CNS) symptoms:** Headache and dizziness can occur with the flu, requiring pain medications and bedrest.

SAFETY STAT!

When a child presents with flulike symptoms (eg, cough, fever, body aches), no matter what the clinical setting, the child and family should be placed away from others and a mask should be placed on the child. Preventing the spread of influenza to vulnerable sick children is a nursing imperative.

Interventions for Influenza

The only medication that is currently approved for treating influenza is Oseltamivir phosphate (Tamiflu). This medication can be administered to children as young as 2.

Nursing Considerations for Influenza

Supportive treatment for influenza is geared toward maintaining adequate hydration and controlling fever. Young children are at risk for febrile seizures as the flu can cause rapid increases in body temperature. Temperature control is particularly important in this patient population.

It is not uncommon to hear "I don't get the flu shot—it gives me the flu." The standard flu vaccine or "flu shot" is an inactivated influenza vaccine that contains the noninfectious killed virus, so it cannot give a child the flu. Antibodies that protect against the illness are produced at about 2 weeks after the vaccination. During this time someone exposed to the flu virus can still become infected. Some experience aches and pains after an injection but these symptoms are mild in comparison to the actual flu symptoms and usually subside in 1 to 2 days. It is important to know if a person has an allergy to eggs that might cause a reaction because the vaccine is produced in an egg product. The flu vaccine is made from inactivated viruses or uses recombinant technology, and has no flu virus that can cause the illness.

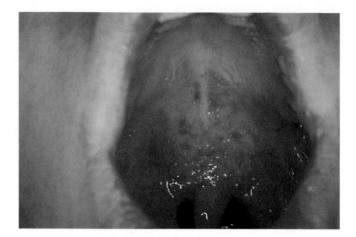

FIGURE 39.1 Koplik's spots.

FIGURE 39.2 Rash caused by rubeola (ie, measles) virus.

One type of influenza vaccine is an intranasal spray that uses a live attenuated influenza virus. These immunizations can give some children adverse side effects that include fever, malaise, muscle pain, and other generalized symptoms.

Flu vaccines are recommended for anyone older than 6 months. Vaccinations are usually started in the fall and contain three viral strains that are likely to be prevalent in the coming winter. Three strains of influenza viruses are common: influenza B viruses, influenza A H1N1 viruses, and influenza A H3N2 viruses. The yearly flu virus is made by using one flu virus from each type.

Measles

Measles is a very contagious respiratory illness caused by the rubeola virus and spread by infected airborne droplets that occur when someone coughs or sneezes. A person is contagious from 4 days before the rash starts until 4 days after the rash appears. The virus is most often spread when one first gets ill, before it is known that the child has become infected. Once exposed, symptoms are displayed within 8 to 12 days. Once a person contracts the illness and recovers, he or she is considered to have lifelong immunity.

Assessment of the Measles

Once contracted, the measles cause fever, a generalized red rash, red eyes (ie, conjunctivitis), runny nose, cough, and general malaise. The development of bluish spots on the buccal mucosa (ie, Koplik's spots) is unique to this disease (Fig. 39.1 and 39.2).

Interventions for the Measles

There are no interventions or treatments for a child who has a measles infection. The viral infection will run its course, which lasts about 4 to 5 days, with a spreading rash and high fevers. The child may require extra fluids and support for fevers and itching.

Postexposure vaccinations may help children who are not yet fully vaccinated against the measles, provided the immunization is administered within 72 hours of exposure to the measles virus. The infection may still develop after the incubation period but it is often a milder infection with less symptoms and a shorter course of infection.

Members of high-risk populations such as pregnant women or children with immune dysfunction diseases may have IV immunoglobulins (ie, antibodies) administered to lessen the measles infection and prevent serious complications.

Vitamin A is also known to reduce the symptoms and severity of the infection for those who have low vitamin A levels.

Nursing Considerations for the Measles

Cases of the measles can be mild to severe. Mild cases of the illness produce self-limiting symptoms that can be treated at home supportively by treating the fever, maintaining hydration, and getting rest. The illness runs its course in children within an approximate 2-week time period.

Moderate cases of this illness can involve secondary ear infections, pneumonia, and high fevers. These cases will require antibiotics and possibly hospitalization, depending on the severity. The child usually recovers without complications.

Serious cases of measles are rare but can involve complications in the brain tissue called *encephalitis* or *encephalopathy*. Pneumonia and respiratory infection can be serious and require hospitalization and intensive care. Very rarely, deaths have been reported caused by measles: about 1 to 2 per 1,000 cases.

PATIENT TEACHING GUIDELINES

Family members can provide comfort for a child who has a significant rash associated with a childhood communicable disease such as the measles or varicella. Ideas for making a child more comfortable and less symptomatic include the following:

- Wear only cotton clothing, no synthetics
- Wear loose-fitting, light-weight clothing
- Keep the rash covered from the sun
- Keep the skin cool and dry
- Provide cool baths or cool compresses on the rash; try oatmeal baths
- Do not allow the child to scratch or itch the rash lesions; cover the hands of infants or young toddlers; apply infant mittens if needed
- Use mild soaps when providing bathing, such as Neutrogena
- Prevent the child from becoming sweaty
- Change linens daily
- Use oral antihistamines if needed to prevent scratching
- Use calamine lotion for topical relief

Mumps

Mumps, also known as *viral parotitis,* is a virus that only affects humans and causes illness that can last from several days to several weeks. Any child who has neither had mumps nor received a vaccination is susceptible. Before the development of the vaccine in 1967, mumps was a common illness in the United States, but this has dramatically decreased to a less than 300 reported cases a year.

Mumps is spread by respiratory droplets, frequently through the coughing and sneezing of an infected person. The usual incubation period is 16 to 18 days; it is contagious from 7 days before to 5 days after salivary swelling begins. The illness usually affects children 5 to 9 years old (mostly school-aged), but can infect adolescents and adults.

Assessments of the Mumps

The characteristic symptom of mumps, salivary gland inflammation (also known as *parotitis*), causes swelling of the glands, cheeks, and jaw, can be unilateral or bilateral, and can last for 1 to 10 days (Fig. 39.3). The fever that accompanies the acute phase of the illness can range up to 40°C for 1 to 6 days. Mumps typically starts with a few days of fever, headache, muscle aches, tiredness, and loss of appetite, and is followed

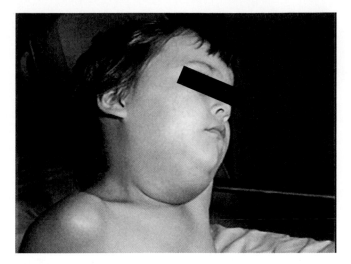

FIGURE 39.3 Child with a mumps infection.

by swelling of salivary glands. Diagnosis is usually made after observation of symptoms or a known mumps exposure. While serological tests are available for definitive diagnosis, the mumps virus can be isolated from throat washings, urine, cerebrospinal fluid (CSF), and other body fluids.

Interventions for the Mumps

Treatment of mumps is supportive and includes analgesics/antipyretics, fluids, rest, scrotal elevation, and ice packs, all focusing on symptom relief. Complicated cases may require hospitalization. Respiratory isolation precautions should be implemented and the child should be kept from school and day care until all manifestations of the symptoms have subsided, about 9 days after parotid swelling.

Nursing Considerations for the Mumps

Mumps is usually a mild disease, but can have complications. Inflammation of the testicles (ie, epididymitis) in males who have reached puberty is the most common complication. Fertility issues are often a concern but are rare. Females may experience inflammation of the ovaries and/or the breast. Other rare complications that have been reported are meningitis and encephalitis. At one time, when mumps was more prevalent, deafness was a significant complication, but is now rarely reported.

Rubella: German Measles

Rubella is an airborne virus spread by coughing and sneezing, or contact with nasopharyngeal secretions, urine, blood, and stool of those infected. The measles cause a fever and rash for 2 to 3 days. The symptoms are usually considered mild in comparison with other illnesses and often are unrecognized. At times there may be body and joint aches, but this illness does not usually cause severe illness in a child who is otherwise healthy. Rubella is considered a highly infectious viral disease that still occurs among children who are not immunized. Children can be infectious up to 10 days before the appearance of the rubella rash (Venes, 2009).

Assessments of Rubella

Children with rubella will present with a 1- to 2-day history of not feeling well, mild fevers, and a sore throat. The child may present with a maculopapular rash that typically begins on the child's forehead or face and progresses downward to the rest of the body (Fig. 39.4).

Interventions for Rubella

Treatment for rubella is usually symptomatic for an individual who has the disease and includes medication for fever and aches; fluids; and rest.

Nursing Considerations for Rubella

The primary risk, and therefore the primary reason for vaccination, is the association of birth defects with women who contract this illness while pregnant. The consequence of this exposure, particularly during the first 12 weeks of pregnancy, can cause serious birth defects such as heart problems, hearing and vision loss, brain damage, and liver or spleen damage. Acquiring a rubella infection during pregnancy can also cause a miscarriage or premature delivery. The vaccine for rubella is usually given with measles and mumps in the form of the MMR.

Roseola

Roseola, also known as *exanthem subitum* or human herpesvirus type 6b (HHV-6b), is a viral infection caused by the HHV-6 pathogen. The transmission of the virus is by saliva of an infected person. The approximate incubation period for roseola is 10 days. Roseola typically presents with low-grade fevers and fussiness for 1 to 2 days, then a sudden elevated fever. The classic roseola rash starts after the last fever (sometimes the day of the last fever) and begins on the child's face and then progresses downward (Fig. 39.5).

Assessments of Roseola

Assessments for a viral roseola infection are based on the identification of the classic rash. The roseola rash is red, pink, and papular in nature. Assessing for a recent history of fevers will also assist in the diagnosis.

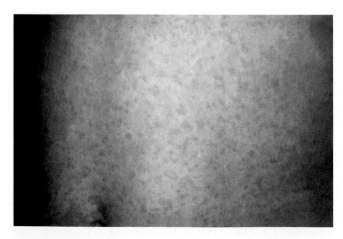

FIGURE 39.4 Rubella.

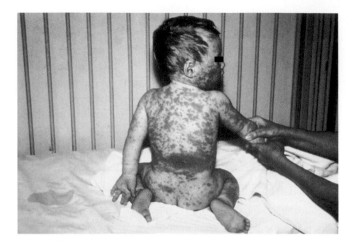

FIGURE 39.5 Roseola rash.

Interventions for Roseola

There are no treatments for the viral infection caused by *Roseolovirus.* Supportive care includes antipyretics such as acetaminophen or ibuprofen, rest, and hydration.

Nursing Considerations for Roseola

The greatest concern with a child who has developed a roseola infection is the spike in temperatures. Rapid high temperatures are associated with febrile seizures.

Varicella: Chickenpox

Varicella, also called *chickenpox,* is a common childhood illness that is highly contagious. Varicella is an airborne virus that is spread through coughing, sneezing, and direct contact with infected lesions. Once someone is infected with the varicella virus, the organism lies dormant and resides within the nerves of the body. The infection can recur in adulthood in the form of shingles, which is an outbreak along nerve tracts that causes significant pain and discomfort.

Assessments of Varicella

The illness begins with a fever, malaise, poor appetite, and lesions, often on the chest or back (Fig. 39.6). The lesions then spread to the body and extremities distally. An individual with varicella begins to be contagious 1 to 2 days before the rash appears. On the second day of illness, the rash lesions turn to blisters and begin to itch; new lesions will continue to develop. By the third day of illness, the blisters crust over. The cycle of new lesions, blisters, and crusting affects the entire body, including the face and extremities, and continues throughout the course of the illness: about 5 days, until all lesions crust over. At the point when all lesions crust over and the patient is no longer febrile, he or she is considered to no longer be contagious. Once someone recovers from a primary varicella infection, he or she usually has immunity for life.

Varicella used to be a very common illness in the United States, with about 3.5 million reported cases of this disease each year (2015). It is estimated that vaccination programs have decreased the incidence of the illness by about 75%.

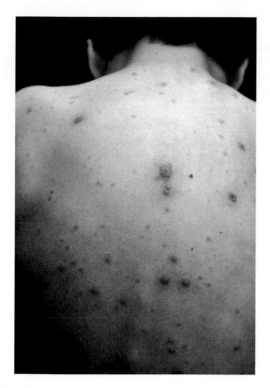

FIGURE 39.6 Lesions caused by varicella infection.

The CDC recommends two doses of chickenpox vaccine for children: the first dose at 12 to 15 months and a second dose at 4 to 6 years. These doses can be given after the age of 1 year, but at least 2 months apart. The vaccine will provide up to 98% immunity to contracting a varicella infection.

Interventions for Varicella

There is no treatment for a viral infection of varicella. Children will need supportive care including fluids, rest, and isolation to prevent the spread to those not vaccinated, or young children who have not completed their two doses of the varicella vaccine. Immunocompromised children, such as those receiving high-dose steroids or those being treated for cancer, may be given the varicella zoster-specific immunoglobulins known as *VZIG*.

Moderate cases of varicella can involve a secondary bacterial infection of the lesions and be more painful, sometimes leaving a scar. Acyclovir, an antiviral medication, is sometimes used in older children and adults within 72 hours of developing a rash to help control the severity of the illness and prevent fever. Acyclovir can limit the outbreak of lesions and the accompanying uncomfortable itching, thus reducing the likelihood of secondary infections.

SAFETY *STAT!*

Severe cases of varicella illness are rare but serious when they occur. Serious complications can include pneumonia, septicemia, toxic shock syndrome, bacterial pneumonia, septic arthritis, encephalitis, viral pneumonia, hemorrhagic conditions, and death.

Nursing Considerations for Varicella

Severe complications from chickenpox for healthy individuals are rare, but chickenpox can be life-threatening to patients who are immunocompromised or who have HIV/AIDS. Using appropriate PPE and infection control measures is very important for a child with confirmed or suspected varicella infection. Contact and airborne precautions are used. Strict hand washing before entering the child's room, again before care, after care, and again after removing PPE is required. Mask, gloves, and gown are worn at all times when providing care. Careful removal of the soiled PPE is warranted and items should be placed in a biological infectious waste container with a tight lid.

Children who have viral infections such as varicella should not be given aspirin; there is an association with viral syndromes, the consumption of aspirin, and the development of Reye's syndrome.

PATIENT TEACHING GUIDELINES

Serious complications can occur in pregnant women who are infected in the first 20 weeks of pregnancy. Approximately 2% of women infected in this period of gestation will have children born with congenital varicella syndrome. This is a syndrome that can result in scarring of the skin, abnormalities in the limbs, brain, and eyes, and low birth weight. If a woman develops a varicella rash from 5 days before to 2 days after delivery, the newborn will be at risk for neonatal varicella. Without immediate antiviral treatment, up to 30% of such newborns may develop severe neonatal varicella infection, which can be life-threatening.

TEAM WORKS

Varicella outbreaks in settings such as child-care centers, schools, institutions, and hospitals can last as long as 4 to 5 months. Outbreaks are monitored by public health departments and the CDC. Outbreaks in community settings can result in significant loss of school for children and work for parents. In hospital settings, varicella identification is a major focus of infectious disease departments because of the vulnerability of hospitalized patients who are immunocompromised.

Polio

Polio is a virus that reached worldwide epidemic outbreaks in the 20th century and was prevalent in the United States as recently as the 1950s. Before the development of the vaccine, each year in the United States thousands of people died and an estimated 35,000 reported people were crippled by the disease. Polio is spread mainly by fecal/oral transmission but less frequently can be spread by direct contact with respiratory secretions or saliva. Polio can be transmitted through poor hand washing, contaminated food and water, unsanitary food preparation, and direct contact with an infected person.

Polio is a disease that mainly affects children under 5 years. The virus spreads between people and can survive in water and sewage. It is often transmitted through contaminated water sources. The incubation period, or the time between exposure and initial symptoms, is usually 6 to 20 days, with a maximum range of 3 to 35 days.

Assessments of Polio

The main assessments for polio are the onset of abrupt symptoms of a cold followed by low-grade fevers. Paralysis can present within 3 days, but this depends on the degree of nerve tissue involvement (Fig. 39.7).

Interventions for Polio

There is no treatment for polio. Once infected, the child will need to be supported through the paralysis. The child may present with paralysis in one extremity, or they may suffer paralysis across all extremities. Mechanical ventilation may be required if the paralysis extends to the trunk and compromises the child's ventilation. Aggressive physical therapy may be ordered to improve the associated muscular hypotonia with the paralysis.

Nursing Considerations for Polio

The majority of children and adults infected with the polio virus may never show symptoms or develop the disease, but may act as carriers and spread the virus. A small percentage of children and adults infected with the virus may develop symptoms classified as nonparalytic, or abortive polio, and have symptoms such as fever, fatigue, nausea, headache, flulike symptoms, stiffness in the neck, back, arms and legs, muscle spasms, and sometimes meningitis. These symptoms can last a few days to a few weeks. There can be complete recovery without further progression of the illness.

A smaller percentage of cases (ie, 1% to 2%) is classified as paralytic polio, which has devastating effects, causing paralysis and, in some cases, death. In these cases, the poliovirus infects the CNS, destroying the motor neurons that control skeletal muscles. Differing degrees of paralysis may develop depending on the nerves involved.

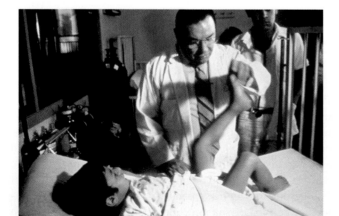

FIGURE 39.7 Paralysis caused by polio infection.

The classifications of paralytic polio are:

- **Spinal polio:** This is the most common form of polio; it attacks motor neurons in the spinal cord, causing paralysis in the arms and legs.
- **Bulbar polio:** This form of polio attacks the cranial nerves affecting sight, vision, taste, swallowing, and breathing.
- **Bulbospinal polio:** This form of polio is a combination of spinal and bulbar polio. It is the most severe form; it affects the ability to swallow and can cause paralysis of the respiratory muscles, leading to death.

Because of vaccination programs, polio is no longer prevalent in the United States. Vaccination is recommended for children under the age of 5. There are two types of vaccines that protect against polio: the inactivated polio vaccine (IPV) and the oral polio vaccine (OPV). Protection includes a series of injections that have been used exclusively in the United States since 2000 and countries where the disease has been eradicated. IPV is given in a four-dose series.

Haemophilus Influenzae Type B

Haemophilus influenzae type B (Hib) is a bacterium that causes meningitis, blood infections, bone infections, epiglottitis, and pneumonia. Before the development of the Hib vaccine, there were about 20,000 cases of serious infections reported in the United States each year. The severity of illness from Hib can vary.

Assessments of Haemophilus Influenzae Type B

Mild cases often start with cold symptoms that sometimes progress to fever, ear infections, and respiratory infections such as bronchitis or pneumonia, and often can be treated with antibiotics.

An infant/child with a moderate case of Hib infection can present as quite ill. Common presentations include respiratory symptoms in addition to secondary infections. The child may appear lethargic and ill, show signs of increased work of breathing and labored respiration, and have signs of mild to moderate dehydration from fever and poor oral intake.

Interventions for Haemophilus Influenzae Type B

Because Hib is caused by bacteria, the child will be treated with antibiotic therapy. A child may be admitted to the hospital for hydration, antibiotics, and monitoring.

Nursing Considerations for Haemophilus Influenzae Type B

Patients with severe cases of Hib can develop meningitis, pneumonia, or epiglottitis. Epiglottitis is a severe infection that can rapidly occlude the child's airway. The classic presentation of epiglottitis includes drooling, dystonia, and dysphagia. The child needs immediate emergency care, airway support, and rapid antibiotics to avoid death. These illnesses can be life-threatening and require immediate medical intervention, hospitalization, and antibiotic treatment; intensive care can sometimes be required. Long-term sequelae of meningitis can involve hearing loss, learning disorders, and/or nerve injury.

SAFETY *STAT!*

A child who presents with symptoms of epiglottitis should not have any type of throat assessment such as a visual inspection with a tongue blade. Touching the site can result in rapid swelling and total occlusion of the child's airway.

Reported cases of serious Hib have decreased to about 25 cases from the 20,000 yearly cases since the development of the Hib vaccine in the 1980s (Sears, 2011). This vaccine is considered relatively safe and is reported to have a low number of side effects compared with other vaccines. Considering the serious illnesses that can arise from Hib infection and the few side effects associated with the vaccine, this vaccine is recommended for all infants.

Pneumococcus

Pneumococcus, also known as *Streptococcus pneumoniae*, is a bacterium that can cause a number of illnesses such as ear infections, serious respiratory infections, pneumonia, and meningitis in children that can range from minor symptoms to severe illness. Blood tests can isolate *S. pneumoniae*; then, oral or IV antibiotics can be given if the patient is hospitalized. Severe causes of pneumococcal disease affect mainly infants and children under the age of 5. These young patients can present with symptoms of meningitis or sepsis and will require treatment with aggressive antibiotics; often they will require intensive care unit (ICU) stays. Infections of this type have a 20% to 30% mortality rate with complications that include brain damage and hearing loss in some children.

Assessments of Pneumococcus

Symptoms of pneumococcus usually begin as similar to cold symptoms and may progress to ear infections, bronchitis, or pneumonia.

Interventions for Pneumococcus

Mild cases are treated on an outpatient basis with antibiotics. In more severe cases, the child may appear lethargic and have increased respiratory distress. Severe cases should be treated in the hospital with IV antibiotics, monitoring, and nursing care.

Nursing Considerations for Pneumococcus

The pneumococcus vaccine is limited in effectiveness because it does not cover all the dozens of strains of pneumococcus that exist—only the most common strains (typically 22 to 23 strains at a time). Many emerging strains of pneumococcus are resistant to antibiotics and may not be covered by current vaccines. The CDC estimates the annual number of cases of this disease has decreased by 75% from 60,000 because of rapid identification and treatment (CDC, 2014).

Approximately 50% of children report local and systemic side effects to the pneumococcal conjugate vaccine (PCV), and 80% may experience fussiness. Fevers are found in 5% of children after the vaccine. Severe reactions have been reported during vaccine trials; 8% of infants experienced pneumonia, chest cold, and gastroenteritis, but this may have occurred unrelated to the vaccine (CDC, 2014).

PATIENT TEACHING GUIDELINES

Child With a Streptococcus A Throat Infection

Symptoms of *Streptococcus* A (ie, strep) throat include:

- Severe sore throat (ie, severe pharyngitis), often rapid onset
- Red, raw, swollen throat tissue with white spots (ie, tonsillar exudates)
- High fevers
- Low energy
- Cervical adenopathy
- Not wanting to swallow (ie, dysphagia)

Antibiotics given to treat this condition after a rapid strep test or throat culture include penicillin and amoxicillin. If the child has an allergy to penicillin, cephalosporin and erythromycin are administered. Protocols for notifying parents of the child's fellow classmates are important because strep infections have a rapid incubation period (ie, 24 to 72 hours) and are easily transmitted to other children in a classroom or child-care setting via respiratory secretions. Prompt identification of the pathogen and rapid notification of schools, after-school programs, and social networks are imperative. The child must finish the entire course of oral antibiotics to prevent the development of resistant strains of bacteria and to make sure the maximal amount of bacteria is killed to prevent a prolonged infection or a recurrence.

Diphtheria

Diphtheria is serious throat infection caused by *Corynebacterium diphtheriae* bacterium. The bacterium secretes a toxin that irritates the respiratory tract, causing severe coughing and breathing difficulty. Diphtheria is spread by respiratory droplets from coughing and sneezing and is contagious 2 weeks after the development of symptoms.

Assessments of Diphtheria

The symptoms can range from mild to serious (Fig. 39.8). Symptoms of diphtheria start as a sore throat and develop into a visible white coating on the tonsils or in the nose. This coating is referred to as a *pseudomembranous coating*.

SAFETY *STAT!*

In moderate to severe cases of diphtheria, the pseudomembranous coating on the tonsils or in the nose becomes so thick it becomes difficult for the child to breathe. This can lead to swelling, swollen neck glands, and airway obstruction.

Interventions for Diphtheria

Diphtheria is a serious infection. The child with a diagnosis of diphtheria must be treated immediately with both antibiotics and an antitoxin that will neutralize the diphtheria

NURSING CARE PLAN for the Child With Pneumococcus Bacteria

Children with pneumococcus bacteria can present with a variety of infections. The following two nursing diagnoses and corresponding goals are appropriate when caring for an infant with bacterial otitis media (bilateral) and infected sore throat from pneumococcus:

Nursing Diagnosis:
- There is pain related to an inner ear infection as evidenced by crying, fever, inconsolability, and hitting the side of the head.

Expected Outcome:
- The patient will demonstrate a 1 or less on a FLACC pain scale 1 hour after the administration of an antipyretic/analgesic.

Nursing Diagnosis:
- There is a potential for infection to others, related to the infected throat, as evidenced by inability to control secretions, drooling, and crying.

Expected Outcome:
- The patient will not spread the bacterial infection to others; all family members will use good hand washing techniques and reduce exposure to the infant's secretions.

toxin spreading in the child's body. Either erythromycin PO or IV, or penicillin G by injection, will be required. The medical team will be aggressive in treating a diphtheria infection, including the IM or IV administration of the antitoxin. Because a severe case of diphtheria can cause respiratory obstruction from the thick throat covering, the child may be treated in an ICU (Mayo Clinic, 2014).

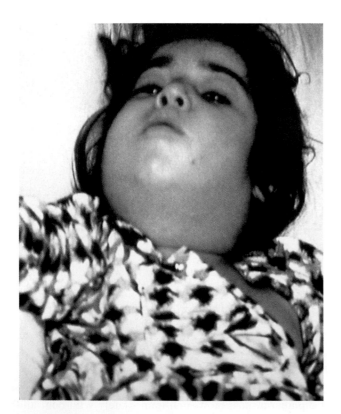

FIGURE 39.8 Diphtheria.

Nursing Considerations for Diphtheria

The toxin secreted from the bacteria can cause heart arrhythmias and sometimes heart failure. The toxin can lead to nerve damage and paralysis. This illness can be fatal for as many as 1 in 5 children under the age of 5.

With the development of the diphtheria vaccine, incidence rates (ie, new cases) of this illness have dropped from about 200,000 cases in the 20th century to five cases a year. There have been no reported cases of diphtheria in the United States since 2003. The vaccine for diphtheria is part of the DTaP vaccination (ie, diphtheria, tetanus, and acellular pertussis). Vaccination does not provide lifetime immunity and boosters are needed every 10 years to maintain immunity.

Tetanus

The tetanus infection is caused by a toxin secreted by the bacterium *Clostridium tetani*. A spore that lives in soil, the intestinal systems of many animals, and contaminated manure, tetanus enters the body through punctures from rusty metal, dirty needles, open wounds, or a break in the skin exposed to contaminated surfaces. Tetanus is transmitted through wounds or injuries that foster anaerobic conditions. Once introduced into the body, the spores germinate at the site of entry and secrete a toxin. This toxin then spreads and begins to bind to the neurons of the CNS, gradually causing paralysis throughout the body. Left untreated, the illness can be fatal.

If a child does not have a vaccine history or his or her parent or caregiver cannot accurately recall or produce documentation of the vaccine history, a vaccine can be given at the time of injury to prevent the development of the disease. If there is a considerably high risk of infection, tetanus immune globulin (TIG) injection can be given to inactivate any tetanus toxin that may develop and spread in the days following the injury.

The incubation period for tetanus is usually about 7 to 8 days, with a range of 3 to 21 days. Once tetanus binds to nerve cells and symptoms begin, there is no cure. Contractions and paralysis can continue for weeks. After the several-week acute period of illness, rehabilitation will be needed for months.

There are two main types of tetanus: localized and generalized. Localized tetanus affects only the nerves near the wound site and causes muscle contractions lasting for several weeks. The more serious form of tetanus, generalized tetanus, spreads to the CNS and progresses in a descending (ie, top to bottom) pattern.

Assessments of Tetanus

Tetanus is often called *lockjaw* because the stiffness usually starts with the jaw muscles and spreads to the neck, causing swallowing difficulty. Within 24 to 48 hours, rigidity and spasms may develop and spread to the trunk and extremities. As the neural blockade of the toxin continues, the child's neck and back become stiff and arched, the abdominal wall becomes rigid, and the severity of the muscle contractions can cause fractures of the spine and long bones (Fig. 39.9). Other symptoms can include fever, tachycardia, high blood pressure, sweating, and cardiac arrhythmias.

Interventions for Tetanus

The treatment for a contaminating injury includes the following:

1. Immediate cleansing of the wound with clean water and a disinfectant
2. Immediate medical attention to prevent the toxin from developing and spreading
3. Antibiotics to kill the bacteria
4. TIG shot to neutralize any toxin that is free-floating and not bound to nerve cells
5. Evaluation of previous immunizations: A person who has received a series of tetanus vaccinations and has received a booster shot within 5 years will already have antibodies and should be protected from developing the disease.

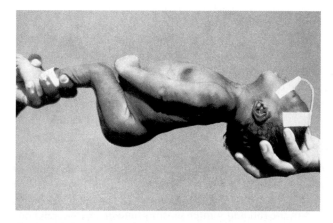

FIGURE 39.9 Tetanus infection.

Nursing Considerations for Tetanus

The severity of this illness is largely determined by how quickly medical treatment is obtained after a contaminated injury. The earlier treatment can be started with TIG and antibiotics, the sooner the toxin can be neutralized and the degree of CNS impairment can be limited. The incidence of tetanus in the United States has only been 25 to 50 cases a year, occurring mostly in adults who have never been vaccinated.

Pertussis: Whooping Cough

Pertussis is a common, serious, and very contagious bacterial infection of the upper respiratory tract, which is especially concerning in infants. The disease is spread by being in close contact with someone coughing and sneezing and can be spread by parents, siblings, and caregivers. Children at greatest risk for serious illness from pertussis are infants less than 6 months.

This is a disease caused by a bacterium that affects the upper respiratory tract and lungs. The bacteria secretes a toxin that causes severe irritation and damages the lining of the throat and lungs. Initially, the symptoms start as upper respiratory symptoms similar to a cold, including runny nose, congestion, and sneezing. After 1 to 2 weeks, the patient has repeated violent, prolonged coughing fits that can last up to 30 to 60 sec. The severity of the coughing spells makes it difficult to inhale, and inhalation only occurs when the respiratory tract has been emptied of air. The characteristic "whooping" sound is the result of trying to inhale through the glottis, which is irritated from the coughing spells and narrowed by spasm and secretions. The patient has an impaired ability to clear secretions because of damage to the cilia of the lung. Thick, tenacious secretions obstruct the bronchi and bronchioles of the lungs, often leading to atelectasis and pneumonia. The incubation period for pertussis is 7 to 10 days, and usually occurs 6 to 20 days after exposure.

Assessments of Pertussis

While at first the symptoms of the illness may be mild with dry cough, within 2 weeks the cough often progresses to the coughing spells characteristic of the disease, which then continue to increase in severity and frequency. With the severe coughing episodes, cyanosis can occur, the eyes can roll back, and the level of consciousness can change. Seizures and, in rare cases, encephalopathy, have been associated with the illness.

Interventions for Pertussis

Hydration and nutrition are important considerations in treating these patients and are particularly important since children, particularly infants, are highly susceptible to dehydration. Posttussive emesis is common with pertussis infections, and oral intake is often difficult because of coughing episodes and difficulty breathing.

While many cases of pertussis can be treated at home, hospitalization is often required when an infant demonstrates apnea, respiratory compromise, and neurological impairment secondary to anoxic episodes. Airway maintenance and maintaining adequate hydration and nutrition are priorities in treatment. These infants can be very ill and sometimes require extended periods of hospitalization.

Nursing Considerations for Pertussis

Pertussis outbreaks are increasingly common with peaks in disease every 3 to 5 years in the United States. Pertussis education and immunization programs are geared to increase awareness of the prevalence and seriousness of the disease. In young infants, particularly those less than 6 months, whooping cough can be life-threatening.

THERAPEUTIC COMMUNICATION

Pertussis infections in young children and infants are very frightening for parents. The characteristic cough is traumatic for the child and scary to witness for the parents. It is important to be supportive and therapeutic in all interactions with the family, especially if the young child was underimmunized or not immunized fully, or was infected by an older sibling who was underimmunized or not immunized. The family will require teaching about the importance of childhood immunizations, but during the course of the acute illness and hospitalization, the parents need support.

Hepatitis A

Hepatitis A is a virus that affects the liver, causing temporary inflammation. The virus is transmitted by stool or blood and is often the result of contaminated objects put in the mouth, poor hand hygiene and food handling, and contaminated water. The infection can easily be transmitted in restaurants and homes if there is poor hand washing and hygiene practices.

Community outbreaks of hepatitis A can be quite common since it is most contagious 1 week before symptoms begin.

Assessments of Hepatitis A

Approximately 4 weeks after exposure, an exposed person starts to feel ill. The severity of the disease varies depending on the age of the infected person. Children under the age of 6 often do not show symptoms and of those who do, the symptoms resemble mild intestinal flu symptoms. Children 6 to 12 years often feel ill but have what are considered mild symptoms. Older children and adults can have severe symptoms that resemble food poisoning or gastroenteritis, but can last up to a few weeks.

Moderate cases of hepatitis A in children can involve abdominal pain, vomiting, diarrhea, and dehydration for several days.

Interventions for Hepatitis A

In cases where there are more pronounced symptoms of abdominal pain, diarrhea, and dehydration, a hospitalization

for antinausea and antidiarrhea medication, as well as IV rehydration, may be needed. In an outbreak of hepatitis A, preventive measures can be taken. Both children and adults can be given an infusion of IV immunoglobulin (IVIG) within 2 weeks of exposure; this has an 85% chance of preventing the development of the disease.

Nursing Considerations for Hepatitis A

Many families will be familiar with hepatitis B but may not be familiar with hepatitis A. Because hepatitis A is transmitted easily via stool; blood; and contaminated objects, food, and water, it is important to teach and reinforce learning about hand hygiene. Parents should be aware of community breakouts of hepatitis A and should perform strict hand hygiene when taking children to visit family in long-term care facilities, hospitals, or other health-care settings where stool and blood are handled.

Hepatitis B

Hepatitis B is a blood/body fluid-borne virus transmitted through sexual activity and use of contaminated (sometimes shared) IV drug needles, tattoo needles, health care–related needle sticks, or at birth when a baby is exposed to contaminated blood and body fluids. The hepatitis B virus is virulent and can survive outside a person on a razor or toothbrush for periods up to a week.

Assessments of Hepatitis B

Symptoms of hepatitis B in teens and adults are nausea, vomiting, abdominal pain, diarrhea, fatigue, and jaundice. Symptom onset occurs within 90 days of exposure.

Interventions for Hepatitis B

In a majority of cases, the immune system can kill the virus, and up to 95% of cases resolve in 1 to 6 months without long-term problems. A small percentage (ie, 5%) of those exposed to hepatitis B become chronic, asymptomatic carriers.

Nursing Considerations for Hepatitis B

The clinical presentation of hepatitis B for infants and children is quite different. At this age, the virus can lie dormant in the body for many years, and patients can be asymptomatic. About 25% of infected infants develop liver cancer or liver failure later in childhood and sometimes require a liver transplant. Children who acquire hepatitis B later in childhood during toddler or preschool years often become chronically infected. The long-term outlook for these children is poor and often results in chronic illness and liver failure.

Rotavirus

Rotavirus is an intestinal virus that is extremely contagious and transmitted through stool, saliva, and poor hand washing and hygiene practices. Rotavirus infections are most common in the fall and winter seasons, and are a frequent cause of illness and hospitalization in young infants and children.

Rotavirus is resistant to disinfectant solutions and antibacterial hand soaps. This virus is easily spread in day-care centers, where frequent diaper changes occur and children share toys and food.

Assessments of Rotavirus

Initial symptoms of rotavirus are similar to gastroenteritis and involve fever, vomiting, and diarrhea. The diarrhea can last more than a few days, up to a few weeks in some cases, and can be more frequent and foul smelling. Infants and young children are at risk for dehydration because of fluid loss from vomiting and severe, prolonged diarrhea.

Interventions for Rotavirus

Treatment involves antinausea medication, rehydration, and sometimes treatment with probiotic powder to decrease diarrhea.

SAFETY *STAT!*

Zinc deficiency has been found to be associated with immune system impairment and greater severity of serious infectious childhood diseases. In childhood communicable or infectious diseases that have associated diarrhea, zinc supplementation has shown to greatly shorten the duration.

Nursing Considerations for Rotavirus

The rotavirus vaccine is a liquid given by mouth. Depending on the brand, it can be given in a two- or three-dose series at 2, 4, and 6 months, with at least 1 month between doses. The vaccine contains whole, live viruses that multiply in the intestines and cause a mild case of the illness to stimulate the body's immune system. A primary point of education with this vaccine is to teach the parents and caregivers that the live virus can be expelled in the diapers up to 15 days after the first dose. It is unclear how contagious postvaccine stool can be, but careful hand washing and hygiene precautions should be taken to prevent transmission of the disease to other children and family members.

Common side effects of the vaccine include fever, vomiting, and diarrhea in 10% of children, and poor feeding in 25% of children. Severe reactions to the vaccine include seizure, Kawasaki's disease, and intussusception.

Human Papillomavirus (HPV)

There is only one form of cancer for which there is a vaccine: cervical cancer caused by the two main strains of cervical cancer-causing HPV. Arguably, this may be one of the most controversial vaccines available because of the recommended age of immunization in the preteen years and the controversy over preteens and teens having sex. Cervical cancer in women is often asymptomatic and is detected on Pap smears. It is the second-leading cause of death in women worldwide. If it is caught early, it can be cured by surgical intervention (CDC, 2014).

HPV is a sexually transmitted virus spread through unprotected genital sex. It is the most commonly sexually transmitted disease in the United States (CDC, 2014). There are 40 strains of the virus and it often goes undetected since there are often no visible signs, such as genital warts. Both women and men can carry the virus; most sexually active women carry the virus by the time they are in their twenties, and most sexually active men will have come into contact with the virus by the same age and can act as carriers. Most HPV infections will clear on their own, but when they do not, health problems such as warts and various cancers can develop (CDC, 2014). HPV is associated with not only cervical cancer, but anal, head, and neck cancer in males, genital warts across the lifespan, and rarely, the presence of warts in the airway of infants and children (healthychildren.org, 2015).

Assessments of Human Papillomavirus

In the newborn period, the infant can be exposed to HPV infection during the birth process via an infected mother with cervical HPV. Newborns can become ill very quickly with high fever and seizures, and may become lethargic. HPV infection in newborns can be very severe (CDC, 2014) and can lead to infant death (New York State Department of Health, 2011).

Interventions for Human Papillomavirus

There is no treatment for HPV during childhood. There are treatments for the complications and problems that arise from having a HPV infection, including treatment for warts, treatment for abnormal Pap smears in teen girls, and surgery of warts that grow into the throat or airway structures (CDC, 2015).

Nursing Considerations for Human Papillomavirus

Pediatric nurses have the opportunity to teach sexually active teenagers how to prevent the spread or acquisition of HPV infections. The use of condoms for sexually active teenagers may decrease the likelihood of infection, and having a regular Pap test can detect if the cervix has precancerous lesions (Mayo Clinic, 2015).

The HPV vaccine is recommended for all teenage girls and boys (CDC, 2014). The vaccine is a three-shot series started at age 11 or 12, usually before sexual activity begins. The second dose is given 2 months after the first, and the third dose is given 6 months after the first dose. The HPV vaccine does not protect against all strains, only the most common ones. The HPV vaccine is genetically engineered. Neither vaccine used to make the HPV is a live virus so there is no way to acquire the disease from the vaccination. Common side effects include injection site reactions, headache, fatigue, muscle aches, and joint pain.

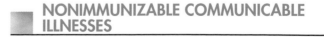

NONIMMUNIZABLE COMMUNICABLE ILLNESSES

There are many infectious diseases and illnesses that do not have an associated childhood immunization. These infections are of particular concern; because there is no way to prevent them, pediatric health-care providers must identify risk factors, common clinical presentations and symptoms, and then determine best treatment options and nursing care.

Developmental aspects of children lead them to be particularly vulnerable to the development of communicable illnesses. During infancy and early childhood, the child's immune system is maturing. Exposures to infectious materials cause the child's immune system to produce immunoglobulins that provide protection. The younger the child, the more vulnerable the child is to the development of diseases and illnesses because they have less circulating immunoglobulins. Table 39.2 provides information on the nonimmunizable communicable illnesses that are found during childhood. Pediatric nurses benefit their patients by being astute in their understanding of these infections so rapid communication of observations can lead to rapid treatments and infection control procedures.

SAFETY *STAT!*

Tick Prevention and Removal
Tick Prevention

Several protective measures are recommended to prevent being bitten and infected by ticks. These measures should be used in areas where there is grass, trees, or brush:

- Tuck pant legs into socks so ticks cannot get inside pants legs.

- Wear a long-sleeved shirt and tuck it inside the pants.
- Spray insecticide containing permethrin on boots and clothing.
- Apply insect repellent containing DEET on your skin and reapply every few hours.
- Inspect for ticks, particularly in hair and on creased areas of the body where ticks may nest.

Tick Removal

If preventing a tick bite is not successful, measures are recommended to remove the tick:

- Use fine-tipped tweezers to grasp the tick as close to the skin's surface as possible.
- Pull upward with steady, even pressure. Do not twist or jerk the tick; this can cause the mouthparts to break off and remain in the skin. If this happens, remove the mouthparts with clean tweezers.

REPORTING MANDATES

Severe reactions are rare but sometimes do occur with childhood immunizations. After a vaccine has been released and administered for use, serious reactions that do occur can be voluntarily reported through the Vaccine Adverse Events Reporting System (VAERS). If a severe reaction is reported enough times, it is listed as a postlicensing–reported reaction in the vaccine information or product insert (PI). Check with the local public health department to find out which reactions or childhood diseases are mandated to be reported.

(Text continued on page 688)

TABLE 39.2 NONIMMUNIZABLE COMMUNICABLE ILLNESSES OF CHILDHOOD

Disease	Definition	Causative Agent	Clinical Presentation	Treatment
Common Cold and Coldlike Illnesses	The common cold is actually a syndrome of several illnesses with overlapping clinical symptoms that can be caused by a variety of different organisms.	Colds are caused by viruses, with rhinoviruses causing over 40% of cases. Other viruses that commonly cause cold symptoms are coronaviruses; respiratory syncytial virus (RSV); parainfluenza-virus (PIV) 1, 2, and 3; adenoviruses; *Mycoplasma pneumoniae*; and group A streptococcus.	The common cold varies in severity and involves nasal congestion and drainage, conjunctivitis, sore throat, cough, and redness of the pharynx and tonsils. The incubation period is short; usually 1–2 days. Symptoms can involve headache, chills, malaise, muscle aches, low-grade fever, and enlarged cervical lymph nodes. The illness can last a week to 10 days.	Supportive care is given to a child with a coldlike illness. Because of the concern with inaccurate dosing, over-the-counter pediatric cold preparations should be used with caution and should be discussed with the child's primary care provider.
Respiratory Syncytial Virus (RSV)	RSV is the most common cause of respiratory illness and lower respiratory tract infections in infants and children, and is a major cause of bronchiolitis, croup, and pediatric pneumonia. RSV in the adult population often causes cold symptoms. The effect on infants and children can be far more significant. At particular risk for severe respiratory complications from RSV infection are infants, especially premature infants.	The RSV occurs regularly, most often between winter and early spring, with a peak between January and March. It is estimated that 50% of children will be infected with RSV within their first year of life during the winter months. By the age of 3, almost 100% of children will have had RSV at least one time, and often more than once. Children can get repeated infections from RSV because the body does not develop immunity even after having the illness. Repeated infections within a year are often milder. RSV is transmitted by direct airborne exposure to large droplets. The virus is shed profusely and may	RSV is a virus that initially produces symptoms in the nasopharyngeal passage and then spreads to the lower respiratory tract. RSV is considered the leading cause of bronchiolitis in children. Inflammation of small airways and sloughing and necrosis of the bronchiolar epithelium occur once the virus migrates to the lower respiratory tract. The increased mucus production and significant inflammatory response often cause narrowing and plugging of the small airways, resulting in atelectasis and airway obstruction. Symptoms initially begin as increased nasal secretions but then progress to increased congestion,	Hospitalization is often required for infants with severe respiratory distress to provide supplemental oxygen, suction secretions, provide hydration, and monitor respiratory status for distress.

Continued

TABLE 39.2 NONIMMUNIZABLE COMMUNICABLE ILLNESSES OF CHILDHOOD—cont'd

Disease	Definition	Causative Agent	Clinical Presentation	Treatment
		survive for 4–7 hours on skin and surfaces, despite routine infection control. The most effective prevention of transmission of RSV is implementing hand washing, protective gear, and infection control precautions. Because droplet precautions are required when within 3 feet of the symptomatic child, gown, gloves, and mask are required to be worn.	coughing, paroxysmal coughing spells, and inability to clear secretions. Infants—under 6 months in particular—can present in moderate to severe respiratory distress with increased work of breathing, decreased oxygen saturation, and fatigue that leads to the inability to clear secretions.	
Croup	Croup is a respiratory condition that is often the result of an acute viral illness that affects the upper airway and results in symptoms of inspiratory stridor, cough, and hoarseness. The cough associated with croup is a harsh barking cough and children often have trouble breathing. Croup is also considered a symptom of a condition called laryngeal tracheal bronchitis (LTB).	Croup most commonly is caused by PIVs 1, 2, and 3, but can be caused by adenovirus, influenza A and B, rhinoviruses, or RSV.	Stridor is a high-pitched wheezing sound resulting from turbulent air flow in the upper airway. Stridor is a physical sign that is produced by a narrowed or obstructed airway path. It can be inspiratory, expiratory, or both. Inspiratory stridor is common. It can indicate serious airway obstruction and should be immediately evaluated for severe respiratory conditions such as epiglottitis, foreign body obstruction of the airway, or PIV 1. Stridor is sometimes present; it can indicate a potential medical emergency and should always be evaluated and treated immediately. Wherever possible, attempts should be made to immediately establish the	The treatment for croup is usually supportive and is aimed at maintaining the airway through humidification, proper positioning of the child for optimal airway maintenance, and supplemental oxygen if necessary.

Epiglottitis	Acute epiglottitis is a life-threatening medical emergency in children. Epiglottitis can progress rapidly, causing a complete airway obstruction.	The causative agent of epiglottitis is bacterial in origin and is usually caused by *H. influenzae.*	Children with epiglottitis present with symptoms of fever, stridor, and drooling, and appear ill. Children with epiglottitis often appear anxious, have inspiratory stridor, and appear more comfortable in a sitting position to breathe. Epiglottitis causes supraglottic obstruction that results in the inability to handle secretions and the drooling that is characteristic of this illness.	Management of epiglottitis is to keep the child as comfortable as possible to reduce anxiety, and preventing agitation and crying, which cause increased airway swelling. Supportive treatment can involve supplemental oxygen, antibiotics, and immediate medical evaluation and treatment to establish an artificial airway. The development of conjugated Hib vaccine has greatly reduced the incidence of these illnesses in children.
Parvovirus B19 and Fifth Disease	Parvovirus B19 is a common viral infection that is associated with several clinical diseases. The most common of these diseases is fifth disease, also known as *erythema infectiosum.* The incubation period for this disease is 4–14 days, but can range to 20 days. Parvovirus B19 is spread through respiratory droplets during coughing and sneezing. The virus can also be spread through blood and blood products. The most contagious period is when there are mild signs of "a cold" but the rash and joint pain has not yet appeared.	Fifth disease is caused by parvovirus B19.	This infection is asymptomatic in about 20% of cases. In those who are symptomatic, the initial symptoms are often a mild and benign fever, runny nose, and headache and upper respiratory symptoms. The symptoms mimic so many other illnesses it is often undiagnosed. However, there is a distinguishing rash that occurs in three phases. The initial face rash is referred to as a "slapped cheek" appearance and is characteristic of this disease. It is followed a few days later by a rash that often spreads to the trunk and extremities. There	Parvovirus usually resolves on its own without specific treatment. Intervention in this illness is symptomatic and supportive. Medications to relieve fever, headache, and joint pain are often given. Nonsteroidal anti-inflammatory drugs (NSAIDs) are often used. Topical medications to control itching and antihistamines are also used. Rest and fluids are encouraged.

cause of the stridor. In cases of epiglottitis, the immunization history of the child is extremely important in determining possible causes.

Continued

TABLE 39.2 NONIMMUNIZABLE COMMUNICABLE ILLNESSES OF CHILDHOOD—cont'd

Disease	Definition	Causative Agent	Clinical Presentation	Treatment
	 (Fifth disease)		is usually itching and joint pain with the rash. When the rash fades, it often appears as a classic lacelike pattern. The rash usually fades in about three weeks. The third stage of the rash may continue for weeks or months and may recur in response to environmental stimuli such as sunlight, heat, exercise, and stress.	
Mononucleosis	Although associated with some specific cancers in which there is a lymphoproliferative process, such as large cell lymphomas, Epstein-Barr virus (EBV) is most commonly associated with infectious mononucleosis. This illness is frequently referred to as the "kissing disease" because the virus is primarily spread through saliva.	Mononucleosis is caused by the EBV, a virus of the herpes family.	Many people exposed to infectious mononucleosis do not develop illness. The virus can exist in a latent state and someone with the virus not exhibiting illness can be a carrier. The illness primarily affects older children, adolescents, and young adults. Adolescents and young adults who are infected with EBV contract infectious mononucleosis 35%–50% of the time. The incubation period for this illness can be 4–6 weeks after exposure. Symptoms can develop suddenly or come on slowly. The acute phase of the illness can last 2–4 weeks. Fatigue is common with this	Most patients recover from infectious mononucleosis with symptomatic and supportive treatment. Rest, fluids, and NSAIDs for fever and pain are recommended for symptom management. Corticosteroids may be used in severe cases of swollen and enlarged lymph nodes that may occlude the airway, or cases that produce neurological or cardiac complications.

Continued

	illness and may persist for months after the acute illness has passed. The characteristic signs of mononucleosis are fever, sore throat, and swollen lymph nodes (ie, lymphadenopathy). The initial signs of the illness, usually fever, chills, loss of appetite, and malaise, are quickly followed by lymph node enlargement, splenomegaly, and tonsillopharyngitis with exudates. The nodes can be enlarged for several days to a period of several weeks.	
Tick-Borne Diseases include: • Lyme Disease • Rocky Mountain Spotted Fever (RMSF) • Southern Tick-Associated Rash Illness (STARI)	A number of vector-borne diseases present serious illness when transmitted to people. Worldwide it is estimated there are more than 850 tick species and at least 30 major tick-borne diseases. It is estimated that there are 10 major tick-borne diseases in the United States, with the most commonly known diseases being Lyme disease and RMSF. Tick-borne diseases are prevalent throughout the United States, usually in the spring and summer. While some diseases are found in certain geographic areas, some are prevalent throughout the United States. As populations move to previously uninhabited areas, tick-borne illnesses are an increasingly severe problem.	Tick-borne diseases can be viruses, bacteria, or parasites. Clinical presentation will vary depending on which specific tick-borne disease results. Treatment will vary based on the specific type of tick-borne disease.

TABLE 39.2 NONIMMUNIZABLE COMMUNICABLE ILLNESSES OF CHILDHOOD—cont'd

Disease	Definition	Causative Agent	Clinical Presentation	Treatment
Lyme Disease	Lyme disease is the most common vector-borne disease in the United States and one that has received much publicity. Although Lyme disease has been reported throughout the United States, the areas with the highest reported cases are New England, New York, New Jersey, Pennsylvania, Minnesota, and Wisconsin. A number of factors can influence whether someone will become infected with Lyme disease from a tick bite. Transmission of the bacteria will depend on how quickly the mouth part of the tick can implant (in this case, it takes hours), and how quickly it takes for the tick to become engorged with blood (in this case, days). Ticks must become engorged with blood before they can transfer the infecting organism to a host. This can take 48–72 hours. This is an important factor in understanding and preventing the transmission of disease. Inspection and removal of ticks after walking in wooded areas or areas where there may be tick exposure is the first line of defense in the prevention of illness.	Lyme disease is caused by a spirochete, *Borrelia burgdorferi*, a bacterium transmitted by the deer tick.	Lyme disease is an inflammatory illness that can affect joints and the nervous system. Clinically there are two different stages to the illness: *Early Stage:* The early stage of the disease is 7–14 days after the initial bite. A localized rash, called *erythema migrans*, originates at the site of the bite and expands as a solid red rash or as a central spot surrounded by a ringed red rash (resembles a bull's-eye). This rash then spreads to multiple areas of the skin. This usually occurs soon after the initial bite. Other symptoms include joint pain, headaches, fatigue, fever, chills, facial palsy, and a stiff and aching neck with swollen lymph glands. CDC (Lyme disease rash)	When caught and treated early, Lyme disease has a very good prognosis for children. Treatment is supportive, as well as the administration of amoxicillin or ceftriaxone antibiotics.

Late Disseminated Disease:
This phase of Lyme disease can occur months after the initial infection and usually involves arthritis (ie, pain and swelling) of large joints. Swelling can last 1 week up to several weeks. In this phase of illness there can be neurological involvement: disorientation, confusion, inability to concentrate, and aseptic meningitis. Numbness of the hands and feet are often present. Fatigue and joint and muscle pain can persist for weeks or months after treatment has been completed for acute illness.

Rocky Mountain Spotted Fever (RMSF)	RMSF is also known as tick-borne typhus. The infection can occur via a bite from the Rocky Mountain wood tick or the dog tick. It is the second most common tick-borne illness in the United States. The disease is only in the western hemisphere and is prevalent in the southeastern United States, although it can be found throughout most states in the country. Over 50% of cases are diagnosed from April–September in states such as Delaware, Maryland, Washington, D.C., Virginia, West Virginia, North Carolina, Missouri, and Oklahoma. Like other tick-transmitted diseases, the	RMSF is a bacterial illness caused by *Rickettsia rickettsii*. RMSF is a serious, sometimes fatal disease, if not treated correctly in the first 8 days of illness.	Initial symptoms are often headache, malaise, and muscle pain. The symptoms of RMSF often worsen with the abrupt onset of chills and fever. Other symptoms may involve a rash 2–5 days after the fever. This begins as maculopapular rash, but within 1–3 days becomes hemorrhagic. Other symptoms of RMSF include headache, nausea and vomiting, abdominal pain, muscle pain, loss of appetite, and reddened eyes. The damage caused by the organism also affects the skin, CNS, heart, lungs, liver, and kidney, as well as larger blood vessels as they become occluded. Vascular occlusion	RMSF can be treated with antibiotics. Tetracycline, doxycycline, and chloramphenicol are the most frequently used drugs. Prognosis is relatively good in patients who are treated within 4 days of the onset of symptoms. Treatment of RMSF often requires hospitalization and time-intensive care for treatment of DIC and other multi-system complications of the illness.

Continued

TABLE **39.2**   NONIMMUNIZABLE COMMUNICABLE ILLNESSES OF CHILDHOOD—cont'd

Disease	Definition	Causative Agent	Clinical Presentation	Treatment
	bacteria from the tick may not be transmitted for 48–72 hours after a tick has implanted; the tick has to engorge with blood before transferring the bacteria, so surveillance and removal of ticks is the best prevention of the illness. The organism multiplies in the endothelium and smooth muscles, causing damage to cells and blood vessels, resulting in occlusion of small blood vessels. Coagulopathies develop and disseminated intravascular coagulation (DIC) has been associated with the illness. The incubation period for RMSF is usually 5–7 days.		leads to necrosis and gangrene of digits and areas of distal perfusion.	
Southern Tick-Associated Rash Illness (STARI)	One of the newest tick-borne diseases identified in the United States is STARI.	The tick responsible for transmission is the lone star tick. The lone star tick is common in southern states, as well as on the East Coast up to Maine.	The symptoms of the disease are similar to those observed in Lyme disease, although it is not known what the infectious organism is that is responsible for the illness.	STARI symptoms are similar to Lyme disease and respond well to a treatment program similar to one used to treat Lyme disease.
Tuberculosis (TB)	TB is a highly contagious airborne droplet bacterial infection spread from person to person through coughing, sneezing, singing, or heavy breathing. The droplets can remain suspended in the air for hours and masks and respiratory isolation precautions are needed to prevent transmission of the bacteria.	TB is caused by the bacteria *Mycobacterium tuberculosis.* A single sneeze can release up to 40,000 droplets. Each one of these droplets may transmit the disease, since the infectious dose of TB is very low.	Once in the body, the organism multiplies and creates an inflammatory exudate. The bacilli are then carried through the local lymphatic system to the nearest group of lymph nodes. The incubation period between the introduction of the bacilli and the development of delayed hypersensitivity is usually	After confirmation of a TB infection by positive skin test, sputum analysis, chest x-ray, identification of associated symptoms, and/or a positive TB blood test, the child is treated for 6–9 months with one of several anti-TB medications such as the isoniazid-rifapentine regimen. (Search the CDC

TB is a worldwide problem and pediatric TB is particularly challenging to diagnose; the disease in the pediatric population clinically differs from adults in significant ways. Pediatric cases of TB occur most frequently in children less than 5 years and in children older than 10 years. Clinically the symptoms of TB present quite differently than adults. Young children are less likely to produce sputum and have a forceful enough cough to be as infectious as adults.

About 50% of infants and children have no physical findings and are diagnosed only when traced through an adult they are in contact with who is suspected to have TB. Older children and adolescents often will show signs and symptoms resembling those of adults, such as fever, night sweats, anorexia, and decreased activity. Infants will often show signs of failure to thrive or poor weight gain. Some infants and children will show signs of wheezing or respiratory distress. Young children, for a number of reasons, are generally considered to be less infectious than adults. In addition to the fact that there are fewer organisms in the pulmonary secretions of children, they do not produce sputum in quantities and with the force necessary to be infectious.

3–12 weeks. The changes to the lung happen mostly at a microscopic level; it can become "calcified" and walled off. Some children will have a febrile illness, mild cough, and respiratory symptoms for 1–3 weeks when the hypersensitivity first develops. Other symptoms of a TB infection include weight loss, lethargy, failure to thrive, night sweats, and prolonged fevers.

Web site for information about populations to gather information about the most current TB treatment in children.)

Continued

TABLE 39.2 NONIMMUNIZABLE COMMUNICABLE ILLNESSES OF CHILDHOOD—cont'd

Disease	Definition	Causative Agent	Clinical Presentation	Treatment
	The age of the child is one of the most important factors in determining whether a TB infection will actually progress to disease. The symptoms and severity of the illness depends largely on the age of the patient when infected and their immune status. Children less than 5 years make up 60%–75% of pediatric cases of TB in the United States. TB infection usually begins in the lungs, although the bacilli can be transmitted less frequently by oral ingestion or direct contact with infected body fluids such as urine, nasal secretions, or sputum. Not everyone infected with TB is symptomatic or develops the disease. Two TB conditions exist: *Latent TB Infection:* A person with latent TB is asymptomatic and noninfectious. They will have a positive skin test but will not spread the bacteria to others. Children with latent TB will often be treated to prevent them from developing active disease. *Active TB Disease:* Someone with active TB will have a			

Continued

positive skin test, become sick from the bacteria actively multiplying, and have active symptoms. Active TB requires treatment. When infants and young children contract TB, they are more likely to develop TB disease and develop life-threatening forms of the illness such as disseminated TB and TB meningitis.

| Cytomegalovirus (CMV) | CMV is a common viral infection, although most with an infection will not know they have the virus because of the lack of symptoms associated with it. Some health-care providers call a CMV infection a silent infection because rarely does one show clinical signs or symptoms. Once infected, the body retains the virus for life. If a child becomes immunocompromised (eg, cancer, HIV, weakened immune system, transplant recipients) then the concern is that the child will develop a CMV infection. There is no vaccine for CMV, but clinical trials on a vaccine continue. | CMV is a virus that is spread through blood, saliva, semen, urine, breast milk, and body fluids. A fetus can acquire CMV through transmission during pregnancy. Newborns will not show CMV (ie, it is undetected) until they are 2–3 weeks old. | There is no treatment or cure known for a CMV infection. If immunocompromised, the child should be treated with immunoglobulin to decrease the chance of a CMV infection. |

TABLE 39.2 NONIMMUNIZABLE COMMUNICABLE ILLNESSES OF CHILDHOOD—cont'd

Disease	Definition	Causative Agent	Clinical Presentation	Treatment
Human Immunodeficiency Virus (HIV)	The vast majority of children who are infected with HIV have become so via pregnancy (ie, vertical transmission), childbirth, or exposure to breast milk of an infected adult. Further modes of transmission include IV drug use, sexual activity, or administration of infected blood products. Detecting HIV in newborns is not considered accurate because antibody tests reflect maternal antibodies for up to 18 months, not the infant's. The most accurate window of time for diagnosis is after 3 months, through the use of HIV viral cultures and a nucleic acid test (NAT). Virological assay for HIV via the bDNA polymerase chain reaction (PCR) and HIV RNA assay tests are recommended for confirmation.	HIV is a lentivirus that replicates via RNA strands. There are HIV subtypes such as HIV type 1 and 2, and HIV subgroups. The HIV virus spreads through the body via fluids and affects specific immune cells.	Clinical presentation of HIV is based on the development of associated conditions, infections, and cancers that are caused by the immunocompromised state of the HIV-infected child. Signs and symptoms of HIV infection in the pediatric population include severe fungal (eg, thrush), bacterial (eg, severe otitis media [OM], pneumonias), or viral infections (eg, CMV retinitis, zoster infections). Wasting syndromes, failure to thrive, and delayed developmental and motor milestones are not uncommon.	There is no cure or treatment for HIV. There is no vaccine for HIV. HIV-associated infections are treated as needed. Antiretroviral medications are administered to children and are based on the child's CD4 cell count. Monitoring a child's immune status should be done by regular analysis of the CD4 T lymphocyte cell count. Typically, a child is placed on one or more of the following pediatric antiretroviral drugs: nucleoside analogue reverse transcriptase inhibitors; nonnucleoside analogue reverse transcriptase inhibitors; protease inhibitors; and/or integrase strand transfer inhibitors (NIH, 2015). Nephrotic toxicity and CNS toxicity are both concerns with HIV antiretroviral medications.

| Clostridium Difficile | *C diff.* is a bacterium that causes severe inflammation of the child's colon called *colitis*. It is very easy to transmit the bacteria to others who touch contaminated surfaces or items touched by the child. This includes food trays, bed or crib rails, toilets and bathroom fixtures, doorknobs, vital sign equipment, and toys. Any item that is contaminated with feces has the potential to cause infection in others. Diapered young children are at particular risk for transmitting the bacteria to others. Fecal/oral routes transmit the bacteria between people. Health-care providers who do not participate in strict hand washing techniques, or have contaminated uniforms, can easily pass the bacteria to other patients. | *C diff.* is a spore-forming, gram-positive, anaerobic bacillus that produces two endotoxins: toxin A and toxin B. | A child with a *C diff.* infection might present with a history of copious watery diarrhea, with or without blood. Fever, abdominal pain, cramps, or tenderness is common; loss of appetite, nausea, and vomiting can all occur. Diseases that can result from a *C diff.* infection include toxic megacolon, sepsis, pseudomembranous colitis (PMC) and rarely, death (CDC, 2015). | Antibiotics are administered to treat a *C diff.* infection. Vancomycin, metronidazole (needs 10-day course of oral treatment, used for mild cases only), and fidaxomicin are approved to treat *C diff.* In 20% of cases, the infection returns after the antibiotic course is complete (CDC, 2015). All staff providing care for the child must ensure meticulous hand washing. House cleaning staff must make sure all contact areas are cleansed for *C diff.* per protocol. This communicable disease situation is very serious and requires contact precautions. Some institutions use the phrase "expanded contact precautions" for *C diff.* because the bacterium is resistant to alcohol-based hand gels and some cleaning products. Hand washing is required! Hospitalized patients are particularly vulnerable to acquire a *C diff.* infection and can become very sick. *C diff.* infections are considered one of the most serious health-care complications, causing diarrhea, dehydration, malnutrition, increased patient frailty, and increased mortality (ie, death). |

Key Points

- During the childhood developmental period, children are at risk for developing common infections such as the cold virus, respiratory syncytial virus (RSV), and strep throat. Other less-commonly encountered childhood infectious diseases such as measles, mumps, and pertussis place children at risk for severe complications.
- Childhood immunizations are an important and life-saving part of a comprehensive health promotion and disease prevention program for children.
- There is no medication or immunization that is 100% guaranteed to be without risks and side effects. The best a pediatric health-care professional can do is rely on available medical research and continue to study the efficacy and safety of vaccines.
- Using reputable Web site such as the CDC and the National Institutes of Health (NIH) to find information about childhood vaccines is an important part of being an informed pediatric nurse. Learning about both illnesses that have vaccines and those that do not is important for rapid identification of infectious processes, rapid treatments, and rapid infection control procedures.
- Childhood infectious diseases covered by a complete vaccine schedule include varicella, measles, mumps, rubella, polio, hepatitis B, diphtheria, pertussis, tetanus, pneumococcus, hepatitis A, Hib, and rotavirus.
- Because immunization schedules change according to public need, it is important to review the recommended schedule of childhood immunizations on a regular basis.

- While the risks of immunizations are present, the risks of contracting vaccine preventable illnesses cannot be underestimated. Many illnesses, such as polio or smallpox, are no longer common because of vaccination programs. The effectiveness of vaccines in eradicating or reducing the incidence of illness may cause parents to falsely believe they do not need to immunize for these serious, sometimes fatal diseases.
- Even vaccine-preventable illnesses that are not typically fatal can have severe consequences if there is a delay or failure in receiving vaccinations. Outbreaks of measles or chickenpox can be a health emergency in institutions such as hospitals or with vulnerable populations such as pregnant women or immunocompromised children.
- Outbreaks such as these in local schools may result in extended absences from school and activities and require parents to take time from work to care for children who need to stay at home.
- Health-care professionals working with children with actual or suspected childhood infectious diseases must participate in use of PPE, infection control precautions, and isolation as needed. Infection control precautions include standard, airborne, droplet, contact, expanded contact, and protective precaution, which is also referred to as reverse or *neutropenic precautions*.
- Severe reactions are rare but sometimes do occur with childhood immunizations. It is important that pediatric nurses understand the need to report serious reactions to the VAERS.

REVIEW QUESTIONS

1. Vaccines are able to produce a desired effect of increasing a child's antibodies to protect him or her from infection if the child is exposed to a communicable disease. How would the nurse describe the effectiveness of childhood vaccines?
   1. They are considered 100% effective in protecting children across the developmental period.
   2. They are only effective if started in infancy and the entire immunization schedule is followed exactly as recommended.
   3. They cannot be "caught up" if doses are missed.
   4. They are useful in the prevention of childhood communicable diseases but are not always 100% effective.

2. What is one difference between the use of the terms *enteric contact precautions* and *contact precautions?*
   1. Enteric precautions refer to PPE and behaviors used to prevent the spread of diarrhea.
   2. Contact precautions are used exclusively for diapered infants who present with diarrhea.
   3. There is no difference between contact precautions and enteric precautions.
   4. Contact precautions are used when there is a likelihood of infection transmission through direct or indirect contact with a patient or his or her care items.

3. While talking to a father of a child who has been admitted for IV antibiotics for methicillin-resistant *Staphylococcus aureus* (MRSA)–positive pneumonia, the father asks about the term *incubation period.* Your reply that:
   1. The incubation period relates to the severity of the illness presented by the child.
   2. The incubation period is the time between exposure to the infection and the first symptoms.
   3. The incubation period is the process of growing the child's blood culture sample.
   4. The incubation period is the time between first exposure and recovery.

4. The anatomical site used for an injection of the hepatitis B vaccine would be:
   1. Abdomen
   2. Deltoid
   3. Gluteal region
   4. Vastus lateralis

5. While providing anticipatory guidance to family of a 9-month-old, the immunization record should demonstrate that the child has received which of the following:
   1. Hepatitis B series only
   2. Measles, mumps and rubella (MMR), diphtheria, tetanus, and pertussis (DTP), and PCV
   3. Measles, mumps, and rubella (MMR), hepatitis B, and Hib
   4. Hepatitis B, diphtheria, tetanus, and pertussis (DTP), Hib, IPV, and PCV

6. Childhood immunizations pose risks. One risk is the development of an allergic reaction. If suspected, allergic reactions will prevent a child from receiving further childhood immunizations.
   1. True
   2. False

7. Although there is no treatment for an HPV infection, there are treatments for complications associated with HPV. Complications include: *(select all that apply)*
   1. Genital warts
   2. Abnormal Pap smears
   3. Encephalopathy
   4. Liver cancer
   5. Hepatitis

8. Attending kindergarten is an important milestone for a young child. Which immunizations, if all prior immunizations are complete, would be needed for a 5-year-old attending kindergarten?
   1. MMR, IPV, and DTP
   2. Hib and DTP
   3. Hepatitis B
   4. Pertussis vaccine

9. Active immunity is obtained by either exposure to a bacterium, virus, or toxin sufficient to stimulate an immune response by the body, or stimulating the body's immune response through vaccination or immunization.
   1. True
   2. False

10. Current science has not found a link between thimerosal and autism, or any serious harm.
    1. True
    2. False

CRITICAL THINKING QUESTIONS

1. How are school-aged children exposed to communicable diseases?
2. What behaviors of preschool children make them at particular risk for communicable diseases? What are common communicable childhood infectious and diseases during the early school-aged child's developmental period?
3. Using the principles of anticipatory guidance, list common means parents can take to reduce the spread of communicable diseases and infections in their children.

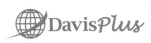 For additional resources and information, visit **www.DavisPlus.com.** Post-Conference Questions and Activities, Answers, and References can be found on DavisPlus.

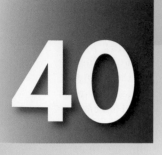

40

Child With an Oncological or Hematological Condition

KEY TERMS

hemophilias
induction
kernicterus
leukemia
maintenance therapy
neutropenia
petechiae
purpura
sickle cell anemia (SCA)
stomatitis
thrombocytopenia
vaso-occlusive episode

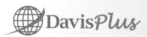
For audio pronunciation guide, visit www.DavisPlus.com

CHAPTER CONCEPTS

Cellular Regulation
Comfort
Communication
Development
Infection
Promoting Health
Safety

LEARNING OUTCOMES

1. Define the key terms.
2. Describe the characteristics of childhood cancer, including the pathology of solid and blood/lymphatic-based malignancies.
3. Describe the composition and function of the components of blood and relate each function to the pathology of hematological and oncological diseases.
4. Analyze the pathology of anemias and relate types of anemia with an anemic child's clinical presentation.
5. State the assessments conducted for a child who presents with iron-deficiency anemia and SCA and describe the required medical and nursing care for each.
6. Review the developmentally appropriate pain scales used for a child during a sickle cell episode (ie, crisis) and review effective pain control measures.
7. Review the nursing care required for a child who is receiving a blood product transfusion: packed red blood cells (PRBCs) and platelets.
8. Differentiate the types and pathology of hyperbilirubinemia, as well as medical care and nursing care for an infant with hyperbilirubinemia.
9. Describe the pathology of idiopathic thrombocytopenia purpura (ITP) and treatment protocols administered across childhood.
10. Analyze the most common forms of hemophilia and describe the teaching needs of families to administer emergency treatments for a child experiencing a bleeding episode.
11. Review the effect of childhood cancer on the functioning and teaching needs of the family caring for a child who is hospitalized for treatments or is home in a neutropenic state.
12. Analyze the issues of safety associated with a child with an oncology disorder, including error reduction, protection from infection, and safe implementation of care.

REAL-WORLD CASE STUDY

Katrina

■ Two-year-old Katrina has been admitted to the pediatric intensive care unit (PICU) for blood transfusions for severe anemia. Her presenting hemoglobin was 4.1 g/dL. She had seen her pediatrician the day before admission for fatigue and pale skin color. The pediatrician drew her laboratory values and determined the severity of her clinical presentation. She was sent to the hospital for a direct admit to the PICU for transfusion therapy and nutrition education. She received two transfusions: the first was 6 mL/kg of packed red blood cells (PRBCs) and the second was 10 mL/kg. She received her transfusions over a course of 6 hours and then demonstrated a rise in hemoglobin to 7.3 g/dL. The etiology of her anemia was determined to be nutritionally based as she continued to take bottles of whole milk throughout the day and evening. Her parents met with the dietician for a long session of teaching on iron-rich foods and she was given a discharge prescription for oral iron supplements.

1. What symptoms would the pediatric nurse expect to find upon admission to the PICU for this severely anemic child?
2. What information should be included in teaching the family about administering oral iron supplements?

CONCEPTUAL CORNERSTONE

Cellular Regulation

Cellular regulation is different for cancer cells than it is for noncancerous cells. Cancer cells do not stop dividing, do not have contact inhibition, and do not perform the original function of the cell. The prolific growth of cancer cells causes the development of childhood cancer. There are 250 different types of childhood cancers in two major categories: solid tumors and bloodborne malignancies. The experience of abnormal cellular regulation leading to the development of cancer causes a variety of symptoms. Nursing care measures include using developmentally appropriate pain assessment tools, providing pharmaceutical and nonpharmaceutical symptom management, and re-evaluating the success of symptom control measures.

Nursing care of children who have an oncological disease (ie, cancer) or a hematological disease (ie, anemia or a blood disease) requires a specific body of knowledge and skill set. The diagnosis of a hematological/oncological condition carries with it the potential for great emotional distress for each member of the family, and yet, the majority of childhood cancers are curable. Rapid diagnosis and timely therapy helps to ensure an optimal chance of a cure. A thorough search for metastatic diseases most often precedes biopsies of suspicious lesions. Histological evaluation of suspected cancer cells allows for the selection of the most appropriate therapies.

Families experiencing both a new diagnosis, as well as ongoing care of a child with a hematological/oncological condition, must learn specific skills to care for their children to prevent what can be life-threatening side effects of treatment or complications of the disease process. This chapter will review the foundations of care required to manage the complexities associated with a diagnosis of childhood cancer, anemias, and hyperbilirubinemia.

INTRODUCTION TO HEMATOLOGICAL CONDITIONS

Caring for a child diagnosed with a blood disorder requires a knowledge base of the composition and function of blood. The capacity of the blood to carry oxygen, fluids, and nutrients, and to collect and transport waste products, becomes interrupted when a child has a condition of the hematological system. Reviewing the normal physiology of the blood system and the function of each component allows the nurse to understand and expect the clinical presentation of the child.

THE DEVELOPMENT OF THE HEMATOLOGICAL SYSTEM AND HEMATOLOGICAL ABNORMALITIES

The development of the hematological system begins early in fetal development and continues to mature throughout early childhood. The content in this section describes the composition of the essential cellular components of the blood, and the fluid portion that provides nutrients and fluids to the body.

The Composition and Function of Blood

The plasma portion of the blood is made up of about 10% solutes and 90% water. The main plasma solutes are albumin, proteins, and electrolytes. These proteins include circulating antibodies, fibrinogen, globulins, and clotting factors. The cellular elements of blood are the white blood cells (WBCs), the red blood cells (RBCs), and the thrombocytes, which produce platelets. All of the formed elements of the blood are thought to originate from the primitive cell called the *stem cell.*

The major organ for the formation of blood is the hematopoietic system found within the bone marrow (ie, myeloid tissue) and lymphatic system (Fig. 40.1). The lymphatic system consists of several components, including the lymphatic vessels, which carry lymph fluid and the lymphoid solid structures of the lymph nodes. The solid structures include the spleen, the thymus, and the tonsils.

Blood contains RBCs, called *erythrocytes;* and white bloods cells, which include neutrophils, eosinophils, basophils, T lymphocytes, and B-lymphocytic plasma cells. All have distinct functions to assist in the maintenance of homeostasis

Cells of the Immune System

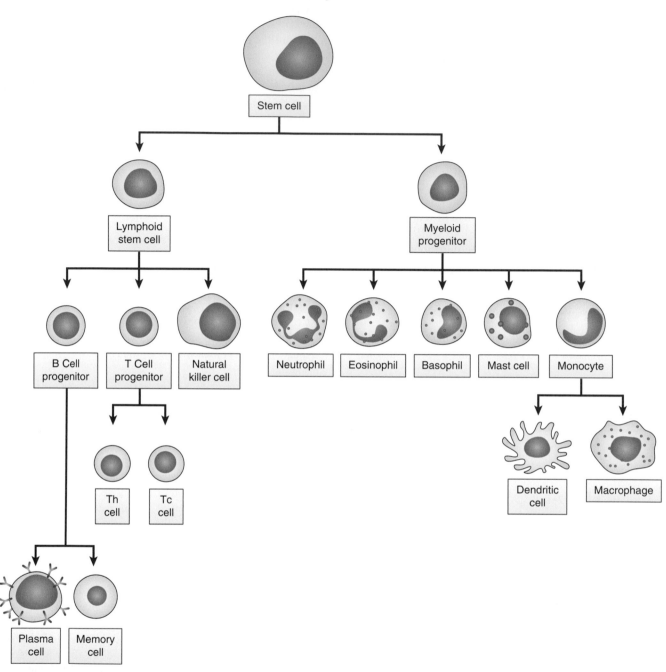

FIGURE 40.1 Bone marrow cells.

within the child's hematological system. See Table 40.1 for information on a complete blood cell count (CBC).

The functions of the components of blood are as follows:

• **Oxygenation:** RBCs contain hemoglobin molecules that attach and release oxygen. The transportation of oxygen to all tissues of the body is essential to provide the foundation of cellular metabolism. When a child presents in a state of anemia, the transportation and release of oxygen throughout the body is compromised.

• **Cellular nutrition:** Blood plasma carries all the essential nutrients for cellular metabolism. Disruptions in

the volume of blood diminish the body's ability to distribute proteins, vitamins, electrolytes, water, and nutrients.

• **Excretion of wastes:** Cellular waste products are collected by the blood and transported to the liver for processing and the kidneys for excretion.

• **Maintenance of acid-base balance:** The vascular system carries bicarbonate concentrated from the kidneys to assist in the balance of pH in the blood.

• **Regulation of body temperature:** Blood circulating through the vascular system distributes and helps to maintain a normal body temperature.

TABLE **40.1** INTERPRETING A COMPLETE BLOOD CELL COUNT WITH A MANUAL DIFFERENTIATION

Cell Component	Function	Expected Values
White Blood Cell	Infection-fighting cell	4,500–11,000 K/uL
RBC	Oxygen-carrying capacity	4.2–5.0 M/uL
Hemoglobin	Molecule to attach oxygen	2 months: 9.0–14.0 g/dL 6–12 years: 11.5-15.5 g/dL
Hematocrit	Percentage of RBCs in blood	< 2 months: 28%–42% 2 months–6 years: 36%–47% 6–12 years: 35%–45%
Reticulocytes	Newly formed RBCs	3.8–5.5 million/mL or 0.5%–2.5% of total number of RBCs
Mean corpuscular volume (MCV)	Average volume or size of RBC	Range from 80–95 fL
Mean corpuscular hemoglobin (MCH)	Average hemoglobin level per cell	Divide hemoglobin by number of RBCs
Segmented neutrophils	Mature infection-fighting cell	15%–32% across childhood
Bands	Immature infection-fighting cell	5%–16% across childhood
Lymphocytes	Immunoglobulin production/delayed hypersensitive reaction	26%–76%
Absolute neutrophil count (ANC)	Determines ability to fight infection	1,500 to 8,000/mm³

- **Defense against foreign antigens:** Blood provides the distribution of immune cells and immunoglobulins to areas of the body experiencing infection.
- **Transport of hormones:** Hormones manufactured in the endocrine glands throughout the body are transported to target cells by circulating blood.

Red Blood Cells

RBCs live about 120 days. After that time, the cell grows old and its cell wall membranes become fragile and rupture. The hemoglobin found within the RBC is then broken down into two components: (1) the hemosiderin (ie, iron), which is recycled, and (2) the bilirubin, which must be processed and excreted in bile. When the body sends a message to the kidneys that there is hypoxia (ie, a state of reduced oxygen), the kidneys produce the hormone erythropoietin, which regulates the production of new RBCs in the bone marrow. This process produces a rise in newly formed RBCs, called *reticulocytes*. The main purpose of the RBC is to transport hemoglobin molecules, which carry oxygen to the cells of the body. Effective oxygen transport is dependent on adequate numbers of circulating RBCs and the amount of hemoglobin found within the RBC. The term *hematocrit* refers to the measurement of the percentage of circulating RBCs within the blood and gives a clinical picture of the severity of certain

anemias. The percentage of the child's hematocrit is about three times that of the total concentration of hemoglobin (in g/dL).

White Blood Cells

WBCs provide the child the ability to launch a response to the presence of an infection. Neutrophils, the most prolific of the WBCs, are considered the primary defense in bacterial infections. After killing the bacteria, the neutrophils then consume (ie, phagocytize) and transport the bacterial cell components to be eliminated. Monocytes are large phagocytic cells involved with an early inflammatory reaction. Lymphocytes provide the body with the production of antibodies and a delayed hypersensitivity response. There are two types of lymphocytes: (1) the T cells, which must circulate through the thymus gland to become mature and then circulate to become sensitized to specific antigens, and (2) the B cells, whose main function is to synthesize and secrete antibodies in response to specific antigens. Some T cells are called "killer" cells because they have the unique ability to produce chemical compounds that are lethal to microbes; they are also called "helper" cells because they assist in a more complex system of the major fight against foreign proteins and microbes. T cells have a very significant role in the body's fight against the presence of cancer cells.

Thrombocytes

Platelets are small pieces of a thrombocyte's cell wall. Their primary function is to assist with clotting. Platelets will adhere to the endothelium lining of the vasculature to form clots (ie, a type of plug) to manage bleeding. Additionally, platelets have two unique properties: (1) they secrete chemicals that then attract other platelets to the damaged cellular site, and, (2) they secrete serotonin, a substance that causes vasoconstriction to prevent further bleeding at the site of injury.

Anemias

Anemias are defined as conditions or diseases that reduce the total circulating hemoglobin within the blood. This reduced hemoglobin then minimizes the body's ability to circulate oxygen to all tissues, including organs and muscles. A reduced oxygen-carrying capacity causes complications in growth, cellular repair, and overall homeostasis. Anemia can be categorized in six ways:

1. Impaired production of hemoglobin or impaired or decreased production of RBCs
2. Nutritional deficiency that impairs the production of RBCs
3. Metabolic condition that causes disturbances of production, including nutritional disorders
4. Increased destruction of erythrocytes
5. Impaired or decreased rate of production of the hormone erythropoietin
6. Excessive blood loss

Clinical manifestations of anemia will depend on the cause of the anemia and the severity of the reduced circulating RBCs. The following are clinical signs and symptoms of anemia:

- **Changes in behavior:** Irritability, fatigue, and reduced play
- **Skin:** Pallor, ulcers, and **petechiae** (ie, very small hemorrhagic purplish spots found on the child's skin when the child's platelets are also low), ecchymoses, and jaundice rashes
- **Cardiopulmonary:** Dizziness, dyspnea, edema, and palpitations
- **Gastrointestinal:** Bleeding, diarrhea, vomiting, anorexia, and melena
- **Genitourinary:** Urinary frequency, and hematuria
- **Nervous system:** Syncope, parenthesis, seizures, decreased mental concentration, and loss of consciousness
- **Endocrine:** Polyphagia, polydipsia, polyuria, and temperature intolerance
- **Eyes, ears, nose, mouth, and head:** Diplopia, visual blurring, cataracts, sclera jaundice, tinnitus, vertigo, epistaxis, **stomatitis** (ie, a state of inflammation of the mouth, often painful), bleeding gums, buccal mucosa ulcerations, and texture changes on tongue

Assessments of Anemias

Children who present with anemia need to have an assessment performed by members of the health-care team who focus on the etiology and the clinical presentation of the disorder. The following list notes aspects that should direct the physical assessment of the child:

- Diet history, especially an assessment of the diversity of food intake and the quantity of milk consumed daily
- General performance status, concentration, level of mental activity, complaints of weakness, exercise, and play intolerance
- General appearance, including height, weight, and rate of physical growth
- Blood values, including a CBC with differentiation of cell lines and peripheral smear to identify abnormal cell morphology
- Urine, emesis, and stool checks for blood
- Skin pallor from tissue hypoxia
- Jaundice and color of nail beds, mucous membranes
- Vital signs (VS), assessing for an increased heart rate (HR), respiratory rate (RR), increased pulsations, heart murmurs, and an assessment of orthostatic hypotension

Interventions for Anemias

Nursing care of the child with anemia includes protecting the child from injury. The child may require oxygen therapy if anemia is severe and the hypoxia is causing difficulty in breathing. The child will need a quiet environment with choices of quiet play activities that continue to promote social, physical, and cognitive development. The child will need to have structured rest periods and naps if developmentally appropriate. A nutritionist should be notified and a referral made for a dietary assessment and a family teaching session, and for the development of a nutritional plan. The child may require blood transfusions if anemia is severe. The family will need education about the need for oxygen therapy and the need to save energy and decrease fatigue. The family will also need to understand the frequency of phlebotomy to check the status of the child's anemia, and the care, benefits, and risks associated with transfusion therapy.

Medical care depends on the type and cause of the anemia. The child may require several medical interventions, including iron therapy, oxygen therapy, transfusion therapy, and frequent follow-up appointments.

Further laboratory assessments and diagnostic studies for anemia may include:

- **Direct Coombs' test** for the presence of antibodies attached to the RBC that cause hemolysis
- **Ferritin** to assess the major iron storage protein (will be decreased in iron deficiency anemia)
- **Serum iron** to measure the amount of iron bound to transferrin
- **Lead levels** to determine if the cause of the anemia is related to lead poisoning
- **Osmotic fragility,** which is associated with hereditary spherocytosis

- **Hemoglobin electrophoresis** to determine which specific type of hemoglobin is reduced if the child has a hemoglobinopathy

Transfusion Therapy

Blood product support is often a cornerstone of hematology and oncology therapy. Many treatments to cure cancer produce periods of severe chemotherapy-induced anemia. Children with **sickle cell anemia (SCA)** require blood product support to optimize the recovery of a sickle cell crisis (ie, episode). RBC deficiency can result from the side effects of medications, an increased loss, or decreased production. The indication for blood product therapy is to restore volume, minimize bleeding, correct coagulopathies, replace plasma proteins, or improve the child's oxygen-carrying capacity.

Sources of Blood Product Therapy

The administration of blood products may be required for a child with a severe anemia. The most commonly administered blood product is PRBC, in which most of the serum and WBCs have been removed. Each transfused product is different and has unique properties. Transfused products and considerations for each are listed below:

- **Whole blood:** Rarely given because of the chance of severe reactions, whole blood is transfused for traumas in which massive volume is lost or sometimes used for blood exchange transfusions. Child and donor blood must be matched for ABO and Rh-compatibility.
- **PRBCs:** These are most commonly used for the improvement of oxygen-carrying capacity. The volume guidelines demonstrate that for every 10–15 mL/kg transfused, an expected rise of hemoglobin is 3 g/dL. Transfusion time should be 3 hours per single transfusion. Filters are required.
- **Platelets:** These are transfused when a child's count is below 20,000/mm^3 or if there is evidence of bleeding. Single donor infusions are preferred as they decrease the exposure to foreign proteins. A single unit should raise the overall platelet count by 10,000/mm^3. Although cross-matching is not required, ABO and Rh-compatible platelets are preferred. The length of the transfusion is as fast as the child can tolerate it.
- **Granulocytes:** These transfusions are rarely performed because of the chances of severe reactions and are saved for children who are experiencing severe neutropenia with documented and resistant infections. Single donor granulocytes are required.
- **Fresh-frozen plasma:** This is transfused to provide a source of stable coagulation factors such as fibrinogen and factor IX (ie, stable), and factor V and factor IX (ie, unstable).

SAFETY *STAT!*

Whole blood transfusion has more side effects than PRBCs because all of the products of the blood remain and can cause a variety of mild to life-threatening side effects.

Because of the potential frequency of transfusion therapy for children with hematological or oncological conditions, it is important to provide components with the following special preparations:

- Irradiated blood products to prevent graft-versus-host disease (GVHD)
- Leukocyte-depleted products for all children with cancer or those who experience repeated febrile reactions
- Cytomegalovirus (CMV)-negative components; ensuring that transfused products are not infected by this virus diminishes the potential of the child becoming infected

Potential Complications of Transfusion Therapy

Children receiving transfusion therapies need to be carefully monitored for side effects and complications. It is imperative that the nursing care team immediately respond to and report on any suspected or actual adverse reaction to transfusion therapy. Various side effects and complications, including how each is treated, include the following:

- **Febrile responses** are manifested by chills, flushing, headache, chest pain, muscle pain, and elevated temperatures. Acetaminophen administration is given to prevent or treat febrile reactions.
- **Urticaria responses** produce hives and itching. Diphenhydramine is given to reduce this reaction. Without treatment, the child may experience wheezing, dyspnea, and respiratory distress.
- **Hemolytic responses** can occur when alloimmunization has taken place. In alloimmunization, the more transfusions the child is exposed to, the greater numbers of antibodies are formed against the transfused foreign proteins. Matching the recipient to the donor decreases the severity of alloimmunization, thus reducing the chances of more and more severe hemolytic reactions.
- **Septic shock** can occur on the rare occasions when the transfused product is contaminated with a type of bacteria that flourishes in cold temperatures such as cold product storage. This type of microbe is called a *halophil.*
- **Circulatory overload** can occur when the total volume of the transfused unit adds volume to the child's vascular space. Transfusions can affect the total vascular volume, potentially causing symptoms of circulatory overload. Symptoms of circulatory overload include hypotension, bradycardia or tachycardia, and cyanosis.

SAFETY *STAT!*

Alloimmunization (ie, antibodies against the blood product are produced) is a sensitization toward transfused foreign protein antigens and is often manifested by fevers. These antigens are found on all components of blood. If alloimmunization takes place, leukocyte depletion of the transfused product is essential. For example, leukocyte-depleted PRBCs would be required for a child who has been exposed previously to transfused products that then lead to alloimmunization.

Nursing Care for Transfusion Therapy

The following steps, in order, provide guidance for the transfusion of blood products.

1. Assess the child's previous transfusion history to anticipate a potential transfusion reaction.
2. Assess the child's laboratory values to confirm the need for a transfusion.
3. Ensure a blood product transfusion consent is signed and in the chart.
4. Assess the child's pretransfusion status, including VS and lung sounds.
5. Assess the need to administer a premedication such as acetaminophen (Tylenol) or diphenhydramine (Benadryl).
6. Verify the physician's precise transfusion order for the type of product and special processing (eg, CMV-negative, irradiated, or leukocyte-depleted components), premedications, filters, and rate/volume. Blood may be ordered as a dose, such as 10 to 15 mL/kg of PRBCs.
7. Reduce errors by making sure the unit is double-checked by two registered nurses (RNs) at the bedside using at least two personal identifiers. These include the patient's name, medical record number, and birthday.
8. Before spiking and hanging the bag, double-check the correct unit by the following:
   • Type of product ordered
   • Special processing or handling
   • Rh type
   • Blood group
   • Medical record number and patient's name
   • Expiration date
   • Unit number
   • Lot number (if provided)
9. Hang the unit only with a 0.9% sterile normal saline IV bag.
10. Monitor the child throughout the transfusion, carefully following institutional policy. The child should be carefully monitored for the first 15 min with VS checks because this is the time period of 90% of all transfusion reactions.
11. Send the tubing, transfused product bag, and normal saline bag all together to the blood bank if a transfusion reaction is suspected.
12. Document carefully all aspects of the transfusion.

SAFETY STAT!

The two medications that members of the pediatric health-care team should have immediate access to if a transfusion reaction is suspected are diphenhydramine and epinephrine.

HEALTH HISTORY AND PHYSICAL ASSESSMENT

It is imperative that the health-care team assesses whether or not a child has received blood products before. As the child is exposed to the foreign proteins found in each transfused product, antibodies against the blood product are produced (ie, alloimmunization). The more antibodies present, the greater the chance the child will have a blood transfusion reaction and therefore require transfusion premedications such as antipyretics, antihistamines, and possibly steroid anti-inflammatories.

Before any transfusion, the pediatric nurse should assist the team in conducting a thorough physical assessment of the child. VS should be assessed, as well as lung sounds, because transfused products may cause fluids to shift.

COMMON HEMATOLOGICAL DISORDERS

Childhood hematological disorders are complex and diverse. Disorders of the hematological system can affect a number of blood products, ranging from blood cells to clotting components, such as platelets, to clotting factors whose deficiency causes **hemophilias** (ie, a group of hereditary bleeding disorders noted by a deficient level of blood-clotting proteins). The following sections describe the most commonly encountered hematological disorders found in childhood.

Iron-Deficiency Anemia

Iron-deficiency anemia is the most common form of anemia affecting children in the United States. After depletion of maternal iron stores, at 6 months the infant must have sufficient iron intake from their nutritional means. Risk factors for iron-deficiency anemia include the introduction of solid foods to an infant before the recommended age of 6 months, the introduction of cow's milk before the child's first birthday, or the excessive consumption of cow's milk during the toddler/early childhood period. The overconsumption of milk causes the young child to feel full, refusing to eat a well-balanced diet, leading to anemia. Cow's milk is an incomplete protein and does not contribute proteins used for the building blocks of blood components.

SAFETY STAT!

Preterm infants are also at risk for developing iron-deficiency anemia. Loss of as little as 1 to 7 mL of blood through chronic gastrointestinal bleeding daily can lead to anemia. An infant with iron-deficiency anemia will display microcytic anemia or small, pale RBCs.

The incidence of iron-deficiency anemia is between 24% and 35% of all infants 6 to 24 months, and 68% of all infants have some level of iron deficiency.

Assessments of Iron-Deficiency Anemia

Iron-deficiency anemia is assessed through symptoms displayed by the child. The symptoms of anemia include:

- Increased need for rest, napping, and sleep hours
- Slow mental processing
- Lethargy
- Tachycardia
- Shortness of breath
- Dizziness
- Pica
- Pallor
- Anorexia, abdominal pain, and vomiting
- Systolic heart murmur and/or heart failure
- Nail bed deformities
- Play or activity intolerance

Laboratory tests are used to assess and confirm a diagnosis of iron-deficiency anemia. Laboratory findings that confirm the diagnosis include:

- Decreased hemoglobin
- Decreased hematocrit
- Decreased serum iron concentration
- Decreased mean corpuscular volume (MCV)
- Decreased mean corpuscular hemoglobin concentration (MCHC)

Interventions for Iron-Deficiency Anemia

Iron-deficiency anemia is corrected by diet, the oral intake of iron supplements, and, if needed in moderate cases, intramuscular injections of iron. Severe cases of iron-deficiency anemia in which the child is symptomatic with fatigue, shortness of breath, and tachycardia, requires blood transfusions. Although mild iron deficiency may be able to be treated with oral iron supplementation, this requires weeks to months to correct the anemic state.

Nursing Considerations for Iron-Deficiency Anemia

Caring for a child with iron-deficiency anemia takes a team approach. Families need to learn about the physiology and pathology of anemia, and how to commit to treatment and prevention. The team should work together in explaining all aspects of care required, taking into consideration the best teaching approach that works for each unique family. The following list includes important points to consider when taking care of an anemic child:

- Teaching the family to make sure the young child rinses his or her mouth after taking oral iron preparations, as the medication can stain the child's teeth
- Teaching families that oral elemental iron should be taken with a source of vitamin C to improve absorption, such as a small amount of orange juice, and taking it either 1 hour before or 2 hours after ingesting milk products or antacids.
- Teaching families that supplemental oral iron can cause the child to become constipated and produce dark stools.

- Educating the family to prevent relapses by encouraging well-balanced meals
- Referring the family to a nutritionist
- Assessing for contributing factors such as a low economic status of the family

---

PATIENT TEACHING GUIDELINES

Educate patients about the long-term effects of chronic iron deficiency anemia, including growth retardation and developmental delays.

Because of the complexities of caring for a child with iron-deficiency anemia, a nursing care plan should be created. The plan should include considerations associated with the needs of the child experiencing anemia. Essential nursing diagnoses include:

- Knowledge deficit
- Fatigue
- Altered nutrition: Less than body requirements
- High risk for altered growth and development

Sickle Cell Anemia

SCA is a group of diseases that leads the child to have abnormal sickle hemoglobin S (HbS). Occurring in one out of every 500 live births of African American babies, this condition is marked by chronic hemolytic anemia and vaso-occlusion. These two outcomes cause pain and fatigue and affect the child's quality of life.

When a child with this genetic disorder experiences a trigger, a sickle cell episode leads to the bone marrow producing rigid, sickle-shaped RBCs, which increases blood viscosity and causes tissue hypoxia because of the obstructed blood flow. Symptoms of the genetic disorder appear after 4 to 6 months of age; before this time, the young infant has the presence of fetal hemoglobin. If the infant does not present with SCA, they will during toddlerhood or preschool when they experience an infection such as in the gastrointestinal or respiratory tract.

Triggers that cause a sickling episode include either an increased demand for oxygen, such as emotional distress, infection, or pain, or a decreased demand for oxygen, such as pulmonary infections. Children who go up to high altitudes where there is less oxygen can also experience sickle cell episodes. The exacerbation of sickle cell episodes leads to the child experiencing pain, often severe and requiring narcotic pain control measures.

Risk factors for the development of SCA include being of African or African American decent. SCA is an autosomal recessive genetic disorder in which the child's normal hemoglobin A (HbA) is either partially or completely replaced with HbS.

A child with SCA is at risk to develop what is known as an *SCA crisis*, also referred to as an *SCA episode*. Here, the child has experienced a trigger that causes his or her bone marrow to rapidly produce larger numbers of dysfunctional sickle-shaped cells. Triggers include infection, dehydration, stress, and hypoxemia, among others. There are four common types of SCA crises. Each can cause significant pain, and may be life-threatening.

The four common types of SCA crisis situations include:

- **Vaso-occlusive crisis:** This type of SCA crisis lasts up to 6 days and presents with severe pain in the joints, bones, and abdomen, and with swollen joints, feet, and hands. The child may experience visual disturbances.
- **Aplastic anemia crisis:** This is a form of extreme anemia caused by the severe destruction and lack of production of the child's RBCs.
- **Sequestration crisis:** This type of SCA crisis is caused by large quantities of blood that collect and pool in the child's spleen and liver, causing tachycardia, weakness, and dyspnea. It may lead to shock as the vascular volume of the child's blood decreases.
- **Hyperhemolytic crisis:** This type of SCA crisis is caused by an increasing rate of RBC destruction, which leads to severe anemia and a state of jaundice.

Newborn screening is imperative for the early identification of children with this disorder. Once identified, teaching must be initiated to prevent, as much as possible, the triggers that lead to painful SCA episodes (ie, crises).

SAFETY *STAT!*

Complications of SCA can be life-threatening. These include:
- Acute chest syndrome, in which microclots form in the lungs, leading to acute respiratory distress
  - Without immediate identification and treatment, the child will experience acute dyspnea, retractions, and severely decreased oxygen saturations. Early interventions may prevent a PICU stay.
- Acute infections, which can be life-threatening
  - Early identification of the infectious microbe and the provision of the correct antibiotic sensitive to the source of infection can save lives.

Assessments of Sickle Cell Anemia

Special considerations should be taken when assisting the health-care team to conduct assessments on the status of a child with SCA. A holistic approach is essential.

- Child's psychosocial status
- Risk for depression or other altered mood states
- Pain level
- Hydration status
- Symptoms of infection

The team should assess each body system, including respiratory, cardiac, musculoskeletal, skin, and neurological/mental status. Laboratory values, such as a CBC, a percentage of sickled cells, fluid status, and electrolytes, are all assessed on a regular basis, especially during an SCA episode.

Laboratory tests include:

- CBC
- Sickledex (ie, sickle cell index or sickle solubility test) to screen for the presence of HbS
- Hemoglobin electrophoresis to separate the various forms of hemoglobin, thus providing a definitive diagnosis

Nursing assessments of a child with SCA include meticulous assessment of pain scores on a consistent validated pain scale appropriate to the child's age (eg, Wong-Baker FACES or numerical scale). Children experiencing a pain episode must be managed with pain medications that provide comfort during a painful crisis situation.

Interventions for Sickle Cell Anemia

Children with SCA who are experiencing an episode of increased sickling will need specific treatments to improve their status rapidly. Interventions for a child experiencing a sickle cell **vaso-occlusive episode** (ie, a SCA exacerbation with a large number of sickled cells produced) include pain control, hydration, oxygenation if needed, and rest. Blood transfusions may be warranted to improve oxygen delivery to cells. Exchange transfusions may be needed to reduce the circulating numbers of sickle cells. Nursing care includes monitoring intake and output (I&O) and providing adequate oral fluids and nutrition when able to tolerate. Many children find comfort in warm packs placed on swollen and painful joints. The administration of oral penicillin is ordered to provide prophylaxis against infections. If a child presents with a fever or any evidence of infection, antibiotics will be ordered.

DRUG FACTS

IV fluids are administered to correct dehydration and improve circulation of the rigid, sickle-shaped cells associated with SCA. Pain medications are administered to decrease the joint pain, headaches, and skeletal pain associated with severe sickling. Antibiotics are started to treat infections that may be causing the sickling episode. The child is encouraged to keep moving to improve circulation, but must balance movement and range of motion with rest to promote healing.

Nursing Considerations for Sickle Cell Anemia

Nursing care of a child with SCA requires specialized considerations. Because SCA is a chronic, lifelong disorder, the child requires special nursing care that promotes independence, self-care to prevent dehydration and infections, and family involvement to provide support to a child who suffers periodic SCA episodes. Because many children require hospitalizations for SCA episodes, it is important to provide care that promotes early identification of potential complications and rapid treatments that minimize the lengths of stay. The nurse should assist the pediatric health-care team in identifying clinical manifestations of a child with SCA during an episode.

Clinical manifestations of child with SCA include:

- Reports of pain, especially in joints where rigid sickle cells form clots, leading to hypoxia
- Abdominal pain, nausea, vomiting, and anorexia
- Shortness of breath
- Fatigue
- Tachycardia
- Jaundice
- Muscle weakness
- Lethargy
- Irritability
- Impaired healing
- Priapism (ie, prolonged and painful erections because of the presence of viscous blood/clots in the penis)

Emotional support is very important for both the child and the family. Knowing painful episodes are a life reality may cause distress, fear, and depression. Encouraging the family to meet with social services, spiritual care providers, and counseling services may help to cope with the disease. Fatigue can also cause a child and their family distress. Refer to Box 40.1 for information about factors concerning fatigue in SCA.

Other nursing concerns surrounding the care of a child with SCA include:

- Maintaining skin integrity to prevent infections
- Avoiding taking aspirin
- Teaching relaxation techniques
- Providing the adolescent with a behavior contract to adhere to medical treatments, nursing care, self-care, and health promotion
- Providing family education and emotional support

Hyperbilirubinemia

Hyperbilirubinemia is a condition of the neonate in which there is an increase in the breakdown of RBCs that release bilirubin. The child presents with jaundice from lipid-soluble unconjugated or indirect bilirubin in tissues. Jaundice occurs when there is a decrease of lipid-soluble bilirubin binding with albumin that should travel to the liver for processing. Conjugated bilirubin is water-soluble, has been processed by the enzyme glucanotransferase, and is typically excreted through the infant's urine and bile.

Hyperbilirubinemia of the newborn most often occurs when there is a physiological immaturity of the liver functions or when there is an increased destruction of the RBCs. Typical onset is by 3 days of age. For normal newborns without a diagnosis of hyperbilirubinemia, slightly elevated levels decrease without interventions by the 10th day of life.

Jaundice can be identified not only in the tissues but also in the sclera and mucous membranes, and by the presence of dark urine. There are two types of hyperbilirubinemia:

1. **Indirect hyperbilirubinemia:** Transient, physiological, or breastfeeding jaundice
2. **Direct hyperbilirubinemia:** Biliary obstruction, metabolic disorders, or neonatal hepatitis syndrome

---

Box 40.1 Biobehavioral Factors of Fatigue in Sickle Cell Anemia

SCA, a disease of global concern, produces a significant level of fatigue during vaso-occlusive episodes (also called *crises*). Although pain is the most frequently associated symptom for a child with this disease, acute and chronic episodes of fatigue highly affect the child's quality of life, including producing a decreased psychological well-being. Nurses can assist the child with SCA by teaching the child and family to prevent or decrease contributing factors:

- **Hypoxemia:** Inflammation and hypoxemia are two key processes of SCA. Hypoxemia is found to be associated with fatigue. Preventing situations in which there is an increased oxygen demand will reduce the severity of hypoxemia-related fatigue. Teaching families about preventing infections will reduce the severity of hypoxemia.
- **Anemia:** Hemoglobin levels should be maintained. Families must be taught to maintain regular healthcare visits so that the child's CBC will be monitored for increasing anemia and the need for transfusion therapy.
- **Hyperviscosity of blood:** Dehydration should be prevented because it leads to an increased viscosity, or thickness, of the blood. Teach the family to provide adequate hydration, especially in hot seasons and with physical exercise.
- **Elevated inflammatory cytokines:** Children in a SCA episode will demonstrate elevated cytokines, which contribute to the experience of fatigue. Families need to be taught to increase rest. Promote adequate sleep because inflammation associated with SCA contributes to the child's fatigue experience.
- **Stress:** A child's experience with a chronic illness such as SCA is associated with stress. Linked with fatigue, stress produces an increased release of cortisol, which then causes an increase in cytokines, producing more fatigue. Families need to be taught to identify stressors in a child's life and to make efforts to decrease perceived stressful situations or events.

Ameringer, S and Smith, W. Emerging biobehavioral factors of fatigue in sickle cell disease. *J Nurs Scholarsh* 43:1, 22-29, 2011.

Assessments of Hyperbilirubinemia

Assessments for hyperbilirubinemia include assessing for the presence of jaundice. Jaundice can be identified by applying light pressure over bony prominences to blanch the skin. The yellow color of the jaundiced tissues will be evident.

Furthermore, the child may present with other conditions associated with hyperbilirubinemia, such as:

- Poor feeding behaviors
- Poor breast feeding
- Lethargy
- Encephalopathy; this life-threatening complication of severe hyperbilirubinemia is caused by the deposition of unconjugated bilirubin in the brain tissues, also referred to as *kernicterus.*

Laboratory values are followed on a regular basis as part of ongoing assessment of the child's status; elevated indirect bilirubin levels will dictate the length of stay under bili lights. Serial bilirubin levels can be drawn by heelstick. Hyperbilirubinemia is determined by values that exceed the expected levels for the child's age. Many pediatricians determine serum bilirubin levels over 13 mg/dL to be elevated.

LABS & DIAGNOSTICS

Expected Bilirubin Values in the Newborn Period
- Cord: Less than 2 mg/dL
- 0 to 1 days: Less than 6 mg/dL
- 1 to 2 days: Less than 8 mg/dL
- 3 to 7 days: Less than 12 mg/dL

Interventions for Hyperbilirubinemia

Hyperbilirubinemia is treated with bili light phototherapy. This therapy draws the bilirubin from the tissues to then be secreted via bile or urine. Time under the bili is determined by the child's serial bilirubin laboratory draws. Bili lights can be ordered as single-, double-, or triple-light therapy. New technology has been developed to allow the child with mild to moderate hyperbilirubinemia to be treated at home with a bilirubin light that is placed on the child's back side, and then both are wrapped in a blanket (Fig. 40.2). Home-care nurses

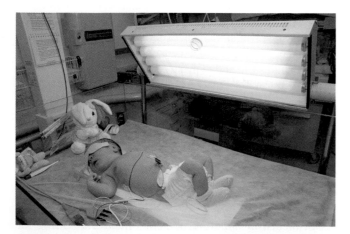

FIGURE 40.2 Infant receiving hyperbilirubinemia phototherapy treatment. The eyes and genitalia of the newborn are always covered to prevent tissue and retinal damage.

or clinic visits will then monitor the child's progress toward clearing the hyperbilirubinemia.

Nursing Considerations for Hyperbilirubinemia

Nursing considerations for a child with hyperbilirubinemia include the following:

- Provide support for the new parents, who are experiencing anxiety from their infant being maintained under the phototherapy lights. They may feel distressed that they have limited bonding time because of the need to keep the infant under the lights as much as possible.
- Provide regular scheduled time intervals for the parents to hold, bond with, and feed the infant.
- If the infant is lethargic or presenting as sleepy because of his or her bilirubin levels, the nurse must provide nutrition by waking up the infant, simulating the child, and feeding the child.
- Protein is essential in processing bilirubin. Proteins bind with the conjugated bilirubin so the infant must be provided with sufficient breast milk or formula. The nursing team must work with the interdisciplinary team to determine adequate intake, especially if the child is lethargic and difficult to feed.
- The phototherapy is damaging to the infant's eyes. The nurse must make sure the infant's eyes are covered with protective shield devices while under the intense bili lights. Teach the parents about the importance of this safety measure. If the parents find their eyes to be sensitive to the phototherapy, especially when the therapy includes triple lights, they can be provided plastic, eye-shielding glasses that have a yellow tint. Overhead florescent lights should be turned on to diffuse the lights.
- Assess the hydration status of the infant under the warm bili lights. Dehydration must be prevented. Assess the child's skin turgor, mucous membranes, capillary refill time (CRT), urine output, HR, and fontanels for evidence of dehydration.
- Check the child's serum bilirubin level at regular intervals until there is an acceptable pattern of reduction in total bilirubin levels. Some physicians may want to check for rebound effects and will monitor the child for 6 to 8 hours after the removal of the phototherapy.

Idiopathic Thrombocytopenia Purpura

Idiopathic thrombocytopenia purpura (ITP) is an acquired hemorrhagic disorder in which the child's total number of circulating platelets is severely reduced. The child will present with bruising, bleeding, or injury, most commonly presenting between 2 and 5 years. The disorder may be acute or chronic and the etiology is unknown. Current theory is that the child is experiencing an autoimmune phenomenon. ITP often follows an acute infection such as an upper respiratory infection or an experience of a childhood communicable disease, such as varicella or the measles. An antiplatelet antibody is produced in the spleen, which rapidly and severely reduces the production of platelets, leading to bleeding into the tissues, which is called *purpura.* Petechiae is seen on the child's skin as tiny pinpoint bruises and the child might present with hematuria and/or blood in the stools. Upon presentation, the child's platelet count is usually under 20,000/mm³. A bone marrow aspiration may be performed to rule out other disorders, such as an oncological diagnosis of **leukemia** (ie, malignancy of the bone marrow's WBCs).

Thrombocytopenia is a decrease in the quantitative number of circulating platelets in the blood, resulting in a count of less than 100,000/mm³. Spontaneous bleeding/hemorrhaging may occur with counts at or less than 10,000/mm³. Thrombocytopenia may be the result of either direct bone marrow invasion of malignant cells, or it may be from the side effects of chemotherapy, both of which cause bone marrow suppression. Radiation therapy and certain pharmacological agents, such as penicillin G, ampicillin, ticarcillin, and amphotericin B, which are often used to treat infections in a child experiencing cancer treatments, have been noted to cause transient platelet dysfunction.

Thrombocytopenia requires the implementation and strict adherence of bleeding precautions. These precautions include:

- Frequently assessing for bruising, petechiae, and bleeding from gums, rectum, and nose
- Regularly assessing for hematuria and occult or frank blood in the stool
- Meticulously monitoring for changes in the mental status or any change in the neurological system for symptoms of intracranial bleeds from low platelet count. A leukemic child who presents with a WBC of 300,000/mm³ is at risk for cerebral injury such as a clot or obstruction caused by massive WBCs.

Assessments of Idiopathic Thrombocytopenia Purpura

Assessments for ITP include the following:

- Bruising and bleeding into the tissues (ie, purpura)
- Petechiae or pinpoint bruising
- Bleeding of the mucous membranes
- Blood found in the child's urine or stool

Laboratory tests for ITP include the following:

- Monitor the child's CBC and platelet counts on a regular basis. The nurse should report drops in the child's overall platelet count or when the count falls below 20,000/mm³.
- Monitor the child's coagulation studies.
- Bone marrow biopsy may be ordered to be performed to rule out leukemia or other severe conditions.

Interventions for Idiopathic Thrombocytopenia Purpura

Treatment for ITP includes the administration of oral or IV corticosteroids. The administration of IV immunoglobulins (IVIG) is considered if the child does not demonstrate improvement. The administration of anti-D antibody in one dose for children with RhD-positive blood types may also be ordered only for those children with no mucosal bleeding, no infections, and a normal WBC count. Actual infusions of donor platelets are not considered generally helpful, but may be considered in cases of ITP that have life-threatening bleeding.

Nursing Considerations for Idiopathic Thrombocytopenia Purpura

Nursing considerations for ITP include the following:

- Because the child is at risk for bleeding, the child should be carefully monitored for signs of internal bleeding. These signs include headache, stomachaches, painful joints, and hematuria.
- Family members should be taught to maintain a safe environment for the child and to choose quiet play activities such as coloring, painting, reading, puzzles, clay work, or crafts.
- Nursing care consists of focusing care and teaching families about maintaining safety until treatment allows a rise in the circulating platelet counts. The nurse will administer IVIG for a goal of a rapid rise in platelets, and prednisone to decrease the formation of antiplatelet antibodies. New treatments include the administration of anti-D antibody (one dose) before the administration of prednisone. Children may be hospitalized for a duration of time required to elevate the platelets. This provides safety and monitoring for the onset of bleeds.

 DRUG FACTS

The administration of IVIG requires meticulous dosage calculation and medication administration. The IVIG solution will come in a glass bottle that requires the use of vented IV tubing. Premedications may be ordered. The healthcare team should work closely with the pharmacy to determine the rate and total volume required based on the child's height and weight. Calculations should be double-checked by two nurses. Infusions should start slowly to check for untoward reactions, and then should be increased every 15 min after repeated VS. Monitor the child for hypotension, fever, and urticaria. All assessments should be carefully documented and any change of condition during the infusion or after completion should be reported immediately.

Hemophilia

Hemophilia A and B, the most common forms of this disorder, are both X-linked recessive disorders in which the child has an impaired ability to control bleeding. Clotting factors are lacking, resulting in extended bleeding times. Typically, the disorder is manifested in infancy as the child begins teething, sitting up, or crawling. The young child presents with unusual bruising with only minor falls or bumps. Hemophilia is categorized as mild or severe, depending on the amount of clotting factor (in percentages) that is present. Mild hemophilia may be seen when the child has 48% of their expected level of clotting factors.

Two types of hemophilia are most common: type A hemophilia, in which the child has a deficiency in factor VIII, and type B hemophilia, in which the child has a deficiency in factor IX. Factor IX deficiency is also referred to as *Christmas' disease* and is less common than factor VIII, which composes 80% of all hemophilia.

Assessments of Hemophilia

Assessments for a child with hemophilia include the following:

- Active bleeding or excessive bleeding with minor cuts
- Reports of joint pain and stiffness
- Impaired mobility
- Bleeding in the mouth or in the gums from teething
- Presentation of hematuria
- History of tarry stools
- History of epistaxis (ie, nose bleeds)

  Laboratory tests for ITP include the following:

- Prolonged partial thromboplastin time (PT)
- Factor-specific assays to determine the type of the child's clotting deficiency
- DNA testing to identify traits in the females

Interventions for Hemophilia

Treatment for hemophilia includes rapid administration of the clotting factor in which the child is deficient. Nurses need to teach families how to store and administer factors via an IV administration. Corticosteroids may be used to treat complications associated with bleeding, such as chronic synovitis, hemiarthrosis, or hematuria. 1-deamino(8-D-arginine) vasopressin (DDAVP) is administered to increase plasma factor VIII, but it is only effective for mild hemophilia diseases. DDAVP is often prescribed before scheduled dental procedures or necessary surgical procedures.

Nursing Considerations for Hemophilia

Nursing care concerns for a child with hemophilia are complex and must be holistic in nature. Having a bleeding disorder for life requires education and support from all health-care team members. Nursing care concerns for a child with hemophilia include:

- Avoiding taking temperatures rectally or administering any medications via rectal suppository
- Avoiding skin puncture procedures or subcutaneous, IM, or ID medications
- Applying pressure for no less than 5 min directly over the site of any required injections, needlesticks, or venipuncture
- Monitoring stool, urine, and nasogastric fluids for hidden or occult blood
- Teaching the family to provide safety and prevent any injuries that may lead to a bleed, including discussing with the family the need for only low-impact, low-contact sports
- Teaching families to monitor for bleeds, including symptoms such as headache or changes in HR
- Teaching families to administer factor replacement therapy via rapid retrieval, preparation, and administration via a rapidly placed butterfly IV needle typically into the antecubital space
- Coordinating comprehensive care and follow-up for the family, including referring the family to a social worker and physical therapist
- Teaching families that the risk of exposure to infectious diseases is now minimized with the production of replacement factors via recombinant products

SAFETY *STAT!*

Complications of hemophilia center on uncontrolled bleeding episodes. The nurse must be prepared to act quickly to prevent or reduce the effect of intracranial hemorrhages, or airway obstruction of bleeding into the throat, neck, or chest. Rapid assessment of any evidence of impending shock includes VS and changes in mental status. The nurse must be able to call for help and rapidly administer factor concentrates during the bleeding episode.

NURSING CARE PLAN for Care of a Child with Hemophilia Disease

Nursing Diagnoses:
- There is a risk for injury.
- There is altered peripheral tissue perfusion.
- There is a knowledge deficit.
- The child is experiencing altered growth and development.

Expected Outcome:
- The child will experience minimal injury from internal bleeding.
- The family will learn rapid administration of the deficient factor.

Interventions:
- Teach the family to provide for a safe home environment:
  - Minimize clutter to prevent tripping and falls.
  - Pad corners of furniture.

NURSING CARE PLAN for Care of a Child with Hemophilia Disease—cont'd

- Dress an older, mobile infant and young child in extra clothes for padding.
- Use child safety gates to prevent falls down stairs.
- Use only soft toothbrushes.
- Select daily activities that are low risk for injury.
- Use well-fitting protective gear and equipment for any recreation or sports in which the potential for injury is a probability.
- Avoid aspirin and aspirin-containing medications.
- Teach the child's school administration and teacher/school personnel about the child's bleeding tendencies and how to respond to a bleed at school.
- Instruct the family about signs and symptoms of bleeding, including tenderness, pain, swelling, warmth, tingling, and decreased mobility of joint or extremity.

Evaluation of Outcome:
- The child experiences minimal consequences of bleeding.
- The child experiences optimal growth and development.

Thalassemia major

Thalassemia major is one of a group of heritable hypochromic (ie, pale color of the RBC) and microcytotic anemias found to have a variety of levels of severity. This condition produces a severe hemolytic anemia, causing severe weakness. Transfusions are required to extend life expectancy. If left untreated, a child can experience growth impairment; delayed or absent puberty; and cardiac complications, including intractable arrhythmias and chronic congestive heart failure. Without transfusions, the child's marrow tries to compensate by expanding, and hypertrophy then occurs, leading to thin bones prone to pathological fractures.

Defects in beta globin production occurs in 1.5% of children of African American decent or those of southeast Asian descent. Thalassemia major is found in populations throughout the Mediterranean, India, and Middle East.

Assessments of Thalassemia Major

Assessments for a child with thalassemia major include the following:

- Anemia with abnormally small, or microcytic, cells
- Fatigue
- Pallor

Interventions for Thalassemia Major

Interventions for a child with thalassemia major are limited. This condition does not have a cure. Interventions to maintain adequate perfusion include:

- Regular transfusions to keep the hemoglobin level above 10 g/dL
- If possible, bone marrow transplantation

Nursing Considerations for Thalassemia Major

Nursing considerations for a child undergoing treatment for thalassemia major are related to the frequency of transfusions required. Nursing care considerations include:

- Assessing transfusion reactions related to the consequences of multiple transfusions
- Understanding that repetitive transfusions can lead to iron overload, which requires treatments to remove stored iron
- Educating the family about the severity of the disease, including educating them about the need for lifelong transfusions

COMMON ONCOLOGICAL DISORDERS

The majority of childhood cancers are considered curable. The oncology team that provides care to the child with cancer and to his or her family has a treatment goal of curing that cancer. The overall prognosis of childhood cancer depends on the tumor type (ie, histology), the extent of the cancer at the time of diagnosis, the rapidity of treatment, and the effectiveness of the therapy. Rapid diagnosis and rapid initiation of appropriate therapy optimizes the chances of a child having a complete cure. Children should be treated by a specialized team with expertise in treating cancer.

There are more than 250 types of childhood cancer, each with a particular clinical presentation and treatment plan. Childhood cancer is considered rare, with less than 2% of all cancers across the lifespan occurring in children. The incidence of childhood cancer is less than 1%, with about only 8,000 new cases of childhood cancer being diagnosed per year in the United States. Although cancer remains the leading cause of death from disease in childhood, the cure rate of all childhood cancers combined now equates to 70% to 90%. See Box 40.2 for a summary of common types of cancer found in children.

No single cause of childhood cancer has been identified. The development of cancer is complex and multifaceted (Fig. 40.3). Attributing the development of a cancer diagnosis solely to genetics or to the environment is misleading. The concept of "ecogenetics" or "multifactorial etiology" is more acceptable as it addresses the *combination* of exposure to toxic environmental carcinogenic substances with variations in genetic factors.

At the cellular level, cancer has unique genetic properties that allow the indiscriminate growth of abnormal cells. These cancer properties include the following:

- An inactivation of the tumor suppressor genes that, under normal circumstances, would shut down the cell during abnormal growth
- A process occurs in which proto-oncogenes (ie, those that help regulate growth) convert to oncogenes, which promote abnormal cellular growth
- The process of apoptosis, the process of programmed cell death, is not functioning; when an abnormal cell that is

---

Box 40.2 Childhood Cancers

Aplastic Anemia

A disorder of the bone marrow, aplastic anemia is characterized by the depletion of all marrow elements. The production of marrow cells is decreased or completely lacking, which results in acute pancytopenia or the severe reduction of thrombocytes, which produce platelets, RBCs, and WBCs. Severe aplastic anemia presents with a granulocyte count of less than 500 mm^3, a platelet count of less than 20,000 mm^3, and a reticulocyte count of less than 1%. This type of cancer can be caused by drugs, chemicals, radiation, or viruses. The overall prognosis of this condition is poor and up to 50% of children with this diagnosis die within the first 6 months. Long-term survival is up to 90% if the child receives a successful bone marrow transplant from a histocompatible donor. Medical treatment is bone marrow transplantation or immunotherapy, such as cyclosporine, if a compatible match is not found.

Hodgkin's Lymphoma

Hodgkin's lymphoma accounts for only 5% of all childhood cancers. This disease is a malignant proliferation of lymphocytes. Hodgkin's lymphoma presents as painless, firm adenopathy (ie, swollen lymph nodes) of the cervical or supraclavicular nodes. Treatment consists of multidrug chemotherapy with supplemental radiation in some cases.

Non-Hodgkin's Lymphoma

Non-Hodgkin's lymphoma is a disease of malignant proliferation of T or B lymphocytes. Children often present with an intrathoracic tumor (ie, mediastinal mass) and dyspnea, chest pain, pleural effusions, and dysphagia. Treatment consists of surgical excision of the tumors and multidrug chemotherapy regimens.

Neuroblastoma

A common tumor of neurological tissue, neuroblastoma appears most commonly along the sympathetic nervous system tissues. Most are located in the child's abdomen and are often discovered as a mass or multiple masses

on plain radiographic imaging. Treatment consists of surgery, irradiation therapy, and chemotherapy.

Nephroblastoma (Wilms' Tumors)

Wilms' tumors are a malignancy of the kidneys in which metastasis is rare. The child with an encapsulated kidney tumor will have a better prognosis. The median age of diagnosis is 3 years old and the most frequent presenting sign is an abdominal mass. Treatment consists of surgical removal of the affected kidney followed by multidrug chemotherapy.

Osteogenic Sarcoma

Osteogenic sarcoma is a tumor found in the diaphysis of a child's long bone, such as the femur, ulna, proximal humerus, ileum, or radius, or in a flat bone such as the skull, spine, or pelvis. Often the child presents with a pathological fracture as an initial symptom. The sequence of the clinical course is that tumor cells replace destroyed normal bone, then the abnormal growth penetrates the bone cortex and extends via radiating spindles, and then finally the tumor extends along the bone marrow cavity through the veins and to the lungs. The peak age of diagnosis is 10 years and the survival rate is 50%. Treatment consists of surgery followed by chemotherapy. Limb salvage is not always an option.

Retinoblastoma

Retinoblastoma presents in a child's eye as a chalky, white intraocular tumor, often with a calcified and necrotic foci. Originating from the posterior side of the retina, the child may present with metastasis spreading to the optic nerve and beyond. A parent may seek health care based on the finding of a particular look to the child's eye, "cat's eye reflex," which is more formally known as *leukocoria*. Treatment consists of cryotherapy, radiation, chemotherapy, and/or enucleation (ie, removal) of the affected eye. This tumor has an excellent prognosis of a 96% survival rate.

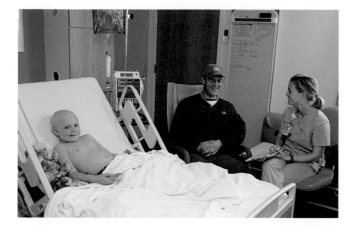

FIGURE 40.3 Child with an oncology diagnosis. Many parents maintain a bedside vigil to support their child during treatment for cancer.

damaged does not die, it leads to the growth and spread of tumor cells
• Chromosome translocation occurs, leading to new cancer genes

A model of carcinogenesis for specific childhood cancers, such as retinoblastoma, is called the *two-hit model.* This model suggests that two mutations are needed for cancer to develop.

Leukemia is the most common form of malignant cancer found in children. For solid tumors, cancer of the central nervous system, such as brain tumors, are those most commonly found in childhood. Some childhood cancers are unique to the pediatric population and are rarely found in adults. These cancers include neuroblastoma, Wilms' tumor, retinoblastoma, Ewing's sarcoma, and osteosarcoma. The most significant improvement of clinical outcomes for children with cancer has been the implementation of chemotherapy protocols with combination drug therapies, and the improvements of supportive care and nursing care. Preventing medication errors, complications, and severe symptoms, as well as providing safe, holistic care, are the most important aspects of pediatric oncology nursing. A specialized body of knowledge is required to provide effective and safe care to children with cancers. Nurses should seek national and institutional certification in chemotherapy administration, biotherapy administration, the care of central lines, and safety promotion such as chemotherapy spill cleanup.

A child will present with either vague symptoms that do not respond to traditional therapies or symptoms that are suggestive of cancer. Vague symptoms may include prolonged fevers, the inability to heal a wound, chronic fatigue, recurring otitis media, or pain. Symptoms that may suggest the presence of a diagnosis of childhood cancer are included in Box 40.3.

Diagnosis of Childhood Cancers

Invasive diagnostic procedures are conducted to rule out the presence of cancer and to determine the exact location, the type of histology, and the severity of the cancer via staging. These

---

Box 40.3 Symptoms Suggestive of Pediatric Cancers

• Significant weight loss
• Recurring febrile states
• Chronic fatigue or malaise
• Presence of petechiae or abnormal bruising or bleeding
• Night sweats
• Prolonged pharyngitis
• Lymphadenopathy
• Abdominal discomfort, masses, and distention
• Headaches and vomiting episodes in the morning
• Cat's eye reflex (see discussion on retinoblastoma)
• Pancytopenia
• Chronic drainage from the ears
• Mobility issues such as limping, arthralgia, or guarding of musculoskeletal structures
• Rectal or abnormal vaginal bleeding
• Significant bone pain
• Visual disturbances
• Periorbital ecchymosis

---

procedures include bone marrow biopsies, lumbar punctures, and surgical procedures for cancer staging or tumor debulking. Further diagnostic studies include computed tomography (CAT) scans with dye via an IV catheter and phlebotomy.

Treatment for childhood cancer is sixfold. Each treatment has been developed to follow particular diagnostic procedures to determine the accurate diagnosis of the type of cancer with the goal of achieving remission and long-term survival. The six forms of therapy for childhood cancer are summarized in Box 40.4.

Psychosocial Aspects of Childhood Cancer

The diagnosis of cancer in a child is a powerful, life-changing event for the entire family. Fear fills the hearts of those who are close to the family and resources are needed to support the well-being of the family structure. Shock, anger, guilt, and disbelief may all appear early in the child's diagnosis and may extend through treatment.

A complete assessment should be conducted for a family whose child was recently diagnosed with cancer, and should be done by a multidisciplinary team of specialists. Coping strategies should be identified and supported. A Child Life Specialist should immediately become involved, providing support, engagement, play, and education for the child and his or her siblings. It is important to help the family meet its basic needs, including education, transportation, and language interpretation services, as well as sleeping, eating, and work/school routines. Great fear about finances and medical coverage may be expressed early in the diagnosis. Financial stressors may be addressed by having a pediatric oncology social worker attend to the family's concerns. The farther away the family lives from the medical center where the child

Box 40.4 Treatments for Childhood Cancers

Chemotherapy

The majority of chemotherapeutic drugs act on the division or multiplication of cancer cells. Unfortunately, the properties of chemotherapy that work effectively on killing cancer cells also affect normal, healthy cells. This process leads to side effects that must be managed. Neutropenia, stomatitis, nausea and vomiting, constipation, and impaired liver function can all occur during chemotherapy treatments. Chemotherapy drugs are in one of several classifications that are either cell-cycle specific or cell-cycle nonspecific. If the chemotherapy works on one aspect of the cell's phase of division, such as the active phase of genetic material division, it is considered cell-cycle specific. Chemotherapy has certain unpleasant side effects that must be managed by meticulous prevention, assessments, and rapid interventions. Side effects include severe nausea and vomiting, myelosuppression, renal impairment, liver function abnormalities, ototoxicity, cardiac toxicity, hypotension, pulmonary fibrosis, peripheral neuropathy, paralytic ileus, mood changes, growth retardation, hyperglycemia, and, rarely, allergic reactions.

Surgery

Surgery is indicated for a child with cancer to diagnose, stage, resect, debulk, debride, or provide relief of mechanical obstruction. Surgery is almost always performed on a child with cancer under general anesthesia. As much as possible, the child with cancer needs to be prepared for the surgery by having adequate hydration, nutrition, platelets and clotting factors, RBCs, and an adequate WBC count to provide healing to the surgical site.

Radiation Therapy

Radiation therapy involves the application of high-energy particles or radiation waves to treat cancer cells by preventing replication. The direction of the radiation beam is such that the goal is to spare those adjacent healthy cells found around the site of the cancer. A total dose of radiation is calculated and then divided into serial radiation therapy sessions. Radiation is used to treat specific types of childhood cancer that are responsive to this type of treatment. Side effects can occur with radiation therapy and include many systems. Common side effects include GI distress, dysphagia, headache, nausea and vomiting, prolonged fatigue, liver tenderness, skin reactions, and pneumonitis.

Biotherapy

Several forms of biological response modifiers are used to help treat childhood cancer. Categories of biotherapy include monoclonal antibodies, cytokines, and investigational substances such as synthetic lipophilics, which have been shown to eradicate osteosarcoma lung metastasis. Side effects of biotherapies include potential allergic reactions, hypotension, headaches, rigors, fever and chills, and flulike syndromes.

Bone Marrow Transplantation

Hematopoietic stem cell transplantation is used with certain cancers to replace a child's damaged, absent, or diseased stem cells. Healthy stem cells from donors (ie, allogenic) are harvested, treated, and infused into the child's circulatory system. The child and donor are matched as close as possible for the best clinical outcomes. Allogenic stem cells harvested from the child may be used in certain circumstances for complete removal of residual tumor cells.

Gene Therapy

Focusing on the cause of the cancer, gene therapy has been investigated to help treat damaged cells. This type of therapy includes the transfer or insertion of new genes into the genome of a cell via a transportation carrier called a *vector*. Vectors are either viruses or nonviral substances such as chemicals. Gene therapy is not conducted on reproductive cells, so that the inserted genes are not passed on to future generations.

---

receives treatment, the more finances are required for transportation, meals, tolls, lodging, and vehicle maintenance.

Oncology team members should provide slow and thoughtful explanations of each step of the process and care requirements for each day. Because of emotional stress, family members may need to have the same topic explained repeatedly to understand complex treatment information.

Culture and spirituality play important roles in the care of the child with cancer and in the communication patterns with family members. Whenever possible and safe, families should be encouraged to implement their cultural or religious practices to provide support to the child. An assessment of cultural or religious/spiritual practices should be conducted early in the treatment process so that family wishes can be provided

for. Decision making, consent procedures, disease definitions, disease and prognosis disclosure, nutrition, hygiene, grieving practices, perspectives on medications, and the use of alternative or complementary practices may all be culturally influenced or bound. Recognizing cultural differences and providing support is paramount for successful cancer treatment and follow-up care.

CULTURAL CONSIDERATIONS

Jehovah's Witnesses and Religious Perspectives About Blood

Families may wish to apply their cultural or religious beliefs in situations concerning the care of a child with cancer. It is very important that the nurse assess these potential influencing factors, support the implementation of the factors if safe, and communicate the factors to other caregivers. One religious organization, Jehovah's Witnesses, also called the *Watchtower Society*, promotes doctrines concerning the avoidance or refusal of transfused blood products. With more than 400 references to blood in the bible, in 1940 Jehovah's Witnesses interpreted the most frequently cited verses as a denouncement of blood transfusion therapy. Many Jehovah's Witnesses believe that, with the violation of a blood transfusion, there may be a loss of salvation and negative spiritual effects, regardless if the recipient actually chooses the transfusion. Other Jehovah's Witnesses disagree and assert that if the recipient is unconscious or the transfusion takes place against the patient's or guardian's will, the soul is not affected.

It is imperative that the caregivers involved in the care of a child with cancer assess cultural or religious beliefs concerning blood and blood product transfusions as these may be medically necessary and life-saving. Investigation into alternative treatments is also important. Few alternatives to transfusion therapies exist but should be contemplated if possible to preserve the integrity of the family's belief systems.

Safe Nursing Care of a Child With Cancer

Because providing care to children with oncology diagnoses includes caring for children receiving chemotherapy, it is imperative that the nurse who is in close contact protect himself or herself from exposure to chemotherapeutic agents. Wearing the appropriate self-protective equipment to prevent exposure, knowing which container is safe for chemotherapy waste, and knowing how to clean up a spill of chemotherapeutic medications are all care imperatives (Fig. 40.4). Check

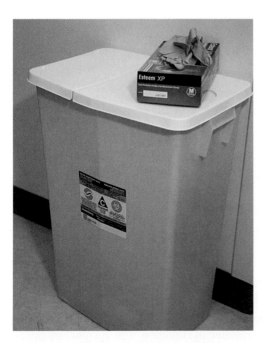

FIGURE 40.4 Chemotherapy waste receptacle.

with institutional policy about specific guidelines for protecting oneself against exposure.

It is imperative to give close attention and meticulous care to the surgically implanted central lines placed in children to administer medications including chemotherapy, and to obtain blood specimens (see Fig. 26.4).

Leukemia

Childhood leukemia is the most common form of cancer found across childhood, accounting for at least 80% of all cancer diagnoses. Leukemia is either lymphocytic or nonlymphocytic in nature. Acute lymphocytic leukemia (ALL) is the most commonly diagnosed leukemia in childhood. An excessive amount of abnormal immature leukocytes is produced in the bone marrow and then invades the blood and various organs of the child's body. There is a displacement of normal cells produced in the bone marrow with these abnormal cells, and therefore insufficient numbers of RBCs, other WBC types, and platelets are formed. The child is at risk for bleeding and infections.

The highest risk for a diagnosis of ALL are in those children between 3 and 5 years of age. The poorest responses to treatment and poorest overall prognoses occur when the child is younger than 1 year, is older than 10, has a total WBC count over 100,000/mm^3 at diagnosis, or is male. Children of African American decent have lower median survival rates.

Assessments of Leukemia

Assessments of a child with a potential diagnosis of leukemia include monitoring for early signs of cancer, including:

• Fever
• Fatigue
• Evidence of bleeding, such as petechiae or hemorrhage
• Bone pain
• Weight loss
• Anorexia

Laboratory tests for leukemia include the following:

• CBC with cellular differentiation
• Bone marrow aspiration for blast cell confirmation
• Lumbar puncture to determine central nervous system involvement/metastasis
• Chest x-ray to detect lung and mediastinal involvement
• Kidney, liver, and spleen scans to detect leukemic cell infiltration
• Bone scans and skeletal surveys to identify the presence of metastasis

Interventions for Leukemia

Leukemia requires medical management through the administration of a chemotherapy drug regimen. The treatment is divided into several progressive phases:

• **Induction** phase, in which treatment focuses on eradicating the disease or inducing a remission, occurs in the first few weeks from the diagnosis. Induction requires that a child experience the administration of multiple drugs in high doses.

- Intensification phase, which is followed by consolidation, in which the goal of treatment is to combat any involvement of the central nervous system or any other vital organ.
- **Maintenance therapy** is the last phase, during which the child receives several months to a year of chemotherapy to sustain the remission.

Review Box 40.5, which depicts the case study of a child with a new diagnosis of ALL.

Nursing Considerations for Leukemia

Nursing care concerns for a child receiving chemotherapy include both the treatments themselves, as well as the child's responses to treatments. Common care concerns include the following:

- The child receiving chemotherapy treatment for leukemia must be monitored for signs of infection. A fever must be reported immediately to the pediatric oncologist so that antibiotics can be started to prevent sepsis.
- The child needs to be monitored for reactions to the chemotherapy medications.
- The child's peripheral and/or central IV site should be monitored for signs of infiltration. Some chemotherapies drugs are vesicants and will cause severe tissue damage and potential cellular death if the drug infiltrates surrounding tissues.
- The child should be offered nutrition only when he or she can tolerate eating. Stomatitis or mucositis is a common side effect of chemotherapy and may make the oral consumption of food or fluids difficult.
- The family needs to be taught how to care for the child's central line, including assessments, flushing, and sterile dressing changes.
- Each family member will have anxiety and concerns that need to be addressed. The diagnosis of childhood cancer provokes powerful emotions and the family will need professional support to maintain a level of functioning that will provide support to the child. Social services and other professionals will need to be involved in the child's care. Spiritual care is important and should be offered to all family members. Twenty-four-hour visitation privileges should be allowed for all family members.
- Nurses must be very careful when they are around children receiving chemotherapy. It is imperative to wear the appropriate safety gear, know how to clean up a chemotherapy spill, and know which waste container in which to place contaminated materials and objects. Follow institutional policy on chemotherapy administration and accidental spill cleanup procedures.
- Nurses must understand that physical changes may occur because of cancer treatments. Some children are very sensitive to these changes. Alopecia, or hair loss, from chemotherapy can cause great distress to a child, especially older school-aged children and teens (Fig. 40.5).

Box 40.5 Case Study

Child With a New Diagnosis of Acute Lymphocytic Leukemia

A 10-month-old infant has been seen in the public health clinic of a large urban health center for ongoing fevers, fussiness, poor nutritional intake, weight loss, and pallor. The child had been seen by clinic pediatricians and treated with antibiotics for bilateral otitis media not responsive to the first course of medication. The mother, a Chinese immigrant, needed to bring two older siblings and use public transportation to attend the infant's doctor's visits. The mother, distressed that her infant was still displaying severe symptoms not seen in her other children, finally brought the infant to an emergency room (ER) of a large teaching hospital. Upon assessment in the ER, the health-care team recognized an abnormally elevated WBC and called a pediatric hematologist/oncologist to consult on the case. Further evaluation was performed on a slide of the child's blood smear. The child was identified as having suspected leukemia and was admitted into the hospital for further diagnostic workup and central line placement. Using a translator, the family was told the child had high-risk ALL and required extensive induction chemotherapy followed by at least a 2-year course of treatment. The family responded to the news with shock and the adults required support and education by several members of the health-care team to adapt to the powerful diagnosis of childhood cancer. The pediatric social worker was called in, the hospital chaplain was asked to provide support, and the hospital-based psychologist and members of the oncology team were all asked to rapidly become involved in the case. Members of the Child Life department were asked to work with the siblings to improve their understanding of the crisis of the new diagnosis.

The hospitalized infant had a Broviac central venous catheter line placed and was started on an alkalizing hydration fluid in anticipation of chemotherapy starting as soon as the diagnosis was confirmed. The child stayed in the hospital for over a month for the first cycle of induction chemotherapy and continued to receive supportive care to adapt to the new diagnosis. Multiple family members brought home-cooked meals to the family while hospitalized and the siblings were allowed to visit provided they had no symptoms of colds, flu, or any infections.

Interventions for Complications Associated With Leukemia

Treatments for leukemia include caring for the complications of bone marrow dysfunction. The dysfunction can be caused by both the cancer within bone marrow, as well as dysfunction

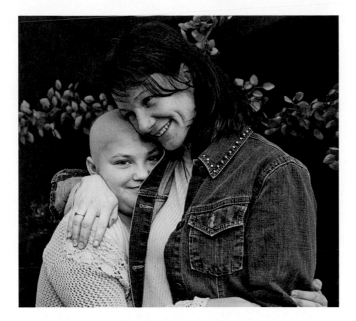

FIGURE 40.5 A child with alopecia. Alopecia is a negative effect associated with cancer treatment that can make the child feel very self-conscious.

caused by chemotherapy suppressing the bone marrow. The complications include neutropenia, thrombocytopenia, and anemia.

ONCOLOGY TREATMENT-RELATED NEUTROPENIA. Neutropenia is a reduction of circulating neutrophils that is measured by a calculation of the child's absolute neutrophil count (ANC). The child is considered neutropenic when the calculated value is less than 1,000 K/uL. When a child is neutropenic, he or she is at risk for a serious bacterial infection. The ANC is calculated by multiplying the total WBC count by the percentage of neutrophils and bands found in the differential.

Example:

Total WBC is 3,500
Segmented neutrophils are 21%
Bands are 2%
= (3,500) (0.21 + 0.02)
= ANC of 805; the child is considered neutropenic

Neutropenia requires the implementation and strict adherence of neutropenic precautions.

HEALTH PROMOTION

Ten Tips to Prevent Sepsis in a Neutropenic Child While Hospitalized

During states of severe myelosuppression from cancer or cancer treatments, children need to be protected from infection to prevent a life-threatening sepsis. Steps that should be considered include:

1. Implementing strict hand washing techniques and hanging signs to remind caregivers and family members to perform meticulous hand washing behaviors
2. Preventing the child from being exposed to ill persons
   • Screen visitors for symptoms of illness and prevent caregivers with any mild illnesses or infections from giving care to the child with neutropenia.
3. Calculating the child's neutropenic state daily (ie, calculated ANC) and planning care according to the severity of the child's myelosuppression
4. Providing adequate nutrition, calories, fluids, and rest to promote bone marrow recovery after chemotherapy
5. Avoiding fresh fruits, vegetables, and flowers in the child's room as they contain bacteria or fungi
6. Providing a mask for the child whenever the child must leave his or her hospital room for diagnostic examinations
7. Promptly reporting any evidence of infection, including any fevers, no matter how high
8. Avoiding any trauma to the rectal mucosa, and avoiding rectal examinations, rectal suppositories, and rectal temperatures
9. Providing the child with his or her own VS assessment equipment to prevent sharing between children who may pass infection to the child with cancer
10. Assessing the child frequently for any breaks in the skin or mucous membranes, such as rashes, cuts, sores, mucositis, hemorrhoids, or any loss of skin integrity

---

To provide safety to a child with an oncology disorder such as leukemia, the health-care team provides the child with safety precautions. Specifically, a child who is neutropenic must be protected by all members of the health-care team from acquiring infection. Neutropenic precautions are required. See Box 40.6 for a list of neutropenic precautions.

ONCOLOGY TREATMENT-RELATED ANEMIA. Children receiving cancer treatment are at risk for the development of anemia because of bone marrow suppression. The child will have daily CBC counts with cellular differentiation to monitor the need for a transfusion of RBCs. Typically, when a child becomes symptomatic from his or her level of anemia, or the hemoglobin count falls below 7 to 8 g/dL, the child will require a PRBC transfusion.

ONCOLOGY TREATMENT-RELATED THROMBOCYTOPENIA. Children receiving cancer treatment are also at risk for developing serious bleeding episodes related to the toxicity of the bone marrow and the reduction of circulating thrombocytes. The child may need to have platelet transfusions to prevent spontaneous bleeds or bleeding episodes related to invasive procedures such as bone marrow aspirations.

Box 40.6 Neutropenic Precautions

- Assess frequently for a fever and immediately report fever to enable the health-care team to implement STAT antibiotic therapy to prevent life-threatening sepsis. Blood cultures should be drawn as ordered, such as every 24 hours. Obtain blood cultures before implementing antibiotic therapy.
- Assess regularly for any signs and symptoms of infection, such as erythema at central line catheter insertion sites and infections at wounds or incision sites. Also assess any other symptoms of impending or actual infection, including diarrhea, mouth pain, anal pain or perirectal irritation, cough, and rhinorrhea. Neutropenic patients may not produce pus because their total WBC count is low. It is imperative to assess for pain, irritation, and redness and to rapidly report any indication of infection, which can be life-saving.
- Maintain a meticulous environment to reduce the possibility of infection. This includes frequent hand washing for the child and family, and preventing exposure to crowds when the child's ANC is less than 500.
- Prevent nosocomial infections by keeping the child in his or her hospital room and not allowing the child to play in the playroom unless the institution has clean "neutropenia" play time only for children with neutropenia.
- To reduce the chance of bleeding and infection, do not use rectal thermometers, conduct rectal examinations, or administer rectal suppositories. Children should only use soft tooth brushes to prevent bleeding.
- Perform meticulous hygiene practices, including daily bathing as tolerated, and strict mouth care to prevent mucositis.
- Teach the family about neutropenia so they can be directly involved with the care of protecting their child and monitoring for signs and symptoms of infection.

Key Points

- Nursing care of children who have an oncology (ie, cancer) or hematology (ie, anemia or blood) disease requires a specific body of knowledge and skill set. The diagnosis of a hematological/oncological condition carries with it the potential for great emotional distress for each member of the family, and yet the majority of childhood cancers are curable.
- Blood product support is often a cornerstone of hematology and oncology therapy. Many treatments to cure cancer produce periods of severe chemotherapy-induced anemia. Children with SCA require blood product support to optimize the recovery of a sickle cell crisis (ie, episode).
- Iron-deficiency anemia is the most common form of anemia affecting children in the United States. After depletion of maternal iron stores, at 6 months the infant must have sufficient iron intake from his or her nutritional means. Risk factors for iron deficiency anemia include the introduction of solid foods to an infant before the recommended age of 6 months, the introduction of cow's milk before the child's first birthday, or the excessive consumption of cow's milk during the toddler/early childhood period.
- SCA is a group of diseases that leads the child to have abnormal sickle HbS. Occurring in one out of every 500 live births of African American babies, this condition is marked by chronic hemolytic anemia and vaso-occlusion.

- Hyperbilirubinemia of the newborn most often occurs when there is a physiological immaturity of liver functions or when there is an increased destruction of the RBCs. Typical onset is by 3 days of age.
- ITP is an acquired hemorrhagic disorder in which the child's total number of circulating platelets is severely reduced. The child will present with bruising, bleeding, or injury, most commonly presenting between 2 and 5 years.
- Hemophilia A and B are both X-linked recessive disorders in which the child has an impaired ability to control bleeding.
- Thalassemia major is one of a group of heritable hypochromic (ie, pale color of the RBC) and microcytotic anemias found to have a variety of levels of severity.
- Leukemia is the most common form of malignant cancer found in children.
- The three most common side effects of cancer treatment that are life-threatening are neutropenia, anemia, and thrombocytopenia. Neutropenia is a reduction of circulating neutrophils and is measured by a calculation of the child's ANC. The child is considered neutropenic when the calculated value is less than 1,000 K/uL. When a child is neutropenic, he or she is at risk for a serious bacterial infection.

REVIEW QUESTIONS

1. What medications would the nurse expect to have on hand to respond to a blood transfusion reaction?
   1. Acetaminophen and diphenhydramine
   2. Morphine and acetaminophen
   3. Steroidal anti-inflammatory drugs and morphine
   4. Diphenhydramine and epinephrine

2. Which developmental stage would be most affected by periods of alopecia associated with chemotherapy treatments?
   1. Late school-aged
   2. Adolescence
   3. Early school-aged
   4. Preschool-aged

3. A registered nurse (RN) will instruct a licensed practical nurse (LPN) to report which of the following behaviors of a preschool child during chemotherapy treatments?
   1. Brushing teeth regularly with a hard toothbrush
   2. Rinsing the mouth out with salt and soda mouthwash tid
   3. Allowing the nurse to check for mouth sores daily
   4. Requesting plain yogurt and oatmeal for breakfast

4. Neutropenic precautions protect an immunosuppressed child during chemotherapy treatments. The following list contains specific precautions for patients with neutropenia: *(select all that apply)*
   1. Positive air pressure isolation room
   2. No fresh flowers or standing water in room
   3. No acetaminophen-containing pain medications
   4. Low-fiber, low-protein diet
   5. Strict hand washing techniques for visitors and caregivers
   6. Mask on child when required to leave room
   7. Daily bathing and complete oral hygiene

5. The developmental time period when a nurse should be concerned about the development of anemia associated with too large quantities of milk is:
   1. Late infancy
   2. Adolescence
   3. Early school-aged
   4. Toddlerhood

6. The nurse is caring for a preschool-aged child with a sickle cell vaso-occlusive crisis. Which of the following physician orders should the nurse question?
   1. Apply oxygen via nasal cannula for 24 hours after all surgical procedures
   2. Offer warm packs to place on painful joints
   3. Give pain medication around the clock (ATC) as needed based on the pain scale score
   4. Restrict oral fluids

7. While discussing the potential complications of chemotherapy treatment for a child with ALL, the nurse would expect the family to describe all of the following *except:*
   1. Anemia
   2. Elevated liver enzymes
   3. Thrombocytopenia
   4. Neutropenia

8. Which test would be performed to demonstrate a definitive diagnosis of childhood leukemia?
   1. A CBC with differential
   2. Serum titer levels
   3. Serum IgG levels
   4. A bone marrow aspiration

9. Which of the following activities would the nurse recommend to the family of a young child with hemophilia? *(select all that apply)*
   1. Soccer
   2. Baseball
   3. Swimming
   4. Fishing
   5. Golfing
   6. Hiking

10. To minimize the effect of chemotherapy-induced nausea for a young child being treated for cancer, the nurse should recommend:
    1. NPO status
    2. Clear liquids
    3. No eating pressures
    4. Full liquid

CRITICAL THINKING QUESTIONS

1. Research the resources a family of a school-aged child with a cancer diagnosis would require to support the child's academic progression and success if the child requires 2 years of chemotherapy treatments.
2. How would a parent best tell friends, family, and neighbors about a cancer diagnosis of testicular cancer for an adolescent boy? Keeping in mind the developmental stage of a teenager, how do you think the child would want his diagnosis shared with others?
3. A child with SCA is being raised by religious parents who are practicing Jehovah's Witnesses. What strengths and barriers would the nurse expect to encounter when providing care for this child? How does this faith view the transfusion of blood products?

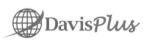

For additional resources and information, visit **www.DavisPlus.com**. Post-Conference Questions and Activities, Answers, and References can be found on Davis*Plus*.

Glossary

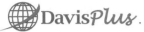
Abortion: A term used to describe a pregnancy loss or termination before the fetus is viable.

Abuse: A form of potential or actual injury or harm inflicted upon a child that may be physical, emotional, or neglectful in nature.

Acanthosis nigricans: A skin disorder in which dark brown or gray plaques appear on the skin, typically on the neck, groin, upper thighs, and under the arms, in patients with insulin excess, such as obesity or type 2 diabetes mellitus (DM).

Acceleration: An abrupt increase in fetal heart rate above the baseline.

[DP] Accidental poisoning: The ingestion of toxic substances or medications by young children who obtain unsafe access to them.

Acidosis: A relative or actual increase in blood acidity because of the accumulation of acids (eg, renal disease or diabetic acidosis) or an excessive loss of bicarbonates (eg, renal disease).

Acme: The peak of the contraction.

Acne neonatorum: Clogged hair follicles or pores in the skin present at birth.

Acne vulgaris: Acne is an inflammatory disease of the sebaceous follicles marked by comedones, papules, and pustules. Acne vulgaris is when there is the presence of cysts, nodules, and scarring.

Acquired immunity: Immunity or resistance to infection or toxicity by the child's natural immune system. Often referred to when a child has experienced an infection and developed antibodies against the infection source or organism.

Acrocyanosis: A blue or purplish discoloration of the hands and feet of the newborn.

Acromegaly: A chronic syndrome of excessive growth hormone, caused by pituitary malfunction, which produces bony enlargement. Acromegaly is diagnosed by an excessive blood level of serum insulin-like growth factor 1 (IGF-1).

Active immunity: Antibodies are formed against specific antigens or foreign substances such as bacteria, viruses, and toxins that stimulate the formation of antibodies.

[DP] Acute distress disorder: A disorder that precedes post-traumatic stress disorder (PTSD), manifested as anxiety; considered a predictor for PTSD.

Addiction: An abnormal dependence and compulsive behavior toward a substance such as alcohol, cocaine, opiates, or tobacco that has adverse emotional, psychological, physical, economic, social, and legal ramifications.

Adventitious breath sounds: Abnormal, acquired, or accidental breath sounds.

Afterpains: The contractions of the uterus for the first few days after childbirth.

Alcohol abuse: An abusive state of alcohol consumption associated with the chronic, frequently progressive, and sometimes fatal disease of impaired control of alcohol consumption.

Alkalosis: A relative or actual increase in blood alkalinity because of the accumulation of alkaloids or because of the reduction of acids.

Alveoli/alveolar sacs: The small air sacs of the lungs where gas exchange takes place.

Amblyopia: Unilateral or bilateral decrease of best-corrected vision in an otherwise healthy eye, often because of asymmetric refractive error (ie, deflection from a straight path or change in direction of light) or the presence of strabismus.

Amenorrhea: Absence of the menstrual period.

Amniocentesis: A procedure in which a thin needle is used to remove amniotic fluid and cells from the amniotic sac surrounding the fetus for testing.

Amnioinfusion: A procedure in which room temperature normal saline is infused into the uterus through an intrauterine pressure catheter to increase the volume of fluid in the uterus. The increase in fluid may relieve the compression of the fetal body on the umbilical cord.

Amniotic band syndrome: A condition in which adhesions between the amnion and fetus occur, causing deformities, such as limb amputation.

Amniotic fluid: Also known as the *bag of waters (BOW),* amniotic fluid provides buoyancy, movement, and protection for the fetus.

Amniotic membrane: A thin membrane formed from the ectoderm layer that surrounds the fetus and amniotic fluid.

Amniotomy: Artificial rupture of the uterine membranes with an amniohook.

Analgesia: The absence of a normal sense of pain that is achieved by the administration of pain relievers or anesthetics.

Anemia: A reduction in circulating red blood cells.

Anesthesia: A drug delivered by gas or injection that causes partial or complete loss of sensation to an area of the body.

Anhedonia: Lack of pleasure in acts that are normally pleasurable.

Animism: A belief that inanimate objects are alive.

Anorexia nervosa: An eating disorder marked by weight loss, disturbance of body image, and eventual emaciation by consciously withholding calorie consumption.

Anoxia: A condition in which no oxygen reaches cells.

Antepartal: The period of pregnancy between conception and onset of labor.

Anthropometric measurements: The measurements of the body, including weight, height, head circumference, and other measurements.

Antigen: Foreign substances such as bacteria, viruses, toxins, and foreign proteins that stimulate the formation of antibodies.

Apgar score: A systematic method of assessing the newborn's heart rate, muscle tone, response to stimuli, and color at 1 min after birth and again at 5 min after birth.

Apnea: A cessation of breathing.

Apparent life-threatening event (ALTE): Also called an *acute life-threatening event,* an ALTE is a sudden, acute, and unexpected change in a young infant's breathing pattern, which leads to a color change, apnea, limpness, and often, choking or gagging.

Areola: The dark area around the nipple.

Artificialism: A belief that everything is made by humans.

Ascites: Edema marked by excess serous fluid accumulating in the peritoneal cavity.

[DP] Asphyxiation: A state of insufficient oxygen intake related to choking, poisoning, shock, trauma, crushing or compression injuries to the chest, drowning, near drowning, or any source of diminished environmental oxygen.

[DP] Assent: The inclusion of the school-aged child in the developmentally appropriate discussions of his or her health-care treatments. This is not a legal form of consent but a respectful inclusion of the child's thoughts, feelings, and desires.

Astigmatism: A visual disorder where the refraction of a ray of light is spread over a diffuse area rather than sharply focused on the retina. This is because of a difference in the curvature of the cornea and lens of the eye.

Atelectasis: A collapsed or airless condition of the lung often caused by an obstruction by mucous plugs.

Atony: Lack of normal uterine muscle tone.

Attachment: The incorporation of the new baby into the family unit.

Attitude: Referring to the positioning of the fetus. The most common fetal attitude and the most successful for a vaginal delivery is when the fetus is in a fully flexed position.

Augmentation: The stimulation of hypotonic uterine contractions once labor has begun but the contractions are ineffective in producing dilation and labor progression.

Autonomy: The sense that one is separate from others and that one has some control over one's environment and interactions; the actual or desired state of independence. May be considered a state of separation from the child's primary caregiver.

Ballottement: A diagnostic maneuver in pregnancy. The fetal part rebounds when touched by an examiner's finger through the vagina.

Battered: A child who has been physically abused by another has lasting marks, erythema, bruises, fractures, or other forms of physical or emotional evidence.

Beneficence: Acting from a spirit of compassion and kindness to benefit others.

Bilirubin: A product of the breakdown of the heme portion of a red blood cell.

Bimanual examination: To determine uterine size and position, the healthcare provider places the gloved middle and index fingers into the vagina to identify the cervix. The other hand is placed midway between the umbilicus and the symphysis pubis and presses downward toward the pelvic hand.

Bishop's score: A tool used to evaluate cervical ripening that is predictive of readiness for labor.

Blastocyst: A maturing embryo in which some cell differentiation has occurred.

Bonding: The emotional and physical attachment between a mother and her newborn that is initiated in the first hour or two after the birth.

Brachial plexus: A network of nerves that originates in the neck area and branches off to form the nerves that control movement and sensation in the shoulders, arms, and hands.

[DP] Brachycephalic: Having a cephalic index of greater than 80%, which demonstrates a short and broad head; considered a short head, but not abnormal.

Braxton Hicks contractions: Irregular, mild contractions that occur in late

pregnancy and do not produce cervical effacement and dilation.

Bronchodilation: A method of opening the airway to ease respiratory distress; often accomplished through the use of bronchodilating medications.

Broselow's tape: Also known as *Broselow's pediatric emergency tape;* a color-coded, length-based system for emergency response based on a child's actual or estimated weight that is used in a variety of settings, including emergency departments, acute and critical care units, and outpatient settings. The system covers both equipment for weight and medications precalculated for weight.

Brown fat: A type of fat found in term newborns in the scapular area, the thorax, and behind the kidneys. It can be used by the newborn to produce body heat.

Bulimia: An eating disorder marked by episodes of binge eating followed by intense emotional distress, including guilt and shame, resulting in self-induced vomiting and diarrhea, as well as excessive exercise and fasting to reverse the effects of the binge eating.

Caput succedaneum: A swelling of the scalp of the newborn caused by pressure from the uterus or vaginal wall during delivery.

[DP] Carbon monoxide: A colorless, odorless, and tasteless poisonous gas often associated with car engine exhaust, broken heaters, sewers, cellars, and mines. Poisoning can result from burning organic fuels in the home or car exhaust without proper ventilation.

Cardiopulmonary: Relating to both the heart and the lungs.

Cardiovascular: Relating to the heart and entire blood vessel system.

Cataract: An opacity (ie, cloudy appearance) of the lens of the eye often caused by trauma, aging, metabolic or endocrine disease, or the side effects of certain medications such as steroids.

Catecholamines: Hormones produced by the adrenal glands, such as dopamine, norepinephrine, and epinephrine.

Centers for Disease Control and Prevention (CDC): Located just outside of Atlanta, Georgia, the CDC operates under the Department of Health and Human Services and is the leading agency for protecting the health of United States residents.

Central cyanosis: Discoloration because of reduced hemoglobin; associated with reduced oxygen saturation measurements.

Cephalic: A medical term of Latin origin referring to the head.

Cephalohematoma: A swelling on the head that does not cross the suture line.

It is caused by birth trauma that causes a rupture of blood vessels between the skull and periosteum.

Cephalopelvic disproportion (CPD): A disproportion or mismatch between the maternal pelvis size and the size or position of the fetal head. This condition occurs when the maternal pelvis is too small for the fetal head.

Cerclage: The use of sutures around the cervix to prevent the opening of the cervix.

Certified nurse midwife (CNM): An advance-practice registered nurse who has graduated from an accredited school of midwifery and passed a national certification examination that allows the nurse midwife to provide health care during the preconception, prenatal, labor, delivery, and postpartum periods.

Cerumen: A substance secreted by glands at the outer third of the ear canal. Although it typically does not accumulate in the ear canal, it may clog the channel.

Cervical incompetence: The inability of the uterine cervix to retain a pregnancy in the second trimester in the absence of uterine contractions.

Cervix: The lower portion of the uterus that projects into the vagina.

Chadwick's sign: A deep blue color of the vagina and cervix because of increased vascularity.

Child Protective Services (CPS): In most states, this is a state-run organization that is a designated social services agency that provides assessment, interventions, and treatment for families who have been identified to have child maltreatment, including various forms of abuse and/or neglect.

Chorioamnionitis: Infection of the fetal amnion and chorion membranes.

Choriocarcinoma: A fast-growing cancer that can develop in the uterus following a molar pregnancy.

Chorion: A thick membrane that develops from the trophoblast and becomes part of the placenta villi.

Chorioretinitis: Inflammation of the choroid and retina of the eye.

Chromosomes: A linear strand of protein DNA that carries genetic material.

[DP] Chronic illness: An illness that lasts a long period of time and significantly affects a person's functioning for at least 3 months out of each year.

[DP] Chronicity: Pertaining to a condition lasting a long time.

Circumcision: The surgical removal of the end of the foreskin of the penis.

Clinical status: A term used to denote the clinical well-being of a child.

Clostridium difficile (C diff.): A gram-positive, anaerobic, spore-forming bacilli that causes watery diarrhea, abdominal pain, fever, and anorexia, and that may produce a pseudomembranous colitis.

Code blue: A phrase used to describe an actual or pending cardiopulmonary arrest.

Collaboration: A process of working together.

Color blindness: An inability to distinguish certain colors or any colors at all.

Colostrum: A fluid rich with antibodies that may be secreted in small amounts during the pregnancy and before milk production. It contains carbohydrates, antibodies, and a small amount of fat.

Communicable: Capable of being transmitted from one individual to another.

Compartment syndrome: A situation in which a traumatic injury causes pressure to build up in a confined space, such as in the rigid fascia surrounding the muscles. If a bleed occurs or there is a buildup of inflammatory fluids, pressure builds up within the muscles, leading to ischemia and necrosis and causing severe tissue damage.

Concrete operations: Created by Dr. Jean Piaget, a Swiss philosopher and psychologist (1896–1980), *concrete operations* refers to the thought processes of the school-aged child who can use and understand logical thinking to interpret his or her world and understand simple and complex phenomena.

Conduction: The transfer of body heat to a cooler surface.

Conductive hearing loss: Form of hearing impairment where the outer ear has been affected or damaged, such as with repeated otitis media, causing scarring on the tympanic membrane.

Congenital: Inherited, or genetic, disorders that are present at birth.

Contactant: A substance that causes an allergic or sensitivity response when the substance is exposed to the skin.

[DP] Contraceptive: A method or device serving to prevent pregnancy.

Convection: The transfer of body heat to the surrounding cool air.

[DP] Coping: Adapting to and managing significant change, illness, work, relocation, pain, death, changes in family structure, or chronic illness.

Corpus luteum: A structure that develops from a ruptured ovarian follicle and that secretes the hormone progesterone.

Couvade syndrome: A syndrome in which the father may experience psychosomatic, pregnancy-simulating symptoms of nausea, fatigue, and backache.

Cranial nerves: Twelve pairs of nerves, numbered by order they contact the brain and that originate in the cranial cavity and that innervate the head.

Crepitus: A crackling sound heard while auscultating the lungs, such as with pneumonia.

Crohn's disease: An inflammatory disease marked by patchy areas of full-thickness inflammation anywhere along the gastrointestinal tract. The condition causes pain, malabsorption, fistulas, and bloody stools.

[DP] Cultural awareness: Developing sensitivity and awareness of another ethnic group (Adams, 1995).

[DP] Cultural competence: Ability of an individual or organization to function effectively within the cultural context of beliefs, behaviors, and needs of the person or community that they serve (Ritter and Hoffman, 2010).

[DP] Cultural sensitivity: The use of neutral language, both verbal and not verbal, in a way that reflects sensitivity and appreciation for the diversity of another. Cultural sensitivity may be conveyed through words, phrases, and categorizations that are intentionally avoided, especially when referring to any individual who may interpret certain language as impolite or offensive (American Academy of Nursing Expert Panel on Cultural Competence, 2007).

[DP] Culture: Learned behavior shared among members of a group; system of shared ideas, concepts, rules, and meanings that underlay and are manifested in ways of life; includes knowledge, beliefs, art, morals, law, customs, and any other capabilities and habits acquired by members of a society (Bird and Osland, 2006; Soderberg and Holden, 2002; Douglas and Pacquiao, 2010).

Cushing's syndrome: Also called *hyperadrenocorticism,* this disorder is related to exposure to excessive glucocorticoid hormones. Cushing's syndrome is a side effect of pharmacological use of steroids in the management of inflammatory illnesses. Symptoms include muscular weakness, thinning of the skin, easy bruising, rounding facial features, and weight gain.

Cyanosis: A blue, gray, slate-colored, or dark purple discoloration of the skin or mucous membranes when deoxygenated or reduced hemoglobin is in the blood. Cyanosis is associated with severe respiratory distress and poor gas exchange. It may start as subtle cyanosis in the lips (ie, circumoral), progressing to the nipples and nail beds, and can be seen on the entire body when severe deoxygenation is present.

Cyberbullying: The use of computer technology and the Internet to bully another. Cyberbullying maybe in the form of defamation, ridicule, intimidation, or threats of violence.

[DP] Cyber threat: A threat made by a person over the Internet. They are prevalent and pose a very real danger to an unsuspecting child.

[DP] Cystocele: A condition in which the bladder drops down and protrudes through the vagina.

Deafness: Inability to process any acoustic sound with or without hearing devices.

Deceleration: A decrease in fetal heart rate from the baseline.

Decibels: A unit of measure of sound.

Deciduous teeth: Primary (ie, baby) teeth are shed to make room for adult or permanent teeth. Deciduous refers to the "falling out" or shedding of the primary teeth.

Decrement: The subsiding of a contraction.

Decubitus: Term used for skin and underlying structures damaged from compression and inadequate perfusion; used synonymously with the term *pressure sore.*

Depression: A mood disorder marked by a loss of interest or pleasure in living, which presents with many symptoms, including poor academic performance, persistent sadness, poor appetite, tearfulness, hopelessness, and loss of energy. Depression is also called *clinical depression, major depressive disorder, dysthymic disorder,* and *unipolar depression.*

Dermal melanosis: Also known as a *Mongolian spot,* this congenital birthmark is caused by melanocytes trapped deep in the skin, appears flat and bluish-gray or brown, and is located on the back or buttocks.

Dermatological: Pertaining to the skin, or study or science of the skin.

Diabetes insipidus (DI): In this disorder, the opposite of syndrome of inappropriate antidiuretic hormone (SIADH) occurs. In DI, there is a reduced production of posterior pituitary secretion of SIADH and the child's urine has a very low specific gravity. DI causes the child to produce copious urine (ie, uncontrolled diuresis).

Diabetes mellitus (DM): A chronic metabolic disorder marked by hyperglycemia that results from either failure to produce insulin (ie, type 1) or insulin resistance with inadequate insulin secretion to sustain metabolism (ie, type 2).

Diabetic ketoacidosis (DKA): An acidotic state caused by an excess of ketone bodies in patients who do not produce adequate insulin.

Diagonal conjugate: The distance from the lower posterior border of the symphysis pubis to the sacral promontory.

Diaphoresis: Profuse sweating.

Diastasis recti: Separation of the abdominal muscles.

Dilation: The opening of the closed cervix to approximately 10 cm.

Dilation and curettage (D&C): A surgical procedure in which the cervix is dilated and the physician scrapes the lining of the uterus to remove the contents of pregnancy.

Direct or conjugated bilirubin: Bilirubin that is broken down into a water-soluble form for excretion.

Disseminated intravascular coagulation (DIC): A coagulation disorder in which the body responds to hemorrhage by overproducing clotting factors that can cause clots that cut off the blood supply to major organs.

Diuresis: The secretion and passage of large amounts of urine.

Diurnal incontinence: Incontinence of urine occurring every day; when it occurs during the day, it usually has a pathological cause.

[DP] Diversity (Cultural Competency): Differences in race, ethnicity, national origin, religion, age, gender, sexual orientation, ability or disability, social and economic status or class, education, and related attributes of groups of people in society (Andrews and Boyle, 2008).

Dizygotic twins: Fraternal twins who develop from two separate sperm and ova.

Doula: A professional who provides physical, emotional, and informational support to the laboring woman.

[DP] Down's syndrome: Present in 1 of 700 births in the United States, the clinical consequence of having three #21 chromosomes (ie, trisomy 21), which results in mild to moderate cognitive impairment and specific physical characteristics, including low-set ears, sloping forehead, single palmar crease, and a tendency to have cardiac disease.

Ductus arteriosus: A blood vessel in the fetus that permits most blood to bypass the lungs.

Ductus venosus: A small blood vessel that allows fetal blood to bypass the liver.

Duration: The actual time that a contraction lasts, from beginning to end.

[DP] Dysmenorrhea: Painful menstrual periods.

Dyspnea: Labored or difficult breathing.

Dysuria: Painful or difficult urination.

Early decelerations: A gradual decrease in fetal heart rate with the onset of deceleration caused by head compression as the fetus moves through the pelvis.

Echocardiography: A test that looks at how blood flows through the heart vessels, valves, and chambers.

Eclampsia: The onset of seizure activity with all the symptoms of severe pre-eclampsia.

Ectopic pregnancy: A situation in which a fertilized ovum implants outside the uterus.

Effacement: The process of thinning of the cervix.

[DP] Emancipation: The granting of legal control over one's decisions or lifestyle. For adolescents who are not yet 18 years of age, emancipation can be the granting of financial independence or related to the granting of rights over health-care decisions.

Embryo: The stage of development between the fertilized ovum and the fetus.

Emesis: Defined as the forceful expulsion or emptying of stomach content caused by either a gastrointestinal disorder or by a nongastrointestinal disorder.

Empowerment: A concept within family-centered care principles that describes assisting a family to feel as though they are supported, listened to, and competent.

Enabling: A concept within family-centered care principles that describes the teaching, supporting, and enabling that allows a family to care for their child.

Encephalopathy: A generalized brain dysfunction of varying degrees that causes an impairment of arousal, orientation, speech, and cognitive processing. It is caused by exposure to toxins, hypoxia, or an infectious process.

Encopresis: Uncontrolled soiling during the day in a child who is 4 years of age or older who had previously mastered toilet training. This condition is associated with stool retention and holding.

[DP] Endemic: A condition or a disease that is found regularly among a certain area.

[DP] Endometrial ablation: A procedure in which the tissues lining the uterus are destroyed.

[DP] Endometriosis: A condition in which uterine tissue is growing outside the uterus.

Endometritis: An infection of the endometrium, which is the lining of the uterus.

Endometrium: The mucous membrane that lines the cavity of the uterus. It is the site where the embryo implants after arriving in the uterus.

Engagement: The entrance of the widest diameter of the presenting part of the fetus into the mother's pelvis.

Engorgement: An over-full breast that occurs at times with breastfeeding.

Engrossment: An attitude of total focus on something.

Enucleation: Surgical removal of an eye from the eye socket.

Enuresis: Involuntary elimination of urine after the age in which the child should have or has had bladder control, but now is lost. Control is usually secured by 5 years of age. Enuresis is multifactorial.

Epidemic: The presence, or prevalence, of a disease within a widespread geographical area. Typically refers to a rapid spread or an increased occurrence of a disease within a widespread geographical area.

Epidural: Anesthesia infused through a catheter between the fourth and fifth vertebrae into the epidural space to decrease pain and perception.

Epiglottitis: A medical emergency in which the child's epiglottis becomes inflamed, mostly caused by a viral infection, and in which the child's airway may become completely closed.

Epiphyseal plate: The center of ossification at the extremity of each of the long bones. Considered the "growth plate" of long bones, where new bone growth occurs.

Episiotomy: An incision into the perineum to enlarge the vaginal opening.

Episodic decelerations: Decelerations of fetal heart rate that are not associated with uterine contractions.

Epispadias: A congenital condition in which the meatus, the opening of the urethra, is located on the dorsum of the penis.

Erythema toxicum neonatorum: Also known as a *newborn rash,* this rash may appear as macules, papules, or vesicles and may appear on any part of the body except the palms and soles of the feet.

Esotropia: Inward deviation of the eye laterally.

Estriol: One of three types of estrogens that occur naturally in the body.

Estrogen: A female hormone secreted by the ovaries.

Ethics: Moral principles that guide a person's behavior.

[DP] Ethnicity: The perception of oneself and a sense of belonging to a particular ethnic group, or to more than one group. Ethnicity includes commitment to cultural customs and rituals. It is not the same as physical traits associated with race (eg, skin or eye color, hair) related to a geographical origin.

[DP] Ethnographic: The scientific description of individual cultures.

Eustachian tubes: Anatomical auditory tubes lined with mucous membranes and located from the middle ear to nasopharynx. Occlusion can lead to otitis media, an infectious process.

Evaporation: The loss of heat as fluid evaporates.

Exanthem: Any type of a reaction or eruption that appears on the skin as opposed to a reaction or eruption that forms on mucous membranes; often used to describe pediatric rashes.

Exfoliation: The shedding or casting off of a body surface.

Exophthalmos: An abnormal protrusion of the eyeball often because of thyrotoxicosis (ie, hyperthyroidism).

Exotropia: Outward deviation of the eye laterally.

External cephalic version: An attempt by the health-care provider to move a malpositioned fetus, such as a breech or transverse lie, into a vertex cephalic presentation.

External version: A procedure in which the health-care provider attempts to change the fetal position externally.

Failure to thrive (FTT): A term used to denote an infant's or child's growth measurements that are below what is expected; may be associated with pathology, neglect, or poor parenting skills.

Family-centered care: A philosophy of family-focused care in which the family is considered the child's constant. Family is given the opportunity to be included in all medical decision making, are empowered to make informed decisions for their child, and are enabled to provide all care for their child.

Fetal: Pertaining to a fetus.

Fetal demise: The death of a fetus at any stage of the pregnancy.

Fetal fibronectin (fFN): A protein that helps the amniotic sac to adhere to the uterine wall. It is detected before 22 weeks' gestation and after 37 weeks' gestation.

Fetal lie: The alignment of the fetus with the mother.

Fetal presentation: The part of the fetus that is first to enter the pelvis.

Fetal station: The measurement in centimeters of the fetal head in relationship to the maternal ischial spine in the pelvis.

[DP] Fibroids: Benign tumors in the uterus.

Fibromyomas: Benign uterine tumors.

Fistula: An abnormal opening between anatomical structures that should not be there, such as between the rectum and the vagina, or between the trachea and the esophagus.

Fluid maintenance calculation: A standard calculation used in pediatrics to determine the daily maintenance of fluids that should be consumed or administered. Based on the child's weight in kilograms, this is not considered as resuscitative fluids, but what should be taken in daily to maintain a balanced fluid status.

Follicle-stimulating hormone (FSH): A hormone that stimulates the development of a follicle in the ovary before ovulation.

Fontanel: Often referred to as the "soft spot" on the baby's head, this fibrous membrane lies between the bones of the cranium.

Food lags and jags: A phrase used to describe how a young child goes through phases of not experiencing hunger and therefore refusing to eat, or taking in a reduced number of calories.

Foramen ovale: The opening in the atria of the fetal heart that allows blood to bypass the lungs.

Forceps: A metal instrument that has two curved spoonlike blades with locking handles that fit on either side of the fetal head and assists with delivery of the baby.

Fore milk: The milk produced and stored between feedings.

Frequency: The time between contractions, which is measured from the beginning of one contraction to the beginning of the next contraction.

Fundus: The upper large part of the uterus.

[DP] Galactorrhea: Inappropriate or excessive production of milk.

Galactosemia: A rare genetic metabolic disorder that makes it difficult for the infant to metabolize milk sugar, which can damage organs.

Gastroenteritis: An inflammatory process that occurs in the stomach, small intestine, or large intestine.

General anesthesia: Medication given IV to cause the patient to lose consciousness, and the subsequent placement of an endotracheal tube in the trachea to allow the administration of oxygen and gas to keep the patient unconscious during a procedure.

Genetics: The study of how genes, chromosomes, and genotypes, or sequencing and combinations of genes, are expressed and responsible for health or disorders.

Genomics: A branch of biotechnology that focuses on genetics and molecular biology to map the DNA sequencing of sets of genes.

Gigantism: The excessive development of the body or of a body part.

Glaucoma: A group of eye diseases that leads to increased intraocular pressure and eventually leads to the atrophy of the optic nerve.

Glomerulonephritis: A condition of inflamed glomerular tissue, nephritis, in which the lesions involve the glomeruli. Also called *acute nephritic syndrome,* this condition frequently follows an infection with particular strains of streptococci.

Glucagon: A polypeptide hormone secreted by the α cells of the pancreas. This hormone stimulates the liver to change stored glycogen to glucose.

Gluten intolerance: The inability to tolerate the consumption of foods with gluten, including wheat, oats, barley, and rye. Consumption of glutens in a child with intolerance can cause inflammation, flatus, cramping, fatigue, and diarrhea. In severe cases, it can cause a failure to thrive (FTT) trajectory.

Glycogen: Glucose stored in the liver until needed for energy.

Goiter: An enlargement of the thyroid gland caused by a variety of reasons, including iodine deficiency, thyroiditis, nodules, or any hyperfunction or hypofunction of the thyroid.

Goodell's sign: Softening of the cervix caused by the increased vascularity of pregnancy.

Grand mal seizure: A type of seizure activity that crosses over the brain's hemispheres and causes full-body neuromuscular seizure activity. It is associated with a loss of consciousness, tonic/clonic movements, urinary and fecal incontinence, amnesia of the event, and an icteric (ie, sleepy) state afterwards.

Grave's disease: A form of hyperthyroidism in which an autoimmune destruction of the thyroid gland takes place. The condition increases production of thyroxine and causes an enlargement of the thyroid gland.

Gravida: The number of times a woman has been pregnant.

Gynecomastia: Enlarged breasts in the newborn caused by maternal hormones.

Hard of hearing: Phrase used to denote the reduced ability to hear but the continued ability to hear and process acoustic sounds at some level.

Health-care disparity: Lack of similarity in access to health care. Many residents of the United States have no access to health care.

[DP] Health literacy: The degree to which individuals have the capacity to obtain, process, and understand basic health information and services needed to make appropriate health-related decisions (Institute of Medicine, 2004).

Healthy People 2020: An initiative created by the Surgeon General's office in 1979 that states major health goals for United States residents in the upcoming decade.

Hegar's sign: A sign of pregnancy; softening of the lower uterine segment.

Hemangioma: Also known as *nevus vascularis,* this growth consists of newly formed and dilated capillaries in the dermal and subdermal layers of the skin.

Hematochezia: The passage of bright red, fresh blood in the stool.

Hematoma: A collection of blood in the tissues outside a blood vessel.

Hematuria: Blood in the urine.

Hemolytic uremic syndrome (HUS): An acute condition in which microangiopathic hemolytic anemia, thrombocytopenia, and acute nephropathy are present. *Escherichia coli* O157:H7 and

E. coli O111 are frequently the causative agents, which are acquired from eating contaminated foods or raw meat.

Hemophilia: A group of hereditary bleeding disorders noted by a deficient level of blood clotting proteins. The two major types are hemophilia A (1 in 10,000 males) and hemophilia B (1 in 30,000 males).

Hemoptysis: The presence of blood in respiratory secretions or mucus.

Hemorrhoids: Enlarged veins in the anus and rectal area.

Hereditary: The transmission of genetic characteristics from the parent to the offspring.

Higher level of care: A phrase used to denote the transfer of a child from a lower level of care, such as a hospital pediatric unit bed, to the pediatric intensive care unit.

Hind milk: Milk that is produced during the breastfeeding session.

[DP] Hirsutism: An excessive growth of hair or the presence of hair in unusual places, particularly in women; can be associated with the side effects of certain anticonvulsant medications.

Human chorionic gonadotropin (hCG): A hormone that is produced by the fertilized egg that supports the development of the embryo.

Human papillomavirus (HPV): A papillomavirus found in humans that is considered a common sexually transmitted disease. The virus causes genital warts and can develop into cervical cancer.

Human placental lactogen: A hormone that assists with milk production and increases the mother's metabolism during pregnancy.

Hydatiform mole: A genetic abnormality that occurs during early placental attachment and fetal development in which the trophoblast cells that would normally attach the ovum to the uterine wall develop abnormally.

Hydrocephalus: An accumulation of excessive quantities of cerebral spinal fluid (CSF) within the ventricles of the brain, which can cause blocking of normal CSF drainage systems and an increasing head circumference.

Hypercapnia: Excessive carbon dioxide in the bloodstream.

Hyperemesis gravidarum: Nausea and vomiting that interferes with adequate intake of fluid and food, and/or that persists past 20 weeks' gestation.

Hyperinsulinemia: A condition of excess insulin circulating in the blood.

Hyperinsulinism: A condition in which the amount of insulin in the blood is higher than normal.

Hyperopia: A defect of vision called *farsightedness* caused by a flattening of the globe of the eye where parallel rays of light come to focus behind the retina.

Hyperthermia: A state in which the body temperature is above the normal range.

Hyperventilation: A state that results from an individual's breathing too fast and too deep, which causes a decrease in carbon dioxide in the blood.

Hypocalcemia: Low levels of calcium in the blood.

Hypoglycemia: A plasma glucose level of less than 30 mg/dL in the first 24 hours of life and less than 45 mg/dL thereafter.

Hypomagnesemia: Low levels of magnesium in the blood.

Hyponatremia: A decreased concentration of sodium in the bloodstream.

Hypoparathyroidism: Decreased level of parathyroid hormone, which can cause deficiencies of calcium and phosphorous in the blood.

Hypospadias: A congenital condition in which there is an abnormal opening of the meatus on the underside of the penis. This term is also used to describe the condition in which the urethral opening is within the vagina.

Hypothermia: A body temperature below normal.

Hypoxemia: An abnormally low level of oxygen in the blood resulting from respiratory compromise that prevents the lungs from adequately performing gas exchange.

Hypoxia: A decrease in oxygen supply to the tissues.

Hypoxic-ischemic encephalopathy: Acute brain injury caused by asphyxia.

Hysterectomy: A surgical procedure to remove the uterus.

[DP] Hysterosalpingography: A diagnostic test that uses dye to visualize the fallopian tubes and uterus.

[DP] Hysteroscopy: Procedure in which a lighted scope is placed through the cervix into the uterus to visualize the uterine cavity.

[DP] Hysterosonography: Procedure in which a saline infusion ultrasound is used to view the uterus.

Imminent justice: A belief that everything has a determined universal code of law and order.

Immunity: A term that refers to the body's response of developing antibodies against specific bacteria, viruses, and toxins that, once developed, can prevent illness to future exposure of the organism.

Immunizations: The protection of an individual or of groups by the administration of a vaccine or an injection of specific immunoglobulins for a specific disease or infectious material.

Immunoglobulin: A protein that functions as an antibody.

[DP] Impaired nurse: A nurse who is not behaving or functioning appropriately because of illness or addiction, or who is incapable of carrying out his or her professional duties.

[DP] Incident report: A legal document used in health care to launch a communication sequence related to a near-miss medical or medication error, or an actual medication or medical error. An incidence report can be used to document and inform hospital administration of an unusual occurrence that could have or that did lead to harm.

Increased intracranial pressure: Increased pressure within the brain's ventricles that is caused by either an overproduction or a lack of absorption of cerebral spinal fluid (CSF).

Increment: The onset and buildup of intensity of a contraction.

Incubation period: The interval of time between exposure to a communicable disease or infection and the presentation of the first symptoms.

Indirect or unconjugated bilirubin: Bilirubin that travels through the bloodstream to the liver.

Induction: A phase of chemotherapy administration often used in pediatric oncology practice that is the first phase in the treatment of many cancers. Induction usually includes one or more drugs administered with the intent of inducing a remission, or having no identifiable (ie, minimal) residual disease (ie, evidence of cancer cells).

Inhaler: A device used to breathe in inhaled medications into the lungs. Usually a hand-held device that can have a mask attached for easier use with children younger than 5.

Insulin resistance: A condition in which the muscle, fat, and liver cells do not respond to insulin and cannot absorb glucose from the bloodstream.

Intensity: The strength of the contraction at the peak, or acme, of the contraction.

Intentional injury: Considered a possible form of physical child abuse, this type of injury is considered an injury that is caused by another person during such activities as discipline. It can include hitting, slapping, pushing, and causing fractures, burns, or severe harm.

Intrathecal space: Something that exists within the spinal canal.

Intrauterine growth restriction (IGR): Decreased fetal growth because of a decrease in placenta perfusion during gestation.

Intrauterine pressure catheter (IUPC): A small flexible tube inserted into the uterus along the uterine wall that provides an exact measurement of contraction length and intensity.

Intuitive thinking: The ability to classify information while becoming more aware of cause-and-effect relationships.

Intussusception: The invagination, or folding, of one section of the bowel into the other, which causes acute bowel obstruction, inflammation, and necrosis if not rapidly treated by low-pressure contrast or water enema.

Inverted nipples: Nipples that do not protrude or stand out from the breast.

Involution: The reduction in size of the uterus after childbirth.

[DP] Ipecac syrup: An over-the-counter medication known to induce vomiting related to toxic ingestion; it is no longer used in health-care settings because it has been replaced with activated charcoal and whole bowel irrigation.

Iron-deficiency anemia: A reduction in the mass of circulating red blood cells caused by a deficiency of dietary iron.

Ischial tuberosity diameter: The smallest dimension of the pelvis. It should be at least 10 cm to allow the head to pass through the ischial spines of the pelvis.

Isoimmunization: The creation of antibodies against Rh-positive blood that occurs in the mother's body after she is exposed to fetal Rh-positive blood.

Jaundice: A yellow discoloration of the skin caused by the breakdown of red blood cells that are not cleared by the liver.

Justice: The ethical principle of acting out of fairness for individuals, groups, organizations, and communities.

Kegel exercise: An exercise for strengthening the muscles of the perineum and vagina. The patient should repeatedly and rapidly contract and relax the muscles of the perineum and vagina for 10 sec then relax for 20 sec, and then repeat the routine. The number of repetitions should be increased gradually to between 50 and 150 per day.

Kernicterus: A form of jaundice occurring in the newborn period (ie, the second to eighth day after birth). The basal ganglia and other areas of the brain and spinal cord are infiltrated with bilirubin, a yellow substance produced by the breakdown of hemoglobin.

Ketogenic diet: A special high-fat, low-carbohydrate diet that is thought to help control seizures in some people who have a documented history of epilepsy.

Ketones: Acids made when the body uses fat instead of carbohydrates for energy.

Kussmaul's respirations: A deep, gasping, repetitive breathing pattern associated specifically with acidosis.

Kyphosis: A condition of exaggerated angulation of the posterior curvature of the thoracic (ie, upper) spine. In lay language, kyphosis is also referred to as "humpback" or "hunchback."

Labor induction: The use of mechanical or chemical methods to start cervical effacement, dilation, and contractions.

Lactoferrin: A protein which has bactericidal and iron-binding properties found in breast milk.

Lactogenesis: Production of milk.

Lanugo: A fine hair that covers the forehead, ears, and body of the newborn.

Large-for-gestational age (LGA): Newborn is an infant whose weight is greater than 90% for gestational age.

Laryngitis: Inflammation of the larynx or laryngeal mucosa and the vocal cords; characterized by hoarseness and aphonia (ie, lost voice).

Late decelerations: Deceleration of fetal heart rate that occurs after the uterine contraction begins; the nadir is noted after the peak of the contraction.

Leading Health Indicators: A list of some of the *Healthy People* objectives that were selected because they are high-priority health issues.

Left-to-right blood flow shunt: A cardiovascular conduit through which blood flows from the left side of the heart, which usually perfuses the systemic circulation, to the right side of the heart, which usually perfuses the pulmonary circulation. This may result in pulmonary congestion and eventual heart failure.

Legal blindness: A term used to note that a child's visual acuity is measured or approximated to be below 20/200.

[DP] Leiomyoma: A benign tumor of smooth muscle.

Leopold's maneuvers: A pattern of maneuvers that can be performed to determine the fetal position in the uterus.

Lethality of attempt: Refers to the determination of the potential threat of suicidal death per the patient's description of plans, methods, reasons, and availability of rescue.

Leukemia: Any class of hematological malignancies (ie, cancer) of bone marrow cells in which immortal clones of immature blood cells multiply, causing a depletion of normal blood cells. Leukemias are categorized as chronic or acute; by the cell type they originated from; and by the genetic, chromosomal, or growth factor aberration present in the malignant cell.

Leukokoria: Also called "cat's eye reflex," it is a white to yellow glow to the retina seen when light hits the retina; a tumor of the eye, retinoblastoma, is present.

Leukorrhea: A white vaginal discharge that is usually increased in pregnancy.

Lightening: The "dropping" of the fetus descending into the mother's pelvis.

Linea nigra: A dark line that runs from the umbilicus to the pubis in pregnant women; caused by hormonal changes.

Lipodystrophy: A disturbance of fat metabolism with a common finding of localized accumulation of fat under the skin, especially over the trunk.

Lithotomy position: A position in which the patient lies on the back, thighs flexed on the abdomen, legs on thighs, and thighs abducted.

Local anesthesia: Medication injected to numb an area of the body that is infused by the needle.

Lochia: The postpartum discharge of blood, mucus, and uterine tissue from the uterus after childbirth.

Lochia alba: The final stage of uterine sloughing. The discharge is yellow-white and may continue up to 6 weeks after delivery.

Lochia rubra: Postpartum, bright red uterine discharge that usually lasts for 1 to 3 days after childbirth.

Lochia serosa: Postpartum, pink or brown uterine discharge that lasts for 4 to 9 days after childbirth.

Lordosis: A condition of anterior convexity of the lumbar spine.

Lund-Browder classification tool: A tool that is used to estimate the extent of a burn, allowing for varying proportion of the body surface; used instead of the "rule of nines" in children because of their larger head.

Luteinizing hormone (LH): A hormone causing ovulation that converts the ruptured follicle into the corpus luteum.

Macrosomia: A newborn with a birth weight greater than 4,000 to 4,500 g.

Macular rash: A rash that has flat spots on the skin; a macule is a flat, nonpalpable lesion less than 1 cm in diameter. Examples are freckles and petechiae.

Magical thinking: The invention of stories and fantasies to process a young child's reality.

Maintenance therapy: A phase of chemotherapy administration often used in pediatric oncology practice that is the end phase of treatment. Maintenance therapy has a goal of keeping the child in remission with no evidence of residual disease.

[DP] Maladaptive behaviors: Responses to stress that are considered unhealthy, such as the consumption of alcohol, drug use, smoking, not sleeping, not eating well, self-harm, and fighting between family members.

[DP] Malpractice: An injury to a patient caused by an action taken by a health-care professional. The action is deemed a failure to meet a reasonable standard of practice.

Mandatory reporters of child abuse and neglect: People who, because of their positions, are legally responsible to report actual or suspected child abuse to authorities. All health-care providers are considered mandatory reporters. Commercial film developers, child-care custodians, and all branches of the law are considered mandatory reporters. Each of these four categories of mandatory reporters has the potential to identify actual or suspected abuse.

Mastitis: An infection in the breast tissue.

Meconium: A newborn's first stool that is composed of secretions from the intestines, bile pigments, mucus, lanugo, epithelial cells, and blood; it is greenish to black in color.

[DP] Mediating process: The process when one consciously or unconsciously reacts to manage a stressful situation.

Medical play: Structured play provided by the Child Life or the nursing staff that provides the opportunity for a child to learn about his or her diagnosis, procedures, surgery, and diagnostic or medical equipment, including lines, tubes, and devices through the use of anatomically correct dolls or other play equipment used for teaching and demonstration.

Melanocytic nevi: Also known as *moles,* a nevus may be flat or raised. The congenital melanocytic nevus is usually evenly pigmented and brown or black in color.

Melasma: Brown facial skin discoloration. It appears on the upper cheeks, upper lip, forehead, and chin. It is related to sun exposure, hormones such as birth control pills, and hormonal changes in pregnancy.

Meningitis: Inflammation of the membranes of the brain or spinal cord, often caused by an infectious process.

Mental illness: A condition that affects behaviors or mood, such as personality disorders, depression, or schizophrenia.

Mesoderm: Laying between the ectoderm and the endoderm, the mesoderm is the middle embryonic germ layer from which the urogenital and circulatory systems develop.

Microencephaly: The state of having a small brain and head.

Milia: Sebaceous glands occluded with keratin that appear as tiny white papules about 1 mm in size located on the nose, chin, cheeks, and forehead.

[DP] Mittelschmerz: A term for the pain that is noticed by a woman during the middle of the menstrual cycle when ovulation occurs.

Monozygotic twins: Identical twins that develop from one fertilized egg.

Morbidity: A disease state.

Mortality: Death.

Munchausen's syndrome by proxy (MSBP): Harm or significant injury to a child by another individual, often the mother, who typically has some health-care knowledge and who inflicts harm to the child to receive attention from others.

Myelination: The process of growth of a myelin sheath around nerve fibers. This sheath, which acts as an electrical insulator, represents maturity of the nerve body and allows for increased velocity of the impulse.

Myoclonic: Clonic spasms or severe twitching of a muscle or group of muscles.

[DP] Myomas: Tumors that contain muscle tissue.

Myometrium: The middle layer of uterine muscle. The function of this layer is to contract and expel the fetus during childbirth.

Myopia: A defect of vision called *nearsightedness* caused by an error of refraction where parallel rays of light come to focus in front of the retina.

Nadir: The lowest point of the fetal heart rate deceleration.

Naegele's rule: The formula used to determine the estimated due date. Subtract 3 months from the first day of the last menstrual period and then add 7 days.

Nasopharyngeal: Relating to the area of the nasopharynx or the area situated above the soft palate.

[DP] National Standards for Culturally and Linguistically Appropriate Services in Health Care (CLAS): The collective set of CLAS mandates, guidelines, and recommendations issued by the Health & Human Services (HHS) Office of Minority Health intended to inform, guide, and facilitate required and recommended practices related to culturally and linguistically appropriate health services (Office of Minority Health Department of Health & Human Services).

[DP] Near drowning: A phrase used to denote a level of survival after an immersion in water. This phrase has often been replaced with the phrase *submersion injury.*

Nebulizer: A device that aerates respiratory medications via a machine used for the ease and effectiveness of instilling medications throughout the lung fields. Considered very effective for the administration and distribution of asthma medications, such as nebulized albuterol or levosalbutamol (Xopenex).

Necrosis: The death of cells, tissues, or organs.

Necrotizing enterocolitis: A serious disease of premature infants characterized by damage to the intestinal tract mucosa.

Negativism: The tendency of being negative in attitude, including resisting suggestions, requests, or commands from others. This behavior of a young child is marked by resistance or retreat, and is often associated with tantrums.

Neglect: The failure of another to provide for a child's most basic needs. Neglect can be emotional, physical, or educational.

[DP] Negligence: The failure of a healthcare team member, or the team itself, to provide care according to his or her professional responsibility. There are four elements of negligence: breach of duty, duty owed, proximate cause, and damages/harm/injuries.

Neonatal sepsis: A blood infection that presents within the first 7 days of life but may occur up to 90 days after birth.

Nephrotic syndrome: A condition marked by an abnormal increase in renal glomerular permeability to serum proteins with subsequent hyperalbuminuria, hypoalbuminemia, and hyperlipidemia.

Neural tube defects: Defects of the spinal cord, spine, or brain.

Neuroleptic: Refers to any medication that is taken to treat psychotic behavior, usually by blocking dopamine receptors in the brain (eg, chlorpromazine, haloperidol, or clozapine).

Neurotransmitter: A chemical molecule released by the axon terminals of a nerve cell that triggers a reaction that excites or inhibits the activity of the target cell. Serotonin, dopamine, and norepinephrine are examples of neurotransmitters.

Neutropenia: The presence of an abnormally small number of circulating neutrophils in the blood, usually less than 1,500 per microliter.

Nevus flammeus: Also known as a *port wine stain,* this reddish purple skin deformity is made up of dilated skin capillaries.

Nevus simplex: Also known as *stork bite, angel kiss,* or *salmon patch,* this type of benign birthmark is a capillary malformation that fades over time.

New morbidity: A phrase used to describe contemporary issues that affect a given population, such as children, and that is related to illness, injury, disease, and death.

Nightmares: Nighttime dreams that have the potential to or that actually frighten a child.

Night terrors: Waking up at night with a strong emotional reaction to a nightmare.

Nocturia: Excessive urination during the night, which can be a symptom of renal or bladder problems.

Nocturnal incontinence: Incontinence of urine that occurs during the night, usually with a pathological cause.

[DP] Nonaccidental poisoning: When a child takes a toxic substance or medication for abuse, suicide gestures/attempts, or successful self-inflicted death.

Nonmaleficence: The ethical principle of "do no harm" or inflict the least possible harm to reach a beneficial outcome.

[DP] Normalcy: The movement toward being normal in one's life; pertains to attaining normal standards in one's life when faced with chronic illness, disability, or impairment.

Nuchal cord: The umbilical cord around the neck of the fetus.

Nystagmus: Involuntary back-and-forth movements of the eyes, most often noticeable when the patient gazes at objects moving by rapidly or at fixed objects.

Obesity: Considered a body mass index of greater than 30 kg/m². It is an unhealthy accumulation of body fat and is the most common metabolic/nutritional disease in the United States, leading to health consequences including diabetes, heart disease, hypertension, stroke, and fatal cancers.

Obstetric conjugate: The diameter from the sacral promontory to the upper inner border of the symphysis pubis; it measures approximately 11 cm.

Oligohydramnios: An abnormally small amount of amniotic fluid.

Ophthalmia neonatorum: An eye infection the newborn receives from exposure to vaginal secretions from untreated sexually transmitted infections.

Orthostatic hypotension: A drop in the blood pressure when a patient stands; caused by low blood volume or low blood pressure.

Osteomyelitis: Inflammation of the bone tissue and the marrow caused by an infection (or other less common sources, such as radiation) that most often occurs in the long bones.

[DP] Osteoporosis: A condition in which the bones become thin and fragile.

[DP] Overflow incontinence: A condition in which an individual is unable to hold urine and then passes urine when the bladder is too full.

Overweight: Having weight in excess of what would be considered normal for a person's height, age, and overall build; person having a body mass index higher than expected for age and height, and at the 95th percentile for others of the same age, height, and body mass.

Oxygenation: The exchange of gases in the lungs that allows oxygen to move into the blood.

Oxytocin: A hormone that is produced in the pituitary gland and secreted into the bloodstream.

Papanicolaou (Pap) smear: A test for cervical cancer.

Papular rash: A rash that has raised bumps or pimples rising above the skin and found of various colors; a papule is an elevated, firm, palpable lesion that is less than 1 cm in diameter. Examples include psoriasis and eczema.

Para: A woman who has produced a viable infant (weighing at least 500 g or more than 20 weeks' gestation), regardless of whether the fetus is alive at birth.

Parallel play: A form of play associated with the toddler developmental stage in which the child does not play with another toddler, but plays close by, often back to back, with separate toys that they do not have to share.

Passive immunity: Temporary immunity acquired by transfusing immune globulins or antitoxins either artificially from another human or from an animal that has been actively immunized against an antigen, or naturally from the mother to the fetus via the placenta.

[DP] Pediatric medical traumatic stress (PMTS): Set of psychological and physiological responses of children and their families to injury, pain, serious illness, medical procedures, and invasive or frightening treatment interventions.

Perfusion: The body's ability to circulate blood through the body to oxygenate tissues.

Perimetrium: A serous membrane that lines the external surface of the uterus.

Periodic decelerations: Decelerations of fetal heart rate associated with uterine contractions.

Peripheral cyanosis: Decreased cardiac output with an accompanying decrease in the peripheral blood flow; peripheral cyanosis may not demonstrate a reduced oxygen saturation measurement.

Personal protective equipment (PPE): Equipment that is made available to health-care professionals to prevent the spread of infections or diseases. This equipment includes gloves, gowns, eye shield/glasses, masks, shoe protectors, hair protective coverings, and disposable equipment such as stethoscopes.

Personality disorder: A pathological disturbance that affects communication, thinking, and perception and can manifest in different types such as antisocial and borderline categories.

Petechiae: Very small hemorrhagic purplish spots found on the child's skin when there is a significant reduction in circulating platelets.

Pfannenstiel's incision: A "bikini cut" incision above the symphysis pubis.

Pica: The practice of eating non-nutritive foods.

Placenta: An organ that provides the fetus with oxygen and nourishment.

Placenta abruptio: The premature separation of the placenta from the wall of the uterus.

Placenta accreta: A situation in which the placenta is attached too deeply into the wall of the uterus, causing complications with removal.

Placenta previa: A complication of pregnancy in which the placenta implants in the lower uterus and covers the cervix.

Pneumonitis: Inflammation of the lungs usually affecting the bronchioles and alveoli.

Pneumothorax: A collection of air or gas in the pleural cavity. Often follows a perforation through the chest wall; a pneumothorax is sudden in onset with severe, sharp pains in the side of the chest and accompanying dyspnea.

Polycythemia: An excess of red blood cells.

Polydipsia: An experience of excessive thirst, often associated with dehydration, hypovolemia, and hyperglycemia.

Polyhydramnios: Excessive amniotic fluid.

Polyphagia: An experience of excessive hunger and eating abnormally large amounts of food.

Polyuria: An excessive secretion and discharge of urine, defined as more than 50 mL of urine per kg of body weight per day.

Post-term: An infant born after 42 weeks' gestation.

[DP] Posttraumatic stress disorder (PTSD): Considered a mental health condition following a traumatic or terrifying event; can be actually experienced or an event that was witnessed. PTSD can last for months to years.

[DP] Posttraumatic stress syndrome (PTSS): Set of symptoms experienced by children and adults after an event that is perceived as being traumatic.

Precipitous delivery: An unusually rapid labor of less than 3 hours and ending with a rapid spontaneous delivery of the infant.

Precocious puberty: The appearance of secondary sex characteristics before 8 years in girls and 9 years in boys. The cause of this condition may be premature secretion of sex hormones not caused by pituitary or hypothalamic action.

Preconceptual thinking: A young child's judgment of their environment by visual experiences.

Pre-eclampsia: Hypertension and proteinuria that is present after 20 weeks' gestation.

Premature rupture of membranes (PROM): Ruptured membranes within the patient that are at least 37 weeks' gestation before the onset of labor.

Prepubescence: The period of growth right before the onset of puberty that is marked by physical changes that denote sexual and reproductive maturation.

Pressure ulcers: Also referred to as *decubitus ulcers,* these skin wounds result from impaired circulation or inadequate perfusion from pressure. They often develop from bedrest without consistent turning. They can vary from a superficial depth, appearing as nonblanching redness, to deep craters that extend into bone tissue. Hospitalized patients with mobility deficits are at high risk.

Preterm: An infant born before 37 weeks' gestation.

Preterm premature rupture of the membranes (PPROM): The rupture of membranes before 37 weeks' gestation.

Probiotics: Intestinal bacteria that aid in breaking down food for digestion.

Progesterone: A hormone that is produced by the corpus luteum and the placenta.

Prolactin: The hormone responsible for milk production.

[DP] Prolapse: To drop down out of place.

Prostaglandins: Hormonelike substances with a variety of effects on tissues, including the contraction and relaxation of smooth muscle.

Pruritic urticarial papules and plaque of pregnancy (PUPP): A dermatitis of itchy plaques and papules with erythematous patches of papules and vesicles.

Pruritus: Intense itching of the skin.

Pseudomenstruation: A mucus- and blood-tinged vaginal discharge that may be present in the newborn female for a few days until the maternal hormone level decreases.

Psychosis: A state in which a person experiences an impairment of reality testing. He or she inaccurately evaluates perceptions and thoughts.

Puberty: The time period or stage in a child's life when he or she becomes sexually mature and able to reproduce. Typically, this occurs during a rapid period of time between 13 and 15 years for boys and 9 and 16 years for girls.

Pudendal block: An anesthetic injected into the pudendal nerve to anesthetize the vulva and perineum.

Puerperium: The postpartum period after childbirth that lasts approximately 6 weeks as the reproductive system returns to the prepregnancy state.

Purpura: Any rash in which blood cells leak into the skin or mucous membranes, usually at multiple sites. Purpuric rashes are often associated with disorders of thrombosis or coagulation.

Pustule: A small raised skin lesion protruding above the skin line and filled with pus (ie, white blood cells); found in many skin disorders, including drug rashes and acne.

Quickening: Fetal movement felt by the mother after 18 to 20 weeks' gestation.

[DP] Race: Genetic physical characteristics that are similar among members of a group, such as skin, hair, and eye color (Purnell and Paulanka, 2008).

Radiation: The transfer of body heat to a cooler object, such as a window.

Rales: Also known as *crackles,* adventitious breath sounds associated with fluid collection in the base of the lungs.

Rapid response team: A designated team designed to rapidly assemble at a child's bedside or clinic room to provide emergency response skills and resuscitation if needed.

[DP] Rectocele: A condition in which the rectum drops down and protrudes into the back wall of the vagina.

Refractory error: A common eye disorder where the eye bends light and is unable to focus because of an abnormal shape of the eye.

Regression: Demonstration of behaviors associated with a previous developmental stage. Usually associated with stress and anxiety; a child will regress to earlier behaviors such as bed wetting, use of diapers, wanting to be fed, or tantrums.

Relaxin: A hormone that works with progesterone to maintain the pregnancy and that causes relaxation of pelvis ligaments to aid in birthing.

Respiratory distress syndrome: A severe impairment of the respiratory function of a preterm newborn caused by immature lungs and lack of surfactant.

Respiratory syncytial virus (RSV): A viral infection associated with winter months that sequesters in the lung and causes severe symptoms of respiratory distress in infants. Children younger than 6 months are often hospitalized for supportive treatment.

Restraints: Devices that prevent patients from hurting themselves or others; may infrequently be warranted, although their use is highly discouraged and left for extreme safety issues. Adhering to strict hospital policy concerning the application for restraints is an imperative. All other forms of care and control should be used, such as family members or sitters being present, or Child Life interventions applied, before the decision to use restraints.

Retained placenta: A placenta that does not detach from the wall of the uterus, or, as the placenta separates from the uterus, small pieces or fragments of the placenta may be left attached to the uterus.

Retinoblastoma: A malignant glioma of the retina, usually unilateral, found in young children and associated with heredity.

Retinopathy of prematurity (ROP): A bilateral disease of the retinal vessels in premature infants leading to neovascularization and retinal detachment in the first few weeks of life. Although the etiology is unknown, ROP is associated with oxygen levels and environmental factors.

Retractions: A pulling in of the skin around the ribs and sternum when inhaling that is observed during respiratory distress.

Reye's syndrome: Acute encephalopathy with brain swelling, and fatty infiltration of the liver, spleen, kidney, pancreas, and lymph that is associated with the use of salicylates (ie, aspirin) following a viral infection such as varicella.

Rhonchi: A low-pitched adventitious breath sound when a mucous plug is within a large airway structure; a rattling sound that moves with coughing.

Right-to-left blood flow shunt: A cardiovascular conduit through which blood flows from the right side of the heart, which usually perfuses the pulmonary circulation, to the left side of the heart, which usually perfuses the systemic circulation. This may result in underperfusion of pulmonary circulation and worsening cyanotic changes.

Rugae: The folds in the wall of the vagina.

Rule of nines: An assessment tool used to estimate the extent of a burn; used in late adolescence and adulthood.

Safety precautions: The use of multiple safety measures to keep children safe, including locking the wheels on the crib or bed; keeping the rails up; using high-top cribs for standing young children; keeping appropriately sized emergency equipment at the bedside, such as suction, oxygen, and a resuscitative bag/mask/valve; preventing aspiration; preventing strangulation with IV tubing or any wires in the crib; preventing burns and electrocution; and teaching parents how to use the rapid response team.

***Salmonella* food poisoning:** Pathogenic bacilli that produce a range of reactions from mild gastroenteritis to fatal food poisoning. There are more than 1,400 species.

Salpingectomy: Removal of the fallopian tube.

Salpingostomy: A small, linear incision made into a fallopian tube that has become occluded or for drainage purposes.

SBAR: A method of organizing oneself for an oral report or telephone call with a primary provider using four components: **S**ituation, **B**ackground, **A**ssessment, and **R**ecommendation.

Schizophrenia: A thought disorder marked by hallucinations, disorganized speech and behavior, and delusions. The child may be withdrawn, socially isolated, and present with a flat affect.

School vision: When a child is considered to be partially sighted with a measured or approximate visual acuity of 20/70 to 20/200.

Scoliosis: A lateral or *S*-shaped curvature of the spine that often presents with two curves: the abnormal curve and a compensatory curve on the opposite side.

[DP] Scope of practice: The boundaries in which a health-care provider can practice as described by the associated professional organization or licensure body; the legal outline of what a nurse can do according to the law of that state.

Selective attention: A demonstration during play, such as reading a book or playing a game, that the child does not hear the voice of a parent or teacher.

[DP] Sentinel events: Unexpected occurences that cause injury or death of a patient.

Separation anxiety: An emotional reaction experienced by an older infant that starts at approximately 8 to 10 months, in which the child expresses anxiety when parents leave or the child is taken from the parents.

Sexual abuse: Inappropriate sexual behavior by an adolescent or adults with a child. This includes fondling the child's genitals, making the child fondle the adult's genitals, incest, intercourse, rape, sodomy, exploitation, exhibitionism, inappropriate sexually oriented photographing of a child, and exposure to pornography.

Sexual latency: A term used to describe the disinterest in the school-aged child's sexuality. This developmental period comes after the phases in infancy and young childhood of "oral" and "anal." The concept was proposed by Dr. Sigmund Freud, an Austrian neurologist and psychoanalyst (1856–1939).

Shock: A clinical syndrome marked by inadequate oxygenation and perfusion of tissues and organs at the cellular level because of markedly low systemic blood pressure; it can be caused by a number of factors, including sepsis, hemorrhage, severe dehydration, heart disease, burns, spinal cord injury, or trauma.

Shoulder dystocia: A situation during birth that occurs when one or both shoulders become wedged in the maternal pelvis after the head has been delivered.

Sickle cell anemia: An autosomal recessive disorder causing an abnormality of the globin genes in hemoglobin, leading to a chronic anemia disorder with a higher incidence in African Americans, native Africans, and Mediterranean people. If the child is exposed to low levels of oxygen, the hemoglobin S becomes viscous and causes the red blood cell to become rigid, fragile, sickle-shaped, and sticky, all of which leads to an increase in destruction called *hemolysis.*

Sitz bath: A warm bath for the perineal area to provide comfort and promote healing.

Small-for-gestational age (SGA): An infant whose weight is less than the 10th percentile for his or her gestational age.

Social determinants: Risk factors in one's living conditions that can influence risk for disease.

Somatic pain: Pain caused by activation of pain receptors in the body surface or musculoskeletal tissues.

[DP] Special needs: A child's state when he or she has a functional limitation or disability that requires special assistance; this construct can pertain to autism, sensory impairment, impaired mobility, technology dependency, or an emotional/psychological disorder.

Spina bifida: A congenital defect of the spine in which part of the spinal cord and meninges are exposed through an opening in the vertebrae.

Spinal anesthesia: The placement of a needle into the intrathecal space to inject anesthetic medication.

[DP] Spiritual distress: A state of disruption in a person's emotional and psychological well-being. An impaired ability to feel connected with self, others, nature, and/or a power greater than oneself.

[DP] Spirituality: An awareness of the metaphysical, sublime, or religious. A practice of spirituality typically includes participation in an organized religion and/or meditation, prayer, contemplation, reflection, and/or other activities that foster self-growth.

Standards of care: A model of established practice that is accepted as the correct way to provide care for a patient.

Status epilepticus (SE): Continued seizure activity (ie, seizures back-to-back) that can rapidly progress to being life-threatening and that require aggressive interventions and medications to prevent injury and death.

[DP] Stereotyping: A conception, opinion, or belief about some aspect of an individual or group (Purnell and Paulanka, 2008).

Stomatitis: A painful inflammation of the mouth that can affect the tongue, mucous membranes, and lips.

Strabismus: Disorder of the eye in which optic axes cannot be directed to the same object; found in approximately 4% of children. The child may squint to deviate the alternative eye to the same extent as the eyes are carried in different directions. Lay term for strabismus is "wall eye."

Stranger anxiety: Anxiety experienced by an older infant or young child when they encounter a new person in his or her environment.

[DP] Stress: A state produced by a change in the environment that is perceived as threatening, challenging, or damaging to an individual's dynamic balance or equilibrium.

[DP] Stress incontinence: Leaking of urine when coughing or laughing.

Striae gravidarum: Stretch marks located on the abdomen and thighs because of weight gain of pregnancy.

Stridor: A high-pitched harsh sound that occurs during inspiration (often heard without the aid of a stethoscope), which denotes the presence of an obstruction in the upper airway.

Subinvolution: A state in which the uterus fails to complete the involution process after giving birth.

Suicidal ideation: The thought process of considering suicide but without any physical attempts to do so. Many people who contemplate killing themselves have seen a health-care professional in the months before an attempt or successful suicide, showing the importance of early screening, identification, and intervention.

Suicidal thinking: When a child or teen is thinking about suicide but has no plan. This is not uncommon, with approximately 3% of the general teen population reporting suicidal thinking at one point of their development.

Suicide: Death associated with taking one's own life via a variety of methods.

Suicide attempt: A situation in which a person attempts to take his or her life via a variety of means, but is unsuccessful.

Surfactant: A mixture of phospholipids and lipoproteins secreted by the lung cells that assists the alveoli to stay open when the newborn begins breathing.

Symbolic functioning: The creation of an image in the mind that represents something as other than it is (eg, a horse for a pillow or a sheet for a tent).

Tachypnea: Rapid breathing.

Tachysystole: The term for contractions occurring more often than five or more contractions in a 10-minute window, averaged over 30 min. This can be caused by overstimulation from oxytocin or it may be a spontaneous occurrence.

Tardive dyskinesia: Considered a neurological syndrome of slow, stereotyped rhythmical movements, generalized or focal, of muscle groups. Associated with psychotropic drugs, it is an unwanted side effect of therapy requiring medical intervention.

[DP] Technology dependent: The dependence on a medical device and or skill to maintain health and wellness.

Temperament: The combination of the mental, physical, and emotional traits of a person; in toddlerhood, it marks the toddler's predisposition to how he or she interacts with others and his or her unique environment.

Teratogen: Any substance that may cause a birth defect.

Testosterone: A male hormone produced in the testes.

Therapeutic hugging: The use of a parent's or a caregiver's hugs to hold a child during a procedure such as injections, IV line placement, wound care, or a dressing change. Not considered a restraint, but a means to protect and comfort a child during an uncomfortable, painful, or frightening procedure.

Thermoregulation: An intrinsic or extrinsic process of maintaining a normal core body temperature.

Thrombocytopenia: The presence of an abnormally small number of circulating platelets in the blood. A platelet count of less than per 50,000/mm³ may increase the risk of a child bleeding.

Thromboembolism: A condition of an inflammation of a vein in conjunction with a thrombus.

Thrombosis: Formation of a blood clot.

Thrombus: A blood clot.

Tocolytic medications: Medications used to decrease uterine activity and stop preterm labor.

Tonic-clonic seizure: Muscle activity associated with grand mal seizures that is marked by rapid contraction and then relaxation of large muscle groups.

[DP] Tort: A wrongful act or injury committed against another that can be pursued in civil court by the party that was injured.

[DP] Toxicology: The study of harmful or poisonous levels of chemicals in the body, including their detection, avoidance, chemistry, pharmacological actions, antidotes, and treatments.

Toxoid: A substance that is chemically modified to retain its antigen properties but is no longer considered poisonous; used to make immunizations.

Traction: A therapy used to help in the healing process of a fracture; it often uses two lines of pull for extension and stabilization.

Trial of labor after Cesarean (TOLAC): Allowing a woman who desires a vaginal birth after a Cesarean birth to begin labor while being closely monitored for progress and complications.

Umbilical cord: The attachment between the fetus and the placenta.

Unintentional abuse or injury: An injury to a child that was unintentionally inflicted. Not considered a form of child abuse, unintentional injury occurs when a child is injured but it was not caused by abuse or neglect.

[DP] Urinary retention: A condition in which the bladder cannot empty completely.

Urticaria: A condition associated with allergic reactions and marked by multiple discrete areas of swelling on the skin (also known as *wheals*); can cause severe itching because of the associated secretion of vasoactive mediators from mast cells.

Uterine inversion: A situation in which the uterus inverts and the uterine fundus prolapses to or through the dilated cervix. The inverted uterine wall may extend to or through the cervix. In severe cases, the entire uterus and vagina may invert and prolapse out of the patient's body.

Uterine rupture: A nonsurgical opening of the uterus that can allow the uterine contents to move into the abdomen.

Vacuum extraction: The use of a cuplike device that attaches to the fetal head with suction, which allows the healthcare provider to assist with the birth.

Vaginal birth after Cesarean (VBAC): Allowing a woman to attempt a vaginal birth after a previous Cesarean birth.

Variability: Fluctuations in the baseline that are irregular in frequency and amplitude because of interactions between the sympathetic and parasympathetic nervous systems.

Variable decelerations: An abrupt decrease in fetal heart rate of 15 beats per minute or more caused by cord compression, which disrupts the oxygenation of the fetus.

Varicose veins: Distended, swollen veins.

Vaso-occlusive episode: During a sickle cell anemia exacerbation, a vaso-occlusive episode (called a *vaso-occlusive crisis* in the past) is when a large number of rigid, sickle-shaped red blood cells infiltrate organs, joints, lung tissue, and the retina, causing hypoxia and damage to the affected tissues. Vaso-occlusive episodes are associated with pain and can be life-threatening if severe.

Vena cava syndrome: Condition when the weight of the uterus on the vena cava causes compression and the reduced blood flow causes hypotension and light-headedness.

Vernix caseosa: A white protective coating on the skin of the newborn.

Vesicle: A small elevation on the skin that is blisterlike and contains serous fluid; varies in diameter and color.

Viability: A newborn weighing at least 500 g at more than 20 weeks' gestation.

Viable: A term used to describe a fetus that is able to live outside the uterus.

Villi: Fingerlike projections in the placenta that are surrounded by the mother's blood.

Visceral pain: Pain in internal organs caused by the activation of receptors in the chest, abdomen, or pelvic area that send signals to the spinal cord and on to the brain.

[DP] Vulvovaginitis: Infection of the vagina and vulva.

Wharton's jelly: A gelatinous substance that provides support and protection for the vessels inside the umbilical cord.

Wheal: A round and elevated lesion, often temporary, that is white in the center and surrounded by red inflammation; often seen with insect bites and urticaria.

[DP] Worldview: A set of explanations used by a group of people to explain life's events and to offer solutions to life's mysteries; also defined as a major thought process of shared cultural backgrounds (Andrews and Boyle, 2008).

Credits

Note: Unless cited below, credits appear within the text.

Figures 3.10 and 3.11: Smith, B.R. (2013). The multidimensional human embryo, Carnegie Stages. Retrieved from http://embryo.soad.umich.edu/carnStages/carnStages.html.

Figure 8.7: Adapted with permission from Wong DL et al. Maternal Child Nursing Care, 2/e. Mosby. Copyright 2002.

Figure 9.7, 9.8, and 14.1: Adapted with permission from Lowdermilk & Perry. Maternity and Women's Healthcare, 8/e. Mosby. Copyright 2004.

Figure 16.12: Reprinted from The Journal of Pediatrics, 119:3, J.L. Ballard, J.C. Khoury, K. Wedig, L. Wang, B.L. Eilers-Walsman, R. Lipp. New Ballard Score, expanded to include extremely premature infants. Copyright 1991, with permission from Elsevier.

Figure 17.3: All images are Copyright ©2015 Medela, Inc.

Figures 18.4, 19.2, 19.3, and 40.2: Courtesy of St. Luke's Hospital, Bethlehem, PA.

Figure 19.1: Courtesy of McLeod Regional Medical Center, Florence, SC.

Figures 20.1, B2.1: Courtesy of the National Institutes of Health, www.nih.gov.

Figures 20.5 and 20.6: PediaSIM pediatric simulation photo courtesy of CAE Healthcare. © 2011 CAE Healthcare.

Figure 20.7: Photo courtesy of the Back to Sleep campaign, Eunice Kennedy Shriver National Institute of Child Health and Human Development, National Institutes of Health and Human Services (www.nichd.nih.gov/sids).

Figures 21.3 and 21.4: From Centers for Disease Control and Prevention. Published by the Centers for Disease Control and Prevention, November 1, 2009. SOURCE: WHO Child Growth Standards (http://www.who.int/childgrowth/en). Retrieved from http://www.cdc.gov/growthcharts/who_charts.htm#The%20WHO%20Growth%20Charts.

Figure 22.7: From National Cancer Institute. Photographer: Linda Bartlett.

Figure 22.8: From the Centers for Disease Control and Prevention, Department of Health and Human Services. Retrieved from http://phil.cdc.gov/Phil/details.asp,ID #3318.

Figure 23.4: From the National Cancer Institute. Photographer, Bill Branson.

Figures 24.2, 24.3, 24.5, and 27.5: From Centers for Disease Control and Prevention Public Health Library. http://phil.cdc.gov

Figure 25.4: From Healthy People 2020 http://www.healthypeople.gov/2020/topicsobjectives2020/overview.aspx?topicid=2

Figure 26.4: Photo from the National Cancer Institute.

Chapter 26 Team Works: Principles of Pain Management, QUESTT Tool: Adapted with permission from Whaley & Wong's Nursing Care of Infants and Children, 6th ed., 1999, Wong et al ed. Copyright Elsevier 1999.

Unnumbered Figure 26.1: © 1983 Wong-Baker FACES Foundation, www.WongBakerFACES.org. Used with permission. Originally published in Whaley & Wong's Nursing Care of Infants and Children. © Elsevier Inc.

Unnumbered Figure 26.2: © 2002, The Regents of the University of Michigan

Unnumbered Figure 26.4: Used with permission of OUCHER!.org; ©The African-American version was developed and copyrighted by Mary J. Denyes, PhD, RN, and Antonia M. Villarruel PhD, RN, USA, 1990. Cornelia Porter PhD, RN and Charlotta Marshall RN, MSN contributed to the development of the scale.

Figure 27.6 (bottom): Permission for use granted by Cook Medical, Bloomington, Indiana.

Table 27.3: Reprinted with permission, 2010 American Heart Association Guidelines, For CPR and ECC, Part 4: CPR Overview, Circulation. 2010;122 [suppl 3]: S676-S684, ©2010, American Heart Association, Inc.

Figure 29.9: Modified from Jennet, B. & Teasdale, G. (1977). Aspects of coma after severe head injury. Lancet. 1: 878; James, H. E. (1986). Neurologic evaluation and support in the child with an acute brain insult. Pediatric Ann. 15:16; Siberry, G., & Iannone, R. (2000). The Harriet Lane handbook (15th ed.).St. Louis, Mosby, p. 14); and Andreoni, C. Klinkhammer, B. (2000). Quick reference guide for pediatric emergency nursing. Saunders, Philadelphia.

Figure 30.2: Gylys & Wedding: Medical Terminology Systems, A body systems approach, 6e. F.A. Davis, Philadelphia.

Figure 30.6: Courtesy of D.M. Kocisko.

Figure 31.1: From the National Cancer Institute. Photographer, Michael Anderson.

Figure 31.4: From Sniffing Markers Destroys Your Brain, reproduced with permission of the National Inhalant Prevention Coalition, 1991.

Figure 31.5: From National Institutes of Health.

Figure 37.3: Adapted from the National Institutes of Health. Retrieved from http://kidney.niddk.nih.gov/kudiseases/pubs/nephrotic/.

Figures 38.4, 39.7, 39.8, 39.9, and Unnumbered Figure 39.1: Courtesy CDC.

Figure 38.8: Courtesy of Dr. Loretta Fiorillo.

Figure 39.1: From the Centers for Disease Control and Prevention, Department of Health and Human Services, Dr. Heinz F. Eichenwald, 1958. Retrieved March 2012 from http://phil.cdc.gov/phil/details.asp?pid=3187, ID #3187.

Figure 39.2: From the Centers for Disease Control and Prevention, Department of Health and Human Services, Dr. Heinz F. Eichenwald, 1958. Retrieved March 2012 from http://phil.cdc.gov/Phil/details.asp, ID #3168.

Figure 39.3: From the Centers for Disease Control and Prevention, Department of Health and Human Services, NIP/Barbara Rice. Retrieved March 2012 from http://phil.cdc.gov/phil/details.asp?pid=130

Figure 39.4: From the Centers for Disease Control and Prevention, Department of Health and Human Services, 1975. Retrieved March 2012 from http://phil.cdc.gov/Phil/details.asp, ID #4514.

Figure 39.5: From the Centers for Disease Control and Prevention, Department of Health and Human Services, 1969. Retrieved March 2012 from http://phil.cdc.gov/phil/details.asp , ID #3318.

Figure 39.6: From the Centers for Disease Control and Prevention, Department of Health and Human Services, 1995. Retrieved March 2012 from http://phil.cdc.gov/phil/details.asp, ID #6121.

Unnumbered Figure 39.2: From the Centers for Disease Control and Prevention, Department of Health and Human Services, 2007. Retrieved from http://phil.cdc.gov/Phil/details.asp, ID #9875.

Figure B3.1: Adapted from World Health Organization (WHO) Department of Reproductive Health and Research, Johns Hopkins Bloomberg School of Public Health/Center for Communication Programs (CCP). Knowledge for health project. Family planning: a global handbook for providers (2011 update). Baltimore, MD; Geneva, Switzerland: CCP and WHO; 2011; and Trussell J. Contraceptive failure in the United States. Contraception 2011;83:397–404. Retrieved from The Centers for Disease Control at http://www.cdc.gov/reproductivehealth/unintendedpregnancy/contraception.htm#.

Unit 1 opening photos
Left: Copyright © Jupiterimages/Stockbyte/Thinkstock.
Middle: Copyright © BananaStock/BananaStock/Thinkstock.
Right: Copyright © Ryan McVay/Photodisc/Thinkstock.

Unit 2 opening photos
Left: Copyright © monkeybusinessimages/iStock/Thinkstock.
Middle: Copyright © szeyuen/iStock/Thinkstock.
Right: Copyright © Feverpitched/iStock/Thinkstock.

Unit 3 opening photos
Left: Copyright © oceandigital/iStock/Thinkstock.
Middle: Copyright © Naomi Bassitt/iStock/Thinkstock.
Right: Copyright © Purestock/Thinkstock.

Unit 4 opening photos
Left: Copyright © Glenda Powers/iStock/Thinkstock.
Middle: Copyright © Photodisc/Photodisc/Thinkstock.
Right: Copyright © v_zaitsev/iStock/Thinkstock.

Unit 5 opening photos
Left: Copyright © Fuse/Thinkstock.
Middle: Copyright © sansara/iStock/Thinkstock.
Right: Copyright © telltam/iStock/Thinkstock.

Unit 6 opening photos
Left: Copyright © DragonImages/iStock/Thinkstock.
Middle: Copyright © MarcelaC/iStock/Thinkstock.
Right: Copyright © BananaStock/BananaStock/Thinkstock.

Unit 7 opening photos
Left: Copyright © monkeybusinessimages/iStock/Thinkstock.
Middle: Copyright © Keith Brofsky/Photodisc/Thinkstock.
Right: Copyright © Creatas Images/Creatas/Thinkstock.

Unit 8 opening photos
Left: Copyright © Fuse/Thinkstock.
Middle: Copyright © Rob Marmion/Hemera/Thinkstock.
Right: Copyright © mtreasure/iStock/Thinkstock.

Index